Encyclopedia of

HUMAN NUTRITION

SECOND EDITION

ENCYCLOPEDIA OF
HUMAN
NUTRITION

SECOND EDITION

Editor-in-Chief
BENJAMIN CABALLERO

Editors
LINDSAY ALLEN
ANDREW PRENTICE

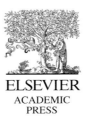

ELSEVIER
ACADEMIC
PRESS

Amsterdam   Boston   Heidelberg   London   New York   Oxford
Paris   San Diego   San Francisco   Singapore   Sydney   Tokyo

Elsevier Ltd., The Boulevard, Langford Lane, Kidlington, Oxford, OX5 1GB, UK

© 2005 Elsevier Ltd.

Second edition 2005

Library of Congress Control Number: 2004113614

A catalogue record for this book is available from the British Library

ISBN 0-12-150110-8 (set)

This book is printed on acid-free paper
Printed and bound in Spain

EDITORIAL ADVISORY BOARD

FOREWORD

Why an encyclopedia? The original Greek word means 'the circle of arts and sciences essential for a liberal education', and such a book was intended to embrace all knowledge. That was the aim of the famous Encyclopedie produced by Diderot and d'Alembert in the middle of the 18th century, which contributed so much to what has been called the Enlightenment. It is recorded that after all the authors had corrected the proofs of their contributions, the printer secretly cut out whatever he thought might give offence to the king, mutilated most of the best articles and burnt the manuscripts! Later, and less controversially, the word 'encyclopedia' came to be used for an exhaustive repertory of information on some particular department of knowledge. It is in this class that the present work falls.

In recent years the scope of Human Nutrition as a scientific discipline has expanded enormously. I used to think of it as an applied subject, relying on the basic sciences of physiology and biochemistry in much the same way that engineering relies on physics. That traditional relationship remains and is fundamental, but the field is now much wider. At one end of the spectrum epidemiological studies and the techniques on which they depend have played a major part in establishing the relationships between diet, nutritional status and health, and there is greater recognition of the importance of social factors. At the other end of the spectrum we are becoming increasingly aware of the genetic determinants of ways in which the body handles food and is able to resist adverse influences of the environment. Nutritionists are thus beginning to explore the mechanisms by which nutrients influence the expression of genes in the knowledge that nutrients are among the most powerful of all influences on gene expression. This has brought nutrition to the centre of the new 'post-genome' challenge of understanding the effects on human health of gene-environment interactions.

In parallel with this widening of the subject there has been an increase in opportunities for training and research in nutrition, with new departments and new courses being developed in universities, medical schools and schools of public health, along with a greater involvement of schoolchildren and their teachers. Public interest in nutrition is intense and needs to be guided by sound science. Governments are realizing more and more the role that nutrition plays in the prevention of disease and the maintenance of good health, and the need to develop a nutrition policy that is integrated with policies for food production.

The first edition of the Encyclopaedia of Human Nutrition established it as one of the major reference works in our discipline. The second edition has been completely revised to take account of new knowledge in our rapidly advancing field. This new edition is as comprehensive as the present state of knowledge allows, but is not overly technical and is well supplied with suggestions for further reading. All the articles have been carefully reviewed and although some of the subjects are controversial and sensitive, the publishers have not exerted the kind of political censorship that so infuriated Diderot.

John Waterlow.

J.C. Waterlow
Emeritus Professor of Human Nutrition
London School of Hygiene and Tropical Medicine
February 2005

INTRODUCTION

The science of human nutrition and its applications to health promotion continue to gain momentum. In the relatively short time since the release of the first edition of this Encyclopedia, a few landmark discoveries have had a dramatic multiplying effect over nutrition science: the mapping of the human genome, the links between molecular bioenergetics and lifespan, the influence of nutrients on viral mutation, to name a few.

But perhaps the strongest evidence of the importance of nutrition for human health comes from the fact that almost 60% of the diseases that kill humans are related to diet and lifestyle (including smoking and physical activity). These are all modifiable risk factors. As individuals and organizations intensify their efforts to reduce disease risks, the need for multidisciplinary work becomes more apparent. Today, an effective research or program team is likely to include several professionals from fields other than nutrition. For both nutrition and non-nutrition scientists, keeping up to date on the concepts and interrelationships between nutrient needs, dietary intake and health outcomes is essential. The new edition of the Encyclopedia of Human Nutrition hopes to address these needs. While rigorously scientific and up to date, EHN provides concise and easily understandable summaries on a wide variety of topics. The nutrition scientist will find that the Encyclopedia is an effective tool to "fill the void" of information in areas beyond his/her field of expertise. Professionals from other fields will appreciate the ease of alphabetical listing of topics, and the presentation of information in a rigorous but concise way, with generous aid from graphs and diagrams.

For a work that involved more than 340 authors requires, coordination and attention to detail is critical. The editors were fortunate to have the support of an excellent team from Elsevier's Major Reference Works division. Sara Gorman and Paula O'Connell initiated the project, and Tracey Mills and Samuel Coleman saw it to its successful completion.

We trust that this Encyclopedia will be a useful addition to the knowledge base of professionals involved in research, patient care, and health promotion around the globe.

Benjamin Caballero, Lindsay Allen and Andrew Prentice
Editors
April 2005

GUIDE TO USE OF THE ENCYCLOPEDIA

Structure of the Encyclopedia

The material in the Encyclopedia is arranged as a series of entries in alphabetical order. Most entries consist of several articles that deal with various aspects of a topic and are arranged in a logical sequence within an entry. Some entries comprise a single article.

To help you realize the full potential of the material in the Encyclopedia we have provided three features to help you find the topic of your choice: a Contents List, Cross-References and an Index.

1. Contents List

Your first point of reference will probably be the contents list. The complete contents lists, which appears at the front of each volume will provide you with both the volume number and the page number of the entry. On the opening page of an entry a contents list is provided so that the full details of the articles within the entry are immediately available.

Alternatively you may choose to browse through a volume using the alphabetical order of the entries as your guide. To assist you in identifying your location within the Encyclopedia a running headline indicates the current entry and the current article within that entry.

You will find 'dummy entries' where obvious synonyms exist for entries or where we have grouped together related topics. Dummy entries appear in both the contents lists and the body of the text.

Example
If you were attempting to locate material on food intake measurement via the contents list:

FOOD INTAKE *see* DIETARY INTAKE MEASUREMENT: Methodology; Validation. DIETARY SURVEYS. MEAL SIZE AND FREQUENCY

The dummy entry directs you to the Methodology article, in The Dietary Intake Measurement entry. At the appropriate location in the contents list, the page numbers for articles under Dietary Intake Measurement are given.

If you were trying to locate the material by browsing through the text and you looked up Food intake then the following information would be provided in the dummy entry:

Food Intake *see* **Dietary Intake Measurement**: Methodology; Validation. **Dietary Surveys. Meal Size and Frequency**

Alternatively, if you were looking up Dietary Intake Measurement the following information would be provided:

DIETARY INTAKE MEASUREMENT

Contents
Methodology
Validation

2. Cross-References

All of the articles in the Encyclopedia have been extensively cross-referenced.

The cross-references, which appear at the end of an article, serve three different functions. For example, at the end of the ADOLESCENTS/Nutritional Problems article, cross-references are used:

i. To indicate if a topic is discussed in greater detail elsewhere.

> *See also*: **Adolescents**: Nutritional Requirements of Adolescents. **Anemia**: Iron-Deficiency Anemia. **Calcium**: Physiology. **Eating Disorders**: Anorexia Nervosa; Bulimia Nervosa; Binge Eating. **Folic Acid**: Physiology, Dietary Sources, and Requirements. **Iron**: Physiology, Dietary Sources, and Requirements. **Obesity**: Definition, Aetiology, and Assessment. **Osteoporosis**: Nutritional Factors. **Zinc**: Physiology.

ii. To draw the reader's attention to parallel discussions in other articles.

> *See also*: **Adolescents**: Nutritional Requirements of Adolescents. **Anemia**: Iron-Deficiency Anemia. **Calcium**: Physiology. **Eating Disorders**: Anorexia Nervosa; Bulimia Nervosa; Binge Eating. **Folic Acid**: Physiology, Dietary Sources, and Requirements. **Iron**: Physiology, Dietary Sources, and Requirements. **Obesity**: Definition, Aetiology, and Assessment. **Osteoporosis**: Nutritional Factors **Zinc**: Physiology.

iii. To indicate material that broadens the discussion.

> *See also*: **Adolescents**: Nutritional Requirements of Adolescents. **Anemia**: Iron-Deficiency Anemia. **Calcium**: Physiology. **Eating Disorders**: Anorexia Nervosa; Bulimia Nervosa; Binge Eating. **Follic Acid**: Physiology, Dietary Sources, and Requirements. **Iron**: Physiology, Dietary Sources, and Requirements. **Obesity**: Definition, Aetiology, and Assessment. **Osteoporosis**: Nutritional Factors. **Zinc**: Physiology.

3. Index

The index will provide you with the page number where the material is located, and the index entries differentiate between material that is a whole article, is part of an article or is data presented in a figure or table. Detailed notes are provided on the opening page of the index.

4. Contributors

A full list of contributors appears at the beginning of each volume.

CONTRIBUTORS

E Abalos
Centro Rosarino de Estudios Perinatales
Rosario, Argentina

A Abi-Hanna
Johns Hopkins School of Medicine
Baltimore, MD, USA

L S Adair
University of North Carolina
Chapel Hill, NC, USA

A Ahmed
Obetech Obesity Research Center
Richmond, VA, USA

B Ahrén
Lund University
Lund, Sweden

J Akré
World Health Organization, Geneva, Switzerland

A J Alberg
Johns Hopkins Bloomberg School of Public Health
Baltimore, MD, USA

L H Allen
University of California at Davis
Davis, CA, USA

D Anderson
University of Bradford
Bradford, UK

J J B Anderson
University of North Carolina
Chapel Hill, NC, USA

R A Anderson
US Department of Agriculture
Beltsville, MD, USA

L J Appel
Johns Hopkins University
Baltimore, MD, USA

A Ariño
University of Zaragoza
Zaragoza, Spain

M J Arnaud
Nestle S.A.
Vevey, Switzerland

E W Askew
University of Utah
Salt Lake City, UT, USA

R L Atkinson
Obetech Obesity Research Center
Richmond, VA, USA

S A Atkinson
McMaster University
Hamilton, ON, Canada

L S A Augustin
University of Toronto
Toronto, ON, Canada

D J Baer
US Department of Agriculture
Beltsville, MD, USA

A Baqui
Johns Hopkins Bloomberg School of Public Health
Baltimore, MD, USA

Y Barnett
Nottingham Trent University
Nottingham, UK

G E Bartley
Agricultural Research Service
Albany, CA, USA

C J Bates
MRC Human Nutrition Research
Cambridge, UK

J A Beltrán
University of Zaragoza
Zaragoza, Spain

A E Bender
Leatherhead, UK

D A Bender
University College London
London, UK

I F F Benzie
The Hong Kong Polytechnic University
Hong Kong SAR, China

C D Berdanier
University of Georgia
Athens, GA, USA

R Bhatia
United Nations World Food Programme
Rome, Italy

Z A Bhutta
The Aga Khan University
Karachi, Pakistan

J E Bines
University of Melbourne
Melbourne, VIC, Australia

J Binkley
Vanderbilt Center for Human Nutrition
Nashville, TN, USA

R Black
Johns Hopkins Bloomberg School of Public Health
Baltimore, MD, USA

J E Blundell
University of Leeds
Leeds, UK

A T Borchers
University of California at Davis
Davis, CA, USA

C Boreham
University of Ulster at Jordanstown
Jordanstown, UK

F Branca
Istituto Nazionale di Ricerca per gli Alimenti e la Nutrizione
Rome, Italy

J Brand-Miller
University of Sydney
Sydney, NSW, Australia

A Briend
Institut de Recherche pour le Développement
Paris, France

P Browne
St James's Hospital
Dublin, Ireland

I A Brownlee
University of Newcastle
Newcastle-upon-Tyne, UK

H Brunner
Centre Hospitalier Universitaire Vaudois
Lausanne, Switzerland

A J Buckley
University of Cambridge
Cambridge, UK

H H Butchko
Exponent, Inc.
Wood Dale, IL, USA

J Buttriss
British Nutrition Foundation
London, UK

B Caballero
Johns Hopkins Bloomberg School of Public Health and
    Johns Hopkins University
Baltimore, MD, USA

E A Carrey
Institute of Child Health
London, UK

A Cassidy
School of Medicine
University of East Anglia
Norwich, UK

G E Caughey
Royal Adelaide Hospital
Adelaide, SA, Australia

J P Cegielski
Centers for Disease Control and Prevention
Atlanta, GA, USA

C M Champagne
Pennington Biomedical Research Center
Baton Rouge, LA, USA

S C Chen
US Department of Agriculture
Beltsville, MD, USA

L Cheskin
Johns Hopkins University
Baltimore, MD, USA

S Chung
Columbia University
New York, NY, USA

L G Cleland
Royal Adelaide Hospital
Adelaide, SA, Australia

L Cobiac
CSIRO Health Sciences and Nutrition
Adelaide, SA, Australia

G A Colditz
Harvard Medical School
Boston, MA, USA

T J Cole
Institute of Child Health
London, UK

L A Coleman
Marshfield Clinic Research Foundation
Marshfield, WI, USA

S Collier
Children's Hospital, Boston, Harvard Medical School,
   and Harvard School of Public Health
Boston, MA, USA

M Collins
Muckamore Abbey Hospital
Antrim, UK

K G Conner
Johns Hopkins Hospital
Baltimore, MD, USA

K C Costas
Children's Hospital Boston
Boston, MA, USA

R C Cottrell
The Sugar Bureau
London, UK

W A Coward
MRC Human Nutrition Research
Cambridge, UK

J M Cox
Johns Hopkins Hospital
Baltimore, MD, USA

S Cox
London School of Hygiene and Tropical Medicine
London, UK

P D'Acapito
Istituto Nazionale di Ricerca per gli Alimenti e la Nutrizione
Rome, Italy

S Daniell
Vanderbilt Center for Human Nutrition
Nashville, TN, USA

O Dary
The MOST Project
Arlington, VA, USA

T J David
University of Manchester
Manchester, UK

C P G M de Groot
Wageningen University
Wageningen, The Netherlands

M de Onis
World Health Organization
Geneva, Switzerland

M C de Souza
Universidad de Mogi das Cruzes
São Paulo, Brazil

R de Souza
University of Toronto
Toronto, ON, Canada

C H C Dejong
University Hospital Maastricht
Maastricht, The Netherlands

L Demeshlaira
Emory University
Atlanta, GA, USA

K G Dewey
University of California at Davis
Davis, CA, USA

H L Dewraj
The Aga Khan University
Karachi, Pakistan

C Doherty
MRC Keneba
The Gambia

C M Donangelo
Universidade Federal do Rio de Janeiro
Rio de Janeiro, Brazil

A Dornhorst
Imperial College at Hammersmith Hospital
London, UK

E Dowler
University of Warwick
Coventry, UK

J Dowsett
St Vincent's University Hospital
Dublin, Ireland

A K Draper
University of Westminster
London, UK

M L Dreyfuss
Johns Hopkins Bloomberg School of Public Health
Baltimore, MD, USA

R D'Souza
Queen Mary's, University of London
London, UK

C Duggan
Harvard Medical School
Boston, MA, USA

A G Dulloo
University of Fribourg
Fribourg, Switzerland

E B Duly
Ulster Hospital
Belfast, UK

J L Dupont
Florida State University
Tallahassee, FL, USA

J Dwyer
Tufts University
Boston, MA, USA

J Eaton–Evans
University of Ulster
Coleraine, UK

C A Edwards
University of Glasgow
Glasgow, UK

M Elia
University of Southampton
Southampton, UK

P W Emery
King's College London
London, UK

J L Ensunsa
University of California at Davis
Davis, CA, USA

C Feillet-Coudray
National Institute for Agricultural Research
Clermont-Ferrand, France

J D Fernstrom
University of Pittsburgh
Pittsburgh, PA, USA

M H Fernstrom
University of Pittsburgh
Pittsburgh, PA, USA

F Fidanza
University of Rome Tor Vergata
Rome, Italy

P Fieldhouse
The University of Manitoba
Winnipeg, MB, Canada

N Finer
Luton and Dunstable Hospital NHS Trust
Luton, UK

J Fiore
University of Westminster
London, UK

H C Freake
University of Connecticut
Storrs, CT, USA

J Freitas
Tufts University
Boston, MA, USA

R E Frisch
Harvard Center for Population and Development Studies
Cambridge, MA, USA

G Frost
Imperial College at Hammersmith Hospital
London, UK

G Frühbeck
Universidad de Navarra
Pamplona, Spain

D Gallagher
Columbia University
New York, NY, USA

L Galland
Applied Nutrition Inc.
New York, NY, USA

C Geissler
King's College London
London, UK

M E Gershwin
University of California at Davis
Davis, CA, USA

H Ghattas
London School of Hygiene and Tropical Medicine
London, UK

E L Gibson
University College London
London, UK

T P Gill
University of Sydney
Sydney, NSW, Australia

W Gilmore
University of Ulster
Coleraine, UK

G R Goldberg
MRC Human Nutrition Research
Cambridge, UK

J Gómez-Ambrosi
Universidad de Navarra
Pamplona, Spain

J M Graham
University of California at Davis
Davis, CA, USA

J Gray
Guildford, UK

J P Greaves
London, UK

M W Green
Aston University
Birmingham, UK

R Green
University of California
Davis, CA, USA

R F Grimble
University of Southampton
Southampton, UK

M Grønbæk
National Institute of Public Health
Copenhagen, Denmark

J D Groopman
Johns Hopkins University
Baltimore MD, USA

S M Grundy
University of Texas Southwestern Medical Center
Dallas, TX, USA

M A Grusak
Baylor College of Medicine
Houston, TX, USA

M Gueimonde
University of Turku
Turku, Finland

C S Gulotta
Johns Hopkins University and Kennedy
Krieger Institute
Baltimore, MD, USA

P Haggarty
Rowett Research Institute
Aberdeen, UK

J C G Halford
University of Liverpool
Liverpool, UK

C H Halsted
University of California at Davis
Davis, CA, USA

J Hampsey
Johns Hopkins School of Medicine
Baltimore, MD, USA

E D Harris
Texas A&M University
College Station, TX, USA

Z L Harris
Johns Hopkins Hospital and School of Medicine
Baltimore, MD, USA

P J Havel
University of California at Davis
Davis, CA, USA

W W Hay Jr
University of Colorado Health Sciences Center
Aurora, CO, USA

R G Heine
University of Melbourne
Melbourne, VIC, Australia

R Heinzen
Johns Hopkins Bloomberg School of Public Health
Baltimore, MD, USA

A Herrera
University of Zaragoza
Zaragoza, Spain

B S Hetzel
Women's and Children's Hospital
North Adelaide, SA, Australia

A J Hill
University of Leeds
Leeds, UK

S A Hill
Southampton General Hospital
Southampton, UK

G A Hitman
Queen Mary's, University of London
London, UK

J M Hodgson
University of Western Australia
Perth, WA, Australia

M F Holick
Boston University Medical Center
Boston, MA, USA

C Hotz
National Institute of Public Health
Morelos, Mexico

R Houston
Emory University
Atlanta, GA, USA

H-Y Huang
Johns Hopkins University
Baltimore, MD, USA

J R Hunt
USDA-ARS Grand Forks Human Nutrition Research Center
Grand Forks, ND, USA

R Hunter
King's College London
London, UK

P Hyland
Nottingham Trent University
Nottingham, UK

B K Ishida
Agricultural Research Service
Albany, CA, USA

J Jacquet
University of Geneva
Geneva, Switzerland

M J James
Royal Adelaide Hospital
Adelaide, SA, Australia

W P T James
International Association for the Study of Obesity/
    International Obesity Task Force Offices
London, UK

A G Jardine
University of Glasgow
Glasgow, UK

S A Jebb
MRC Human Nutrition Research
Cambridge, UK

K N Jeejeebhoy
University of Toronto
Toronto, ON, Canada

D J A Jenkins
University of Toronto
Toronto, ON, Canada

G L Jensen
Vanderbilt Center for Human Nutrition
Nashville, TN, USA

I T Johnson
Institute of Food Research
Norwich, UK

P A Judd
University of Central Lancashire
Preston, UK

M A Kalarchian
University of Pittsburgh
Pittsburgh, PA, USA

R M Katz
Johns Hopkins University School of Medicine and Mount
   Washington Pediatric Hospital
Baltimore, MD, USA

C L Keen
University of California at Davis
Davis, CA, USA

N L Keim
US Department of Agriculture
Davis, CA, USA

E Kelly
Harvard Medical School
Boston, MA, USA

C W C Kendall
University of Toronto
Toronto, ON, Canada

T W Kensler
Johns Hopkins University
Baltimore, MD, USA

J E Kerstetter
University of Connecticut
Storrs, CT, USA

M Kiely
University College Cork
Cork, Ireland

P Kirk
University of Ulster
Coleraine, UK

S F L Kirk
University of Leeds
Leeds, UK

P N Kirke
The Health Research Board
Dublin, Ireland

G L Klein
University of Texas Medical Branch at Galveston
Galveston TX, USA

R D W Klemm
Johns Hopkins University
Baltimore, MD, USA

D M Klurfeld
US Department of Agriculture
Beltville, MD, USA

P G Kopelman
Queen Mary's, University of London
London, UK

J Krick
Kennedy–Krieger Institute
Baltimore, MD, USA

D Kritchevsky
Wistar Institute
Philadelphia, PA, USA

R Lang
University of Teeside
Middlesbrough, UK

A Laurentin
Universidad Central de Venezuela
Caracas, Venezuela

A Laverty
Muckamore Abbey Hospital
Antrim, UK

M Lawson
Institute of Child Health
London, UK

F E Leahy
University of Auckland
Auckland, New Zealand

A R Leeds
King's College London
London, UK

J Leiper
University of Aberdeen
Aberdeen, UK

M D Levine
University of Pittsburgh
Pittsburgh, PA, USA

A H Lichtenstein
Tufts University
Boston MA, USA

E Lin
Emory University
Atlanta, GA, USA

L Lissner
Sahlgrenska Academy at Göteborg University
Göteborg, Sweden

C Lo
Children's Hospital, Boston, Harvard Medical School, and
  Harvard School of Public Health
Boston, MA, USA

P A Lofgren
Oak Park, IL, USA

B Lönnerdal
University of California at Davis
Davis, CA, USA

M J Luetkemeier
Alma College
Alma, MI, USA

Y C Luiking
University Hospital Maastricht
Maastricht, The Netherlands

P G Lunn
University of Cambridge
Cambridge, UK

C K Lutter
Pan American Health Organization
Washington, DC, USA

A MacDonald
The Children's Hospital
Birmingham, UK

A Maqbool
The Children's Hospital of Philadelphia
Philadelphia, PA, USA

M D Marcus
University of Pittsburgh
Pittsburgh, PA, USA

E Marietta
The Mayo Clinic College of Medicine
Rochester, MN, USA

P B Mark
University of Glasgow
Glasgow, UK

V Marks
University of Surrey
Guildford, UK

D L Marsden
Children's Hospital Boston
Boston, MA, USA

R J Maughan
Loughborough University
Loughborough, UK

K C McCowen
Beth Israel Deaconess Medical Center and Harvard
  Medical School
Boston, MA, USA

S S McDonald
Raleigh, NC, USA

S McLaren
London South Bank University
London, UK

J L McManaman
University of Colorado
Denver, CO, USA

D N McMurray
Texas A&M University
College Station, TX, USA

D J McNamara
Egg Nutrition Center
Washington, DC, USA

J McPartlin
Trinity College
Dublin, Ireland

R P Mensink
Maastricht University
Maastricht, The Netherlands

M Merialdi
World Health Organization
Geneva, Switzerland

A R Michell
St Bartholomew's Hospital
London, UK

J W Miller
UC Davis Medical Center
Sacramento, CA, USA

P Miller
Kennedy–Krieger Institute
Baltimore, MD, USA

D J Millward
University of Surrey
Guildford, UK

D M Mock
University of Arkansas for Medical Sciences
Little Rock, AR, USA

N Moore
John Hopkins School of Medicine
Baltimore, MD, USA

J O Mora
The MOST Project
Arlington, VA, USA

T Morgan
University of Melbourne
Melbourne, VIC, Australia

T A Mori
University of Western Australia
Perth, WA, Australia

J E Morley
St Louis University
St Louis, MO, USA

P A Morrissey
University College Cork
Cork, Ireland

M H Murphy
University of Ulster at Jordanstown
Jordanstown, UK

S P Murphy
University of Hawaii
Honolulu, HI, USA

J Murray
The Mayo Clinic College of Medicine
Rochester, MN, USA

R Nalubola
Center for Food Safety and Applied Nutrition,
US Food and Drug Administration, MD, USA

J L Napoli
University of California
Berkeley, CA, USA

V Nehra
The Mayo Clinic College of Medicine
Rochester, MN, USA

B Nejadnik
Johns Hopkins University
Baltimore, MD, USA

M Nelson
King's College London
London, UK

P Nestel
International Food Policy Research Institute
Washington, DC, USA

L M Neufeld
National Institute of Public Health
Cuernavaca, Mexico

M C Neville
University of Colorado
Denver, CO, USA

F Nielsen
Grand Forks Human Nutrition Research Center
Grand Forks, ND, USA

N Noah
London School of Hygiene and Tropical Medicine
London, UK

K O O'Brien
Johns Hopkins University
Baltimore, MD, USA

S H Oh
Johns Hopkins General Clinical Research Center
Baltimore, MD, USA

J M Ordovas
Tufts University
Boston, MA, USA

S E Ozanne
University of Cambridge
Cambridge, UK

D M Paige
Johns Hopkins Bloomberg School of Public Health
Baltimore, MD, USA

J P Pearson
University of Newcastle
Newcastle-upon-Tyne, UK

S S Percival
University of Florida
Gainesville, FL, USA

T Peters
King's College Hospital
London, UK

B J Petersen
Exponent, Inc.
Washington DC, USA

J C Phillips
BIBRA International Ltd
Carshalton, UK

M F Picciano
National Institutes of Health
Bethesda, MD, USA

A Pietrobelli
Verona University Medical School
Verona, Italy

S Pin
Johns Hopkins Hospital and School of Medicine
Baltimore, MD, USA

B M Popkin
University of North Carolina
Chapel Hill, NC, USA

E M E Poskitt
London School of Hygiene and Tropical Medicine
London, UK

A D Postle
University of Southampton
Southampton, UK

J Powell-Tuck
Queen Mary's, University of London
London, UK

V Preedy
King's College London
London, UK

N D Priest
Middlesex University
London, UK

R Rajendram
King's College London
London, UK

A Raman
University of Wisconsin–Madison
Madison, WI, USA

H A Raynor
Brown University
Providence, RI, USA

Y Rayssiguier
National Institute for Agricultural Research
Clermont-Ferrand, France

L N Richardson
United Nations World Food Programme
Rome, Italy

F J Rohr
Children's Hospital Boston
Boston, MA, USA

A R Rolla
Harvard Medical School
Boston, MA, USA

P Roncalés
University of Zaragoza
Zaragoza, Spain

A C Ross
The Pennsylvania State University
University Park, PA, USA

R Roubenoff
Millennium Pharmaceuticals, Inc.
Cambridge, MA, USA and Tufts University
Boston, MA, USA

D Rumsey
University of Sheffield
Sheffield, UK

C H S Ruxton
Nutrition Communications
Cupar, UK

J M Saavedra
John Hopkins School of Medicine
Baltimore, MD, USA

J E Sable
University of California at Davis
Davis, CA, USA

M J Sadler
MJSR Associates
Ashford, UK

N R Sahyoun
University of Maryland
College Park, MD, USA

S Salminen
University of Turku
Turku, Finland

M Saltmarsh
Alton, UK

J M Samet
Johns Hopkins Bloomberg School of Public Health
Baltimore, MD, USA

C P Sánchez-Castillo
National Institute of Medical Sciences and Nutrition
Salvador Zubirán, Tlalpan, Mexico

M Santosham
Johns Hopkins Bloomberg School of Public Health
Baltimore, MD, USA

C D Saudek
Johns Hopkins School of Medicine
Baltimore, MD, USA

A O Scheimann
Johns Hopkins School of Medicine
Baltimore, MD, USA

B Schneeman
University of California at Davis
Davis, CA, USA

D A Schoeller
University of Wisconsin–Madison
Madison, WI, USA

L Schuberth
Kennedy Krieger Institute
Baltimore, MD, USA

K J Schulze
Johns Hopkins Bloomberg School of Public Health
Baltimore, MD, USA

Y Schutz
University of Lausanne
Lausanne, Switzerland

K B Schwarz
Johns Hopkins School of Medicine
Baltimore, MD, USA

J M Scott
Trinity College Dublin
Dublin, Ireland

C Shaw
Royal Marsden NHS Foundation Trust
London, UK

J Shedlock
Johns Hopkins Hospital and School of Medicine
Baltimore, MD, USA

S M Shirreffs
Loughborough University
Loughborough, UK

R Shrimpton
Institute of Child Health
London, UK

H A Simmonds
Guy's Hospital
London, UK

A P Simopoulos
The Center for Genetics, Nutrition and Health
Washington, DC, USA

R J Smith
Brown Medical School
Providence, RI, USA

P B Soeters
University Hospital Maastricht
Maastricht, The Netherlands

N Solomons
Center for Studies of Sensory Impairment, Aging and
 Metabolism (CeSSIAM)
Guatemala City, Guatemala

J A Solon
MRC Laboratories Gambia
Banjul, The Gambia

K Srinath Reddy
All India Institute of Medical Sciences
New Delhi, India

S Stanner
British Nutrition Foundation
London, UK

J Stevens
University of North Carolina at Chapel Hill
Chapel Hill, NC, USA

J J Strain
University of Ulster
Coleraine, UK

R J Stratton
University of Southampton
Southampton, UK

R J Stubbs
The Rowett Research Institute
Aberdeen, UK

C L Stylianopoulos
Johns Hopkins University
Baltimore, MD, USA

A W Subudhi
University of Colorado at Colorado
Colorado Springs, CO, USA

J Sudagani
Queen Mary's, University of London
London, UK

S A Tanumihardjo
University of Wisconsin-Madison
Madison, WI, USA

J A Tayek
Harbor–UCLA Medical Center
Torrance, CA, USA

E H M Temme
University of Leuven
Leuven, Belgium

H S Thesmar
Egg Nutrition Center
Washington, DC, USA

B M Thomson
Rowett Research Institute
Aberdeen, UK

D I Thurnham
University of Ulster
Coleraine, UK

L Tolentino
National Institute of Public Health
Cuernavaca, Mexico

D L Topping
CSIRO Health Sciences and Nutrition
Adelaide, SA, Australia

B Torun
Center for Research and Teaching in Latin
 America (CIDAL)
Guatemala City, Guatemala

M G Traber
Oregon State University
Corvallis, OR, USA

T R Trinick
Ulster Hospital
Belfast, UK

K P Truesdale
University of North Carolina at Chapel Hill
Chapel Hill, NC, USA

N M F Trugo
Universidade Federal do Rio de Janeiro
Rio de Janeiro, Brazil

P M Tsai
Harvard Medical School
Boston, MA, USA

K L Tucker
Tufts University
Boston, MA, USA

O Tully
St Vincent's University Hospital
Dublin, Ireland

E C Uchegbu
Royal Hallamshire Hospital
Sheffield, UK

M C G van de Poll
University Hospital Maastricht
Maastricht, The Netherlands

W A van Staveren
Wageningen University
Wageningen, The Netherlands

J Villar
World Health Organization
Geneva, Switzerland

M L Wahlqvist
Monash University
Victoria, VIC, Australia

A F Walker
The University of Reading
Reading, UK

P A Watkins
Kennedy Krieger Institute and Johns Hopkins
   University School of Medicine
Baltimore, MD, USA

A A Welch
University of Cambridge
Cambridge, UK

R W Welch
University of Ulster
Coleraine, UK

K P West Jr
Johns Hopkins University
Baltimore, MD, USA

S Whybrow
The Rowett Research Institute
Aberdeen, UK

D H Williamson
Radcliffe Infirmary
Oxford, UK

M-M G Wilson
St Louis University
St Louis, MO, USA

R R Wing
Brown University
Providence, RI, USA

C K Winter
University of California at Davis
Davis, CA, USA

H Wiseman
King's College London
London, UK

M Wolraich
Vanderbilt University
Nashville, TN, USA

R J Wood
Tufts University
Boston, MA, USA

X Xu
Johns Hopkins Hospital and School of Medicine
Baltimore, MD, USA

Z Yang
University of Wisconsin-Madison
Madison, WI, USA

A A Yates
ENVIRON Health Sciences
Arlington, VA, USA

S H Zeisel
University of North Carolina at Chapel Hill
Chapel Hill, NC, USA

X Zhu
University of North Carolina at Chapel Hill
Chapel Hill, NC, USA

S Zidenberg-Cherr
University of California at Davis
Davis, CA, USA

T R Ziegler
Emory University
Atlanta, GA, USA

CONTENTS

VOLUME 1

VOLUME 4

R

S

I

IMMUNITY

Contents
Physiological Aspects
Effects of Iron and Zinc

Physiological Aspects

A T Borchers, C L Keen and M E Gershwin,
University of California at Davis, Davis, CA, USA

Immunity can be defined as the ability of an organism to resist or eliminate potentially harmful foreign organisms and materials or abnormal cells. Any substance capable of eliciting an immune response is called an antigen (antibody generator). Immune responses can be classified as innate or adaptive. Innate immune responses are also called nonspecific because they can be elicited by a wide range of foreign substances and are the same regardless of the exact nature of the substance and whether it had been encountered before. The major mechanisms of innate immunity include phagocytosis, inflammation, complement activation, and induction of cell death. Neutrophils and macrophages are the main cell types responsible for phagocytosis, and the chemical messengers that they and some other cell types produce play an important role in the initiation of an inflammatory response. The induction of apoptosis (programmed cell death) as part of the innate immune response is accomplished by natural killer (NK) cells.

In contrast to innate immune responses, adaptive immune responses are highly specific for a particular antigen and become stronger and more rapid over time. B cells and T cells represent the two types of lymphocytes responsible for adaptive immune responses. The main function of B cells is to produce antibodies, which neutralize pathogens or stimulate their elimination by other cell types through opsonization or complement activation. There are two major classes of T cells, namely helper T cells and cytotoxic T cells. One subclass of helper T cells provides help to macrophages in killing pathogenic microorganisms they have engulfed. The other subclass of helper T cells is vital for the induction of antibody production by B cells. Cytotoxic T cells directly eliminate infected cells by inducing them to undergo apoptosis. T cells also play a central role in self-tolerance (i.e., the ability not to respond to self antigens).

Initial exposure to pathogens (i.e., disease-producing microorganisms such as viruses and bacteria) most commonly occurs at the interfaces of host tissues and the external environment. Such tissues include the outer cells of the skin and, since the vertebrate body is essentially a 'tube within a tube,' the layers of cells and mucous lining the digestive, reproductive, and respiratory tracts. These cell layers and their secretions constitute nonimmunological physical and chemical barriers that provide a first line of defense against invasion by pathogenic microorganisms. Their barrier function is often reinforced by a variety of bacteria that generally do not harm the host but, on the contrary, provide additional protection from pathogens via competition, production of toxic substances, and stimulation of the immune system.

The main function of the immune system is to provide protection from invading pathogens, primarily viruses and bacteria but also fungi and parasites. For this purpose, the ability to discriminate between self or harmless non-self and potentially harmful non-self is absolutely crucial. Also important is the capability to recognize whether pathogens are extracellular (outside of the host's cells), such as fungi, certain bacteria, and some parasites, or intracellular, such as other bacteria and parasites and all viruses. Other activities of the immune system include the removal of worn-out cells, the identification and destruction of mutant or otherwise abnormal cells and also such inappropriate responses as allergies and autoimmune diseases, and graft rejection after organ transplantation.

Immune Cells and Organs

Immune cells are leukocytes (white blood cells) and, together with red blood cells, are ultimately derived from the same precursor or progenitor cells in the bone marrow. As illustrated in **Figure 1**, these stem cells give rise to either lymphoid or myeloid progenitors that subsequently differentiate into the different immune cells. A few other types of immune cells, including NK cells and mast cells, also arise from these pluripotent stem cells, but the pathways of their development are not fully known.

The differentiation of lymphocytes takes place in the central (also called primary) lymphoid organs—that is, bone marrow in the case of B cells and thymus in the case of T cells. After puberty, the thymus gradually atrophies and the production of new T cells decreases. After their maturation in the primary lymphoid organs, both types of lymphocytes migrate from these tissues

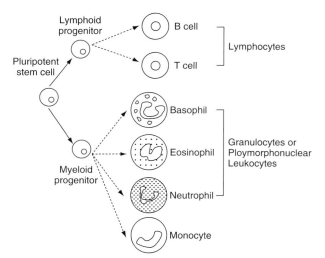

Figure 1 Immune cells give rise to either lymphoid or myeloid progenitors, which subsequently differentiate into the different immune cells.

Table 1 Functions of myeloid and lymphoid immune cells

Cell progenitor	Cell type	Function
Myeloid		
	Basophil	Unknown
	Eosinophil	Killing of antibody-coated parasites
	Neutrophil	Phagocytosis and activation of bactericidal mechanisms
	Macrophage[a]	Phagocytosis
	Mast cell	Release of histamine and other vasoactive and inflammatory mediators
Lymphoid		
	B cell	Antibody production
	T cell	
	Cytotoxic	Killing of virus-infected cells
	Helper (Th1 and Th2)	Activation of other cells such as B cells and macrophages
	Natural Killer cells	Killing of virus-infected cells and cancer cells

[a]This cell type circulates as monocytes in the bloodstream and matures into macrophages when taking up residence in a tissue.

through the bloodstream into the peripheral, or secondary, lymphoid tissues. These include the lymph nodes, spleen, and lymphoid tissues associated with mucosa, and they constitute the main sites at which the reaction of B and T lymphocytes with foreign antigens takes place. Lymph then carries circulating lymphocytes from the peripheral lymphoid tissues to the thoracic duct, where they reenter the bloodstream. The functions of the various immune cells are summarized in **Table 1**.

Innate (Nonspecific) versus Adaptive (Specific) Immunity

Immune responses can be divided into two broad categories: innate and adaptive. Innate immune responses are also called nonspecific since they do not discriminate between most foreign substances. They are also not enhanced by previous exposure to a pathogen. In contrast, adaptive (also called acquired) immunity is highly specific to a particular pathogen and becomes more rapid and stronger with subsequent exposure to an antigen. Upon the initial encounter with an antigen, the adaptive immune response takes 4 or 5 days to become fully effective. During this period, the innate immune response plays a critical role in limiting and controlling infections. In addition, it is crucial in stimulating and directing the subsequent adaptive immune responses.

Innate or Nonspecific Immunity

Phagocytosis Pathogens can cause infection only after they have breached the nonimmunological barriers of skin or mucosal surfaces. Generally, the first immune cells they come in contact with are macrophages. Among the many chemicals macrophages start to produce are chemokines, small proteins involved in the recruitment and activation of immune cells. The first cells to be recruited to the site of infection are neutrophils. Macrophages along with neutrophils are the major cell types involved in phagocytosis (i.e., the ingestion of foreign materials, including entire microorganisms). Phagocytosis is triggered via receptors on the surface of macrophages and neutrophils that recognize common cell wall components of bacteria. Killing of the ingested bacteria occurs via several different mechanisms involving the production of reactive oxygen and nitrogen species as well as the release of a variety of preformed antimicrobial substances.

Inflammation   In addition to stimulating phagocytosis, the encounter of macrophages and neutrophils with bacteria frequently initiates an inflammatory response. The characteristics of inflammation are pain, redness, swelling, and heat. These symptoms are the consequence of the activities of cytokines and chemokines along with a variety of other vasoactive and inflammatory mediators, such as histamine, prostaglandins, and leukotrienes. They act mostly on local blood vessels, where their combined effect is to enhance blood flow, induce vasodilation, and increase the permeability of blood vessels. These changes allow leakage of fluids and plasma proteins, such as immunoglobulins, complement, and acute phase proteins, into the affected tissue. Cytokines also induce the expression of molecules that make it possible for immune cells to adhere to, and eventually pass between, the cells lining the blood vessels. Together, these alterations result in the infiltration of the site of inflammation by immune cells.

The major inflammatory cytokines are tumor necrosis factor-α (TNF-α), interleukin-1 (IL-1, IL-6, and IL-12, all of which are produced mostly by macrophages. Among these, TNF-α, IL-1, and IL-6 are central to mediating the acute phase response, which is characterized by elevation of the body temperature (fever) and a marked shift in the types of proteins secreted by the liver into the bloodstream. Whereas the synthesis of some liver proteins, called acute phase proteins, is dramatically increased, that of others is decreased. Among the acute phase proteins, C-reactive protein, mannose-binding protein, and serum amyloid P component undergo the most striking increase in synthesis, whereas only moderate increases are observed in a number of other acute phase proteins. It appears that the diverse activities of these proteins are ultimately beneficial to the host since they not only enhance the inflammatory response and other immune cell activities, thereby boosting host resistance, but also promote tissue repair.

Natural killer cells   All viruses are intracellular pathogens since they lack the ability to replicate on their own and need to penetrate cells of the host in order to take over their replication machinery. The killing of such infected cells before the virus has had a chance to reproduce can be accomplished by a variety of cell types but is one of the major functions of NK cells. NK cells are large granular lymphocytes with a morphology and lineage that are distinct from those of B and T lymphocytes. They are known to be able to distinguish between normal cells and virally infected or tumorous cells, but the exact mechanisms by which they do so remain to be fully established. The granules of NK cells contain perforin, a protein that can polymerize and form transmembrane pores in the infected cell, possibly providing an entry route for a variety of enzymes also stored in the granules. As a result, the infected cell initiates an active suicide program called programmed cell death or apoptosis.

Interferons   Interferon-α and interferon-β are proteins produced by many cells types in response to viral infection. They reduce the spread of viruses to uninfected cells by inhibiting protein synthesis and DNA replication in virus-infected cells and activating NK cells. In addition, they increase the expression of certain molecules and enhance certain cellular processes that are of great importance in activating components of the adaptive immune system involved in eliminating virally infected cells.

Complement   The complement system consists of a group of proteins synthesized by the liver and released into the bloodstream in inactive form. It is part of the nonspecific immune response but can also be triggered by antigen–antibody complexes (i.e., it forms part of the humoral response in adaptive immunity). The latter pathway of activation is called the classical pathway and constitutes one of the three different pathways of complement activation. All three pathways involve a series of cleavage reactions converting inactive proteins into their active forms and ultimately converge at the formation of C3 convertase, an enzyme that cleaves complement component C3 into the large fragment C3b, on the one hand, and a group of smaller peptides consisting of C3a, C4a, and C5a, on the other hand. These smaller peptides mediate certain inflammatory processes and participate in the recruitment of phagocytes. C3b binds to the surface of pathogens and, in the presence of simultaneous coating with antibodies, stimulates phagocytes to engulf and ultimately destroy the microorganism. In addition, further cleavage of C3b yields a group of terminal complement components that form a membrane attack complex able to damage the cell membrane and causing the lysis of certain pathogens.

Adaptive or Acquired Immunity

The cells of the innate immune system are vital as a first line of defense, but they are not always able to completely neutralize or eliminate infectious organisms. The adaptive immune system is thought to have evolved later in evolutionary history and now provides not only more specificity and versatility but also has added immunological memory as a further level of protection against reinfection with the same pathogen.

Adaptive immune responses can be classified as either antibody- or cell-mediated. Antibody-mediated, or humoral, responses are accomplished by plasma cells derived from B cells; cellular immune responses are mediated by activated T lymphocytes. Although they use vastly different effector mechanisms, the activation and subsequent differentiation of B and T lymphocytes nonetheless have many features in common.

In adaptive immunity, antigen alone is generally insufficient to activate naive antigen-specific lymphocytes. Naive T cells require a costimulatory signal from antigen presenting cells; naive B cells usually require accessory signals from an activated helper T cell, but in some cases the signal can be provided directly by microbial constituents. T cell help for B cells has to come from activated helper T cells that respond to the same antigen as the B cell, although the epitope—the specific part of the antigen that is recognized—is generally not identical. Upon recognition of its specific antigen in the context of the appropriate costimulatory signals, the previously small lymphocyte enlarges and undergoes a variety of changes in preparation for vastly increased RNA and protein synthesis. The activated cell is called a lymphoblast. This lymphoblast then begins to divide, duplicating every 6–12 h, thereby giving rise to ~1000 daughter cells, each exhibiting specificity that is identical to that of the parent. Thus, this group of cells constitutes a clone, defined as a population of identical cells that derive from the same ancestral line. Note that most antigens stimulate many different lymphocyte clones, making the resulting response polyclonal. The process of clonal expansion is followed by differentiation into either effector cells or memory cells.

Memory cells, unlike effector cells, do not participate in the initial immune response but can become activated cells when they encounter the same antigen at a later time point, in some cases years or even decades later. This, along with other changes in memory cells compared to virgin (or naïve) cells, accounts for the fact that the primary immune response is characterized by a lag phase of several days (the period during which lymphocytes undergo clonal expansion and differentiation) and is relatively weak, whereas a second exposure to the same antigen results in a much more rapid and stronger response.

B cells   The primary function of B cells is the production of antibodies, or immunoglobulins. There are five major classes (isotypes) of antibodies: IgA, IgD, IgE, IgG, and IgM, with IgA and IgG having two and four subclasses, respectively. Resting B cells express IgM and IgD on their cell surface as antigen receptors. Their function is to capture antigen so that it can then be processed and displayed to helper T cells specific for peptide fragments of the same antigen. In response to binding antigen and receiving the necessary accessory signal from helper T cells in the form of cell–cell interactions along with secreted molecules, B cells start to produce a secreted version of IgM. Under the influence of certain cytokines produced predominantly by activated helper T cells, B cells undergo isotype switching, also called class switching, meaning that they start to produce other types of immunoglobulins. The types and combinations of immunoglobulin isotypes depend on the nature and relative amounts of these cytokines. In B cell activation and initiation of antibody production, a subclass of helper T cells called Th2 plays the major role; the Th1 subclass of helper T cells, however, participates in isotype switching via the production of interferon-γ, a cytokine that induces switching to specific subclasses of IgG, namely IgG2a and IgG3.

Antibody structure and diversity   It is estimated that even in the absence of antigen stimulation, the human body contains B cells capable of producing approximately 10^{15} different antibody molecules. This enormous diversity is generated through a variety of mechanisms.

The basic structure of an antibody is a Y shape (**Figure 2**) consisting of two heavy chains and two light chains, with each arm containing a specific antigen binding site formed by parts of the respective heavy and light chain. The light and the heavy chain each have a constant region and a variable region. Within the variable region three small

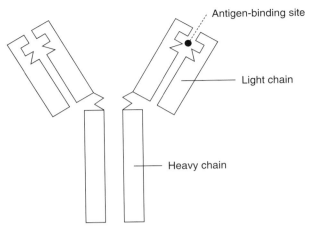

Figure 2 Basic structure of immunoglobulins.

hypervariable regions containing 5–10 amino acids form the antigen binding site. A different pool of gene segments encodes the constant and variable regions and, in addition, there is another pool for joining (J) segments for both heavy and light chains and a pool for diversity (D) segments in the case of heavy chains. The exact number of gene segments in these pools is not known, but the mouse genome is estimated to contain approximately 300 variable (V) segments for one of the two possible light chains, and these can be joined to any of 4 different J segments, yielding at least 1200 different V regions. In addition, there are approximately 500 V segments in the heavy-chain pool of the mouse, which can be combined with 4 J segments and at least 12 D segments to encode 24 000 different heavy-chain V regions. Thus, a total of at least 2.5×10^7 different antigen binding sites can be generated by combinatorial diversification, as the combining of V, J, and D segments is called.

The joining process further increases this diversity via two mechanisms. One operates in heavy- and light-chain segments and is the loss of 1 or more nucleotides from the ends of recombining gene segments. Heavy-chain gene segments can additionally be modified through the random insertion of up to 20 nucleotides. Although it is not uncommon for this junctional diversification to result in the production of nonfunctional genes, it nonetheless increases the number of different B cells in the mouse to an estimated 5×10^8.

After the assembly of functional antibody genes is completed, an additional mechanism for increasing diversity takes place when a B cell is stimulated by antigen. This process is called somatic hypermutation since it involves the insertion of point mutations at a rate that is approximately 1 million times greater than the spontaneous mutation rate in other genes. A few of these point mutations confer increased affinity for the antigen to the antigen receptors, ultimately resulting in the production of antibodies with progressively increasing affinity during the course of an immune response.

The function of antibodies The coating of pathogens and toxins with antibodies helps protect the host from infection in three main ways: neutralization, opsonization, and complement activation. Neutralization refers to the ability of antibodies to inhibit the adherence of pathogens to cells they might invade and destroy. Opsonization is defined as the coating of pathogens with antibodies in order to increase their susceptibility to ingestion by phagocytes. As discussed previously, antibodies complexed with antigen can also trigger the classical pathway of complement, thereby either enhancing opsonization or directly killing some bacteria through the formation of membrane attack complexes. Not all of the secreted antibody isotypes participate in all of these functions, and the extent to which they do so also differs. Certain additional functions are restricted to specific isotypes. For example, only some IgG subclasses can bind to certain viral proteins displayed on virally infected cells and, through interaction with specific receptors, signal NK cells to destroy these cells. Another example is IgE, which is the only isotype capable of sensitizing mast cells, resulting in a local inflammatory response mediated by the release of histamine and other inflammatory mediators. Allergic reactions are the consequence of such a response directed against innocuous antigens.

T cells Whereas B cells recognize and bind directly to extracellular antigens, generally native protein structures, T cells recognize partially degraded protein antigens—that is, peptide fragments that result from intracellular processing and are then carried to the cell surface for display there. The generation of peptide fragments is called antigen processing and the display is called antigen presentation.

Intracellular pathogens can be located in two different compartments of a cell, the cytosol or the vesicular compartment, which is separated from the cytosol by membranes. Depending on the cellular location of the microorganism, one of two different classes of T cells is activated, either cytotoxic T cells or helper T cells. Cells infected with cytosolic pathogens, such as viruses and some bacteria, are eliminated by cytotoxic T cells via mechanisms closely resembling those described for NK cells. Cells containing foreign material or microorganisms in their vesicular compartment stimulate helper T cells.

These do not kill cells but enhance the activity of the very cells stimulating them (i.e., macrophages and B cells). Although macrophages can phagocytose and kill many infectious agents without T cell help, there are certain situations in which such help is indispensable. For example, the mycobacteria responsible for tuberculosis and leprosy have developed mechanisms to survive the process of phagocytosis and can replicate inside vesicular structures. However, they can be eliminated when the macrophage is activated by a helper T cell. T lymphocytes providing help for macrophages belong to a subclass of helper T cells characterized mainly by the types of cytokines it produces and designated as Th1. Another subclass, Th2, activates B cells to make antibody.

Cytotoxic and helper T cells have the same kind of antigen receptors, designated as T cell receptors. This indicates that the ability of the different classes of T cells to distinguish between peptide fragments coming from the cytosolic or the vesicular compartment must involve other molecules. The most important of these are major histocompatibility complex (MHC) molecules.

The MHC is a cluster of genes encoding not only two different classes of MHC molecules but also a variety of other proteins that participate in immune responses. 'Histo' means tissue, and the name 'major histocompatibility complex' reflects the fact that the proteins encoded by this group of genes were first identified as the target of the immune reaction that can result in graft rejection after organ transplantation. In humans, MHC molecules are called human leukocyte-associated antigen (HLA) molecules. In addition to being polygenic (having several genes encoding proteins with the same function), the MHC genes are strikingly polymorphic, meaning that there are multiple alleles, or copies, of each gene.

T cells recognize antigen only when presented as peptide fragments by a MHC molecule. Furthermore, a T cell recognizing a peptide fragment bound by a MHC molecule encoded by a particular allele will not recognize the same peptide bound to another type of MHC molecule, an effect called MHC restriction. Together with the polymorphism of the MHC genes, this limits the ability of a pathogen to put entire populations or even species at risk since the individuals within the population will vary in their susceptibility to the pathogen.

There are two classes (I and II) of MHC molecules that are structurally similar, though distinct, but differ functionally. Class I MHC molecules present foreign peptides to cytotoxic T cells; class II MHC molecules present foreign peptides to helper T cells.

Since viruses can infect any cell containing a nucleus, virtually all nucleated cells express MHC class I molecules, although the levels at which they do so can differ considerably. In contrast, the main function of helper T cells is to activate other cells of the immune system. Thus, MHC class II molecules are constitutively expressed on B lymphocytes, macrophages, and other antigen presenting cells, but they are inducible on many other cell types via certain cytokines.

Since MHC molecules insert themselves into the cell membrane once they have picked up processed antigen fragments inside the cell and the T cell receptor is also a cell surface molecule, T lymphocytes must make direct contact with their target cells. This cell–cell interaction is enhanced by so-called coreceptors, designated CD4 on helper T cells and CD8 on cytotoxic T cells. CD4 proteins recognize an invariable part of the class II MHC molecule, whereas CD8 proteins bind to a nonvariable region of the class I MHC molecule, and both play a vital role in ensuring that a T cell recognizes only those target cells bearing the correct type of MHC molecule.

As in the case of B cells, antigen alone is insufficient to activate T cells. For helper T cells, the accessory signal is provided either by a secreted signal such as IL-1 or by a specific plasma membrane molecule on the surface of an antigen presenting cell. The major cell type presenting antigen to T cells is the dendritic cell found in lymphoid organs, but macrophages and, under certain conditions, B cells can also act as antigen presenting cells. Antigen presenting cells with strong costimulatory activity also provide the secondary signal for cytotoxic T cells, but in some cases the presence of CD4 T cells seems to be required as well.

Tolerance

Many immune responses can be destructive to host tissue; hence, it is vital that they be restricted to pathogens and not be raised against innocuous substances. The devastating consequences of autoimmune diseases, which result from immune responses that are inappropriate in that they are directed against self, illustrate the crucial need for self-tolerance. It is now known that the immune system has the inherent capability of responding not only to foreign but also to self antigens. During development, it 'learns' not to respond to self antigens. The two major mechanisms for establishing self-tolerance are clonal deletion, the killing of self-reactive lymphocytes, and clonal anergy, the functional inactivation of self-reactive lymphocytes involving antigen stimulation in the absence of accessory signals. These processes are focused mainly on T lymphocytes since most B cells require helper T cells to respond to antigen so that the elimination of self-reactive helper T cells also ensures the inactivation of self-reactive B cells.

Interactions between Nutrition and Immunity

There are considerable interactions between nutrition and immunity; that is, not only does nutrition affect immune functions but also immune responses have profound effects on metabolism and nutritional status. Essentially every aspect of immunity can be affected by undernutrition, and there is growing evidence that overnutrition also has detrimental effects on immune responses. Protein–energy malnutrition during childhood leads to stunted development of many of the immune organs. In subjects of all ages suffering from protein–energy malnutrition, almost all immune functions are considerably impaired, resulting in increased severity and prolonged duration of most infectious diseases. However, protein–energy malnutrition rarely occurs in the absence of inadequate intake of other essential nutrients, and deficiencies in virtually every vitamin and essential mineral or trace element are associated with reductions in one or more functions of innate and adaptive immunity. The amount of fat and types of fatty acids in the diet are also known to influence certain immune functions, such as phagocytosis, the ability of cells to move to the site of inflammation, and the production of proinflammatory cytokines and other inflammatory mediators. In addition, evidence is beginning to accumulate that many other dietary constituents (e.g., carotenoids, flavonoids, other plant-derived chemicals, and probiotics (beneficial bacteria)) can also modulate a variety of immune responses, but their effects in humans remain largely unexplored.

Infection, in turn, is associated with profound effects on nutritional status resulting from decreased nutrient intake due to loss of appetite, decreased nutrient absorption as a result of intestinal damage and malabsorption, and nutrient losses arising from diarrhea and increased urinary excretion. Moreover, the inflammatory processes following infection can cause oxidative damage to host cells, and the prevention of such damage increases the demand for antioxidant defenses, including the vitamins C and E and a variety of enzymes that depend on trace metals for their function. In addition to its effects on nutritional status, the acute phase response is accompanied by marked changes in a variety of metabolic processes, with priority being shifted to the synthesis of all the different proteins involved in protecting the host from the invading pathogen. Another protective mechanism involves the redistribution of iron away from the bloodstream into the cells that participate in the phagocytosis and killing of invading pathogens. The removal of iron from the blood is accomplished by lactoferrin, an iron-binding protein that is produced in greatly increased amounts during the inflammatory response. By sequestering iron from pathogens that require this trace element for growth, lactoferrin can prevent such organisms from multiplying. Note that supplementation of iron-deficient subjects may reduce the resistance to malaria and may increase the short-term risk of certain infections. In general, however, correction of nutritional deficiencies via supplementation results in the partial or even full restoration of the compromised immune functions.

See also: **Cytokines. Immunity**: Effects of Iron and Zinc. **Infection**: Nutritional Interactions. **Prostaglandins and Leukotrienes**.

Further Reading

Gershwin ME, German JB, and Keen CL (eds.) (2000) *Nutrition and Immunology: Principles and Practice*. Totowa, NJ: Humana Press.

Janeway CA Jr and Travers P (1996) *Immunobiology: The Immune System in Health and Disease*. London/New York: Current Biology Limited/Garland.

Roitt IM (1994) *Essential Immunology*. Oxford: Blackwell Scientific.

Weir DM and Stewart J (1993) *Immunology*. New York: Churchill Livingstone.

Effects of Iron and Zinc

C Doherty, MRC Keneba, The Gambia

Introduction

Iron and zinc have achieved prominence among the micronutrients due to the wealth of research detailing their fundamental importance to a multitude of basic cellular physiological mechanisms. The complexity of the immune system ensures that both divalent cations are necessary for normal function. The effects of deficiency and supplementation on the immune functioning of both deficient and replete individuals have provided valuable clues to the specific immune processes in which they are involved. However, single nutrient deficiencies rarely occur alone and the effects of coexisting macro- and micronutrient deficiencies have contributed to the continuing debate on individual nutrient importance. Individuals and populations respond differently to supplementation. The basis of this variability is poorly understood but key to the improved targeting of supplementation. Specific mechanisms to explain the immune effects of zinc supplementation of deficient individuals have been particularly difficult to characterize as zinc is involved in so many cellular processes.

These nutrients are also important for prokaryotes and their acquisition by invading microbes is an important step in the development of a potential pathogen. The host action of micronutrient withdrawal is recognized as a mechanism of immune defense. In the era of genomic medicine the characterization of the molecular determinants of acquisition, storage, flux, and excretion of iron have increased our understanding and illustrated the complexity of iron homeostasis. In this article the evidence for the immune importance of both iron and zinc from *in vitro* experimentation and *in vivo* studies of human deficiency and supplementation is considered. The objective of supplementation, dose, route, preexisting level of deficiency, immunocompetence, coexistent deficiencies, genetic determinants, and the presence of infection should all be considered in the decision of who to supplement and when.

Iron and Zinc Homeostasis

Iron is the most abundant element on Earth. Despite this it is the most common micronutrient deficiency on Earth with up to 50% of all children under 5 years and pregnant women in developing countries affected. The ability of iron to both bind oxygen and to donate and accept electrons ensures that it has a central role in cellular energy metabolism. The utility of this redox potential is, however, counterbalanced by the propensity of iron to generate free radicals and damage cell membranes through lipid peroxidation. Genomic investment and redundancy in mechanisms to control iron availability at the cellular level illustrates both its importance and potential for toxicity.

Iron homeostasis depends on the regulation of iron absorption from the intestine as there are no pathways for iron excretion. On average, 1–2 mg enters the adult human body on a daily basis and a variable amount leaves via sloughing of skin and mucosal cells. Diets rich in heme iron and vitamin C promote iron absorption. Meat and nonanimal

foods such as legumes and green leafy vegetables combine readily available heme iron with promoters of absorption and utilization of non-heme iron. Phytate-containing foods, e.g., cereals, inhibit absorption. Non-heme iron is reduced and solubilized to the ferrous form in the proton rich environment of the proximal duodenum and actively transported across the enterocyte. The transport of ferrous iron through the enterocyte represents the primary site of iron homeostasis – it can be stored as ferritin, lost through sloughing of intestinal cells, or exported systemically.

Transferrin binds and solubilizes ferric iron exported from the enterocyte with high affinity and transports it to cells. Uptake and internalization of iron-transferrin by endocytosis is followed by its dissociation at lower intracellular pH and storage of iron in cytoplasmic ferritin molecules. Iron absorption, however, does not fulfil the majority of daily hemopoietic requirement. Senescent red blood cells are phagocytosed by reticuloendothelial macrophages, which recycle the iron from heme – they load the ferric iron back onto transferrin for reuse and this recycling of heme iron accounts for 80% of hemopoietic requirement.

Hemoglobin and intracellular ferritin, in the liver, bone marrow and spleen, account for over 99% of total body iron. Iron is more readily available than zinc and we have developed strategies to manage large fluxes of iron. Conditions characterized by hemolysis demonstrate the complex adaptive mechanisms that protect cells from episodes of flux.

Zinc is the twenty-fifth most abundant element comprising less than 0.01% of the earth's crust. Its single oxidant state enables it to hydolyze bonds involving carboxyl and amino groups and its ability to form stable complexes with sulfur and nitrogen atoms is utilized in stabilizing proteins. It has structural and regulatory roles in numerous enzymes, signaling pathways, and gene transcription systems essential for growth, reproduction, and metabolism. Up to 2 g of zinc is present in an adult man but most (95%) is locked away in pools from which it cannot rejoin the circulation and influence plasma levels, e.g., muscle and bone. Small plasma and liver pools are accessible and labile and act as the only reserve available in dietary deficiency. Zinc homeostasis is thus dependent on dietary intake and the average man has an intake of $10 \, mg \, day^{-1}$. Meat is a good source of zinc but plant sources (e.g., lentils and cereals) are often compromised by the presence of phytate, which inhibits absorption.

Plasma zinc is 99% bound to albumin and other low molecular weight proteins. Plasma zinc makes up only a small percentage of body zinc. The control of zinc flux at the cellular level is much less well characterized than that of iron.

Metallothionens are a group of intracellular monomeric polypeptides that bind zinc and serve as homeostatic modulators of zinc availability. Relatively little is known of how zinc enters immune cells and how it influences function. Recently, a family of zinc transport genes (ZnT 1–4) has been cloned. ZnT 1 is associated with zinc efflux and expression of this gene is regulated by zinc intake. Further work is needed to clarify the role of this family in zinc transport and its possible regulatory influences, e.g., zinc status and inflammation. Zinc deficiency is difficult to identify both clinically and biochemically and only in the last decade has the widespread nature of this deficiency been recognized particularly in children in developing countries.

Deficiency

Iron and especially zinc deficiency are difficult to diagnose and differing diagnostic criteria contribute to the confusion surrounding deficiency and immune dysfunction. Plasma levels of either micronutrient are not adequate to define status, however they commonly have been used for such. Deficiency of iron can be quantified at individual and community levels using a combination of indices, e.g., hemoglobin/mean cell volume combined with an index of storage iron, ferritin plus an index of iron supply to tissues, or serum transferrin receptor concentration. Plasma zinc level decreases with inflammation and currently the best method of assessment for deficiency is response to supplementation. Alternatively, plasma zinc levels can be interpreted with caution in conjunction with a marker of the acute phase response. In developing countries iron and zinc deficiency are widespread and often occur together. Meat is the most important dietary source for both micronutrients; however, in many countries with predominately vegetarian diets phytate-containing cereals inhibit absorption of both.

Deficiency and Immunity

Proliferation of cells requires iron, as the DNA synthetic enzyme ribonucleotide reductase is iron dependent. Impaired T cell proliferation and impaired delayed type hypersensitivity have been consistently reported in iron deficiency. Phagocytosis is accompanied by the generation of toxic oxygen intermediates to kill ingested bacteria and both neutrophils and macrophages require iron for this process – nitroblue tetrazolium reduction and

hydrogen peroxide production are reduced in neutrophils and macrophages if made iron deficient. In contrast, excessive iron results in decreased phagocytosis by neutrophils possibly due to increased free radical production and consequent lipid peroxidation damage of the phagosome membrane. Iron overload and saturation of transferrin also inhibits lymphocyte proliferation. When assessing the effect of iron on the immune system macrophages deserve special attention, as they are responsible for recycling heme iron back to the bone marrow. Iron thus fluxes through macrophages en route to fulfil hemopoietic need and is also utilized to kill intramacrophagal microbes. Macrophage activation and intracellular killing are dependent on the generation of toxic oxidant molecules such as the hydroxyl radical; however, these same free radicals can damage host cell membranes through lipid peroxidation. The control of intracellular iron in macrophages is thus important to hemopoiesis, microbial killing, and cell membrane stability within the macrophage itself. Iron overloading of macrophages impairs normal function and may increase risk of disease. Iron overloading of the macrophage causes oxidant damage to the phagocyte and an impaired ability to kill intracellular pathogens via IFNγ-mediated pathways. Iron has a direct inhibitory effect on the actions of IFN-γ, e.g., formation of tumor necrosis factor apha (TNF-α), expression of major histocompatibility factor (MHC) class II antigens, formation of neopterin, and nitric oxide synthesis.

Studies of immune function in iron-deficient human populations are frequently confounded by coexisting nutritional deficiencies, prevailing socioeconomic conditions, and differing diagnostic criteria, which make them difficult to interpret and compare. Increased morbidity from infectious disease has been reported in iron-deficient populations; however, it is not clear whether this is due to iron deficiency alone or at what level of deficiency the immune system is functionally compromised. In studies of children in predominately malarious areas a definite increase in mortality has only been demonstrated in anemic patients with less than $50 \, \mathrm{g \, l^{-1}}$ hemoglobin, whereas in those children with milder anemia the evidence for increased risk of mortality is inconclusive.

Zinc promotes mRNA stability, regulates gene expression, and influences DNA replication ensuring an essential role in cell division and activation. These processes are central to the immune response and zinc deficiency affects immune function at many levels both in the innate and specific arms. Zinc deficiency rarely occurs alone and has no pathognomonic clinical features. Cell-mediated immunity is profoundly affected in zinc deficiency. Lymphopenia is common, as are defects in specific T and B lymphocyte function. Lymphoid atrophy, decreased delayed cutaneous hypersensitivity responses, reduction in numbers of CD4 helper cells, B cell dysfunction, impairment of phagocytosis, and deficient thymic hormone activity have all been described. Secretion and function of cytokines and the potentiation of apoptosis are affected by zinc deficiency. Gastrointestinal barrier function, polymorphonuclear and natural killer cell function, and complement activity are also affected. Zinc may also prevent free radical-induced injury through its antioxidant and cell membrane stabilizing properties. Mild zinc deficiency resulted in an imbalance between TH1 and TH2 functions in male volunteers – reduced serum thymulin activity, reduced CD4/CD8 lymphocyte ratio, and reduced interleukin-2 (IL-2) production but production of IL-4, IL-5, IL-6, and IL-10 was unaffected. Influencing TH1/TH2 balance is a potentially important pathway by which zinc deficiency affects cell-mediated immunity.

Supplementation

Studies of the effect of iron supplementation or food fortification on morbidity from infection have been inconsistent in showing evidence of benefit. Morbidity is difficult to measure accurately and populations differ in relative deficiency, dietary supply of iron, and prevalent infectious agents. Individuals will also differ in their response to supplementation and the causes of population and individual variation are not well defined. Whilst some populations have shown a decline in infectious disease morbidity some observational evidence that iron supplementation leads to increased morbidity and mortality from infection has been reported. Supplemental oral iron given to septic kwashiorkor children was associated with increased risk of death. Prophylactic iron dextran given intramuscularly to Polynesian newborns in New Zealand caused increased neonatal sepsis that declined on stopping supplementation. In a controlled trial of prophylactic iron given intramuscularly to 2-month-old infants in Papua New Guinea supplementation was associated with a significant increase in hospital admissions for pneumonia.

Malaria is associated with hemolysis and fluxing of iron through the reticuloendothelial macrophages back to the bone marrow. Malaria-associated anemia is therefore not necessarily associated with iron deficiency (though it commonly can coexist) but with iron delocalization in macrophages. The effect of supplemental iron on iron delocalization is unclear. An increase in the prevalence of malaria parasites in thick blood films, splenomegaly, and

malaria-associated hospital admissions were reported in the Papua New Guinea study. Other trials of oral iron supplementation in children in areas where malaria is endemic have reported mixed findings but concerns persist as to possible increased morbidity from malaria due to iron supplementation. Current guidelines favor the continued use of iron supplementation in malarious regions as benefit to the host is felt to outweigh possible benefits to the parasite. Avoidance of parenteral administration and usage of lower supplementation doses has been advocated.

The study of conditions of chronic iron overload, e.g., hemochromatosis, chronic renal failure or hereditary hemolytic anemia requiring repeated blood transfusions, has provided further insights into how disturbed iron homeostasis affects immunity and infectious disease morbidity. Impaired phagocytic function inversely correlates with ferritin concentration and impaired natural killer cell function from iron overloaded thalassemic patients correlated with their degree of iron overload. Iron-overloaded patients are more susceptible to infections and the excess free iron encourages bacterial growth and pathogenicity. *Yersinia* infection has been reported in patients with hemochromatosis and those treated for acute iron toxicity with desferrioxamine. This bacterium can only acquire free iron and is therefore more likely to be invasive in its presence.

Zinc supplementation has been clearly demonstrated to improve immune function. Marasmic children given zinc supplementation demonstrate enlarged thymic shadows, increased conversion of delayed hypersensitivity skin reactions, enhanced lymphoproliferative response to PHA, and increased salivary IgA concentrations. Supplementation of malnourished children was associated with significantly larger delayed type hypersensitivity skin reactions and significantly decreased incidence of fever, cough, and upper respiratory tract infections. Zinc-supplemented infants also demonstrated significantly better serum IgA and significantly reduced incidence of pyoderma and anergy. Zinc supplementation decreased the percentage of children under 3 years who remained anergic to skin tests of delayed hypersensitivity associated with a significant rise in CD3, CD4, and the CD4/CD8 ratio.

The last decade has provided a wealth of studies detailing benefit from zinc supplementation in populations of under 5s in developing countries despite the difficulties in diagnosing zinc deficiency and understanding zinc homeostasis. By implication widespread deficiency exists. The evidence for immune benefit of zinc supplementation is much stronger than that for iron. There is now clear evidence that malnourished children and children with chronic diarrhea benefit from therapeutic zinc supplementation and that prophylactic zinc supplementation reduces diarrheal disease morbidity. Studies continue on the use of zinc to prevent and treat acute respiratory tract infection but any benefit to malaria morbidity or mortality has not been clearly established. There is good evidence for zinc deficiency in certain population subgroups, e.g., stunted/wasted children and children with chronic diarrhea. Population-based supplementation rather than targeting specific patient groups has also demonstrated benefit but recognition of appropriate populations to supplement is problematic. Populations with high rates of stunting may well have a high likelihood of zinc deficiency and thus be considered as potential candidates for supplementation. Knowledge of local dietary supply of zinc and results of local intervention studies should guide targeting to zinc-deficient populations.

Population-based supplementation approaches assume the safety of supplementation of individuals within populations who are not deficient. In general zinc supplementation is safe; however, individual variability in response exists and supplementation of replete individuals is not beneficial. There may be subgroups within the population for which supplementation may be detrimental. Zinc supplementation during sepsis has caused clinical problems particularly in the presence of a compromised immune system. Marasmic infants have demonstrated reduced phagocytic and fungicidal monocytic activity and a significantly increased number and duration of episodes of impetigo. High-dose zinc supplementation ($6 \, mg \, kg^{-1} day^{-1}$) given early in rehabilitation to severely malnourished children led to increased sepsis and mortality compared to low-dose supplementation ($1.5 \, mg \, kg^{-1} day^{-1}$). *In vitro* evidence points to free zinc ion concentration as a determinant of effects on monocytes and lymphocytes. Excess zinc induces the release of IL-1β and IL-6 and TNF-α from monocytes and inhibits IL-1-dependent T cell stimulation. Granulocyte phagocytosis is also impaired by zinc in a concentration-dependent manner. Supplemental zinc in rats decreased mobilization of polymorphonuclear cells and macrophages into the peritoneal cavity and phagocytic function. In adult men administration of 150 mg of elemental zinc twice a week for 6 weeks was associated with a reduction in lymphocyte stimulation response to phytohemagglutinin as well as chemotaxis and phagocytosis of bacteria by polymorphonuclear leukocytes. *In vitro* evidence points to a concentration-dependent effect of zinc on immune function.

Inflammation and Micronutrient Flux

The acute inflammatory reaction is a coordinated and complex series of physiological and immune adaptations designed to optimize protection to an invading pathogen. Immune cells are activated and cytokines released (e.g., IL-1 and TNF) to increase endothelial permeability and chemotaxis and activate complement. Effector immune cells are thus brought to a site of tissue injury and activated. Cytokines mediate the dramatic changes in the micronutrient milieu that accompanies inflammation. Plasma levels of both iron and zinc fall as both micronutrients are withdrawn from readily available pools and diverted to the reticuloendothelial system so as to both optimize immune response and deny access to invading pathogens. Decreased iron absorption, decreased iron release from reticuloendothelial macrophages, and increased transferrin catabolism contribute to iron withdrawal. Macrophagal sequestration of iron is mediated by inflammatory cytokines. Cellular iron homeostasis is a post-transcriptional event and expression of the transferrin receptor limits acquisition of iron. Iron-response proteins (IRP) 1 and 2 bind to iron-responsive elements (IRE) in transferrin receptor and ferritin mRNA and thus regulate expression of these genes and uptake, utilization, and storage of intracellular iron. Inflammatory cytokines modulate intracellular iron status by regulating the IRP/IRE network. Proinflammatory cytokines released during inflammation, e.g., TNF-α and IL-1, increases ferritin transcription and induce a diversion of metabolically available iron into the storage compartment in macrophages thus limiting iron availability for erythropoiesis. This diversion of iron underlies the anemia of inflammation/chronic disease.

Zinc is also diverted to the reticuloendothelial system during inflammation and lower plasma zinc concentrations are associated with both optimal phagocytic function and decreased microbial virulence. Calprotectin is an acute phase zinc-binding protein produced by polymorphonuclear leucocytes that sequesters zinc from invading pathogens. IL-1 released in inflammation increases the expression of metallothionen 1 and 2 in the liver, bone marrow, and thymus, which accompanies the increased uptake of zinc in these organs.

Iron and zinc are essential for microbial survival as cofactors for both superoxide dismutase and catalase redox enzyme systems. These enzymes neutralize the reactive oxygen intermediates integral to phagosomal killing. Both iron and zinc are also cofactors for bacterial enzymes required for DNA

Table 1 Immune effects of iron and zinc deficiency.

Iron	Zinc
Effect of deficiency	**Effect of deficiency**
Impaired lymphocyte proliferation	Lymphopenia
Impaired delayed type hypersensitivity	Impaired T & B lymphocyte function
Impaired phagocytic function	Impaired phagocytic function
	Impaired gastrointestinal barrier function
	Impaired natural killer cell function
	Impaired complement function
	Impaired TH1/TH2 balance
Effect of overload	**Effect of overload**
Impaired lymphocyte proliferation	Impaired lymphocyte stimulation
Impaired phagocytic function	Impaired phagocytic function
Impaired natural killer cell function	

synthesis. Intracellular pathogens, e.g., tuberculosis, must acquire iron and polymorphic variants of host NRAMP1 (natural resistance-associated macrophage protein), which influence intramacrophagal flux of iron, can determine susceptibility to intracellular pathogens. The host macrophage uses iron to generate free radicals to kill *Mycobacterium tuberculosis* – the competition for essential micronutrients between the host and the invading microbe continues within immune cells. The control of iron flux during malaria may be important in determining the severity of malaria, the severity of postmalarial anemia, and the propensity to bacterial

coinfection and may underlie the protective effect of hemoglobin, haptoglobin, and red cell enzyme variants. Oxidant stress accompanying the hemolysis of malaria is driven by free hemoglobin and is detrimental to both invading parasite and red blood cell membrane. The intraerythrocytic parasite degrades hemoglobin within its food vacuole and controls the resultant generation of free radicals by polymerizing free hemoglobin to hemozoin. Antimalarials, e.g., chloroquine, prevent this process and the parasite succumbs to its own waste. Hemoglobin, haptoglobin, or red cell enzyme variants that offer a more pro-oxidant environment can offer protection from severe malaria by ensuring earlier immune destruction of parasitized red cells. Strategies to manipulate hemolysis, oxidant stress, and iron flux during malarial episodes are key to the intraerythrocytic battle between host and parasite.

Correction of micronutrient deficiencies associated with defined functional consequences is a worthy goal. Iron and zinc deficiency are commonplace, particularly in children in developing countries, and have a significant effect on public health. Supplementation trials of zinc have been associated with significantly reduced infectious disease morbidity and mortality and there is good rationale for using targeted zinc supplementation to reduce infectious disease morbidity. Iron supplementation would not be advocated solely on the basis of its effect on infectious disease morbidity but this effect should be considered in supplementation programs. A recent meta-analysis showed

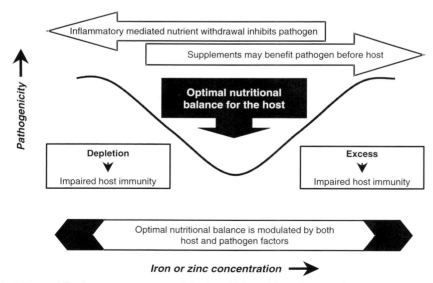

Figure 1 Micronutrient flux and the immune response to infection. (Adapted from Doherty CD, Weaver LT, and Prentice AM (2002) Micronutrient supplementation and infection: a double edged sword? *Journal of Pediatric Gastroenterology and Nutrition* **34**: 346–352.)

no harmful effect of iron supplementation on overall infectious disease incidence. However, if micronutrient withdrawal is a deliberate immune defense strategy and the control of micronutrient flux is worthy of such genomic investment then interference with blanket micronutrient supplementation will likely have adverse effects for subgroups within those populations. Understanding host variability in response to supplementation, the effect of supplementation during infection and nutrient–gene interactions in both host and potential pathogen is key to identifying these subgroups and improving micronutrient targeting.

The objective of supplementation, dose, route, pre-existing level of deficiency, immunocompetence, coexistent deficiencies, genetic determinants, and the presence of infection should all be considered in the decision of who to supplement and when.

See also: **Anemia**: Iron-Deficiency Anemia. **Bioavailability**. **Cytokines**. **Food Fortification**: Developed Countries; Developing Countries. **Infection**: Nutritional Interactions. **Iron**. **Supplementation**: Dietary Supplements; Role of Micronutrient Supplementation; Developing Countries; Developed Countries. **Zinc**: Physiology; Deficiency in Developing Countries, Intervention Studies.

Further Reading

Aggett PJ (1994) Zinc. *Annales Nestle* 52: 94–106.
Andrews NC (2000) Iron homeostasis:insights from genetics and animal models. *Nature Reviews Genetics* 1: 208–213.
Black RE (2003) Zinc deficiency, infectious disease and mortality in the developing world. *Journal of Nutrition* 133: 1485S–1489S.
Destro Bisol G (1999) Genetic resistance to malaria, oxidative stress, and hemoglobin oxidation. *Parasitologia* 41: 203–204.
Gera T (2002) Effect of iron supplementation on incidence of infectious illness in children: systematic review. *British Medical Journal* 325: 1142–1151.
Ibs KH (2003) Zinc-altered immune function. *Journal of Nutrition* 133: 1452S–1456S.
Oppenheimer SJ (2001) Iron and its relation to immunity and infectious disease. *Journal of Nutrition* 131: 616S–635S.
Rink L (2000) Zinc and the immune system. *Proceedings of the Nutrition Society* 59: 541–552.
Sherwood RA (1998) Iron homeostasis and the assessment of iron status. *Annals of Clinical Biochemistry* 35: 693–708.
Weinberg E (2000) Modulation of intramacrophagal iron metabolism during microbial cell invasion. *Microbes and Infection* 2: 85–89.
Weiss G (1995) Linkage of cell-mediated immunity to iron metabolism. *Immunology Today* 16: 495–499.
Weiss G (2002) Iron and immunity: a double-edged sword. *European Journal of Clinical Investigation* 32(supplement 1): 70–78.
Wyllie S (2002) The natural resistance-associated macrophage protein S1c11a1 (formerly Nramp1) and iron metabolism in macrophages. *Microbes and Infection* 4: 351–359.

INBORN ERRORS OF METABOLISM

Contents
Classification and Biochemical Aspects
Nutritional Management of Phenylketonuria

Classification and Biochemical Aspects

D L Marsden, Children's Hospital Boston, Boston, MA, USA

Introduction

Garrod identified the first inborn error of metabolism in 1902 when he described the symptoms that had been observed in patients with alkaptonuria as being due to an inherited enzyme deficiency. Since that time over 400 disorders have been described that are due to an enzyme deficiency in the catabolic pathways of proteins, fatty acids, and carbohydrates. The resulting accumulation of toxic intermediates and, in some cases, the depletion of a necessary end product cause a variety of metabolic derangements, often with significant neurological sequelae. The severity and the age of onset of symptoms usually, although not always, depend on the amount of residual enzyme activity.

The vast majority of these disorders are inherited in an autosomal recessive fashion. While the individual inborn errors of metabolism are rare, based on recent results of expanded newborn screening programs (in which over 30 disorders can be detected), the overall incidence is approximately 1 in 5000 live births worldwide. The incidence of disorders may vary across populations because of the 'founder effect', where a specific mutation arises and is maintained in subsequent generations, and may be higher where there is a higher incidence of consanguinity.

With a few exceptions, infants are normal at birth because the placenta efficiently eliminates the toxic metabolites.

Newborn Screening

Mass population screening of newborns was introduced in the 1960s, initially for phenylketonuria (PKU), after the development of the bacterial inhibition assay (BIA) for phenylalanine by Robert Guthrie. This simple method, popularly referred to as the Guthrie test, is still the mainstay of screening for PKU in much of the world. Essentially, it entails the addition of a solution of *B. subtilis* to an agar well, to which is added a standardized punched sample from the newborn screening filter paper, from which the blood is then eluted. High levels of phenylalanine inhibit growth of the bacteria, and the laboratory technician can easily visually identify this 'no-growth' zone as abnormal. Quantification is necessary, using a follow-up method such as high-performance liquid chromatography. BIA has been adapted to screen for elevated levels of leucine (for maple syrup urine disease; MSUD) and for methionine (for homocystinuria).

The most significant advance in newborn screening since its inception has been the adaptation of tandem mass spectrometry (MS/MS). With this technology, multiple compounds can be identified (both amino-acids and acylcarnitine species) from the same dried blood filter-paper sample after a simple preparation. Over 30 different inborn errors of metabolism can now be identified. The major drawbacks, however, are the relative expense of the equipment and the lack of long-term outcome data on infants detected and treated presymptomatically. Further modification of MS/MS will enable future screening for many more disorders, for example steroid profiling for congenital adrenal hyperplasia and the identification of lysosomal storage disorders.

Disorders of Protein Metabolism

Amino-Acid Disorders

Amino-acidopathies are due to an enzyme deficiency early in the catabolic pathway of one or more amino-acids that results in the accumulation of the amino-acid(s); they are detected by amino-acid analysis of serum or plasma. Symptoms may be due to the chronic accumulation of toxic amino-acid(s) or due to acute metabolic decompensation, for which aggressive intervention is necessary to prevent death or severe morbidity. Treatment is dietary restriction of the toxic amino-acid by limiting the intake of whole protein and supplementing with special modular amino-acid formulas to provide the appropriate nutrients for normal growth and development. All disorders are inherited in an autosomal recessive fashion.

The classic example is PKU. In PKU, a deficiency of the phenylalanine hydroxylase (PAH) enzyme (**Figure 1**) results in a high level of phenylalanine, which, if not treated with dietary restriction of phenylalanine in the early newborn period, causes severe irreversible mental retardation. The diagnosis is confirmed by a phenylalanine level of more than $1200\,\mu\text{mol}\,\text{L}^{-1}$ in an infant on unrestricted protein intake. The incidence of PKU is approximately 1 in 20 000 in Caucasians. Although PKU is pan-ethnic, the incidence varies in certain populations. The level of phenylalanine can vary between individual patients because of variations in the amount of residual enzyme activity, which, in turn, depends on the specific mutations. There are currently over 400 known mutations. Most patients are compound heterozygotes (i.e., have one copy each of two different mutations). Prior to the introduction of newborn screening, PKU was the commonest cause of inherited mental retardation. Early recognition of presymptomatic infants allows for the institution of a phenylalanine-restricted diet, with the

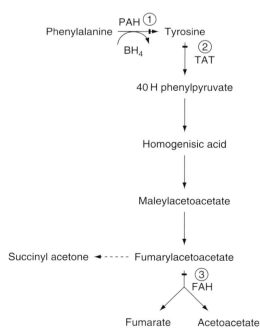

Figure 1 Catabolic pathway of phenylalanine. PAH, phenylalanine hydroxylase; TAT, tyrosine aminotransferase; FAH, fumarylacetoacetase; 1, PKU; 2, tyrosinaemia type II; 3, tyrosinaemia type I.

best outcomes achieved when recommended phenylalanine levels are attained by 2 weeks of age.

Untreated patients develop progressive severe mental retardation, often with seizures and Parkinson-disease-like neurological symptoms. The primary pathogenesis is due to the toxic effect of phenylalanine on the central nervous system; secondary symptoms may be due to a deficiency of tyrosine, which is an important precursor for the synthesis of some neurotransmitters. These symptoms include anxiety and depression.

Benign or mild hyperphenylalaninemia is due to allelic variants of PAH that result in greater residual enzyme activity. On an unrestricted diet, levels are typically in the range 120–360 μmol L^{-1}, and no dietary treatment is necessary.

Moderate elevation of phenylalanine is also present in patients with defects of tetrahydrobiopterin (BH$_4$), the cofactor for PAH. BH$_4$ is also the cofactor for other enzymes, tryptophan hydroxylase and tyrosine hydroxylase. These amino-acids are important precursors of the neurotransmitters 5-hydroxytryptophan and dopamine. A deficiency causes a neurological syndrome characterized by hypotonia, seizures, and movement disorder (dystonia).

MSUD has an incidence of approximately 1 in 185 000 births. It is due to a deficiency of the branched chain ketoacid dehydrogenase enzyme and the resulting accumulation of the branched chain amino-acids (BCAAs) leucine, isoleucine, and valine, which are detected by plasma amino-acid analysis. Elevation of alloisoleucine (a derivative of isoleucine) is pathognomonic. In classic MSUD, symptoms typically occur in the first week of life and, if untreated, rapidly progress to cerebral oedema, coma, and death. Toxicity is due

primarily to high levels of leucine. The characteristic maple syrup (or burnt sugar) odour is due to the presence of sotolone, a metabolite of isoleucine or alloisoleucine. It is detectable only when the BCAAs are significantly elevated; the ester is concentrated in the urine and the earwax of affected patients.

Variant forms of MSUD also occur. Intermediate MSUD typically presents in infancy with developmental delay; seizures may occur. Moderate levels of the BCAAs (including alloisoleucine) are present. Intermittent MSUD is associated with intermittent symptoms during acute infections or periods of prolonged fasting. Typical symptoms include ataxia, vomiting, and seizures. Acute severe decompensation may occur, similar to the classic form of MSUD. The BCAAs are elevated only during the episode of acute symptoms. Other disorders are listed in **Table 1**.

Urea cycle defects are due to enzyme deficiencies associated with the elimination of waste nitrogen produced by the normal catabolism of protein. There are six enzymatic steps involved in this process (**Figure 2**): a deficiency in any of the first five enzymes causes accumulation of nitrogen, in the form of ammonia (NH$_3$), and increased levels of the amino-acids glutamine and glycine.

Symptoms typically occur in the newborn period, except in the case of arginase deficiency, but milder late-onset variants have been well described. Symptoms include lethargy, poor feeding, vomiting, tachypnea, and progressive encephalopathy. Routine biochemical testing shows respiratory alkalosis and hyperammonemia. The liver transaminases are usually elevated. Hypoglycemia is not typical.

Plasma amino-acid and urine organic acid analyses are necessary to make a presumptive diagnosis.

Table 1 Disorders of amino-acid metabolism

Disorder (Deficient enzyme)	Elevated analyte	Clinical features	Treatment
Tyrosinemia type I (fumarylacetoacetase)	Tyrosine SA	Cirrhosis Liver failure Failure to thrive Renal tubular acidosis Rickets Hepatocellular Carcinoma (late)	NTBC (inhibits SA production) Tyrosine restriction
Tyrosinemia type II (tyrosine aminotransferase)	Tyrosine ($\uparrow\uparrow$)	Keratoconjunctivitis Palmar keratosis Mental retardation	Tyrosine restriction
Homocystinuria (cystathionine β synthase)	Methionine Total homocysteine Free homocystine+ Mixed disulfides	Mental retardation Thromboembolism Lens dislocation Osteoporosis	Vitamin B$_6$ (50% respond) Methionine restriction
Nonketotic hyperglycinemia (glycine cleavage enzyme deficiency)	Glycine ($\uparrow\uparrow$) (plasma and CSF)	Seizures Developmental delay	Sodium benzoate (decreases glycine)

CSF, cerebrospinal Fluid; SA, Succinylacetone; NTBC, 2-(2-nitro-4-trifluoro-methylbenzoyl)-1,3-cyclohexanedione.

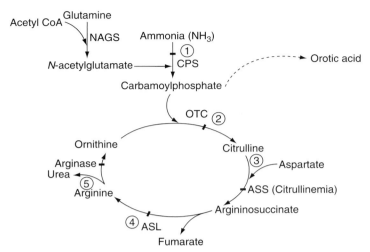

Figure 2   The urea cycle. NAGS, *N*-acetylglutamine synthetase; CPS, carbamoylphosphate synthetase; OTC, ornithine transcarbamoylase; ASS, argininosuccinate synthetase; ASL, argininosuccinate lyase; 1, CPS deficiency; 2, OTC deficiency; 3 citrullinemia; 4, argininosuccinic aciduria; 5, arginase deficiency.

In argininosuccinate synthetase (ASS) deficiency citrulline is elevated, in argininosuccinate lyase (ASL) deficiency argininosuccinic acid and citrulline are elevated, and in arginase deficiency, arginine is elevated. In ornithine transcarbamoylase (OTC) deficiency, on the other hand, citrulline is very low or absent. In each of these disorders, orotic acid is also present (found on urine organic acid analysis); it is produced via the pyrimidine cycle from the excessive carbamoylphosphate that accumulates owing to each enzyme defect. In carbamoylphosphate synthetase (CPS) deficiency, however, the amino-acid and orotic acid levels are normal, so the diagnosis is essentially one of exclusion in a patient who presents with the typical symptoms and severe hyperammonemia in which no other cause is determined. Confirmation of the diagnosis requires a liver biopsy for enzyme analysis of CPS and OTC. Skin fibroblasts can be assayed for ASS and ASL deficiencies, and red blood cells can be assayed for arginase deficiency; mutation analysis may be possible in some cases.

OTC deficiency is the most common urea-cycle defect. It is inherited in an X-linked fashion (all other disorders are autosomal recessive); symptomatic females can present with variable symptoms ranging from acute hyperammonemia to recurrent episodes of nausea, vomiting, and headache. The severity of the symptoms in female patients depends on the degree of lyonization (the normal random inactivation of one of the X chromosomes) and the resultant residual enzyme activity. Some women may remain asymptomatic, and a diagnosis is made only after the birth of a symptomatic son.

Patients with ASL deficiency also have progressive cirrhosis of the liver, possibly owing to the direct toxic effect of the argininosuccinic acid. In arginase deficiency, hyperammonemia is rare (most of the urea has already been eliminated), but arginine itself is toxic to the central nervous system, causing progressive spastic quadriplegia and developmental delay; seizures are common.

The toxicity of these disorders is primarily due to the accumulation of ammonia (NH_3) and glutamine, which is increased because of the transfer of excess ammonium ions (transamination). Acute severe hyperammonemia in the newborn period is catastrophic and often fatal. Survivors have variable neurological deficits.

Acute treatment of hyperammonemia due to a urea cycle defect involves the elimination of dietary protein, elimination of ammonia (by hemodialysis or peritoneal dialysis), administration of a high concentration of dextrose to reverse catabolism, arginine (except in arginase deficiency) to regenerate the cycle, and the nitrogen scavenging drugs sodium benzoate (which conjugates with glycine to form hippurate) and sodium phenylacetate (which conjugates with glutamine to form sodium phenylacetylglutamine). Early reintroduction of limited dietary protein is necessary to provide a substrate for anabolism and prevent further catabolism. This should consist of whole protein and a special formula to provide enough essential amino-acids to ensure normal weight gain, without producing excessive amounts of nitrogen for ammonia production. Chronic treatment involves similar dietary protein restriction, arginine, and an oral

Table 2 Organic acidemias

Disorder (Deficient enzyme)	Elevated analyte(s)	Clinical features	Treatment
Methylmalonic acidemia (methylmalonyl CoA Mutase)	Methylmalonic acid	Metabolic acidosis Hyperammonemia Failure to thrive Vomiting	Protein restriction Carnitine
Isovaleric acidemia (isovaleryl CoA dehydrogenase)	Isovalerylglycine	Metabolic acidosis Vomiting	Protein restriction Glycine
Glutaric aciduria type I (glutaryl CoA dehydrogenase)	3-Hydroxyglutaric acid Glutaric acid	Metabolic acidosis Vomiting Macrocephaly Developmental delay	Protein restriction Carnitine
3-Methylcrotonyl glycinuria (3-methylcrotonyl CoA carboxylase)	3-Hydroxyisovaleric acid 3-Methylcrotonylglycine	Metabolic acidosis Hypoglycemia Hyperammonemia Seizures (Some patients asymptomatic)	Protein restriction Carnitine
Mitochondrial acetoacetyl CoA thiolase deficiency	2-Methyl-3-hydroxybutyrate acid 2-Methylacetoacetic acid Tiglylglycine	Metabolic acidosis Vomiting	Protein restriction Carnitine

form of nitrogen-scavenging medication (sodium phenylbutyrate). For arginase deficiency, dietary protein restriction and formula is usually adequate.

Organic acidemias (**Table 2**) are due to enzyme deficiencies further along the catabolic pathway, usually of several amino-acids, resulting in the accumulation of the toxic products of intermediary metabolism (organic acids). In some cases, there is a functional defect of the enzyme owing to a deficiency of the enzyme cofactor, rather than of the enzyme itself. Examples of this are biotinidase deficiency and defects of cobalamin (vitamin B_{12}) metabolism.

The accumulation of large amounts of organic acids causes severe metabolic acidosis and ketosis. Hyperammonemia is often present, owing to secondary inhibition of the urea cycle. Hypoglycemia may be variably present, owing to secondary inhibition of fatty-acid oxidation. Symptoms are often present in the newborn period; recurrent episodes of metabolic decompensation can occur because of excessive protein intake or because of catabolism (and therefore an increased load of amino-acids endogenously released from muscle) associated with acute infections or prolonged periods of fasting. Morbidity and mortality is due to acute acidosis and the associated neurologic sequelae.

The diagnosis is made by finding high levels of the characteristic organic acids in the urine. Newer analytic methods, such as MS/MS, can detect even small elevations of characteristic plasma acylcarnitine and urine acylglycine conjugates of the intermediary metabolites. Confirmation is by enzyme analysis, usually in skin fibroblasts; DNA mutation analysis is available for many disorders.

Propionic acidaemia is a typical organic acidaemia. It is due to an isolated defect of the enzyme propionyl CoA carboxylase in the catabolic pathways of the amino-acids isoleucine, valine, methionine, and threonine as well as cholesterol and odd chain fatty acids (**Figure 3**). The resulting accumulation of the intermediary metabolites 3-hydroxypropionic acid, methylcitric acid, propionyglycine, and tiglyglycine can cause severe metabolic acidosis, ketosis, coma, and death. Other associated symptoms can include hyperammonemia, hypoglycemia, and pancytopenia, owing to bone marrow suppression by the accumulated toxic organic acids.

Symptoms can occur within days of birth in the classic disease or later in infancy or childhood in the milder variant forms. The later-onset form may be associated with persistent vomiting, failure-to-thrive,

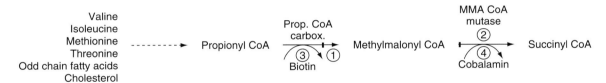

Figure 3 The catabolic pathways of isoleucine, valine, methionine, threonine, cholesterol, and odd chain fatty acids. 1, propionic aciduria; 2, methylmalonic aciduria; 3, multiple carboxylase deficiency; 4, cobalamin disorders.

and developmental delay, but often does not involve severe episodes of metabolic acidosis. Dystonia may occur owing to infarction of the basal ganglia.

Cofactor Deficiencies

Biotin is an essential cofactor for the four carboxylase enzymes propionyl CoA carboxylase, methylcrotonyl CoA carboxylase, pyruvate CoA carboxylase, and acetyl CoA carboxylase. It is endogenously derived from lysine and also present in its protein-bound form in small amounts in many foods. Holocarboxylase synthetase (HCS), which forms the inactive parent apoenzyme, is also biotin dependent. Enzyme activation requires free biotin, which is released by the action of biotinidase; this enzyme also plays an essential role in the recycling of biotin for further use. A deficiency of biotinidase, therefore, results in depletion of biotin and a functional defect of the carboxylases. Symptoms include hypotonia, lethargy, vomiting, and ataxia. Recurrent metabolic acidosis may occur. Alopecia and a generalized erythematous rash are common. The symptoms are more severe in HCS deficiency. The characteristic pattern of organic acids is present in both disorders. The diagnosis is made by measuring biotinidase activity in plasma or carboxylase-enzyme activity in leucocytes or fibroblasts. Treatment with pharmacologic doses of biotin is effective.

Multiple defects of cobalamin (vitamin B_{12}) metabolism can occur, involving the transport of vitamin B_{12} into the cell (defects of the transporter proteins transcobalamin I and II) or subsequent intracellular utilization of the different biologically active forms. These disorders are classified into complementation groups, depending on whether the defect is in adenosylcobalamin (Cbl A and B), methylcobalamin (Cbl G and E), or both (Cbl C and D).

Adenosylcobalamin is the cofactor for methylmalonyl CoA mutase; a defect results in a milder form of methylmalonic acidaemia than that found with a defect of the enzyme itself. Methylcobalamin is the cofactor for methionine synthase; a defect results in low methionine and homocystinuria (distinct from classic homocystinuria due to a defect of cystathionine β synthase). A defect of both adenosylcobalamin and methylcobalamin causes both methylmalonic acidaemia and homocystinuria.

Symptoms vary with the complementation group, but can include metabolic acidosis, hypotonia, developmental delay, macular degeneration, and megaloblastic anemia. Treatment with hydroxocobalamin corrects some of the biochemical derangements, especially in Cbl A and B. Treatment is less successful in the other groups.

A syndrome similar to Cbl C has been described in the breast feeding infants of strict vegetarian (vegan) mothers and in mothers with pernicious anemia, who are vitamin B_{12} deficient.

Disorders of Fatty-Acid Oxidation

Disorders of fatty-acid oxidation have been recognized only since the early 1980s, but as a group they represent the most common inborn errors of metabolism. Fat provides a significant source of energy in the form of glucose and ketone bodies during times of metabolic stress (such as febrile illness) or during prolonged fasting. Free fatty acids, released from the adipose tissue, are transported into the mitochondria via the carnitine shuttle system, where they undergo β-oxidation (**Figure 4**), the progressive cleavage from an 18-carbon very long-chain fatty acid to the two-carbon aceto-acetyl CoA, the substrate for glucose (via the TCA (Tricarboxylic acid) cycle) and ketones. A deficiency of any of the enzymes in this pathway can cause symptoms of hypoketotic hypoglycemia and hepatic encephalopathy, with hyperammonemia (due to secondary inhibition of the urea cycle) and sudden death. Many cases of what would previously have been diagnosed as Reye syndrome are now known to be due to defects of fatty-acid oxidation. Symptoms can occur at any time, from the newborn period to adulthood.

Carnitine has a dual role: in addition to its critical role in the transport of free fatty acids into mitochondria, it conjugates with the fatty acyl CoA intermediates that accumulate proximal to an enzyme block, forming acylcarnitine species that can be excreted by the kidneys. They can also be measured in plasma for diagnostic purposes and in the newborn-screening dried blood spot. Increased use of carnitine owing to an enzyme defect causes a secondary depletion, further impairing fatty-acid oxidation.

Long-chain fatty-acid (carnitine palmityl transferase (CPT) oxidation defects I and II, very long-chain acyl CoA dehydrogenase (VLCAD), TFP (Trifunctional protein), and long-chain 3-hydroxy acyl CoA dehydrogenase (LCHAD)) may present in the newborn period or later in infancy with severe hypoketotic hypoglycemia, cardiomyopathy, and hepatic encephalopathy, due to deposition of fat in the heart and liver. Rhabdomyolysis (lysis of muscle cells) is common. Pigmentary degeneration of the retina may be present in LCHAD and is thought to be due to impaired endogenous production of docosahexanoic acid (DHA), which is necessary for normal retinal function. Milder variant forms of CPT II and VLCAD may present in adolescence or adulthood with muscle cramping and rhabdomyolysis, which may be severe enough to cause

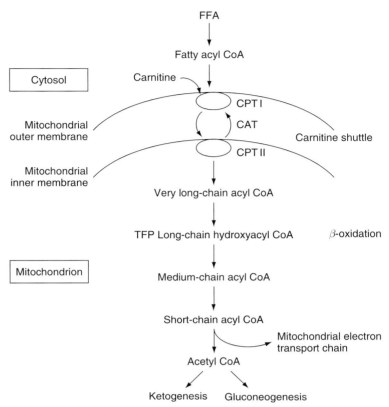

Figure 4   Fatty-acid oxidation. FFA, free fatty acids; CPT I, carnitine palmitoyltransferase type I; CPT II, carnitine palmitoyltransferase type II; CAT, carnitine acylcarnitine translocase; TFP, trifunctional protein.

acute renal failure owing to the deposition of the muscle pigment myoglobin in the renal tubules.

Treatment of these disorders, which can reverse the cardiac and liver disease, includes frequent feeding and avoidance of fasting, together with limitation of dietary fat and supplementation with medium-chain triglycerides (MCT), which bypass the metabolic block. There is no clear consensus on the amount of MCT needed; the general recommendation is to provide 20–40% of total calories from fat, with about half of these calories coming from MCT. Special formulas can provide the MCT requirements, but some are deficient in some essential fatty acids, such as linoleic and linolenic acids and DHA. Addition of oil, such as canola oil, provides most of the essential fatty acids. DHA is not currently commercially available, but fish oil may provide an alternative source. Uncooked cornstarch can provide an alternative source of complex carbohydrate (especially for overnight fasting) after the age of about 9 months. Normal pancreatic amylase activity is necessary and may not be adequate prior to this age.

Treatment of the medium-chain and short-chain defects is simpler, involving avoidance of fasting and early intervention during acute illness to prevent hypoglycemia. Carnitine supplementation is frequently used to prevent secondary depletion. The dietary-fat recommendation is approximately 30% of total calories, or a 'heart healthy' diet.

Disorders of Carbohydrate Metabolism

Galacatosemia

Galactose is derived primarily from dietary lactose, which is the major disaccharide in dairy products, human breast milk, and many fruits and vegetables. There is also a small contribution from endogenous production. There are three known enzyme deficiencies in the pathway that oxidizes galactose to glucose (**Figure 5**); all are autosomal recessive genetic disorders.

Classic galactosemia is due to the almost complete absence of galactose-1-phosphate uridyltransferase (GALT) activity. Symptoms generally occur in the first few weeks of life, with poor weight gain, lethargy, hypotonia, liver disease (hyperbilirubinemia, coagulopathy, and hepatomegaly), and renal tubular acidosis. Hypoglycemia can occur. *Escherichia coli* sepsis may also be a complication: elevated

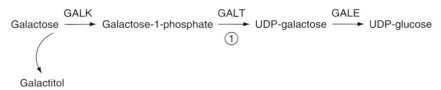

Figure 5 Galactose oxidation. GALK, galactokinase; GALT, galactose-1-phosphate uridyl transferase; GALE, uridine diphosphate galactose 4-epimerase; 1, galactosemia; UDP, uridine diphosphate.

galactose is thought to impair leucocyte bactericidal activity, allowing the bacteria to invade the red blood cells more easily with subsequent dissemination. Mental retardation is a long-term complication.

The underlying pathogenesis of galactosemia is not fully understood; despite compliance with a lactose-restricted diet, speech delay is almost universal, some patients have learning disorders, and female patients have ovarian failure.

Treatment is by restriction of lactose in the diet, primarily by eliminating dairy products and other foods known to be high in galactose.

Variant forms of galactosemia occur owing to mutations in the GALT gene that result in greater residual enzyme activity. The commonest variant is the Duarte variant, in which there is usually one copy of a classic galactosemia mutation (e.g., Q188R) and one copy of the variant N314D. This combination results in approximately 25% residual enzyme activity. There is varying opinion as to whether or not dietary treatment is necessary: some clinicians consider that the residual enzyme activity is sufficient to prevent the pathologic sequelae, others elect to treat the patient with lactose restriction for the first year of life. There are no long-term outcome data to support either approach.

Galactokinase deficiency causes an excessive accumulation of galactitol, which is oxidized from galactose by an alternative pathway. High levels of galactitol cause cataract formation, which is the only symptom of this disorder. Lactose restriction is necessary.

Epimerase deficiency is very rare. There are two isoforms of the enzyme, one isolated to red blood cells and one in the liver. The most common disorder is due to an isolated deficiency of the red-blood-cell isoform, which will be detected incidentally by newborn screening programs that measure total galactose. There are no clinical symptoms and no treatment is necessary. A defect of both isoforms will cause symptoms similar to those of classic galactosemia and should be treated similarly.

Glycogen Storage Disorders

Glycogen is a complex carbohydrate stored primarily in the liver and muscle. Liver glycogen provides glucose to maintain blood-sugar levels between normal feeding; defects of the liver enzymes for glycogen

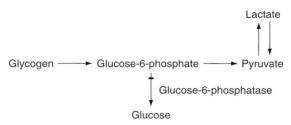

Figure 6 Glycogen storage disease type I.

degradation lead to hypoglycemia and/or liver disease because of excessive accumulation of glycogen. Muscle glycogen is an important substrate for energy production for normal muscle function, so disorders are usually indicated by cramping with exercise.

Glycogen storage disease (GSD) type I (GSD I) (**Figure 6**), the most common disorder, is due to a deficiency of glucose-1-phosphatase in the liver, kidney, and intestinal mucosa. Symptoms typically occur in infancy when the frequency of feeding decreases. Profound hypoglycemia can occur; progressive hepatomegaly and liver dysfunction are due to storage of glycogen. Other metabolic derangements include lactic acidaemia, which is due to increased pyruvate production; increased fatty-acid synthesis causes hypertriglyceridemia and hypercholesterolemia (causing xanthomas); hyperuricemia (causing gout and renal calculi) is due to decreased renal excretion (lactate is preferentially excreted) and increased uric-acid production owing to phosphate depletion. Other long-term complications include progressive renal disease (proteinuria) and hepatocellular carcinoma. Treatment involves frequent meals and continuous nocturnal feeding (in infants); supplemental uncooked cornstarch provides exogenous glucose.

Other GSDs are summarized in **Table 3**.

Disorders of Fructose Metabolism

There are three disorders of fructose metabolism, all inherited in an autosomal recessive fashion. Fructose is widely distributed in the diet as the primary sugar in fruits, vegetables, and honey. It is also derived from sucrose and sorbitol, which are found in large variety of products, including infant formulas and intravenous fluids. The toxic effect of fructose is due to inhibition

Table 3 Glycogen storage disorders

Disorder	Deficient enzyme	Primary affected tissue	Symptoms	Treatment
GSD O	Glycogen synthase	Liver	Hypoglycemia	Uncooked cornstarch, frequent feeds
GSD I	Glucose-6-phosphatase	Liver, muscle	Hypoglycemia, hepatomegaly, growth retardation, proteinuria, lactic acidemia, hyperlipidemia, hyperuricemia (gout), hepatocellular carcinoma	Uncooked cornstarch, frequent feeds
GSD II (Pompe disease)	Acid maltase (α glucosidase)	Lysosomes of muscle (skeletal and cardiac)	Cardiomyopathy, skeletal myopathy, cardiorespiratory failure	Enzyme replacement (in clinical trial)
GSD III	Debranching enzyme (amylo-1, 6-glucosidase)	Liver, muscle	Hypoglycemia (mild), hepatomegaly, myopathy, hyperlipidemia	Uncooked cornstarch, frequent feeds
GSD IV (amylopectinosis)	Branching enzyme	Liver	Hepatomegaly, cirrhosis, liver failure, myopathy	Liver transplant, Uncooked cornstarch
GSD V (McArdle disease)	Myophosphorylase	Muscle	Muscle cramping (with exercise)	Oral glucose, high-protein diet
GSD VI (Hers disease)	Liver phosphorylase	Liver	Hepatomegaly, hypoglycemia, myopathy	Frequent feeds
GSD VII (Tarui disease)	Phosphofructokinase	Muscle	Fatigue exercise intolerance, cramping	Avoidance of strenuous exercise
GSD IX	Phosphorylase kinase	Liver, muscle	Hepatomegaly, growth retardation	Frequent feeds

GSD, glycogen storage disorder.

of gluconeogenesis by high levels of fructose-1-phosphate and subsequent depletion of inorganic phosphate and, thus, adenosine triphosphate.

Essential fructosuria is a benign disorder due to a defect of the enzyme fructokinase. Patients have increased urinary excretion of fructose, which is usually an incidental finding on routine testing for reducing substances.

Hereditary fructose intolerance is due to a deficiency in aldolase B, which splits fructose-1-phosphate into glyceraldehyde and dihydroxyacetone. Symptoms occur only after exposure to fructose, usually from dietary ingestion although they are more severe after intravenous infusion. The symptoms include gastrointestinal discomfort, vomiting, and hypoglycemia. Chronic exposure causes failure-to-thrive, liver disease, and renal tubular acidosis. Affected patients are often misdiagnosed as having behavioral problems or an eating disorder. Treatment involves elimination of fructose from the diet.

Fructose-1,6-bisphosphatase deficiency is a defect of gluconeogenesis and not dependent on exposure to fructose. Symptoms, including recurrent episodes of vomiting, lactic acidosis, tachypnea, seizures, and apnea, occur when dietary glucose and glycogen stores are depleted, for example during periods of fasting or febrile illness. Approximately 50% of patients are symptomatic in the newborn period. Treatment involves the prevention of fasting and supplementation with uncooked cornstarch to provide a source of complex carbohydrate. Acute episodes respond to intravenous infusions of dextrose.

Abbreviations

ASL	Argininosuccinate lyase
ASS	Argininosuccinate synthetase
BCAA	Branched chain amino-acids
BH_4	Tetrahydrobiopterin
BIA	Bacterial inhibition assay
CPS	Carbamoyl synthetase
CPT	Carnitine palmityl transferase
GALT	Galactose-1-phosphate uridyl transferase
GSD	Glycogen storage disorder
HCS	Holocarboxylase synthetase
LCHAD	Long-chain 3-hydroxy acyl CoA dehydrogenase
MCAD	Medium-chain acyl CoA dehydrogenase
MS/MS	Tandem mass spectrometry
MSUD	Maple syrup urine disease
OTC	Ornithine transcarbamylase

PAH	Phenylalanine hydroxylase
PKU	Phenylketonuria
SCAD	Short-chain acyl CoA dehydrogenase
VLCAD	Very long-chain acyl CoA dehydrogenase

See also: **Inborn Errors of Metabolism**: Nutritional Management of Phenylketonuria.

Further Reading

Burton BK (1998) Inborn errors of metabolism in infancy: a guide to diagnosis. *Pediatrics* **102**: E69.

Chace DH, Kalas TA, and Naylor EW (2003) Use of tandem mass spectrometry for multianalyte screening of dried blood specimens from newborns. *Clinical Chemistry* **49**: 1797–1817.

Fernandes J, Saudubray J-M, and van den Berghe G (eds.) (2000) *Inborn Metabolic Diseases*, 3rd edn. Berlin: Springer-Verlag.

Gillingham MB, Connor WE, Matern D *et al.* (2003) Optimal dietary therapy of long-chain-3-hydroxyacyl-CoA dehydrogenase deficiency. *Molecular Genetics and Metabolism* **79**: 114–123.

Holme E and Lindstedt S (1998) Tyrosinemia type I and NTBC (2-(2-nitro-4-trifluoromethylbenzoyl)-1,3-cyclohexanedione). *Journal of Inherited Metabolic Disease* **21**: 507–517.

Kahler SG and Fahey MC (2003) Metabolic disease and mental retardation. *American Journal of Medical Genetics* **117C**: 31–41.

Levy HL, Sepe SJ, Walton DS *et al.* (1978) Galactose-1-phosphate uridyl transferase deficiency due to the Duarte/galactosemia combined variation: clinical and biochemical studies. *Journal of Pediatrics* **92**: 390–393.

Podebrad F, Heil M, Reichert S *et al.* (1999) 4,5-Dimethyl-3-hydroxy-2[5H]-furanone (sotolone)—the odour of maple syrup urine disease. *Journal of Inherited Metabolic Disease* **22**: 107–114.

Vockley J, Singh RH, and Whiteman DA (2002) Diagnosis and management of defects of mitochondrial beta-oxidation. *Current Opinion in Clinical Nutrition and Metabolic Care* **5**: 601–609.

Walter JH, Collins JE, and Leonard JV (1999) Recommendations for the management of galactosemia. UK Galactosemia Steering Group. *Archives of Disease in Childhood* **80**: 93–96.

Zytkovicz TH, Fitzgerald EF, Marsden D *et al.* (2001) Tandem mass spectrometric analysis for amino, organic and fatty acid disorders in newborn dried blood spots: a two-year summary from the new England Newborn Screening Program. *Clinical Chemistry* **47**: 1945–1955.

Nutritional Management of Phenylketonuria

D L Marsden, F J Rohr and K C Costas, Children's Hospital Boston, Boston, MA, USA

Introduction

Phenylketonuria (PKU) is a disorder of amino acid metabolism caused by a deficiency in the enzyme phenylalanine hydroxylase, which converts the essential amino acid phenylalanine to tyrosine. High levels of phenylalanine are toxic to the central nervous system, resulting in severe irreversible mental retardation. Details of the biochemistry are discussed elsewhere in this encyclopedia.

PKU is often considered a paradigm for the nutritional therapy for metabolic disorders. It was the first inborn error of metabolism identified by newborn screening, thus allowing for early dietary treatment. Early treatment was successful in preventing the mental retardation associated with untreated PKU. Since the advent of successful dietary treatment of PKU four decades ago, the field has expanded greatly, but the principle of treating phenylketonuria remains the same – to control the intake of the amino acid that is not metabolized normally. This principle applies to all amino acidopathies, but PKU is used here as an example.

Dietary treatment is started as soon as the diagnosis is confirmed in a newborn. Outcomes are best when the diet is implemented and the phenylalanine levels are within the recommended guidelines by 2 weeks of age. Diet is now recommended to be life-long. Adult and adolescent patients who have resumed an unrestricted diet, while intellectually normal, have been shown to have an increased incidence of neuropsychiatric illness, such as increased anxiety and depression. Others report poor concentration, headaches, and sleep disturbance.

The pathophysiology of PKU is not well understood, although recent focus has been on the role of amino acids in the brain. Phenylalanine competes with other large neutral amino acids for transport across the blood–brain barrier, and it is theorized that high levels of brain phenylalanine and low levels of other amino acids, specifically tyrosine and tryptophan, may impede neurotransmitter synthesis in the brain and be responsible for the symptoms associated with untreated PKU. While the ideal brain level of phenylalanine has not been established, treatment guidelines have been established for blood levels at various ages, although these guidelines differ slightly in different countries. In the US, recommendations have been developed by an expert panel convened under the direction of the National Institutes of Health (NIH) and the American Academy of Pediatrics (**Table 1**).

The goal of nutritional therapy is to keep blood phenylalanine controlled while providing a nutritionally sound diet. This necessitates the use of a special medical food (most often as a formula) that provides amino acids other than phenylalanine. A medical food is required because the phenylalanine restriction needed to maintain blood levels within the desired range is so severe that the amount of natural protein

Table 1 Treatment goals for PKU

Age (years)	Phenylalanine level ($\mu mol\,l^{-1}$)
0–12	120–360
12–adult	120–900
	(120–600 preferred in adolescents)
Maternal PKU	120–360

Adapted from NIH Consensus Development Conference Statement (2001) Phenylketonuria, screening and management. *Pediatrics* **108**(4): 972–982.

allowed in the diet would not support normal growth and development. Several medical foods are currently available. When PKU was first treated, only one medical food was commercially available: a protein hydrolysate from which most of the phenylalanine had been removed. Now, medical foods for PKU use synthetic L-amino acids (other than phenylalanine) as the protein source and are phenylalanine free. The medical foods vary in the amount of amino acids that they contain; in addition, most also provide carbohydrate and fat, vitamins and minerals, but others do not. The amount of medical food prescribed is intended to meet protein needs at various ages in the life cycle (see **Table 2**).

Introduction of Dietary Therapy

Infant formulas for PKU come in a powdered form and are mixed with water and taken as a substitute for regular infant formula or breast milk. In some clinics, only phenylalanine-free formula is given for a few days so that blood phenylalanine will quickly decrease to an acceptable level. A prescribed amount of breast milk or standard infant formula, however, should be shortly introduced into the diet. Whole protein is needed to meet phenylalanine requirements and prevent phenylalanine deficiency, which will lead to muscle protein catabolism and inadequate weight gain. For formula-fed infants, both standard infant formulas and PKU medical foods are used in prescribed amounts and are bottle fed. Breast-feeding of an infant with PKU is possible and, as with all infants, should be encouraged whenever possible. Mature breast milk contains approximately $46\,mg\;100\,ml^{-1}$ of phenylalanine compared to approximately $59\,mg\;100\,ml^{-1}$ in cows' milk protein-based formula and approximately $88\,mg\;100\,ml^{-1}$ in soy-based formulas. Therefore, breast-fed infants may initially have slightly lower plasma phenylalanine levels. If a mother chooses to continue breast-feeding, she is advised about the proper ratio of breast milk to PKU medical food to feed her infant. The key to either method is frequent monitoring of blood phenylalanine and adjusting the diet based on phenylalanine intake, weight gain, and blood levels. Guidelines for the frequency of monitoring were also recommended by the NIH consensus panel (**Table 3**). The method used for monitoring varies

Table 2 Recommended daily nutrient intakes (ranges) for infants, children, and adults with PKU

Age	Nutrient				
	PHE	TYR	Protein	Energy	Fluid
Infants	($mg\,kg^{-1}$)	($mg\,kg^{-1}$)	($g\,kg^{-1}$)	($kcal\,kg^{-1}$)	($ml\,kg^{-1}$)
0 to <3 months	25–70	300–350	3.50–3.00	120 (145–95)	160–135
3 to <6 months	20–45	300–350	3.50–3.00	120 (145–95)	160–130
9 to <12 months	15–35	250–300	3.00–2.50	110 (135–80)	145–125
7 to <9 months	10–35	250–300	3.00–2.50	105 (135–80)	135–120
Girls and boys	($mg\,day^{-1}$)	($g\,day^{-1}$)	($g\,day^{-1}$)	($kcal\,day^{-1}$)	($ml\,day^{-1}$)
1 to <4 years	200–400	1.72–3.00	≥30	1300 (900–1800)	900–1800
4 to <7 years	210–450	2.25–3.50	≥35	1700 (1300–2300)	1300–2300
7 to <11 years	220–500	2.55–4.00	≥40	2400 (1650–3300)	1650–3300
Women					
11 to <15 years	140–750	3.45–5.00	≥50	2200 (1500–3000)	1500–3000
15 to <19 years	230–700	3.45–5.00	≥55	2100 (1200–3000)	1200–3000
≥19 years	220–700	3.75–5.00	≥60	2100 (1400–2500)	2100–2500
Men					
11 to <15 years	225–900	3.38–5.50	≥55	2700 (2000–3700)	2000–3700
15 to <19 years	295–1100	4.42–6.50	≥65	2800 (2100–3900)	2100–3900
≥19 years	290–1200	4.35–6.50	≥70	2900 (2000–3300)	2000–3300

PHE, phenylalanine; TYR, tyrosine.
Reproduced with permission from Acosta PB and Yanicelli S (2001) *Nutrition Support Protocols*, 4th edn. Abbott Laboratories. Columbus, OH, USA.

Table 3 Monitoring for PKU

Age (years)	Frequency of testing for phenylalanine
0–1	Weekly
1–12	Twice monthly
12–adult	Monthly
Maternal PKU	Twice weekly

Adapted from NIH Consensus Development Conference Statement (2001) Phenylketonuria, screening and management. *Pediatrics* **108**(4): 972–982.

depending on the resources available at individual PKU clinics: either frequent visits to the clinic for blood drawing or filter paper samples (as used for newborn screening) that can be collected at home and then mailed to the clinic or, in some cases, to the newborn screening program, for analysis. Because of the time delay in the latter method, it is more suitable for use after the initial stabilization period.

When an infant with PKU is 4–6 months old, solid food is introduced. Since nearly all food contains some phenylalanine, it must be measured and counted. Lists of the phenylalanine content of foods are available and are essential to diet management. The phenylalanine content of foods is listed in milligrams; in some clinics, an exchange system is used where one exchange is equal to a given amount of phenylalanine (often 15 mg per exchange, but in some cases 20 or 50 mg). Since the total amount of phenylalanine taken daily remains the same (adjusted for weight gain), adjustments are made in the amount of regular infant formula or breast milk given to the infant once solid foods are started. This process continues until all of the phenylalanine requirement is provided as food. In general, infants with PKU begin with fruit and small amounts of infant cereal. As the infant's appetite increases, other foods are added, but the choices are limited to fruits, vegetables and, in some cases, small portions of bread and cereal products. For some individuals with PKU, the phenylalanine restriction is severe enough to preclude any regular grain products. Instead, specialty low-protein foods are available, often through mail order. A whole array of low-protein breads, cereals, crackers, bagels, pasta, cakes, cookies, and even low-protein cheeses and peanut butter are critical to proper diet management. These foods provide much needed variety and calories to the diet. High-protein foods such as meat, fish, poultry, dairy, nuts, eggs, and legumes are not allowed on a PKU diet. Thus, the phenylalanine-free medical food continues to be the main source of protein for life.

A wide variety of medical foods are now available for children and adults with PKU in order to meet different tastes and caloric needs. Some of the medical foods for children, teens, and adults are packaged in pouches or sachets for convenience, and several are available in bar, capsule, or tablet form to promote ease of use. Nevertheless, many individuals with PKU struggle with this aspect of the diet. If the full amount of medical food is not taken, nutritional intake is inadequate and may lead to catabolism of lean body mass, which in turn leads to poor control of blood phenylalanine.

Once established, the amount of dietary phenylalanine an individual is allowed remains the same, except for periods of rapid growth, when more phenylalanine may be necessary. A typical phenylalanine intake for a child with severe PKU is $250 \, \text{mg day}^{-1}$, and for a child with moderate PKU is $400 \, \text{mg day}^{-1}$. Thus, in addition to achieving the correct amount of medical food, the crux of the diet is to provide the prescribed amount of phenylalanine while making the diet taste and appear as appetizing and socially acceptable as possible. Families require a good deal of support in doing this. Internet-based support groups, newsletters, regional networks, family gatherings, as well as camps for children with PKU provide a link for families and a forum for exchange of practical information and emotional support. PKU clinic personnel are another source of support and reliable information on medical advances in treating PKU.

All patients with PKU should have their blood phenylalanine and other amino acids monitored regularly as long as they remain on the diet; they should have regular physical examinations, especially for assessment of growth parameters in children and adolescents, and review of the dietary intake since the previous visit. Extensive dietary counseling is an ongoing process. It is also recommended that adult patients who are not following phenylalanine-restricted diets with prescribed medical foods should be seen at least once a year for nutritional assessment, as they often tend to self limit their protein intake and may have inadequate diets.

Adequacy of Nutritional Therapy

Carefully executed diet therapy for individuals with PKU is widely considered to be safe as well as efficacious in preventing mental and neurological impairment. However, it cannot be assumed that largely synthetic diets supplemented with individual vitamins, minerals, and trace elements will confer the same benefits as diets composed of whole foods. Synthetic diets may have an inherent inability to supply all essential nutrients. In addition, patients who are noncompliant or partially compliant with their intake of medical food are at increased nutritional risk. Formerly treated patients who are 'off diet' tend to select high-carbohydrate diets and continue their habit of avoiding high-protein foods such as meat, milk, and eggs. Micronutrients previously supplied by the medical food, such as vitamin B_{12}, zinc, and iron, may not be replaced in adequate amounts on such a self-selected diet.

Growth

A strict PKU diet supplies 80–90% of its prescribed protein via a phenylalanine-free medical food. Most of the nitrogen in medical foods is supplied via essential amino acids. Meals that supply most of the protein as L-amino acids result in more rapid absorption and oxidation than observed after consumption of whole-protein meals. L-amino acids also may not be as efficiently absorbed as whole protein. Owing to these reasons, protein requirements for patients with PKU are considered to be greater than those given in the WHO guidelines and recommended daily intakes (RDIs). Normal growth and protein status has been observed in infants consuming at least 3 g protein $kg^{-1} day^{-1}$. Long-term inadequate protein intake will result in impaired growth in infants and children, low plasma prealbumin concentrations, radiological bone changes (osteopenia), and reduced phenylalanine tolerance. Because phenylalanine is an essential amino acid, it is crucial to prevent its deficiency. Phenylalanine deficiency will result in catabolism of body protein stores and subsequent elevation of blood phenylalanine levels, anemia, and mental retardation as well as the above symptoms accompanying overall inadequate protein intake.

Fatty Acids

Diet-treated children and adults with PKU consume very small amounts of animal fats, including fish-derived oils and long-chain polyunsaturated fatty acids (LC PUFAs.) In infants, small amounts of cows' milk-based formula are typically used to supply phenylalanine requirements. The majority of fatty acids supplied are typically not longer than 18 carbons long. While many standard infant formulas in Europe and the US are now supplemented with docosohexanoic acid (DHA) and arachadonic acid (ARA), metabolic formulas are not. Fatty acids are a structural component of all cell membranes. Alpha linolenic acid-derived compounds are essential for proper development of the central nervous system and retina. Linoleic acid-derived compounds play a role in promoting normal growth, skin, and reproduction. Breast milk contains formed DHA and ARA, and some studies indicate that breast-fed infants have better visual and cognitive development than unsupplemented formula-fed infants. The diets of children with PKU provide similar energy, higher carbohydrate, and lower lipid (with high unsaturated/saturated ratio) and cholesterol content than controls. Circulating plasma lipid levels of treated PKU patients contain lower concentrations of arachadonic acid (ARA), docosahexanoic acid (DHA), and eicosapentanoic acid than controls. Erythrocyte membranes of patients contain relatively high amounts of ARA and relatively low amounts of DHA. In theory, patients receiving adequate amounts of the essential fatty acid precursors linoleic and alpha linolenic acids would be able to synthesize LC PUFAs via elongation and desaturation reactions. It is unclear whether the amount of LC PUFAs synthesized would be adequate for optimal tissue function. Especially in infants, DHA and ARA may be partially essential nutrients. Trials of LC PUFA supplementation in PKU patients are underway. A number of widely available PKU formulas for older children and adults do not supply fat. Patients prescribed these formulas are presently advised to regularly include good sources of linoleic and alpha-linolenic acids in their diets. Flax, canola, and walnut oils are good sources.

In theory, patients with poorly controlled phenylalanine levels cannot efficiently build reserves of DHA and ARA from precursors. Carnitine-dependent mitochondrial enzymes that also use a cofactor, alpha tocopherolquinone, perform elongation and desaturation reactions. Phenyllactate and phenylpyruvate, metabolic byproducts of phenylalanine, may inhibit the synthesis of the cofactor alpha tocopherolquinone. This process may be at least partly responsible for the mental retardation and microcephaly observed in untreated PKU patients and poorly controlled maternal PKU.

Iron, Zinc, Vitamin A, and selenium

Some diet-treated patients with PKU have exhibited altered iron, zinc, vitamin A, and selenium status. With the exception of selenium, aberrations have been demonstrated even when patients consumed close to or greater than the RDI levels of the vitamin/mineral in question. The mechanisms of these changes are unclear and may be multifactorial. The actual impact of these changes on the health of the individual patients is unknown.

Low serum ferritin but appropriate hemoglobin and mean erythrocyte volumes have been noted, even in patients consuming close to three times the recommended dietary allowance (RDA) for iron. Iron absorption or bioavailability may be inhibited by the presence of calcium and phosphorous salts, diets high in PUFAs, and dietary fiber. The presence of alterations in the PUFA composition of gut cell membranes could affect iron absorption. In vitamin A-deficient rats, anemia occurred, which was not remedied by the administration of oral iron. This suggests that vitamin A deficiency in PKU patients could result in anemia unresponsive to iron therapy. The iron status of diet-treated patients should be serially monitored.

Low serum zinc has occurred in infants and children receiving greater than or equal to 70% of the RDA for zinc. Low serum zinc occurred more often in patients receiving casein hydrolysates than in patients receiving L-amino acids alone. Serum zinc may not be an accurate marker for assessment of zinc deficiency. Zinc absorption in general is inhibited by a PUFA-rich diet, fiber, phosphorous, and large amounts of iron. Competitive inhibition between calcium and zinc also occurs.

Low plasma retinol levels have been observed in infants and young children despite consumption of up to three times the RDA for vitamin A. Retinol is transported on retinol-binding protein (RBP); zinc is needed for the synthesis of RBP. Prealbumin is a carrier for RBP. RBP and zinc levels have been normal in nearly all patients with low retinol levels. Low prealbumin levels or abnormal release of RBP from prealbumin may be responsible for the low serum retinol levels. In fact, a number of children have low prealbumin levels despite receiving adequate protein and energy intakes.

Until recently, selenium was not routinely added to PKU formulas. In the past it was supplied to patients via contamination of foods grown in selenium-containing soil. Low serum, whole blood, urine, and hair levels of selenium have been observed in some patients with PKU on strict diet therapy. Low activity of the selenium-containing enzyme glutathione peroxidase also occurs. Clinical symptoms of selenium deficiency in the patients studied have not been reported.

Bone mineral density

Osteopenia is prevalent in diet-treated persons with PKU from early life. Reduced bone mineral density and/or bone mass has been detected in up to approximately 50% of patients screened by various methods. These methods have included DEXA (dual energy X-ray absorptiometry), pQCT (peripheral quantitative computed tomography), and SPA (single photon absorptiometry). The defect seems to be characterized by a reduction in the speed of bone mineralization, especially after 8 years of age. Osteoporosis is an important cause of morbidity and mortality in older adults in the general population. Reduction in bone mass increases the risk of fracture. A reduction of one standard deviation in spine bone mass is associated with a bone fracture rate of 2.0–2.5. Some authors have reported an increased fracture rate in children over 8 years of age with PKU.

The pathogenesis of osteopenia in PKU is under study. Discrepant associations have been reported between osteopenia and blood phenylalanine levels, serum vitamin and mineral levels, protein, vitamin and mineral intakes, serum markers of bone formation and PTH, and ratio of urinary minerals, to creatinine. One theory is that impaired mineralization is a direct effect of the lifelong disease process of PKU. The total and the bone-specific fraction of alkaline phosphatase are reduced in some patients. This reduction may affect osteoblast activity and impact bone formation and turnover. High blood phenylalanine levels have not been consistently correlated with osteopenia. High blood levels of phenylalanine and phenylalanine metabolites would result in their increased urinary excretion. Chelating of minerals with phenylalanine and phenylalanine derivatives could theoretically result in significant mineral losses.

Osteopenia may be an accumulated result of lifelong diet treatment or poor diet compliance at vulnerable stages of bone development. Compliant patients tend to have low variation in their lifelong intake of whole protein, as controlled amounts of whole protein are required to maintain good metabolic control. Compliant patients tend to have similar trends in overall intakes. Lack of adequate trace elements, whole protein, vitamins, and/or minerals may be culprits. Impaired absorption of the synthetic diet or the type of medical food used (hydrolysate versus elemental formulation) may exert an independent effect. Inadequate intakes of calcium and phosphorous are known risk factors for the development of osteoporosis in nonaffected persons. Tailoring medical foods to specifically deliver the amounts of calcium and phosphorous recommended in the new RDIs may help to prevent osteopenia.

Trials of calcitriol (1-25 (OH)2 D) supplementation in estrogenic patients with PKU are in progress. Calcitriol has been chosen as most patients already receive expected sun exposure from participating in normal outdoor activities, and their intakes of dietary vitamin D generally meet or exceed the RDA. Clairol has been shown to be a useful treatment; treated patients require close monitoring of urinary calcium excretion and blood calcium levels.

Maternal PKU

For women with PKU who intend to become pregnant, following a strict phenylalanine-restricted diet and controlling blood phenylalanine to $120–360\,mol\,l^{-1}$ is critical to offspring health. Women with PKU who have high blood phenylalanine levels are at high risk of having children with microcephaly, mental retardation, low birth weight, and congenital heart anomalies. In an International Study of Maternal PKU, women who had good metabolic control by 10 weeks' gestation had babies with good birth outcomes and development. In women with poor control, the degree of microcephaly and mental retardation was proportional to the level of blood phenylalanine. Congenital heart disease, on the other hand, was not directly related to the degree of metabolic control, suggesting that etiology is multifactorial, although in this study, no serious heart defects occurred when mothers were in good metabolic control by 10 weeks' gestation. The recommendation is for women to be on the diet for PKU and in good metabolic control before conceiving in order to prevent damage to the fetus. Nevertheless, many women come to medical attention during pregnancy, indicating the need for better strategies for keeping women on the diet for life or helping them return to the diet before pregnancy. While blood phenylalanine during pregnancy was the best predictor of outcome in maternal PKU in the Collaborative Study, other nutritional factors, including sufficient energy, protein, vitamin B_{12} and fat, also played an important role.

Alternative Therapies

Tetrahydrobiopterin (BH4)

Tetrahydrobiopterin (BH4) is the cofactor for phenylalanine hydroxylase. Some mutations for PAH are considered to be relatively milder than others; a number of studies have shown that certain of these mutations result in enzyme activity that may be improved by the addition of BH4 to the diet. In these cases, the degree of phenylalanine restriction needed to maintain good control could be liberalized, although not eliminated altogether.

Large Neutral Amino Acid Supplementation

The large neutral amino acids (LNAAs), phenylalanine, tyrosine, tryptophan, and the branched-chain amino acids share the same L-amino acid transport system across the blood–brain barrier. Therefore,

high levels of phenylalanine in the blood impede the transport of these other amino acids into the central nervous system (CNS). Tyrosine and tryptophan are important neurotransmitter precursors, relative deficiency or imbalance of which may contribute to the neuropsychiatric symptoms seen in some adult PKU patients who have resumed an unrestricted diet. Treatment with supplemental LNAAs (in tablet form) theoretically will increase the competition with phenylalanine for transport into the CNS. A net reduction in phenylalanine and an increase in CNS tyrosine and tryptophan may result in improvement in symptoms. Long-term outcome data are not yet available. This treatment is not suitable for children or women in the childbearing years who might be contemplating pregnancy.

See also: **Bone**. **Brain and Nervous System**. **Breast Feeding**. **Osteoporosis**. **Selenium**. **Supplementation**: Role of Micronutrient Supplementation. **Vitamin A**: Physiology; Biochemistry and Physiological Role; Deficiency and Interventions. **Vitamin K**. **Zinc**: Deficiency in Developing Countries, Intervention Studies.

Further Reading

Acosta PB (1996) Nutrition studies in treated infants and children with phenylketonuria: vitamins, minerals, and trace elements. *European Journal of Pediatrics* 155(supplement 1): S136–139.

Acosta PB, Matalon K, Castiglioni L *et al.* (2001) Intake of major nutrients by women in the maternal PKU (MPKU) study and effects on plasma phenylalanine concentrations. *American Journal of Clinical Nutrition* 73: 792–796.

Al-Qadreh A, Schulpis K, and Athanasopoulou H (1998) Bone mineral status in children with phenylketonuria under treatment. *Acta Pediatrica* 87(11): 1162–1166.

Giovanni M, Biasucci G, Agostini C *et al.* (1995) Lipid status and fatty acid metabolism in phenylketonuria. *Journal of Inherited Metabolic Diseases* 18: 265–272.

Koch R, Fishler K, Azen C, Guldberg P, and Guttler F (1997) The relationship of genotype to phenotype in phenylalanine hydroxylase deficiency. *Biochemistry and Molecular Medicine* 60(2): 92–101.

Koch R, Hanley W, Levy H *et al.* (2003) The Maternal Phenylketonuria International Study: 1984–2002. *Pediatrics* 112(6 part 2): 1523–1529.

NIH Consensus Development Conference Statement (2001) Phenylketonuria, screening and management. *Pediatrics* 108(4): 972–982.

Perez-Duenas P, Cambra F, and Vilaseca M (2002) New approach to osteopenia in phenylketonuric patients. *Acta Pediatrica* 91(8): 899–904.

Przyrembel H and Bremer H (2000) Nutrition, physical growth, and bone density in treated phenylketonuria. *European Journal of Pediatrics* 159(supplement 2): S129–S135.

INFANTS

Contents
Nutritional Requirements
Feeding Problems

Nutritional Requirements

S A Atkinson, McMaster University, Hamilton, ON, Canada

Optimal nutritional support of infants in the first year of life is essential to attain normal trajectories of growth and development. Additionally, evidence supports the thesis that during critical periods of early development nutrition may be key to 'programming,' possibly through modification of gene expression or differential cell proliferation, that subsequently impacts on risk for chronic diseases in later life. Information on early nutrition programming is not sufficient to be used as a basis to set dietary standards for infants. However, the importance of adopting the quantity and quality of nutrients in human milk as a gold standard in the determination of nutrient recommendations has been reinforced by several agencies worldwide, such as the pioneering partnership between the Food and Nutrition Board of the Institute of Medicine in the United States and Health Canada.

Recommended nutrient intakes or dietary standards are produced by many countries as well as key international agencies such as the FAO/WHO. For infants, the recommended intakes are usually intended for term-born, healthy, and normally growing infants who have a birth weight of more than 2500 g (and thus not small for gestational age). In this article, the nutrient requirements outlined reflect recent reports of the Dietary Reference Intakes (DRIs) for the United States and Canada as published by the Institute of Medicine. For a summary of the range of recommended nutrient intakes for infants that reflect a review of several international reports, the reader is referred to the March of Dimes document, *Nutrition Today Matters Tomorrow* (Appendix D-2).

The key changes in the derivation of the DRIs for infants compared to previous dietary standards from the United States and Canada include adoption of human milk as the reference model for setting recommended nutrient intakes for infants; simplification of age groupings within the first year; no specific provision of dietary recommendations for formula-fed infants; and gender-specific DRI values for fewer nutrients and only where data were available to support such gender specificity. Another major change from previous dietary standards is that upper levels (ULs) for nutrient intake were defined for the first time. Unfortunately, for infants, few ULs were established due to a paucity of pertinent knowledge; even for ages 1–18 years, the UL values were mostly extrapolated from adult values.

This article provides an overview of key concepts and examples of the DRIs specific for infants, future needs for additional research, and practical aspects of meeting the dietary recommendations for infants.

Dietary Reference Intakes for Infants

For infants, evaluation of evidence to establish the DRIs consistently revealed a paucity of appropriate studies on which to base an Estimated Average Requirement (EAR) or UL. A Recommended Dietary Allowance (RDA) could not be calculated if a value for the EAR was not established, in which case the recommended intake was based on an Adequate Intake (AI). The nutrient recommendations for infants from birth through 6 months of age for all nutrients except for energy and vitamin D were set as an AI, a value that represents "the mean intake of a nutrient calculated based on the average concentration of the nutrient in human milk from 2 to 6 months of lactation using consensus values from several reported studies," multiplied by an average volume (0.780 l/day) of human milk. The predicted daily volume of breast milk ingested by an infant was based on observational studies that used test weighing of full-term infants. For infants aged 7–12 months, the AI for many nutrients was based on mean observed nutrient intake from human milk in the second 6 months (0.6 l/day) in addition to published values for intake of nutrients from complementary or weaning foods if such data were available.

Assuming an adequate intake of milk for all infants was considered a valid approach since there is evidence that the volume of milk produced during the early months of lactation is very consistent among women irrespective of racial, cultural, or nutritional diversity or variations in body size. The volume of milk produced increases with greater size of the infant, when twins are nursing, and in response to greater frequency of nursing.

Using consensus values for the nutrient content of human milk was deemed appropriate since for many nutrients—energy, macronutrients, and macrominerals—maternal diet does not influence the nutrient content of the milk. The exceptions to this include the fatty acid profile, selenium, iodine, and the water-soluble vitamins. Although human milk is known to contain many nonnutrient bioactive factors, such as immune and growth factors and live enzymes, these were not considered to impact on nutrient needs *per se*.

For nutrients for which intake data were not available for ages older than 6 months, the EAR or AI was derived by extrapolation from estimates of intakes from older children or adults using the formula with adjustments for metabolic body size, growth, and variability:

$$EAR_{infant \text{ or } child} = EAR_{child \text{ or } adult} \times (F)$$

where $F = (weight_{infant \text{ or } child}/weight_{child \text{ or } adult})^{0.75}$ $(1 + growth\ factor)$; or occasionally by extrapolating up from intake of breast-fed infants with similar adjustments using the formula

$$AI\ 6 - 11\ months = AI\ 0 - 5\ months \times F$$

where $F = (weight_{6-11\ months}/weight_{0-5\ months})^{0.75}$

For a few nutrients, such as iron and zinc, sufficient metabolic data were available to derive an EAR using modeling or factorial methods.

Because no specific AIs were derived for formula-fed infants, it is incumbent upon industry to design formulas with a quantity and quality of nutrients that when fed will provide an amount of nutrients that meets the RDA or AI. An approach to establishing the amount of nutrient needed by formula-fed infants is addressed under the section titled "Special Considerations" in each DRI report.

When possible, a DRI called the tolerable upper level was defined as "the highest level of daily nutrient intake that is likely to pose no risk of adverse health effects for almost all individuals in the general population" (Institute of Medicine, 2002). Chronic consumption of nutrients above the UL increases the potential risk of adverse effects, the latter varying by nutrient. For infants, data were only available to reliably estimate ULs for vitamins A and D and the minerals fluoride, selenium, zinc, and iron. Although adequate data were not available to define a UL for infants for other nutrients, it

is important to note that intake for nutrients for which a UL does not exist should only be consumed from food or formula and not from supplements. Also notable is that the UL for iron for infants is only relevant to intake from supplements and not foods.

Summary of DRIs for infants

Macronutrients: Energy, Carbohydrate, Fat, Protein, and Amino Acids

Energy The estimated energy requirement (EER) for infants was derived by summing predicted total energy expenditure (TEE) and energy deposition for growth. Because the energy needs for growth decelerate with advancing age, an equation for EER was established for three age intervals during the first year of life (**Table 1**). The TEE is calculated using an equation (**Table 1**) based on energy expenditure measured by doubly labeled water and adjusted for weight of the child. The EER is then the sum of TEE for an individual child plus the predicted energy deposition for age (**Table 1**). No adjustment for physical activity was included in the EER for infants. Examples of the EER for males and females using reference weights are shown in **Table 1** for infants at five ages during the first year. At most ages beyond the first 2 months of life, the values for EER exceed the average energy provided (500 kcal) by human milk assuming a volume of intake (0.780 l/day) from human milk.

Table 1 DRI estimated energy requirement (EER) for infants[a]

Equations

0–3 months	(89 × weight of infant (kg) − 100) + 175 (kcal for energy deposition)
4–6 months	(89 × weight of infant (kg) − 100) + 56 (kcal for energy deposition)
7–12 months	(89 × weight of infant (kg) − 100) + 22 (kcal for energy deposition)

Calculated EER for age using reference weights for age

Age (months)	Males (kcal/day)	Females (kcal/day)
1	472	438
3	572	521
6	645	593
9	746	678
12	844	768

[a]From the Institute of Medicine (2002) *Dietary Reference Intakes for Energy, Carbohydrates, Fiber, Fat, Protein, and Amino Acids (Macronutrients)*. Washington, DC: National Academy Press.

Carbohydrate The AI for carbohydrate for infants through 1 year of age is based on the average carbohydrate intake from human milk and complementary foods for the 7- to 12-month age group (**Table 2**). Although the carbohydrate from human milk is almost exclusively lactose and that from infant formula may be lactose, sucrose, or glucose polymers alone or in combination, there is no evidence that non-lactose-containing formulas vary from lactose contained in human milk with regard to available energy.

Fat As for other nutrients, the AI for fat intake is based on the average intake of fat from human milk alone or in addition to complementary foods after 7 months of age (**Table 2**). Although infant formulas are designed to contain a percentage of energy as fat similar to human milk (approximately 50%), the type of fat in formulas varies widely, including such sources as safflower, sunflower, soybean oil, and coconut and palm oils, usually in some combination.

Linoleic acid (n-6) and α-linolenic acid (n-3) The n-6 fatty acids are essential for infants, and in extreme long-term deficiency skin lesions and delayed growth may develop. Linoleic acid serves as a precursor of arachidonic acid (AA), which is required for synthesis of prostaglandins and other eicosanoids. The n-3 fatty acids are also essential as a precursor of docosahexenoic acid (DHA), which comprises a large percentage of the fatty acids incorporated into developing brain and retina, and of eicosapentenoic acid, which is the substrate for eicosanoid synthesis. Human milk is a natural source of both fatty acid families, including the long-chain polyenoic derivatives DHA and AA. The pattern of all fatty acids in human milk, including the polyenoic fatty acids, is dependent on maternal diet. The

AI established for infants for n-6 and n-3 fatty acids is based on the average content in human milk reported for North American women with the addition of that from complementary foods during months 7–12 (**Table 2**).

Feeding of mother's milk compared to cow milk-based infant formula has been associated with a positive benefit to developmental outcomes (cognitive, motor, and vision) in both retrospective and prospective studies (but not randomized trials for obvious ethical reasons). To date, investigations of the nutrient(s) possibly responsible for the observed benefits of mother's milk on neurodevelopment have focused on the long-chain polyenoic fatty acids DHA and AA. These fatty acids represent the greatest proportion of polyenoic fatty acids contained in phospholipids of neural and retinal tissues, and they are present naturally in human milk. Until very recently, DHA and AA were not provided in infant formulas, but such formula is now marketed globally.

A positive benefit of breast-feeding compared to formula feeding on short-term visual and developmental outcomes in term and premature infants has been observed in several studies. However, the evidence for a benefit is more consistently observed in premature than in term infants, perhaps due to a greater immaturity of their enzymatic pathway to convert α-linolenic and linoleic acids to the long-chain polyenoic derivatives. Due to the conflicting evidence, specific requirements for DHA and AA for term infants were not included in the recent DRI report.

Protein For infants age 0–6 months, the AI for protein is based on the intake from human milk (**Table 2**). For infants age 7–12 months, sufficient information was available from nitrogen balance studies and protein deposition to derive an EAR based on the factorial method. For both males and females, this averaged 1.1 g protein/kg body weight/day. The RDA was set as the EAR + 2 standard deviations (based on coefficients of variation observed in adults), which yielded a value for protein intake of 1.5 g/kg/day. Because the absorption and digestibility of protein contained in infant formula may be less efficient than from human milk, the quantity of protein contained in infant formulas may have to be adjusted depending on the protein source used.

Amino acids The DRI for the essential (indispensable) amino acids for infants was derived from the content of human milk for ages 0–6 months. For older infants, an EAR was derived for these amino acids using a factorial estimate that was based on

Table 2 DRI for macronutrients for infants—carbohydrate, protein, fat, and essential fatty acids[a]

Nutrient[b]	0–6 months	7–12 months
Carbohydrate, AI (g/day)	60	95
Protein		
AI (g/day)	9.1	—
RDA (g/day)	—	13.5
Total fat, AI (g/day)	31	30
Linoleic acid (n-6), AI (g/day)	4.4	4.6
α-Linolenic acid (n-3), AI (g/day)	0.5	0.5

[a]From the Institute of Medicine (2002) *Dietary Reference Intakes for Energy, Carbohydrates, Fiber, Fat, Protein, and Amino Acids (Macronutrients)*. Washington, DC: National Academy Press.
[b]No upper levels of nutrients were set for any macronutrients.
AI, Adequate Intake; RDA, Recommended Dietary Allowance.

Table 3 DRI for indispensible (essential) amino acids[a]

Amino acid[b]	0–6 months[c]	7–12 months
	AI (mg/kgday)	RDA (mg/kg/day)
Histidine	23	32
Isoleucine	88	43
Leucine	156	93
Lysine	107	89
Methionine + cysteine	59	43
Phenylalanine + tyrosine	135	84
Threonine	73	49
Tryptophan	28	13
Valine	87	58

[a]From the Institute of Medicine (2002) *Dietary Reference Intakes for Energy, Carbohydrates, Fiber, Fat, Protein, and Amino Acids (Macronutrients)*. Washington, DC: National Academy Press.
[b]No upper levels were set for any of the indispensable amino acids.
[c]AI values shown as amino acid in mg/kg/day can be converted to mg amino acid/day by multiplying by the reference weight of 6 kg for infants 0–6 months of age.

Table 4 DRI for minerals for infants—calcium, phosphorus, magnesium, and fluoride[a]

Nutrient	0–6 months	7–12 months
Calcium		
AI (mg/day)	210	270
UL	ND	ND
Phosphorus		
AI (mg/day)	100	275
UL	ND	ND
Magnesium		
AI (mg/day)	30	75
UL	ND	ND
Fluoride		
AI (mg/day)	0.01	0.5
UL (mg/day)	0.7	0.9

[a]From the Institute of Medicine (1997) *Dietary Reference Intakes for Calcium, Phosphorus, Magnesium, Vitamin D and Fluoride*. Washington, DC: National Academy Press.
AI, Adequate Intake; ND, not determinable due to lack of data of adverse effects in infants; RDA, Recommended Dietary Allowance; UL, upper limit.

the amino acid needs for growth or protein deposition, with adjustments for efficiency of protein deposition and maintenance requirement. The RDA was determined by adding the coefficient of variation derived for maintenance and protein deposition to the value for the EAR. No values were set for UL for any of the amino acids. A summary of the AI and RDA for the indispensable amino acids of infants is provided in **Table 3**.

Other macronutrients For infants, no DRI was set for saturated fat, monounsaturated fat, *trans* fatty acids, and cholesterol or dietary fiber. Although some dietary fiber is present in the diet after solid foods are introduced, there are no data on fiber intakes in such young age groups and no theoretical basis exists on which to establish a need for fiber at less than 1 year of age.

Macrominerals: Calcium, phosphorus, magnesium, and fluoride The AI for infants for the "bone" minerals are summarized in **Table 4**. The content of human milk was used as the basis to derive the AI for calcium, phosphorus, and magnesium for infants age 0–6 months and with the addition of intake from complementary foods for those age 7–12 months. For fluoride, intake from human milk was the reference for the first 6 months only. After 6 months, the AI for fluoride was set at 0.05 mg/kg/day and adjusted to a reference weight for age, based on the well-documented evidence of the benefit of fluoride intake for the prevention of dental caries (**Table 4**).

Microminerals/trace elements The AI for iron for ages 0–6 months is based on the concentration of iron in human milk albeit low (approximately 0.35 mg/l) but assumes the infant is born with maximal iron stores due to transplacental transfer of iron from an iron-replete mother. If the latter conditions do not apply, then an exogenous source of iron such as iron drops may be required. For infants age 7–12 months, an EAR and RDA were developed based on a factorial modeling method that summed basal loss of iron with needs for growth, increasing hemoglobin mass, and iron stores. This value was then adjusted for iron bioavailability using a factor of 10% for infants due to a medium bioavailability of iron from infant cereals, which are generally the major dietary source of iron in weaning foods before meats are introduced (**Table 5**). A UL was established (**Table 5**) for iron based on the risk of adverse gastrointestinal side effects from supplemental (not food) iron.

For zinc, an AI was based on the human milk model only for the 0- to 6-months age group (**Table 5**). The zinc content of human milk declines rapidly during the first 6 months (from 4 to 1.2 mg/l), so the AI was based on a milk zinc concentration of 2.5 mg/l. This value cannot be directly applied to infants being fed cow milk- or soy-based infant formulas because zinc absorption is significantly lower from these compared to human milk. The EAR for the 7- to 12-months age group was set using a factorial method that summed obligatory losses with requirements for growth and adjusted for fractional absorption of dietary zinc from human milk and complementary foods. The RDA

Table 5 DRI for micronutrient/trace minerals for infants—chromium, copper, fluoride, iodine, iron, manganese, molybdenum, selenium, and zinc[a]

Nutrient	0–6 months	7–12 months
Chromium		
AI (μg/day)	0.2	5.5
UL	ND	ND
Copper		
AI (μg/day)	200	220
UL	ND	ND
Iodine		
AI (μg/day)	110	130
UL	ND	ND
Iron		
AI (mg/day)	0.27	—
RDA (mg/day)	—	11
UL (mg/day)	40	40
Manganese		
AI (μg/day)	30	75
UL	ND	ND
Molybdenum		
AI (μg/day)	2	3
UL	ND	ND
Selenium		
AI (μg/day)	15	20
UL (μg/day)	45	60
Zinc		
AI (mg/day)	2	—
RDA (mg/day)	—	3
UL (mg/day)	4	5

[a]From the Institute of Medicine (2001) *Dietary Reference Intakes for Vitamin A, Vitamin K, Arsenic, Boron, Chromium, Copper, Iodine, Iron, Manganese, Molybdenum, Nickel, Silicon, Vanadium and Zinc*. Washington, DC: National Academy Press. AI, Adequate Intake; ND, not determinable due to lack of data of adverse effects in infants; RDA, Recommended Dietary Allowance; UL, upper limit.

was derived by adding twice the coefficient of variation of 10% to the EAR (2.5 mg/day of zinc) for infants 7–12 months (**Table 5**). A UL was set for zinc on the basis of the possibility of an adverse effect of high zinc intakes on copper status.

For the trace elements chromium, copper, iodine, manganese, molybdenum, and selenium, an AI was set for infants age 0–6 months based on the human milk model (**Table 5**). For the age group 7–12 months, data on intake from complementary foods were only available to set an AI for chromium, copper, and selenium (**Table 5**). For iodine and molybdenum, the AI represents an extrapolation up from the AI values for the age group 0–6 months based on differences in metabolic body weight ($kg^{0.75}$). For manganese, the AI represents an extrapolation down from the AI for adults as described previously (**Table 5**). Due to lack of relevant information no UL values for infants younger than 1 year of age were established for chromium, copper, iodine, manganese, or molybdenum, but intakes of these nutrients should be limited to foods and not supplements. A UL was established for selenium due to the known toxicity of chronic excess selenium ingestion, which presents clinically as brittleness and loss of nails and hair. The UL was set for infants based on the highest known intake of selenium from human milk and adjusting for a reference infant weight (**Table 5**). The UL value pertains to intake from both foods and supplements.

The trace elements arsenic, boron, nickel, silicon, and vanadium are recognized as having a role in human metabolism, but due to lack of information DRI values, including UL, could not be established for infants.

Globally, deficiencies of iron, iodine, and zinc in infants are still widespread despite international efforts to develop sustainable food fortification and supplementation programs. In North America, the prevalence of iron deficiency anemia is relatively low at 4–5% owing to the promotion of breast feeding and the widespread fortification of infant formulas and cereals with iron. In developing countries, prevalence of anemia can be 50% or more by one year of age. Premature and/or low birth weight (<2.5 kg) infants represent a particular risk group for iron deficiency owing to a major reduction in transplacental transfer of iron when birth occurs during the third trimester of pregnancy, the period when most iron is transferred to the fetus as long as the mother is not iron deficient. Infants of low birth weight require iron supplementation in a liquid form until complementary foods containing iron can be introduced. Use of weaning foods that are not iron-fortified and that often contain phytic acid, a strong inhibitor of iron absorption, is a key causative factor for high rates of anemia in many developing countries.

Fat-soluble vitamins A, K, E, and D For vitamins A, K, and E, the AI for infants 0–6 months of age was based on the human milk model as previously described (**Table 6**). For vitamins A, K, and E, the AI for infants 7–12 months of age was extrapolated up from the values for 0–6 months using a reference weight for infants at this age. There are two important points with respect to the AI established for vitamin K. First, the AI was set assuming infants had received a prophylactic injection of vitamin K just after birth. Since vitamin K is not readily transferred to the fetus while *in utero*, and human milk is relatively low in vitamin K, newborn infants, at least in North America, routinely receive an injection of vitamin K within a few hours after birth. Second, the AI set for ages 7–12 months may be lower than the actual intake of vitamin K once a child's diet of

Table 6 DRI for fat-soluble vitamins[a]

Nutrient	0–6 months	7–12 months
Vitamin A		
AI (µg/day)	400	500
UL (µg/day)	600	600
Vitamin D		
AI (µg/day)	5	5
UL (µg/day)	25	25
Vitamin E		
AI (mg/day)	4	5
UL	ND	ND
Vitamin K		
AI (µg/day)	2.0	2.5
UL	ND	ND

[a]From the Institute of Medicine (1997) *Dietary Reference Intakes for Calcium, Phosphorus, Magnesium, Vitamin D and Fluoride.* Washington, DC. National Academy Press; Institute of Medicine (2000) *Dietary Reference Intakes for Vitamin C, Vitamin E, Selenium, and Carotenoids.* Washington, DC: National Academy Press; and Institute of Medicine (2000) *Dietary Reference Intakes for Vitamin A, Vitamin K, Arsenic, Boron, Chromium, Copper, Iodine, Iron, Manganese, Molybdenum, Nickel, Silicon, Vanadium and Zinc.* Washington, DC: National Academy Press. AI, Adequate Intake; ND, not determinable due to lack of data of adverse effects in infants; UL, upper limit.

complementary food becomes varied. Any evaluation of dietary intake of vitamin K should use the recently updated vitamin K values for raw and cooked foods available from the USDA National Nutrient Database for Standard Reference, Release 17 (http://www.nal.usda.gov/fnic/foodcomp/Data/SR17/wtrant/wt_rank.html). Although carotenoids are present in human milk, a factor to calculate their bioconversion to vitamin A is not known so their contribution to vitamin A was not included.

For vitamin D, it was determined that a dietary (or supplement) intake of 100 IU would likely prevent rickets but not maintain normal circulating concentrations of 25-hydroxyvitamin D. Thus, assuming that most infants obtain minimal or no vitamin D via exposure to sunlight, an AI of 200 IU (5 µg) was established. This amount of vitamin D was also recommended for infants 7–12 months of age assuming most infants could maintain normal vitamin D status with this intake. The AI for vitamin D set by the Institute of Medicine was adopted by the American Academy of Pediatrics (AAP). The AAP recommended a minimum intake of 200 IU vitamin D per day for all infants beginning during the first 2 months of life in recognition of the risk in vitamin D-deficiency rickets in the United States, especially among infants who are breast fed for a number of months without vitamin D supplementation. In Canada, a recent recommendation by Health Canada (2004) was for

all breast fed infants to receive 10 µg (400 IU)/day of vitamin D from birth until their diet included equal amounts of vitamin D from other food sources. Considerations for this recommendation (rather than 5 µg (200 IU)/day of the DRI) included lack of sun exposure owing to Canada's northern geographic latitude, current practices related to protection from the sun, and an increasing prevalence of vitamin D deficiency rickets in infants.

Water-soluble B vitamins, folate, choline, and vitamin C The AIs for infants age 0–6 months for most water-soluble vitamins were based on the content of human milk (**Table 7**). This approach may be problematic for water-soluble B vitamins, in which milk content is dependent on maternal intake of vitamins. An example of clinical relevance is the vegan mother

Table 7 DRI for water-soluble vitamins[a]

Nutrient	0–6 months	7–12 months
Vitamin C		
AI (mg/day)	40	50
UL	ND	ND
Thiamin		
AI (mg/day)	0.2	0.3
UL	ND	ND
Riboflavin		
AI (mg/day)	0.3	0.4
UL	ND	ND
Niacin		
AI (mg/day)	2	4
UL	ND	ND
Vitamin B$_6$		
AI (mg/day)	0.1	0.3
UL	ND	ND
Folate		
AI (µg/day)	65	80
UL	ND	ND
Vitamin B$_{12}$		
AI (µg/day)	0.4	0.5
UL	ND	ND
Pantothenic acid		
AI (mg/day)	1.7	1.8
UL	ND	ND
Biotin		
AI (µg/day)	5	6
UL	ND	ND
Choline		
AI (mg/day)	125	150
UL	ND	ND

[a]From the Institute of Medicine (1998) *Dietary Reference Intakes for Thiamin, Riboflavin, Niacin, Vitamin B$_6$, Folate, Vitamin B$_{12}$, Pantothenic Acid, Biotin, and Choline.* Washington, DC: National Academy Press; and Institute of Medicine (2000) *Dietary Reference Intakes for Vitamin C, Vitamin E, Selenium, and Carotenoids.* Washington, DC: National Academy Press. AI, Adequate Intake; UL, upper limit.

who may have subclinical vitamin B_{12} deficiency and produce B_{12}-deficient milk. For vitamin C, the effect of maternal supplementation on milk content remains uncertain, but available reports do not indicate that excessive amounts of vitamin C are secreted in milk, even in mothers taking supplements of 1000 mg or more. For age 7–12 months, the AI for thiamin, riboflavin, niacin, folate, pantothenic acid, and choline was derived by extrapolation down from values for older children or adults due to a lack of information of dietary intake of these nutrients from solid foods. Tolerable ULs for infants were not established for any of the water-soluble vitamins.

Water and electrolytes Optimal water intake in infants is more critical than at any other period of life. Not only do infants have higher total body water content per body mass than children or adults but also they have a higher water turnover rate, a less well-developed sweating mechanism, and little ability to indicate when they are thirsty. The AI for water intake of infants age 0–6 months is 0.7 l/day and is based on the water content of human milk. Assuming infants are breast-fed on demand, infants will drink to meet thirst needs; thus, even in hot and humid climates supplemental water should not be required. The AI for water intake of 0.8 l/day set for 7–12 months is based on the sum of the water content of human milk, complementary foods, and beverages, the latter obtained from reported food intakes from surveys in the United States.

For sodium and potassium, the AI of 0.12 g/day and 0.4 g/day, respectively, is based on the human milk model. For 7–12 months, the AI for sodium is 0.37 g/day and for potassium is 0.7 g/day based on the sum of observed intakes from human milk and complementary foods. No ULs were established for infants due to lack of data on adverse effects of these nutrients on infant health. However, particularly because the renal excretory capacity of young infants may not be able to handle excess amounts of ingested electrolytes, the DRI report notes that intake of sodium, chloride, and potassium should be limited to human milk (or infant formula) and solid foods appropriate for age.

Assessment of Growth as an Indication of Adequate Nutrition

Assessment of growth in weight, length and head circumference is an internationally accepted measure of health and nutritional status of infants, albeit not an indicator that is nutrient specific. The interpretation of growth measures requires comparison with reference data from normal populations of infants that have been complied into growth charts with centiles indicated. The growth charts from the Center for Disease Control in the United States as revised in 2000 (http://www.cdc.gov/nchs/about/major/nhanes/growthcharts/charts.htm), were adopted for use in the USA and Canada as well as by the World Health Organization (WHO) for use internationally. The growth charts as shown in **Figures 1–6** may be downloaded from the CDC website and copied. Weight gain of exclusively breast fed infants is more rapid than formula-fed infants in the first 2 to 3 months but they weigh less from 6 to 12 months. The longitudinal data that form the basis of the growth charts for infants from birth to 36 months growth represent a mix of both breast and formula fed infants from the American population. A Working Group of WHO has undertaken a project to develop growth charts specifically for exclusively or predominantly breast fed infants but these are not yet available.

Research Needs

The paucity of sound evidence on which to provide a substantial basis for estimating the nutrient requirements for infants is highlighted at the end of each chapter in the DRI reports. Since infants and children are not just "little adults," the DRI values must be carefully defined for the specific stages of growth and development and with consideration for nutritional programming that occurs in early life in response to dietary exposures as our knowledge of this area becomes more complete.

Practical Aspects of Meeting the Nutrient Needs of Infants

Adequate amounts of breast milk meet the nutrient needs of most infants for the first 6 months of life. However, there is not universal agreement on the optimal duration of exclusive breast feeding and the precise timing or the order of introduction of complementary foods. Internationally, recommendations from most health agencies state that the ideal feeding of infants is exclusive breast feeding for the first 6 months of life with appropriate introduction of foods from 6 months onward including partial breast feeding through 2 years of age or beyond. When assessing intakes of infants fed marketed formulas, it must be kept in mind that intakes of most nutrients will exceed the new DRI values for AI given that these are based on the composition of human milk. In many cases, the greater concentration of nutrients in infant formula is appropriate due

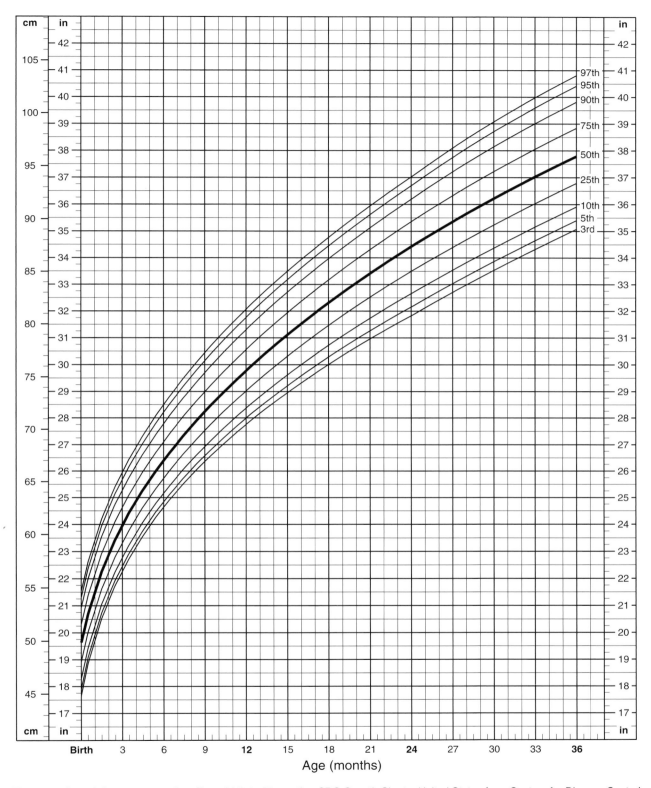

Figure 1 Length-for-age percentiles: Boys, birth to 36 months. CDC Growth Charts: United States from Centers for Disease Control and Prevention, National Center for Health Statistics. Source: Developed by the National Center for Chronic Disease Prevention and Health Promotion (2000).

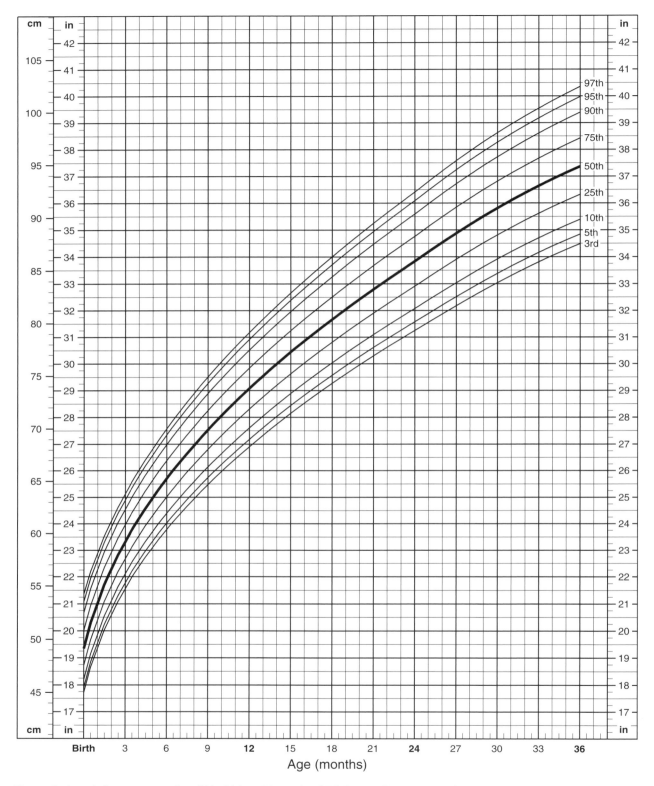

Figure 2   Length-for-age percentiles: Girls, birth to 36 months. CDC Growth Charts: United States from Centers for Disease Control and Prevention, National Center for Health Statistics. Source: Developed by the National Center for Chronic Disease Prevention and Health Promotion (2000).

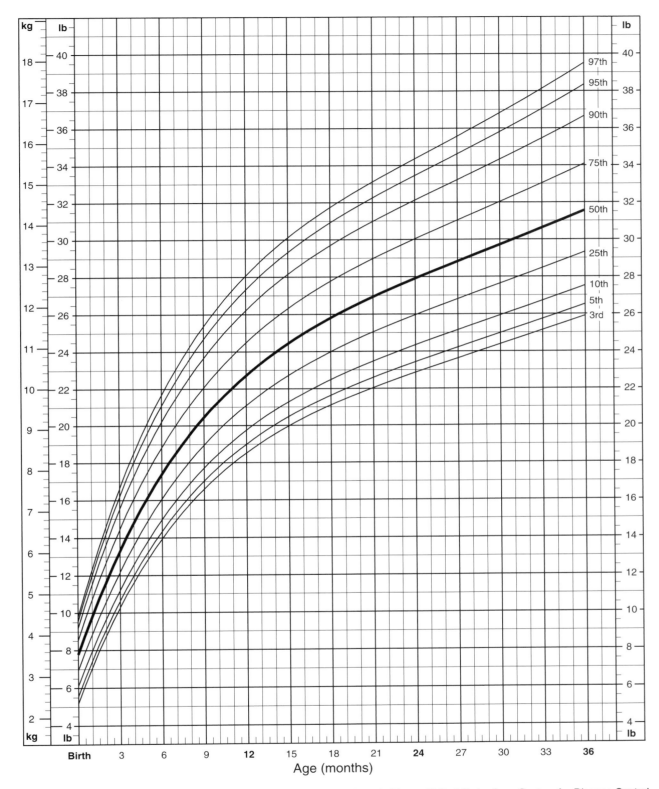

Figure 3 Weight-for-age percentiles: Boys, birth to 36 months. CDC Growth Charts: United States from Centers for Disease Control and Prevention, National Center for Health Statistics. Source: Developed by the National Center for Chronic Disease Prevention and Health Promotion (2000).

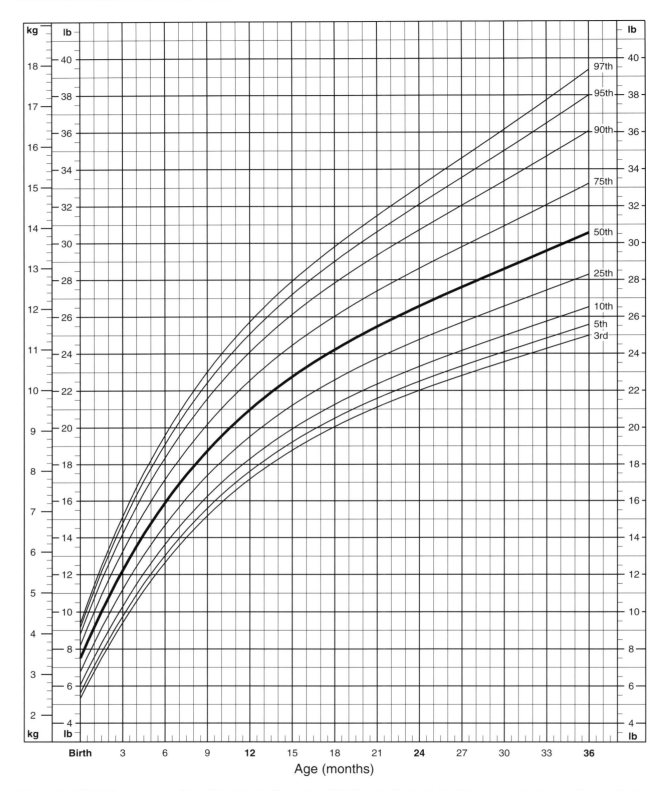

Figure 4 Weight-for-age percentiles: Girls, birth to 36 months. CDC Growth Charts: United States from Centers for Disease Control and Prevention, National Center for Health Statistics. Source: Developed by the National Center for Chronic Disease Prevention and Health Promotion (2000).

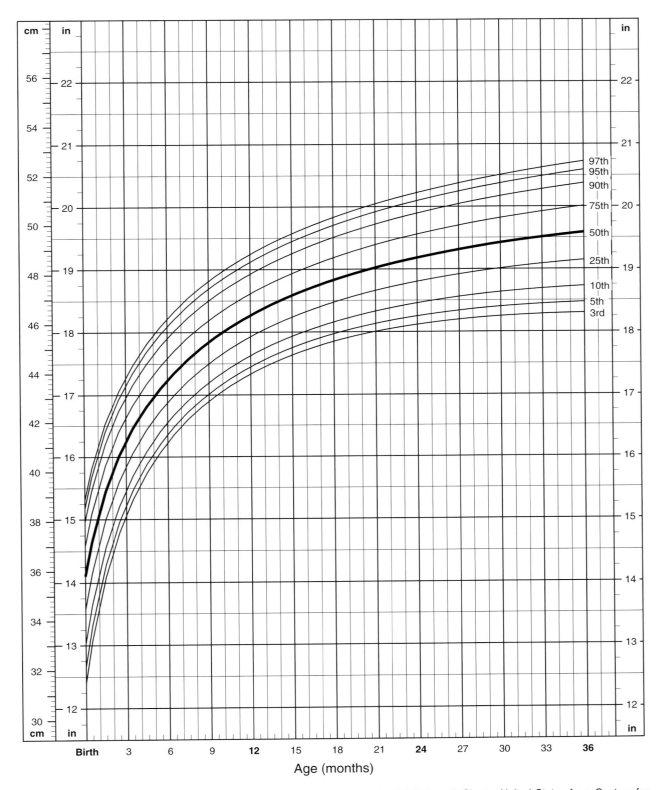

Figure 5   Head circumference-for-age percentiles: Boys, birth to 36 months. CDC Growth Charts: United States from Centers for Disease Control and Prevention, National Center for Health Statistics. Source: Developed by the National Center for Chronic Disease Prevention and Health Promotion (2000).

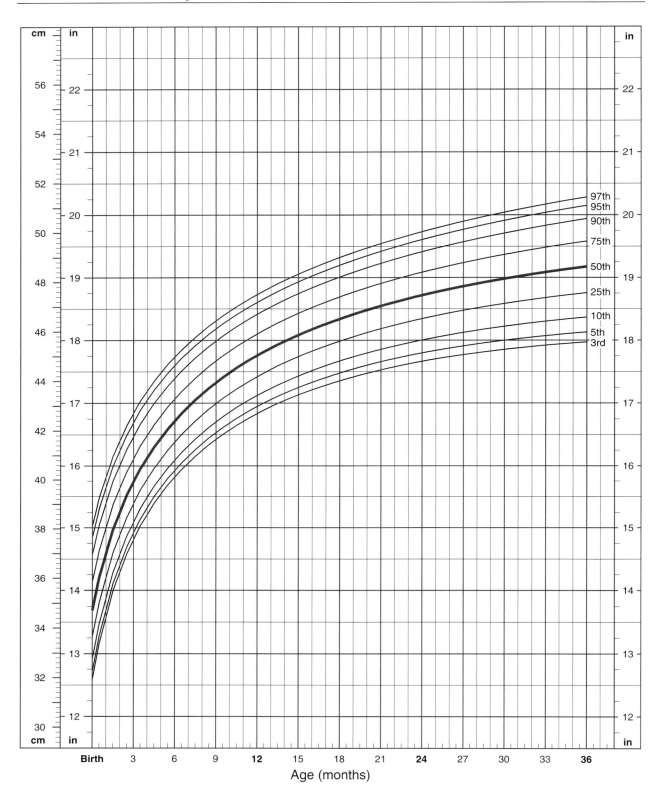

Figure 6 Head circumference-for-age percentiles: Girls, birth to 36 months. CDC Growth Charts: United States from Centers for Disease Control and Prevention, National Center for Health Statistics. Source: Developed by the National Center for Chronic Disease Prevention and Health Promotion (2000).

to lower digestibility or bioavailability of nutrients from cow milk- or soy-based protein in formulas compared to human milk.

The introduction of complementary foods, especially solids and eventually finger foods, is important for infants to develop normal oral and motor skills related to eating and to attain adequate intakes of nutrients that may be low in breast milk (e.g., protein or iron). In a report by the March of Dimes, three common inappropriate complementary feeding practices were delineated: (i) introducing foods too early or too late, (ii) introducing foods of low nutrient density, and (iii) feeding contaminated foods. It is noted in the report that early introduction of foods may reduce the intake of breast milk due to limited gastric capacity of very young infants or precipitate an allergic reaction in infants with a family history of food allergy or atopy. By delaying introduction of foods beyond 6 months, there is increasing risk of deficiencies of nutrients known to be relatively low in breast milk and yet essential to support rapid growth of infants, such as iron and zinc. The choice of first foods is important so that they contain adequate energy and micronutrients to meet the needs of infants. For example, reduced-fat cow milk (skim 2%, and 1% fat) should not be fed to infants before 2 years of age. Excessive amounts of fruit juices or 'empty calorie' fast foods should not be fed to infants. To achieve adequate intakes of micronutrients such as iron, choice of nutrient-fortified foods (e.g., iron-fortified infant cereal or other weaning food) may be required in areas where natural sources of micronutrients are not available. Finally, both solid and liquid foods offered to infants need to be free of contamination since the transmission of infections through food is thought to be a primary cause of diarrhea in young infants, particularly in developing countries.

The March of Dimes report (2002) outlined three key recommendations for ensuring optimal nutrition of term-born infants through breast-feeding and complementary feeding practices. The rationale for each recommendation and suggestions for implementation strategies on a global basis are provided in the report. The three key recommendations are as follows:

Recommendation 1: Promote and support exclusive breast feeding for 6 months, with the introduction of complementary foods and continued breast feeding thereafter—up to 2 years of age or longer as mutually desired by the mother and infant.

Recommendation 2: Promote and support programs to ensure that pregnant women and breast feeding mothers receive adequate nutrient intakes.

Recommendation 3: Promote the appropriate introduction of safe, nutritionally adequate, and developmentally appropriate complementary foods.

The recommendations from the March of Dimes report are universally applicable and will ensure that infants attain nutrient intakes that match the nutrient requirements as set out in dietary standards such as the DRI reports.

See also: **Amino Acids**: Chemistry and Classification; Metabolism. **Ascorbic Acid**: Physiology, Dietary Sources and Requirements. **Breast Feeding**. **Calcium**. **Carbohydrates**: Requirements and Dietary Importance. **Complementary Feeding**. **Electrolytes**: Water–Electrolyte Balance. **Fats and Oils**. **Fatty Acids**: Omega-3 Polyunsaturated. **Folic Acid**. **Infants**: Nutritional Requirements. **Iron**. **Lactation**: Dietary Requirements. **Magnesium**. **Phosphorus**. **Protein**: Requirements and Role in Diet. **Vitamin A**: Biochemistry and Physiological Role. **Vitamin B₆**. **Vitamin D**: Rickets and Osteomalacia. **Vitamin E**: Metabolism and Requirements. **Vitamin K**. **Zinc**: Physiology.

Further Reading

Atkinson SA (2004) Nutritional requirements for fetal & neonatal bone health & development. In: Holick M and Dawson-Hughes B (eds.) *Nutrition & Bone Health*, pp. 157–172. Clifton, NJ: Humana Press.

Atkinson SA and Zlotkin S (1997) Recognizing deficiencies and excesses of zinc, copper and other trace elements. In: Tsang R, Zlotkin S, Nichols B, and Hansen J (eds.), *Nutrition during Infancy: Birth to Two Years*, pp. 635–641. Cincinnati OH: Digital Education Publishing, Inc.

Institute of Medicine (1997) *Dietary Reference Intakes for Calcium, Phosphorus, Magnesium, Vitamin D and Fluoride.* Washington, DC: National Academy Press. Available at http://www.nap.edu/catalog/5776.html.

Institute of Medicine (1998) *Dietary Reference Intakes for Thiamin, Riboflavin, Niacin, Vitamin B₆, Folate, Vitamin B₁₂, Pantothenic Acid, Biotin, and Choline.* Washington, DC: National Acadamy Press. Available at http://www.nap.edu/catalog/6015.html.

Institute of Medicine (2000) *Dietary Reference Intakes for Vitamin C, Vitamin E, Selenium, and Carotenoids.* Washington, DC: National Acedemy Press. Available at http://www.nap.edu/catalog/9810.html.

Institute of Medicine (2001) *Dietary Reference Intakes for Vitamin A, Vitamin K, Arsenic, boron, Chromium, Copper, Iodine, Iron, Manganese, Molybdenum, Nickel, Silicon, Vanadium and Zinc.* Washington, DC: National Acedemy Press. Available at http://www.nap.edu/catalog/10026.html.

Institute of Medicine (2002) *Dietary Reference Intakes for Energy, Carbohydrates, Fiber, Fat, Protein, and Amino Acids (Macronutrients).* Washington, DC: National Academy Press. Available at http://www.nap.edu/catalog/10490.html.

Institute of Medicine (2004) *Dietary Reference Intakes for Water, Potassium, Sodium, Chloride and Sulfate.* Washington, DC: National Acadamy Press. Available at http://www.nap.edu/catalog.

Jain A, Concato J, and Levanthal J (2002) How good is the evidence linking breastfeeding and intelligence? *Pediatrics* **109**: 1044–1053.

Lawrence M, Gartner MD, Frank R, Greer MD and the Section on Breastfeeding and Committee on Nutrition (2003) Prevention of rickets and vitamin D deficiency: new guidelines for vitamin D intake. *Pediatrics* 111(4): 908–910.

March of Dimes, Task Force on Nutrition and Optimal Human Development (2002) *Nutrition Today Matters Tomorrow.* White Plains, NY: Education Services, March of Dimes.

Raiten DJ, Talbot JM, and Waters JH (eds.) (1998) Executive summary for the report Assessment of nutrient requirements for infant formulas. *Journal of Nutrition* 11(supplement).

Feeding Problems

R M Katz, Johns Hopkins University School of Medicine and Mount Washington Pediatric Hospital, Baltimore, MD, USA
L Schuberth, Kennedy Krieger Institute, Baltimore, MD, USA
C S Gulotta, Johns Hopkins University and Kennedy Krieger Institute, Baltimore, MD, USA

Feeding is the process by which growing children accept and digest food in amounts adequate to meet their nutritional needs. What seems at first glance to be a simple intuitive act is actually a complex process requiring successful caregiver interaction, adequate oral motor skills, and intact gastrointestinal motility and absorption. The term 'feeding disorder' is applied to situations in which young children are unable or unwilling to eat enough to maintain their nutritional needs. The *Diagnostic and Statistical Manual of Mental Disorders*, a compendium of diagnoses and the related criteria, more specifically defines pediatric feeding disorders as "persistent failure to eat adequately as reflected in significant failure to gain weight or significant weight loss over at least one month." Feeding disorders are surprisingly common in children, and it has been reported that 25–35% of normal children will have mild feeding disorders and up to 70% of premature infants will have more severe feeding problems. Clinical manifestations include food refusal/selectivity, gagging, vomiting, swallowing difficulty, poor weight gain, or failure to thrive. These can be grouped into medical, oral motor, and behavioral categories, although many children have overlapping problems.

Certain groups may be at a higher risk for feeding difficulties. For example, children with food allergy may have accompanying gastroesophageal reflux and motility disorders, which then result in food refusal. A variety of medical conditions, such as cardiopulmonary, genetic, and metabolic disorders, can lead to poor appetite and slow weight gain. Oral motor and/or swallowing problems are commonly seen in children with congenital and acquired neurologic conditions such as cerebral palsy, structural abnormalities, or traumatic brain injury. Premature and medically fragile infants may miss sensitive periods of oral motor development resulting in delayed acquisition of feeding skills. This early interruption of feeding skills can lead to serious feeding disorders and food refusal due to lack of experience and impaired oral sensitivity.

Lastly, behavioral difficulties such as food refusal or selectivity are not always isolated problems. More often, they develop when medical illness adversely affects feeding patterns and caregiver interactions. If a child is failing to thrive, the most immediate solution to address the lack of weight gain and growth is to start nasogastric or gastrostomy tube feeding. However, this supplemental feeding often results in a decrease in oral intake, which ultimately impacts on hunger, experience, and endurance. Medical issues (i.e., reflux, cleft palate, etc.) that occur very early in infancy can be the initial cause for food refusal. Consequently, for the majority of children with a feeding disorder, an early avoidance pattern is established. The parent–child interaction usually exacerbates this pattern. For example, because of severe reflux the child learns to associate eating with pain. Consequently, when the parent tries to feed the child, he or she will often encounter severe refusal behavior, which leads most parents to terminate the meal prematurely. At this point, the child not only has associated food with pain but also has learned that by having severe food refusal the meal will be terminated. Even when the reflux is medically managed, the child will still have the learned history of pain associated with eating, and the child will also have the new history of having refusal behaviors to escape the meal.

Normal Development of Feeding and Swallowing

In order to understand feeding and swallowing disorders, one must recognize that there are dynamically changing developmental skills and social abilities in the growing child. Progression through the normal stages of feeding (**Table 1**) requires the attainment of physical abilities such as postural stability, oral motor coordination, and sensory awareness. In addition, factors such as emerging cognitive skills and

Table 1 Normal infant feeding

Age	Stage
Birth–12 months	Suck/swallow liquids (breast or bottle)
4–6 months	Pureed solids by spoon (cereal, fruits, vegetables, and meats)
8–9 months	Cup drinking liquids
	Ground or junior foods by spoon
	Finger feeding soft dissolvables
10–12 months	Soft table food
24 months	Self-feed with utensils

socialization play an important role in an effective caregiver–child feeding interaction.

The Swallowing Process

Understanding the mechanisms involved in eating can also be useful in understanding why a child is refusing to eat. The swallowing process is usually divided into three phases: oral, pharyngeal, and esophageal. In the newborn and young infant, all phases are driven reflexively by typical rooting and sucking behavior. As children age, the oral phase of chewing and managing food comes under more voluntary control, requiring cortical integration of sensory/motor input to coordinate the complex patterns of jaw, tongue, and oral movements. Factors such as smell, taste, and emotion become increasingly important. Once the process of chewing is completed, the tongue and soft palate propel the bolus toward the pharynx, initiating the pharyngeal phase of swallowing. As food progresses through the pharynx, a complex sequence of movements allows the safe passage of food around the airway into the esophagus. Closure of the mouth and nasal/laryngeal passages prevents aspiration while elevation and anterior displacement of the larynx opens the upper esophageal sphincter. This automatically generates a pressure gradient, which propels the bolus toward the esophageal opening. Once the food progresses to the esophageal phase, the subsequent movements are almost entirely automatic and no longer subject to cortical control. After passing the lower esophageal sphincter, food normally enters the stomach, beginning the gastrointestinal and absorptive phase of feeding. Food is emptied from the stomach based on the volume, nutrient composition, and caloric density of the meal.

Classification of Feeding Disorders in Children

A single underlying cause for why children refuse to eat enough to sustain normal growth is rarely

Table 2 Common feeding disorder symptoms

Food refusal—partial/total
Liquid dependent
Enteral tube dependent
Food selectivity
Texture
Type

evident, and therefore this problem presents a significant diagnostic and therapeutic challenge to clinicians and parents. Given the complexity of this challenge, numerous attempts at classifying feeding disorders have been made based on the apparent etiology, physical condition, or associated behaviors. Because most feeding disorders are the result of multiple factors (i.e., physical, motivational, skill, and parent/child relationships), a more functional classification has been developed that allows differentiation of patient types by symptoms rather than an arbitrary disease-based diagnostic approach (**Table 2**).

Children with food refusal who require any kind of enteral tube feed would be categorized as 'food refusal—enteral tube dependent,' whereas a child who drinks more than 80% of his or her calorie requirement would be considered 'food refusal—liquid dependent.' Another feeding problem category is 'food selectivity—type.' In this category, children would eliminate 75% of the four basic food groups. Typically, a child with this categorization would have the skill to eat but would choose to only eat one or two different foods and restrict all other foods. The child may or may not be able to sustain normal growth with this kind of diet. 'Food selective—texture' describes a child who does not eat an age-appropriate texture of food due to lack of skill or oversensitivity to a particular food texture—for example, a 5-year-old child who only eats pureed foods when he or she should be able to handle regular textured food. Again, the child may or may not sustain normal growth.

Assessment

An appropriate assessment of a child's feeding disorder is a critical first step in initiating treatment. The management of complicated feeding disorders usually requires a multidisciplinary team devoted to establishing diagnosis, assessment of need, and developing a thorough treatment plan. This team may include a variety of pediatric specialists, including physicians (e.g., general pediatricians, developmental pediatricians, pediatric gastroenterologists, allergists, and otolaryngologists), nurse practitioners, nutritionists, occupational therapists, speech therapists, psychologists, and social workers. The assembled team must begin its approach to diagnosis and therapy with complete history taking by all interested parties. This includes a careful prenatal, birth, and neonatal history. In addition to determining the nutritional and medical status of the child, an appropriate psychological and developmental pediatric evaluation must be performed.

Physicians

An important goal of the physician history taking is to assess for any comorbid conditions that would require treatment prior to the implementation of a therapeutic treatment program for the food refusal (**Table 3**). As part of the initial evaluation, an observation of a feeding session between the child and

Table 3 Medical conditions associated with pediatric feeding disorders

Disorders of the oral and pharyngeal phases of swallowing
Anatomic lesions
– Cleft lip and/or palate
– Pierre–Robin sequence
– Choanal atresia
– Laryngeal clefts
– Macroglossia
– CHARGE association
Acquired structural abnormalities
– Dental caries
– Tonsillar hypertrophy
– Viral/inflammatory stomatitis
– Retropharyngeal mass
– Candida stomatitis
Cardiopulmonary effects
– Chronic lung disease
– Complex congenital heart disease
– Reactive airway disease
– Tachypnea
Neuromuscular disorders
– Familial dysautonomia
– Cerebral palsy
– Pseudo-bulbar palsy
– Bulbar atresia or palsy
– Cranial nerve anomalies
– Muscular dystrophic disorders
– Arnold–Chiari malformation
– Myelomeningocele
– Intracranial mass lesions

Disorders of the esophageal phase of swallowing
Anatomic lesions
– Esophageal atresia
– Cricopharyngeal achalasia
– Tracheoesophageal fistula
– Esophageal mass
– Esophageal stricture
– Esophageal web
– Esophageal rings
– Vascular rings/aberrant vessels
– Foreign bodies

Disorders of the lumen
– Peptic esophagitis
– Candida esophagitis
– Viral esophagitis
– "Pill" esophagitis
– Inflammatory bowel disease
– Behcet syndrome
Motility disorders
– Achalasia
– Diffuse esophageal spasm
– Chronic pseudo-obstruction
– Systemic lupus erythematosis
– Polymyositis
Genetic disorders
– Prader–Willi syndrome
– Trisomy 21
– Cornelia de Lange syndrome
– Velocardiofacial syndrome
– Rett syndrome
Metabolic disorders
– Urea cycle abnormalities
– Hereditary fructose intolerance
– Hypothyroidism
Miscellaneous
– Gastroesophageal reflux
– Constipation
– Gas-bloat syndrome
– Dumping syndrome
– Food allergies
– Sensory loss (visual/auditory impairment)

primary caregiver will often provide insight into the feeding problem, especially from an oral motor/sensory and behavioral perspective. Clinical signs of oral motor dysfunction, length of meals, and nature of the caregiver–child interaction are all noted. Observation of the muscle tone, posture, and positioning as well as special seating systems and feeding devices is routine because this can provide insight into the child's overall neurological functioning. Physical examination of the child includes a general survey examination for the determination of any underlying medical disorders that may preclude safe feeding. This includes evaluation of tongue and jaw movement, dentition, airway sounds, speech, and oral cavity assessment. Additionally, a complete physical examination including cardiac, pulmonary, and abdominal exams is mandatory.

Diagnostic Testing

Diagnostic evaluations may be warranted to better assess swallowing and anatomy (**Table 4**). The modified barium swallow study (MBS) is the procedure of choice to assess oral, pharyngeal, and upper esophageal phases of swallowing. Seat positioning, food texture, and rate and amount of food presented can be manipulated during the performance of the MBS

Table 4 Diagnostic evaluation for patients with feeding disorders

Detailed history and physical examination
Upper gastrointestinal contrast radiography
– Esophogram
– Small bowel follow-through
Videofluoroscopic swallow study
Gastric emptying study
pH monitoring
Esophagogastroduodenoscopy with biopsies
Antroduodenal manometry
Fiberoptic endoscopic evaluation of swallowing
CBC
Comprehensive metabolic panel
Thyroid function
RAST analysis for food allergies
Skin test for food allergies
Plasma amino acids
Urine organic acids
Karyotype

to determine the safest and most efficient method of feeding. Clinical evaluation prior to the MBS is essential so that appropriate food textures and liquid consistencies are available at the time of the study. Changes in head and neck position, such as chin tuck, should be tried before the actual study is performed to better correlate clinical and radiologic findings.

Additionally, a standard upper gastrointestinal contrast series utilizing barium is required for assessment of anatomy of the gastrointestinal tract. Children with repetitive vomiting or abdominal pain require endoscopic evaluation, and many will also need colonoscopy to rule out the possibility of underlying inflammatory bowel disease. Some children will need cranial imaging, such as computed tomography or magnetic resonance imaging, to search for evidence of intracranial mass lesions, hydrocephaly, or posterior fossa anomalies such as the Chiari malformation. Fiberoptic endoscopic evaluation of swallowing (FEES) allows for direct visualization of the hypopharynx and larynx during swallowing by use of a flexible laryngoscope. This will allow evaluation of the valleculae and pyriform sinuses as well as the assessment of anatomy during swallowing and potential aspiration problems. This procedure, however, does not provide information on the oral phase of swallowing. FEES may also be combined with sensory testing to induce a laryngeal adductor response. Lastly, increasingly important is the need for allergy evaluation, including consultation by an allergist. Appropriate skin testing may be necessary as well as appropriate RAST testing to search for response to food allergy.

Feeding Specialist

The generic term 'feeding specialist' refers to the team member whose responsibilities include assessing and treating oral motor and swallowing dysfunction and performing MBS studies when warranted. This may be either an occupational therapist or a speech/language pathologist depending on the training and local facility. Occupational therapists can also evaluate fine motor, sensorimotor, and visual motor function as well as positioning and the need for adaptive equipment. Speech/language pathologists can evaluate and make recommendations for communication skills when necessary.

Nutritionists

Nutritionists dedicated to pediatric care are also essential in the diagnostic team functioning. The role of the nutritionist in the assessment of current nutritional status, anticipated growth, and recommended caloric intake that would be age and diagnosis appropriate is essential.

Psychologists/Behavioral Therapists

Behavioral therapists help to provide detailed observation and an analysis of variables that may be contributing to food refusal behaviors. An integral part of the therapist's approach is performing an in-depth assessment of the child's behavior patterns with regard to eating. The goal of an assessment is to help the therapist identify what behaviors have been shaped in a child with regard to eating patterns and to help identify rewards preferred by the child to help reinforce or shape new eating patterns. The behavioral therapist then designs a treatment plan oriented toward shaping new child behaviors, and ultimately the therapist teaches the parents how to implement these strategies in the home environment.

Social Workers

Because the medical issues, behavioral needs, and family psychodynamics play a central role in the development of abnormal feeding patterns, a clinical social work evaluation is necessary for assessment and treatment of underlying familial interactions and support systems. These assessments and planning help to ensure continued success once the child has returned to the home environment.

Treatment of Feeding Disorders

The goal of all therapy is directed toward allowing parents to safely feed their children in a developmentally appropriate manner. The physician in the treatment team must ensure that all appropriate diagnostic studies have been performed to determine if an underlying medical condition has predisposed a child to developing an unusual feeding pattern. This includes appropriate utilization of consultants and diagnostic modalities (Table 4). Once these studies have been performed, the physician must coordinate all the resources and direct care so that feeding therapy may proceed with minimal risk to the patient—keeping the child safe from aspiration and other complications.

The initial, and perhaps most important, part of any therapeutic approach to introducing or increasing oral food intake is to establish the safety of eating as well as the types and textures of food the child can consume most efficiently. Approaches to therapy are often described as nutritive or nonnutritive. Nonnutritive oral stimulation is performed to decrease hypersensitivity, facilitate management of secretions, establish or retrain the swallowing mechanism, maintain coordination of breathing and swallowing, and develop oral movement for sound production and communication.

Objectives for a nutritive approach include increasing oral intake, advancing food texture, transitioning to utensil use, and improvement of self-feeding. Oral motor techniques to improve muscle tone and postural control as a foundation for feeding and swallowing are largely based on a neuro-developmental framework. The use of adaptive seating systems is a key component to feeding a child with physical disabilities that require external devices to provide head, neck, and trunk support. Attention must be paid to how positioning affects the feeding process because a change in head and neck posture and oral motor structures may affect oral motor control.

Once airway safety, positioning, and sensitivity have been controlled, a variety of treatment approaches have been suggested for children with pediatric feeding disorders. These range from individual child psychotherapy to interactional therapy between child and caregiver. However, the most widely employed treatments for feeding disorders are behavioral interventions usually included within an interdisciplinary team approach that also addresses physiology, oral motor functioning, parent–child interactions, and community or social support.

Behavioral interventions for pediatric feeding disorders are the most common modality of therapy and are often a mixture of antecedent and consequence-based treatment packages. Antecedent interventions include the establishment of a systematic feeding routine (i.e., the same time and place to eat), reducing or increasing the level of texture of food

(i.e., puree vs chopped fine), and presenting a preferred food along with a nonpreferred food. Consequence-based treatments include rewarding appropriate eating behavior and/or ignoring (i.e., escape extinction) or punishing food refusal behavior. Thus, if a child accepts a bite, he or she is rewarded with attention or an arbitrary reinforcer, such as a toy or music. If the child engages in food refusal behavior, such as batting at the spoon or turning his or her head away from the food, the consequence is to ignore or extinguish the food refusal behavior and continue to present the bite to the child until it is accepted. If the child continues to refuse by expelling the food, this refusal behavior is ignored/extinguished by re-presenting the expelled bite of food to the child. In some cases, a child refuses food by holding the bite of food in his or her mouth. This form of food refusal behavior can also be ignored or extinguished by moving or redistributing the food from between the child's cheek and teeth onto the tongue, where it is more likely to be swallowed. Finally, training the parents in the use of the various feeding techniques is critical in maintaining long-term treatment gains. Skill-based parent training involving step-by-step criteria-based training has been shown to be superior to didactic methodology. Parent training, including instruction, discussion, handouts, role-playing, feedback, and the practice of techniques with a trained clinician, can result in increased parent treatment integrity.

Conclusion

Despite the increased awareness of feeding disorders in young children, there remain many challenges in implementing the specialized treatment necessary for these children. Foremost among these challenges is the financial burden associated with diagnosis and therapy. Children who cannot or will not eat require a systematic diagnostic and therapeutic approach by a team of dedicated professionals. The goal of safe oral feeding is attainable in most children when those involved in the care of children understand the complexity of eating and the associated medical and psychological conditions that comprise a feeding disorder. Helping these children to eat will allow independence from artificial sources of nutrition, such as gastrostomy feeds and parenteral nutrition, and ultimately reduce the total cost of health care for these children.

See also: **Dietetics**. **Food Allergies**: Etiology; Diagnosis and Management. **Infants**: Nutritional Requirements.

Further Reading

American Psychiatric Association (1994) *Diagnostic and Statistical Manual*, 4th edn. Washington, DC: American Psychiatric Association.

Babbitt RL, Hoch TA, Coe DA *et al.* (1994) Behavioral assessment and treatment of pediatric feeding disorders. *Journal of Developmental and Behavioral Pediatrics* 15: 278–291.

Burklow K, Phelps A, Schultz J, McConnell K, and Rudolph C (1998) Classifying complex pediatric feeding problems. *Journal of Pediatric Gastroenterology and Nutrition* 27: 143–147.

Dellert S *et al.* (1993) Feeding resistance and gastroesophageal reflux in infancy. *Journal of Pediatric Gastroenterology and Nutrition* 17: 66–71.

Kerwin ME (1999) Empirically supported treatments in pediatric psychology: Severe feeding problems. *Journal of Pediatric Psychology* 24(3): 193–214.

Logemann J (1983) *Evaluation and Treatment of Swallowing Disorders*. San Diego: College Hill Press.

Manikam R and Perman J (2000) Pediatric feeding disorders. *Journal of Clinical Gastroenterology* 30(1): 34–36.

Morris SE and Klein MD (2000) *Pre Feeding Skills. A Comprehensive Resource for Mealtime Development*. Tucson, AZ: Therapy Skill Builders.

Munk DD and Repp AC (1994) Behavioral assessment of feeding problems of individuals with severe disabilities. *Journal of Applied Behavior Analysis* 27: 241–250.

Piazza CC, Fisher WW, Brown KA *et al.* (2003) Functional analysis of inappropriate mealtime behaviors. *Journal of Applied Behavior Analysis* 37: 187–204.

Rommel N, DeMeyer AM, Feenstra L, and Veereman-Wauters G (2003) The complexity of feeding problems in 700 infants and young children presenting to a tertiary care institution. *Journal of Pediatric Gastroenterology and Nutrition* 37: 75–84.

Rudolph C and Link D (2002) Feeding disorders in infants and children. *Pediatric Clinics of North America* 49: 97–112.

Sevin BM, Gulotta CS, Sierp BJ, Rosica LA, and Miller LJ (2002) Analysis of a response class hierarchy of food refusal behavior. *Journal of Applied Behavior Analysis* 35(1): 65–68.

Shore BA and Piazza CC (1992) Pediatric feeding disorders. In: Konarski EA and Favell JE (eds.) *Manual for the Assessment and Treatment of the Behavior Disorders of People with Mental Retardation*. Morgantown NC: Western Carolina Center Foundation.

Tuchman D (1994) *Physiology of the Swallowing Apparatus*. San Diego: Singular Publishing.

Wolf LS and Glass R (1992) *Feeding and Swallowing Disorders in Infancy—Assessment and Management*. Tucson, AZ: Therapy Skill Builders.

INFECTION

Contents
Nutritional Interactions
Nutritional Management in Adults

Nutritional Interactions

H Ghattas, London School of Hygiene and Tropical Medicine, London, UK

Introduction

Immunological competence (the ability of the immune system to mount a response in the presence of a pathogen) and nutritional status are major determinants of morbidity and mortality, particularly in children of the world's least developed countries. Communicable and nutritional deficiency diseases are often grouped together in mortality statistics, as many infection-related deaths occur in individuals who are also malnourished, making it difficult to disentangle infectious causes from malnutrition-related causes of death. It is estimated that infectious and nutritional deficiency diseases are responsible for 32% of global mortality and up to 59% of deaths in the world's poorest countries (World Health Organization 2004).

The relationship between malnutrition and infection has often been described as synergistic, and is the result of multifaceted interactions between nutritional intake, nutritional status, immunity, and vulnerability to infections. However, the role of nutrition in host resistance to infection is such that both nutrient deficiencies and excesses can increase susceptibility to infection.

The Cycle of Malnutrition and Infection

Malnutrition and infection interact in a cycle of adverse events (**Figure 1**) whereby malnutrition impairs immunocompetence by affecting both nonimmunological defense mechanisms (such as epithelial membrane integrity) and immunological defenses (e.g., cytokine activity, neutrophil function, T-cell maturation) thereby increasing host

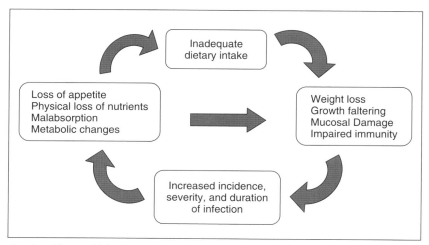

Figure 1 The cycle of malnutrition and infection. (Reproduced from Tomkins A and Watson F (1989) *Malnutrition and Infection: A Review. Nutrition Policy Discussion Paper No.5 (ACC/SCN State of the Art Series)*. Geneva: United Nations.)

susceptibility to infection. Conversely, infection can affect energy requirements and appetite, and can lead to weight loss in adults and growth faltering in children. This occurs through a simultaneous increase in energy requirements during the acute phase response of an infection, anorexia (primarily mediated by interleukin (IL)-1 released by infected macrophages), physical loss of nutrients from the intestine, and malabsorption. The resulting deterioration in nutritional status is associated with additional mucosal damage, which can in turn further prolong and increase the severity of the infection as well as leaving the individual susceptible to further pathogenic invasion, thus bridging the vicious cyclical relationship between malnutrition, impaired immunity, and infection.

The Effect of Infection on Nutritional Status

Infection triggers several processes that lead to the deterioration of nutritional status (**Figure 2**). The innate response to an acute infection induces a catabolic response that increases basal metabolism (therefore increasing energy expenditure), places individuals in negative nitrogen balance (as a result of amino acid mobilization from peripheral muscle for gluconeogenesis), and leads to loss of body weight. This primarily occurs in the febrile stage of an infection during which the increase in body temperature is accompanied by an increase in basal energy requirements. This energy is required to fuel the increased rates of enzymatic reactions that occur when body temperature is elevated and to provide energy for the synthesis of proteins involved in the

response to infection, e.g., acute phase proteins and immunoglobulins. The latter explains why energy metabolism can also be increased in subclinical non-febrile infections.

The acute phase reaction is mainly driven by cytokines produced by infected leucocytes. Interleukin-1 (IL-1) is the primary mediator of the acute phase response and stimulates endocrine changes that lead to amino acid mobilization as well as the initiation of anorexia (loss of appetite). This can be compounded by physical discomfort associated with eating or swallowing that can occur in certain infections. For example, dehydration due to diarrhea can lead to mouth dryness, and opportunistic oral infections may occur following acute infections. Nutritional intake can be further reduced as a result of the cultural practice of withdrawal of food from individuals with signs of infection (such as fever or diarrhea).

Amino acid mobilization during the acute phase response to infection is also accompanied by redistribution of other nutrients among tissues as well as vitamin (e.g., retinol, folate, riboflavin, ascorbic acid) and mineral (e.g., potassium, zinc, copper) losses from the body. These changes reflect a shift in the transport of nutrients by nutrient transport proteins, the synthesis of which is reduced in response to infection, in order to prioritize the synthesis of acute phase proteins by the liver. Consequently, plasma nutrient concentrations fall due to reduced circulating levels of nutrient transport proteins.

Reductions in circulating levels of iron also occur through the sequestration of iron by the reticuloendothelial system as well as the release of the iron-binding protein lactoferrin by neutrophils, increased storage of iron as ferritin in the liver and spleen, and reduced intestinal iron absorption. This is

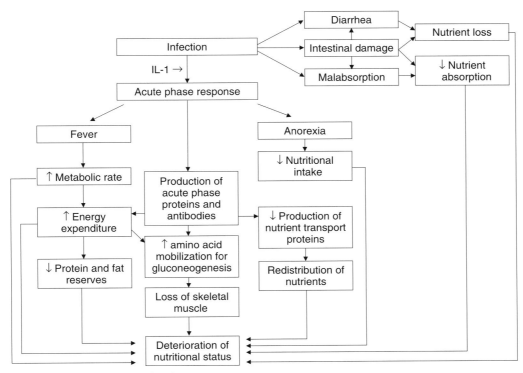

Figure 2 The effect of infection on nutritional status.

a protective mechanism that deprives microorganisms of the iron required for microbial growth and replication, therefore restricting further spread of infection.

Serum retinol levels are also reduced in a range of infections including acute respiratory infections, gastroenteritis, measles, malaria, pneumonia, and hookworm infection. Retinol depletion in measles infection has been shown to be closely related to the severity of infection.

Direct nutrient losses also occur in infection through diarrhea and nutrient malabsorption. Various infections of the gastrointestinal (GI) tract can cause diarrhea including viral, bacterial, protozoan, and helminthic infections, although non-GI infections such as malaria may also precipitate diarrheal episodes. GI infections can damage the gastrointestinal epithelium leading to flattening of microvilli, this decreases the absorptive surface area of the intestine resulting in malabsorption and electrolyte imbalance.

Table 1 lists examples of major infections, how they affect nutritional status, and the ways in which these infections may be modulated by certain nutrients.

The Effect of Nutrition on Immunity and Infection

In nutritionally compromised individuals with infection, a persistent catabolic state prevails, impairing the capacity for recovery from infection, as several recovery processes are dependent on active protein synthesis, for example, tissue repair, replacement of structural and functional proteins, and synthesis of immunoproteins. Additionally, the coexistence of malnutrition and infection increases susceptibility to secondary infection.

Severe Malnutrition and Reductive Adaptation

The acute phase response to an infection is muted in severe protein-energy malnutrition in part of a process referred to as 'reductive adaptation,' whereby the structure and function of cells or tissues cannot be maintained due to the limited supply of energy resulting from decreased nutritional intake. Protein synthesis from amino acids is highly energy-dependent and proteins have a wide variety of structural and functional roles in the body, including the cytokines that initiate the acute phase reaction (IL-1, Il-6, tumor necrosis factor (TNF-α)). Severely malnourished individuals are therefore immunocompromised, in that they cannot produce an adequate immune response to infection. The generalized responses to infection such as fever and increased pulse, as well as localized responses such as inflammation and delayed cutaneous hypersensitivity, may also not manifest. Silent infections must therefore always be suspected and treated in severe malnutrition.

Table 1   Major infections: their effect on nutritional status and ways in which these infections may be modulated by nutrition

Nutritional modulation	Infection	Nutritional effects
• Zinc: ↓ incidence and morbidity • Ascorbic acid: may have protective effect (conflicting results)	Acute Respiratory infections (ARI)	• Anorexia • Dysphagia
• Vitamin A: ↓ incidence of diarrhea • Breast feeding: ↓incidence of diarrhea • Malnutrition → ↓ epithelial integrity and ↑ diarrhea • Zinc: ↓ duration and mortality	Diarrheal diseases	• Nutrient losses • Intestinal damage and malabsorption • Dehydration • Electrolyte imbalance • Nutrient deficiencies (e.g., vitamin A)
• Vitamin A: ↓ morbidity and mortality in HIV + children • ↓ plasma selenium associated with ↑ HIV severity • Ascorbic acid: may ↓ HIV viral load • Zinc supplementation → conflicting results in HIV • Vitamin A: in lactation may ↑ MTCT[a]	Human immunodeficiency virus (HIV)	• Anorexia • Wasting syndrome • When treated with HAART[b] can lead to metabolic changes and lipodystrophy
	Intestinal parasites	• Nutrient losses • Malabsorption • Anorexia • Anemia (in hookworm and *Trichuris*) • Impaired growth and weight loss
• Vitamin A: ↓ malaria-anemia • Iron: ↓ malaria-anemia but may ↑ morbidity	Malaria	• Anemia • ↑ Protein metabolism • Anorexia • Fever → ↑ energy needs • ↓ Plasma retinol • Malaria in pregnancy → low-birth-weight baby
• Vitamin A: ↑ measles specific Ab in response to measles vaccination • Vitamin A: ↓ morbidity	Measles	• Anorexia • Buccal mucosal lesions → ↓ intake • ↑ Catabolism → growth faltering and weight loss • ↓ Plasma retinol
	Tuberculosis (TB)	• ↑ Energy metabolism • ↑ Protein breakdown • Anorexia • Anemia

[a]MTCT: mother to child transmission.
[b]HAART: highly active anti-retroviral therapy.

Malnutrition and the Breakdown of Defenses

The skin and mucous membranes provide the first layer of physical and chemical defense against an invading pathogen, and the mucosae are the major sites of entry of infectious agents into the host. The structural integrity of these barriers is compromised in malnutrition through the reduced production of mature epithelial cells, and the decreased secretion of mucin, gastric acid, lysozyme, and secretory immunoglobulins. This results in reduced gastric acidity and intestinal villous atrophy, which facilitate pathogen entry into the host. The host gut-associated lymphoid tissue (GALT) is the principal site of stimulation of mucosal immune responses and the gastrointestinal epithelium functions in the transport of nutrients as well as in immunological surveillance. Reduced epithelial integrity therefore impairs mucosal immune function and can further exacerbate nutritional status.

Lymphoid organs and cell-mediated immunity are also affected by malnutrition. In the context of malnutrition-related immunodeficiency, changes in both thymic morphology and function have been observed. These include thymic involution, thymus atrophy, circulation of immature lymphocytes, and increased thymocyte apoptosis. Similar changes occur in the spleen and lymph nodes. Where innate immunity is an organism's first level of defense in response to an infective agent, adaptive immunity and hence thymic involvement may be considered to be less crucial in the short term. The case has therefore been made that when faced with a stress such as malnutrition, adaptive immunity becomes less of a priority and is shut down in order to prioritize other more critical organ functions. It has been suggested that critical periods in lymphoid organ development, such as the fetal and neonatal phases of development, may be particularly susceptible to malnutrition-induced changes, which may be irreversible and have long-term consequences on host resistance to immunity.

Cell-mediated immunity depends on thymus-derived T lymphocytes, which may be reduced in both number (lymphopenia) and function (impaired maturation) in malnutrition. This may result from reduced production of thymocytes by the thymus or from impaired T-cell differentiation and proliferation. Lymphocyte response to mitogens is undermined in both protein-energy and specific micronutrient deficiencies.

Moreover, neutrophil activity and bactericidal capacity are decreased in undernutrition. The neutrophil respiratory burst (which involves the production of toxic metabolites including hydrogen peroxide, superoxide anion, and nitric oxide that cause direct damage to bacteria) is impaired.

Complement proteins are also reduced in malnutrition. However, B-lymphocyte function and humoral immunity appear unaffected and normal antibody response to infectious agents is seen (except antibody responses that are highly dependent on T-cell help). However, secretory immunoglobulin (Ig) A responses may be decreased in malnutrition, possibly due to reduced secretion of IgA from damaged or atrophied mucosal surfaces.

Low Birth Weight

Low birth-weight babies are born with low nutrient reserves, an immature immune system, and small sized lymphoid organs. Studies have also linked low birth weight to reductions in T-cell counts, altered proportions of lymphocyte subsets, and reduced *in vitro* lymphocyte proliferation in infants and children. Additionally, mucosal surfaces (of the gastrointestinal and respiratory tract) are underdeveloped, thereby weakening the first layer of defense against an invading pathogen. Low birth-weight infants have increased neonatal mortality, mainly from diarrhea, pneumonia, and measles, and there is evidence that they remain at an increased risk of infection past the first year of life.

Breast feeding and Immunity to Infection

Human milk is the first form of nutrition for a neonate. Mammary glands are part of the integrated mucosal immune system and produce antibodies against mucosal pathogens that the mother is exposed to and which the infant is most likely to encounter. Breast milk contains several factors that protect against infections in the breast-fed infant either through passive immunity or by activating the infant's immune system. These include secretory IgA and IgM antibodies specific to maternal pathogenic encounters, short-chain fatty acids (SCFA), which can inhibit bacterial growth, block bacterial toxins and activate eosinophils, bactericidal lactoferrin, lysozymes, and mucins, as well as lymphocytes (both T cells and B cells), which may transfer primed immunity to the infant.

Additionally, cytokines and other growth factors in human milk contribute to the activation of the lactating infant's immune system, rendering breast-fed infants less susceptible to diarrheal diseases, respiratory infections, otitis media, and other infections and may impart long-term protection against diarrhea. Breast feeding also reduces mortality from diarrhea and respiratory infections. However, human immunodeficiency virus (HIV) infection (and other viral infections) can be transmitted from a virus-positive mother to her child through breast milk, and breast-feeding is responsible for a significant proportion of childhood HIV infection.

Key Nutrients Involved in Host Resistance to Infection

Ascorbic acid (vitamin C)   Ascorbic acid is rapidly mobilized and utilized in infection and high levels of ascorbic acid are found in leucocytes. Studies in humans and animals have found a reduced T-cell response, delayed cutaneous hypersensitivity, and reduced epithelial integrity in vitamin C deficiency. Vitamin C supplementation is associated with increased lymphocyte proliferation in response to mitogen, increased phagocytosis by neutrophils, and decreased serum lipid peroxides. A role for vitamin C has been suggested in the treatment of autoimmune diseases as well as in delaying the progression of HIV to AIDS; however, further research is required to confirm such a role. The effectiveness of ascorbic acid in preventing and reducing the duration of acute respiratory infection also remains controversial. Claims that high intakes of vitamin C can prevent the common cold have not been corroborated, although there is evidence of a decrease in duration and alleviation of symptoms of the common cold.

Iron   The effects of iron on infection are bipolar, with both deficiency and excess leading to increased susceptibility to infection. Iron deficiency has been found to impair cell-mediated immunity (CMI), neutrophil function, natural killer (NK) cell activity, and bactericidal activity of macrophages, and to delay the development of CMI. The assessment of iron status in infection is however complicated by the redistribution of iron-binding proteins in the inflammatory response, making it difficult to interpret studies that find associations between measures of iron deficiency and infection.

Excess iron has immunosuppressive effects and can promote bacterial growth. Iron overload (hemochromatosis) decreases the phagocytic capacity of macrophages, alters lymphocyte subset distribution, and increases incidence of infection. Free iron acts as a catalyst in the production of reactive oxygen species (ROS) thereby increasing lipid peroxidation and cell membrane damage (of both host and microbial cells).

Invading organisms compete with the host for available iron necessary for cell function and proliferation. Pathogen replication and virulence is increased when iron supplements are administered to individuals with both iron deficiency and infection, leading to increased morbidity and mortality from infection (there is accumulating evidence for such an effect in malaria, tuberculosis, and HIV). In malaria, iron supplementation reduces malaria anemia but some studies have found increased incidence and severity of the disease, although this may be related to mode and dosage of iron administration.

The detrimental effect of iron supplementation in infection remains controversial; however, the variation in the response to supplementation may be explained by polymorphisms in genes that affect iron metabolism. For example, studies have shown poorer prognosis in HIV-infected patients with the haptoglobin (Hp) 2-2 phenotype (characterized by high serum iron, transferrin saturation and ferritin levels).

Retinol (vitamin A) Vitamin A is essential for the maintenance of mucosal surfaces and plays a role in cytokine regulation. Vitamin A supplementation has been reported to reduce child mortality from diarrheal diseases and HIV/AIDS, and to decrease the prevalence, severity, and duration of diarrheal episodes (particularly in nonbreastfed infants). Vitamin A is also involved in increasing levels of long-term measles-specific antibodies in response to measles vaccination and in reducing measles-related morbidity.

However, vitamin A does not necessarily play a beneficial role in all infections and supplementation may not always achieve the desired outcome; for example, the role of vitamin A supplementation in reducing malaria morbidity and increasing resistance remains contentious. Despite evidence for reductions in malaria-anemia, supplementation studies in respiratory infections have found no beneficial effect and a recent study found increased mother to child transmission of HIV when HIV-infected mothers were supplemented with vitamin A.

Selenium The role of selenium in resistance to infection mainly derives from its antioxidant function, but an increasing number of studies have shown that selenium also functions in both cell-mediated immunity and humoral immunity. Selenium containing proteins (selenoproteins) are the major modulators of the effects of selenium on immunity. Of these, the selenium-dependent glutathione peroxidases have an antioxidant function, and play a regulatory role in the synthesis pathways of both anti-inflammatory and proinflammatory eicosanoids.

Selenium deficiency leads to impaired antioxidant capacity, resulting in cell damage as well as a diminished respiratory-burst reaction (a microbicidal reaction in neutrophils and monocytes/macrophages). Low serum selenium levels are associated with severity of HIV, and selenium supplementation may be beneficial in HIV infection where it has been shown to reduce oxidative stress and to modulate cytokine production. Keshan disease, a juvenile cardiomyopathy with a viral etiology, is precipitated by selenium deficiency.

Selenium appears to be able to modulate pathogens as well as the immune response, as demonstrated by the increased virulence of Coxsackie virus and influenza A in response to selenium deficiency.

Zinc Zinc acts as a cofactor for many enzymes and plays a role in cellular DNA synthesis, RNA transcription, cell division, and activation. Zinc modulates both humoral and cell-mediated immunity and zinc deficiency is marked by lymphoid organ atrophy, lymphopenia, decreased T-helper 1 cell function, impaired B-cell function, and reduced phagocytic capacity.

Zinc supplementation has been found to improve infectious morbidity in individuals with sickle cell disease. In malnourished children, zinc supplementation improves epithelial integrity, decreases the duration of diarrheal episodes and mortality from diarrhea, decreases the incidence of respiratory tract infection respiratory morbidity, and improves T-cell-mediated immunity. Maternal zinc deprivation results in small thymus and spleen size in the neonate.

Results of zinc supplementation studies in HIV-positive individuals are conflicting with both benefits and adverse effects reported. The role of zinc in reducing the severity and duration of the common cold is also still contested. High doses of zinc however have been associated with increased mortality in severe malnutrition and sepsis indicating a potential detrimental effect associated with pharmacological (versus physiological) doses of zinc.

Multiple micronutrients Much of the research in the field of nutrition–infection interactions has focused on the effect of single nutrient deficiencies on immunity, and how single nutrient supplementation may modulate infectious outcomes. However, micronutrient deficiencies often occur concurrently and significant interactions exist between different micronutrients, whereby large supplementation doses of one nutrient may inhibit uptake of another. Recent studies have shown beneficial effects of a multiple micronutrient supplement including vitamins B-complex, C, E, and folate on lymphocyte counts and birth outcomes of pregnant HIV-positive women. Few other studies have investigated the effects of multiple micronutrient supplementation on infectious outcomes, although these are warranted in populations where multiple micronutrient deficiencies coexist with infection.

The effects of nutrition on immune function are mainly modulated through the action of nutrients as essential cofactors and substrates in biosynthetic pathways or as antioxidants; with cell-mediated immunity and mucosal immunity being the most cited immunological outcomes affected by nutrition. **Table 2** lists the key nutrients involved in host defense against infection and their major effects on infectious outcomes.

Confounding Factors in the Nutrition-Infection Relationship

Infection and malnutrition are interdependent indices; however, the nature of the interaction between nutrition and immunity is complex and is confounded by factors that affect both nutritional status and immunocompetence (**Figure 3**).

Despite the clinical evidence for increased frequency and severity of infections in malnourished individuals, the major factor confounding the relationship between nutrition and immune status is that the environmental conditions of poverty simultaneously lead to both malnutrition and increased exposure to infections. The increase in morbidity and mortality from infectious diseases in malnourished children is often attributed to mucosal and epithelial damage caused by malnutrition, whereas this damage may be caused by the infection itself, making it difficult to confirm a causal path in the malnutrition–infection paradigm.

Furthermore, studies investigating the effects of single nutrient deficiency on infection are often confounded by coexisting nutritional deficiencies, and although nutrition can modulate immunocompetence, susceptibility to secondary opportunistic infection can be independent of nutritional status.

Additionally, the assessment of nutritional status is complicated by the presence of infection, as is the diagnosis of infection in malnourished individuals. During the acute phase response to infection, the plasma concentrations of many micronutrients are altered making it difficult to assess nutritional status, whereas the metabolic and physiological changes (reductive adaptation) that occur in severe malnutrition impair immune responses, making it difficult to diagnose infection.

Table 2 Role of key nutrients in host defense against infection

Nutrient	Effect on infection
Ascorbic acid	• Prevents oxidative damage in infection • Role in reducing ARI is controversial • May improve HIV outcome
Iron	• ↓ Malaria-anemia • Supplementation may ↑ morbidity from malaria, TB, and HIV
Retinol (vitamin A)	• ↓ Child mortality from diarrhea and AIDS • ↓ Prevalence of diarrhea • ↑ Measles-specific antibodies, ↓ measles morbidity • Benefits in malaria controversial • ↑ Mother-to-child transmission of HIV
Selenium	• Deficiency can precipitate Keshan disease • Deficiency ↑ virulence of Coxsackie virus and influenza A • Deficiency may ↑ severity of HIV
Zinc	• ↑ Epithelial integrity • ↓ Diarrheal duration and mortality • ↓ Incidence of and morbidity from respiratory tract infection • High doses associated with ↑ mortality in severe malnutrition and sepsis

Conclusions

Owing to the complex nature of the interaction between nutritional status and host-susceptibility to infection, establishing a better understanding of the underlying mechanisms behind the nutrition–infection relationship is crucial to the formulation of intervention strategies to reduce morbidity and mortality from communicable and nutritional deficiency diseases in developing countries.

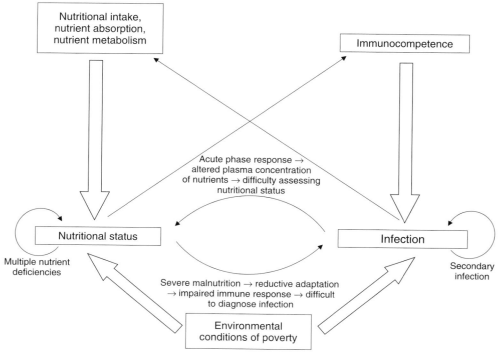

Figure 3   Confounding factors in the nutrition–infection paradigm.

See also: **Breast Feeding**. **Diarrheal Diseases**. **Fatty Acids**: Omega-3 Polyunsaturated. **Immunity**: Physiological Aspects; Effects of Iron and Zinc. **Infection**: Nutritional Management in Adults. **Lung Diseases**. **Malnutrition**: Primary, Causes Epidemiology and Prevention; Secondary, Diagnosis and Management. **Parasitism**. **Tuberculosis**: Nutrition and Susceptibility; Nutritional Management.

Further Reading

Calder PC, Field CJ, and Gill HS (2002) *Nutrition and Immune Function.* Oxon: CAB International.

Dreyfuss ML and Fawzi WW (2002) Micronutrients and vertical transmission of HIV-1. *American Journal of Clinical Nutrition* 75(6): 959–970.

Doherty CP, Weaver LT, and Prentice AM (2002) Micronutrient supplementation and infection: a double-edged sword? *Journal of Pediatric Gastroenterology and Nutrition* 34(4): 346–352.

Field CJ, Johnson IR, and Schley PD (2002) Nutrients and their role in host resistance to infection. *Journal of Leukocyte Biology* 71(1): 16–32.

Gershwin ME, Nestel P, and Keen CL (2004) *Handbook of Nutrition and Immunity.* New Jersey: Humana Press.

Harbige LS (1996) Nutrition and immunity with emphasis on infection and autoimmune disease. Nutrition and Health 10: 285–312.

Powanda MC and Beisel WR (2003) Metabolic effects of infection on protein and energy status. *Journal of Nutrition* 133(1): 322S–327S.

Scrimshaw NS, Taylor CF, and Gordon JF (1968) *Interactions of Nutrition and Infection.* Monograph Series 57. Geneva: World Health Organization.

Scrimshaw NS and SanGiovanni JP (1997) Synergism of nutrition, infection and immunity: an overview. *American Journal of Clinical Nutrition* 66: 464S–477S.

Suskins MS and Tontisirin K (2001) *Nutrition, Immunity and Infection in Infants and Children.* Philadelphia: Lippincott Williams and Wilkins.

Tomkins A and Watson F (1989) *Malnutrition and Infection: A review. Nutrition Policy Discussion Paper No.5 (ACC/SCN State of the Art Series).* Geneva: United Nations.

Nutritional Management in Adults

J A Tayek, Harbor–UCLA Medical Center, Torrance, CA, USA

Metabolic and Nutritional Changes in Patients with Infection

An increased blood glucose concentration is the most common abnormality in the infected hospitalized patient. This section discusses the metabolic abnormalities in glucose, protein, and fat metabolism as well as abnormalities in specific nutrients in this population. Specific nutritional treatment plans are presented. In addition, the host response to injury and why patients may not be able to become anabolic with conventional nutritional support are discussed. The acute phase response typifies the host's response to infection. Mechanisms to blunt the catabolic state are important because the extent of muscle wasting and weight loss is inversely correlated with long-term survival. The potential uses of conventional nutritional support and newer nutritional adjunctive techniques utilized for patients are discussed.

Glucose Utilization in Injury and Infection

In nearly all studies of glucose metabolism in patients with infection, injury, or cancer, there is a significant reduction in glucose utilization. This occurs even when the insulin concentrations are in the physiological range. This effect is not overcome even with administration of supraphysiological insulin concentrations. In sepsis, the insulin resistance associated with injury is due to defective insulin-mediated activation of the glycogen storage pathway. By approximately 7 h after the onset of injury, there is a reduction in glucose utilization via the nonoxidative pathway. This injury response persists until the source of injury, infection, or tumor is removed.

Hepatic Glucose Metabolism

During infection, the liver increases glucose production to defend against hypoglycemia. In fact, the increase in hepatic glucose production is the major reason why patients with infection have an elevated blood glucose concentration. For example, patients with active malaria can have an increase in fasting glucose concentration due to an increase in gluconeogenesis and overall glucose production. Approximately 75% of cancer patients, like patients with infection, also have an elevated rate of glucose production. Cancer patients also have a mild form of injury; approximately 75% have an elevated rate of hepatic glucose production. In 18 studies, hepatic glucose production for normals ranges between 1.6 and 3.0 mg/kg/min, with an average of 2.1 mg/kg/min. Glucose production for cancer patients without weight loss ranges from 1.7 to 5.1 mg/kg/min, with a mean of 2.75 mg/kg/min. This is a 30% increase in the fasting rate of hepatic glucose production. For cancer patients with weight loss, glucose production ranges from 2.3 to 3.3 mg/kg/min, with a mean of 2.96 mg/kg/min. This represents a 41% increase in the rate of hepatic glucose production. Not all cancer types have an elevation in hepatic glucose production. For example, head and neck cancer patients may not have an elevation in fasting hepatic glucose production, but it is commonly elevated in lung cancer patients, probably because they have an increased injury response. In

cancer patients, the etiology for the elevated rate of fasting hepatic glucose production is not known. Early studies tested whether excessive growth hormone (GH) release in cancer patients might be responsible. However, there was no direct correlation between GH secretion pattern and hepatic glucose production. Furthermore, the administration of GH to cancer patients for a 3-day period failed to increase the rate of glucose production. Koea and Shaw suggested that the rate is related to the bulk of the tumor, and others have suggested it is related to cytokines or other factors. Earlier studies on normal volunteers demonstrated that the loss of the first-phase insulin response causes a delay in the normal inhibition of glucose production. Although the latter effect may explain postprandial hyperglycemia, it is an unlikely explanation for fasting hepatic glucose production.

Gluconeogenesis is elevated in head and neck cancer patients and also in lung cancer patients. Gluconeogenesis accounts for approximately 50% of the overall glucose production after an overnight fast. It was demonstrated that glucose carbon recycling was elevated in five of seven published studies. Glucose carbon recycling is an indicator of increased gluconeogenesis. The ability to measure gluconeogenesis was not possible in humans until recently, when a method using $[U-^{13}C]$ glucose and isotopomer analysis was developed. The Cori cycle is increased in cancer patients and has been estimated to account for 300 kcal of energy loss per day. In 70% of published studies, cancer patients have a significant elevation in the rate of gluconeogenesis compared to normal weight-matched controls. Gluconeogenesis was directly related to the morning blood cortisol concentration in both the normal volunteers ($r = 0.913$, $p < 0.01$) and the cancer patients ($r = 0.595$, $p < 0.05$). In the septic host, the increase in glucose production is likely due to an elevation of multiple counterregulatory hormones (cortisol, GH, catecholamines, and glucagon) and cytokines (interleukin-1 (IL-1), tumor necrosis factor-α (TNF-α), etc.).

It is important to note that unlike diabetic patients with an elevated blood glucose concentration, cancer patients with an elevated glucose production rate frequently have a normal blood glucose concentration. Fasting glucose concentrations may be 110–120 mg/dl, which may be overlooked as a subtle indicator of an elevated glucose production rate. The increased rate may contribute to an increased energy cost. Data indicate that the resting energy expenditure is elevated in lung cancer patients and those with other types of cancer compared to weight-matched controls. As expected, energy expenditure is increased in most critically ill patients a few days after admission. However, the precise measurement of energy expenditure is difficult in this setting. Early in the course of critically ill patients, one should focus on excellent blood glucose control. A total caloric intake of 20–25 kcal/kg/day should be provided to the nonthermal injured patient. Protein intake should be 1.5 g/kg body weight/day.

Unlike the normal fasting blood glucose that is seen in cancer patients, patients with injury or infection most commonly have an increase in blood glucose. This has been associated with a large increase in hospital mortality (**Table 1**). Hyperglycemia as a marker of intensive care unit (ICU) mortality may be greater in surgical patient compared to medical ICU patients. In a prospective randomized clinical trial in which intravenous insulin was provided to surgical patients, preventing the increase in blood glucose associated with injury and infection, there was significantly reduced mortality.

Protein Metabolism

Sepsis is associated with an increase in skeletal muscle catabolism and a reduction in the rate of skeletal protein synthesis. Both contribute to a large loss of lean body mass during injury and infection. Skeletal protein breakdown occurs more in the fast-twitch or white muscle fibers than in the red fibers. In addition to sepsis, injury and cancer are also associated with muscle wasting and malnutrition. The etiology is multifactorial, including poor dietary intake, insulin resistance, elevated resting energy expenditure, and other unknown factors. Muscle wasting is due to a combination of increased skeletal muscle protein catabolism and reduced skeletal muscle protein synthesis. For example, in an experimental model of cancer cachexia, protein synthesis was reduced in rats with several tumor types and it occurred at small tumor burdens. In humans with renal cell cancer, the rate of muscle protein synthesis was reduced. In this cancer host, the loss of skeletal muscle appears to be due in part to a reduced protein synthesis and in part to a

normal rate of protein catabolism. This can occur even in the face of an adequate dietary intake.

Whole body protein metabolism can be measured in many ways. The most common isotope is that of the essential amino acid leucine. In the majority of studies on cancer, injury, and infected patients, the rate of plasma amino acid appearance or turnover is elevated. This rate of plasma appearance is a reflection of multiple sites of protein metabolism. The most important are the skeletal muscle, liver, and gastrointestinal (GI) mucosa. Other sites also play an important role, as does the tumor. Studies have demonstrated that the rate of plasma amino acid appearance is related to the bulk of the tumor mass. Measurements of protein metabolism in tumor tissue have demonstrated that the tissue has a very high fractional protein synthesis rate of 50–90% per day. This is similar to that of the liver, and it contrasts with a rate of 1–3% for the skeletal muscle. However, since the body is composed mostly of skeletal muscle, its overall contribution to whole body amino acid metabolism is large and it contributes to a significant proportion of plasma amino acid appearance rates. Data suggest that the increase in the protein catabolism in humans is via the effect of cytokines (IL-1, IL-6, and TNF) and the glucocorticoids, which are known to stimulate the ubiquitin–proteasome pathway of skeletal muscle protein catabolism. Earlier work demonstrates that TNF administration reduces skeletal muscle amino acid content by 20%, but it has no effect on skeletal muscle protein synthesis. The loss of amino acids without stimulation of protein synthesis suggests that TNF stimulates protein catabolism via a loss of amino acids from inside the skeletal muscle. This effect of TNF wanes after 6 h since animals studied at 60 h have a 30% increase in the rate of protein synthesis and a normal skeletal muscle amino acid content. The increased rate of protein synthesis probably reflects the recovery of the depleted amino acid pool due to

Table 1   Mean blood glucose concentrations, hospital mortality

Patients	Controls		IV insulin		Reference
	Glucose (mg/dl)	Mortality (%)	Glucose (mg/dl)	Mortality (%)	
1600 mixed ICU	152	20.9	131	14.8[*]	Krinsley (2004)
1548 C-T surgery	153	10.9	103	7.2[*]	Van den Berghe et al. (2001)
139 DM with acute MI	162	26.1[a]	153	18.6[*]	Malmeberg (1995)
620 DM with acute MI	162	43.9[b]	148	33.3[*]	Malmeberg (1999)
3554 DM with C-T surgery	213	5.3	177	2.4[*]	Furnary (2003)
Mean ± SEM	168 ± 11	21.4 ± 6.7	142 ± 12	15.3 ± 5.3	

[a]One-year mortality.
[b]Three-year mortality.
[*]p < 0.01 vs mortality at baseline.

earlier administration of TNF. The increased intracellular concentration of amino acids in the skeletal muscle may stimulate synthesis. The direct effect of TNF 60 h after a single administration is not likely since it has a short half-life. Chronic administration results in a reduction in whole body protein synthesis and a net loss of skeletal muscle protein but an increase in liver protein synthesis. An increase in the thyroid hormone triiodothyronine also plays an important role in promoting protein breakdown in both the ubiquitin–proteasome pathway and the lysomal pathway. However, under most conditions, patients with malignancy have either a normal or a reduced triiodothyronine concentration. Similar processes are responsible for the loss of protein seen in infection.

Data suggest that humans make and break down approximately 300 g of protein per day, which is exchanged and reused. This is meditated by the flow of amino acids into and out of cells. Since the amino acid pool is small (only 60 g), the turnover is large. An average person ingests approximately 70 g of protein per day and loses approximately 70 g per day in the form of nitrogen. The cellular proteins, including muscle and extracellular proteins, are approximately 10 400 g. These proteins are broken down and reused at various rates. The key to a small intake of amino acids in the diet is the reutilization of amino acids locally inside the cell and the maintenance of the plasma amino acid pool. The amino acid pool is only 0.6% of the whole body amino acid content, but it plays a vital role in the maintenance of protein synthesis.

Cancer patients who have an elevated plasma amino acid appearance rate survive and those with a normal rate have a worse survival. In one study, stage D colorectal cancer patients who were able to sustain an increased whole body protein metabolism over a 3-month period, as measured by amino acid kinetics, survived and those who had a normal or reduced rate died. Although fasting plasma glucose concentrations were greater in the survivors (100 ± 2 vs 92 ± 3 mg/dl), there was no difference in glucose production rate, age, and body weight. Carcinoembryonic Antigen (CEA) concentrations were higher in the patients who died, which suggests that they had a larger tumor burden. There may be subgroups of patients who are able to mount an acute phase response, which may improve survival. It is not known why some patients mount an increased amino acid appearance rate with cancer, and further research is needed to confirm that it may predict survival. Historically, an elevated plasma amino acid appearance rate was believed to represent protein wasting, but recent data suggest that an elevated rate of whole body protein metabolism may

not reflect a maladaptive processes but rather a healthy response to the tumor. An adequate acute phase response to tumor may reflect a greater fight against cancer. The absence of a response may be unfortunate, as data from patients with colorectal carcinoma suggest. Unfortunately, there are no similar data from infected patients for this comparison.

Lipid Metabolism

Energy in the body is stored mainly in body fat, which is depleted during the wasting process. This process is normally increased during fasting without tumor or injury. When the patient has a tumor, there is a metabolic response to the injury that also promotes lipid mobilization. Several authors have implicated a lipid mobilization factor as being responsible for this process, which is believed to occur in both infection and cancer. Data suggest that this factor may also be responsible for the depletion of liver glycogen in cancer cachexia. This factor(s) increases lipolysis and plasma triglyceride concentrations. The former effect may be due to an increase in the hormone-sensitive lipase and the latter effect due to inhibition of lipoprotein lipase activity. However, the exact factor(s) that is responsible for these effects is not known.

Cancer patients with weight loss have an increase in whole body lipid turnover measured by radioactively labeled fatty acids. However, when weight loss is prevented, there is no increase in the rate of lipolysis. Similarly, the rates of lipid oxidation are normal in cancer patients compared to weight-matched controls. In more severe injury, as seen in sepsis, the rate of lipolysis is increased.

Hormonal Response to Injury, Infection, and Cancer

Infection, cancer, or any injury to the body result in an increase in counterregulatory hormones as well as insulin concentration. As a result of cancer, sepsis, or injury, many patients develop the syndrome of insulin resistance even though they had no history of diabetes prior to cancer. In cancer patients, when the overall injury is smaller, many studies have failed to demonstrate an elevation in counterregulatory hormones. Mild elevations in cortisol concentrations may contribute to the protein catabolism and increased gluconeogenesis. When serum insulin is measured with a sensitive assay, cancer patients demonstrate a small but significant elevation in serum insulin concentration. This is consistent with the observation that these patients have insulin resistance. Cancer patients, like diabetics, have a reduced glucose utilization and loss of the first-phase insulin response, and many have an increased fasting hepatic glucose production rate. As mentioned previously, underweight cancer patients frequently have increased fatty acid oxidation and plasma fatty acid appearance rates. Triglyceride hydrolysis involves much more than fat oxidation, so albumin-bound fatty acids are used partially for energy but many are utilized for reesterification or substrate cycling back to triglyceride.

The rise in serum cortisol as the host's response to the tumor is one of many factors that are responsible for the development of insulin resistance. Insulin resistance is easy to diagnosis because the patient's fasting glucose will be elevated. An elevated fasting glucose level of approximately 110 mg/dl is a good marker of insulin resistance. This is not likely seen in mild injury alone unless the patient has a predisposition to the development of diabetes mellitus. Although insulin resistance is present, the presence of frank diabetes (blood glucose level >126 mg/dl or >7 mm) is not common in cancer or mild injury. It is more common in patients with severe infection or injury. Although most of the counterregulatory hormones are usually normal, serum cortisol and/or glucagon can be mildly elevated. Newer glucagon assays measure the normal value as 35–45 ng/ml, so a significant increase in injury can be detected, which was difficult to do with the older Unger assay. Recent data from pancreatic cancer patients have shown elevated glucagon concentrations, which may be contributing to the development of diabetes. Earlier work found that GH secretion was increased in cancer patients by 24-h analysis and by random sampling. However, after careful study, the increase in GH does not appear to have a major influence on hepatic glucose metabolism. Although there may be a small effect on glycogen breakdown, the major effect is likely via inhibition of glucose utilization in the skeletal muscle.

The sick euthyroid state, in which total triiodothyronine (T_3) concentrations are reduced in severely injured and infected patients, is common. This is likely a normal response to conserve energy in the injured person as the body's ability to convert the stored form of a thyroid hormone (thyroxine (T_4)) into the active form of thyroid hormone, T_3, becomes impaired. T_4 is converted to an inactive thyroid hormone known as reverse-T_3 hormone (rT_3). This event may have evolved as a necessary energy-saving response during a severe injury or illness to reduce the known contribution of T_3 to resting energy expenditure. The low T_3 syndrome is an adaptive way to reduce the normal day-to-day effect of T_3 on resting energy expenditure. This process can occur in the aggressive cancers,

for which the patient's response is similar to that of an injury response.

In septic and injured patients, all counterregulatory hormones are routinely elevated, contributing to an increase in protein catabolism, glucose production, gluconeogenesis, and glycogen breakdown and a major reduction in glucose utilization and anabolism.

Acute Phase Response

The development of injury, infection, or cancer cachexia elicits an acute phase response. This is one of the most basic responses of the body to defend itself against injury. Phylogenetically, this response could be considered the most primitive response of the body. This stereotypical response is similar for injury from an accident, burn, infection, foreign objects, and, in some cases, from a tumor. Unfortunately, this response does not occur for most tumors, but it is seen when the malignancy presents with infection, such as in lung cancer, or in other more aggressive malignancy, such as seen in leukemia. The host develops a response that includes reductions in serum iron and zinc levels, increased serum copper and ceruloplasmin levels, alterations in amino acid distribution and metabolism, an increase in acute phase globulin synthesis, and gluconeogenesis. Although not common, fever can occur, and a negative nitrogen balance results. The tumor can elicit a sequence of events that include changes in cytokine levels as well as several classical hormone levels. For example, a malignant process in the lung will attract monocytes that will be transformed into macrophages at the tissue site of tumor. These macrophages will secrete proteins known as cytokines and other peptides that can attract other white blood cells and initiate an inflammatory response common to many types of injury. Cytokines include TNF-α and IL-1 to IL-20. TNF and other cytokines circulate to the liver, inhibit albumin syntheses, and stimulate the synthesis of acute phase proteins. Acute phase proteins include C-reactive protein, which promotes phagocytosis, modulates the cellular immune response, and inhibits the migration of white blood cells into the tissues; α_1-antichymotrypsin, which minimized tissue damage due to phagocytosis and reduces intravascular coagulation; and α_2-macroglobulin, which forms complexes with proteases and removes then from circulation, maintains antibody production, and promotes granulopoiesis and other acute phase proteins. Unfortunately, the majority of tumors do not elicit a large acute phase response. This limited response may result in a decreased inflammatory and tumorcidal effect.

Urine Urea Nitrogen Loss as a Marker of Catabolism

As part of the host response to injury, infection, or tumor, patients frequently lose protein in the urine in the form of nitrogen. For example, 16 g of urea nitrogen in the urine per day represents a 1-lb loss of lean body mass, such as muscle tissue. In some aggressive cancers, urea nitrogen loss can be as high as 24 g per day. The loss of 1 g of urinary urea nitrogen is equal to 6.25 g of dry protein. A total of 6.25 g of dry protein is equal to approximately 1 oz. of lean body mass. A loss of 16 g of urinary urea is equal to the loss of 1 lb of skeletal muscle or lean body mass per day. Specific areas of lean body mass loss that may result in a functional impairment of the respiratory muscles include the diaphragm, heart muscle, and GI mucosa. The loss of lean body mass in these areas can contribute to the development of respiratory failure, heart failure, and diarrhea, respectively. The rapid development of malnutrition can occur in patients with infection due to large losses of lean body mass per day.

Vitamin Deficiencies

Reduced serum concentrations of several vitamins, including vitamins C and E, have been reported in patients with sepsis. In one study, the administration of additional vitamin E and C resulted in a significant reduction in 28-day mortality (67.5 vs 45.7). Clearly, cancer patients with a poor intake can have deficiencies of many vitamins. For example, cancer patients have been noted to have significant reductions in plasma levels of many of vitamins, especially folate, vitamin A, and vitamin C.

Vitamin C and Vitamin A   Patients with a premalignant lesion called leukoplakia also have reductions in plasma levels of retinol (vitamin A), β-carotene, and vitamin C. A study of healthly elderly demonstrated that approximately 20% had a reduced vitamin C level (<0.5 mg/dl) and 10% had a reduced serum vitamin A level ($<33\,\mu$g/dl). The replacement of multiple vitamins and minerals with 80 mg of vitamin C and 15 000 IU of vitamin A per day for 1 year resulted in a significant reduction in the number of days associated with an infection-related illnesses (48 ± 7 to 23 ± 5 days per year). The multiple vitamin and mineral supplement improved the lymphocyte response to phytohemagglutin and the natural killer cell activity. In another study, the administration of a multivitamin for 1 year demonstrated a 41% reduction in infectious illnesses. In addition, there was a 63% reduction in infection-related absenteeism compared to that of placebo-treated individuals. The administration a MVI to pregnant HIV mothers also reduced HIV progression and mortality (24.7 vs 31.1% mortality, $p < 0.05$).

Vitamin deficiency states are difficult to diagnose. Plasma levels of vitamins are not the best way to assess deficiency. Vitamin C decreases during injury. Although plasma vitamin C concentrations reflect whole body stores, the measurement of plasma vitamin A (retinol) is not the best marker of an actual deficiency state. Liver vitamin A measurements may be a better marker. Patients who die of cancer and subsequent infections have an 18% incidence of moderate liver deficiency of vitamin A at autopsy. Serum vitamin A (retinol) levels are low in up to 92% of patients with serious infections. This depletion of liver stores of vitamin A may be due to excessive loss of retinol in the urine in patients with sepsis. In contrast to what is noted in patients with cancer or serious infections, trauma patients who die within 7 days of hospitalization only have a 2% incidence of severe liver vitamin A deficiency. Vitamin A can be provided by supplementation dietary intake, parenteral intake, or intramuscular vitamin A administration. In addition to the changes in folate, vitamin A, and vitamin C mentioned previously, excessive losses of several vitamins have been observed in patients receiving medications that interfere with normal utilization or elimination (**Table 2**).

Table 2 Drug-induced nutrient deficiencies

Drug	Nutrient(s) affected
Steroids	Vitamin A, potassium
Phenothiazines	Vitamin B$_2$
Tricyclic antidepressants	Vitamin B$_2$
Hydralazine	Vitamin B$_6$
Isoniazid	Vitamin B$_6$, niacin
Penicillamine	Vitamin B$_6$
Ammonium chloride	Vitamin C
Aspirin	Vitamin C
Phenobarbital and phenytoin	Vitamin C, vitamin D
Tetracycline	Vitamin C
Coumadin	Vitamin K
Estrogen and progesterone compounds	Folic acid, vitamin B$_6$
Aminoglycoside	Magnesium, zinc
Platinum	Magnesium, zinc
Diphenylhydantoin	Niacin
Antacid	Phosphorus, phosphates
Diuretics	Sodium, potassium, magnesium, zinc
Laxatives	Sodium, potassium, magnesium
Cholestyramine	Triglycerides, fat-soluble vitamins

Mineral Deficiencies

Multiple elevated cytokines are likely responsible for the commonly observed reduction in serum mineral concentrations. This is known as part of the cytokine-mediated inflammatory response. In addition, in patients with injury, infection, or cancer, the reduced mineral content may also occur secondary to poor oral intake, increased requirements, and excessive urinary and stool losses.

Magnesium   Total body stores are 2028 g of magnesium. Communications with several experts on magnesium and current work on the antiarrhythmic actions of magnesium suggest a that the commonly used normal values for serum magnesium levels should be increased from 1.7–2.3 mg/dl to 2.0–2.6 mg/dl. Large losses can occur in conditions such as diarrhea, in which the stool may have up to 12 meq of magnesium per liter and the urine may have up to 25 meq per day. Large urinary losses can occur in cancer patients given aminoglycides, diuretics, and ketoconazole. Furthermore, large losses can occur in some of the intestinal fluids (**Table 3**) in cancer and other operative patients who develop GI fistulas.

Zinc   Total body stores are only 2 or 3 g of zinc. Zinc concentration in the blood decreases as an early response to cytokines. This is commonly seen in many different types of injury as well as in cancer patients. There are minor tissue stores of zinc in skin, bone, and intestine. Zinc is redistributed to liver, bone marrow, thymus, and the site of injury or inflammation. This redistribution is mediated by IL-1 and the other cytokines secreted from macrophages. In hospitalized cancer patients, a reduced serum zinc concentration ($<70\,\mu g/dl$) is not uncommon. The administration of approximately 50 mg of zinc per day is associated with a normalization of the zinc level after 3 weeks of feeding. Fifteen percent of healthy elderly have been found to have reduced serum zinc levels ($<67\,\mu g/dl$). The replacement of a multivitamin with 14 mg of zinc per day for 1 year resulted in a significant reduction in the number of days associated with infection-related illnesses (48 ± 7 to 23 ± 5 days per year). This vitamin and mineral supplementation improved the lymphocyte response to phytohemagglutin and the natural killer cell activity. There was no change in the placebo-treated group. Zinc supplementation in hospitalized patients may help with normal immune response for minor infection and wound healing. Zinc is needed for cell mitosis and cell proliferation. It has also been demonstrated to improve wound healing in patients provided 600 mg of zinc sulfate (136 mg of elemental zinc) orally per day who had a serum zinc level on admission of less than $100\,\mu g/dl$. In this double-blind study, the healing rate increased more than twofold in those randomized to receive zinc supplementation. In addition, large losses of zinc can occur via intestinal losses (**Table 3**). It is important to note that intestinal fluids can contain up to 17 mg of zinc per liter, so the replacement rate of zinc should take into account the abnormal sources of zinc loss as well as the routine nutritional requirements.

Copper   Total body stores are very small at 60–80 mg. Serum copper status is normal or increased compared to that of serum zinc, and cytokines are also believed to be responsible for these changes. The benefits of or rational for these increased concentrations are not known.

Iron   Total body stores are 3.5–4.5 g of iron. An increase in cytokines also contributes to the observed decrease in serum iron concentration. This is a mediated response to cancer, injury, or infection. The exact mechanism is not known, but iron is stored in Kupffer cells of the liver until the injury wanes. This is probably a beneficial effect

Table 3   Electrolyte contents of body fluids

Body fluid	Electrolyte and mineral concentration (meq/l)					
	Sodium	Potassium	Chloride	Bicarbonate	Magnesium	Zinc (mg)
Bile	145	5	100	15–60	1–2	—
Colonic fluids	50	30–70	15–40	30	6–12	17
Diarrheal fluids	50	35	40	45	1–13	17
Duodenum	130	5–10	90	10	1–2	12
Ileal fluids	140	10–20	100	20–30	6–12	17
Pancreatatic juice	140	5	75	70–115	0.5	—
Saliva	10	20–30	15	50	0.6	—
Stomach fluids	100	10	120	0	0.9	—
Urine	60–120	30–70	60–120	—	5	0.1–0.5
Urine post Lasix	15× normal	2× normal	—	—	20× normal	—

since many microbes use iron as a source of energy. Iron administration should be restricted in patients who have a serious infection because it has been shown to cause harm with fungal, parasitic, malarial, or other types of low-grade or quiescent infections.

Summary

Vitamins and minerals act as cofactors for essential processes in health and in illness. The requirements for the healthy person have been well established and are published as the recommended daily requirements (**Tables 4** and **5**). The exact needs for the infected, injured, or cancer patient are not well documented and evaluations are in progress. Reduced levels of vitamin C, vitamin A, copper, manganese, and zinc have been observed, and all of these are associated with poor wound healing. Wound dehiscence is eight times more common with decreased vitamin C levels. This is probably due to the fact that vitamin C enhances capillary formation and decreases capillary fragility, is a necessary component of complement, and is key to the hydroxylation of proline and lysine in collagen synthesis. Vitamin A enhances collagen synthesis and crosslinking of new collagen, enhances epithelialization, and antagonizes the inhibitory effects of glucocorticoids on cell membranes. Manganese is a cofactor in the glycosylation of hydroxylysine in procollagen. Copper acts a cofactor in the polymerization of the collagen molecule and as a cofactor in the formation of collagen crosslinks.

Table 4 Adult daily vitamin nutritional requirements (RDA, 1989)

Nutrient	Oral	Intravenous	Special requirements (diagnosis)
Vitamin A	3300 IU/day	3300 IU/day (1 mg)	5000+ IU/day (serious infections)
Vitamin B (Biotin)	100 µg/day	60 µg/day	
Vitamin B (Folic acid)	0.2 mg/day	0.4 mg/day	5 mg/day (ICU patients/thrombocytopenia)
Vitamin B (Niacin)	20 mg/day	40 mg/day	
Vitamin B$_1$ (Thiamin)	1.5 mg/day	3 mg/day	50 mg/day (alcoholics/Wernike–Korsakoff)
Vitamin B$_2$ (Riboflavin)	1.8 mg/day	3.6 mg/day	
Vitamin B$_6$ (Pyridoxine)	2 mg/day	4 mg/day	
Vitamin B$_{12}$	2 µg/day	5 µg/day	
Vitamin C	60 mg/day	100 mg/day	
Vitamin D	400 IU/day	200 IU/day (5 µg)	
Vitamin E	10 mg/day	10 mg	
Vitamin K	80 µg/day	[a]	
Pantothenic acid	7 mg/day	15 mg/day	

[a]Vitamin K is routinely given as 10 mg SQ on admission and then every Monday.

Table 5 Daily nutritional requirements

Nutrient	Adult daily nutritional requirements		
	Oral	IV	Special requirements (diagnosis)
Macronutrients			
Protein	1.5–2.0 g/kg	1.5–2.0 g/kg	2–3 g/kg (thermal injury)
Glucose	20–25 kcal/kg	20–25 kcal/kg	3000 kcal goal in alcoholic liver disease patients
Lipid	4% of kcals	4% of kcals	Can administer up to 60% of calories to prevent hyperglycemia
Micronutrients			
Sodium	60–150 meq	60–150 meq	
Potassium	40–80 meq	40–80 meq	
Chloride	40–100 meq	40–100 meq	
Acetate	10–40 meq	10–40 meq	
Phosphorus	10–60 mmol	10–60 mmol	
Calcium	5–20 meq	5–20 meq	100 meq or more severe hypocalcemia and hungry bone syndrome
Magnesium	10–20 meq	10–20 meq	50–100 meq (cardiac arrthymias, diarrhea)
Zinc	3 mg	2.5–4 mg	10–100 mg (diarrhea, fistula, wounds)
Copper	1.5–3 mg	1–1.5 mg	
Chromium	50–200 µg	10–15 µg	40 µg (diarrhea, gastrointestinal losses)
Molybdenum	75–250 µg	100–200 µg	
Manganese	2–5 mg	150–800 µg	
Selenium	40–120 µg	40–120 µg	120–200 µg (thermal injury, wounds)

Nutritional Assessment and Predictors of Hospital Outcome

Markers of Nutritional Assessment

Conventional nutritional assessment in injured, infected, or cancer patients is of clinical value. Body weight and history of weight loss is one of the best indicators of survival in patients with infection or cancer. In addition, serum albumin concentration upon admission is probably one of the best predictors of hospital survival (Table 2). Serum albumin is commonly used as an indicator of nutritional status. Its level provides the clinician with an index of visceral and somatic protein stores for most medical illnesses. A level less than 3.0 is considered malnutrition and may also be called hypoalbuminemic malnutrition or protein malnutrition. Exceptions to this include the isolated starved state such as anorexia nervosa, severe edema, and the rare case of congenital analbuminemia. Serum albumin has a 21-day half-life, and this can reflect processes that have been ongoing for a few weeks. The benefit of serum albumin is that it is also an inverse acute phase reactant. The further it declines, the more severe the injury response on top of the severity of malnutrition at the time of the injury or cancer.

Predictors of Clinical Outcome

The best marker of injury is serum albumin concentration. It is an excellent predictor of survival in patients with cancer and other types of illnesses (Table 6). More than 20 studies have shown that a serum albumin level below normal can be used to predict disease outcomes in many groups of patients. One of the first studies in this area was a Veterans Administration study in which 30-day mortality rates were evaluated for a total of 2060 consecutive medical and surgical admissions. Investigators found that 24.7% of the patient population had a low albumin level defined as 3.4 g/dl or lower. The 30-day mortality rate for hypoalbuminemia patients was 24.6% compared to 1.7% for patients with a normal albumin level. These investigators demonstrated an excellent correlation between serum albumin levels and 30-day mortality rates. A 1-g decrease in serum albumin levels (3.5 to 2.5 g/dl) translated into a 33% increase in mortality. Patients with an average albumin level of 1.8 g/dl had a mortality rate of 65%. It is interesting to note that of 15 hypoalbuminemia patients in this study who were provided with total parenteral nutrition, only 1 died (7% mortality).

Protein malnutrition is associated with a greater risk for infection, especially fungal infections. In one

Table 6 Serum albumin and mortality

Patient population	Mortality				
	With normal albumin		With low albumin (%)	Increased risk (-fold)	Albumin cutoff level (g/dl)
	n	%			
VA hospital	2060	1.7	24.7	14.7	3.5
Medical and surgical patients	500	1.3	7.9	6.1	3.5
Hodgkins	586	1.0	10	10.0	3.5
Lung CA	59	49	85	1.7	3.4
VA hospital	152	3.3	25.8	7.8	3.5
Surgical patients	243	4.7	23	4.9	3.5
Malnutrition	92	8.0	40	5.0	3.5
Surgery (colorectal)	83	3.0	28	9.3	3.5
ETOH hepatitis	352	2.0	19.8	9.9	3.5
Pneumonia	38	0	100	—	3.0
Cirrhosis	139	32	52	1.6	2.9
ICU patients	55	10	76	7.6	3.0
Cardiovascular disease	7735	0.0	2.0	—	4.0
Trauma	34	15.4	28.6	1.9	3.5
Sepsis	199	0.7	15.9	22.7	2.9
Pneumonia	456	2.1	8.3	4.0	3.5
Multiple meyloma	23	25	50	2.0	3.0
CABG/cardiac valve surgery	5156	0.2	0.9	5.7	2.5
Preoperative (VA hospital)	54 215	2.0	10.3	5.1	3.5
Beth Israel Hospital	15 511	4.0	14.0	3.5	3.4
Hemodialysis	13 473	8.0	16.6	2.1	4.0
Average ± SEM	4275	7.8 ± 2.8	31 ± 7	15 ± 2-fold risk	3.4 ± 0.1
Total No. of patients	101 178				

study, the most important risk factor for the development of candidemia was malnutrition. A reduced serum albumin level is an independent risk factor for nosocomial infections. The greater the protein malnutrition, the greater the risk for nosocomial infections.

In summary, serum albumin concentrations provide the clinician with a tool to help predict recovery or mortality. Albumin levels should be monitored at regular intervals (every 3 or 4 days) for hospitalized patients who are ill and at risk for malnutrition. Once hypoalbuminemia is documented, it is not an ideal indicator of nutritional rehabilitation since it returns to normal slowly (21-day half-life) and lags behind other indices of nutritional status, such as transferrin (7-day half-life), prealbumin (1-day half-life), or retinol binding protein (4-h half-life). Albumin replacement does not reverse the metabolic process that the hypoalbuminemia state represents. The reduced level of protein reserves in the patient and the severity of the metabolic injury or cancer are the two most important determinants of serum albumin level.

Nutritional Diagnoses Commonly Seen in Hospitalized Patients

The diagnosis of malnutrition is made by taking a good history and obtaining a physical exam. It is important to ask the patient if he or she has been able to maintain his or her appetite and body weight during the past several months. A history of a recent hospitalization is also important to note due to the common development of protein malnutrition during hospital stay. The physical exam involves inspection of the muscle mass, especially noting a loss of temporals muscle, 'squaring off' of the deltoid muscle, and loss of the thigh muscles. Obtaining a measured body weight should be standard on all admissions, and this weight should be followed on a daily basis.

Up to 50% of hospitalized surgical and medical patients have either hypoalbuminemia or marasmic-type malnutrition. Hypoalbuminemia or protein malnutrition can be diagnosed with the measurement of reduced albumin, transferrin, prealbumin, or retinol binding protein levels. Albumin levels are most commonly used to make the diagnosis. Marasmic malnutrition is the diagnosis for anyone who has lost 20% of usual body weight during the preceding 3–6 months or who is less than 90% of ideal body weight. Of these two types of malnutrition, protein malnutrition is most common. The presence of hypoalbuminemia malnutrition in one study was

associated with a 4-fold increase in dying and a 2.5-fold increased risk of developing a nosocomial infection and sepsis. As indicated in **Table 6**, a low serum albumin level predicts a significant increase in mortality across many diseases.

Loss of Lean Body Mass

The use of body weight as an index of muscle mass in the cancer patient is very difficult due to the possible fluid shifts that occur in the extracellular compartment. Body weight can be divided into three compartments: extracellular mass, lean body mass, and fat mass. Extracellular mass is known to increase in malnutrition and as a result of hypoalbuminemia. An increase in extracellular fluid occurs more commonly in the malnourished patient. A large portion of the fluid shift noted in cancer patients is due to a reduction in the plasma colloid oncotic pressure. Lean body mass is the mixture of skeletal muscle, plasma proteins, skin, skeleton, and visceral organs. The skin and skeleton account for 50% of the lean body mass. Currently, there are no convenient markers to determine the loss of nitrogen from either skin or skeleton. The plasma proteins account for only 2% of the lean body mass, but albumin measurement can reflect the overall status of the lean body mass. The viscera accounts for 12% of the lean body mass, and decreases in some of visceral sizes (gut atrophy and cardiac atrophy) are noted in cancer patients. Unfortunately, there is no convenient marker of loss of lean body mass that originates from the visceral organs. On the other hand, urine creatinine is a marker of skeletal muscle mass. The skeletal muscle accounts for 35% of the lean body mass, and it provides the major storage area for amino acids needed during illness. The standard way to assess the size of the skeletal mass is to determine the creatinine height index by collecting 24-h urine and comparing the value to normal values of creatinine excretion for age, sex, and height. A simplified way is to collect 24-h urine and divide the total amount by the ideal body weight based on the patient's height. The normal value for an adult male is 23 mg/kg of ideal body weight, and that for a female is 18 mg/kg. A value of 10% less than normal would be consistent with a 10% loss in the muscle mass for unit height. A value of 20% less than the lower range of normal would classify patients as having mild muscle loss. A 20–40% loss would classify them as having a moderate loss, and a 40% or greater reduction in the creatinine per weight would document severe muscle loss. The most accurate estimate is to obtain urine creatinine over a 3-day period and to repeat at intervals to document the loss of muscle mass over an extended period of time. Dietary creatine and creatinine intake has only a minor influence ($<20\%$) on urinary creatinine in the normal eating individual. Changes in dietary intake may influence the accuracy of the collection, but repeating the values over 3 days will help average variations in dietary intake. Impairment of renal function reduces the normal creatinine excretion and excludes the creatinine height index as a marker of muscle mass.

Elevated Resting Energy Expenditure

Resting energy expenditure (REE) is directly linked to the size of the lean body mass. REE is difficult to determine accurately in volunteers since the method of indirect calorimetry has variations when the same individual is restudied. Several studies have demonstrated an elevated rate of energy expenditure when compared to controls of similar weight. The use of D_2O^{18} has helped in the estimate of energy expenditure and will improve our understanding of energy expenditure in the future.

Nutritional Feeding of the Patient: Enteral versus Parenteral

Vitamins and Minerals

The standard oral and intravenous vitamin intake and what is currently being given at Harbor-UCLA Medical Center and UCLA Medical Center are listed in **Table 4**. Also included are the few exceptions to the routine intravenous amounts for both **Tables 4** and **5**. The mineral and trace element requirements are listed in **Table 5**. These vitamin, mineral, and trace mineral recommendations are for hospitalized cancer patients and noncancer patients who are hospitalized. They should not have oliguric renal failure or cholastatic liver disease. In acute oliguric renal failure, vitamins A and D should be reduced or eliminated from the enteral or parenteral solutions. Potassium, phosphorus, magnesium, zinc, and selenium should be reduced or eliminated. Iron and chromium are known to accumulate in renal failure and should be removed from the parenteral or enteral formulations. In cholastatic liver disease, the trace elements copper and manganese are excreted via the biliary tree in the bile and should be reduced or eliminated to prevent toxicity. In comparison, large amounts of electrolytes and minerals can be lost in gastrointestinal fluids and in urine (**Table 3**). It is essential to replace the estimated amounts lost on a daily basis in the parenteral nutrition.

Enteral versus Parenteral Feeding

In all situations, if the gut is functional, then it should be used as the route of calorie administration. Gut atrophy predisposes bacterial and fungal colonization and subsequent invasion associated with bacteremia. Sepsis due to microbial or toxin translocation into the portal system is a frequent source of fever evaluations that do not indicate an obvious source of infection. Utilization of the GI track can reduce the incidence of bacterial translocation.

Enteral Products

Enteral nutrition is best taken by mouth if the patient can ingest the required amount. If the patient cannot, then either supplements or full tube feeding is the method of choice. Protein in the peptide form is better absorbed than the free amino acid form due to specific transporters in the small intestines for amino acids, dipeptides, and tripeptides. Feeding tube placement is best in the small bowel up to the ligament of Treitz. This can be obtained best by the direct use of fluoroscopy or may be obtained by the passage of the feeding tube into the small bowel by a corkscrew technique, in which the distal tip of the feeding tube is bent at an approximately $30°$ angle with the wire stilet in place. Upon placement into the stomach, the tube is rotated so that the tip may pass via the pylorus into the small bowel. The infusion of enteral products into the small bowel will reduce the incidence of aspiration because the infusion is below the pylorus. Intubated patients have a low risk for aspiration due to the endotracheal cuff, so placement of a feeding tube into the small bowel is less essential.

Supplementation of enteral products with higher than standard amounts of the amino acid arginine has been done to enhance immune function. Published data on its beneficial effect in surgical patients have demonstrated some benefit; however, data from nonsurgical patients suggest harm. Immunonutrition should not be given to patients with severe infection, especially patients with pneumonia.

Branched-chain amino acid-enriched enteral products are available and have been shown to improve mental function and mortality in patients with hepatic encephalopathy. Albumin synthesis is also stimulated by branched-chain-enriched amino acid solutions. However, additional branched-chain amino acids did not improved morbidity or mortality in trauma or septic patients randomized to receive branched-chain-enriched amino acids compared to conventional feeding.

Glutamine-enriched enteral formulas are very common. There are many enteral products used in hospitalized patients and for home enteral nutritional support. These can be found at several enteral nutrition pharmaceutical Web sites.

The choice of lipid composition in enteral products is a field that is rapidly evolving, and this is an important decision to be made by the clinician depending on the type of disease being treated. The use of omega-3-enriched fatty acids in the enteral product (fish oil-enriched) has been associated with an ability to modify the inflammatory response that may be related to the increased arachondic acid metabolism and a decrease in the omega-6 pathway fatty acid metabolism. Unfortunately, most commercially available enteral products that have omega-3 fatty acids also have other additives, such as arginine, glutamine, and nucleotides, so that the benefits attributed to the use of an omega-3-enriched fatty aid enteral diet await future clinical studies.

Energy Intake for Patients with Malnutrition

The diagnosis of protein malnutrition can be made when the serum albumin level is less than 2.8 g/dl. Many of these patients have a 20% weight loss during the preceding 3 months, or they have a reduced ideal body weight (<90% for height). Patients at high risk for the development of malnutrition are those who are unlikely to ingest a minimum of 1500 kcal by day 5.

There are currently only three studies that support the importance of energy intake in malnourished patients. Elderly hospitalized patients who consume less than 50% of their estimated maintenance caloric requirement have an 8-fold increase in hospital mortality (11.8 vs 1.5%). This suggests that an intake of less than 1000 kcal may not be helpful. In a prospective study providing approximately 400 additional calories as 'sip feeds,' reduced mortality was seen in severely malnourished (body mass index <5th percentile), medically ill elderly patients. In this study, patients were randomized to receive 120 ml of enteral supplements provided by the registered nurse three times per day or provided no additional sip feeds. Patients who received the sip feeds had a significantly better energy intake (1409 kcal) than nonsupplemented patients (1090 kcal), and they had an increased overall weight gain compared with a loss in the controls. Patients in the severely undernourished group who received intervention had a significant reduction in mortality compared to controls (15 vs 35%, $p < 0.05$). The less

malnourished or normals did not demonstrate the same benefit. In the third study, patients with less than 25% of recommended calorie intake (<600 kcal) had a 3.7-fold increased rate of nosocomial bloodstream infections. Candida and coagulase-negative *Staphylococcus* accounted for 63% of the nosocomial infections, with candida accounting for 29%.

See also: **Anemia**: Iron-Deficiency Anemia. **Ascorbic Acid**: Physiology, Dietary Sources and Requirements; Deficiency States. **Cancer**: Epidemiology of Gastrointestinal Cancers Other Than Colorectal Cancers; Epidemiology of Lung Cancer. **Carbohydrates**: Regulation of Metabolism. **Cholesterol**: Sources, Absorption, Function and Metabolism. **Copper**. **Cytokines**. **Diabetes Mellitus**: Etiology and Epidemiology; Classification and Chemical Pathology; Dietary Management. **Fatty Acids**: Metabolism. **Glucose**: Chemistry and Dietary Sources; Metabolism and Maintenance of Blood Glucose Level; Glucose Tolerance. **Iodine**: Deficiency Disorders. **Iron**. **Lipids**: Chemistry and Classification. **Magnesium**. **Malnutrition**: Secondary, Diagnosis and Management. **Nutritional Assessment**: Anthropometry; Biochemical Indices; Clinical Examination. **Nutritional Support**: Adults, Enteral; Adults, Parenteral. **Protein**: Deficiency. **Vitamin A**: Physiology; Deficiency and Interventions. **Zinc**: Deficiency in Developing Countries, Intervention Studies.

Further Reading

Barringer TA, Kirk JK, Santaniello AC, Foley KL, and Michielutte R (2003) Effect of multivitamin and mineral supplement in infection and quality of life. *Annals of Internal Medicine* **138**: 365–371.

Carson GL (2004) Insulin resistance in human sepsis: Implications for nutritional and metabolic care of the critically ill surgical patient. *Annals of the Royal College of Surgeons* **86**: 75–81.

Christiansen C, Tolf P, Jorgensen HS, Andersen SK, and Tonnesen E (2004) Hyperglycemia and mortality in critically ill patients. *Intensive Care Medicine* **30**: 1685–1688.

Fawzi WW, Msamanga GI, Spiegelman D et al. (2004) A randomized trial of multivitamin supplements and HIV disease progression and mortality. *New England Journal of Medicine* **35**: 23–32.

Koea J and Shaw JFH (1992) The effect of tumor bulk on the metabolic response to cancer. *Annals of Surgery* **215**: 282–288.

Plank LD and Hill GL (2003) Energy balance in critically illness. *Proceedings of the Nutrition Society* **62**: 545–552.

Ramaswamy G, Rao VR, Kumaraswamx SV, and Anantha N (1996) Serum vitamin status in oral leucoplakia: A preliminary study. *European Journal of Cancer* **328**(2): 120–122.

Rubinson L, Diette GB, Song X, Grower RG, and Krishnan JA (2004) Low calorie intake is associated with nosocomial bloodstream infections in patients in the medical intensive care unit. *Critical Care Medicine* **32**: 350–357.

Scjmeoder SM, Veyres P, Pivot X et al. (2004) Malnutrition is an independent factor associated with nosocomial infections. British Journal of Nutrition 92: 105–111.

Tayek JA (1992) A review of cancer cachexia and abnormal glucose metabolism in humans with cancer. Journal of the American College of Nutrition 11: 445–456.

Tayek JA and Brasel JA (1995) Failure of anabolism in malnourished cancer patients receiving growth hormone. Journal of Clinical Endocrinology & Metabolism 80: 2082–2087.

Tayek JA and Katz J (1996) Glucose production, recycling, and gluconeogenesis in normals and diabetics; Mass isotopomer U-13C glucose study. American Journal of Physiology 270: E709–E717.

Tayek JA and Katz J (1997) Glucose production, recycling, Cori cycle and gluconeogenesis in humans with and without cancer: Relationship to serum cortisol concentration. American Journal of Physiology 272: E476–E484.

Van den Berghe G, Wouters P, Weekers F et al. (2001) Intensive insulin therapy in critically ill patients. New England Journal of Medicine 345: 1359–1367.

Ziegler TR (1992) Clinical and metabolic efficacy of glutamine-supplemented parenteral nutrition after bone marrow transplantation. Annals of Internal Medicine 116: 821.

Intestine see **Small Intestine**: Structure and Function; Disorders. **Microbiota of the Intestine**: Probiotics; Prebiotics

---

IODINE

Contents
Physiology, Dietary Sources and Requirements
Deficiency Disorders

Physiology, Dietary Sources and Requirements

R Houston, Emory University, Atlanta, GA, USA

A relevant thing, though small, is of the highest importance

MK Gandhi

Iodine is classified as a nonmetallic solid in the halogen family of the Periodic Table of the elements and therefore is related to fluorine, chlorine, and bromine. The halogen family lies between the oxygen family and the rare gases. Iodine sublimates at room temperature to form a violet gas; its name is derived from the Greek *iodes*, meaning 'violet-colored.' Iodine was discovered by Bernard Courtois in Paris in 1811, the second halogen (after chlorine) to be discovered. It took nearly 100 years to understand its critical importance in human physiology. In 1896, Baumann determined the association of iodine with the thyroid gland, and in 1914 Kendall, with revisions by Harrington in 1926, described the hormone complexes synthesized by the thyroid gland using iodine that are so integral to human growth and development.

As the biochemistry of iodine and the thyroid was being established, the scarcity of the element in the natural environment became evident and the link between deficiency and human disease was revealed. Enlargement of the thyroid, or goitre, is seen in ancient stone carvings and Renaissance paintings, but it was not until years later that the link with lack of iodine was firmly established. Even with this knowledge, many years passed before preventive measures were established. From 1910 to 1920 in Switzerland and the USA work was done on the use of salt fortified with iodine to eliminate iodine deficiency, with classic work being done by Dr David Marine in Michigan. Recently the linkage of iodine deficiency with intellectual impairment has brought iodine into the international spotlight.

Recent work has demonstrated that the halogens, including iodine, are involved through the halo-peroxidases in enzymatic activity and production of numerous active metabolites in the human body. While the importance of iodine for the thyroid has been known for some time, recent research on halogen compounds in living organisms suggests additional more complex roles including antibiotic and anticancer activity. Yet it is the critical importance of iodine in the formation of the thyroid hormones thyroxine (T_4) and triiodothyronine (T_3) that makes any discussion of this element and human physiology of necessity bound up with a review of thyroid function.

Existence of Iodine in the Natural Environment

The marine hydrosphere has high concentrations of halogens, with iodine being the least common and chlorine the most. Halogens, including iodine, are concentrated by various species of marine organisms such as macroalgae and certain seaweeds. Release from these organisms makes a major contribution to the atmospheric concentration of the halogens. Iodine is present as the least abundant halogen in the Earth's crust. It is likely that in primordial times the concentration in surface soils was higher, but today the iodine content of soils varies and most has been leached out in areas of high rainfall or by previous glaciation. Environmental degradation caused by massive deforestation and soil erosion is accelerating this process. This variability in soil and water iodine concentration is quite marked, with some valleys in China having relatively high iodine concentrations in water, and other parts of China with negligible amounts in soil and water. Table 1

Table 1 Relative abundance of halogens in the natural environment

Element	Abundance in oceans (ppm)	Abundance in Earth's crust (ppm)	Abundance in human body (mol)
Fluorine	1.3	625	0.13
Chlorine	19 400	130	2.7
Bromine	67	2.5	0.0033
Iodine	0.06	0.05	0.00013

shows the relative abundance of various halogens in the natural environment, while **Figure 1** illustrates the cycle of iodine in nature.

Commercial production of iodine occurs almost exclusively in Japan and Chile, with iodine extracted from concentrated salt brine from underground wells, seaweed, or from Chilean saltpetre deposits.

Absorption, Transport, and Storage

Iodine is usually ingested as an iodide or iodate compound and is rapidly absorbed in the intestine. Iodine entering the circulation is actively trapped by the thyroid gland. This remarkable capacity to concentrate iodine is a reflection of the fact that the most critical physiological role for iodine is the normal functioning of the thyroid gland. Circulating iodide enters the capillaries within the thyroid and is rapidly transported into follicular cells and on into the lumen of the follicle. This active transport is likely to be based on cotransport of sodium and iodine, allowing

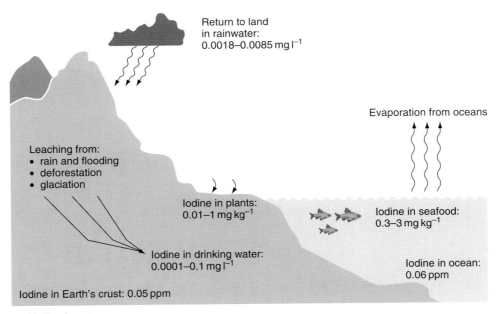

Return to land in rainwater: 0.0018–0.0085 mg l^{-1}

Evaporation from oceans

Leaching from:
- rain and flooding
- deforestation
- glaciation

Iodine in plants: 0.01–1 mg kg^{-1}

Iodine in seafood: 0.3–3 mg kg^{-1}

Iodine in drinking water: 0.0001–0.1 mg l^{-1}

Iodine in ocean: 0.06 ppm

Iodine in Earth's crust: 0.05 ppm

Figure 1 Cycle of iodine in nature.

iodine to move against its electrochemical gradient. Several anions, such as thiocyanate, perchlorate, and pertechnetate, inhibit this active transport. There is evidence that the active transport clearly demonstrated in the thyroid gland is also true for extra-thyroidal tissues, including the salivary glands, mammary glands, and gastric mucosa.

In addition to trapping iodine, follicular cells also synthesize the glycoprotein, thyroglobulin (Tg), from carbohydrates and amino acids (including tyrosine) obtained from the circulation. Thyroglobulin moves into the lumen of the follicle where it becomes available for hormone production. Thyroid peroxidase (TPO), a membrane-bound hem-containing glycoprotein, catalyzes the oxidation of the iodide to its active form, I_2, and the binding of this active form to the tyrosine in thyroglobulin to form mono- or diiodotyrosine (MIT or DIT). These in turn combine to form the thyroid hormones tri-iodothyronine (T_3) and thyroxine (T_4). Thyroglobulin is very concentrated in the follicles through a process of compaction, making the concentration of iodine in the thyroid gland very high. Only a very small proportion of the iodine remains as inorganic iodide, although even for this unbound iodide the concentration in the thyroid remains much greater than that in the circulation. This remarkable ability of the thyroid to concentrate and store iodine allows the gland to be very rapidly responsive to metabolic needs for thyroid hormones. **Figure 2** shows the structures of the molecules tyrosine and thyroxine.

Formation of thyroid hormones is not restricted to humans. Marine algae have an 'iodine pump' that facilitates concentration; invertebrates and all vertebrates demonstrate similar mechanisms to concentrate iodine and form iodotyrosines of various types. Although the function of these hormones in invertebrates is not clear, in vertebrates these iodine-containing substances are important for a variety of functions, such as metamorphosis in amphibians, spawning changes in fish, and general translation of genetic messages for protein synthesis.

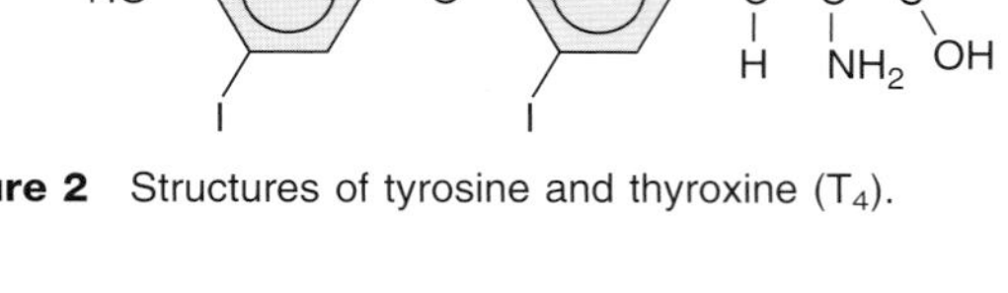

Metabolism and Excretion

Once iodine is 'captured' by the thyroid and thyroid hormones formed in the lumen of the follicles, stimulation of the gland causes release of the hormones into the circulation for uptake by peripheral tissues. Both production and release of the hormones are regulated in two ways. Stimulation is hormonally controlled by the hypothalamus of the brain through thyroid releasing hormone (TRH) which stimulates the pituitary gland to secrete thyroid stimulating hormone (TSH), which in turn stimulates the thyroid to release T_3 and T_4. In addition to the regulation of thyroid hormones by TSH, iodine itself plays a major role in autoregulation. The rate of uptake of iodine into the follicle, the ratio of T_3 to T_4, and the release of these into the circulation, among other things, are affected by the concentration of iodine in the gland. Thus, an increase in iodine intake causes a decrease in organification of iodine in the follicles and does not necessarily result in a corresponding increase in hormone release. Recent research suggests that this autoregulation is not entirely independent of TSH activity and that several other factors may contribute. However, regardless of the mechanism, these regulatory mechanisms allow for stability in hormone secretion in spite of wide variations in iodine intake.

When stimulated to release thyroid hormones, thyroglobulin is degraded through the activity of lysosomes and T_3 and T_4 are released and rapidly enter the circulation. Iodide freed in this reaction is for the most part recycled and the iodinated tyrosine reused for hormone production. Nearly all of the released hormones are rapidly bound to transport hormones, with 70% bound to thyroxine binding globulin (TBG). Other proteins, such as transthyretin (TTR), albumin, and lipoproteins, bind most of the remainder; with significant differences in the strengths of the affinity for the hormones, these proteins transport the hormones to different sites.

This remarkable ability of the thyroid to actively trap and store the iodine required creates a relatively steady state, with daily intake used to ensure full stores. T_4, with a longer half-life, serves as a reservoir for conversion to the more active hormone, T_3, with a much shorter half-life of 1 day. Target organs for thyroid hormone activity all play a role in the complex interplay between conversion of T_4 to T_3 deiodination, and metabolism of various other proteins involved with thyroid function. The liver,

Figure 2 Structures of tyrosine and thyroxine (T_4).

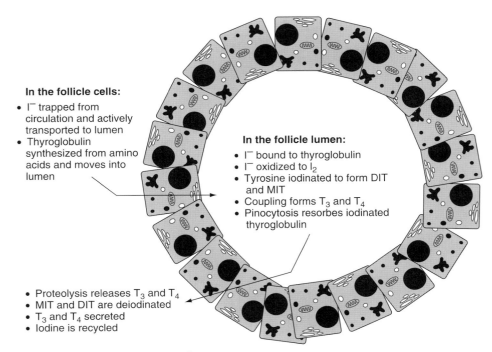

In the follicle cells:

- I⁻ trapped from circulation and actively transported to lumen
- Thyroglobulin synthesized from amino acids and moves into lumen

In the follicle lumen:

- I⁻ bound to thyroglobulin
- I⁻ oxidized to I_2
- Tyrosine iodinated to form DIT and MIT
- Coupling forms T_3 and T_4
- Pinocytosis resorbes iodinated thyroglobulin

- Proteolysis releases T_3 and T_4
- MIT and DIT are deiodinated
- T_3 and T_4 secreted
- Iodine is recycled

Figure 3 Thyroid follicle (courtesy of Kiely Houston).

which is estimated to contain 30% of the extrathyroidal T_4, is responsible, through the activity of the liver cell enzyme, deiodinase, for ensuring adequate supply of T_3 to peripheral tissues and degradation of metabolic by-products. The kidney demonstrates a strong ability to take up the iodothyronines. Iodine is ultimately excreted in the urine, with average daily excretion rates of approximately 100 µg per day. This accounts for the vast majority of iodine excretion, with negligible amounts excreted in feces. **Figure 3** illustrates a thyroid follicle and summarizes iodine transport.

Metabolic Functions

Separating the role of iodine from the complex and pervasive function of the thyroid gland is difficult since iodine is a critical component of the hormones that mediate these functions, and whatever other roles iodine may have are poorly understood. Thyroid hormones affect a wide range of physiological functions, from liver and kidney to heart and brain. Earlier work supported a role for thyroid hormones in affecting the energy generating capacity of cells through biochemical changes in mitochondria. More recent work has shown, however, that these hormones act on specific genetic receptors in cell nuclei, and perhaps through other extranuclear mechanisms. The nuclear receptors belong to a large family of receptors that bind other extranuclear molecules

including vitamins A and D and steroids. Through this interaction, along with a number of other proteins, thyroid hormones modify genetic expression. A great deal of research currently focuses on these thyroid hormone receptors, and the effect primarily of T_3 on the physiological function of the target organ through genetic transcription. These receptors are present in pituitary, liver, heart, kidney, and brain cells.

In the pituitary gland, thyroid hormones, along with many cofactors, regulate the synthesis and secretion of growth hormone by increasing gene transcription. Similarly, as part of the feedback loop for hormone regulation and release, thyroid hormones affect transcription of TSH in the pituitary. In cardiac and skeletal muscle, thyroid hormones affect production of the muscle tissue myosin in a variety of ways, depending on the stage of life and specific muscle tissue affected. In addition, the hormones affect muscle contraction through genetic alteration of calcium uptake within the cell. Carbohydrate metabolism and formation of certain fats (lipogenesis) are affected through hormone-induced changes in gene transcription in liver cells.

In the adult brain, receptors have been identified, but the specific genes affected by thyroid hormones have not yet been located. However, in the developing brain of the fetus and neonate, the effects of thyroid hormones are significant even though the

Table 2 Estimated iodine concentrations in selected organs

Total body	Thyroid gland	Brain	Liver	Blood
15–20 mg	8–12 mg (for a 15–25 g gland)	0.02 μg g^{-1} (wet weight)	0.2 μg g^{-1} (wet weight)	0.08–0.60 μg dl^{-1} (plasma inorganic iodide)

exact mechanisms are still not fully understood. The effects of thyroid hormones on brain development are suggested by failure in development of the nerve elements, failure of differentiation of cerebellar cells, and reduced development of other brain cells, in hypothyroid states. It is this early effect that has recently elevated the status of iodine from an element whose deficiency caused goitre to one whose deficiency is the leading cause of mental impairment worldwide.

In addition to these nuclear mechanisms, several alternative pathways have been suggested, some based on earlier historical studies. The thermogenic effects of thyroid hormones were originally felt to be a direct action on mitochondria, though this has recently been questioned. Thyroid hormones stimulate glucose transport, and again though originally attributed to a direct action on the plasma membrane, recent evidence suggests a genetic mechanism. There may also be a direct effect of thyroid hormones on brain enzymatic activity.

The overall effect of these cellular and systemic actions is to stimulate respiratory and other enzyme synthesis, which results in increased oxygen consumption and resultant increased basal metabolic rate. This affects heart rate, respiratory rate, mobilization of carbohydrates, cholesterol metabolism, and a wide variety of other physiological activities. In addition, thyroid hormones stimulate growth and development and, as noted earlier, are critical for the normal proliferation, growth, and development of brain cells. **Table 2** shows the estimated iodine concentration in selected organs.

Iodine Deficiency and Excess

Iodine Deficiency

Iodine deficiency is the most common cause of preventable mental retardation in the world. This fact, along with the recognition that iodine deficiency is not limited to remote rural populations, has stimulated agencies and governments to mobilize resources to eliminate this problem. This global effort, focusing primarily on iodization of salt for human and animal consumption, is slowly succeeding in eliminating a hidden set of disorders that have plagued mankind for centuries.

Unlike many nutritional deficiencies that are more directly related to socioeconomic status, insufficient intake of iodine is a geographical disease, related to lack of iodine in the environment. Iodine originally present in soil was subjected to leaching by snow and rain, and while a portion of the iodine in the oceans evaporates and is returned to the soil in rainwater, this amount is small. Thus, many areas have insufficient iodine in the environment, and this is reflected in plants grown in that environment. The diets in many developing countries are limited in variability and contain few processed foods. This places large populations at risk of iodine deficiency. The World Health Organization (WHO) estimates that at least 1572 million people are at risk in 118 countries, with 43 million affected by 'some degree of mental impairment.'

In the most simplistic physiological model, inadequate intake of iodine results in a reduction in thyroid hormone production, which stimulates increased TSH production. TSH acts directly on thyroid cells, and without the ability to increase hormone production, the gland becomes hyperplastic. In addition, iodine trapping becomes more efficient, as demonstrated by increased radioactive iodine uptake in deficient individuals. However, this simplistic model is complicated by complex adaptive mechanisms which vary depending on the age of the individual affected. In adults with mild deficiency, reduced intake causes a decrease in extrathyroidal iodine and reduced clearance, demonstrated by decreased urinary iodine excretion, but iodine concentration in the gland may remain within normal limits. With further reduction in intake, this adaptive mechanism is overwhelmed, and the iodine content of the thyroid decreases with alterations in iodination of thyroglobulin, in the ratio of DIT to MIT, and reduction in efficient thyroid hormone production. The ability to adapt appears to decrease with decreasing age, and in children the iodine pool in the thyroid is smaller, and the dynamics of iodine metabolism and peripheral use more rapid. In neonates, the effects of iodine deficiency are more directly reflected in increased TSH. Diminished thyroid iodine content and increased turnover make neonates the most vulnerable to the effects of iodine deficiency and decreased hormone production, even with mild deficiency.

A number of other factors influence iodine balance. Active transport of iodide is competitively inhibited by several compounds, including complex ions such as perchlorate, and by thiocyanate, a metabolic product of several foods. Other compounds, such as propylthiouracil, affect coupling reactions and iodination, doing so regardless of iodine intake, e.g., without blocking iodide transport. Several pharmaceuticals affect peripheral hormone action. Dietary goitrogens, as these compounds have been called, include cassava, lima beans, sweet potatoes, cabbage, and broccoli; these contain cyanide compounds that are detoxified to thiocyanate, which may inhibit iodide transport. Cabbage and turnips, and other plants of the genus *Brassica*, also contain thionamide compounds which block iodination. Certain industrial waste products, such as resorcinol from coal processing, contain phenols that cause irreversible inhibition of TPO and block iodination. In some countries the staple diet includes such goitrogens, and iodine deficiency may be exacerbated, as has been well documented for cassava. While this may be a significant problem in some geographical areas, in most instances adequate dietary iodine can reverse the goitrogenic effect.

The most important clinical effect of deficiency relates to the fact that thyroid hormone is required for the normal development of the brain in both humans and other animals. Numerous studies have demonstrated reduced psychomotor skills and intellectual development in the presence of iodine deficiency, and most experts now believe that there is a continuum of deficits, from mild impairment in IQ to severe mental retardation. Studies in China demonstrated shifts in IQ point distributions in rural communities that were deficient, suggesting an impact of deficiency of 10–15 IQ points. In Europe, where mild deficiency still exists, studies have demonstrated decreased psychomotor, perceptual integrative motor ability as well as lower verbal IQ scores in schoolchildren. Studies in Iran showed similar findings. A recent meta-analysis of 18 studies demonstrated a strong relationship, with an overall 13.5 IQ point difference between deficient and non deficient populations. These findings, coupled with the high prevalence of deficiency in many countries, have major implications for development.

The most severe effect of iodine deficiency is cretinism, which is rare in areas of mildly endemic deficiency but may have reached 5–10% or more in areas with severe deficiency. There are general classifications of cretinism, the symptoms of which frequently overlap. Neurological cretinism presents as extreme mental retardation, deaf-mutism, and impaired motor function including spastic gait.

Myxoedematous cretinism presents as disturbances of growth and development including short stature, coarse facial features, retarded sexual development, mental retardation, and other signs of hypothyroidism. It appears likely that severe deficiency resulting in decreased maternal T_4 may be responsible for the impaired neurological development of the fetus occurring early in pregnancy. The effect of deficiency on the fetus after 20 weeks' gestation may result in hyperstimulation of the developing fetal thyroid, with the extreme manifestation being thyroid failure causing myxoedematous cretinism. Other factors may affect thyroid hormone metabolism. Selenium deficiency, when present with iodine deficiency, may alter the clinical manifestations. Selenium deficiency decreases the activity of the enzyme, glutathione peroxidase (GPX), which, along with thyroid hormone synthesis, reduces hydrogen peroxide (H_2O_2). Combined with iodine deficiency and reduced hormone synthesis, it has been speculated that selenium deficiency may contribute to accumulation of H_2O_2 which may in turn lead to cell damage and contribute to thyroid failure. Selenium is also essential for the deiodinase enzyme activity affecting thyroid hormone catabolism, and deficiency may actually increase serum thyroxine. The balance between these two effects is still not fully understood. The study of cretinism has been critical to the evolution of our understanding of the critical role of iodine for normal mental development.

Iodine deficiency has a number of other effects, including development of goitre, clinical or subclinical hypothyroidism, decreased fertility rates, increased stillbirth and spontaneous abortion rates, and increased perinatal and infant mortality. This spectrum of clinical effects, collectively called 'iodine deficiency disorders,' underlines the importance of iodine in human health.

The most effective method to eliminate iodine deficiency in populations is through iodization of salt. The most classic success of salt iodization was demonstrated in Switzerland. Salt is universally consumed, and in most countries the amount consumed is relatively constant between 5 and 10 g per person per day. Iodine is usually added as iodide or iodate (which is more stable) to achieve 25–50 ppm iodine at consumption. This provides about 150–250 μg of iodine per person per day.

The challenge for national iodine deficiency elimination programs is to mobilize the various sectors that must be involved in a sustainable national program, including education, industry, health, and the political arena. There must be an appropriate regulatory environment, effective demand creation, adequate production to make iodized salt available, and quality assurance of both the product and all program elements to ensure that the program is sustained forever. Success in these efforts has the potential to have a greater impact on development than any public health program to date.

Iodine Excess

Iodine is used in many medications, food preservatives, and antiseptics with minimal adverse effects on populations. Pure iodine crystals are toxic, and ingestion can cause severe stomach irritation. Iodine is allergenic, and acute reactions to radiographic contrast media are not rare. Yet because of the thyroid's unique ability to regulate the body's iodine pool, quite a wide range in intake is tolerated without serious effects, particularly when the exposure is of limited duration.

When ingestion of iodine is in excess of the daily requirement of approximately 150 µg per day, changes in thyroid hormones can occur. A variety of clinical problems can occur, and these differ depending on the dose, the presence of thyroid disease, and whether the individual has been deficient in the past. In iodine-replete individuals without thyroid disease, goitre can result, and rarely, hypothyroidism, although the latter is more common in individuals with other illnesses such as lung disease or cystic fibrosis. The relationship of iodine excess to other diseases such as Hashimoto's thyroiditis remains controversial. In the US iodine levels were quite high from 1960 to 1980, with estimates for adult males as high as 827 µg per day. There was no immediate evidence of an impact on thyroid disease, although longer term longitudinal data are lacking. Effects usually remain subtle and transient, even with ingestion of up to 1500–4500 µg per day.

In the presence of thyroid disease, and in areas with endemic iodine deficiency, suddenly raising daily iodine intake may precipitate hyperthyroidism, and this has been the subject of some concern as salt iodization efforts proceed with fledgling quality assurance. This effect is felt to be related in part to autonomous nodules in the gland that synthesize and release excess thyroid hormone. The exact prevalence of iodine-induced hyperthyroidism in deficient areas is not clear. Many countries initiating salt iodization programs have reported increases in the incidence of toxic nodular goitre and iodine-induced thyrotoxicosis, usually in older people. While this may be a significant clinical problem, the risk is estimated to be between 0.01 and 0.06% and must be considered in the light of the benefit from correction of deficiency.

Assessment of Iodine Status

A standard set of indicators of iodine status has been established by the WHO in response to the need to determine prevalence in countries with endemic deficiency. These indicators reflect iodine status as mediated through the response of the thyroid gland to fluctuations in iodine intake. There are several additional indicators that are used to assess thyroid function, such as T_4 and T_3, but these are less accurate in reflecting iodine status since conversion of T_4 to T_3 and cellular uptake is so responsive to peripheral need.

Urinary iodine reflects iodine sufficiency, and output decreases with diminished intake. Since this indicator reflects the amount of iodine per unit volume of urine, its accuracy is impaired by variable fluid intake and factors affecting the concentration of the urine. Therefore, as a measure of iodine status in an individual, it is less accurate than as a measure of iodine status of a population. Median urinary iodine values are used extensively to assess population prevalence of iodine deficiency.

Thyroid size, either estimated by palpation or using ultrasound volume determination, reflects iodine status since deficiency results in thyroid enlargement, or goitre. Due to the relative ease of palpation, that measure has been a traditional standard to assess populations for iodine deficiency and has been particularly useful in schoolchildren. In adults, where long-standing thyroid enlargement from iodine deficiency may be minimally responsive to corrected iodine intake, palpation may be misleading and could overestimate the current level of iodine sufficiency. In children, palpation becomes increasingly difficult and significantly less accurate when deficiency is mild. Ultrasound volume determination provides a more accurate estimate of thyroid size. For any measure of thyroid size, other factors besides iodine deficiency can cause enlargement, including iodine excess, carcinoma, and infection. In areas of the world where deficiency is a problem, the prevalence of these other diseases compared with goitre from iodine deficiency is negligible.

TSH is produced in response to decreased iodine intake and diminished thyroid hormone production and is used as a measure of iodine status. TSH is best measured in neonates—in the developed world for surveillance against congenital hypothyroidism, and in endemic countries to estimate the magnitude of iodine deficiency. Neonatal TSH has been a useful advocacy tool to demonstrate to policy makers that iodine deficiency is not limited to rural remote populations but affects children born in big city

Table 3 WHO criteria for iodine deficiency as a public health problem in populations

Indicator	Population assessed	Mild deficiency (%)	Severe deficiency (%)
Goitre by palpation	Schoolchildren	5–19.9	≥30
Thyroid volume by ultrasound (>97th percentile)	Schoolchildren	5–19.9	≥30
Median urinary iodine ($\mu g\,l^{-1}$)	Schoolchildren	50–99	<20
TSH (>5 mU l^{-1} whole blood)	Neonates	3–19.9	≥40

Table 4 Recommended dietary intake

Age	WHO recommended intake (μg per day)	US RDA 1989 (μg per day)
0–6 months	40	40
6–12 months	50	60 (at age 1 year)
1–10 years	70–120	60–120
11 years–adult	120–150	150
Pregnancy	175	175
Lactation	200	200

hospitals. However, with the complexity of the interactions between TSH and other hormones, TSH has not been shown to be as useful in older children or adults in estimating prevalence of iodine deficiency. Also, use of iodine containing antiseptics affects TSH distributions in neonates.

Uptake of radioactive iodine isotopes can be used to scan the gland, and determine the affinity of the gland to introduced iodine, and is a measure of deficiency. The most common isotope used is ^{123}I because of its relatively short 13-h half-life and γ photon emission. Uptake is increased in iodine deficiency. Isotopes can also be used to examine the organification of iodine in the formation of thyroid hormones. This is an impractical method for surveying populations. **Table 3** provides the WHO criteria for defining iodine deficiency as a public health problem.

Requirements and Dietary Sources

The daily requirement for iodine in humans has been estimated based on daily losses, iodine balance, and turnover, with most studies ranging from 40 to 200 μg per day, depending on age and metabolic needs, as shown in **Table 4**.

Natural sources of iodine include seafood, seaweeds, and smaller amounts from crops grown on soil with sufficient iodine, or from meat where livestock has grazed on such soil. The contribution of the latter two is small, and in most countries other sources are required. Iodine added to salt, as noted above, is the primary source for many populations. **Table 5** shows sample iodine content for various sources.

In the US and Britain, as well as in other developed countries, most dietary iodine comes from food processing. Intake can vary, as illustrated in **Table 6**. Iodophors used as antiseptics in the dairy and baking industries provide residual iodine in milk and processed foods. In addition, iodine is present in several vitamin and pharmaceutical preparations.

Iodine as a trace element in low concentrations in most environments plays a critical role in the normal growth and development of many species. In humans, iodine is critical for brain development and correction of global deficiencies is an unparalleled opportunity to improve the well-being of our global community.

Table 6 Iodine intake from average US and British diets

Country	Milk (μg per day)	Grains (μg per day)	Meat, fish, and poultry (μg per day)
US	534	152	103
Britain	92	31	36

Table 5 Sample iodine content for various sources

Water	Cabbage	Eggs	Seafood	Sugar	Iodized salt
0.1–2 $\mu g\,l^{-1}$ in endemic area	0–0.95 $\mu g\,g^{-1}$	4–10 μg egg^{-1}	300–3000 $\mu g\,kg^{-1}$	<1 $\mu g\,kg^{-1}$ in refined sugar	20–50 ppm (at household level, depending on climate, and currently subject to review)
2–15 $\mu g\,l^{-1}$ in nonendemic area				30 $\mu g\,kg^{-1}$ in unrefined brown sugar	

See also: **Fruits and Vegetables**. **Iodine**: Deficiency Disorders. **Legumes**.

Further Reading

Braverman LE and Utiger RD (eds.) (1996) *Werner and Ingbar's The Thyroid, A Fundamental and Clinical Text*. Philadelphia: Lippincott-Raven.

Burgi H, Supersaxo Z, and Selz B (1990) Iodine deficiency diseases in Switzerland one hundred years after Theodor Kocher's survey: A historical review with some new goitre prevalence data. *Acta Endocrinologica (Copenhagen)* **123**: 577–590.

Gaitan E (1990) Goitrogens in food and water. *Annual Review of Nutrition* **10**: 21–39.

Hall R and Kobberling J (1985) *Thyroid Disorders Associated with Iodine Deficiency and Excess*. New York: Raven Press.

Hetzel BS (1994) Iodine deficiency and fetal brain damage. *New England Journal of Medicine* **331**(26): 1770–1771.

Hetzel BS (1989) In *The Story of Iodine Deficiency: An International Challenge in Nutrition*. Oxford: Oxford University Press.

Hetzel BS and Pandav CS (eds.) (1994) *SOS for a Billion—The Conquest of Iodine Deficiency Disorders*. Delhi: Oxford University Press.

Mertz W (1986) *Trace Elements in Human and Animal Nutrition*, 5th edn. New York: Academic Press.

Patai S and Rappoport Z (eds.) (1995) *The Chemistry of Halides, Pseudo-halides and Azides*, Supplement D2: part 2. New York: John Wiley & Sons.

Stanbury JB (ed.) (1994) *The Damaged Brain of Iodine Deficiency*. New York: Cognizant Communication Corporation, The Franklin Institute.

Sullivan KM, Houston RM, Gorstein J, and Cervinskas J (1995) *Monitoring Universal Salt Iodization Programmes* Ottowa: UNICEF, MI, ICCIDD, WHO publication.

Thorpe-Beeston JG and Nicolaides KH (1996) *Maternal and Fetal Thyroid Function in Pregnancy* New York: The Parthenon Publishing Group.

Todd CH, Allain T, Gomo ZAR et al. (1995) Increase in thyrotoxicosis associated with iodine supplements in Zimbabwe. *Lancet* **346**: 1563–1564.

Troncone L, Shapiro B, Satta MA, and Monaco F (1994) *Thyroid Diseases: Basic Science Pathology, Clinical and Laboratory Diagnosis*. Boca Raton: CRC Press.

WHO, UNICEF, and ICCIDD (1994) *Indicators for Assessing Iodine Deficiency Disorders and Their Control through Salt Iodization*, (limited publication). Geneva: WHO, UNICEF, ICCID.

Wilson JD and Foster DW (eds.) (1992) *Williams Textbook of Endocrinology*. Philadelphia: WB Saunders.

Deficiency Disorders

B S Hetzel, Women's and Children's Hospital, North Adelaide, SA, Australia

Iodine deficiency is discussed as a risk factor for the growth and development of up to 2.2 million people living in iodine-deficient environments in 130 countries throughout the world. The effects of iodine deficiency on growth and development, called the iodine deficiency disorders (IDD), comprise goiter (enlarged thyroid gland), stillbirths and miscarriages, neonatal and juvenile thyroid deficiency, dwarfism, mental defects, deaf mutism, and spastic weakness and paralysis, as well as lesser degrees of loss of physical and mental function.

Iodine deficiency is now accepted by the World Health Organization as the most common preventable cause of brain damage in the world today.

Since 1990, a major international health program to eliminate iodine deficiency has developed that uses iodized salt. The progress of this program and the continuing challenge are discussed as a great opportunity for the elimination of a noninfectious disease, which is quantitatively a greater scourge than the infectious diseases of smallpox and polio.

History

The first records of goiter and cretinism date back to ancient civilizations, the Chinese and Hindu cultures and then to Greece and Rome. In the Middle Ages, goitrous cretins appeared in the pictorial art, often as angels or demons. The first detailed descriptions of these subjects occurred in the Renaissance. The paintings of the madonnas in Italy so commonly showed goiter that the condition must have been regarded as virtually normal. In the seventeenth and eighteenth centuries, scientific studies multiplied and the first recorded mention of the word 'cretin' appeared in Diderot's *Encyclopédie* in 1754. The nineteenth century marked the beginning of serious attempts to control the problem; however, not until the latter half of the twentieth century was the necessary knowledge for effective prevention acquired.

Mass prophylaxis of goiter with iodized salt was first introduced in Switzerland and in Michigan in the United States. In Switzerland, the widespread occurrence of a severe form of mental deficiency and deaf mutism (endemic cretinism) was a heavy charge on public funds. However, following the introduction of iodized salt, goiter incidence declined rapidly and cretins were no longer born. Goiter also disappeared from army recruits.

A further major development was the administration of injections of iodized oil to correct iodine deficiency in Papua New Guinea for people living in inaccessible mountain villages. These long-lasting injections corrected iodine deficiency and prevented goiter for 3–5 years, depending on the dosage.

Subsequently, the prevention of cretinism and stillbirths was demonstrated by the administration of iodized oil before pregnancy in a controlled trial in the Highlands of Papua New Guinea. This proved the causal role of iodine deficiency.

To further establish the relation between iodine deficiency and fetal brain development, an animal model was developed in the pregnant sheep given an iodine-deficient diet. Subsequently, similar models were developed in the primate marmoset monkey and in the rat.

Studies with animal models confirmed the effect of iodine deficiency on fetal brain development (as already indicated by the results of the field trial with iodized oil in Papua New Guinea). The combination of the controlled human trials and the results of the studies in animal models clearly indicated that prevention was possible by correction of the iodine deficiency before pregnancy.

This work led Hetzel to propose the concept of the IDD resulting from all the effects of iodine deficiency on growth and development, particularly brain development, in an exposed population that can be prevented by correction of the iodine deficiency. Iodine deficiency is now recognized by the World Health Organization (WHO) as the most common form of preventable mental defect.

Although the major prevalence of iodine deficiency is in developing countries, the problem continues to be very significant in many European countries (France, Italy, Germany, Greece, Poland, Romania, Spain, and Turkey) because of the threat to brain development in the fetus and young infant.

Ecology of Iodine Deficiency

There is a cycle of iodine in nature. Most of the iodine resides in the ocean. It was present during the primordial development of the earth, but large amounts were leached from the surface soil by glaciation, snow, or rain and were carried by wind, rivers, and floods into the sea. Iodine occurs in the deeper layers of the soil and is found in oil well and natural gas effluents, which are now a major source for the production of iodine.

The better known areas that are leached are the mountainous areas of the world. The most severely deficient soils are those of the European Alps, the Himalayas, the Andes, and the vast mountains of China. However, iodine deficiency is likely to occur to some extent in all elevated regions subject to glaciation and higher rainfall, with runoff into rivers. It has become clear that iodine deficiency also occurs in flooded river valleys, such as the Ganges in India, the Mekong in Vietnam, and the great river valleys of China.

Iodine occurs in soil and the sea as iodide. Iodide ions are oxidized by sunlight to elemental iodine,

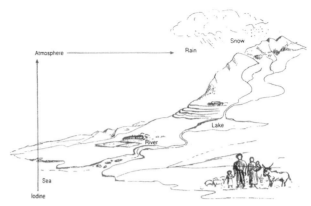

Figure 1 The iodine cycle in nature. The atmosphere absorbs iodine from the sea, which then returns through rain and snow to mountainous regions. It is then carried by rivers to the lower hills and plains, eventually returning to the sea. High rainfall, snow, and flooding increase the loss of soil iodine, which has often been already denuded by past glaciation. This causes the low iodine content of food for man and animals. (Reproduced from Hetzel BS (1989) *The Story of Iodine Deficiency: An international Challenge in Nutrition.* Oxford: Oxford University Press.)

which is volatile so that every year approximately 400,000 tons of iodine escapes from the surface of the sea. The concentration of iodide in the seawater is approximately $50–60\,\mu g/l$, and in the air it is approximately $0.7\,\mu g/m^3$. The iodine in the atmosphere is returned to the soil by rain, which has a concentration of $1.8–8.5\,\mu g/l$. In this way, the cycle is completed (**Figure 1**).

However, the return of iodine is slow and the amount is small compared to the original loss of iodine, and subsequent repeated flooding ensures the continuity of iodine deficiency in the soil. Hence, no natural correction can take place and iodine deficiency persists in the soil indefinitely. All crops grown in these soils will be iodine deficient. The iodine content of plants grown in iodine-deficient soils may be as low as $10\,\mu g/kg$ compared to $1\,mg/kg$ dry weight in plants in a non-iodine-deficient soil.

As a result, human and animal populations that are totally dependent on food grown in such soil become iodine deficient. This accounts for the occurrence of severe iodine deficiency in vast populations in Asia that live within systems of subsistence agriculture in flooded river valleys (India, Bangladesh, Burma, Vietnam, and China).

Iodine Deficiency Disorders

The effects of iodine deficiency on the growth and development of a population that can be prevented by correction of iodine deficiency, denoted by the term IDD, are evident at all stages, including

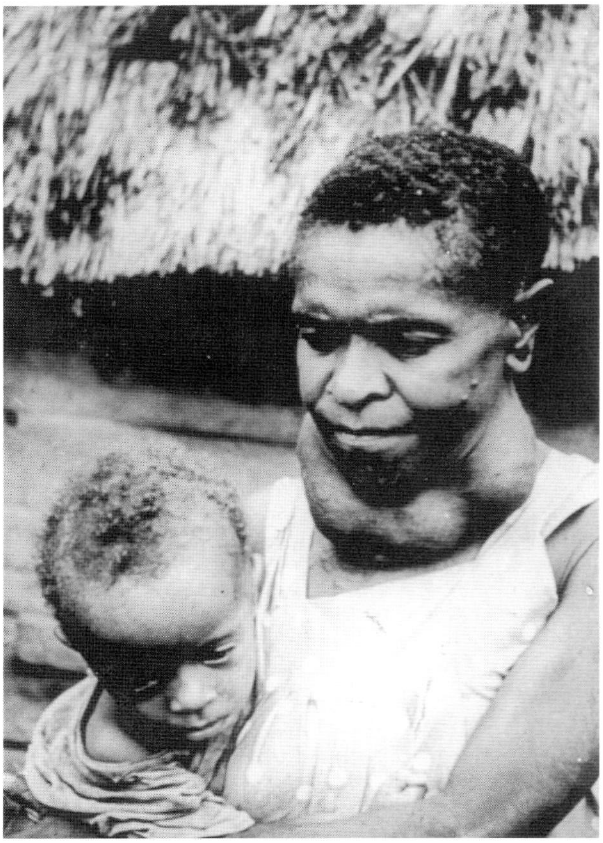

Figure 2 A mother and child from a New Guinea village who are severely iodine deficient. The mother has a large goiter and the child is also affected. The larger the goiter, the more likely it is that she will have a cretin child. This can be prevented by eliminating the iodine deficiency before the onset of pregnancy. (Reproduced from Hetzel BS and Pandav CS (eds.) (1996) *SOS for a Billion: The Conquest of Iodine Deficiency Disorders*, 2nd edn. Oxford: Oxford University Press.)

particularly the fetus, the neonate, and in infancy, which are periods of rapid brain growth. The term goiter has been used for many years to describe the enlarged thyroid gland caused by iodine deficiency (**Figure 2**). Goiter is indeed the obvious and familiar feature of iodine deficiency, but knowledge of the effects of iodine deficiency on brain development has greatly expanded in the past 30 years so that the term IDD was introduced to refer to all the effects of iodine deficiency on growth and development, particularly brain development, in a population that can be prevented by correction of the deficiency (**Table 1**).

The following sections discuss in detail the IDD at various stages of life: the fetus, the neonate, the child and adolescent, and the adult (**Table 1**).

The Fetus

Iodine deficiency of the fetus is the result of iodine deficiency in the mother (**Figure 2**). The condition is

Table 1 Spectrum of Iodine Deficiency Disorders

Fetus	Abortions
	Stillbirths
	Congenital anomalies
	Neurological cretinism
	Mental deficiency, deaf mutism, spastic diplegia, squint
	Hypothyroid cretinism
	Mental deficiency, dwarfism, hypothyroidism
	Psychomotor defects
Neonate	Increased perinatal mortality
	Neonatal hypothyroidism
	Retarded mental and physical development
Child and adolescent	Increased infant mortality
	Retarded mental and physical development
Adult	Goiter with its complications
	Iodine-induced hyperthyroidism
All ages	Goiter
	Hypothyroidism
	Impaired mental function
	Increased susceptibility to nuclear radiation

Reproduced with permission from Oxford University Press and the World Health Organization, WHO/UNICEF/ICCIDD (2001).

associated with a greater incidence of stillbirths, abortions, and congenital abnormalities, which can be prevented by iodization.

Another major effect of fetal iodine deficiency is the condition of endemic cretinism, which is quite distinct from the condition of sporadic cretinism or congenital hypothyroidism due to a small or absent thyroid gland.

Endemic cretinism-associated with an iodine intake of less than 25 μg per day, in contrast to a normal intake of 100–150 μg per day, has been widely prevalent, affecting up to 10% of populations living in severely iodine-deficient regions in India, Indonesia, and China. In its most common form, it is characterized by mental deficiency, deaf mutism, and spastic diplegia (**Figure 3**). This form of cretinism is referred to as the nervous or neurological type, in contrast to the less common hypothyroid or myxedematous type characterized by hypothyroidism with dwarfism (**Figure 4**).

In addition to Asia, cretinism also occurs in Africa, (Zaire, now the Republic of the Congo), South America in the Andean region (Ecuador, Peru, Bolivia, and Argentina), and the more remote areas of Europe. In all these areas, with the exception of the Congo, neurological features are predominant. In the Congo, the hypothyroid form is more common, probably due to the high intake of the root vegetable cassava, which contains substances inhibiting the function of the thyroid gland.

However, there is considerable variation in the clinical manifestations of neurological cretinism,

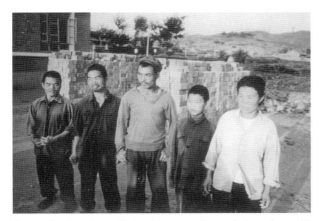

Figure 3 A mother with her four sons, three of whom (ages 31, 29, and 28 years) are cretins born before iodized salt was introduced, and the fourth is normal (age 14 years), born after iodized salt became available in Chengde, China. (Reproduced from Hetzel BS and Pandav CS (eds.) (1996) *SOS for a Billion: The Conquest of Iodine Deficiency Disorders*, 2nd edn. Oxford: Oxford University Press.)

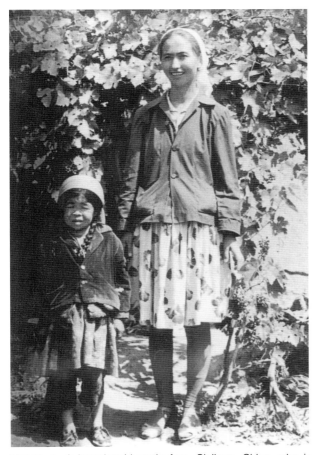

Figure 4 A hypothyroid cretin from Sinjiang, China, who is also deaf mute. This condition is completely preventable. (Right) The barefoot doctor of her village. Both are approximately 35 years old. (Reproduced from Hetzel BS (1989) *The Story of Iodine Deficiency: An international Challenge in Nutrition*. Oxford: Oxford University Press.)

which include isolated deaf mutism and mental defect of varying degrees. In China, the term cretinoid is used to describe these individuals, who may number 5–10 times those with overt cretinism.

The Neonate

Apart from the question of mortality, the importance of the state of thyroid function in the neonate relates to the fact that at birth the brain of the human infant has only reached approximately one-third of its full size and continues to grow rapidly until the end of the second year. The thyroid hormone, dependent on an adequate supply of iodine, is essential for normal brain development, as has been confirmed by animal studies.

Data on iodine nutrition and neonatal thyroid function in Europe confirm the continuing presence of severe iodine deficiency. This affects neonatal thyroid function and hence represents a threat to early brain development. These data have raised great concern about iodine deficiency, which is also heightened by awareness of the hazard of nuclear radiation with carcinogenic effects following the Chernobyl disaster in the former Soviet Union (**Table 1**).

These observations of neonatal hypothyroidism indicate a much greater risk of mental defects in iodine-deficient populations than is indicated by the presence of cretinism. Apart from the developing world, there has been a continuing major problem in many European countries, such as Italy, Germany, France, and Greece, and Romania, Bulgaria, and Albania still have very severe iodine deficiency with overt cretinism.

The Child

Iodine deficiency in children is characteristically associated with goiter. The goiter rate increases with age and reaches a maximum at adolescence. Girls have a higher prevalence than boys. Goiter rates in schoolchildren over the years provide a useful indication of the presence of iodine deficiency in a community.

In a review of 18 studies, a comparison was made between IQ scores in iodine-deficient children and carefully selected control groups. The iodine-deficient group had a mean IQ that was 13.5 points lower than that of the non-iodine-deficient control group. Detailed individual studies demonstrating these defects in Italian and Spanish schoolchildren as well as those from Africa, China, Indonesia, and Papua New Guinea have been published. There is a serious problem in Europe as well as in many developing countries.

The Adult

Long-standing large goiter may require surgery to reduce pressure in the neck. Long-standing goiter may also be associated with iodine-induced hyperthyroidism (IIH) due to an increase in iodine intake. IIH is associated with nervousness, sweating, and tremor, with loss of weight due to excessive levels of circulating thyroid hormone. This condition no longer occurs following correction of iodine deficiency and therefore is within the spectrum of IDD.

In northern India, a high degree of apathy has been noted in whole populations living in iodine-deficient areas. This may even affect domestic animals such as dogs. It is apparent that reduced mental function is widely prevalent in iodine-deficient communities, with effects on their capacity for initiative and decision making. This is due to the effect of hypothyroidism on brain function. This condition can be readily reversed by correction of the iodine deficiency, unlike the effects on the fetus and in infancy, so that villages can come to life.

Thus, iodine deficiency is a major block to the human and social development of communities living in an iodine-deficient environment. Correction of the iodine deficiency is indicated as a major contribution to economic development. An increase in physical and mental energy leads to improved work output, improved learning by children, and improved quality of life. Improved livestock productivity (chickens, cattle, and sheep) is also a major economic benefit.

Magnitude of the Problem

The number of cases of IDD throughout the world was estimated by WHO in 1990 to be 1.6 billion, including more than 200 million cases with goiter and more than 20 million cases with some degree of brain damage due to the effects of iodine deficiency in pregnancy. Recent estimates of the population at risk have been increased to 2.2 billion, with the recognition that even mild iodine deficiency in the mother has effects on the fetus. There are now estimated to be 130 IDD-affected countries, including the most populous: Bangladesh, Brazil, China, India, Indonesia, and Nigeria. Therefore, there is a global scourge of great magnitude, which provides one of the major challenges in international health today.

Correction of Iodine Deficiency

Iodized Salt

Since the successful introduction of iodized salt in Switzerland and the United States in the 1920s, successful programs have been reported from a number of countries, including those in Central and South America (e.g., Guatemala and Colombia) and Finland and Taiwan. However, there has been great difficulty in sustaining these programs in Central and South America mainly due to political instability. Following the breakup of the Soviet Union, iodine deficiency recurred in the Central Asian republics.

The difficulties in the production and quality maintenance of iodized salt for the millions who are iodine deficient, especially in Asia, were vividly demonstrated in India, where there was a breakdown in supply. These difficulties led to the adoption of universal salt iodization (USI) for India and subsequently for many other countries. This policy includes legislation to provide for compulsory iodization of all salt for human and animal consumption, and this legislation makes it illegal for noniodized salt to be available for human or animal consumption.

In Asia, the cost of iodized salt production and distribution is on the order of 3–5 cents per person per year. This must be considered cheap in relation to the social benefits that have already been described.

However, there is still the problem of the iodine in the salt actually reaching the iodine-deficient subject. There may be a problem with distribution or preservation of the iodine content: It may be left uncovered or exposed to heat. Thus, it should be added after cooking to reduce the loss of iodine.

Potassium iodate is the preferred vehicle compared to potassium iodide because of its greater stability in the tropical environment. A dose of 20–40 mg iodine as potassium iodate per kilo is recommended to cover losses to ensure an adequate household level. This assumes a salt intake of 10 g per day; if the level is below this, then an appropriate correction can readily be made by increasing the concentration of potassium iodate.

Iodized Oil

Iodized oil by injection or by mouth is singularly appropriate for isolated communities characteristic of mountainous endemic goiter areas. The striking regression of goiter following iodized oil administration, with improved well-being from correction of hypothyroidism, ensures general acceptance of the measure (**Figure 5**).

Iodized oil is more expensive than iodized salt but is used especially for severe iodine deficiency in remote areas. It provides instant correction of the deficiency and the consequent prevention of brain damage.

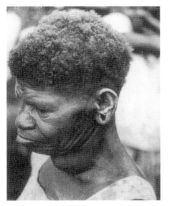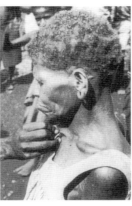

Figure 5 Subsidence of goiter in a New Guinea woman 3 months after the injection of iodized oil. This is accompanied by a feeling of well-being due to a rise in the level of the thyroid hormone in the blood. This makes the injections very popular. (Reproduced from Hetzel BS (1989) *The Story of Iodine Deficiency: An international Challenge in Nutrition*. Oxford: Oxford University Press.)

In a suitable area, the oil (1 ml contains 480 mg iodine) should be administered to all females up to the age of 40 years and all males up to the age of 20 years. A dose of 480 mg will provide coverage for 1 year by mouth and for 2 years by injection.

Iodized Milk

This is particularly important for infants receiving formula milk as an alternative to breast-feeding. An increase in levels from 5 to 10 μg/dl has been recommended for full-term infants and 20 μg/dl for premature infants. However, breast-fed infants will be iodine deficient if the mother is iodine deficient.

Iodized milk has been available in the United States, the United Kingdom and Northern Europe, Australia, and New Zealand as a result of the addition of iodophors as disinfectants by the dairy industry. This has been a major factor in the elimination of iodine deficiency in these countries. However, in most countries of Southern Europe and Eastern Europe, this has not occurred and the risk of iodine deficiency continues. Recently, the use of iodophors has been phased out, with a substantial decrease in the level of urine iodine excretion. Recurrence of iodine deficiency has been confirmed in Australia and New Zealand.

The Role of the United Nations

In 1990 the United Nations Sub-Committee on Nutrition recognized IDD as a major international public health problem and adopted a global plan for the elimination of IDD by the year 2000 proposed by the International Council for Control of Iodine Deficiency Disorders (ICCIDD) working in close collaboration with UNICEF and WHO.

The ICCIDD, founded in 1986, is an independent multidisciplinary expert group of more than 700 professionals in public health, medical, and nutritional science, technologists, and planners from more than 90 countries.

In 1990, the World Health Assembly and the World Summit for Children both accepted the goal of elimination of IDD as a public health problem by the year 2000. These major meetings included government representatives, including heads of state at the World Summit for Children, from 71 countries, and an additional 88 countries signed the plan of action for elimination of IDD as well as other major problems in nutrition and health.

Since 1989, a series of joint WHO/UNICEF/ICCIDD regional meetings have been held to assist countries with their national programs for the elimination of IDD. The impact of these meetings has been that governments now better realize the importance of iodine deficiency to the future potential of their people.

A dramatic example is provided by the government of the People's Republic of China. As is well-known, China has a one child per family policy, which means that an avoidable hazard such as iodine deficiency should be eliminated. In China, iodine deficiency is a threat to 40% of the population due to the highly mountainous terrain and flooded river valleys—in excess of 400 million people at risk. In recognition of this massive threat to the Chinese people, in 1993 the government held a national advocacy meeting in the Great Hall of the People sponsored by the Chinese Premier, Li Peng. The commitment of the government to the elimination of iodine deficiency was emphasized by Vice Premier Zhu Rongyi to the assembly of provincial delegations led by the provincial governors and the representatives of international agencies.

In 1998, an international workshop was held in Beijing by the Ministry of Health of China with the ICCIDD. Dramatic progress was reported, as indicated by a reduction in mean goiter rate (from 20 to 10%) with normal urine iodine levels. Severe iodine deficiency has persisted in Tibet due to difficulty in the implementation of salt iodization. In other provinces, excess iodine intake was noted in 10% of the population. The need for continuation of monitoring with urine iodine was emphasized at the meeting. Tibet is now receiving special assistance with a program supported by WHO, UNICEF, and the Australian Aid Program (AusAID).

Elimination of Iodine Deficiency Disorders at the Country Level

It is now recognized that an effective national program for the elimination of IDD requires a multisectoral approach as shown in **Figure 6**, which provides a model in the form of a wheel.

This wheel model represents the continuous feedback process involved in the national IDD control (elimination) program. All actors in the program need to understand the whole social process. The wheel must keep turning to maintain an effective program.

The wheel model also shows the social process involved in a national IDD control program. The successful achievement of this process requires the establishment of a national IDD control commission, with full political and legislative authority to carry out the program.

The program consists of the following components:

1. Assessment of the situation requires baseline IDD prevalence surveys, including measurement of urinary iodine levels and an analysis of the salt economy.
2. Dissemination of findings implies communication to health professionals and the public so that there is complete understanding of the IDD problem and the potential benefits of elimination of the most common preventable cause of brain damage.
3. Development of a plan of action includes the establishment of an intersectoral task force on IDD and the formulation of a strategy document on achieving the elimination of IDD.

4. Achieving political will requires intensive education and lobbying of politicians and other opinion leaders.
5. Implementation requires the complete involvement of the salt industry. Special measures, such as negotiations for monitoring and quality control of imported iodized salt, will be required. It will also be necessary to ensure that iodized salt delivery systems reach all affected populations, including the neediest. In addition, the establishment of cooperatives for small producers, or restructuring to larger units of production, may be needed. Implementation will require training in management, salt technology, laboratory methods, and communication at all levels.

   In addition, a community education campaign is required to educate all age groups about the effects of iodine deficiency, with particular emphasis on the brain.
6. Monitoring and evaluation require the establishment of an efficient system for the collection of relevant scientific data on salt iodine content and urinary iodine levels. This includes suitable laboratory facilities.

Striking progress with USI has occurred, as indicated by the WHO/UNICEF/ICCIDD report to the 1999 World Health Assembly. Data show that of 5 billion people living in countries with IDD, 68% now have access to iodized salt. Of the 130 IDD-affected countries, it was reported that 105 (81%) had an intersectoral coordinating body and 98 (75%) had legislation in place.

Criteria for tracking progress toward the goal of elimination of IDD have been agreed on by ICCIDD, WHO, and UNICEF. These include salt iodine (90% effectively iodized) and urine iodine in the normal range (median excretion, 100–200 µg/l).

The major challenge is not only the achievement but also the sustainability of effective salt iodization. In the past, a number of countries have achieved effective salt iodization, but in the absence of monitoring the program lapsed with recurrence of IDD. To this end, ICCIDD, WHO, and UNICEF offer help to governments with partnership evaluation to assess progress toward the goal and also provide help to overcome any bottlenecks obstructing progress.

The Global Partnership

Since 1990, a remarkable informal global partnership has come together composed of the people and countries with an IDD problem, international agencies (particularly UNICEF, WHO, and

Wheel model for IDD Elimination Program

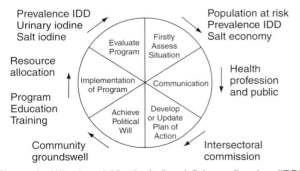

Prevalence IDD
Urinary iodine
Salt iodine

Population at risk
Prevalence IDD
Salt economy

Resource
allocation

Evaluate Program

Firstly Assess Situation

Implementation of Program

Communication

Health profession and public

Program
Education
Training

Achieve Political Will

Develop or Update Plan of Action

Community
groundswell

Intersectoral
commission

Figure 6 Wheel model for the iodine deficiency disorders (IDD) elimination program. The model shows the social process involved in a national IDD control program. The successful achievement of this process requires the establishment of a national IDD control commission, with full political and legislative authority to carry out the program. (Reproduced from Hetzel BS (1989) *The Story of Iodine Deficiency: An international Challenge in Nutrition.* Oxford: Oxford University Press.)

ICCIDD), bilateral aid agencies (Australia (AusAID) and Canada (CIDA)), the salt industry (including the private sector), and Kiwanis International. Kiwanis International is a world service club with 500,000 members throughout the world that has achieved a fundraising target of $75 million toward the elimination of IDD through UNICEF.

This partnership exists to support countries and governments in their elimination of IDD.

A more recent development is the establishment of the Global Network for the Sustainable Elimination of Iodine Deficiency, in collaboration with the salt industry.

The achievement of the global elimination of iodine deficiency will be a great triumph in international health in the field of noninfectious disease, ranking with the eradication of the infectious diseases smallpox and polio.

However, the goal of elimination is a continuing challenge. Sustained political will at both the people and the government level is necessary to bring the benefits to the many millions who suffer the effects of iodine deficiency.

Nomenclature

Endemic Occurrence of a disease confined to a community

Endemic Cretinism A state resulting from the loss of function of the maternal thyroid gland due to iodine deficiency during pregnancy characterised by mental defect, deaf-mutism and spastic paralysis in its fully developed form

Goiter An enlarged thyroid gland most commonly due to iodine deficiency in the diet

Hypothyroidism The result of a lowered level of circulating thyroid hormone causing loss of mental and physical energy

Hyperthyroidism The result of excessive circulating thyroid hormone with nervousness, sweating, tremor, with a rapid heart rate and loss of weight

ICCIDD International Council for Control of Iodine Deficiency Disorders-an international non-government organization made up of a network of 700 health professionals from more than 90 countries available to assist IDD elimination programs in affected countries

IDD Iodine Deficiency Disorders referring to all the effects of iodine deficiency in a population that can be prevented by correction of the iodine deficiency

IIH Iodine Induced Hyperthyroidism-due to increase in iodine intake following long standing iodine deficiency. The condition is transient and no longer occurs following correction of iodine deficiency

Iodization The general term covering fortification programs using various agents (iodide, iodate) or various vehicles (salt, oil, bread and water)

Iodized Oil Iodine in poppy seed oil-lipiodol is extensively used in radiology as a radio-contrast medium to demonstrate holes (cavities) in the lung. Available both by injection (lipiodol) and by mouth (oriodol) for the instant correction of iodine deficiency

Iodized Salt Salt to which potassium iodate or potassium iodide has been added at a recommended level of 20–40 milligrams of iodine per kilogram of salt

Kiwanis International A World Service Group including more than 10,000 clubs and over 500,000 members based in the USA

Thyroid size Measured by ultrasound-a much more sensitive and reproducible measurement than is possible by palpation of the thyroid

Thyroxine Thyroid Hormone (T_4) an amino acid which includes four iodine atoms

Triiodothyronine A more rapidly active thyroid hormone (T_3) which includes 3 iodine atoms on the amino acid molecule

UNICEF United Nations Children's Fund

USI Universal Salt Iodization-iodization of all salt for human and animal consumption which requires legislation and has been adopted by a number of countries

WHO World Health Organization-the expert group on health within the UN System

See also: **Food Fortification**: Developing Countries. **Iodine**: Physiology, Dietary Sources and Requirements. **Supplementation**: Role of Micronutrient Supplementation. **World Health Organization**.

Further Reading

Buttfield IH and Hetzel BS (1967) Endemic goiter in Eastern New Guinea with special reference to the use of iodized oil in prophylaxis and treatment. *Bulletin of the World Health Organization* 36: 243–262.

Delange F, Dunn JT, and Glinoer D (eds.) (1993) *Iodine Deficiency in Europe: A Continuing Concern*, NATO ASI Series A: Life Sciences vol. 241. New York: Plenum.

Hetzel BS (1983) Iodine deficiency disorders (IDD) and their eradication. *Lancet* 2: 1126–1129.

Hetzel BS (1989) *The Story of Iodine Deficiency: An International Challenge in Nutrition*. Oxford: Oxford University Press.

Hetzel BS and Pandav CS (eds.) (1996) *SOS for a Billion: The Conquest of Iodine Deficiency Disorders*, 2nd edn. Oxford: Oxford University Press.

Hetzel BS, Pandav CS, Dunn JT, Ling J, and Delange F (2004) *The Global Program for the Elimination of Brain Damage Due to Iodine Deficiency*. Oxford: Oxford University Press.

Ma T, Lu T, Tan U et al. (1982) The present status of endemic goiter and endemic cretinism in China. *Food and Nutrition Bulletin* 4: 13–19.

Pharoah POD, Buttfield IH, and Hetzel BS (1971) Neurological damage to the fetus resulting from severe iodine deficiency during pregnancy. *Lancet* 1: 308–310.

Stanbury JB (ed.) (1994) *The Damaged Brain of Iodine Deficiency*. New York: Cognizant Communication Corporation.

Stanbury JB and Hetzel BS (eds.) (1980) *Endemic Goiter and Endemic Cretinism*. New York: John Wiley.

World Health Organization (1990) *Report to the 43rd World Health Assembly*. Geneva: World Health Organization.

World Health Organization (1996) *Recommended Iodine Levels in Salt and Guidelines for Monitoring Their Adequacy and Effectiveness*, WHO/NUT/96.13. Geneva: WHO/UNICEF/ICCIDD.

World Health Organization (1999) *Progress towards the Elimination of Iodine Deficiency Disorders (IDD)*, WHO/NHD/99.4. Geneva: World Health Organization.

WHO/UNICEF/ICCIDD (2001) Assessment of Iodine Deficiency Disorders and their Elimination: A guide for Program Managers WHO/NHD/01.1.

IRON

J R Hunt, USDA-ARS Grand Forks Human Nutrition Research Center, Grand Forks, ND, USA

Iron, the Earth's most abundant metal and fourth most common element, is also the essential nutrient that is most commonly deficient in human diets. At the beginning of the 21st century, the World Health Organization recognizes iron deficiency as one of the 10 greatest global health risks, ranked according to the number of lost healthy life years. Iron deficiency impairs reproductive performance, cognitive development, and work capacity. Effectively resolving this problem with preventative nutritional strategies remains an unmet challenge.

Iron Chemistry and Physiology

Body Content, Forms, and Function

Iron, the 26th element of the periodic table, has a molecular weight of 55.85. Two common aqueous oxidation states, ferrous (Fe^{2+}) and ferric (Fe^{3+}), enable iron to participate in oxidation/reduction reactions that are essential to energy metabolism by accepting or donating electrons. However, this property also enables free iron to catalyze oxidative reactions, resulting in reactive and damaging free radicals. Accordingly, body iron must be chemically bound to facilitate appropriate physiological function, transport, and storage, with minimal opportunity for free ionic iron to catalyze harmful oxidative reactions.

Most of the body's iron functions in heme protein complexes that transport oxygen as hemoglobin and myoglobin. Approximately two-thirds of the body iron is in hemoglobin, a 68,000 MW structure containing four subunits of heme, a protoporphyrin ring with iron in the center (**Figure 1**), and four polypeptide chains (two chains each of α- and β-globin). For transport by hemoglobin, oxygen bonds directly to the iron atom, stabilized in a Fe^{2+} oxidation state surrounded by the protoporphyrin ring and histidine

residues. Hemoglobin iron easily binds and releases oxygen, circulating in blood erythrocytes. Myoglobin, consisting of a single heme molecule and globin, enables oxygen transfer from erythrocytes to cellular mitochondria in muscle cytoplasm.

Smaller quantities of iron in the heme form function in mitrochondrial cytochromes involved with electron transfer, oxygen utilization, and the production of ATP. A small fraction of body iron functions in heme-containing hydrogen peroxidases such as catalase that protect against excessive hydrogen peroxide accumulation by catalyzing its conversion to hydrogen and oxygen.

Iron also functions in non-heme proteins that contain an iron–sulfur complex, a cubical arrangement of four iron and four sulfur atoms. This is the principal form of iron in mitochondria, functioning in enzymes of energy metabolism such as aconitase, NADH dehydrogenase, and succinate dehydrogenase. In both mitochondria and cytosol, aconitase

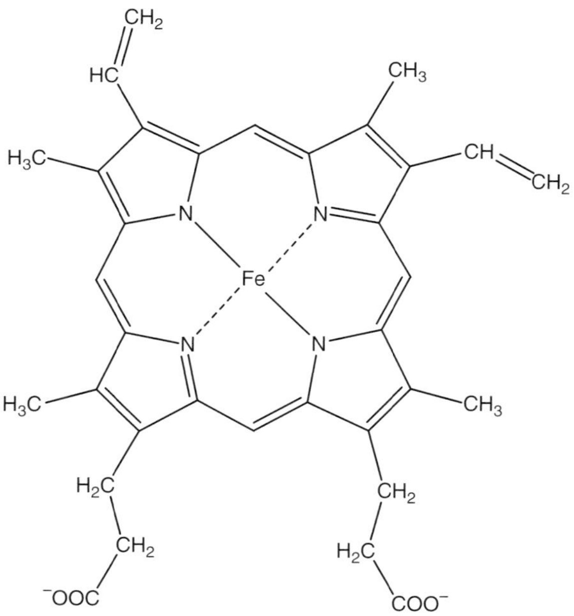

Figure 1 Heme (ferroprotoporphyrin 9).

is sensitive to iron concentrations. When iron is abundant, the aconitase enzyme assumes the full iron–sulfur cubic structure that is associated with carbohydrate metabolism. However, when iron concentrations are reduced, the protein loses aconitase activity and functions as an iron binding protein (IRP). IRPs interact with iron response elements (IREs) of the mRNA to regulate the synthesis of proteins involved with iron transport, storage, and use, in response to changes in cellular iron concentrations.

Absorption, Excretion, Transport, and Storage

Absorption Both heme and non-heme (inorganic) iron are absorbed in an inverse proportion to body iron stores (indicated by serum ferritin; **Figure 2**). Heme iron is absorbed more efficiently than the non-heme form. Non-heme iron absorption can vary from 0.1 to >35% and that of heme iron from 20 to 50%, depending on body iron status (stores, erythropoiesis, and hypoxia) and dietary bioavailability. These ranges indicate greater control of non-heme compared to heme iron absorption. When iron stores are high, absorption of non-heme iron can be minimized more completely, and when iron stores are low, non-heme iron is absorbed nearly as efficiently as heme iron. Because there is considerably more non-heme iron in the diet (~85–100%), this form accounts for most of the physiological control of iron absorption in relation to iron needs.

The upper portion of the duodenum, with its low pH luminal conditions, is the primary site for both heme and non-heme iron absorption (**Figure 3**). Non-heme iron absorption is better understood

than heme iron absorption, and only receptors for mucosal uptake of non-heme iron have been identified. The globin proteins of hemoglobin are proteolytically digested in the intestinal lumen, producing peptide remnants that may enhance the absorption of the heme molecule by preventing heme polymerization. The heme molecule is absorbed as an intact porphyrin structure, possibly involving endocytosis. In the mucosal cell, heme iron is split into ferrous iron and bilirubin by heme oxygenase, adding to a common pool of cellular iron for transport into plasma or intracellular storage and exfoliation.

Non-heme iron is best absorbed if presented to the intestinal villi as soluble ions (preferably reduced, ferrous ions) or as low-affinity, low-molecular-weight iron ligands. Stomach acid facilitates these conditions. Ascorbic acid concurrently ingested with iron helps to maintain the iron in a soluble, reduced, low-molecular ligand form in the intestinal lumen. Mucin, an intraluminal protein, has been proposed to bind iron and facilitate duodenal uptake.

Proteins involved in mucosal uptake and transfer of non-heme iron as well as possible regulatory molecules have been identified (**Figures 3 and 4**). These include duodenyl cytochrome b (Dcytb), which converts ferric to ferrous iron at the apical mucosal surface. A divalent metal transporter (DMT-1) transfers ferrous iron into the mucosal cell. Mutations in DMT-1 impair iron absorption and produce microcytic anemia in rodents. Ferrous iron has the highest affinity for DMT-1, but it will also transport other divalent ions, such as manganese, lead, cadmium, zinc, and copper. This may contribute to competitive inhibition observed in the absorption of these metals. Ferric iron is transported into the mucosal cell by mobilferrin, followed by ferroreduction with the protein paraferritin. Iron transported into the enterocyte may be further transported to the body at the basolateral membrane, completing absorption, or may be held and returned to the intestinal lumen with cellular desquamation. Ireg-1, or ferroportin, is involved in efflux of iron from the mucosal cell at the basolateral membrane. A mutation in Ireg-1 results in an uncommon form of hemochromatosis, an iron storage disorder. The mRNA for both DMT-1 and Ireg-1 contain an IRE, enabling regulation of mRNA translation by intracellular iron concentrations. Dcytb, DMT-1, and Ireg-1 are all upregulated in iron deficiency. Intestinal transfer of iron to the circulation also involves hephaestin, an intestinal ferroxidase with a protein sequence similar to that of ceruloplasmin (a copper-containing ferroxidase in serum). A defective hephaestin gene in mice results in anemia and

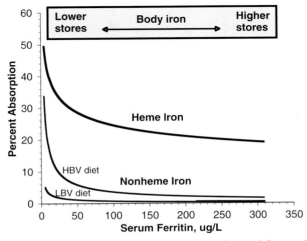

Figure 2 Heme and non-heme iron absorption as influenced by body iron stores and dietary bioavailability. HBV and LBV indicate high and low dietary bioavailability, respectively.

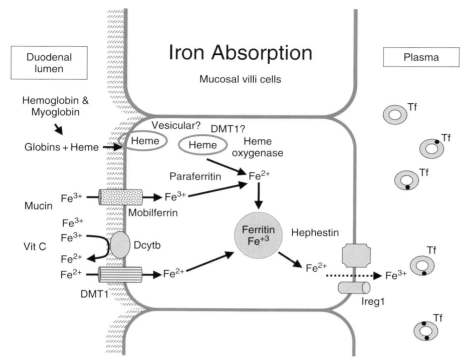

Figure 3 Absorption of iron in the intestinal mucosa.

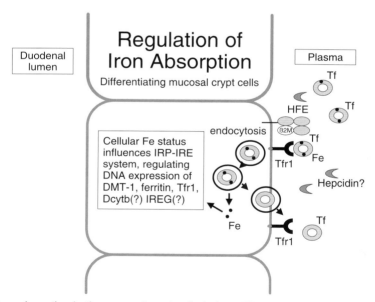

Figure 4 Regulation of iron absorption in the mucosal crypt cells before differentiation and development into actively absorbing intestinal villi cells.

accumulation of iron in intestinal cells. However, unlike Dcytb, DMT-1, or Ireg-1, hephaestin is not preferentially expressed in the duodenum, the main site of iron absorption.

Iron absorption is responsive to recent iron intake, iron stores, erythropoiesis, hypoxia, pregnancy, and inflammation. A newly identified peptide, hepcidin, may be related to several of these stimuli of regulatory control. Hepcidin is an antimicrobial peptide found in human blood and urine that apparently serves as a signal for limiting iron absorption. Control of absorption also likely involves the HFE protein located in the basolateral membrane of intestinal crypt cells. A specific point mutation in the HFE gene is associated with the most common form of hemochromatosis, a disorder involving excessive iron absorption and accumulation. The HFE protein interacts with β_2-microglobin and transferrin receptor, apparently influencing iron uptake from serum transferrin, the primary protein involved in serum iron transport (**Figure 4**). Knowledge of the control of iron absorption is growing rapidly.

Transport Transferrin transports essentially all of the 3 or 4 mg of iron in blood serum, including dietary iron absorbed from the duodenum as well as iron from macrophages after the degradation of hemoglobin. Each transferrin molecule binds two iron atoms; the transferrin in serum is normally approximately one-third saturated with iron. The amount of iron that can be bound by transferrin is measured as the total iron binding capacity (TIBC). In iron deficiency, serum iron is reduced, and TIBC is elevated; expressing serum iron as a fraction of the TIBC defines the transferrin saturation, which is reduced in iron deficiency. As iron deficiency develops, these measures of iron transport signal iron deficiency before the functional pool of circulating hemoglobin is reduced (**Figure 5**).

Membrane transferrin receptors enable the cellular uptake of iron. Transferrin receptors complex with transferrin, the complex is internalized by endocytosis, and the iron is released to the cell from transferrin upon vesicular acidification (**Figure 4**). Transferrin receptors are abundant in erythrocyte precursors, placenta, and liver, and the number of receptors changes inversely with cellular iron status. Serum transferrin receptors are a soluble, truncated form of the cellular receptors, present in proportion to the cellular receptors, which serve as a clinical indicator of cellular iron status that is useful in distinguishing between iron deficiency and other causes of anemia.

Other proteins involved in iron transport include lactoferrin, which is structurally similar to transferrin and occurs in body fluids such as milk and semen. Haptoglobin and hemopexin proteins clear hemoglobin and heme, respectively, from circulation as they are released from senescent red blood cells.

Storage Iron is primarily stored in liver, spleen, and bone marrow in the form of ferritin or hemosiderin. Ferritin is a water-soluble protein complex of 24 polypeptide subunits in a spherical cluster with a hollow center that contains up to 25% iron by weight, or 4000 atoms of iron per molecule.

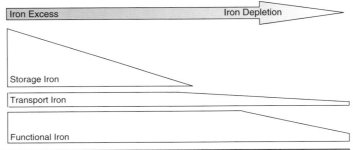

	Excessive Body Iron	Adequate Iron	Low Iron Stores	Iron Deficiency	Iron Deficiency Anemia
Serum Ferritin	↑	---	↓	↓↓	↓↓
Transferrin Receptor (sTfR)	---	---	---	↑	↑↑
Index: Log (sTfR/ferritin)	↑	---	↓	↓↓	↓↓↓
Transferrin Saturation	↑↑	---	---	↓	↓
Serum Iron	↑↑	---	---	↓	↓
Total Iron Binding Capacity	---	---	---	↑	↑
Erythrocyte Protoporphyrin	---	---	---	↑	↑↑
Hemoglobin, Hematocrit	---	---	---	---	↓

Figure 5 Clinical indicators of body iron status.

Hemosiderin is a water-insoluble complex, immuno-logically similar to ferritin, containing up to 35% iron. Ferritin and hemosiderin each account for approximately half of the storage iron in liver.

Excretion The approximately 1 mg of iron lost daily by men and postmenopausal women represents mainly obligatory fecal losses from exfoliated mucosal cells, bile, and extravasated red cells, with minor additional amounts in desquamated skin cells and sweat. Urine contains minimal amounts of iron.

Adolescent girls and premenopausal women excrete considerable amounts of iron through menstruation. The menstrual losses of individual women vary considerably; half of women lose less than 14 mg of iron per menstrual period, but the distribution is highly skewed, and 5% lose 50 mg or more. Iron deficiencies among women in prosperous countries are commonly attributable to these high iron excretion rates rather that to differences in dietary intakes.

Body iron balance The body contains 2–4 g of total iron, or approximately 50 mg/kg in men and 40 mg/kg in women. Red blood cells contain approximately two-thirds of body iron and have an average life span of 120 days; consequently, approximately 20 mg of iron daily is efficiently recycled from senescent to newly formed erythrocytes through the reticuloendothelial system.

In contrast to other nutrients, controlled through both absorption and excretion, body iron balance is controlled almost exclusively by absorption. Approximately 10–20 mg iron is consumed daily from food. Average absorption and excretion of iron for adult men or postmenopausal women is approximately 1 mg daily. Menstruation can more than double iron losses in women of child-bearing age, increasing their requirement for absorbed iron. Iron balance is also challenged by the growth demands of pregnancy and early childhood.

Clinical Assessment of Iron Status

With adequate iron status, there is sufficient iron to meet all of iron's functional roles and a small reserve of storage iron that can be mobilized when needed (**Figure 5**). Excessive body iron, stored in liver and bone marrow, is marked by elevated serum ferritin and also serum iron and transferrin saturation. Ferritin in plasma corresponds well with body iron stores, but its use as an indicator is limited under inflammatory conditions. Iron deficiency occurs when iron stores are depleted and the iron transported for physiological function is reduced. Iron

deficiency without anemia is commonly detected from abnormal values for two out of three blood indices, usually serum ferritin, transferrin saturation, and free erythrocyte protoporphyrin (**Figure 5**). As iron deficiency becomes more severe, iron deficiency anemia results, with small, pale erythocytes and reduced blood hemoglobin and hematocrit. Measurement of hemoglobin in reticulocytes, or immature red blood cells, is a possible new tool to assess developing anemias. The ratio of serum transferrin receptor to serum ferritin provides a single, sensitive indicator of iron status across the full range of body iron status, except under conditions of inflammatory stress.

Iron Nutrition

Iron Deficiency

Iron deficiency is the most common of nutrient deficiencies, affecting as many as two-thirds of all children and women of child-bearing age worldwide. Iron deficiency severe enough to cause anemia affects 20–25% of infants and as many as 40% of women and 25% of men. Iron deficiency occurs in industrially developed as well as developing populations. In the United States, 9–11% of toddlers, adolescent girls, and women of child-bearing age have iron deficiency, and 2–4% have iron deficiency anemia. The prevalence of iron deficiency is approximately doubled in US black and Hispanic women.

Consequences of Iron Deficiency

Iron deficiency adversely affects pregnancy, impairs early childhood development and cognitive function, and reduces the ability to do physical work. These serious problems are almost exclusively associated with iron deficiency severe enough to cause anemia; however, small reductions in exercise capacity, detectable in a laboratory setting, are also detectable in women with low iron stores and no anemia.

Physical work capacity Iron deficiency anemia adversely affects physical work capacity, reflecting the element's key role in oxygen and energy utilization. Maximal oxygen consumption during exercise is reduced, in association with decreased muscle myoglobin and other iron-containing enzymes. Iron supplementation has improved productivity among Guatemalan sugar and coffee plantation workers, Indian tea pickers, and Indonesian road construction workers and rubber tappers. Iron supplementation programs are clearly cost-effective in addition to providing a positive impact on human health and well-being.

Cognitive development In infants, iron deficiency anemia has been associated with reduced mental and motor test scores and behavioral changes such as being more hesitant and wary. This impaired mental and motor functioning appears to persist after treatment with iron, emphasizing the need for early detection and treatment and preferably prevention of iron deficiency during early development.

Reproduction Iron deficiency anemia has been associated with greater perinatal maternal and infant mortality, premature birth, and low birth weight. Iron supplementation during pregnancy has not been completely effective in preventing maternal anemia, leading to suggestions for promoting adequate iron stores in all women of child-bearing age prior to conception.

Other Iron deficiency increases the susceptibility to lead poisoning. It may also impair resistance to infection and regulation of body temperature. Iron deficiency has been associated with the eating of non-food material (pica) or ice (pagophagia). Clinical signs may include spoon-shaped fingernails and abnormalities of the mucosa of the mouth and gastrointestinal tract.

Recommended Dietary Intakes

The US and Canadian recommended iron intakes are intended to meet the requirements of 97.5% of the healthy population, replacing excreted iron and maintaining essential iron functions with a minimal supply of body iron stores. They also assume a relatively high bioavailability of the dietary iron. The recommended 8 mg daily for adult men and postmenopausal women can easily be met with varied Western-style diets. More careful food choices are needed to obtain the 18 mg recommended to meet requirements for 97.5% of adult menstruating women. This higher recommendation reflects the high menstrual iron losses of some women; the median iron requirement is 8.1 mg for menstruating women.

During pregnancy, dietary iron recommendations are increased to 27 mg daily, based on the iron content of the fetus and placenta (approximately 320 mg) as well as the expanded blood volume associated with a healthy pregnancy. Meeting this recommendation generally requires iron supplementation. Supplementation with 30–60 mg daily is commonly recommended. Lactation has minimal impact on maternal iron balance and recommendations.

The high iron requirements of early growth put infants and toddlers at risk of iron deficiency.

Breast-feeding is recommended for the first year of life. Although iron in breast milk is relatively low (0.35 mg/l, or 0.27 mg daily), it is well absorbed, possibly because of lactoferrin. Breast milk alone is assumed to be adequate for the first 6 months of infancy, with the addition of iron-rich foods in the next 6 months. When prepared formula is used, iron fortification of the formula is recommended.

Dietary recommendations at other ages reflect the increased needs of active growth periods, such as adolescence. Western dietary recommendations have been based on mixed diets with a relatively high bioavailability of iron and may need to be increased twofold or more for low meat, plant-based diets with greater phytic acid content (see Bioavailability).

Other factors that may increase dietary requirements include achlorhydria, which decreases iron absorption, hookworm or other parasites that increase gastrointestinal blood loss, or intrauterine contraceptive devices that may increase menstrual losses by 30–50%. In contrast, hormonal contraceptives reduce iron requirements by reducing menstrual losses by approximately 50%.

Dietary Iron

Food Sources

Typical Western diets contain approximately 6 mg iron per 1000 kcal. Men and women consume approximately 16–18 and 12–14 mg daily, respectively. In the United States, 24% of dietary iron is supplied by breads, pasta, and bakery products. An additional 21% comes from (mostly fortified) cereal products. Other abundant dietary sources are red meats (9% from beef), poultry, legumes, and lentils. In countries such as the United States, fortification practices increase the influence of grain and cereal products as sources of iron. In countries without fortification to at least replace the iron lost during milling, the refinement of grain products considerably reduces dietary iron content. The populations of developing countries that eat little meat and do not include legumes or lentils as a dietary staple are at increased risk of inadequate iron intake.

Bioavailability

In underdeveloped countries, diets may be inadequate in both iron content and bioavailability (the amount that is absorbed and utilized by the body). However, the bioavailability of iron can be more important than the iron content in determining the amount of iron absorbed from food. Diets with similar total iron contents can differ 8- to 10-fold in the amount of absorbable iron. Dietary iron bio-availability is high from refined Western diets containing meat, poultry, and fish and abundant sources of ascorbic acid with low consumption of phytic acid from whole grains and legumes and limited drinking of coffee and tea with meals. On average, men absorb 1 mg daily from such diets, and women, with their lower iron stores, absorb approximately 2 mg. Individuals may absorb considerably more or less, depending on their body iron stores (**Figure 2**).

Despite the considerable differences in dietary iron bioavailability observed with absorption measurements, dietary changes are slow to influence biochemical indices of iron status. However, people following vegetarian diets for years have lower iron stores than their omnivorous counterparts, and consumption of red meat is often a predictor of iron status in epidemiological studies.

Heme iron Approximately 10%, or 1 or 2 mg, of the iron in a mixed, Western diet is in the well-absorbed heme form. Heme iron accounts for approximately 40% of the iron in meat, poultry, or fish flesh. There is little to no heme iron in organ meats, dairy products, or foods of plant origin. Heme iron is absorbed as an intact porphyrin structure. Heme iron absorption is enhanced by meat, poultry, or fish and is reduced by calcium consumed concurrently, but it is not influenced by the other enhancers and inhibitors of non-heme iron absorption.

Non-heme iron Non-heme iron accounts for 85–100% of dietary iron. In contrast to heme iron, the absorption of non-heme iron is substantially influenced by dietary enhancers and inhibitors consumed concurrently. These factors appear to affect the solubility of a single exchangeable pool of non-heme iron absorbed from the intestinal digestate.

Absorption of non-heme iron is enhanced by ascorbic acid, which reduces ferric iron to ferrous iron, resulting in a soluble iron–ascorbic acid complex. Enhanced absorption has been demonstrated with synthetic as well as several food sources of ascorbic acid. The enhancement increases logarithmically with the dose, approximately doubling absorption with as little as 25 mg of ascorbic acid and increasing absorption by nearly 10-fold with 1000 mg of ascorbic acid.

Non-heme iron absorption is also enhanced by concurrently consuming meat, poultry, or fish. Despite intensive study, the factor responsible for this enhancement by animal flesh has not been identified and may involve the general matrix of low-molecular-weight peptides released during digestion.

Non-heme iron absorption is reduced by phytic acid (inositol hexaphosphate), present in legumes, rice, and grains, that binds iron and makes it insoluble. Both phytate and iron are concentrated in the aleurone layer and germ of grains, and they are reduced with milling, which increases the bioavailability of the remaining iron. An additional unidentified factor in soy beans, independent of the phytic acid, also impairs iron absorption. Polyphenols in grains, fruits, and vegetables, and including the tannins in tea and coffee, also inhibit non-heme iron absorption. Ascorbic acid consumed concurrently can partially reduce the inhibition of non-heme iron absorption by both phytic acid and polyphenols. Calcium in supplemental quantities inhibits both heme and non-heme iron absorption from foods. Supplemental zinc also inhibits non-heme iron absorption.

Supplementation and Fortification

The serious international problem of iron deficiency has been met with poor success by supplementation and fortification efforts. Both approaches suffer from difficulties in delivery and acceptance. Supplements that readily ionize into the ferrous form, such as ferrous sulfate, ferrous fumerate, or ferrous gluconate, are highly bioavailable but may cause gastrointestinal discomfort. Iron injections are poorly tolerated and can result in serious infections. Because daily supplementation reduces the physiological efficiency of iron absorption, routine weekly iron supplementation with 60 mg iron has been suggested in developing countries for women of childbearing age, beginning in adolescence. Menstruating women in more prosperous countries are advised to obtain assessment from a health professional before taking iron supplements in excess of 20 mg daily.

Fortification of staple foods with 3–10 mg iron daily, depending on the needs of the population, is a long-term preventative strategy. In the United States, bread and cereal products are routinely fortified with 20 mg iron per pound (460 g) of flour, and additional fortification at the option of food suppliers is common. However, fortification is difficult when food processing is decentralized, as is common in poor populations. Food fortification carries the additional challenge that the chemical forms of iron most bioavailable also tend to be the most reactive with the food fortified, resulting in adverse changes in flavor, color, and shelf life. Promising approaches include the fortification of food sauces with iron chemically bound with amino acids or with EDTA (sodium iron ethylenediaminetetraacetic acid), which are well absorbed even in the presence of phytic acid. Elemental iron powders, commonly referred to as carbonyl, electrolytic, and reduced forms of iron, are relatively inert in foods and inexpensive, but their bioavailability may be 30–80% less than iron from ferrous sulfate, depending on the dissolution in the gastrointestinal tract. Ferric orthophosphate and ferric pyrophosphate do not adversely affect foods but are poorly bioavailable; however, efforts are under way to enhance their bioavailability by reducing the particle size and encapsulating the particles with various lipids or carbohydrates to prevent agglomeration.

Excessive Intakes

An extensive biological control system limits the occurrence of free ionic iron that can readily participate in toxic, free radical-producing reactions. Large quantities of ingested iron are acutely toxic, and accidental ingestion of medicinal iron preparations is a leading cause of poisoning deaths in young children. Iron supplementation is also associated with gastrointestinal irritation. Iron supplements adversely affect absorption of zinc. Iron absorption is well controlled, but iron overload can result from excessive parenteral iron administration or blood transfusions. Dietary iron overload, possibly exacerbated by genetic factors, occurs in sub-Saharan tribes that consume a high-iron traditional beer prepared and stored in iron containers. Genetic factors can substantially influence body iron retention, as indicated by hemochromatosis, a relatively frequent iron storage disorder of northern European descendants characterized by excessive iron absorption and leading to life-threatening iron damage of organs in adulthood. The possible association of high iron stores with increased risk of diseases related to oxidative stress, including cardiovascular disease, diabetes, and cancer, is an area of epidemiological investigation.

See also: **Adolescents**: Nutritional Requirements. **Anemia**: Iron-Deficiency Anemia. **Bioavailability**. **Breast Feeding**. **Food Fortification**: Developed Countries; Developing Countries. **Pregnancy**: Nutrient Requirements. **Supplementation**: Dietary Supplements; Role of Micronutrient Supplementation; Developing Countries; Developed Countries.

Further Reading

Brugnara C (2003) Iron deficiency and erythropoiesis: New diagnostic approaches. *Clinical Chemistry* **49**: 1573–1578.

Centers for Disease Control and Prevention (1998) Recommendations to prevent and control iron deficiency in the United States. *MMWR Recommendations and Reports* **47**: 1–29.

Eisenstein RS and Ross KL (2003) Novel roles for iron regulatory proteins in the adaptive response to iron deficiency. *Journal of Nutrition* **133**: 1510S–1516S.

Institute of Medicine, Food and Nutrition Board (2001) *Dietary Reference Intakes for Vitamin A, Vitamin K, Arsenic, Boron, Chromium, Copper, Iodine, Iron, Manganese, Molybdenum, Nickel, Silicon, Vanadium, and Zinc.* Washington, DC: National Academy Press.

Knutson M and Wessling-Resnick M (2003) Iron metabolism in the reticuloendothelial system. *Critical Reviews in Biochemistry and Molecular Biology* **38**: 61–88.

Mielczarek EV and McGrayne SB (2000) *Iron, Nature's Universal Element: Why People Need Iron and Animals Make Magnets.* New Brunswick, NJ: Rutgers University Press.

Miret S, Simpson RJ, and McKie AT (2003) Physiology and molecular biology of dietary iron absorption. *Annual Review of Nutrition.*

Ischemic Heart Disease *see* **Coronary Heart Disease**: Lipid Theory

KETOSIS

D H Williamson[†], Radcliffe Infirmary, Oxford, UK

This article is a revision of the previous edition article by D H Williamson, pp. 1160–1167, © 1999, Elsevier Ltd.

The two ketone bodies, acetoacetate ($CH_3COCH_2COO^-$) and D-3-hydroxybutyrate ($CH_3CHOHCH_2COO^-$), are the only freely soluble lipids in the circulation.

The name ketone bodies originates from the German *Ketonkörper* (literally, ketones excreted from the body) and refers to their discovery in the urine of diabetic patients in the latter half of the nineteenth century. In reality, the term is a misnomer because 3-hydroxybutyrate is not a ketone. It arose because the reagent originally used reacted positively with ketones in diabetic urine. Acetone (CH_3COCH_3), the product of the spontaneous decarboxylation of acetoacetate, is also a ketone and is present in blood and urine when the plasma concentration of acetoacetate is elevated. It is excreted via the kidneys and lungs and is responsible for the sweet smell on the breath in ketotic states.

The association of ketone bodies with the pathology of diabetes resulted in the view that they were toxic waste products. It is only in the past 30 years that this view has been convincingly reversed. Two factors led to this change, namely the development of an enzymatic method for the determination of acetoacetate and 3-hydroxybutyrate, which in turn allowed the dramatic finding of Cahill and colleagues in 1967 that adult human brain removed appreciable amounts of ketone bodies from the circulation in prolonged starvation.

The aim in this contribution is to review (a) the formation of ketone bodies in physiological and pathological situations, and (b) the function of ketone bodies as physiological substrates and signals.

Formation of Ketone Bodies

It is well established that in humans and other mammals the only organ that contributes significant amounts of ketone bodies to the blood is the liver; this organ, unlike peripheral tissues, is unable to utilize ketone bodies to any appreciable extent. More recently it has been found that during the suckling period (high-fat diet) the intestine also has the capacity (about 10% of the liver) to produce ketone bodies. Whether ketone bodies are used *in situ* or are transported via the portal blood to supplement the existing hyperketonemia is an open question.

The main blood-borne substrates for the synthesis of ketone bodies (ketogenesis) are the nonesterified fatty acids; others of lesser importance are the branched-chain amino acids, leucine and isoleucine. In addition, acetate (sources: intestinal fermentation, in vinegar or an oxidation product of ethanol) is a ketogenic substrate.

Long-chain fatty acids contained in dietary lipids do not enter the portal blood directly but are esterified in the intestinal cells, packaged with proteins and phospholipids to form chylomicrons (large lipoproteins), and transported via the lymphatic system to the thoracic duct where they enter the blood. In contrast, the short- and medium-chain fatty acids (below C_{14}) contained in dairy products or in clinical medium-chain triacylglycerol preparations are directly absorbed as the respective fatty acids and are transported to the liver via the portal blood (**Figure 1**). The long-chain

[†]Deceased.

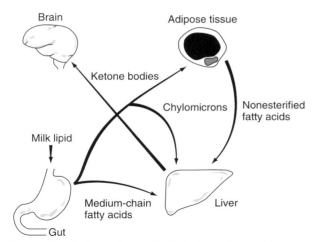

Figure 1 Intertissue fluxes of substrates in the suckling neonate. Thickness of line denotes rate of flux.

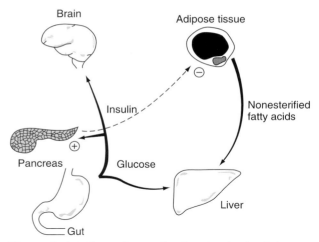

Figure 2 Intertissue fluxes of substrates in the fed state. Thickness of line denotes rate of flux.

fatty acids in the plasma are bound to albumin and are released from adipose tissue triacylglycerol stores by the process of lipolysis.

Extrahepatic Regulation

A key factor in the regulation of ketogenesis is the availability of nonesterified long-chain fatty acids to the liver, which in turn is controlled by their release from adipose tissue. The enzyme responsible for the initiation of the hydrolysis of stored triacylglycerols to fatty acids is hormone-sensitive lipase. As its name implies, this enzyme is exquisitely sensitive to hormones: adrenaline (in the plasma) and noradrenaline (released from sympathetic nerve endings) are activators, whereas insulin inhibits the activity. In small mammals glucagon is also an activator of the enzyme, but this does not seem to be the case in the human.

Insulin has an additional effect on the net release of long-chain fatty acids from adipose tissue in that it stimulates their reesterification to triacylglycerols. Thus after a high-carbohydrate meal, when insulin secretion and its concentration in the plasma is high, the release of fatty acids from adipose tissue is suppressed and their concentration in the plasma is low (**Figure 2**). In contrast, during stress, when adrenaline and noradrenaline are elevated, the release of fatty acids is increased and their plasma concentration is high.

In experimental animals increased plasma ketone body concentrations (hyperketonemia) can inhibit adipose tissue lipolysis (a) indirectly by increasing the secretion of insulin or (b) by a direct effect on the tissue (**Figure 3**). This can be viewed as a feedback mechanism for controlling the rate of ketogenesis via fatty acid supply to the liver, but whether

this is important in the human is not known. In contrast, the supply of short- and medium-chain fatty acids to the liver is mainly dependent on the dietary intake and on the proportion that escapes further metabolism in the intestinal tract; there is no known involvement of hormones in the process.

Intrahepatic Regulation

There are situations (e.g., stress) where the supply of fatty acids to the liver may be increased, but there is no necessity to increase the availability of ketone bodies to the peripheral tissues. Consequently, there is a requirement that the rate of hepatic ketogenesis should be controlled independently of the supply of fatty acids. However, it must be stressed that without an increase in the supply of fatty acids the rate of ketogenesis cannot increase.

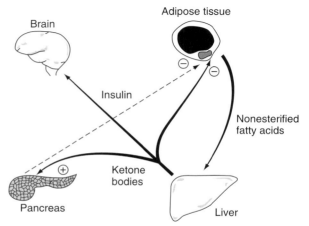

Figure 3 Role of ketone bodies as feedback regulators.

Much of the current interest is concerned with how the intrahepatic metabolism of fatty acids (**Figure 4**) is regulated. Long-chain fatty acids entering the liver have three main fates:

1. They can be re-esterified to phospholipids and triacylglycerols and then be secreted as very low-density lipoproteins (VLDL).
2. They can be oxidized via the mitochondrial β-oxidation complex to acetyl-CoA. The latter can combine with another molecule of acetyl-CoA in the reaction catalysed by acetoacetyl-CoA thiolase and then enter the hydroxymethylglutaryl-CoA pathway to form acetoacetate.
3. The acetyl-CoA derived from the fatty acids can be completely oxidized in the tricarboxylate cycle.

The short- and medium-chain fatty acids cannot be re-esterified to any appreciable extent in mammalian liver and therefore they are either metabolized to ketone bodies or completely oxidized. In addition, unlike the long-chain fatty acids, they are transported directly into the mitochondrial matrix without the need to be converted first to the corresponding acyl-CoA derivatives.

The role of malonyl CoA The entry of free long-chain fatty acids into the hepatocyte is via a specific carrier on the plasma membrane. Once inside the cytosol the long-chain fatty acids are bound to binding proteins, converted to the acyl-CoA derivatives, and then can either be esterified or enter

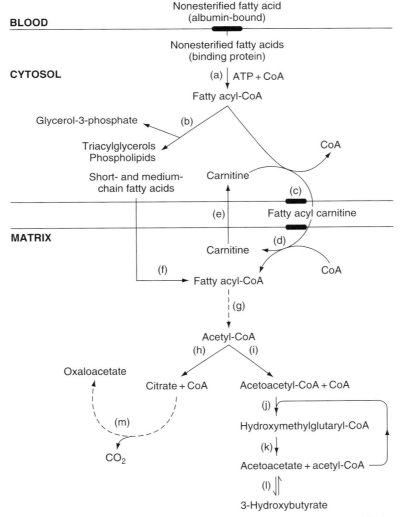

Figure 4 Pathway of fatty acid catabolism in liver. Enzymes involved: (a) long-chain fatty acyl-CoA synthetase; (b) glycerol-3-phosphate acyl-CoA transferase; (c) CAT I; (d) CAT II; (e) carnitine exchange; (f) short- and medium-chain fatty acyl-CoA synthetase; (g) fatty acid oxidation complex; (h) citrate synthase; (i) acetoacetyl-CoA thiolase; (j) hydroxymethylglutaryl-CoA synthase; (k) hydroxymethylglutaryl-CoA lyase; (l) hydroxybutyrate dehydrogenase; (m) tricarboxylate cycle.

the mitochondria via a complex transport system, the carnitine–acyl-CoA transferase (CAT) system. This consists of two proteins: CAT I located on the outer mitochondrial membrane and CAT II on the inner mitochondrial membrane (**Figure 5**). The overall action of the two enzymes results in the transfer of a long-chain fatty acyl-CoA to the mitochondrial matrix and the return of free carnitine to the cytosol via an exchange mechanism. Although carnitine is not consumed in the reaction, the available concentration can be critical. In nutritional carnitine deficiency there is impairment of long-chain fatty acid oxidation and ketogenesis.

The activity of CAT I is the key to the intrahepatic regulation of fatty acid metabolism in most situations. Its activity increases in ketogenic situations. More importantly, CAT I is inhibited by malonyl-CoA and the sensitivity of CAT I to this inhibitor changes in various pathophysiological situations such as fasting or diabetes.

As malonyl-CoA is a key intermediate in the synthesis of fatty acids (lipogenesis) from products (pyruvate and lactate) of glucose metabolism, this interaction provides a regulatory link between lipid and carbohydrate metabolism (**Figure 5**). Thus on high-carbohydrate diets, when the rate of hepatic lipogenesis, and consequently the cytosolic concentration of malonyl-CoA, is high, the activity of CAT I will be inhibited and fatty acids will be diverted to esterified products and secretion as VLDL rather than oxidation and conversion to ketone bodies. Conversely, on high-fat diets or in starvation, when

lipogenesis is inhibited, malonyl-CoA concentration is low and CAT I is active. The sensitivity of CAT I to malonyl-CoA generally correlates with the prevailing concentration of the latter.

The short- and medium-chain fatty acids do not utilize the CAT I and II system to enter the mitochondrial matrix and therefore their oxidation is not greatly influenced by the prevailing 'carbohydrate status' (amount of glycogen, direction of carbohydrate flux, glycolysis, or gluconeogenesis) of the liver (**Figure 5**).

Insulin can rapidly depress the rate of ketogenesis *in vitro*. This effect is thought to result mainly from its stimulatory action on a key enzyme of lipogenesis, acetyl-CoA carboxylase, which in turn increases the concentration of malonyl-CoA. Glucagon and the catecholamines have the opposite effect. Thus hormonal effects can be exerted at both the extrahepatic (lipolysis) and intrahepatic (modulation of lipogenesis) levels.

Intramitochondrial regulation Once the fatty acyl-CoA molecule is attached to the mitochondrial β-oxidation complex there appears to be little regulation exerted until release of the acetyl-CoA fragments. As indicated above, the acetyl-CoA can enter the tricarboxylate cycle and be oxidized to CO_2 or can be converted to ketone bodies via the hydroxymethylglutaryl-CoA pathway.

It appears that in most experimental situations the complete oxidation of fatty acids proceeds at a low, but relatively similar, rate and it is the activity of the

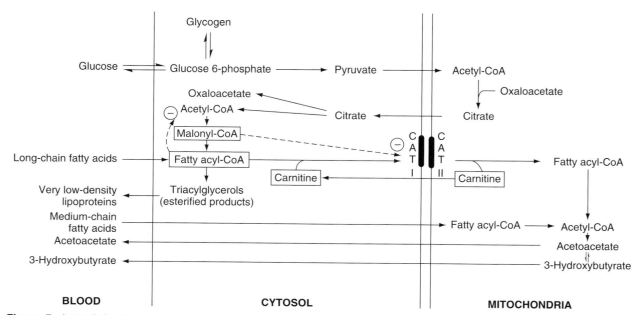

Figure 5 Interrelationship between hepatic carbohydrate metabolism, lipogenesis, and ketogenesis. Circled minus signs indicate inhibition by the metabolite.

hydroxymethylglutaryl-CoA pathway that shows larger changes. This has led to the view that the pathway might be regulated by mechanisms other than substrate supply.

Studies on the expression of 3-hydroxy-3-methylglutaryl-CoA (HMG-CoA) synthase have shown that both the mRNA coding for the protein and the amount of protein increase during the onset of ketogenic states (fasting, diabetes) and that these changes are rapidly reversed (refeeding, insulin treatment). However, the finding that rates of ketogenesis from medium-chain fatty acids (CAT I and II) do not alter greatly with change in physiological state, if the rate of fatty acid supply is held constant, would seem to rule out appreciable regulation within the hydroxymethylglutaryl-CoA pathway. Indeed, current thinking suggests that the activity of CAT I is the primary intrahepatic site for the regulation of fatty acid oxidation and ketogenesis. If there is another important site, particularly during situations associated with the reversal of ketogenesis, it is likely to be proximal to the step catalysed by this protein (e.g., the supply of fatty acids to the liver). Thus *in vivo* there is little doubt that the primary step that controls ketogenic flux is the rate of long-chain fatty acid release from adipose tissue.

Function of Ketone Bodies

The major role of ketone bodies is to supply an alternative oxidizable substrate to glucose for the brain in situations where the availability of the latter is impaired (e.g., starvation). In addition, ketone bodies can act as precursors for the acetyl-CoA required in neural lipid synthesis (myelin). Other mammalian tissues, including heart, skeletal muscle, kidney, and lactating mammary gland, can utilize ketone bodies but, in contrast to glucose utilization, no energy can be obtained in the absence of oxygen. In these tissues metabolism of ketone bodies results in the inhibition of glucose utilization and inhibition of the oxidation of pyruvate. The net result is a sparing of carbohydrate for the brain and the strictly glycolytic tissues (erythrocytes, retina).

Pathways of Ketone Body Utilization

Mitochondrial pathway The major site of ketone body utilization in peripheral tissues is the mitochondria (**Figure 6**). Although transporters for ketone bodies have been described on the plasma and inner mitochondrial membranes of some tissues, these do not appear to limit the flux. The initiating enzyme for acetoacetate metabolism is 3-oxoacid-CoA transferase:

$$\text{Acetoacetate} + \text{succinyl-CoA} \rightleftharpoons \text{acetoacetyl-CoA} + \text{succinate}$$

The resulting acetoacetyl-CoA is cleaved to two molecules of acetyl-CoA by acetoacetyl-CoA thiolase; they are then oxidized in the tricarboxylate cycle.

3-Hydroxybutyrate is converted to acetoacetate by 3-hydroxybutyrate dehydrogenase:

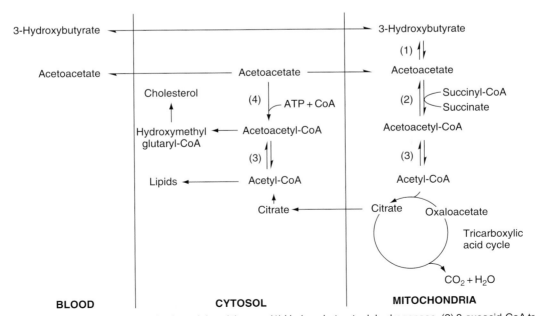

Figure 6 Pathways of ketone body utilization in peripheral tissues. (1) Hydroxybutyrate dehydrogenase, (2) 3-oxoacid-CoA transferase; (3) acetoacetyl-CoA thiolase; (4) acetoacetyl-CoA synthetase.

$$3\text{-Hydroxybutyrate} + NAD^+ \rightleftharpoons \text{acetoacetate}$$
$$+ NADH + H^+$$

The ready reversibility of the three enzymes of the mitochondrial pathway (**Figure 6**) means that if the overall system is near equilibrium within the cell *in vivo*, the utilization of the ketone bodies will be dependent on their respective concentrations and on the rate of removal of the products. Thus acetoacetate utilization will be promoted when mitochondrial acetyl-CoA is decreased, whereas an increase in the latter will have the opposite effect. Similarly, oxidation of hydroxybutyrate will increase if the concentrations of $NADH_2$ and acetoacetate fall. Unlike the hepatic hydroxymethylglutaryl-CoA pathway for ketogenesis, which is essentially irreversible, the free reversibility of this pathway in peripheral tissues can be viewed as means of buffering the mitochondrial acetyl-CoA pool and hence energy production. Some of the acetyl-CoA can be transported to the cytosol in the form of citrate to act as a precursor for lipogenesis (**Figure 6**).

Cytosolic pathway The cytosol of tissues where active lipogenesis occurs (adipose tissue, developing brain, lactating mammary gland, and liver) contains an enzyme, acetoacetyl-CoA synthetase, which converts acetoacetate to acetoacetyl-CoA (**Figure 6**):

$$\text{Acetoacetate} + ATP + CoA$$
$$\rightarrow \text{acetoacetyl-CoA} + AMP + \text{pyrophosphate}$$

Its activity is at least an order of magnitude lower than that of the mitochondrial 3-oxoacid-CoA transferase, whereas its affinity for acetoacetate is appreciably higher. The presence of acetoacetyl-CoA thiolase in the cytosol allows the conversion of acetoacetate to acetyl-CoA and then to lipids without the involvement of the mitochondria.

Brain cytosol also contains 3-hydroxy-3-methylglutaryl-CoA synthase, allowing acetoacetate to act as a direct precursor for sterol synthesis. Evidence from *in vivo* experiments with ^{14}C-labelled acetoacetate has confirmed the existence of this pathway in developing brain and liver. The cytosolic route for acetoacetate utilization can be seen as a mechanism for directing this substrate to lipid or sterol synthesis rather than to oxidation.

Ketosis

The concentration of ketone bodies in the blood at any time represents a balance between the rate of hepatic ketogenesis and the rate of utilization by peripheral tissues. It is generally assumed that an increase in ketogenesis leads to a rise in blood ketone bodies, which in turn results in their increased utilization. In rare situations, such as congenital absence of key enzymes involved in ketone body utilization (e.g., 3-oxoacid-CoA transferase) or inhibition of these enzymes by pharmacological agents, blood ketone bodies may increase without any concomitant increase in ketogenesis.

The concentration of ketone bodies in the blood is exquisitely sensitive to changes in pathophysiological state. It is therefore useful to define *normoketonemia* in mammals as a concentration of total ketone bodies in blood below $0.2\,mmol\,l^{-1}$, *hyperketonemia* as above this level, and *ketoacidosis* (ketosis; by analogy to the definition of lactic acidosis) as above $7\,mmol\,l^{-1}$. In adult mammals there are small but characteristic diurnal variations in ketone body concentrations. Larger increases in concentration occur in man in response to change in pathophysiological state (**Table 1**). The concentrations span a 200-fold range and it is this which underlines the important role of ketone bodies as substrates and signals.

Physiological Ketosis

Physiological hyperketonemia is found in the suckling neonate (high-fat diet of the milk; **Figure 1**), postexercise (depletion of hepatic glycogen reserves), and after prolonged fasting (more than 24 h; **Figure 7**). All these situations have in common a low hepatic carbohydrate status (depletion of glycogen and/or activation of gluconeogenesis) and therefore from a physiological standpoint one would expect an increased rate of ketogenesis. Comparison of the factors which can influence ketogenesis in suckling and fasting (**Table 2**) shows the expected broad agreement.

Table 1 Range of blood ketone body concentrations in humans

Situation	Ketone body concentration $(mmol\,l^{-1})$
Fed normal diet	about 0.1
Fed high-fat diet	up to 3
Fasted: 12–24 h	up to 0.3
Fasted: 48–72 h	2.0–3.0
Postexercise	up to 2
Late pregnancy	up to 1
Late pregnancy: fasted 48 h	4.0–6.0
Neonate: 0–1 days	0.2–0.5
Neonate: 5–10 days	0.7–1.0
Hypoglycemia	1.0–5.0
Untreated diabetes mellitus	up to 25

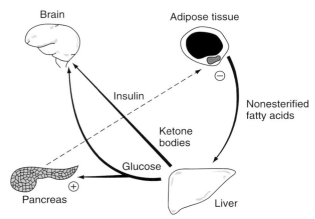

Figure 7 Intertissue fluxes of substrates in the starved state. Thickness of line denotes rate of flux.

More detailed information on the hierarchy of the regulatory factors during onset and reversal of ketogenesis has been obtained for the fasting state by measurements at short time intervals. The first event after withdrawal of food is a lowering of plasma insulin accompanied by an increase in plasma fatty acids (stimulation of lipolysis). However, for an appreciable period (8–10 h) there is no increase in blood ketone bodies or in the *in vitro* rates of hepatic ketogenesis (measured with saturating fatty acid concentrations). The major increment in ketogenic rate occurs at the nadir of the hepatic malonyl-CoA concentrations and when the sensitivity of CAT I to malonyl-CoA is starting to increase rapidly. This long time lag before a change in sensitivity of the protein to malonyl-CoA inhibition is thought to be due to the time required to bring about alterations to the lipid environment of the outer mitochondrial membrane.

Confirmation of this view is that on refeeding, when insulin rapidly increases and plasma fatty acids decrease with a parallel decrease in blood ketone bodies, there is again a time lag before malonyl-CoA concentrations rise and a longer one before sensitivity returns. In physiological and

Table 2 Comparison of factors influencing ketogenesis in suckling and fasted states

Factor	Suckling	Fasted
Plasma nonesterified fatty acids	Increased	Increased
Plasma insulin	Decreased	Decreased
Plasma glucagon	Increased	Increased
Hepatic carnitine	Increased	Increased
Hepatic lipogenesis	Decreased	Decreased
Hepatic malonyl-CoA	Decreased	Decreased
Hepatic CAT I activity	Increased	Increased
Sensitivity to malonyl-CoA	Decreased	Decreased

nutritional terms this delay of return to the normal fed settings of intrahepatic regulation makes excellent sense. It is only when the refeeding consists primarily of large amounts of carbohydrate that the starved liver needs to inhibit the activity of CAT I to prevent the oxidation of newly synthesized fatty acids. If the meal consists mainly of lipid with little carbohydrate the activity of CAT I needs to remain high to allow oxidation of the excess fatty acids. Thus the liver must sense a prolonged increase in plasma insulin before the high activity of CAT I is suppressed.

Pathological ketosis

The major example of pathological ketosis is of course insulin-dependent or type 1 diabetes. Essentially the changes in this condition are similar to those that occur during fasting, but they are more pronounced. Insulin is absent or very low in the plasma and therefore there is no antagonistic action to restrain the opposing hormones, adrenaline, noradrenaline, and glucagon. Consequently, lipolysis in adipose tissue is greatly stimulated and plasma fatty acids increase to high levels.

The lack of insulin and the large flux of fatty acids to the liver means that lipogenesis is inhibited at the level of acetyl-CoA carboxylase and there is the expected decrease in malonyl-CoA concentration. In addition, the sensitivity of CAT I to inhibition by malonyl-CoA is considerably decreased. The level of expression of hepatic CAT I and II proteins also increases several-fold in diabetes. Thus the liver is in the ideal mode for producing excessive amounts of ketone bodies.

It has been suggested that diversion of oxaloacetate to hepatic glucose synthesis (which is also increased in insulin deficiency) may also play a role in the increased rate of ketogenesis by diverting acetyl-CoA from the tricarboxylate cycle. However, present evidence suggests that this makes a minor contribution. Although the excessive output of ketone bodies by the liver undoubtedly makes the major contribution to their high levels in the blood, it is likely that there is also a degree of underutilization by peripheral tissues. The net result is ketoacidosis and excretion of large amounts of energy as ketone bodies in the urine.

A rare, but intriguing, example of pathological ketosis (ketone bodies up to $10 \, \text{mmol} \, \text{l}^{-1}$) is the inborn error of hepatic glycogen synthase deficiency (**Figure 8**). Here glycogen is virtually absent from the liver so that after short-term fasting (5–10 h) the glucose falls to hypoglycemic levels, plasma insulin is decreased, plasma fatty acids increase, and

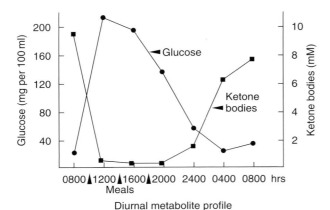

Diurnal metabolite profile

Figure 8 Diurnal blood metabolite profile of a child with glycogen synthetase deficiency. Values taken from Aynsley-Green A, Williamson DH and Gitzelmann R (1977) *Archives of Disease in Childhood* **52**: 573–579. (With permission from BMJ Publishing Group.)

ketogenesis is switched on. On consuming a meal the pattern is reversed until the blood glucose falls again. This case illustrates the importance of hepatic glycogen (and its mobilization) in the smooth transition of substrate supply from the fed to the fasted state. Treatment in this case was to recommend the consumption of more frequent high-carbohydrate snacks. It is of interest that this particular child suffered no ill effects from the daily exposure to high concentrations of ketone bodies, underlining their role as normal substrates for the brain when available.

Metabolic Acidosis

The great disadvantage of ketone bodies is that both acetoacetate and hydroxybutyrate are relatively strong acids. When they increase to high concentration there is the expected decrease in the blood pH, the plasma hydrogen carbonate concentration, and the partial pressure of carbon dioxide in blood and body fluids. The symptoms of acidosis include malaise, weakness, anorexia, and vomiting and these may eventually lead to coma. Treatment of diabetic ketoacidosis is to give insulin as soon as possible, usually as a continuous intravenous infusion. This rapidly decreases the raised plasma fatty acids and more slowly lowers the blood glucose and ketone bodies. Prolonged starvation, where the blood ketone bodies may reach $8-10 \, \mathrm{mmol \, l^{-1}}$, does not usually cause a serious disturbance of the acid–base balance. Loss of ketone bodies via the urine occurs but is not excessive. The nonenzymic decarboxylation of acetoacetate to acetone and carbon dioxide can be seen as a primitive mechanism for removing the potential acidotic effects of

ketone bodies. The fact that acetone can be converted to glucose by the liver at low rates is an extra bonus.

The other common form of metabolic acidosis is lactic acidosis. This can arise because of infection, tissue hypoxia (anaerobic glycolysis), can be drug induced (ethanol, hypoglycemic biguanides), or can arise because of a congenital defect (pyruvate dehydrogenase or pyruvate carboxylase deficiency). In addition to the acidosis caused by lactic acid or ketone bodies there is a group of organic acidurias (some 25–30 different types) in which an inborn error results in the accumulation of an organic acid in the blood and urine. However, frank acidosis is not always associated with these conditions. The key investigation is chromatographic identification of the organic acid.

See also: **Adipose Tissue**. **Carbohydrates**: Regulation of Metabolism. **Cholesterol**: Sources, Absorption, Function and Metabolism. **Fatty Acids**: Metabolism. **Lactation**: Physiology. **Starvation and Fasting**.

Further Reading

Bach AC, Ingenbleek Y, and Frey A (1996) The usefulness of dietary medium-chain triglycerides in body weight control: fact or fancy? *Journal of Lipid Research* **37**: 708–726.

Girard JR, Ferré P, Pégorier JP, and Duée PH (1992) Adaptations of glucose and fatty acid metabolism during perinatal period and suckling–weaning transition. *Physiological Reviews* **72**: 507–562.

Krebs HA, Woods HF, and Alberti KGMM (1975) Hyperlactataemia and lactic acidosis. *Essays in Medical Biochemistry* **1**: 81–103.

McGarry JD and Foster DW (1980) Regulation of hepatic fatty acid oxidation and ketone body production. *Annual Review of Biochemistry* **49**: 395–420.

Nehlig A and de Vasconcelos AP (1993) Glucose and ketone body utilization by the brain of neonatal rats. *Progress in Neurobiology* **40**: 163–221.

Owen OE, Morgan AP, Kemp HG *et al.* (1967) Brain metabolism during fasting. *Journal of Clinical Investigation* **46**: 1589–1595.

Page MA and Williamson DH (1971) Enzymes of ketone body utilisation in human brain. *Lancet* **2**: 66–68.

Porter R and Lawrenson G (eds.) (1982) Metabolic acidosis. *Ciba Foundation Symposium*, **87**. London: Pitman.

Robinson AM and Williamson DH (1980) Physiological roles of ketone bodies as substrates and signals in mammalian tissues. *Physiological Reviews* **60**: 143–187.

Williamson DH (1982) The production and utilization of ketone bodies in the neonate. In: CT Jones (ed.) *The Biochemical Development of the Fetus*, pp. 621–650. Amsterdam: Elsevier Biomedical.

Williamson DH (1987) Brain substrates and the effects of nutrition. *Proceedings of Nutrition Society* **46**: 81–87.

Zammit VA (1996) Role of insulin in hepatic fatty acid partitioning: Emerging concepts. *Biochemical Journal* **314**: 1–14.

L

LACTATION

Contents

Physiology

J L McManaman and M C Neville, University of Colorado, Denver, CO, USA

Lactation is a uniquely mammalian physiological process in which the caloric and nutrient reserves of the mother are transformed into a complex fluid capable of supporting the nutritional demands of newborns for sustained periods. Milk, the product of lactation, is a mixture of solutes whose composition reflects the activities of distinct secretion and transport processes of the mammary gland and mirrors the differing nutritional requirements of mammalian neonates. In humans, this fluid is capable of providing the full-term infant with all the nutrients required for the first 4–6 months of life as well as offering significant protection against infectious disease. Although artificial formulas are widely utilized for human infant nutrition in developed countries, many components of human milk, including critical growth factors, long-chain polyunsaturated fatty acids, antiinfectious oligosaccharides and glycoconjugates, and the protein lactoferrin, are not duplicated in formula. Although it is likely that such substances are beneficial even to healthy infants in well-protected environments, they are particularly important to infants living in conditions of inadequate sanitation, as well as to preterm infants and infants with feeding problems. Despite the obvious importance of milk to neonatal nutrition and the selective advantage of lactation in mammalian evolution, the physiological mechanisms underlying milk secretion and utilization are not well understood and the molecular mechanisms involved in the production of individual milk components are still poorly characterized. In this article, the functional anatomy of the mammary gland is described, followed by a brief description of human milk composition and a review of the transport mechanisms involved in the secretion of individual milk components. We then summarize the functional differentiation of the mammary gland and the initiation of lactation—a process that involves a series of carefully programmed functional changes that transform a prepared, but nonsecretory, gland into a fully functioning organ during the first week postpartum in humans.

Functional Anatomy of Lactation

The lactating mammary gland consists of an arborizing ductal network that extends from the nipple and terminates in grape-like lobular clusters of alveoli forming the lobuloalveolar unit, which is the site of milk secretion. A stylized diagram of these structures is shown in **Figure 1**. Alveoli are composed of a single layer of polarized secretory epithelial cells that possess specialized features indicative of highly developed biosynthetic and secretory capacities, including numerous mitochondria, an extensive rough endoplasmic reticulum network, and a well-developed Golgi apparatus. Secretory components including lipid droplets and casein containing secretory vesicles are found juxtaposed to the apical membrane of these cells. The epithelial cells are connected to each other through a junctional complex composed of adherens and tight-junctional elements that function to inhibit transfer of extracellular substances between the vascular system and milk compartments during lactation (**Figure 2**). The basal portion of alveolar epithelial cells is surrounded by a meshwork of myoepithelial cell processes that contract to bring about milk

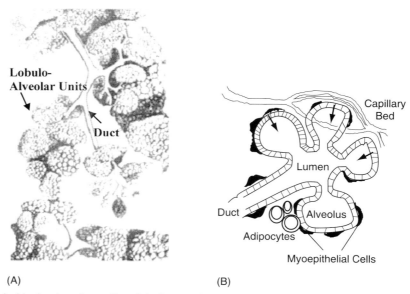

(A)   (B)

Figure 1   (A) Camera lucida drawing of a section of the breast of a woman who died 2 days after last suckling her infant. The drawing clearly shows collecting ducts and the grape-like lobuloalveolar units, which are engorged with milk. (From Dabelow A (1941) *Morphology Journal* **85**: 361–416.) (B) Cross-sectional diagram showing the relationship of the lobuloalveolar unit composed of milk secreting alveoli and ducts to the other cellular compartments of the mammary gland. Arrows indicate milk secretion by the alveolar epithelial cells into the lumen.

ejection and by a connective tissue stroma that supports and separates the lobules. The stromal component also contains lymphatics and becomes extensively vascularized during lactation to sustain

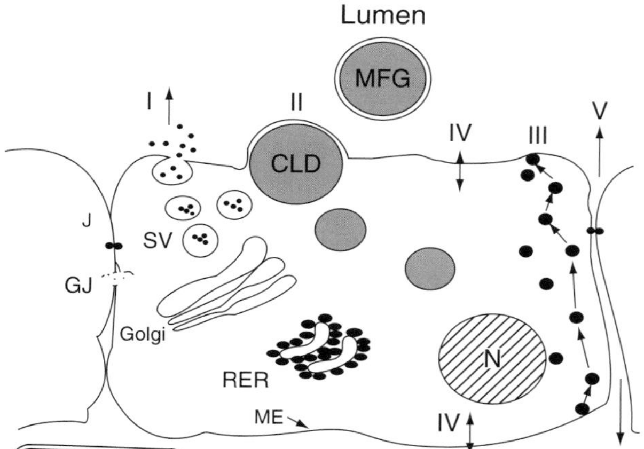

Figure 2   Diagram of a mammary epithelial cell showing pathways for milk secretion described in the text. SV, secretory vesicle; RER, rough endoplasmic reticulum; BM, basement membrane; N, nucleus; PC, plasma cell; FDA, fat-depleted adipocyte; J, junctional complex containing the tight and adherens junctions; GJ, gap junction; ME, myoepithelial cell; CLD, cytoplasmic lipid droplet; MFG, milk fat globule. (Redrawn from Neville MC, Allen JC and Watters C (1983) The mechanisms of milk secretion. In: Neville MC and Neifert MR (eds.) *Lactation: Physiology, Nutrition and Breast-Feeding*, p. 50. New York: Plenum Press.)

the biosynthetic demands of alveolar epithelial cells. In nonpregnant, nonlactating animals the stroma contains a large adipose component.

The nipple, which is the termination point of the mammary ductal network, is innervated by the fourth intercostal nerve. Afferent sensory stimuli from suckling are transmitted to the spinal cord and the brain, resulting in release of prolactin and oxytocin from the pituitary. Prolactin, secreted from the anterior pituitary, acts directly on alveolar epithelial cells to foster synthesis and secretion of milk components. Oxytocin, secreted from the posterior pituitary, stimulates contraction of the myoepithelial cells that surround the alveoli and ducts. This process, called the 'letdown reflex,' forces the milk from the alveoli through ductules into ducts draining several clusters of alveoli. In the human, the small ducts converge into 15–25 main ducts that drain sectors of the gland and open directly on the nipple. The secretory product is stored in the alveolar space until myoepithelial cell contractions force it through the ducts toward the nipple, where it is available to the suckling infant.

Milk Composition

The major macronutrients in milk are lactose (a disaccharide unique to milk); lipids; proteins, including casein, α-lactalbumin, lactoferrin, secretory immunoglobulin A (sIgA), and many others present at much lower concentrations; and minerals such as sodium, chloride, calcium, and magnesium. Minor nutrients in milk are enzymes, vitamins, trace elements, and growth factors. The lipid content of milk varies considerably between species. In human and cow's milk, the fat accounts for approximately 4% of milk volume, whereas in whales and seals it can account for as much as 60% of milk volume. Milk fat is primarily composed of triglycerides, a major source of neonatal calories, but it also contains cholesterol and phospholipids, essential for early neonatal development. Casein micelles form a separate phase that can be pelleted by high-speed centrifugation or acidification. These micelles have a high calcium and phosphate content. The aqueous fraction of milk, often called whey, is a true solution that contains all the milk sugar as well as the major milk proteins lactoferrin, α-lactalbumin, and sIgA and nonprotein nitrogen compounds (mostly urea); the monovalent ions sodium, potassium, and chloride; citrate; calcium; free phosphate; and most of the water-soluble minor components of milk.

The casein fraction from cow's milk, usually obtained by rennin precipitation, is used in cheese making, whereas the whey has a multiplicity of uses, most notably as the base for infant formula. Urea and other nonprotein nitrogen components of milk are a source of nitrogen for amino acid and protein synthesis. Isotope utilization studies indicate that on average 10–20% of urea nitrogen is converted into protein by breast-fed infants. Significantly higher utilization rates, however, have been measured in children recovering from infection, suggesting that alterations in urea nitrogen utilization may be a homeostatic response. Human and bovine milk differ primarily in their concentrations of lactose, mono- and divalent ions, and casein levels and the existence of antiinfectious agents in human milk (**Table 1**). These differences are related to the specific needs of these species. Human milk, for example, possesses higher concentrations of lactose and lower divalent ion concentrations than cow's milk. The high lactose concentration provides a large amount of 'free water,' via osmotic regulation, that serves as a reserve for temperature regulation via sweating in human infants. Human milk also contains a number of agents that protect against gastrointestinal and respiratory infections, including oligosaccharides that interact specifically with pathogen receptors, lactoferrin and sIgA. Bovine milk, on the other hand, contains high concentrations of casein, which provides protein and associated calcium and phosphate needed to support rapid growth of young calves.

Table 1 Comparison of the macronutrient contents of human and bovine milk

Component	Human milk	Bovine milk
Carbohydrates (g/dl)[a]		
Lactose	7.3	4.0
Oligosaccharides	1.2	0.1
Proteins (g/dl)[a]		
Caseins	0.2	2.6
α-Lactalbumin	0.2	0.2
Lactoferrin	0.2	Trace
Secretory IgA	0.2	Trace
β-Lactoglobulin	0	0.5
Nonprotein nitrogen (NPN) (g/l)		
Total NPN	0.42[b]	0.29[c]
Urea	0.16[b]	0.14[c]
Milk lipids (%)[a]		
Triglycerides	4.0	4.0
Phospholipids	0.04	0.04
Minerals and other ionic constituents (mM)[a]		
Sodium	5.0	15
Potassium	15.0	43
Chloride	15.0	24
Calcium	7.5	30
Magnesium	1.4	5
Phosphate	1.8	11
Bicarbonate	6.0	5

[a]Data from Neville MC (1998) Physiology of lactation. *Clinical Perinatology* **26**: 251.
[b]Data from Atkinson SA and Lonnerdal B (1995) In: Jensen RG (ed.) *Handbook of Milk Composition*. San Diego: Academic Press.
[c]Data from Alston-Mills B (1995) In: Jensen RG (ed.) *Handbook of Milk Composition*. San Diego: Academic Press.

Synthesis and Secretion of Milk Components

Solutes enter milk through five general pathways (**Figure 2**). Endogenously generated substances, including the major milk proteins, oligosaccharides, and nutrients such as lactose, citrate, phosphate, and calcium, are secreted through an exocytotic pathway (pathway I). Lipids and lipid-associated proteins are secreted by a process that is unique to mammary epithelial cells (pathway II). The transcytosis pathway (pathway III) transports a wide range of macromolecular substances derived from serum or stromal cells, including serum proteins such as immunoglobulins, albumin, and transferrin; endocrine hormones such as insulin, prolactin, and insulin-like growth factor-1; and stromal-derived agents such as IgA, cytokines, and lipoprotein lipase. In addition, various membrane transport pathways (pathway IV) exist for the transfer of ions and small molecules, such as glucose, amino acids, and water, across basal and apical plasma membranes. Finally, there is a paracellular pathway (pathway V) that provides a direct route for entry of serum and interstitial substances into milk. This pathway, however, closes during the first few days of lactation in the human. Transport through these pathways is affected by the functional state of the mammary gland and regulated by direct and indirect actions of hormones and growth factors. The general cellular and physiological properties of these pathways are summarized next.

Exocytotic Pathway (I)

Like exocytotic secretion mechanisms found in other cells, proteins, oligosaccharides, and nutrients such as lactose and citrate are packaged into secretory vesicles within the Golgi that are then transported to the apical region of the cell, where they fuse with the apical plasma membrane, discharging their contents into the extracellular space. A unique feature of this pathway in the mammary gland is the presence of high concentrations of lactose, phosphate, citrate, and calcium within the vesicles. Lactose is synthesized in the Golgi from UDP-galactose and glucose, which have entered from the cytoplasm using specific transporters, by the enzyme β-galactosidase, with α-lactalbumin acting as a cofactor. The high concentration of lactose present in the Golgi during lactation osmotically stimulates the influx of water that contributes to the fluidity of milk. Casein micelle formation begins in the terminal Golgi with condensation, and simultaneous phosphorylation, of casein molecules. Addition of calcium, possibly in the secretory vesicle, leads to maturation of casein micelles into particles sufficiently dense to be seen in the electron microscope. This complex thus delivers an efficient package of protein, calcium, and phosphate that provides the nutrients necessary for bone growth, among other things. Calcium enters the cytoplasm from the plasma by a poorly defined transport process. Cytoplasmic calcium is then transported into secretory vesicles by an ATP-dependent Ca^{2+} pump localized on Golgi and secretory membranes. The phosphate in secretory vesicles is derived from the hydrolysis of UDP-galactose during the synthesis of lactose. Citrate is generated endogenously within the cytoplasm of alveolar epithelial cells and transported into the Golgi lumen by an undefined process.

Lipid Secretion Pathway (II)

Estimates of the quantity of milk lipid secretion during lactation in humans and rodents indicate that in many species the lactating mammary gland may be one of the most lipogenic organs in the body. In a fully lactating woman secreting 800 ml/day of milk containing 4% fat, the mammary gland synthesizes approximately 32 g of triglyceride daily or approximately 6 g, 10% of the weight of the woman, in a typical 6-month lactation. The fatty acids for triglyceride synthesis are synthesized from glucose or derived from the plasma lipids by the action of lipoprotein lipase. Once available in the mammary alveolar cells, fatty acids are either bound to a fatty acid binding protein or activated by combination with coenzyme A (CoA) and then bound to an acyl-CoA binding protein. Activated fatty acids are joined with glycerol-3-phosphate by transacylases located in the endoplasmic reticulum to form triglycerides, which enter the cytoplasm as protein-coated structures called cytoplasmic lipid droplets. These structures are translocated to the apical membrane, where they are enveloped by a novel budding process that leads to their release as membrane-bound lipid droplets known as milk fat globules.

The fatty acid composition of milk triglycerides reflects differences in maternal diet. Medium-chain (C_{8-14}) fatty acids are synthesized only in the mammary gland using glucose (or acetate in ruminants) as substrate, whereas long-chain fatty acids are derived from the plasma. Nigerian women who have high-carbohydrate, low-fat diets have significantly more medium-chain fatty acids in their milk than Western women who consume a high-fat diet (**Table 2**).

Transcytosis Pathway (III)

Transport of proteins and other macromolecules by transcytotic pathways involves endocytic uptake of substances at the basal membrane, formation and maturation of endosomes, and sorting to lysosomes for degradation or to the apical recycling compartment for exocytosis at the apical membrane. The best studied molecule in this regard is immunoglobulin A (IgA). IgA is synthesized by plasma cells in the interstitial spaces of the mammary gland or elsewhere in the body and binds to receptors on the basal surface of the mammary alveolar cell; the entire IgA–receptor complex is endocytosed and transferred to the apical membrane, where the extracellular portion of the receptor is cleaved and secreted together with the IgA. It is thought that many other proteins, hormones, and growth factors that find their way into milk from the plasma are secreted by a similar mechanism.

Transmembrane Pathway (IV)

Transport processes for sodium, potassium, and chloride exist on the basal and apical plasma

Table 2 Major fatty acids of human and bovine milk (wt%)

Fatty acid	Human milk		Bovine milk
	Western diet	Nigerian diet	
Saturated fatty acids			
Medium and intermediate chain (formed in mammary gland)			
8:0, octanoic acid	0.46		1.3
10:0, decanoic acid	1.03	0.54	2.7
12:0, lauric acid	4.40	8.34	3.0
14:0, myristic acid	6.27	9.57	10.6
Long chain			
16:0, palmitic acid	22.0	23.35	28.2
18:0, stearic acid	8.06	10.15	12.6
Monounsaturated fatty acids			
16:1 n-7 (*cis*), palmitoleic acid	3.29	0.91	1.6
18:1 n-9 (*cis*), oleic acid	31.3	18.52	21.4
18:1 n-9 (*trans*), oleic acid	2.67	0.86	1.7
Polyunsaturated fatty acids (PUFA) (essential fatty acids)			
18:2 n-6, linoleic acid	10.76	11.06	2.9
18:3 n-3, linolenic acid	0.81	1.41	0.3
Long-chain PUFA (n-6)			
18:3 n-6, γ-linolenic acid	0.16	0.12	2.9
20:2 n-6,	0.34	0.26	0.03
20:3 n-6, dihomo-γ-linolenic acid	0.26	0.49	0.1
20:4 n-6, arachadonic acid	0.36	0.82	0.2
Long-chain PUFA (n-3)			
20:5 n-3, eicosapentenoic acid	0.04	0.48	0.08
22:5 n-3	0.17	0.39	
22:6 n-3, docashexenoic acid	0.22	0.93	0.09

Data from Jensen RG (1995) *Handbook of Milk Composition*. San Diego: Academic Press.

membranes of alveolar epithelial cells. Uptake mechanisms for calcium, phosphate, and iodide, however, are thought to be limited to the basal membrane. The mammary epithelial cells possess a GLUT1 glucose transporter and a sodium-dependent glucose transporter. The GLUT1 transporter is thought to mediate glucose transport at the basal and Golgi membranes, but it does not contribute to glucose transport at the apical membrane. Both sodium-dependent and sodium-independent amino acid transport mechanisms analogous to those found in other organs are located in the basolateral component of the mammary epithelium. It is unclear if apical membranes have similar transport mechanisms for amino acids, and it is unknown how amino acids get into milk.

Paracellular Transport Pathway (V)

Pathway V (**Figure 2**) involves passage of substances between epithelial cells rather than through them, and for this reason it is designated the paracellular pathway. During full lactation the passage of even low-molecular-weight substances between alveolar cells is impeded by the gasket-like tight junction structures that join the epithelial cells tightly, one to another. During pregnancy, with mastitis and after involution the tight junctions become leaky and allow components of the interstitial space, such as sodium and potassium, to pass unimpeded into the milk, a fact that is sometimes useful in diagnosing breast-feeding problems.

Regulation of Milk Synthesis, Secretion, and Ejection

Milk volume production is a primary indicator of lactational function; the most precise methods for measuring the volume of milk produced involve weighing infants before and after each feed for 24 h or longer or using an isotope dilution technique with stable isotopes. Clinically, the amount of milk that can be expressed with a breast pump or the change in infant weight after a single feed can be used as a rough index. The volume of milk secreted by women exclusively breast-feeding a single infant at 6 months postpartum is remarkably constant at approximately 800 ml/day in populations throughout the world. Mothers of twins, and occasionally even triplets, are able to produce volumes of milk sufficient for complete nutrition of their multiple infants,

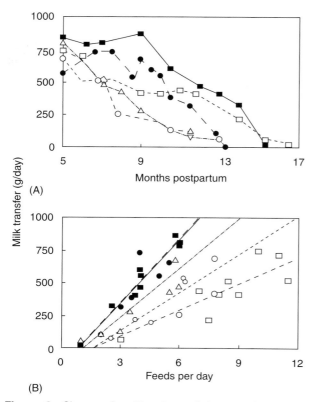

(A)

(B)

Figure 3 Changes in milk volume during weaning and in response to increased feeding frequency. (A) Milk volume transfer as a function of time postpartum. (B) Relation between feeding frequency (feeds/day) and the milk volume. Data are from five breast-feeding dyads; each symbol represents an individual dyad. (Reproduced with permission from Neville MC *et al.* (1991) *American Journal of Clinical Nutrition* **54**: 81–92.)

and studies of wet nurses indicate that at least some women are capable of producing up to 3.5 l of milk per day. On the other hand, if infants are supplemented with foods other than breast milk, milk secretion is proportionately reduced. This point is illustrated in **Figure 3**, which shows that milk volumes gradually decline during weaning and increase as feeding frequency increases. These observations illustrate the important principle that the volume of milk secretion in lactating women is regulated by infant demand. If milk cannot be removed from the breast, local mechanisms bring about an inhibition of milk secretion and downregulation of milk synthetic machinery. With partial removal of milk on a consistent basis, these local factors adjust milk secretion to a new steady-state level. If milk removal ceases for extended periods, involution sets in and the gland loses its competency to secrete milk.

Hormonal Control of Milk Synthesis and Secretion

In most species, the presence of high levels of plasma prolactin appears to be essential for lactation. In rats,

the ergot alkaloid bromocriptine (an inhibitor of prolactin release from the pituitary) inhibits lactation, and in women it inhibits the onset of lactation when given in appropriate doses. How prolactin influences lactation is not known in any detail. However, it appears to promote mammary epithelial cell survival. In addition, it is an osmoregulator in some species of fish, birds, and amphibians and may function to maintain solute transport in the mammary gland.

Local Control of Synthesis and Secretion

Two local mechanisms have been postulated to regulate milk volume production. In one, it is thought that buildup of a specific inhibitory substance occurs in milk as it accumulates in the lumen of the mammary gland. However, the identity of this factor, called feedback inhibitor of lactation, has not been defined. In the second, it is thought that a stretch response of alveoli regulates milk production. Understanding this regulation may be very important in helping women to increase their milk supply, particularly in the postpartum period; therefore, further research is needed.

Regulation of Milk Ejection

When the infant is suckled, afferent impulses from sensory stimulation of nerve terminals in the areolus travel to the central nervous system, where they promote the release of oxytocin from the posterior pituitary. This neuroendocrine reflex can be conditioned, and in the woman oxytocin release is often associated with such stimuli as the sight or sound, or even the thought, of the infant. The oxytocin is carried through the bloodstream to the mammary gland, where it interacts with specific receptors on myoepithelial cells, initiating their contraction and expelling milk from the alveoli into the ducts and subareolar sinuses. The passage of milk through the ducts is facilitated by longitudinally arranged myoepithelial cell processes whose contraction shortens and widens the ducts, allowing free flow of milk to the nipple. Milk is removed from the nipple not so much by suction as by the stripping motion of the tongue against the hard palate. This motion carries milk through the teat into the baby's mouth. The letdown response is decreased by psychological stress or pain, which interfere with oxytocin release. Oxytocin also appears to be involved in regulating maternal behavior in laboratory animals and may play a similar role in humans.

Initiation of Lactation

Pregnancy transforms the mammary gland from a simple ductal tree into a highly efficient exocrine organ with expansive lobuloalveolar structures. This transformation is hormonally regulated and involves changes in the cellular composition of the mammary gland and alterations in the structural, cellular, and biochemical properties of alveolar cells that are critical to development of efficient solute transport and secretory functions. Alveolar epithelial cells begin to differentiate into secretory cells at midpregnancy in most species. The differentiation process occurs heterogeneously and has been divided into initiation and activation phases based on differences in the composition of mammary secretions, gene expression, and structural and functional properties of alveolar cells. Alveolar cells become capable of limited secretion of some milk components during the initiation phase, which in humans is detected by measurement of increased concentrations of lactose and α-lactalbumin in the plasma. Copious milk secretion, however, is induced during the secretory activation phase (sometimes called lactogenesis II) that occurs in response to the decrease in serum progesterone levels. In rodents and ruminants, this decrease is closely associated with parturition; in humans it occurs after parturition.

Changes in Milk Composition during Secretory Activation

Secretory activation is reflected in dramatic modifications of the solute composition of milk and increased secretory volume, which in turn reflect the maturation of secretory mechanisms and transport pathways during this period. In women, there are three temporally distinct changes in milk composition at the onset of lactation. The earliest is a decrease in sodium and chloride concentrations and an increase in the lactose concentration of milk (**Figure 4**). These modifications occur immediately after delivery and are largely complete by 72 h postpartum. They precede increases in milk volume by at least 24 h and can be explained by closure of the tight junctions that block the paracellular pathway. Blocking this pathway prevents lactose, made by the epithelial cells, from passing from the lumen of the alveolus to the plasma, and it prevents sodium and chloride from directly entering the lumen from the interstitial space. These changes result in decreased concentrations of sodium and chloride and increased concentrations of lactose in the mammary secretion. The increased lactose concentration is reflective of decreased water entering the lumina as monovalent ion secretion decreases rather than an increase in the lactose secretion rate.

Secondarily, there are transient increases in the rates of secretion of sIgA and lactoferrin into milk of women soon after delivery. The concentrations of these two important protective proteins remain high, comprising

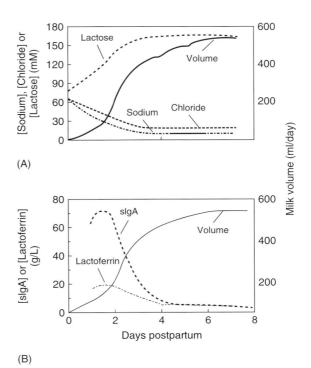

Figure 4 Changes in milk composition and volume in women during secretory activation and early lactation. (Reproduced with permission from McManaman JL and Neville MC (2003) *Advanced Drug Delivery Reviews* **55**: 630–641.)

as much as 10% of milk, for the first 48 h after birth. The concentration of each protein decreases rapidly after day 2, both from dilution as milk volume secretion increases and from actual decreases in their rates of secretion, particularly of immunoglobulins. Although both these proteins are found at high concentrations in colostrum, they are likely to be secreted by different mechanisms; lactoferrin, an endogenous protein of alveolar cells, is secreted by the exocytotic pathway (pathway I), whereas sIgA, a plasma-derived protein, is secreted by receptor-mediated transcytosis (pathway III). In addition, the peak secretion rate of lactoferrin occurs at the same time as that of lactose and the major milk proteins, whereas sIgA secretion peaks 1 day earlier, indicating the possibility that the exocytotic and transcytosis pathways are regulated differently during early lactation.

The third phase occurs approximately 36 h postpartum and is associated with massive and concerted increases in milk volume and the rates of synthesis and/or secretion of almost all the components of mature milk, including, but not limited to, lactose, protein (mainly casein), lipid, calcium, sodium, magnesium, potassium, citrate, glucose, and free phosphate. Considering that the secretion of these substances involves the actions of several distinct transport pathways and biosynthetic processes, such tightly synchronized increases imply the presence of a common activation switch for coordinating their activities.

Hormonal Control of Secretory Activation

The decrease in progesterone around parturition is generally agreed to be required for the onset of milk secretion. In humans, it is known that removal of the placenta, the source of progesterone, is necessary for the initiation of milk secretion. In swine, timing of the increase in milk lactose correlates closely with timing of the decrease in plasma progesterone at parturition. Exogenous progesterone prevents lactose and lipid synthesis in mammary glands of pregnant rats and sheep after removal of their ovaries, the source of progesterone in these species. Progesterone also suppresses β-casein expression in the rat mammary gland during pregnancy and the decrease in progesterone levels is linked to increased β-casein synthesis at parturition. Receptors for progesterone are not detected in lactating mammary tissues, which explains why progesterone does not inhibit established lactation. It is likely that the decline in progesterone is insufficient to activate secretion and that the actions of other hormones, including prolactin and glucocorticoids, are necessary to complete this process. In all *in vitro* mammary systems, insulin and corticoids, in addition to prolactin, are necessary to maintain synthesis of milk components. Further more, cortisol replacement is required for maintenance of milk production in adrenalectomized animals. An early notion that a surge of glucocorticoids is the initiator of lactation is likely incorrect since the increase in cortisol seen in unanesthetized women associated with the stress of labor is complete by the time milk volume begins to increase to any extent. Because secretory activation proceeds at parturition in severely diabetic rats, a role for insulin in lactogenesis as opposed to metabolic adjustments during lactation seems improbable. In summary, the most reasonable interpretation of the data from both animal and human studies is that the hormonal trigger for lactogenesis is a decrease in progesterone in the presence of maintained prolactin. Since postpartum prolactin levels are similar in both breast-feeding and non-breast-feeding women, the basic process appears to be initiated whether or not breast-feeding occurs. The caveat, of course, is that the mammary epithelium must be sufficiently prepared by the hormones of pregnancy to respond with milk synthesis.

Delays in Secretory Activation

A delay in the onset of milk secretion is a problem for the initiation of breast-feeding in a significant number of parturient women. A number of pathological conditions may delay secretory activation in women, including cesarean section, diabetes, obesity, and stress during parturition. The role of cesarean section is controversial, but if there is one it is likely to have only a modest effect. However, poorly controlled diabetes, stress from delivery, or obesity are associated with significant decreases in early milk production. Because each of these conditions is related to higher blood glucose, hyperglycemia may be an underlying factor in the delay in lactation. However, once it is established, diabetics do not have a problem in maintaining lactation. Thus, compensatory factors may override initiation defects to ensure infant nutrition in these disorders.

See also: **Breast Feeding. Fatty Acids**: Omega-3 Polyunsaturated; Omega-6 Polyunsaturated. **Lactation**: Dietary Requirements. **Lipids**: Chemistry and Classification. **Pregnancy**: Energy Requirements and Metabolic Adaptations.

Dietary Requirements

N M F Trugo and C M Donangelo, Universidade Federal do Rio de Janeiro, Rio de Janeiro, Brazil

Introduction

Milk secretion imposes a considerable nutritional demand on lactating women. The challenge to the maternal organism to sustain milk production and nutrient composition while maintaining an adequate nutritional status is high and must be met by increased dietary intake of energy and nutrients. Otherwise, maternal nutrient depletion may occur due to excessive mobilization of maternal stores. Owing to the major gaps in the knowledge on maternal nutrient requirements and the impact of lactation on maternal nutrient status, and the quantitative and qualitative importance of milk production for the incremental nutrient requirements, the recommended nutrient intakes for lactating women are based mainly on the volume of milk secreted and its nutritional content. The high nutritional demands for milk production result in recommended intakes of most nutrients for lactation that are higher (10%–90%) than in nonreproductive stages.

The dietary recommendations for lactating women considered in this article are those of the FAO/WHO Reports on fats (1994) and micronutrients (2001), and the Dietary Reference Intakes (DRIs) of the Institute of Medicine (US) on micronutrients (1997, 1998, 2000, 2001) and macronutrients (2002). The rationale for recommended nutrient intakes, and the nutrient requirements and dietary recommendations for energy, fat, protein, calcium, zinc, folate, and vitamin A are specifically addressed.

Rationale for Recommended Nutrient Intakes

Recommendations on dietary nutrient intakes for lactating women by different scientific authorities are typically based on the estimated total amount of each nutrient secreted daily into breast milk, taking into account, where known, the efficiency of milk synthesis and the bioavailability of the nutrient in the maternal diet. This estimate for each nutrient is then added to the recommended nutrient intake for non-pregnant, non-lactating women.

The onset of lactation after parturition is brought about by the major hormonal changes that occur in this period. During the first 2–7 days post-partum a thick yellow fluid (colostrum) is secreted. With the progress of lactation, the volume of milk secreted increases and its nutrient composition changes, with an increase, decrease or no change in concentration, depending on the nutrient. After about 21 days the milk secreted is considered mature milk. The volume of breast milk secreted daily increases rapidly in the first post-partum days, being ∼500 ml on day 5, ∼650 ml at 1 month, and ∼750 ml at 3 months, remaining relatively stable during full lactation but decreasing during weaning. In industrialized countries, the average volume of breast milk produced is 750–800 ml day^{-1} in the first 4–5 months post-partum and decreases to 600 ml day^{-1} during 6–12 months after delivery. In this period, the volume of milk produced may be even lower and more variable, depending on the weaning practices adopted.

The FAO/WHO and DRI committees considered 750 and 780 ml, respectively, as the average milk volume produced during full lactation and the basis for recommendations. For most nutrients, average concentration in mature milk multiplied by the average milk volume was used to estimate the total amount of nutrient secreted daily into breast milk. A correction factor was then applied to account for the nutrient bioavailability in the maternal diet and, where known, for the anabolic cost of milk synthesis, and the final value was added to the recommended intake of nonpregnant, nonlactating women. The stage of lactation was considered to be a factor for some nutrients and, where applicable, separate values were given according to the period of time post-partum.

The volume of milk secreted during lactation is not influenced by maternal nutritional status, unless maternal undernutrition is severe. The composition of breast milk for most nutrients is adequate to support infant growth and development in a wide range of maternal nutritional status. However, maternal diet and nutritional status do have an influence on the concentration of some micronutrients such as vitamin A, thiamin, riboflavin, vitamins B_6 and B_{12}, iodine, and selenium. Also, the fatty acid composition of breast milk can be affected by maternal diet.

An important step taken by the DRI committees when setting recommendations was taking maternal age into account, thus giving separate values for adolescent (≤18 years) and adult (19–50 years) lactating women. For some nutrients, adolescent lactating women may have greater requirements than adult women because they are still growing and they need to cover their own nutrient demands. Recommendation of intakes during lactation of calcium, phosphorus, magnesium, iron, and zinc are higher for adolescent than for adult women.

In general, there is considerable uncertainty in establishing dietary nutrient recommendations for lactation due to high intra- and interindividual variability in breast milk volume output and in several specific nutrient concentrations in breast milk, and to temporal changes in milk volume and nutrient concentrations during the lactation period. The composition of breast milk is affected by several factors depending on the nutrient, such as stage of lactation, changes during nursing, diurnal rhythm, maternal diet, gestational age at birth, and parity. Moreover, the total amount of nutrients secreted into breast milk depends on the extent and duration of breast feeding. In addition, physiological adaptation to the increased nutrient lactation demands such as increased nutrient absorption and conservation, and use of maternal nutrient stores, which are quite specific for each nutrient and not easily quantified, contributes to the degree of uncertainty. Maternal age and maternal nutritional status during pregnancy and lactation may influence the homeostatic adaptations during lactation such as the efficiency of nutrient absorption and the degree of mobilization of maternal nutrient stores. These factors are not well known and are difficult to quantify.

Requirements and Dietary Recommendations

Macronutrients

Energy The dietary energy intake recommended for healthy adults of normal weight (body mass index between 18.5 and $25\,kg\,m^{-2}$) is the energy required to maintain energy balance, considering gender, age, weight, height, and level of physical activity. The energy requirements of lactating women include the additional energy that is necessary for milk production. The stage and extent of breastfeeding affect the incremental energy requirements for lactation.

The energy density of human milk is mainly determined by its fat content, which represents 50–60% of the total energy in mature milk and is the most variable energy-yielding component. Protein and lactose contribute to approximately 5% and 38% of energy, respectively. The mean energy density of representative 24-h pooled mature milk samples from well-nourished women ranges from 0.64 to $0.74\,kcal\,g^{-1}$ ($2.7–3.1\,kJ\,g^{-1}$).

The estimated energy requirements (EER) for lactating women by the DRI committee are based mainly on studies done in the 1990s, using the doubly labeled water method. The main findings in women who were fully breastfeeding their infants up to 6 months of age were: total energy expenditure of $2109–2580\,kcal\,day^{-1}$ ($8860–10840\,kJ\,day^{-1}$) or $35.8–41.0\,kcal\,kg^{-1}\,day^{-1}$ ($150–172\,kJ\,kg^{-1}\,day^{-1}$), milk energy output of $483–538\,kcal\,day^{-1}$ ($2030–2260\,kJ\,day^{-1}$), and energy mobilization from tissue stores of $72–287\,kcal\,day^{-1}$($300–1200\,kJ\,day^{-1}$). It was concluded that the energy requirements of lactating, well-nourished women are met primarily from the diet and partially by mobilization of tissue stores, without evidence for adaptations in basal metabolism and physical activities. The EER for lactating adult women during the first 6 months of lactation is calculated as the sum of the EER obtained from the equation for adult nonlactating women (using current age, weight, and physical activity level), and the milk energy output ($500\,kcal\,day^{-1}$ or $2100\,kJ\,day^{-1}$), subtracting the energy derived from tissue mobilization during lactational weight loss ($170\,kcal\,day^{-1}$ or $714\,kJ\,day^{-1}$). The committee considered a milk production rate of $0.78\,l\,day^{-1}$ from birth through 6 months of age, with a milk energy density of $0.67\,kcal\,g^{-1}$ ($2.8\,kJ\,day^{-1}$), and an average maternal weight loss of $0.8\,kg\,month^{-1}$. For the second 6 months of lactation, the incremental EER is calculated considering a milk energy output of $400\,kcal\,day^{-1}$ or $1680\,kJ\,day^{-1}$ (milk production rate of $0.61\,l\,day^{-1}$) and no maternal weight loss.

The EER for lactating adolescents (14–18 years) is calculated in the same manner as for adult lactating women, but using the appropriate equation to estimate the EER of nonlactating adolescents.

The acceptable macronutrient distribution ranges as percentage of total dietary energy for lactating women are the same as for the general adult population: 10–35% protein, 20–35% fat, and 45–65% carbohydrates. Natural simple sugars, such as those present in fruit, and complex carbohydrates (polysaccharides), such as in cereals (rice, wheat), cereal products (flour, pasta) and starchy roots, should be the preferred sources of carbohydrates in the diet. Added sugars, usually sucrose, should not be higher than 25% of dietary energy. Many of the energy-yielding carbohydrate food sources are also sources of dietary fiber, which are beneficial in reducing the risk of coronary heart disease, ameliorating constipation, and other ways. A total fiber intake of $29\,g\,day^{-1}$ is recommended for lactating women. Whole grain cereals, nuts, legumes, and fruit are good fiber and energy sources, and are also nutrient-rich foods. Restriction of energy intake during lactation to values below $1800\,kcal$ ($7500\,kJ$) per day may lead to low intakes of several micronutrients such as calcium, magnesium, zinc, folate, vitamin B_6, and vitamin A.

Fat Total fat content in human milk is affected by several factors, including stage of lactation, moment of feeding, and parity, but maternal intake of energy, fat, and fatty acids and maternal status have little influence, except when there is a long-term or severe maternal undernutrition. Milk fat content is highly variable, being on average $35–40\,g\,l^{-1}$ in mature milk from well-nourished women delivering at term gestation. The content of individual fatty acids in milk is also highly variable, especially for the long-chain polyunsaturated fatty acids (LCPUFA; mainly C_{20} and C_{22}), and more dependent on maternal diet than total fat. Fatty acid intake and relative contribution of carbohydrate and fat to the total energy intake, as well as maternal body stores and endogenous synthesis, influence the fatty acid composition of human milk. In well-nourished mothers, the polyunsaturated essential fatty acids (EFA) linoleic acid (18:2n-6) and α-linolenic acid (18:3n-3) represent approximately 11 and 1% (wt/wt), respectively, of the total fatty acids in milk. LCPUFA of the n-6 and n-3 series account for 1.2 and 0.6%, respectively.

The adequate transfer of polyunsaturated fatty acids from maternal circulation to milk and the maternal synthesis of LCPUFA, especially arachidonic acid (20:4n-6), dihomo-γ-linolenic acid (20:3n-6), eicosapentenoic acid (EPA, 20:5n-3), and docosahexenoic acid (DHA, 22:6n-3), from their respective EFA precursors, are important for infant growth, neurodevelopment, and visual function. These polyunsaturated fatty acids are structural components of all cell membrane phospholipids. Arachidonic acid and DHA are the two quantitatively most important LCPUFA in the brain and retina, and the LCPUFA with 20 carbon atoms are precursors for the synthesis of eicosanoids, a group of signaling molecules. The major part of the polyunsaturated fatty acids in human milk (70–85% in women on omnivorous diet) is derived from maternal body stores, which reflects long-term intake, and not from direct dietary transfer.

The metabolic fate of individual fatty acids depends on dietary energy and on energy balance. Therefore, the intake and requirements for fat, EFA, and LCPUFA are usually expressed as a percentage of the total energy in the diet (en %), rather than total intake (g). The fat intake recommended for lactating women is in the range of 20–35 en %, which is the same range as recommended for the adult population. Concerning the fatty acid intake, FAO/WHO recommends an additional maternal intake of 1–2 en % as EFA (3–4 g day^{-1}) during the first 3 months of lactation, and up to 4 en % (about 5 g day^{-1}) thereafter due to depletion of maternal fat stores. Based on the median linoleic and α-linolenic acid intakes of lactating women in the US, the DRI committee recommends an intake of 5–10 en % (average 13 g day^{-1}) of n-6 (as linoleic acid) and of 0.6–1.2 en % (average 1.3 g day^{-1}) of n-3 (as α-linolenic acid) polyunsaturated fatty acids throughout lactation, with a 10% contribution of LCPUFA of the n-6 and n-3 series to these ranges. The ratio of n-6:n-3 unsaturated fatty acids in the diet is important because these fatty acids are desaturated and elongated using the same series of enzymes. Increased intakes of linoleic acid result in decreased conversion of α-linolenic acid to EPA and DHA, whereas the conversion of linoleic acid to arachidonic acid is inhibited by EPA and DHA, and also by arachidonic acid, α-linolenic acid, and linoleic acid itself. The n-6:n-3 ratio recommended for adults by both DRI and FAO/WHO committees is 5:1 to 10:1. Vegetable oils are the main sources of n-6 fatty acids in the diet and also of n-3 fatty acids, although in lower amounts. Fish such as herring, mackerel, and salmon are good sources of n-3 fatty acids.

The intake of *trans* fatty acids (*trans* isomers of oleic and linoleic acid) present in hydrogenated food fats and oils, deep-fried foods, and meats are of special concern in lactating women when their intake is excessively high or when EFA intake is low during pregnancy and lactation. An inverse correlation of arachidonic acid and DHA with *trans* fatty acids in plasma lipids has been reported in infants, suggesting impairment in LCPUFA synthesis and metabolism.

Protein The average protein content in colostrum is 15–20 g l^{-1} decreasing to approximately 8–10 g l^{-1} in mature human milk during the first 6 months of lactation. The protein concentration in human milk is not affected by diet, body composition, or maternal undernutrition.

The recommended dietary allowance (RDA) of protein for adolescent and adult lactating women by the DRI committee is 1.1 g per kg of body weight per day. This corresponds to an increment of 25 g day^{-1} of protein intake above the RDA for nonlactating women, and it is the same as for pregnant women. Recent data have shown that protein intakes of 1 g kg^{-1} day^{-1} are able to maintain good milk production, and promote conservation of maternal skeletal muscle apparently by downregulating protein metabolism. The recommended range of percentage of energy from dietary protein is the same as for the general adult population (10–35%).

The factorial approach was used to estimate the protein RDA for lactation, assuming that the maintenance protein requirement of the lactating women is not different from that of the nonlactating women, and that the additional protein and/or amino acid requirements are proportional to milk production. The additional protein requirement for lactation is defined as the output of total protein and nonprotein nitrogen (converted in protein by multiplying by 6.25) in milk. Nonprotein nitrogen represents 20–25% of total milk nitrogen, mainly as urea. It is taken into account because it is assumed that the nitrogen needed to cover the total nitrogen loss in milk should be derived from dietary protein. The total nitrogen output in milk is converted to total protein output (approximately 10 g day^{-1}) and divided by the incremental efficiency of nitrogen utilization (0.47), which is assumed to be the same in adult and adolescent lactating women. The additional estimated average requirement due to milk production is 21.2 g day^{-1}. After correction by the coefficient of variation and rounding off, the RDA for lactation amounts to +25 g day^{-1}, which corresponds to +0.46 g protein kg^{-1} day^{-1} (based on a reference woman of 57 kg), above the RDA for nonlactating women.

Recommendations for individual indispensable amino acids for lactation by the DRI committee assume that the incremental needs correspond to the amino acids secreted in milk, since there are no specific data on the amino acid requirements in lactating women. Therefore, the RDA of amino acids for lactation are calculated by adding the average amounts of amino acids in human milk in the first 6 months of lactation (expressed as milligrams per kilogram per day) to the respective RDA for the nonlactating women. Recommendations of indispensable amino acids for the lactating women are 36% (histidine) to 80% (tryptophan) higher than those for nonlactating women. The intake of good-quality protein such as in eggs, milk, meat, and fish provide the requirements for all indispensable amino acids. Individuals who restrict their diets to plant proteins (cereals, legumes, nuts, starchy roots, vegetables, and fruits) may be at risk of not getting adequate amounts of certain indispensable amino acids. However, adequate complementary mixtures of plant proteins, with increased digestibility through processing and preparation, can provide high-quality protein.

Micronutrients

Daily requirements for several micronutrients (riboflavin, vitamin B_{12}, vitamin C, vitamin A, vitamin E, copper, iodine, manganese, selenium, and zinc) are higher during lactation than during pregnancy, indicating that lactation is a very demanding process. The only micronutrient needed in lower amounts during lactation is iron, due to the small amount of iron secreted into breast milk and to the usual amenorrhea of nursing women. However, iron requirements may be high post-partum for women who need to replace major blood losses during delivery.

The recommended intakes for micronutrients during lactation established by FAO/WHO and DRI committees are summarized in **Table 1**. The

Table 1 Daily recommended micronutrient intakes for adult lactating women

Nutrient	FAO/WHO[a]		IOM[b]	
	Recommended value	Per cent change[c]	Recommended value	Per cent change[c]
Vitamin A (μg RAE day^{-1})	–	–	1300	↑ 86%
Vitamin A (μg RE day^{-1})	850	↑ 70%	–	–
Vitamin D (μg day^{-1})	5	No change	5	No change
Vitamin E (mg α-TE day^{-1})	7.5	No change	19	↑ 27%
Vitamin K (μg day^{-1})	55	No change	90	No change
Thiamin (mg day^{-1})	1.5	↑ 36%	1.4	↑ 27%
Riboflavin (mg day^{-1})	1.6	↑ 45%	1.6	↑ 45%
Niacin (mg NE day^{-1})	17	↑ 21%	17	↑ 21%
Vitamin B_6 (mg day^{-1})	2.0	↑ 54%	2.0	↑ 54%
Pantothenate (mg day^{-1})	7.0	↑ 40%	7.0	↑ 40%
Biotin (μg day^{-1})	35	↑ 17%	35	↑ 17%
Folate (μg DFE day^{-1})	500	↑ 25%	500	↑ 25%
Vitamin B_{12} (μg day^{-1})	2.8	↑ 17%	2.8	↑ 17%
Vitamin C (mg day^{-1})	70	↑ 55%	120	↑ 60%
Calcium (mg day^{-1})	1000	No change	1000	No change
Iodine (μg day^{-1})	200	↑ 82%	290	↑ 93%
Iron (mg day^{-1})	15^d	↓ 49%	9	↓ 50%
Zinc (mg day^{-1})	9.5^e	↑ 94%	12	↑ 50%
	8.8^f	↑ 80%		
Magnesium (mg day^{-1})	270	↑ 23%	310	No change
Selenium (μg day^{-1})	35	↑ 35%	70	↑ 27%
Chromium (μg day^{-1})	–	–	45	↑ 80%
Copper (μg day^{-1})	–	–	1300	↑ 44%
Fluoride (mg day^{-1})	–	–	3	No change
Manganese (mg day^{-1})	–	–	2.6	↑ 44%
Molybdenum (μg day^{-1})	–	–	50	↑ 11%
Phosphorus (mg day^{-1})	–	–	700	No change

[a]FAO/WHO (2001) *Human Vitamin and Mineral Requirements*. Report of a Joint FAO/WHO Expert Consultation. Rome: Food and Agriculture Organization.
[b]Institute of Medicine (IOM) (2001) *Dietary Reference Intakes for Vitamin A, Vitamin K, Arsenic, Boron, Chromium, Copper, Iodine, Iron, Manganese, Molybdenum, Nickel, Silicon, Vanadium, and Zinc*. Washington, DC: National Academy Press.
[c]Changes from recommendations for nonpregnant nonlactating women: ↑, per cent increase; ↓, per cent decrease.
[d]Considering 10% bioavailability.
[e]0–3 months post-partum, considering moderate bioavailability.
[f]4–6 months post-partum, considering moderate bioavailability.
RAE, retinol activity equivalent; α-TE, alpha-tocopherol equivalent; NE, niacin equivalent; DFE, dietary folate equivalent.

percentages of change from the recommendations for nonpregnant nonlactating women are also shown. In order to meet these intakes, lactating women should be guided to consume daily a large variety of foods rich in micronutrients, since food diversification contributes to improve the intake of limiting nutrients. Micronutrients most commonly at risk of inadequate intakes by lactating women are calcium, zinc, folate, and vitamin A.

Calcium It is estimated that lactating women secrete an average of 200 mg of calcium per day into mature breast milk although this amount is variable among women, usually ranging from 150 to 300 mg day^{-1}. The maternal diet does not affect the milk calcium concentration except when maternal calcium intake is very low (<300 mg day^{-1}). The primary source of calcium for milk production appears to be the increased mobilization of calcium from maternal bone due to the increased bone resorption that occurs during lactation favored by the low estrogen concentration. This results in a net loss of maternal bone mass during lactation that is regained after weaning upon return of ovarian function. The decreased urinary calcium excretion during lactation also contributes to the calcium economy for milk secretion. The efficiency of intestinal calcium absorption is not increased during lactation and, therefore, does not contribute to the extra calcium needed for milk production.

Several studies have shown that the adaptive changes in calcium homeostasis during lactation are independent of maternal calcium intake. It was demonstrated that the loss of bone mass during lactation was not affected by calcium supplementation (1000 mg day^{-1}) of nursing women with habitual dietary calcium intakes of 300 mg day^{-1}, 800 mg day^{-1}, and 1200 mg day^{-1}. Since the loss of maternal bone calcium that occurs during lactation is not prevented by increased dietary calcium, and the calcium lost appears to be regained after weaning, the recommended intake of calcium of lactating women is the same as for nonpregnant nonlactating women of the same age, being 1000 mg day^{-1} and 1300 mg day^{-1} for adult and adolescent women, respectively. Even if not increased during lactation, the recommended calcium intake may be difficult to obtain by women with low habitual intake of dairy products. Therefore, lactating women should be guided to consume dairy products such as milk, yogurt, and cheese, and other calcium-rich foods such as fish with edible bones, broccoli, and kale.

Lactating adolescents are a group of special concern regarding calcium intake due to the already high calcium requirements of nonpregnant nonlactating adolescents. These young women are still increasing their own bone density besides the increased calcium requirement to support lactation. Studies are needed to investigate if these women are able to regain bone after weaning to the same level as when they were nonpregnant nonlactating and if they would benefit from increased calcium intake.

Zinc Zinc concentrations in human milk are highest in colostrum, decrease rapidly during the first 3 months post-partum, and more gradually at later stages of lactation. Typical milk zinc concentrations are 4 mg l^{-1} at 2 weeks, 3 mg l^{-1} at 4 weeks, 2 mg l^{-1} at 8 weeks and 1.2 mg l^{-1} at 24 weeks. These concentrations are not influenced by either maternal dietary intake or zinc supplementation at least in well-nourished women. Less is known about the effect of low maternal zinc intakes on milk zinc concentrations, but the available data indicate that concentrations in developing countries may be lower than those in developed countries at comparable times post-partum.

Average losses of zinc via the mammary gland range from 2.2 mg day^{-1} during the first month post-partum to 1 mg day^{-1} at 6 months. The average estimate of daily output of zinc in milk during the first 3 months of lactation is 1.6 mg day^{-1}, which would theoretically double the minimum endogenous zinc losses in lactating women compared to those of non-lactating nonpregnant women. However, maternal homeostatic mechanisms such as enhanced zinc absorption and reduced urinary zinc excretion contribute to compensate for the secretion of zinc into human milk, independent of maternal zinc intake. Intestinal conservation of endogenous fecal zinc appears to contribute to zinc homeostasis during lactation at low zinc intakes (<8 mg day^{-1}). Involution of the uterus, decreased maternal blood volume and increased resorption of trabecular bone in the post-partum period also contribute to mobilizable zinc pools to compensate for the increased needs. These sources appear to provide up to 0.5 mg day^{-1} of zinc during the first 3 months of lactation. Taking all these adaptation mechanisms into account, the average estimate of increased requirement for absorbed zinc during the first 6 months of lactation is 1.35 mg day^{-1}. Therefore, dietary zinc requirements during lactation are substantially increased compared to nonpregnant nonlactating women, both in adults and adolescents.

Bioavailability is an important factor in setting dietary zinc recommendations since the efficiency of dietary zinc utilization may vary up to fivefold depending on the overall composition of the diet, particularly the balance between promoters (animal protein) and antagonists (phytic acid and possibly calcium, iron, and copper) of zinc absorption.

Dietary zinc recommendations during lactation are set at $12\,mg\,day^{-1}$ for adult lactating women consuming a mixed diet, but recommended intake may be as high as $19\,mg\,day^{-1}$ for nursing women with habitual diets of low zinc bioavailability, such as those based mainly on unrefined cereals and legume seeds, with high phytate:zinc ratio (>15), and low in animal protein. This high-zinc intake may be difficult to obtain using plant-based diets. Therefore, nursing women in developing countries and strict vegetarian women worldwide may be at risk of inadequate zinc status during lactation. Red meat, poultry, eggs, and seafood provide highly available zinc, and their consumption should be encouraged in lactating women.

Folate Concentration of folate in breast milk increases during the lactation period, with lower values for colostrum ($10-40\,\mu g\,l^{-1}$) than for mature milk ($79-133\,\mu g\,l^{-1}$). These concentrations are several-fold higher than in maternal plasma, independent of maternal folate status, suggesting that the mammary gland actively transports and regulates the secretion of this vitamin into milk. Folate concentration in breast milk is maintained with the concomitant depletion of maternal folate when maternal dietary intake is low. Maternal supplementation during lactation has little effect on milk folate but it benefits maternal folate status. Folate deficiency has been implicated in disorders such as neural tube defects, low infant birth weight, aborption, cervical dysplasia, atherosclerosis, and colon cancer.

Dietary folate requirements during lactation are based on the average milk folate concentration of $85\,\mu g\,l^{-1}$ and assume a 50% dietary absorption factor from a mixed diet, to account for dietary bioavailability. The average extra amount of dietary folate needed to cover the lactation needs is thus estimated as $133\,\mu g\,day^{-1}$, an increase of about 40% of the nonpregnant nonlactating average folate requirements. Dietary folate recommendations during lactation are set at $500\,\mu g\,day^{-1}$, as dietary folate equivalents (DFEs). A DFE is defined as $1\,\mu g$ of food folate, or $0.6\,\mu g$ of folic acid from fortified food or as a supplement taken with meals, or $0.5\,\mu g$ of folic acid as a supplement taken on an empty stomach. Thus, in order to meet lactation requirements, much less of this vitamin is needed when given as pure folic acid than as natural food folate.

Present recommendations are very difficult to meet by dietary means and most nursing women worldwide appear to have a much lower dietary folate intake and, therefore, to be at risk for folate deficiency. Although folate is found in a variety of foods, such as fresh green vegetables, oranges, legumes and nuts, it is present in relatively small amounts, and several servings per day of these foods are needed to meet recommended intake. Moreover, considerable losses of folate occur during food harvesting, storage, and cooking. Fortification of cereal grains with folate has become mandatory or encouraged in many countries in order to reduce the risk of folate deficiency.

Vitamin A Vitamin A is present in human milk, primarily as retinyl esters (95%) and free retinol. Vitamin A activity is also provided as carotenoid precursors, mainly as beta-carotene, which accounts for up to 30% of total carotenoids in breast milk. Concentration of vitamin A in human milk is high in early lactation ($600-2000\,\mu g\,l^{-1}$) and declines thereafter ($200-1100\,\mu g\,l^{-1}$), being responsive to maternal intake, particularly in nursing women with poor vitamin A status. These women are at risk of providing insufficient amounts of vitamin A to their infants, as is often the case in developing countries.

Dietary recommendations of vitamin A during lactation are based on replacement of the amount of vitamin A secreted into breast milk during the first 6 months of lactation, while preserving maternal vitamin A stores. Because the bioconversion of carotenoids in human milk and in infants is still unknown, the contribution of maternal carotenoids in breast milk to meeting the vitamin A lactation requirement cannot yet be established.

Based on the average vitamin A milk concentration of $485\,\mu g\,l^{-1}$, an extra intake of $400\,\mu g$ of retinol activity equivalents (RAE) per day is recommended for lactating women, which represents an increase of over 70% of recommended intakes for nonpregnant nonlactating adolescent and adult women. RAE is defined as $1\,\mu g$ all-*trans*-retinol, $12\,\mu g$ beta-carotene, and $24\,\mu g$ alpha-carotene or beta-cryptoxanthin. The amounts of carotenoids equivalent to 1 RAE are double the equivalent to 1 RE (retinol equivalents). The new equivalency value (RAE) is based on recent studies demonstrating that bioconversion of carotenoids to vitamin A is 50% less than previously thought.

The vitamin A intake recommended for lactating women can be obtained as the preformed vitamin from foods of animal origin (primarily milk products, eggs, and liver) and as the carotenoid precursors by regular consumption of green leafy vegetables and ripe, colored fruits. However, meeting the recommended intake by consumption of plant foods alone, as is the case in many developing countries, may be difficult.

See also: **Adolescents**: Nutritional Requirements.
Breast Feeding. **Calcium**. **Dietary Guidelines,
International Perspectives**. **Energy**: Requirements.
Fatty Acids: Metabolism. **Folic Acid**. **Lactation**:
Physiology. **Nutrient Requirements, International
Perspectives**. **Protein**: Requirements and Role in Diet.
Vitamin A: Biochemistry and Physiological Role. **Zinc**:
Physiology.

Further Reading

Allen LH (2001) Pregnancy and lactation. In: Bowman A and Russell RM (eds.) *Present Knowledge in Nutrition*, 8th edn., pp. 403–415. Washington, DC: International Life Science Institute Press.

Donangelo CM and Trugo NMF (2003) Lactation/human milk: composition and nutritional value. In: Caballero B, Trugo LC, and Finglas PM (eds.) *Encyclopedia of Food Sciences and Nutrition*, 2nd edn., vol. 6, pp. 3449–3458. London: Academic Press.

FAO/WHO (1994) *Fats and Oils in Human Nutrition*. Report of a Joint FAO/WHO Expert Consultation. Rome: Food and Agriculture Organization.

FAO/WHO (2001) *Human Vitamin and Mineral Requirements*. Report of a Joint FAO/WHO Expert Consultation. Rome: Food and Agriculture Organization.

Haskell MJ and Brown KH (1999) Maternal vitamin A nutriture and the vitamin A content of human milk. *Journal of Mammary Gland Biology and Neopllasia* 4: 243–257.

Institute of Medicine (IOM) (1997) *Dietary Reference Intakes for Calcium, Phosphorus, Magnesium, Vitamin D, and Fluoride*. Washington, DC: National Academy Press.

Institute of Medicine (IOM) (1998) *Dietary Reference Intakes for Thiamin, Riboflavin, Niacin, Vitamin B$_6$, Folate, Vitamin B$_{12}$, Panthothenic Acid, Biotin, and Choline*. Washington, DC: National Academy Press.

Institute of Medicine (IOM) (2000) *Dietary Reference Intakes for Vitamin C, Vitamin E, Selenium, and Carotenoids*. Washington, DC: National Academy Press.

Institute of Medicine (IOM) (2001) *Dietary Reference Intakes for Vitamin A, Vitamin K, Arsenic, Boron, Chromium, Copper, Iodine, Iron, Manganese, Molybdenum, Nickel, Silicon, Vanadium, and Zinc*. Washington, DC: National Academy Press.

Institute of Medicine (IOM) (2002) *Dietary Reference Intakes for Energy, Carbohydrate, Fiber, Fat, Fatty Acids, Cholesterol, Protein and Amino Acids*. Washington, DC: National Academy Press.

Krebs NF (1998) Zinc supplementation during lactation. *American Journal of Clinical Nutrition* 68(suppl): 509S–512S.

O'Connor DL (1994) Folate status during pregnancy and lactation. In: Allen L, King J, and Lonnerdal B (eds.) *Nutrient Regulation during Pregnancy, Lactation, and Infant Growth*. pp. 157–172. New York: Plenum Press.

Prentice A (2000) Calcium in pregnancy and lactation. *Annual Review of Nutrition* 20: 249–272.

Prentice AM, Goldberg GR, and Prentice A (1994) Body mass index and lactation performance. *European Journal of Clinical Nutrition* 48(suppl 3): S78–S86; discussion S86–S89.

LACTOSE INTOLERANCE

D M Paige, Johns Hopkins Bloomberg School of
Public Health, Baltimore, MD, USA

Lactose maldigestion and intolerance result from an inability to digest varying amounts of the milk sugar lactose. This is a result of an inadequate amount of the genetically regulated milk sugar enzyme lactase. The most common reason for lactose maldigestion is a decline of lactase activity with increasing age. Lactose maldigestion may also occur secondary to intestinal tract infection and diarrhea. A rare form of alactasia, an absence of the milk sugar enzyme, can occur at birth. The symptoms associated with lactose maldigestion are a result of the incomplete hydrolysis, or splitting, of the disaccharide lactose into its absorbable monosaccharide components, glucose and galactose. Lactose maldigestion may result in abdominal bloating and/or pain, flatulence, loose stools, and diarrhea, singly or in combination.

The symptoms associated with lactose maldigestion result in lactose intolerance. The most common form of lactose maldigestion and lactose intolerance, as observed in the majority of the world's adult population, is due to genetically determined low lactase levels. Lactase deficiency due to genetic nonpersistence is reported in approximately 70% of the world's adult population.

The prevalence is lowest in people of Northern European descent (15%) and highest in many Asian populations (near 100%). The prevalence of lactase deficiency in individuals of African descent is approximately 70–80%. Similar levels are reported for Latinos and those of Eastern European and South American ancestry. Not all individuals with a reduced level of the enzyme lactase exhibit symptoms with the ingestion of dietary lactose. The presence or absence of symptoms varies with the amount and type of food consumed, intestinal transit time, and level of residual intestinal lactase. Individuals with low lactase levels may tolerate a moderate intake of lactose. Lactase deficiency can generally be identified by a breath hydrogen test measuring the level of undigested lactose reaching the colon. Bacterial fermentation of the undigested lactose is responsible for the volume of breath hydrogen production. A lactose tolerance test measuring blood sugar rise has also been used. Individuals experiencing discomfort with lactose ingestion can elect to consume commercially hydrolyzed milk that is readily available, milk substitutes, or alternative food sources equally rich in calcium.

Historical and Geographic Perspective

The first herd animal kept by humans, sheep, seems to have been domesticated in approximately 10 000 BC. Herd animals were primarily used for meat and perhaps certain other purposes. The historical record suggests that herd animals during this period were not milked. Evidence that humans milked domesticated animals dates to approximately 4000 to 3000 BC in northern Africa and southwest Asia. Following that time, dairying spread across Eurasia and into sub-Saharan Africa. However, dairying was not adopted by all groups in Asia and Africa who had suitable herd animals. Even as late as 1500 AD, the beginning of the great European overseas expansion, there were sizable areas occupied by nonmilking groups. In Africa, the zone of nonmilking centered on the Congo Basin but extended beyond to cover approximately one-third of the continent. In Asia, the zone of nonmilking covered the bulk of the eastern and southeastern portions of the continent, including Thailand, Vietnam, China, and Korea, as well as the islands to the east. Moreover, dairying remained unknown in the Pacific region and in the Americas in pre-European times. In those days, the nonmilking peoples of Asia, Africa, and the Americas consumed mother's milk as infants but normally ingested no milk after weaning. Animal milk was not part of their diet.

It was striking that adults of all groups whose origins lay in the traditional zone of nonmilking were predominantly maldigesters, usually 70–100% of the individuals tested. Also striking was the fact that the peoples with low prevalences of lactose maldigestion (northwest Europeans and certain East African pastoral groups) came from a long tradition of consuming milk, much of it in lactose-rich forms. This suggested the geographic or culture–historical hypothesis. By that hypothesis, in the hunting and gathering stage, human groups everywhere were like most other land mammals in their patterns of lactase activity. That is, in the normal individual lactase activity would drop at weaning to low levels, which prevailed throughout life. With the beginning of dairying, however, significant changes occurred in the diets of many human groups. In some of these, moreover, there may have been a selective advantage for those aberrant individuals who experienced high levels of intestinal lactase throughout life. That advantage would have occurred only in certain situations: Where milk was a specially critical part of the diet, where the group was under dietary stress, and where people did not process all their milk into low-lactose products such as aged cheese. Under these conditions, most likely to occur among pastoral groups, such aberrant individuals would drink more milk, would benefit more nutritionally as a result, and would enjoy increased prospects of survival, well-being, and bearing progeny and supporting them. In a classical Mendelian way, the condition of high intestinal lactase activity throughout life, or lactase persistence, would come to be typical of such a group.

Lactase Nonpersistence

In its pure form, lactose cannot be transported across the mucosa of the small intestine. To be absorbed, it must be hydrolyzed by lactase to free glucose and galactose. These two simple sugars are rapidly and completely absorbed in the normal small intestine. The rate of lactase synthesis is high from birth until ages 3–5 years. Between ages 5 and 14 years, many people undergo a genetically programmed reduction in lactase synthesis that results in a lactase activity level only 5–10% of that of infancy. This reduction, known as lactase nonpersistence or primary lactase deficiency, is not related to the continued intake of milk or lactose. As noted, less than one-third of the world's adult population is genetically predisposed to maintaining a high degree of lactase activity or lactase persistence throughout adulthood.

Lactase persistence in the human population is inherited as a dominant genetic trait. It has been observed that lactose intolerance is 'ancient and globally distributed,' predating the appearance of a persistent lactase variant that was naturally selected in dairying regions. Hollox *et al.* report, "the continued adult production of lactase results from the persistent expression of the protein lactose–phlorizin hydrolase which is encoded by the lactase gene (LCT) on chromosome 2." Swallow notes, "the distribution of different lactase phenotypes in human populations is highly variable and is controlled by a polymorphic element *cis-* acting to the lactase gene. A putative causal nucleotide change has been identified and occurs on the background of a very extended haplotype that is frequent in Northern Europeans, where lactase persistence is frequent."

Lactose Digestion and Gastrointestinal Function

Lactose is hydrolyzed at the intestinal jejunal brush border by the enzyme lactase into its absorbable monosaccharides glucose and galactose. Lactase activity is robust during infancy and, as is the case in humans and most mammals, declines after weaning. Accordingly, the general pattern of lactase nonpersistence is a continuous decline in genetically programmed populations. A shifting pattern of lactose digestion and gastrointestinal function is a result of lactase nonpersistence. The pattern can be described and monitored during three distinct clinical phases.

First, there is a decreasing ability to digest the large lactose load consumed during the screening test. It is important to recognize that this is not an all-or-none phenomenon but rather a slowly progressive decline in available lactase activity, and that this decline, as noted previously, can be influenced by transit time, the vehicle in which the lactose is consumed, and/or the intake of additional foods along with lactose.

Next, with the continued decline of lactase activity, a point is reached when available lactase activity is no longer sufficient to hydrolyze more modest levels of lactose. Therefore, the consumption of a glass of milk or another product containing the equivalent level of lactose will result in incomplete hydrolysis of the lactose consumed. The individuals so tested frequently do not recognize signs or symptoms associated with the incomplete digestion of lactose.

Finally, with the continued decline of lactase activity with increasing age, individuals become symptomatic as a result of the undigested lactose. The decline in available lactase activity reaches a recognizable clinical threshold with increasing age (**Figure 1**).

Initially, many reports treated the population studied as a single unit and paid incomplete attention to age-specific considerations. Distinctions between secondary lactose malabsorption due to short-term intestinal injury and primary lactose malabsorption that has a genetic basis were not always made. This introduced additional confounding variables. Differences in an individual's capacity to hydrolyze and tolerate a lactose challenge dose compared to his or her ability to utilize lesser amounts of lactose found

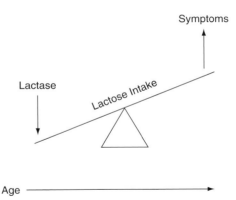

Figure 1 Symptoms associated with lactose maldigestion result from the decline in lactase levels with age and increase with the amount of lactose consumed.

in usually consumed amounts of milk created additional areas of confusion.

When attention is paid to the many factors associated with lactose digestion from infancy to old age, it is possible to place many of the seeming contradictions into perspective. What may have appeared to be incongruities in reported data appear to merge into a relatively predictable pattern of lactose digestion.

Lactose maldigestion and intolerance are influenced by age, infection, size of the lactose bolus, gastric emptying time, intestinal transit time, individual sensitivities, eating habits, genetics, environment, food ideologies, and cultural patterns. Furthermore, symptoms of lactose malabsorption may also be the result of bacterial fermentation of undigested carbohydrate in the colon. The type and extent of the colonic bacterial profile and the absorption of hydrogen and the volatile fatty acids will influence individual reports of symptoms associated with lactose intolerance. Clearly, lactose malabsorption is not a homogeneous event. Neither is it an all-or-none phenomenon having its origins in a single etiology. Clinical expressions of lactose malabsorption, lactose intolerance, and milk rejection find their origins in one or more of the causes outlined previously (**Table 1**).

Prevalence

Children

A review of reported data on diverse populations supports the conclusion that in later childhood and adolescence an important transition in lactose digestion occurs. Older children and young adults are increasingly unable to digest even modest amounts of lactose. This results in increased symptom

Table 1 Patterns of lactose digestion by lactase status

Lactase status	Test results	Symptoms	Lactose intolerance	Milk consumption
Adequate	Normal (−)	0	0	Average (+)
Marginal lactase Deficiency	+ −	0/+	0/+	+ −
Moderate lactase Deficiency	+	0/+	0/+	+ −
Severe lactase Deficiency	+++	++	++	−

Adapted from Paige DM, Davis L, Bayless TM *et al.* (1979) The effects of age and lactose tolerance on blood glucose rise with whole cow and lactose hydrolyzed milk. *Journal of Agriculture and Food Chemistry* **27**(4): 667.

production, recognition of discomfort, and avoidance of lactose-containing products that provoke symptoms.

A progressive decrease in lactase is noted from approximately 1 to 5 years of age through adolescence. Reported rates in US African American children ranged from 27% lactose maldigestion following lactose testing using a lactose load equivalent to two 8-oz. glasses of milk at 1 or 2 years to 74% in 11- or 12-year-old children. The progressive decrease in the ability to hydrolyze a lactose challenge was observed in children of both high and low socioeconomic status. Studies of white children 1–12 years of age identified only 17% of children maldigesting a lactose challenge. Signs and symptom production associated with a reduction in lactose digestion in a child population is difficult to measure due to the nature of the symptoms being reported, the signs observed, and the subjective nature of the reports. This is reinforced by a report on 21 African American girls 11–15 years of age indicating 82% had evidence of lactose maldigestion with reports of gastrointestinal symptoms being negligible, and breath hydrogen excretion, while remaining high, varied between two time periods. Consistent with the previous data, milk consumption

studies, both observed and reported, suggest a progressive decline in milk intake with increasing age in the African American population of children and parallel reports of children from other populations with a high prevalence of lactose maldigestion.

Adults

The progressive increase in prevalence of lactose maldigestion increases with age, reaching reported adult levels of approximately 70% of the world's adult population. The exceptions are populations of Northern and Central Europeans and some Middle Eastern populations as well as groups of primarily European descent in Australia, New Zealand, and North America. Thus, minority populations in North America and Europe, as well as adult populations in most developing countries, are lactose maldigesters (**Table 2**).

Reported milk drinking patterns of individuals classified as maldigesters vary considerably in adults. Data range from 50% reporting symptoms with one 8-oz. glass of milk to 75% reporting symptoms with two 8-oz. glasses of milk and 30% reporting not drinking any milk. Nevertheless, caution

Table 2 Prevalence of lactose maldigestion in selected populations

Population	Country	% Lactose maldigestion	Population	Country	% Lactose maldigestion
African American, 18–54 years	US	75	General, 21–65 years	Finland	15
Asian, 23–39 years	US	100	General, 20.3 years	Germany	70
Native American, 18–54 years	US	81	General, 16–54 years	Chile	80
African American, 13–19 years	US	69	Non-Caucasian	Peru	94
Mexican, 18–94 years	US	53	General, 38–49 years	Brazil	80
Vietnamese, 22–63 years	US	100	Arab adult	Israel	81
Sicilian, 25 years average	Italy	71	General, male 14–34 years	Egypt	73
Northern, 28.7 years average	Italy	52	General, 15–78 years	Greece	45
Central, 36 years average	Italy	18	Bantu, 13–43 years	Uganda	100
Romai	Hungary	56	Yoruba, 13–70 years	Nigeria	83
Austrian, 22 years average	Austria	20	General, adult	India	61
General, 20.3 years average	Finland	17	General, 17–83 years	Korea	75
Aboriginal	Australia	84	General, 15–64 years	Japan	100

must be exercised in interpreting reported symptoms and making the diagnosis of lactose intolerance. There can be considerable crossover between individuals who self-identify as intolerant to lactose and are not diagnosed as lactose intolerant versus those in whom the diagnosis was carefully established. More attention to identifying and categorizing symptoms better may help. A Finnish study noted flatulence as the most severe symptom in maldigesters, whereas abdominal bloating was most frequently reported by individuals self-identifying as lactose digesters. Moreover, microbiota may play a role in the presence and intensity of lactose-related symptoms. Data suggest that increased levels of colonic bacteria, as well as their diversity, may play a role as a result of increased fermentative capacity in reducing the symptoms associated with lactose intolerance.

Pregnant Women

The role of lactose digestion in pregnant women is of special interest. Despite the nutritional value of milk during pregnancy, the lactase levels in some individuals in a number of racial and ethnic groups may be insufficient to hydrolyze commonly consumed amounts of lactose, resulting in lactose maldigestion and possibly milk intolerance. The Institute of Medicine report notes that "lactose intolerance among pregnant African American women may result in their subsequent avoidance of milk." Other populations may also experience lactose maldigestion and intolerance to milk during pregnancy.

Studies of lactose maldigestion in pregnant women, as measured by breath hydrogen response to 240 ml of low-fat (1%) milk, reinforce the Institute of Medicine's concern with lactose digestion among pregnant African American women. The prevalence of lactose maldigestion in early (13–16 weeks), late (30–35 weeks), and 8 weeks postpartum was 66, 69, and 75%, respectively, and that of nonpregnant control women was 80% (**Table 3**).

Accordingly, health care providers instructing African American women on the optimal dietary

Table 3 Lactose maldigestion[a] in pregnant and nonpregnant African American women

African American women	% Lactose maldigestion
Early pregnancy (13–16 weeks)	66
Late pregnancy (30–35 weeks)	69
Postpartum (8 weeks)	75
Nonpregnant	80

[a]Breath hydrogen increase >20 ppm following the consumption of 240 g of low-fat (1%) milk containing 12 g of lactose following an overnight fast.

pattern during pregnancy need to be mindful of a high rate of lactose maldigestion. Implications for fetal growth and development remain to be determined by further study. Also, health providers need to be aware that the presence or absence of symptoms may be unevenly reported by pregnant African American women, and symptoms do not represent a reliable guide to lactose digestion. Less than 25% of pregnant lactose maldigesting women reported any symptoms with 240 ml of low-fat (1%) milk. Symptoms may be further reduced when milk is consumed with other foods. Unanswered is the level of digestion and absorption of a range of nutrients in the consumed milk. Health care providers should discuss with the pregnant woman her ability to tolerate milk and, when appropriate, should educate her as to other food options. In this regard, Kingfisher and Millard report that "Euro-American staff tended to give advise that was biologically appropriate for them but not for many of their patients, a process reflecting biocentrism."

Age-Specific Prevalence

Age-Specific prevalence data suggest a progressive decrease in lactose absorption with age in African American children studied in the United States. This progressive decrease was seen in a study of 409 African American children 13 months to 12 years of age. The population was stratified by age to have approximately equal representation in each 12-month category. The mean age of the children studied was 6.6 years. The study subjects were drawn from four well child clinic sites and a private pediatrician's office in Baltimore, Maryland. All subjects were in good health as determined by history and a review of recent clinic visits. The children were free of any overt intestinal or allergic disorders and had no recent history of gastroenteritis.

Secondary Lactase Deficiency

Secondary lactase deficiency is distinct from genetically determined loss of lactase with age. Secondary lactase deficiency is frequently associated with diseases of the small intestine. Enteric viruses, such as rotavirus and Norwalk agent, can induce lactase deficiency by penetration of the enterocyte in the small intestine Rotaviruses are a principal cause of diarrhea and lactose intolerance in infancy. Denudation of the brush border of the jejunal mucosa associated with diarrhea can lead to the loss of the other two disaccharides, maltase and sucrose. Continued diarrhea may also lead to severe complications such as monosaccharide intolerance. Giardiasis have also been implicated as contributing to lactose maldigestion. An additional infection resulting in an interference with lactose digestion is *Ascaris lumbricoides*. Severe protein malnutrition is frequently associated with lactose maldigestion. Other disease conditions that give rise to secondary lactose maldigestion are celiac disease, gluten-induced enteropathy, and tropical and nontropical sprue. The mucosal brush border of the small intestine is severely damaged in each case.

Lactose Digestion and Diet

Calcium

Dietary calcium is an important element in skeletal development. Dairy products can account for up to three-fourths of dietary calcium in some populations. Milk is a rich source of calcium. Nevertheless, many minorities in the United States and population groups throughout the world drink decreasing amounts of milk after early childhood and little milk as adults. Given the high prevalence of lactose intolerance, alternatives to cow's milk should be identified for those who need them. Lactose-intolerant individuals ultimately attribute their discomfort to lactose-containing foods and voluntarily reduce or eliminate their milk intake. Data from national studies in the United States indicate that African American and Hispanic women have lower intakes of calcium compared to non-Hispanic women. An Institute of Medicine report concludes that the disparity in calcium intake "may be explained in part by the much higher prevalence of lactose intolerance among African Americans and Hispanics, sometimes resulting in their subsequent avoidance of milk." In general, populations at risk for lactose intolerance report a lower calcium intake as a result of the decline in the intake of milk and milk products. One solution to this problem is to educate lactose-intolerant groups about alternative calcium-containing foods, reinforce appropriate cultural patterns and dietary practices that include alternatives to milk, and identify other culturally acceptable calcium-containing foods. Meeting the calcium requirement with an alternative diet is a challenge but nevertheless is required for many in the community. Although milk may serve as a primary source of calcium, appreciable quantities of calcium can be found in nondairy foods.

Clearly, it is more difficult to meet the published calcium recommendation with a diet low in whole cow's milk. A review of the tables of food composition reveals a variety of foods that contain acceptable levels of calcium per 100 g portion or other standard portions (**Table 4**). Other lactose-modified dairy products, including hard cheeses, yogurts, and lactose-modified milk, are good calcium sources.

Table 4 Calcium content in milligrams per 100-g portion or as noted

Food	mg
Canned sardines (3 oz.)	372
Buckwheat pancakes	249
Kale (raw)	225
Mustard greens	220
Muffins[a]	206
Waffles[a]	192
Figs (dry)	186
Canned salmon (3 oz. with bones)	167
Collard greens	162
Oat breakfast cereal[a]	160
Wheat pancakes	158
Almonds	152
Tofu (8 oz.)	143
Egg yolk	147
Corn bread[a]	139
Kale (frozen)	134
Filberts	120
Beet greens	118
Oysters (1/2 cup)	113
Whole cow's milk (100 g)	113
Swiss chard	105
Rhubarb (cooked 1/2 cup)	105
Canned shrimp (3 oz.)	98
Okra	92
Soy beans (1 cup)	90
Sunflower seeds	88
Broccoli	88
Sauerkraut (1 cup)	85
Potato salad (1 cup)	80
Peanut butter	74
Spinach	73
Dates (dry)	72
Brewer's yeast (2 tbs)	66
Lobster	65
Green beans	63
Flounder	61
Bran flakes	61
Canned apricots (1 cup)	57
Gingerbread (1 piece)	57
Plain rolls[a]	55
Toaster pastry (1 piece)[a]	54
Prunes (dry)	54
Orange	54
Whole egg	54
Peanuts	54
Artichokes	51
Cod	50
Brussels sprouts	50
Clams (3 oz.)	47
Lima beans	47
Puffed wheat[a]	46
Whole wheat bread (2 slices)	46
Sweet potato	46
Fruit cocktail (1 cup)	46

Continued

Table 4 Continued

Food	mg
Raisins (1/2 cup)	45
Apricots	44
Farina (1 cup)	44
Fig bars (4 cookies)	44
Pecans	43
White bread (2 slices)	42
Pecans	43
White bread (2 slices)	42
Tangerine	40
Raspberries (raw)	40
Apple sauce	21

[a]Enriched, fortified, or restored to legal standard when one exists. From Oski FA and Paige DM (1994) Cow's milk is a good food for some and a poor choice for others: Eliminating the hyperbole. *Archives of Pediatric and Adolescent Medicine* **148**: 104–107.

In addition, lactose digestive aids are available and are increasingly used, including lactase tablets, lactase preparations, lactose-free milk, and prehydrolyzed milk. Live culture yogurt is another alternative to milk. Lactose in yogurt is better digested than lactose in milk. Tolerance to yogurt is thought to be due to the microbial β-galactosidase activity that digests the lactose.

Osteoporosis

The role of lactose maldigestion, calcium intake, and osteoporosis has been studied. Osteoporosis and osteoporitic fractures are major public health problems. The role of lactose maldigestion and osteoporosis remains unsettled. For example, minority populations consuming small amounts of milk should be at greater risk for osteoporosis. Nevertheless, African American and Hispanic populations in the United States appear to have a lower risk of developing osteoporosis. Caucasian and Asian women were found to have the highest risk for osteoporosis, with fracture rates of 140.7/100 000 and 85.4/100 000, respectively. Hispanic and African American females had lower age-adjusted rates at 49.7/100 000 and 57.3/100 000, respectively. The paradox reinforces the complexity of the disease and the importance of biologic, genetic, and as yet undetermined factors in the eitology of osteoporosis.

Nutrition Policy

Apart from the nutritional implications outlined previously, there are policy considerations that require attention. Clearly, milk has important economic, nutritional, and emotional significance in Western culture, a culture strongly committed to the concept that milk is an ideal food. However, lactose digestion should be an important consideration in developing a suitable policy regarding the use of milk and dairy products by the lactose malabsorber and by ethnic or racial groups, among whom high rates of malabsorption prevail. Accordingly, a balance must be struck between dietary guidance and the interests of a diverse population with a large number of lactose maldigesters. For many, the continued use of a limited amount of milk may be appropriate and comfortable. For others, dietary modification and lactose reduction or elimination may be warranted. The substitution of low-lactose products or alternative foods may be nutritionally beneficial. The successful introduction of a lactose-reduced milk, Lact-Aid, into the US market in the 1970s by Alan Kligerman is one important example of a well-accepted milk product alternative. Traditional diets among lactose-maldigesting populations, using little or no milk or dairy products, should be respected.

Summary

The principles of genetics and evolution help to explain the emergence of the aberrant phenomenon of lactose tolerance. Darwin referred to food as a major factor in selective pressures. Lactose digestion is most effective in illustrating how a certain food, by indirectly favoring the survival of those able to digest that substance, can influence the evolutionary process of man.

Clinical and nutritional consequences of lactose digestion in adults must be examined in relation to malabsorption, intolerance, milk rejection, and symptoms and their recognition. Estimates of how frequently milk intolerance will be a clinically significant problem in adults vary with the nature of the associated gastrointestinal disorders and the format of the individual studies.

There is a series of interrelated physiologic events affecting the amount of undigested sugar and fluid that the small intestine, and subsequently the colon, must metabolize or reabsorb. A balance of these factors tends to prevent symptoms when the stomach, small intestine, and colon can compensate for the increased solute load, but abdominal discomfort or diarrhea occur when these small intestinal and colonic physiologic mechanisms are loaded beyond their capacity. The role of the colonic flora in metabolizing unabsorbed sugar and the importance of colonic salvage of unabsorbed carbohydrate are important variables in the symptom complex. Secondary lactase deficiency due to infectious gastroenteritis and malnutrition represents a distinct clinical syndrome and must be distinguished from lactose intolerance.

Dietary recommendations must take account of lactose maldigestion. Milk and dairy product consumption will vary among lactose-maldigesting and milk-intolerant individuals. Lactose-reduced or lactose-free products are available to lactose-intolerant individuals who wish to drink milk and milk-based products. Nevertheless, dietary recommendations must be modified and respectful of those who do not drink milk. Accordingly, appropriate alternatives to milk and other lactose-containing foods must be identified and guidance provided in developing nutritionally equivalent diets.

See also: **Calcium**. **Celiac Disease**. **Dairy Products**. **Osteoporosis**. **Pregnancy**: Nutrient Requirements.

Further Reading

Enattah NS, Sahi T, Savilahti E *et al.* (2002) Identification of a variant associated with adult-type hypolactasia. *Nature Genetics* 30(2): 233–237.

Hollox EJ, Poulter M, Zvarik M *et al.* (2001) Lactase haplotype diversity in the Old World. *American Journal of Human Genetics* 68(1): 160–172.

Institute of Medicine (US) Subcommittee on Nutritional Status and Weight Gain During Pregnancy (1990) *Nutrition During Pregnancy*. National Academy of Sciences.

Kingfisher CP and Millard AV (1998 Dec) Milk makes me sick but my body needs it: conflict and contradiction in the establishment of authoritative knowledge. *Med Anthropol Q* 12(4): 447–66.

Labayen I, Forga L, Gonzalez A *et al.* (2001) Relationship between lactose digestion, gastrointestinal transit time and symptoms in lactose malabsorbers after dairy consumption. *Alimentary Pharmacology and Therapeutics* 15(4): 543–549.

Oski FA and Paige DM (1994) Cow's milk is a good food for some and a poor choice for others: Eliminating the hyperbole. *Archives of Pediatric and Adolescent Medicine* 148: 104–107.

Paige DM (1981) Lactose malabsorption in children: Prevalence, symptoms, and nutritional considerations. In: Paige DM and Bayless TM (eds.) *Lactose Digestion: Clinical and Nutritional Implications*, pp. 151–161. Baltimore: Johns Hopkins University Press.

Paige DM, Davis L, Bayless TM *et al.* (1979) The effects of age and lactose tolerance on blood glucose rise with whole cow and lactose hydrolyzed milk. *Journal of Agriculture and Food Chemistry* 27(4): 667.

Paige DM, Witter F, Bronner YL *et al.* (2003) Lactose intolerance in pregnant African-Americans. *Public Health Nutrition* 6(8): 801–807.

Perman JA, Barr RB, and Watkins JB (1978) Sucrose malabsorption in children; Non-invasive diagnosis by interval breath hydrogen determination. *Journal of Pediatrics* 93: 17–22.

Pribila BA, Hertzler SR, Martin BR, Weaver CM, and Savaiano DA (2000) Improved lactose digestion and intolerance among African-American adolescent girls fed a dairy-rich diet. *Journal of the American Dietetic Association* 100(5): 524–528.

Rao DR, Bello H, Warren AP, and Brown GE (1994) Prevalence of lactose maldigestion. *Digestive Diseases and Sciences* 39: 1519–1524.

Scrimshaw NS and Murray EB (1988) The acceptability of milk and milk products in populations with a high prevalence of lactose intolerance. *American Journal of Clinical Nutrition* 48: 1083–1159.

Suarez F, Savaiano D, and Levitt M (1995) A comparoson of symptoms after the consumption of milk or lactose-hydrolyzed milk by people with self-reported severe lactose intolerance. *New England Journal of Medicine* 333: 1–4.

Swallow DM (2003) Genetics of lactase persistence and lactose intolerance. *Annual Review of Genetics* 37: 197–219.

Tursi A (2004) Factors influencing lactose intolerance. *European Journal of Clinical Investigation* 34: 314–315.

Vonk RJ, Priebe MG, Koetse HA *et al.* (2003) Lactose intolerance: Analysis of underlying factors. *European Journal of Clinical Investigation* 33: 70–75.

LEGUMES

M A Grusak, Baylor College of Medicine, Houston, TX, USA

Published by Elsevier Ltd.

Legumes have been an important component of the human diet for several millennia and are used throughout the world today. They are a diverse group of plants that belong to the Fabaceae family (sometimes also referred to as the Leguminosae) and are estimated to include approximately 20,000 species in 700 genera. However, only a handful of these species have been developed as crops that are in common culture. Some of the more extensively grown legumes are listed in **Table 1**.

Legumes are consumed primarily as seed foods, but pods, leaves, and roots or tubers of various species are also eaten. The pod is an enveloping structure that protects the seeds as they develop and mature, and it is a characteristic feature of this group of plants. In fact, the name legume comes from the Latin word *legumen*, which means seeds that are harvested from pods. Other names used for legume seeds are pulse, which is derived from the Latin word *puls*, meaning pottage, or the phrase grain legume, used in reference to leguminous seeds. The more general phrase, food legume, is used to represent any vegetative or reproductive structures from legume plants that are utilized for human food.

An important nutritional aspect of legume foods is their high concentration of protein, which in most

Table 1 Commonly cultivated legume species

Scientific name	Common names
Arachis hypogea L.	Peanut, groundnut
Cajanus cajan (L.) Millsp.	Pigeon pea, red gram, Congo pea
Cicer arietinum L.	Chickpea, garbanzo, Bengal gram
Glycine max (L.) Merr.	Soybean, soya, edamame
Lablab purpureus (L.) Sweet	Hyacinth bean, Indian bean, Egyptian bean
Lathyrus sativus L.	Grass pea, chickling pea
Lens culinaris Medik.	Lentil
Lupinus albus L.	White lupine
Macrotyloma uniflorum (Lam.) Verdc.	Horse gram, Madras gram
Phaseolus lunatus L.	Lima bean, butter bean
Phaseolus vulgaris L.	Common bean, black bean, kidney bean, pinto bean, snap bean, string bean, French bean
Pisum sativum L.	Pea, garden pea, English pea
Psophocarpus tetragonolobus (L.) DC.	Winged bean, Goa bean, four-angled bean
Vicia faba L.	Broad bean, fava bean
Vigna aconitifolia (Jacq.) Marechal	Moth bean, mat bean
Vigna mungo (L.) Hopper	Urd bean, black gram
Vigna radiata (L.) Wilczek	Mung bean, green gram, golden gram
Vigna subterranea (L.) Verdc.	Bambara groundnut
Vigna umbellata (Thumb.) Ohwi and Ohashi	Rice bean, Mambi bean
Vigna unguiculata (L.) Walp. ssp. unguiculata	Cowpea, black-eyed pea, southern pea

Source: Rubatzky VE and Yamaguchi M (1997) *World Vegetables: Principles, Production, and Nutritive Values.* New York: Chapman & Hall.

legume seeds is at least twice that of cereal seeds. Legumes can produce more protein because the plants are generally well nourished with nitrogen, even in soils with limited inorganic nitrogen. Legume roots have the ability to form symbiotic associations with particular microbial species, in a structure called the root nodule. This symbiosis allows the plant to readily acquire atmospheric nitrogen and use it for the synthesis of amino acids. These protein precursors are transported to the developing seeds and are deposited there for later use. Legume seeds also contain a broad mix of energy reserves (starch or oil), minerals, and various phytochemicals—all of which are stored in seeds to provide nourishment to the young developing seedling.

As omnivores, humans have been able to take advantage of the nutrient and phytochemical reserves in legume seeds for dietary requirements and health benefits. This is especially important in the developing world, where malnutrition is an ever-present concern, and legumes can provide an inexpensive source of dietary protein (relative to animal food products), among other nutrients. The protein in legume seeds, although somewhat lacking in sulfur amino acids and tryptophan, is still an important complement to energy-rich carbohydrate staples, such as rice, wheat, maize, and various root and tuber crops. However, when eating legumes, we also must deal with the various antinutrients and toxic compounds found in seeds. These seed components include various enzyme inhibitors, tannins, phenolics, alkaloids, and neurotoxins. Some of these can cause debilitating consequences in humans, although cooking and other processing techniques can be used to reduce or alleviate their negative effects.

Legume Types

Legumes are grown throughout the world, with some adapted to warmer tropical and subtropical climates and others preferring temperate to cooler climates. The 20 species listed in **Table 1** are some of the more commonly cultivated legumes and include those whose annual production reaches levels that allow for worldwide marketing. In developing countries, many locally adapted legume species are cultivated on a small scale or are harvested from wild sources. These less cultivated legumes are usually harvested as mature seeds, but immature pods, leaves, roots, or tubers can also be collected.

Most of the common legume species are grown agronomically and harvested as mature seeds. These can be cooked and consumed in their entirety, or they are cracked and used as split seeds with the hulls (seed coats) removed. Seeds of some species are milled to produce a flour product, or they can be processed to yield protein isolate (e.g., soybean and lupine), extracted oils (e.g., soybean and peanut), or starch (e.g., pea).

For those legumes also cultivated as vegetable crops, immature seeds or immature pods can be harvested. These are canned, frozen, or sold as fresh products. Immature pods are nutritionally similar to leafy vegetables in that they contain various carotenoids and other phytochemicals; however, they also contain immature seeds that can provide a modest amount of protein. For some species, young tender leaves or whole shoots are also collected and used as vegetable greens that are eaten fresh or cooked. More detailed information is given on some of the common legume types in the following sections.

Bambara Groundnut

Bambara groundnut (*Vigna subterranea* (L.) Verdc.) is indigenous to west central Africa. Most of its current production is in Africa, but the plant is also cultivated in India, Southeast Asia, Australia, and Central and South America. The plant has an interesting growth habit in that after pollination, the developing pod and seeds are pushed into the ground, where they grow until full maturity. Plants are typically uprooted at harvest to collect the seeds and pods; because of this subterranean growth, they have acquired the common name groundnut. Mature seeds are boiled and consumed as a cooked seed, prepared as porridge, or milled into a flour to form cakes. Immature seeds are also harvested and cooked as a fresh vegetable.

Broad Bean

Broad bean (*Vicia faba* L.), also known as fava bean, is grown from tropical to temperate regions, with production occurring in North and South America, Europe, Africa, and China. This legume is grown for its enlarged, succulent, immature seeds that are removed from its thick, fleshy pod. Mature dry seed is also harvested. Although broad beans are widely consumed, they do contain storage proteins (vicine and convicine) whose metabolites can lead to acute hemolytic anemia in individuals with a deficiency in glucose-6-dehydrogenase (found predominantly in people of Mediterranean or African descent). Additionally, broad beans contain high levels of L-DOPA, a phenolic compound that can be converted to dopamine. Because of their L-DOPA content, broad beans should be avoided by individuals using monoamine oxidase inhibitors (MAOI-type drugs). The use of these drugs, in combination with high intakes of dopamine (or dopamine precursors), can lead to dangerous increases in blood pressure.

Chickpea

Chickpea (*Cicer arietinum* L.) is grown worldwide and is best adapted to cool, dry climates. Thus, it is a winter crop in some regions of the world. Two seed types are recognized: the large-seeded kabuli type, characterized by its beige-colored seed coat and ram's head shape, and the desi type, with its smaller size and dark-colored irregularly shaped seeds. Kabuli varieties are preferred for consumption as whole seeds, whereas desi types are typically processed into flour. Immature green pods and young tender leaves are also cooked and eaten as vegetables, especially in India.

Common Bean

Common bean (*Phaseolus vulgaris* L.) is grown in temperate zones as well as in temperate regions within the subtropics. As a dry seed, it is an important crop in Africa and in Central and South America. Many bean types are cultivated that exhibit vast differences in seed coat coloration and pod characteristics. Mature seeds are harvested as dry beans (e.g., black bean, pinto bean, and kidney bean); immature pods are used as a vegetable (e.g., snap bean and French bean). Pod types have been bred to have few fibers in the pod wall.

Cowpea

Cowpea (*Vigna unguiculata* (L.) Walp. ssp. *unguiculata*) is grown throughout the tropics and subtropics. It is an important crop in Africa, its probable center of origin, but is also grown in Brazil, India, Southeast Asia, and the United States. There are three major subspecies of *V. unguiculata*; in addition to ssp. *unguiculata*, there is appreciable production of ssp. *cylindrica* (common names: catjang cowpea and Bombay cowpea) and ssp. *sesquipedalis* (common names: yardlong bean and asparagus bean), especially in Asia. All types are harvested as vegetables (shoots, leaves, and immature pods) or as dry, mature seeds.

Grass Pea

Grass pea (*Lathyrus sativus* L.) is a hardy, cool-weather adapted legume that is cultivated in India, Africa, the Middle East, and South America. It is harvested primarily as a dry, mature seed, although young leaves and immature pods are edible. Grass pea is quite tolerant of limited moisture and does well in nutrient-poor soils; thus, in times of drought it is one of the few legumes that produces a harvest, and it is widely consumed by low-income populations during times of famine. Unfortunately, excessive or prolonged consumption of grass pea can lead to lathyrism, a debilitating muscle paralysis that is caused by a neurotoxin in the seeds.

Hyacinth Bean

Hyacinth bean (*Lablab purpureus* (L.) Sweet) is grown in India and in many tropical regions of the world. Mature seeds are consumed as a cooked food or a sprouted seed. The immature pods and seeds are also harvested as vegetable foods. Although this plant is cultivated as an annual, it will persist as a perennial, and when cultivation is extended it will form large, starchy roots that can be eaten. Some varieties (mostly dark-seeded types) contain high levels of a cyanogenic glycoside in their seeds.

When cyanogenic glycosides are hydrolyzed by plant enzymes during cooking, or possibly by intestinal enzymes after ingestion, cyanide can be released and lead to cyanide poisoning.

Lentil

Lentil (*Lens culinaris* Medik.) is another of the world's important pulse crops, especially for populations in developing countries. The plant is adapted to cool climates; Canada, India, and Turkey account for nearly 70% of its production. Lentils are harvested primarily as a dry, mature seed, but immature pods are also used as a vegetable in India.

Mung Bean

Mung bean (*Vigna radiata* (L.) Wilczek) is grown in tropical climates and is an important legume in India, China, and other Asian countries. Dry seeds are harvested and consumed as split, whole, boiled, or roasted forms. Immature pods are eaten, and there has been interest in developing the tuberous root as a food because of its high protein content (nearly 15%).

Pea

Pea (*Pisum sativum* L.) is grown primarily in cooler regions of the world. Different varieties have been developed to produce mature, dry seeds; succulent, well-developed immature seeds; or succulent, immature edible pods. Dry seed varieties are sometimes referred to as field peas. The names garden pea and English pea are used for the varieties harvested as immature seeds, whereas the edible pod types are commonly known as snow pea or sugar snap pea. In some Asian cuisines, the shoots of pea plants are also used as vegetable greens.

Peanut

Peanut (*Arachis hypogea* L.) is grown throughout the tropics, much of the subtropics, and even in some temperate zones. As with Bambara groundnut, its pods have a subterranean growth habit, and thus it also has acquired the common name, groundnut. Peanut is one of the few commonly grown legumes whose seeds contain high levels of oil. Most legume seeds have less than 5% oil, but for some peanut cultivars seed oil content is as high as 40–50%. Roasted seed and extracted oil is used and marketed worldwide; in some regions, young shoots and leaves of the plant are used as greens, and immature pods are consumed as a cooked vegetable. Although a nutritious legume, peanut has recently gained much attention and scientific interest due to the low, but nonetheless significant, incidence of individuals who are allergic to peanut proteins. For those extremely hypersensitive to this food, violent and life-threatening reactions can occur in response to exposure to as little as 0.1 mg of peanut. In fact, peanut is believed to be the most common cause of death due to foods.

Pigeon Pea

Pigeon pea (*Cajanus cajan* (L.) Millsp.) is broadly adapted to many climatic regions and soil types, and thus its production occurs over a huge area of crop land. It is an important food legume in India, other Asian countries, Africa, and South America. Mature grains are usually consumed as split, dehulled seeds. Immature seeds and pods are also consumed in large quantities.

Soybean

Soybean (*Glycine max* (L.) Merr.) is undoubtedly the most important food legume today, being a major source of protein and extracted oil. Soybean is believed to have originated in eastern Asia as a subtropical plant, but plant breeders have helped develop varieties adapted to several climatic zones. The crop is grown in many countries, but more than 70% of the world's production comes from the United States, Brazil, and China. Most soybeans are harvested as dry seed; a typical variety contains 20% seed oil and 35% protein (although some varieties can be as high as 45% protein). Both soy oil and soy protein isolate are found as ingredients in many processed foods. In eastern Asia, the immature seed is also harvested extensively and used as a vegetable.

Winged Bean

Winged bean (*Psophocarpus tetragonolobus* (L.) DC.) is adapted to tropical conditions and is grown in Southeast Asia, Papua New Guinea, various Pacific Islands, and Africa. The tender pods are the most widely consumed part of the plant, especially throughout Asia, but the leaves, stems, flowers, seeds, and tuberous roots are all nutritionally valuable and are used as food. Winged bean is another of the legumes with elevated seed oil content; varieties typically average 15% oil, with protein levels of 30–37%. The tuberous roots are a good source of energy in the form of starch, and they contain 8–10% protein.

Grain Legume Nutritional Value

As noted previously, many parts of legume plants are consumed by humans. However, the seeds are the predominant food type across all species, and their nutritional value is discussed in the following sections.

Protein

Protein content in legume seeds is governed both by genotype and by environment. Seed protein levels can vary across varieties of a given species and even among seeds on an individual plant. In general, however, food legumes contain 20–30% protein by proximate analysis (**Table 2**). The exceptions to this are soybean and winged bean, which contain up to 37 and 45% protein, respectively.

Legume proteins are primarily of two types: storage proteins, which account for approximately 70% of total seed nitrogen, and enzymatic, regulatory, and structural proteins, which are present for normal cellular activities, including the synthesis of storage proteins. Legume storage proteins are soluble in dilute salt solutions but insoluble in water and therefore fall into the classical globulin group of protein fractions. Legume protein types are further characterized by their sedimentation coefficients, which in most species approach 11S and 7S; these are commonly referred to as the legumins and vicilins, respectively. Most legumes contain both types of storage protein, but the proportion of the two types varies from species to species.

In terms of protein quality, as defined by an optimal proportion of amino acids required by humans, legume proteins are deficient in the sulfur-containing amino acids and tryptophan but are rich in lysine. Cereals, on the other hand, are relatively deficient in lysine; thus, the combination of legumes with cereals often can improve the overall protein quality of the mixed foods. The nutritive value (or biological value) of legume proteins has been investigated quite extensively and has been shown to be rather low in some legumes, with the amount of utilizable protein ranging from 32 to 78%. In other words, not all of the protein available in a given legume (see **Table 2**) is converted into new protein when consumed by humans. The reasons for this are the general deficiency of essential amino acids (sulfur-containing and tryptophan) and the presence of many inhibitors of protease activity that are found in legume seeds. These enzyme inhibitors are primarily proteinaceous in character, and many have an effect on the digestive enzymes trypsin or chymotrypsin. The inhibition of these enzymes leads to a reduction in protein digestibility and thus the gut's ability to absorb amino acids. Fortunately, because many of these inhibitors are proteinaceous, cooking, heating, fermenting, and, in some cases, germination can inactivate and significantly lower their inhibitory effect. However, not all of the inhibitors found in legume seeds are proteins (e.g., other inhibitors include tannins and polyphenols).

Lipids

Grain legumes generally contain higher concentrations of lipids than cereals. In legumes, lipids are stored in oil bodies in the cotyledons (the bulk of the seed), whereas most oils in cereals are limited to the outer bran layer. Most common legumes contain 1–7% lipid, based on proximate analysis. Exceptions to this range are soybean, peanut, and winged bean, which average 20, 45, and 15%, respectively. Legumes are good lipid sources for humans because they contain high amounts of essential fatty acids. Although composition varies across species, most legumes contain some quantity of oleic, linoleic, and linolenic acids. Phospholipids and glycolipids are also found in legume seeds.

Carbohydrates

Legume seeds contain starch, mono- and oligosaccharides, and other polysaccharides. Total carbohydrates range from 25 to 65% across the commonly grown legume species. Starch is the predominant carbohydrate in most cases, with exceptions in the oilseeds soybean and peanut. Legumes generally contain low amounts of monosaccharides (usually 1% or less) and only slightly higher amounts of

Table 2 Protein contents of food legume seeds

Legume	Protein range (% dry weight)
Broad bean	22.9–38.5
Chickpea	14.9–29.6
Common bean	21.1–39.4
Cowpea	20.9–34.6
Grass pea	22.7–29.6
Horse gram	18.5–28.5
Lentil	20.4–30.5
Moth bean	21.0–31.3
Mung bean	20.8–33.1
Pea	21.2–32.9
Peanut	23.5–33.5
Pigeon pea	18.8–28.5
Rice bean	18.4–27.0
Soybean	33.2–45.2
Urd bean	21.2–31.3
Winged bean	29.8–37.4

Source: Salunkhe DK, Kadam SS and Chavan JK (1985) *Postharvest Biotechnology of Food Legumes*. Boca Raton, FL: CRC Press.

disaccharides, such as sucrose (1–3%). However, some soybean varieties have been reported to contain as much as 7% sucrose.

Various oligosaccharides have been characterized in legume seeds, including raffinose, stachyose, and verbascose, which are galactosides of sucrose. Because humans do not express the enzyme α-galactosidase, these compounds remain undigested in the small bowel and pass through to the large bowel, where they can be fermented by anaerobic microbes. This leads to flatulence, or gas production, which is experienced following the consumption of some legumes. The concentration of raffinose-type oligosaccharides varies among legume species and, not surprisingly, the capacity to induce flatulence also varies.

Fiber

Legume seeds are a source of dietary fiber, containing both crude fiber and neutral detergent fiber. Most legumes contain 3–5 g of fiber per 100 g of dry seed, with most of the fiber found in the seed coat fraction. Exceptions are grass pea and hyacinth bean, which contain 8 and 10 g of fiber, per 100 g of dry seed, respectively. Compositionally, legume seeds contain varying quantities of lignin, cellulose, hemicelluloses, pectins, gums, and mucilage.

Minerals

Legume seeds contain a broad mix of minerals, many of which are essential both for plants and for animals. In fact, almost all essential minerals for humans can be found stored in the seeds. In comparison to cereals, legumes tend to have higher concentrations of calcium and potassium, as well as the micronutrients iron, zinc, and copper. Most of the calcium is sequestered as calcium oxalate crystals, however, and this form of calcium has extremely low bioavailability. Also, the majority of phosphorus in legume seeds is stored as phytic acid, which can complex calcium, iron, and zinc and thereby diminish their bioavailability. Other compounds found in legume seeds, including tannins, phenols, organic acids, protein, and fiber, can also interact with minerals and lower their bioavailability. Fortunately, certain processing procedures, such as fermenting or sprouting seeds, can reduce the levels of some of these mineral chelators. Due to these various problems, there is a significant effort under way in the plant science community to increase the absolute mineral levels in various legume seeds as well as to lower the levels of several major inhibitory compounds.

Vitamins

Most food legumes are good sources of thiamin, riboflavin, and niacin but are poor sources of ascorbic acid. This vitamin is present at only low levels in newly harvested dry seeds, and it disappears after long storage. In some species, varieties exist that produce green- or orange-colored cotyledons, and β-carotene, a pro-vitamin A carotenoid, can be found in some cases. The amounts of this vitamin precursor, however, are generally quite low. Tocopherols (vitamin E) are also found in some legume seeds, and folate, which is present in all legumes, can be quite high in certain species (e.g., lentil). Because folate is important in the prevention of neural tube defects, legume consumption is recommended for women of childbearing age, especially in regions of the world where folate fortification is limited.

Health-Promoting Phytochemicals

There is much interest in the role of various phytochemicals to promote good health and to reduce the risk of various cancers. As with many plant foods, legume seeds contain a number of these types of compounds. Prominent in this group are the isoflavonoids, such as genistein and daidzein, which are found at high levels in soybeans. Epidemiological studies have suggested a positive association between the consumption of soy isoflavones and reduced risk of breast and prostate cancer in humans. These and other related isoflavones are found in seeds of most of the commonly grown legumes. In addition, various saponins, catechins, epicatechins, and anthocyanidins have been measured in various legume seeds, and these compounds have also been suggested to have health-promoting qualities. Plant biochemists and human nutritionists are actively working to manipulate the levels of these and other compounds in legumes.

See also: **Bioavailability**. **Cereal Grains**. **Protein**: Quality and Sources. **Vegetarian Diets**. **Whole Grains**.

Further Reading

Aykroyd WR (1982) *Legumes in Human Nutrition* Rome: Food and Agriculture Organization of the United Nations.

Deshpande SS, Salunkhe DK, Oyewole OB *et al.* (2000) *Fermented Grain Legumes, Seeds and Nuts: A Global Perspective* Rome: Food and Agriculture Organization of the United Nations.

Duke JA (1981) *Handbook of Legumes of World Economic Importance* New York: Plenum Press.

Duranti M and Gius C (1997) Legume seeds: Protein content and nutritional value. *Field Crops Research* 53: 31–45.

Hedley CL, Cunningham J, and Jones A (2000) *Carbohydrates in Grain Legume Seeds: Improving Nutritional Quality and Agronomic Characteristics* New York: CABI.

Rubatzky VE and Yamaguchi M (1997) *World Vegetables: Principles, Production, and Nutritive Values* New York: Chapman & Hall.

Salunkhe DK and Kadam SS (1989) *CRC Handbook of World Food Legumes: Nutritional Chemistry, Processing Technology, and Utilization*, vols. 1–3. Boca Raton, FL: CRC Press.

Salunkhe DK, Kadam SS, and Chavan JK (1985) *Postharvest Biotechnology of Food Legumes* Boca Raton, FL: CRC Press.

Summerfield RJ and Roberts EH (1985) *Grain Legume Crops* London: Collins.

Wang TL, Domoney C, Hedley CL *et al.* (2003) Can we improve the nutritional quality of legume seeds? *Plant Physiology* **131**: 886–891.

LIPIDS

Contents
Chemistry and Classification
Composition and Role of Phospholipids

Chemistry and Classification

J L Dupont, Florida State University, Tallahassee, FL, USA

Lipids are generally known as fats and oils in food and nutrition. They are unique in nutrition, as they are in all of biology, in that they are not soluble in water. Early work on the chemistry of living organisms led to the discovery that fatty substances were soluble in organic solvents, such as chloroform, ethyl ether, alcohols, and hydrocarbons. Those solubility characteristics are dependent on the neutral or polar attributes of particular lipids and define the structural and functional aspects of lipids in living systems. This article presents the classification of lipids in their chemical groupings, their characteristic chemical and physical properties, and their nomenclature. Major groups of lipids include fatty acids, acylglycerols, phospholipids and sphingolipids, and sterols. Some lipid compounds, such as fat-soluble vitamins and waxes, are not included.

Fatty Acids and Acylglycerols

Nomenclature

Fatty acids are hydrocarbons of chain length two or greater with a carboxyl group at one end. Hydrocarbon chains are termed acyl lipids, and fatty acids occur most abundantly esterified to glycerol as triacylglycerols (**Figure 1**). Nomenclature for fatty acids has evolved from studies of food or organ sources of

the lipid, extraction and identification methods, and attempts at classification. **Table 1** lists fatty acids important in food and nutrition. The accepted shorthand description shows the number of carbons: number of double bonds, location of double bonds from the carbon at the methyl (n or omega) position, and *cis* or *trans* configuration (**Figure 2**). Saturated fatty acids (SFAs) have hydrogen atoms at every possible carbon site, and unsaturated fatty acids have double bonds. Fatty acids with double bonds may occur in isomeric forms. Geometric isomers are referred to as *cis* and *trans* rather than the convention Z and E preferred by chemists. For example, linoleic acid is 18:2 n-6, having 18 carbons, two double bonds located at the n (or omega) minus 6 and n minus 9 positions on the chain. Conventional carbon numbering is from the carboxyl end; therefore, linoleic acid can be written as *cis* 18:2 $\Delta^{9,12}$. Delta indicates numbering from the carboxyl carbon and the atom number from the carboxyl is sometimes used (C-9). Desaturase enzymes are named according to the delta number (i.e., Δ-9-desaturase). Commonly, the *cis* configuration is not noted because almost all natural fatty acids are in the *cis* configuration. Also, unless otherwise specified, the

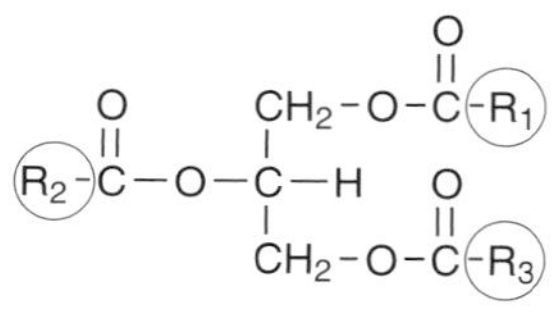

Triacylglycerol

Figure 1 Stereochemical numbering of lipids derived from glycerol. R_1, R_2, and R_3 refer to *sn* nomenclature.

Table 1 Fatty acids important in nutrition

Symbol[a]	Systematic name[b]	Common name	Melting point (°C)	Sources
Saturated fatty acids (SFAs)				
2:0	n-Ethanoic	Acetic	16.7	Many plants
3:0	n-Propanoic	Propanoic	−22.0	Rumen
4:0	n-Butanoic	Butyric	− 7.9	Rumen and milk fat
6:0	n-Hexanoic	Caproic	− 8.0	Milk fat
8:0	n-Octanoic	Caprylic	12.7	Milk fat, coconut
10:0	n-Decanoic	Capric	29.6	Milk fat, coconut
12:0	n-Dodecanoic	Lauric	42.2	Coconut, palm kernel
14:0	n-Tetradecanoic	Myristic	52.1	Milk fat, coconut
16:0	n-Hexadecanoic	Palmitic	60.7	Most common SFA in plants and animals
18:0	n-Octadecanoic	Stearic	69.6	Animal fat, cocoa butter
20:0	n-Eicosanoic	Arachidic	75.4	Widespread minor
22:0	n-Docosanoic	Behenic	80.0	Minor in seeds
24:0	n-Tetracosanoic	Lignoceric	84.2	Minor in seeds
Monounsaturated (monoenoic) fatty acids				
10:1 n-1	cis-9-Decenoic	Caproleic		Milk fat
12:1 n-3	cis-9-Dodecenoic	Lauroleic		Milk fat
14:1 n-5	cis-9-Tetradecenoic	Myristoleic		Milk fat
16:1 n-7t	trans-Hexadecenoic	Palmitelaidic		HVO[c]
16:1 n-7	cis-9-Hexadecenoic	Palmitoleic	1	Most fats and oils
18:1 n-9	cis-9-Octadecenoic	Oleic	16	Most fats and oils
18:1 n-9t	trans-9-Octadecenoic	Elaidic	44	Ruminant fat, HVO[c]
18:1 n-7t	trans-11-Octadecenoic	trans Vaccenic	44	Ruminant fat
20:1 n-11	cis-9-Eicosaenoic	Gadoleic		Fish oils
20:1 n-9	cis-11-Eicosaenoic	Gondoic	24	Rapeseed, fish oils
22:1 n-9	cis-13-Docosaenoic	Erucic	24	Rapeseed, mustard oil
Polyunsaturated (polyenoic) fatty acids				
Dienoic				
18:2 n-9	cis,cis-6,9-Octadecadienoic		−11	Minor in animals
18:2 n-6	cis,cis-9,12-Octadecadienoic	Linoleic	− 5	Most plant oils
Trienoic				
18:3 n-6	All-cis-6,9,12-octadecatrienoic	γ-Linolenic		Evening primrose, borage oils
18:3 n-3	All-cis-9,12,15-octadecatrienoic	α-Linolenic	−11	Soybean and Canola oils
20:3 n-6	All-cis-8,11,14-eicosatrienoic	Dihomogammalinolenic		
Tetra; penta; hexaenoic				
20:4 n-6	All-cis-8,11,14-eicosatetraenoic	Arachidonic	−49.5	Meat
20:5 n-3	All-cis-5,8,11,14,17-eicosapentaenoic	EPA, Timnodonic		Fish oils
22:4 n-6	All-cis-7,10,13,16-docosatetraenoic	Adrenic		Brain
22:5 n-6	All-cis-7,10,13,16,19-docosapentaenoic	DPA, Clupanodonic		Brain
22:6 n-3	All-cis-4,7,10,13,16,19-docosahexaenoic	DHA		Fish

[a]Number of carbons:number of double bonds, location of first double bond from the methyl carbon.
[b]Geometric isomer-Δ positions of double bonds.
[c]HVO, hydrogenated vegetable oil.
t, trans.

double bonds are 3 carbons apart, referred to as 'methylene interrupted,' as contrasted with conjugated double bonds (**Figure 3**).

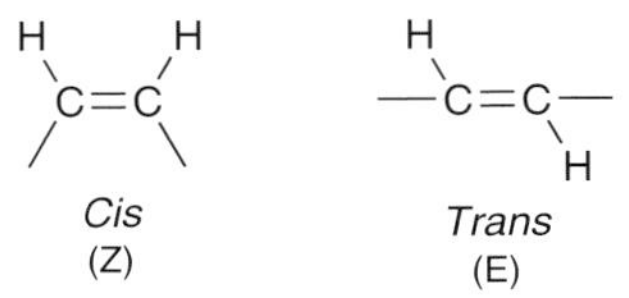

Figure 2 Structure of cis and trans double bonds.

Physical and Chemical Properties

Nonesterified fatty acids or free fatty acids have a polar (acidic) component and a neutral hydrocarbon component. The ratio of carbon to oxygen depends on the chain length and accounts for the solubility properties as well as the energy density of the lipid molecule. The hydrocarbon chain of the fatty acid is hydrophobic and the carboxyl end is hydrophilic, making the molecule amphipathic. This causes a dispersion of oil in water to form a mono molecular

Fatty acid models

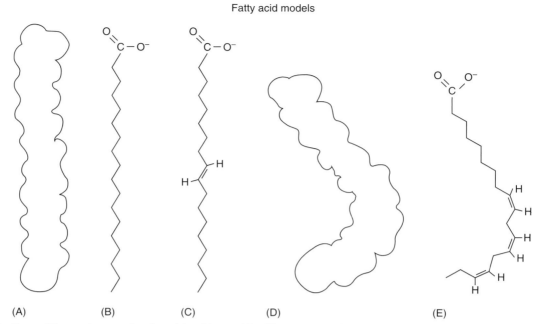

(A)   (B)   (C)   (D)   (E)

Figure 3 Space-filling and conventional models of fatty acids: (A) stearic acid (18:0), space-filling; (B) stearic acid, conformational; (C) elaidic acid (18:1n-9t) *trans*, conformational; (D) α-linolenic acid, all-*cis*, space-filling; (E) α-linolenic acid, conformational.

layer at the surface with the carboxyl end in contact with water and the hydrocarbon extending out of the water. The fatty acids may form a micelle (**Figure 4**) to separate the oil and water phases. These orientations of fatty acids and more complex lipids are a primary aspect of their participation in biological structures and functions. Furthermore, there is free rotation about the carbon–carbon bonds so the fatty acids and acylglycerols are capable of assuming a number of configurations.

Differences in the physical characteristics of fatty acids, particularly saturated compared with unsaturated, are extremely important in food and nutrition. SFAs with a chain length longer than 12 carbons are solid at usual ambient temperatures. As the chain lengthens, the melting point increases.

On the contrary, mono- and polyunsaturated fatty acids (PUFAs) are liquid at room temperatures. Uses of fats in food products are based on these properties. Salad oils, margarines, and shortenings are examples of such differences. Hydrogenation of oils containing PUFAs was introduced to provide food fats that are resistant to rancidity and of a desirable plasticity. The chemical hydrogenation process yields mixtures of *cis* and *trans* fatty acids (**Figure 5**). The physical conformation of *trans* fatty acids is important for their functions in foods and nutrition (**Figure 3**). The melting points are similar to those of SFAs of similar length and their shapes are linear rather than bent as forced by the *cis* configuration. These physical characteristics affect their space-filling functions and the mobility of the molecule.

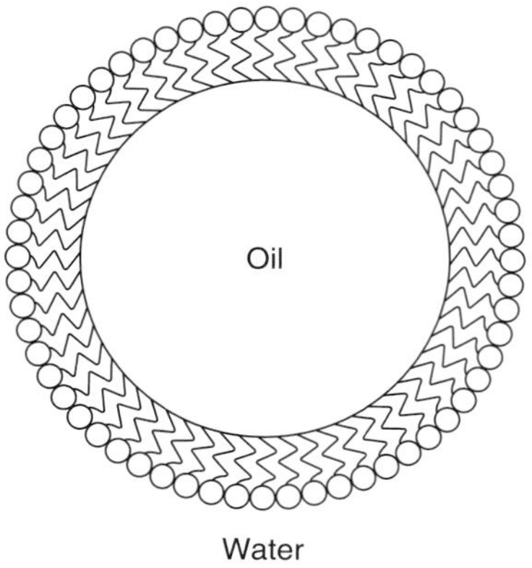

$$CH_3(CH_2)_n-CH=CH-\underset{\underset{H}{|}}{\overset{\overset{H}{|}}{C}}-CH=CH-\underset{\underset{H}{|}}{\overset{\overset{H}{|}}{C}}-CH=CH-(CH_2)_nCOOH$$

Polyunsaturated fatty acid

$\downarrow$ H$_2$ (hydrogenation)
Ni (catalyst)

$$CH_3(CH_2)_n-CH_2-CH_2-CH_2-\underset{\underset{H}{|}}{\overset{\overset{H}{|}}{C}}=C-CH_2-CH_2-C(CH_2)_nCOOH$$

Trans fatty acids

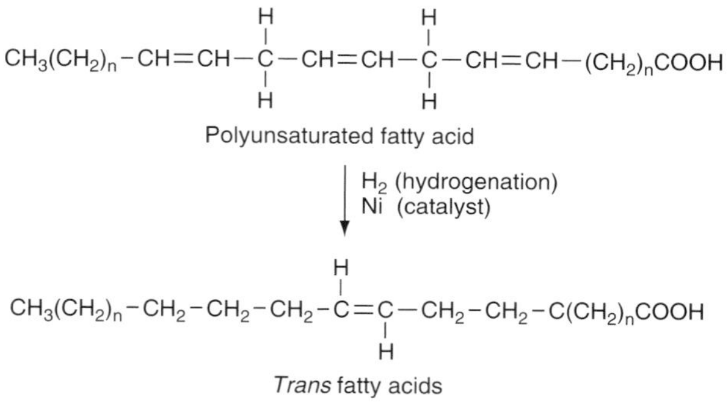

Figure 5 Hydrogenation of polyunsaturated fatty acids. *trans* fatty acids are produced when hydrogenation results in incomplete saturation of double bonds during chemical processing.

Oil

Water

Figure 4 Micelle formed by oil dispersion in water.

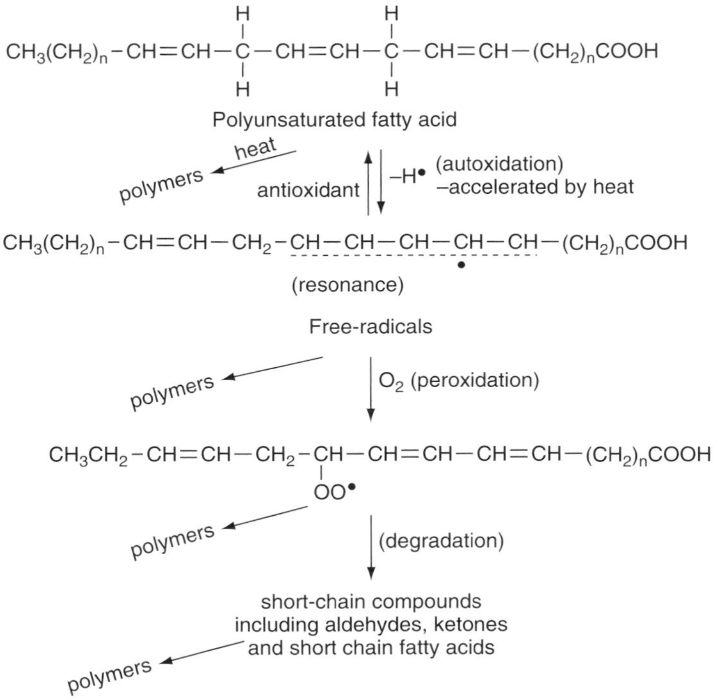

$$CH_3(CH_2)_n - CH=CH - \underset{\underset{H}{|}}{\overset{\overset{H}{|}}{C}} - CH=CH - \underset{\underset{H}{|}}{\overset{\overset{H}{|}}{C}} - CH=CH - (CH_2)_nCOOH$$

Polyunsaturated fatty acid

heat

polymers ← antioxidant | −H• (autoxidation) −accelerated by heat

$$CH_3(CH_2)_n - CH=CH - CH_2 - CH-CH-CH-CH-CH - (CH_2)_nCOOH$$
•

(resonance)

Free-radicals

polymers ← | O₂ (peroxidation)

$$CH_3CH_2 - CH=CH - CH_2 - \underset{\underset{OO•}{|}}{CH} - CH=CH - CH=CH - (CH_2)_nCOOH$$

polymers ← | (degradation)

short-chain compounds
including aldehydes, ketones
and short chain fatty acids

polymers ←

Figure 6 Autoxidation is caused by removal of a hydrogen from the methyl group between double bonds in polyunsaturated fatty acids. Resonating free radicals are produced and propagate peroxidation, degradation, and formation of polymers.

Polyunsaturated fatty acids with the methylene-interrupted double bond are also susceptible to oxidation (**Figure 6**). The hydrogen atoms on the methyl group between double bonds are susceptible to sequestration by oxidizing agents, such as iron or free radicals. This autoxidation results in a resonating free radical that is self-propagating and, with exposure to oxygen, yields peroxides. The peroxides may polymerize or degrade to smaller molecules. In foods, this process results in the condition of rancidity characterized by off flavors. In living systems, the products of peroxidation may cause reactions that damage proteins, membranes, and DNA resulting in pathological processes. Antioxidants are compounds that are capable of interrupting free radical propagation by reducing the peroxide to an alcohol without itself becoming a free radical. Tocopherols are a major antioxidant group in living systems and chemical antioxidants such as BHT (3,5-di-*t*-butyl-4-hydroxytoluene) are used in food products.

Another primary characteristic of naturally occurring PUFAs is that they cannot be synthesized by animals but are necessary for metabolism; therefore, they are an essential component of the diet. Animal organisms can introduce a double bond at the C-9 position but lack the enzymes to insert double bonds between the C-9 position and the methyl terminal carbon. The fatty acids are therefore considered to be in three families in relation to their biological functions: the mono-unsaturated (n-9 or omega-9) family and the polyunsaturated n-6 (omega-6) and n-3 (omega-3) families.

Phospholipids

The glycerol backbone is the central structure of phospholipids, as it is for acylglycerols. They are characterized by a phosphate group at the *sn*-3 position making phosphatidic acid (**Figure 7**).

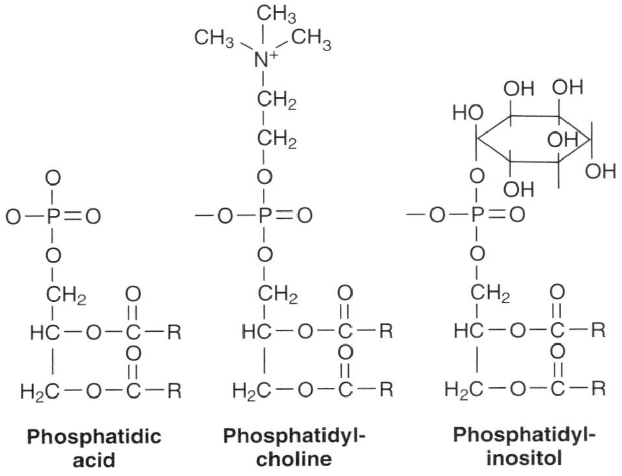

Phosphatidic acid

Phosphatidyl-choline

Phosphatidyl-inositol

Figure 7 Structures of phospholipids.

Phosphoglycerides have fatty acids esterified at the 1 and 2 positions. A number of compounds may be esterified to the phosphate moiety, including choline, ethanolamine, serine, and *myo*-inositol. The compounds are called phosphatidylcholine, etc. These molecules are obviously amphipathic, having very polar constituents at the *sn*-3 position and acyl chains at the 1 and 2 positions. This attribute is very important to their function in biological membranes.

Sphingolipids

A group of acyl lipids has a sphingosine-based structure (**Figure 8**). The derivatives of sphingosine are cerebrosides and ceramides. They are characterized by having sugar molecules as part of their structure and thus are called glycosphingolipids. The most common sugar moiety is galactose. There is a large family of mono-, di-, and triglycosyl ceramides. Some of the glycosphingolipids have sialic (*N*-acetyl neurominic) acid linked to one or more of the sugar residues of a ceramide oligosaccharide. These are called mono-, di-, and trisialogangliosides and are abundant in membranes, particularly in nervous tissue. Their amphipathic structures are functional in membranes and in the water impermeability of skin.

Steroids

Sterols

Sterols are monohydroxy alcohols with a four-ring core structure or steroid nucleus (**Figure 9**). Cholesterol is the most abundant sterol in animal tissues. The tetracyclic structure is uniquely compact and rigid. The unesterified molecule has only one

polar site, the hydroxyl on the number 3 carbon. When it is esterified to an acyl group, usually oleic acid, the cholesteryl ester is extremely hydrophobic. The free hydroxyl enables the cholesterol molecule to orient in membranes, a major function of

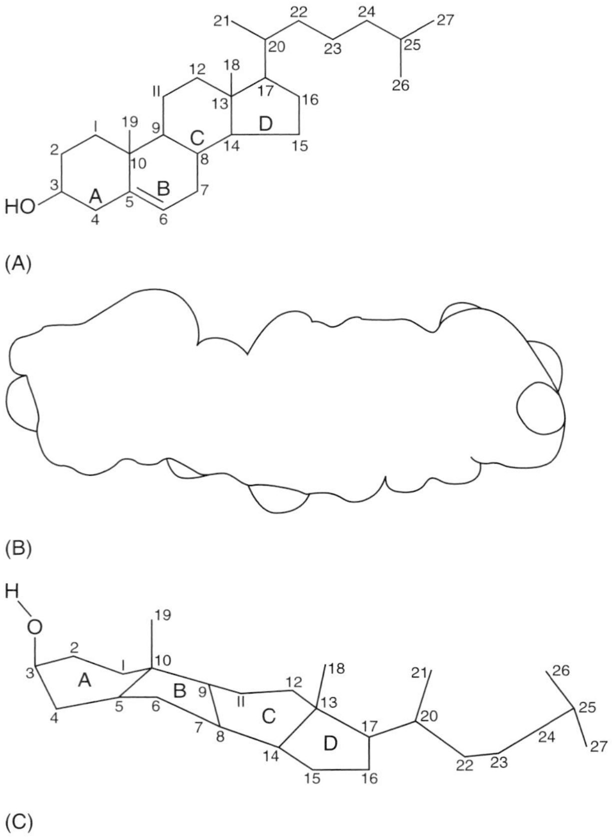

(A)

(B)

(C)

Figure 9 Cholesterol structural models: (A) conventional, (B) space-filling, and (C) conformational.

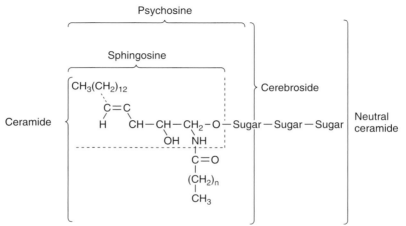

Figure 8 Structure of a sphingolipid.

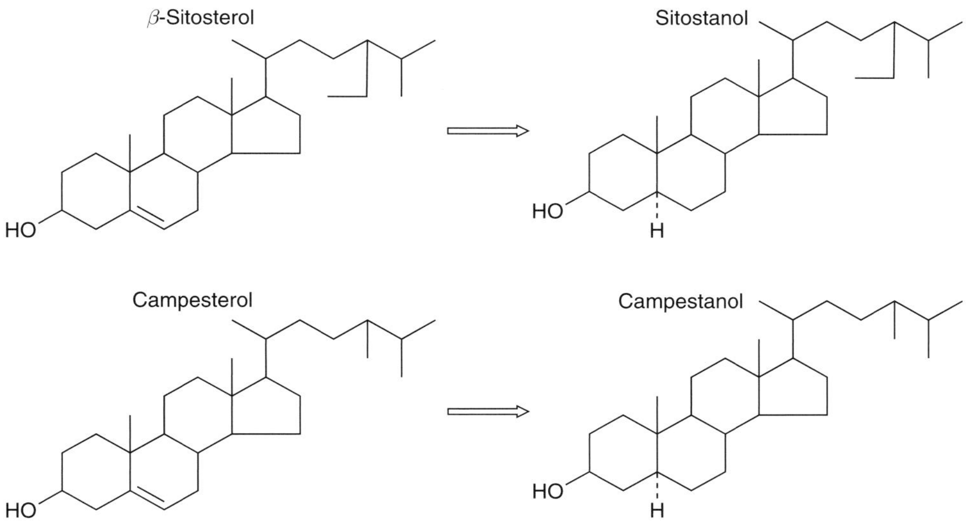
β-Sitosterol
Sitostanol
HO
HO
H
Campesterol
Campestanol
HO
HO
H

Figure 10 Plant sterols.

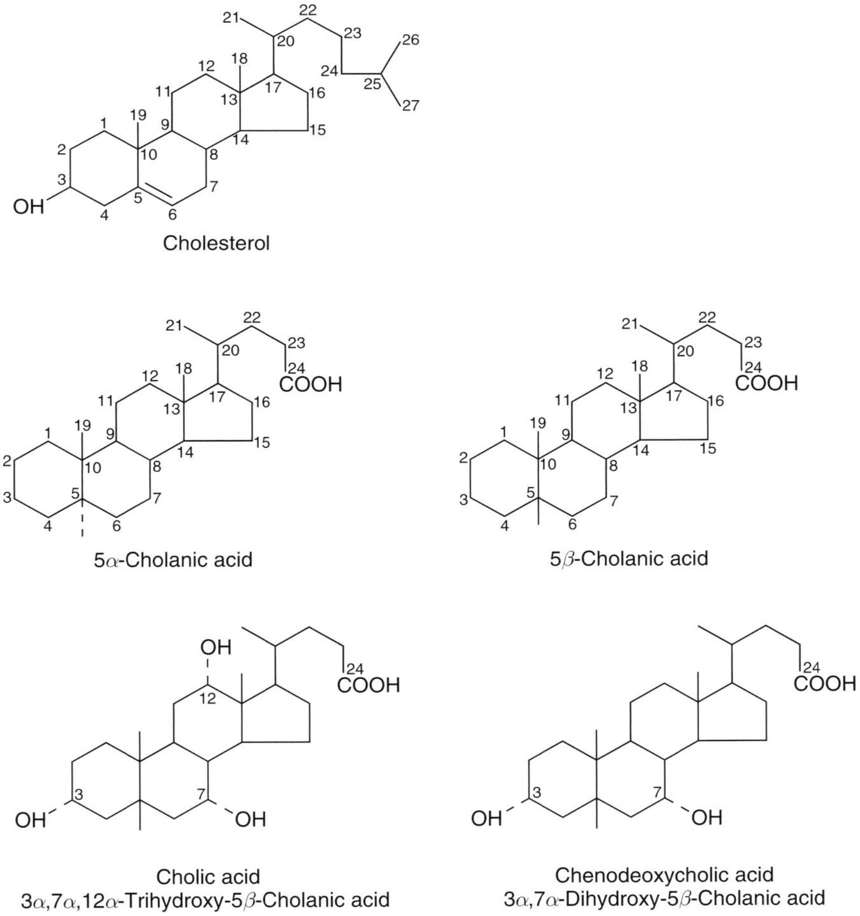
OH
Cholesterol
COOH
5α-Cholanic acid
COOH
5β-Cholanic acid
OH
COOH
OH
OH
Cholic acid
3α,7α,12α-Trihydroxy-5β-Cholanic acid
COOH
OH
OH
Chenodeoxycholic acid
3α,7α-Dihydroxy-5β-Cholanic acid

Figure 11 Bile acid synthesis from cholesterol.

cholesterol. In brain and other nervous tissues, free cholesterol is the major component of myelin and renders the myelin sheath impermeable to electron transfer (dielectric).

Phytosterol and campesterol are the major sterols in plant tissues (**Figure 10**). The plant sterols and their stanol derivatives (saturated at the 5–6 carbons) along with cholesterol are active in regulating cholesterol absorption. All these sterols are consumed in the diet, and some are being added to foods as positive adjuncts to regulation of cholesterol metabolism.

Bile Acids

The most abundant derivatives of cholesterol are bile acids. Cholesterol is important in metabolism and is biosynthesized as well as consumed in the diet. It is the precursor for vitamin D (cholecalciferol) and for the adrenocortical hormones, such as estrogen, androgens, and progesterone. These compounds require very small amounts of the cholesterol precursor. The sterol nucleus cannot be broken by mammalian enzymes, except for the formation of cholecalciferol. Bile acids constitute approximately 50% of the excretion products of cholesterol metabolism and perform essential functions in digestion and absorption of dietary lipids. They are synthesized in the liver (**Figure 11**) and exist in metabolism as conjugates with taurine and glycine (**Figure 12**). As with other lipids in metabolism, the amphipathic properties of the compounds characterize their functions. The planar sterol moiety with an acid group at the 24 carbon is capable of separating water and lipid interfaces and is important in facilitating interaction between lipids and enzymes in digestion. The even greater contrast of polar and neutral within the same molecule is exemplified by the conjugated bile acids. They are also active in digestion and exist in all tissues, so they may have additional functions as amphipathic facilitators between enzymes and lipids.

$$\overset{+}{H_3N}-CH_2CH_2SO_3^-$$

Taurine

$$\overset{+}{H_3N}-CH_2COO^-$$

Glycine

Figure 12 Structures of taurine and glycine.

See also: **Cholesterol**: Sources, Absorption, Function and Metabolism; Factors Determining Blood Levels. **Fats and Oils**. **Fatty Acids**: Metabolism; Monounsaturated; Omega-3 Polyunsaturated; Omega-6 Polyunsaturated; Saturated; *Trans* Fatty Acids. **Fertility**. **Hyperlipidemia**: Overview; Nutritional Management. **Lipids**: Composition and Role of Phospholipids.

Further Reading

Dupont J (1990) Lipids. In: *Present Knowledge of Nutrition*, pp. 56–66. New York: International Life Sciences Institute/Nutrition Foundation.

Dupont J, White PJ, and Feldman EB (1991) Saturated and hydrogenated fats in food in relation to health. *Journal of the American College of Nutrition* 10: 577–592.

Gropper SS, Smith JL, and Groff JL (2005) *Advanced Nutrition and Human Metabolism*, 4th edn., pp. 128–171. Belmont, CA: Thomson Wadsworth.

Gurr ML, Harwood JL, and Frayn KN (2002) *Lipid Biochemistry*, 5th edn. Oxford: Blackwell Science.

Composition and Role of Phospholipids

A D Postle, University of Southampton, Southampton, UK

Phospholipids are amphipathic (amphipathic describes molecules with regions that are both water seeking (hydrophillic) and water repellent (hydrophobic). This is the fundamental physical property that drives the formation of biological membranes) lipids consisting of hydrophobic and hydrophilic regions. This amphipathic nature, which enables phospholipid molecules to assemble into bilayer and hexagonal membrane structures, is critically important for the functional viability of all eukaryote cells. Cellular membranes, composed primarily of phospholipid, separate the intracellular milieu from the extracellular environment and facilitate the formation of specialised intracellular organelles. For many years, phospholipids were considered to be important but relatively inert structural components of the cell. Recently, the central role of membrane phospholipid composition and turnover in the regulation of a wide range of cellular functions has become widely recognized. For instance, all membrane receptor events take place within a phospholipid-rich environment, and it is therefore not surprising that cells have adopted hydrolysis of membrane phospholipids as a major signaling mechanism. Phospholipids have multiple roles, including the following:

1. They provide a structural framework to maintain cellular integrity and to compartmentalize diverse events within the cell.
2. They provide the appropriate physicochemical environment to optimize the activities of membrane-associated receptors, enzymes, and proteins.
3. They act as substrate molecules for a variety of phospholipase enzymes involved in signaling mechanisms.
4. They provide sites for binding of proteins involved in cellular signaling processes.
5. They exert a physicochemical detergent-like action to facilitate the physiological function of a variety of tissues, including the lungs, stomach, and synovial surfaces.
6. They regulate the synthesis and secretion of lipoproteins from the liver.

Phospholipid Structures

There are two major classes of phospholipid, depending on whether they contain a glycerol or sphingosyl backbone. Glycerophospholipids are molecules based on phosphatidic acid (3-*sn*-phosphatidic acid); the nature of the esterified group X defines the class of phospholipid (**Figure 1**). The most common substituent groups include nitrogenous bases, such as choline and ethanolamine, and polyalcohols, such as myoinositol and glycerol. Sphingophospholipids contain sphingosine (*trans*-D-erythro-1,3-dihyroxy 2-amino-4-octadecene). Sphingomyelin is the most abundant sphingophospholipid class, and it is the phosphorylcholine ester of *N*-acylsphingosine, also called ceramide. Sphingophospholipids are important components of all cell membranes and are structurally and metabolically closely related to glycosphingolipids such as glycosylceramides, gangliosides, and cerebrosides. Sphingomyelin is recognized as a major substrate for sphingomyelinase enzymes involved in generating intracellular ceramide and sphingosine, which are intimately involved in the regulation of programmed cell death (apoptosis). Sphingophospholipids contain principally saturated and monounsaturated fatty acids; little information is available on the nutritional effects on sphingophospholipid composition, and sphingomyelin metabolism has been recently reviewed.

The distribution of phospholipids is heterogeneous within any cell both between different subcellular membranes and within individual membranes. For instance, mammalian cells maintain an enriched distribution of neutral lipids, such as phosphatidylcholine (PC) and sphingomyelin, in the outer leaflet of the plasma membrane and hence present an uncharged surface to the exterior of the cell (**Figure 2**). It is critically important to restrict the distribution of uncharged phospholipids to the interior of the cell because increased concentration of phosphatidylserine (PS) in the outer leaflet of the plasma membrane is the initial signal for both programmed cell death (apoptosis) and the clotting cascade.

Classification and Nomenclature of Glycerophospholipids

Glycerophospholipid classes are commonly referred to as phosphatidylcholine, phosphatidylethanolamine, etc. They are composed of a spectrum of molecular species (phospholipid molecular species are the individual different molecules within any different class of phospholipid determined by the combination of fatty acids esterified to the glycerol backbone. Any given mammalian cell contains up to 1000 individual phospholipid molecular species) defined by the substituent fatty acid groups attached to the *sn*-1 and *sn*-2 positions of the glycerol backbone. For example, the individual molecular species palmitoyloleoyl phosphatidylcholine can be named formally as either glycerol 1-hexadecanoate 2-9-octadecaenoate 3-phosphocholine or 1-hexadecanoyl-2-octadeca-9-enoyl-3-glycerophosphocholine. One shorthand designation for this molecule, adopted in this article, is PC16:0/18:1, where PC designates the phospholipid class, in this case phosphatidylcholine, and 16:0 and 18:1 (fatty acid nomenclature is based on total number of carbon atoms in the acyl chain, followed by total number of double bonds. For instance, 16:0 is saturated 16-carbon palmitic acid, whereas 20:4 is poplyunsaturated 20-carbon arachidonic acid) designate the fatty acids esterified at the *sn*-1 and *sn*-2 positions.

For phospholipids from cell membranes, saturated fatty acids are generally located at the *sn*-1 and unsaturated fatty acids at the *sn*-2 position, with notable exceptions. For instance, dipalmitoyl PC (PC16:0/16:0) is a major component of lung and surfactant PC, whereas significant amounts of didocosahexaenoyl phosphatidylethanolamine (PE22:6/22:6) are present in retinal PE. In addition, PC species with 18:1n-9 at the *sn*-1 position are minor components of many cells.

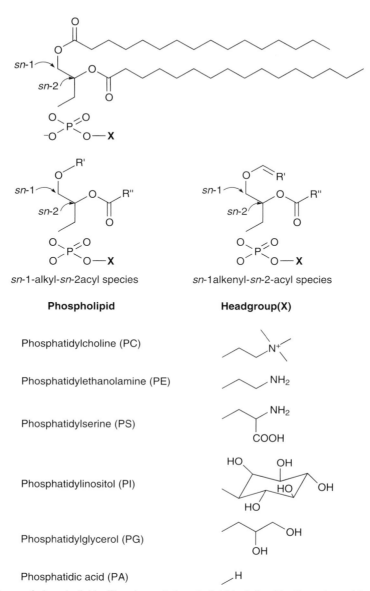

Figure 1   Molecular structures of phospholipids. The class of phospholipid is defined by the nature of the nitrogenous base or polyol esterified to the phosphate group (X). The species distribution within any phospholipid class is determined by the fatty acyl substituents at the *sn*-1 and *sn*-2 positions of the glycerol backbone. The dipalmitoyl species would be designated PC16:0/16:0 if X was choline. If arachidonic acid was esterified at *sn*-2, then the molecule would be designated as PC1 6:0/20:4. In the diacyl species, fatty acids are attached by ester linkages. For *sn*-1-alkyl-*sn*-2-acyl species, the *sn*-1 fatty acid is attached by an ether bond. For *sn*-1-alkenyl-*sn*-2-acyl species, the *sn*-1 fatty acid is attached by a vinyl ether linkage.

In addition to diacyl species, with both fatty acids attached by ester bonds, there are a number of species with ether-linked fatty acids, principally in the *sn*-1 position. These ether phospholipids include 1-alkyl-2-acyl species, largely present in PC, and 1-alk-1-enyl species (plasmalogens), largely present in PE. These ether lipids are major components of many cell membranes, particularly neuronal and inflammatory cells, and there have been significant advances in understanding the biochemical pathways for their synthesis and catabolism. Some alkyl acyl PC species are substrates for the generation of the potent bioactive lipid platelet-activating factor (1-alkyl-2-acetyl-glycero-3-phosphocholine (PAF)), but the function of most ether lipids is largely unclear. One possibility is that generation of 1-alkyl-2-acyl-glycerol as a second messenger rather than diacylglycerol may contribute to differential regulation of protein kinase C isoforms, and antioxidant properties have been reported for plasmalogens.

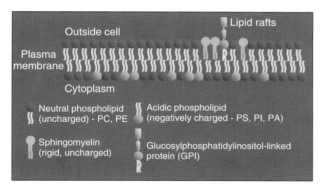

Figure 2 Topology of distribution of phospholipids within the plasma membrane of eukaryotic cells. The outer leaflet of the membrane bilayer is enriched in neutral PC and rigid components, such as sphingolipids and glucosylphosphatdylinositol-linked proteins. The distribution of charged acidic phospholipids, such as PS and PI, to the inner leaflet of the membrane is actively regulated by a combination of enzymes called flipases and scramblases.

Phospholipid Analysis

Historically, phospholipid compositions have been determined by thin-layer chromatography of different classes followed by gas chromatography of fatty acids. Such traditional analysis provides no direct information about the individual molecular species compositions of phospholipids, which are the functional, biologically relevant molecules. For instance, a fatty acid analysis of a phospholipid mixture as 50% 16:0, 50% 18:1 could represent either 16:0/18:1 or an equivalent combination of 16:0/16:0 and 18:1/18:1, which all have very different physical and functional properties. A variety of techniques have been established to provide such information, including high-performance liquid chromatography (HPLC), nuclear magnetic resonance, and mass spectrometry. In this article, compositional data are provided in terms of individual molecular species largely determined by sensitive electrospray ionization mass spectrometry (ESI-MS) methodologies. (Electrospray ionization mass spectrometry is a soft ionization technique that resolves intact molecular ions with minimal fragment formation. Best known for proteomic analysis, when applied to lipid analysis ESI-MS provides direct, very sensitive analysis of molecular species composition with a high degree of resolution.)

Phospholipid Composition

The glycerophospholipid composition of most cell types in the body is regulated within relatively restricted limits and is often specialized for the function of the cell involved. Moreover, most cells maintain distinct and different compositions of the various phospholipid classes. For example, ESI-MS analysis of total lipid extracts from a variety of mouse tissues shows that PC exhibits a wide variation of composition but that of phosphatidylinositol (PI) is relatively constant (**Figure 3**). PC species range from predominantly polyunsaturated in liver (**Figure 3A**) to disaturated and monounsaturated in lungs (**Figure 3B**) and brain (**Figure 3C**). Liver PC contains substantial amounts of species with either n-6 fatty acids (20:4n-6) or n-3 fatty acids (22:6n-3), whereas PC from pancreas, for instance, is essentially composed solely of species containing n-6 fatty acids (**Figure 3D**). This inherent variation in PC composition is emphasised by that of spleen (**Figure 3E**), which, like lung, is dominated by PC16:0/16:0 but also contains increased concentrations of monounsaturated and polyunsaturated species. In contrast, PI from all tissues measured was dominated by the single polyunsaturated stearoyl arachidonoyl species (PI18:0/20:4) (**Figures 3F–3J**). This diversity of composition is mirrored for the distinctive and different compositions of all the other phospholipid classes in most cell types and emphasizes the highly specific mechanisms that regulate phospholipid compositions *in vivo*. PE is typically enriched in arachidonoyl-containing species, whereas PS is generally dominated by the monounsaturated species PS18:0/18:1. It is important to recognize, for nutritional studies *in vitro*, that many of these tissue-specific distributions are lost or reduced for cells maintained in cell culture supplemented with fetal calf serum.

Phospholipid Synthesis

These compositions are mediated by interactions between phenotypic expression and cellular nutrition, which determine the specificities of the enzymes of phospholipid synthesis and hydrolysis and of the transfer proteins that exchange phospholipid species between different membranes. Regulation of synthesis is best characterized for the formation of PC in rat hepatocytes, where PC synthesis is essential for assembly and secretion of very low-density lipoprotein particles, and in the lung epithelial cells responsible for synthesis of pulmonary surfactant phospholipid. Phosphatidylcholine species synthesized *de novo* from diacylglycerol by the enzyme cholinephosphotransferase are subsequently modified by acyl remodeling mechanisms involving sequential actions of phospholipase and acyltransferase activities. The rate of PC synthesis is thought to be dependent on the activity of CTP:choline phosphate cytidylyltransferase (CCT), which is subject to complex regulatory mechanisms involving phosphorylation and reversible enzyme

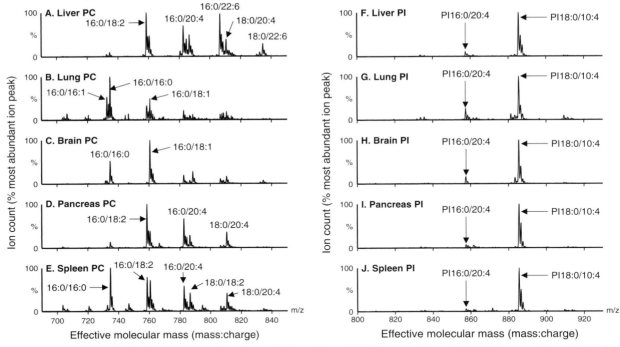

Figure 3 Electrospray ionization mass spectrometry analysis of phospholipid compositions of selected mouse tissue. Total lipids were extracted from liver, lungs, pancreas, and spleen using chloroform:methanol and then analyzed for PC (A–E) and PI (F–J) using diagnostic mass spectrometry scans. The distribution of the phospholipid molecular species in these illustrative spectra is given by the response of the individual ions, presented relative to the predominant ion on display. The identities of the major PC and PI species identified were confirmed by diagnostic fragmentation analysis by tandem MS/MS. (Dombrowsky H, Bernhard W, Rau G, Clark G and Postle A, unpublished results.)

translocation between cytosol and membrane fractions of the cell. In this context, CCT acts as a sensor for the physical structure of the endoplasmic reticulum membrane. Hydrolysis of PC alters the inherent curvature of the membrane and decreases its stored elastic energy, enabling CCT to bind and thus replenish membrane PC.

The spatial pathway of phospholipid synthesis is illustrated schematically in **Figure 4** for the type 2 epithelial cell of the lung alveolus, which synthesizes and secretes lung surfactant. Initial synthesis of phospholipids on the endoplasmic reticulum is followed by a complex series of events that include modification of esterified fatty acid groups by a process of acyl remodeling, selective transport between different intracellular membranes, and uptake of selected phospholipids into lamellar bodies. These lamellar bodies are intracellular stores of surfactant that, when secreted in response to cell stretch, are actively secreted into the alveolar space where they adsorb to the air–liquid interface, oppose surface tension forces within the lungs, and prevent alveolar collapse. In addition, inactive surfactant is recycled by type 2 cells into endosomes that fuse into multivesicular bodies and subsequently into lamellar bodies.

Although the phospholipid metabolism of the type 2 cell is complex compared to that of most cell types, it demonstrates very well the various stages in phospholipid synthesis, transport, and metabolism with potential for modification of molecular compositions.

A limited number of conditions are known in which alterations to the processes of phospholipid synthesis and metabolism have profound effects on health and survival. In human subjects, the inability to synthesise the major phospholipids, such as PC and PE, is incompatible with life, so most genetic abnormalities have been identified in abundances of more minor phospholipids. For instance, Barth's syndrome is an X-linked recessive disorder characterised by childhood onset of cardiomyopathy, neutropenia, and abnormal mitochondrial structure and function. The gene affected is the *tafazzin* gene, responsible for acyl remodeling in cardiolipin synthesis. Cardiolipin is a minor phospholipid enriched within the heart and in mitochondria that contains four fatty acid and two phosphate moieties and is synthesised on the endoplasmic reticulum predominately with four oleoyl ($C_{18:1}$) chains. Patients with Barth's syndrome are unable to convert this tetraoleoyl form into the more functional tetralinoleoyl ($C_{18:2}$) cardiolipin species. This is the only condition

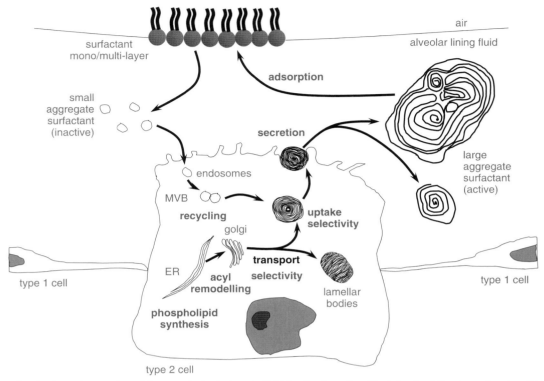

Figure 4 Synthesis and secretion of lung surfactant phospholipid by the type 2 epithelial cell of the lung alveolus. Phospholipid synthesized in the endoplasmic reticulum (ER) is routed through the Golgi apparatus for uptake and packaging into intracellular storage vesicles called lamellar bodies. In response to cell stretch, lamellar bodies fuse with the plasma membrane and secrete their contents into the alveolar space. After processes of adsorption and desorption from the air–liquid interface, inactive surfactant is recycled into lamellar bodies via endosomes and multivesicular bodies (MVB). Metabolically active type 2 cells occupy only approximately 5% of the surface area of the alveolus, with the thin type 1 cells responsible for gas exchange contributing the other 95%.

identified in which the inability to synthesize a precise composition of an individual phospholipid class is apparently responsible for clinical symptoms.

In addition to modification of synthetic mechanisms, alterations to transport and uptake processes can result in severe disease and mortality. ABCA3 is a membrane protein member of the ATP-binding cassette (ABC) family of proteins, which includes the multidrug resistance protein and the ABCA1 protein responsible for reverse cholesterol transport. ABCA3 is though to be involved in the selective uptake and processing of phospholipids destined for lung surfactant assembly within lamellar bodies. Mutations in the *ABCA3* gene cause fatal surfactant deficiency in newborn infants and have been recognized as major contributors to lung disease and respiratory failure in infants delivered full term.

Phospholipid Breakdown

There is also a considerable diversity of specificity of phospholipase enzymes responsible for phospholipid

hydrolysis, in terms of both positional and molecular species selectivity. Phospholipase A activity in rat liver will act selectively to remove sn-1 16:0 from PC species containing sn-2 18:2, whereas cytosolic phospholipase A_2 (PLA_2) is specific for species containing sn-2 20:4n-6. In contrast, secretory PLA_2 must be bound to negatively charged phospholipids for activation, but it is not acyl specific. Mammalian phospholipase Cs (PLCs) act preferentially on phosphatidylinositol-4,5-bisphosphate rather than on PI or PC, whereas agonist-stimulated phospholipase Ds (PLDs) are selective for PC species. However, although the distribution of phospholipases is tissue specific, the contribution of their activities to the regulation of phospholipid compositions in most tissues has not been well defined.

Phospholipid Composition in Development

The most extensive changes to phospholipid composition occur during fetal and neonatal development and have been best characterized for PC in liver, lung, and brain. These changes illustrate clearly the limitations of dietary manipulation on phospholipid composition. During human pregnancy, the polyunsaturated fatty acids (PUFAs) 20:4n-6 and 22:6n-3 are supplied across the placenta from maternal to fetal circulations in increasing quantities toward term. At birth, the onset of milk feeding is characterized by increased intake of the PUFA precursor 18:2n-6. This sequence of nutritional supply is reflected in fetal and neonatal liver PC composition. Immature fetal human liver contains a high proportion of monounsaturated PC species, particularly PC16:0/18:1, and tends to become enriched with species containing 20:4n-6 and 22:6n-3 toward term (Table 1).

Postnatally, the content of 18:2n-6 species increases, and fetal and neonatal plasma PC composition directly mirrors this changing pattern. However, these alterations in development are regulated primarily by metabolic and hormonal rather than by nutritional considerations. The increased supply of PUFA from mother to fetus in later gestation is independent of any change in maternal dietary lipid intake and instead is a consequence of hormonal effects on the specificity of PC synthesis and lipoprotein export by the maternal liver. Similarly, although switching from placental to enteral feeding is the major factor causing the dramatic changes to plasma PC at birth, this composition is still dependent on the metabolic regulation of the specificity of hepatic PC synthesis. The programmed nature of this regulation is shown clearly by food restriction in newborn guinea pig pups, which still display equivalent postnatal alterations to plasma and liver PC composition as

their fed litter mates, even in the total absence of enteral nutrition.

In contrast, immature fetal lung PC also contains a high concentration of PC16:0/18:1 but becomes more, rather than less, saturated with progression of gestation due to increased synthesis of the disaturated species PC16:0/16:0 and PC16:0/14:0. PC16:0/16:0 is a major component of pulmonary surfactant that acts to oppose surface tension forces in the lungs and prevent alveolar collapse. Infants who are born preterm with immature surfactant are at high risk of death and disability caused by neonatal respiratory distress syndrome. In contrast to fetal liver, the phospholipid composition of fetal lung is only marginally affected by the changes to lipid nutrition in utero. Nevertheless, some nutritional influence is evident, even though PUFA-containing species are minor components of lung PC. Comparison of PC compositions in prenatal human lung shows a postnatal increase in the content of PC16:0/18:2, which reflects the increased dietary supply of 18:2n-6. The situation in developing lung reflects that of most other tissues in the body, in which dietary lipid modulation causes relatively modest changes to the specificity of phospholipid compositions. Such subtle alterations to membrane composition, however, can exert profound effects on cellular function.

Finally, adult brain PE contains approximately 50% of 22:6n-3 species, enriched in neuronal synapses and possibly involved in synaptic transmission. Failure to acquire sufficient 22:6n-3 in brain PE during neuronal differentiation in early development can lead to permanent suboptimal neurological function. Many of the changes to maternal lipid metabolism in pregnancy represent adaptations to ensure adequate supply of PUFA to the developing fetal brain. Increased synthesis and secretion of PC16:0/22:6 in livers of pregnant rats and guinea pigs correlates with the period in fetal brain growth of maximal accumulation rate of 22:6n-3 into brain PE. Once incorporated into brain or retinal PE, 22:6n-3 is retained throughout life, even in periods of prolonged nutritional deprivation. Infants who are born preterm and with inadequate reserves of 22:6n-3 are recognized to be in danger of nutritional deficiency if fed milk formula lacking preformed long-chain PUFA. For instance, 22:6n-3 content of brain PE was decreased in infants fed such formula and who had died suddenly from sudden infant death syndrome. For this reason, supplementation of preterm infant milk formula with preformed PUFA has been recommended by the European Society for Pediatric Gastroenterology and Nutrition.

Table 1   Phosphatidylcholine molecular species composition of human liver during fetal and postnatal development[a]

Molecular species	Liver phosphatidylcholine concentration (nmol/pg wet weight)		
	Fetal (15 weeks of gestation, n = 4)	Stillborn (term, n = 4)	Infant (43–64 weeks old, n = 6)
16:0/16:0	992 ± 156	1004 ± 81	538 ± 121
16:0/18:1	2007 ± 250	2240 ± 173	2353 ± 496
16:0/18:2	466 ± 52	1259 ± 139	2202 ± 273
16:0/20:4	1402 ± 98	1784 ± 38	1062 ± 219
16:0/22:6	431 ± 110	953 ± 82	614 ± 512
18:0/18:2	308 ± 56	443 ± 68	1239 ± 252
18:0/20:4	1298 ± 288	953 ± 89	448 ± 403
18:0/22:6	115 ± 31	210 ± 50	221 ± 267

[a]Molecular species were analyzed by reverse-phase HPLC and quantified by postcolumn fluorescence detection with 1,6-diphenyl-1,3,5-hexatriene. Concentrations expressed as mean ± SD.

Phospholipid Composition in Adult Tissues

Information about the detailed molecular species compositions of phospholipids from adult human tissues is surprisingly haphazard. There have been many isolated reports of extensive characterizations of selected phospholipid classes in individual tissues, but such studies have generally measured compositions of bulk preparations from relatively large tissue samples. Very few clinical or nutritional studies have characterized phospholipid compositions in molecular terms. In reality, each cell type contains in excess of 1000 glycerophospholipid species, with differential compositions between different membranes in the same cell and even between different regions in the same membrane. Such regions of microheterogeneity may occur either because of the physical properties of the lipids themselves (e.g., forming hexagonal rather than bilayer structures) or because of sequestration by membrane proteins. Phase transitions within the membrane can also exert significant effects, and interactions of cytoskeletal components of the cell have been described with relative solid gel-phase phospholipids in the plasma membrane. One additional important factor is the transmembrane phospholipid distribution between the two leaflets of the cell bilayer. For practically all cell types, PC is relatively more concentrated in the outer leaflet, whereas PE is located primarily in the inner (cytoplasmic) leaflet. Importantly, PS is almost totally restricted to the side of the plasma membrane facing the cytoplasm, where it acts as an activator of protein kinase C. Redistribution of PS to the outer leaflet of the plasma membrane is a signal of cell senescence and is a potent activator of the clotting cascade. Finally, there has been considerable interest in the concept of lipid rafts, subfractions of membranes that are resistant to extraction with detergent and have been extensively implicated in transmembrane signaling particularly in immune cells. The compositional aspects of many such studies must be interpreted with caution; recent analyses have indicated that detergent solubility is more an intrinsic property of individual lipids than a property dependent on membrane organization.

Examples of recent ESI-MS analyses of phospholipid molecular species compositions of a variety of human tissues are summarized in **Figure 5**, which compares ESI-MS spectra of PC from human blood lymphocytes, monocytes, and neutrophils. As for most hematopoeic cell types and in contrast to the mouse compositions shown in **Figure 2**, the PC composition of these cells is dominated by monounsaturated PC

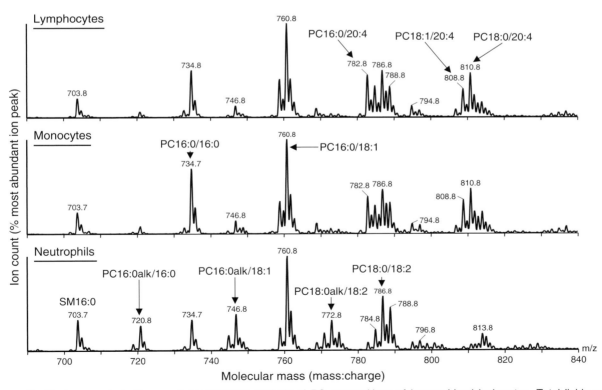

Figure 5 Electrospray ionization mass spectrometry analysis of PC compositions of human blood leukocytes. Total lipids were extracted from lymphocytes, monocytes, and neutrophils and analyzed as described in the legend for **Figure 2**. (Madden J, Wright S, Clark G and Postle A, unpublished observations.)

species, especially PC16:0/18:1 (m/z = 760), but the distribution of polyunsaturated species is considerably variable between cell types. Both lymphocytes and monocytes are relatively enriched in species containing 20:4n-6 (PC16:0/20:4 m/z = 782; PC18:0/20:4 m/z = 810), with an increased content of PC16:0/16:0 (m/z = 734). In contrast, neutrophils are relatively depleted in both PC16:0/16:0 and arachidonoyl species, but they contain considerably higher proportions of sn-1-alkyl-sn-2-acyl species (PC16:01alk/16:0 m/z = 720; PC16:0alk/18:1 m/z = 746; PC18:0alk/18:2 m/z = 772). This comparison illustrates an important role for phenotypic expression as one contributor toward the specificity of cell PC composition.

Different phospholipid classes from the same tissue generally exhibit considerable variation in composition, shown in **Figure 2** for mouse tissues and also in the analysis of the white matter of human brain. Although brain PC was highly enriched in monounsaturated species, diacyl PE was enriched in species containing PUFA. The distribution of such species, however, was highly asymmetric, with 22:6n3 and 20:4n-6 species containing 16:0 at the sn-1 position being present in much lower abundance than the same species containing sn-1 18:0. In contrast, both alkenylacyl PE and PS were characterized by a predominance of monounsaturated species. However, whereas PC was enriched in PC16:0/18:1, alkenylacyl PE was enriched in PE18:1alk/18:1 and PS was enriched in PS18:0/18:1. This comparison illustrates the tight regulation of the composition of individual phospholipid classes and emphasizes potentially important differences in molecular compositions that could not be predicted from total fatty acid analysis.

Nutritional Effects on Phospholipid Molecular Species

Practically all nutritional studies of dietary lipid effects on cellular phospholipid compositions have reported fatty acid compositions, with no molecular information. Due to significant differences in the detailed regulation of their phospholipid composition and metabolism, nutritional data obtained from laboratory animals generally have only a restricted application to human nutrition. The data in **Figure 6** are from one study in which human volunteers were fed fish oil supplements for 4 weeks and the change in their erythrocyte PE molecular species composition was measured. Of interest, the extent of increase in species containing

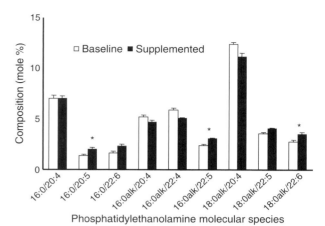

Figure 6 Dietary lipid and the composition of human erythrocyte phosphatidylethanolamine. Erythrocyte PE species were analyzed from six volunteers before and after consumption of fish oil containing 9 g eicosapentaenoic acid (22:5n-3) and 6 g docosahaexenoic acid (22:6n-3) per day for 4 weeks. Results are expressed as mean $\pm$ SEM; *$p < 0.05$. (From Knapp HR, Hullin F and Salem N Jr (1994) Asymmetric incorporation of dietary n-3 fatty acids into membrane aminophospholipids of human erythrocytes. *Journal of Lipid Research* **35**: 1283–1291.)

n-3 fatty acids was variable, and the extent of such changes was modest. This comparison illustrates a general observation that although manipulation of cultured cell phospholipid compositions by medium lipid supplementation is relatively easy, phospholipid compositions of similar cell types in vivo are considerably more resistant to dietary manipulation.

Functions of Phospholipids

Phospholipid composition is a significant factor in most cellular processes. This section, however, is restricted to selected examples of the role of molecular species composition with regard to physiological functions.

Membrane Structure

One frequently addressed role of phospholipids is to maintain an appropriate membrane structure for optimal cell function. The term 'membrane fluidity' is often used but is imprecise. It generally describes the combined effects of lateral and rotational movement of lipids within the plane of the membrane. Other concepts are perhaps more useful, such as the stress, termed 'stored elastic energy,' when phospholipids are prevented by their location within the membrane from assuming their lowest energy configuration. Typically, phospholipids such as PC prefer to adopt a convex membrane curvature, whereas molecules such as PE and PA will spontaneously adopt a concave configuration. In these paradigms, alterations to dietary lipid intake may exert their modulatory effect on cell function by changing phospholipid molecular composition and hence altering these physiochemical properties. Although such effects are evident in model systems, extensive measurement by fluorescence polarization suggests that processes of homeoviscous adaptation restrict the extent of adaptations observed *in vivo*. For instance, increased incorporation of PUFA into membrane phospholipid, which would be expected to have a fluidizing effect, is invariably balanced by compensatory increases in the membrane content of cholesterol and more rigid phospholipid molecules.

Lung Surfactant

Maintenance of the essential composition of lung surfactant phospholipid is critical for the survival of all mammalian species. Lung surfactant is secreted from specialized type 2 epithelial cells in the lung alveolus and forms a continuous lining layer at the air–liquid interface throughout the lungs. To provide adequate gas exchange surface area in the lungs to support respiration, alveolar diameters must be very small, giving a large surface area:volume ratio. One consequence of the small dimensions of the alveolus is that surface tension forces contribute significantly to the dynamics of lung function. Surfactant opposes surface tension in the lungs. It is the absence of adequate surfactant that leads directly to lung collapse and the high incidence of morbidity and mortality associated with neonatal respiratory distress syndrome.

Lung surfactant has a unique phospholipid composition, containing PC16:0/16:0 as 40–60% of total PC and monounsaturated phosphatidylglycerol (PG) species as 10–15% of total phospholipid. Phosphatidylglycerol is not found at such high concentration in any other membrane of the body. PC16:0/16:0 is the principal surface-active component of lung surfactant, has a gel:liquid crystalline transition temperature of $41\,^\circ$C, and consequently is, in effect, solid at a body temperature of $37\,^\circ$C. It has been suggested that the compressed PC16:0/16:0 monolayer at the air–liquid interface survives the high surface pressures within the lungs by forming a solid monomolecular sheet, and it thus prevents any surface tension effects. At the same time, PC16:0/16:0 is metabolically inert, and one proposed specialized role for PG is to fluidise PC16:0/16:0 and facilitate its metabolic processing, secretion, and adsorption to the air–liquid interface.

This composition of lung surfactant is restricted to air-breathing animals. Comparative studies with reptiles, amphibia, and lower vertebrates have shown that concentration of PC16:0116:0 in surfactant correlates with the ratio of lung:body surface area as a measure of an animal's reliance on lung-mediated respiration. Lung surfactant from amphibia, by comparison, also contains phospholipid, but this is largely cholesterol and unsaturated PC, which is thought to serve an antiglue function. By analogy with lung surfactant, phospholipid-rich surfactants have been described for other epithelial surfaces, including the stomach, eustachian tube, and synovial surfaces, where they are thought to create a protective hydrophobic lining layer. The comparison with lung surfactant is somewhat misleading, however, because the PC fraction of these other epithelial secretions contains minimal PC16:0/16:0 and high contents of mono- and diunsaturated species.

Signal Transduction

Phospholipids are substrate molecules for a wide range of lipid-derived signaling molecules, including diacylglycerol (DAG), phosphatidic acid (PA), 20:4n6, eicosanoid products, PAF, and lysophosphatidic acid, generated by the action of PLA_2, PLC, and PLD. The activation of these enzymes is complex, partly because of the large number of isoforms present within a cell and also because of the interdependence and coordination of their regulation. For instance, the bacterial peptide formyl-methionyl-leucyl phenylalanine (FMLP) binds to its receptor on neutrophils and activates the G-protein-regulated PLCβ. PLCβ hydrolyses PI-4,5-P_2 to form DAG, an activator of traditional Ca^{2+}-dependent PKC isoforms, and inositol trisphosphate, which stimulates intracellular Ca^{2+} mobilisation. In addition, FMLP activates PC-specific PLD and cytoplasmic PLA_2. PLD generates PA, which also has signaling responses, including stimulation of NADPH oxidase activity, but which is also readily interconverted with DAG. Alkenyl species of PE are probably the major substrates for cytoplasmic PLA_2, which is specific for molecular species containing 20:4n-6. This multitude of responses to a single agonist is highly coordinated and is typical of lipid signaling mechanisms in general. The activation of the various phospholipase enzymes is tightly regulated by a variety of protein kinases, phosphatases, and regulatory proteins, such that their responses are sequential rather than simultaneous.

Evidence suggests that phospholipid structure contributes to the coordinated regulation of phospholipase activation. PI-4,5-P_2, the substrate for PLC, is an obligate activator of ADP ribosylation factor-dependent PLD; consequently PI-4,5-P_2 must be regenerated after the transient activation of PLC, before maximal activation of PLD can be achieved. In addition, individual phospholipids can act as binding sites for a wide range of signaling proteins and enzymes, enabling their coordinated regulation at the membrane. Perhaps the best characterised of these systems is the generation of trace amounts of 3-phosphorylated PI, typically PI-3,4,5-P_3, when PI-3-kinase is activated by insulin and growth factors. Signaling proteins containing appropriate binding motifs (plecstrin homology or PH domains) then bind to PI-3,4,5-P_3 and initiate signaling cascades. The prototype of such protein is protein kinase B (PKB) also know as Akt. PKB undergoes a conformational change when bound to PI-3,4,5-P_3, becomes phosphorylated, and then is active in the regulation of cell proliferation.

The mechanisms of action of dietary lipid modulation on these signaling pathways are largely unknown. There is good evidence that eating a diet rich in fish oil (containing 22:6n-3 and 22:5n-3) attenuates neutrophil-mediated inflammatory reactions. Part of this antiinflammatory nutritional effect may be to reduce the content of phospholipid species containing 20:4n-6, thus decreasing available substrate for synthesis of eicosanoid and leukotriene products derived from 20:4n-6. Alternatively, it may also result in part from the modulation of the spectrum of molecular species of DAG and PA generated by the various PLC and PLD enzymes. In this paradigm, altering the composition of substrate phospholipid will result in the formation of different DAG or PA species, which then have differential actions on target kinase enzymes. Because inositol phospholipids are generally composed of the 18:0120:4 species, activation of PLC1 will form DAG18:0/20:4, whereas hydrolysis of PC will generate predominately monounsaturated DAG species. It has been suggested, for instance, that individual isoforms of protein kinase C can be differentially regulated in response to different molecular species of DAG, thus providing a molecular basis for many nutritional effects on a wide range of cellular functions.

Despite extensive studies since the 1960s, remarkably little is understood about the fundamental reasons why cells expend considerable energy maintaining lineage-specific molecular species compositions of membrane phospholipids. Even for cell lines in culture, which can be grown successfully over many generations with grossly nonphysiological membrane phospholipid compositions, a degree of lineage specificity is maintained. The detailed metabolic processes that control membrane phospholipid composition are slowly being defined, and studies of the specificities and activities in intact cells of acyltransferase and phospholipid synthetic enzymes using gene transfection and sensitive analytical techniques such as ESI-MS will increase understanding of the fundamental mechanisms involved.

See also: **Brain and Nervous System**. **Fatty Acids**: Metabolism; Monounsaturated; Omega-3 Polyunsaturated; Omega-6 Polyunsaturated; Saturated. **Lipids**: Chemistry and Classification.

Further Reading

Gunstone FD, Harwood JL, and Padley FB (1994) *The Lipid Handbook*, 2nd edn. London: Chapman & Hall.

Han X and Gross RW (2003) Global analyses of cellular lipidomes directly from crude extracts of biological samples by ESI mass spectrometry: A bridge to lipidomics. *Journal of Lipid Research* **44**: 1071–1079.

Hazel JR and Williams EE (1990) The role of alterations in membrane lipid composition in enabling physiological adaptations of organisms to their physical environment. *Progress in Lipid Research* **29**: 167–227.

Lee AG (1991) Lipids and their effects on membrane proteins: Evidence against a role for fluidity. *Progress in Lipid Research* **30**: 323–348.

Neuringer ME, Anderson GJ, and Connor WE (1988) The essentiality of n-3 fatty acids for development and function of the retina and brain. *Annual Review of Nutrition* **8**: 517–541.

Shulenin S, Nogee LM, Annilo T *et al.* (2004) ABCA3 gene mutations in newborns with fatal surfactant deficiency. *New England Journal of Medicine* **350**: 1296–1303.

Spiegel S and Merrill AH Jr (1996) Sphingolipid metabolism and cell growth regulation. *FASEB Journal* **10**: 1388–1397.

Valianpor RF, Wanders RJA, Barth PG, Overmars H, and van Geenup AH (2002) Quantitative and compositional study of cardiolipin in platelets by electrospray ionisation mass spectrometry: Application for the identification of Barth syndrome patients. *Clinical Chemistry* **48**: 1390–1397.

LIPOPROTEINS

J M Ordovas, Tufts University, Boston, MA, USA

Cholesterol and triacylglycerol are transported in blood as lipoproteins. Lipoproteins are generally spherical particles, with a surface layer composed of phospholipid with the fatty acids oriented toward the core of the particle. Included in this phospholipid layer are specific proteins known as apolipoproteins and free cholesterol. The core of the lipoprotein particles is made up of cholesteryl ester and triacylglycerol molecules.

The classification of serum lipoproteins has evolved historically through several phases corresponding with the development of different laboratory methodologies, including electrophoretic, ultra-centrifugal, and immunological techniques. By using these techniques, lipoproteins can be classified based on their electrophoretic mobility, hydrated density, and protein content.

Classification of Lipoproteins

Classification of Serum Lipoproteins According to Their Electrophoretic Mobilities

With the development of techniques to separate proteins according to their electrophoretic behavior, it could be demonstrated that most of the lipid present in serum was associated with proteins migrating with α_1- and β-globulin mobilities. This resulted in the first classification of lipoproteins as α_1- and β-lipoproteins. The ratio of lipid to protein on the α_1-lipoproteins was approximately 1:1, whereas the β-lipoproteins had a greater relative content of

lipids. Application of more advanced electrophoretic techniques resulted in further discrimination among the lipoprotein classes and for many years lipoproteins were classified as β-, pre-β-, and α-lipoproteins. Careful observation of the electrophoretic lipoprotein profiles in normals and subjects with familial lipoprotein disorders gave rise to the first classification of lipoprotein disorders by Fredrickson and colleagues. The equivalence between electrophoretic and ultracentrifugal separation is presented in **Table 1**.

Several electrophoretic supports have been used to separate plasma lipoproteins. These include paper, cellulose acetate, agarose, and polyacrylamide. Agarose gel electrophoresis remains the most commonly used for easy and rapid assessment of lipoprotein patterns in the clinical laboratory. This technique is especially useful for identifying the presence of a broad β band in the diagnosis of type III hyperlipidemia. Gradient agarose-polyacrylamide gel electrophoresis under nondenaturing conditions has been an essential tool to analyze low-density lipoprotein (LDL) and high-density lipoprotein (HDL) subclasses, providing a greater resolution than ultracentrifugation. LDL subfractions have been resolved by nondenaturing polyacrylamide gradient gel electrophoresis (2–16%) in up to seven LDL subclasses with densities ranging from 1.020 to 1.063 g ml^{-1} and diameters ranging from 22.0 to 28.5 nm. Usually a major subpopulation and several (one to four) minor LDL subpopulations are found in most subjects examined. A predominance of smaller, more dense LDL, versus larger, more buoyant LDL particles in plasma has been associated with increased coronary heart disease (CHD) risk. There is evidence supporting the genetic origin of the

Table 1 Classification of plasma lipoproteins

Lipoprotein	Diameter (nm)	Density (g ml^{-1})	Electrophoretic mobility	Major lipids	Major apolipoproteins
Chylomicrons	80–500	<0.95	Origin	Dietary triacylglycerols, cholesteryl esters	A-I, A-II, A-IV, B-48, C-I, C-II, C-III, E
Remnants	>30	<1.006	Origin	Dietary cholesteryl esters	B-48, E
VLDL	30–80	<1.006	pre-β	Endogenous triacylglycerols	B-100, C-I, C-II, C-III, E
IDL	25–35	1.006–1.019	pre-β and β	Cholesteryl esters, triacylglycerols	B-100, E
LDL	18–28	1.019–1.063	β	Cholesteryl esters	B-100
HDL$_2$	9–12	1.063–1.125	α	Cholesteryl esters, phospholipids	A-I, A-II
HDL$_3$	5–9	1.125–1.210	α	Cholesteryl esters, phospholipids	A-I, A-II

distribution of LDL subfractions; however, age, gender, and environmental factors strongly influence the penetrance. HDL subfractions have been resolved using a similar technique, with a polyacrylamide gradient ranging from 4 to 30%, into five subclasses (HDL_{3c}, HDL_{3b}, HDL_{3a}, HDL_{2a}, and HDL_{2b}). More recently 11–14 subclasses have been described, including β-migrating particles, using an improved electrophoresis technique. The clinical importance of these subfractions is still under investigation.

Classification of Serum Lipoproteins According to Their Ultracentrifugal Characteristics

The presence of lipids within the lipoprotein particles confers these macromolecular complexes with a lower density compared with other serum proteins. With the arrival of the analytical ultracentrifugation in the 1940s, this characteristic allowed its initial separation as a discrete peak using this technique. During the following years, it was demonstrated that this fraction was made up of a wide spectrum of particle sizes and densities (d) ranging from 0.92 to $1.21\,g\,ml^{-1}$.

Lipoproteins were classically separated into four major classes designated as chylomicrons (exogenous triacylglycerol-rich particles of $d < 0.94\,g\,ml^{-1}$), very low-density lipoproteins (VLDL, endogenous triacylglycerol-rich particles of $d = 0.94$–$1.006\,g\,ml^{-1}$), LDL (cholesteryl ester-rich particles of $d = 1.006$–$1.063\,g\,ml^{-1}$), and HDL (particles containing approximately 50% protein of $d = 1.063$–$1.21\,g\,ml^{-1}$). With subsequent improvements to the ultracentrifugation techniques, further heterogeneity was detected within each of those major lipoprotein classes; this resulted in the need for further subdivision into several density subclasses such as HDL_{2a} ($d = 1.10$–$1.125\,g\,ml^{-1}$), HDL_{2b} ($d = 1.063$–$1.10\,g\,ml^{-1}$), and HDL_3 ($d = 1.125$–$1.21\,g\,ml^{-1}$).

There is no doubt that the separation of lipoproteins by ultracentrifugation has been esential for the advances in this field; however, this technique is very labor intensive and the isolated lipoproteins are usually modified due to the high g force and salt concentrations used in this process. The development of new vertical and near vertical rotors has shortened considerably the runs and thus diminished some of these negative effects.

Classification of Serum Lipoproteins According to Their Apolipoprotein Composition

Recent interest on the study of lipoprotein subfractions has resulted in an increased use of methods of separation based on affinity chromatography, specially those using immunoaffinity. By using columns containing antibodies against specific apolipoproteins (**Table 2**), a large number of HDL subpopulations have been resolved. Similarly, this technique

Table 2 Classification and properties of apolipoproteins

Apolipoprotein	Amino acids	Tissue expression	Chromosomal localization	Functions
apo A-I	243	Liver Intestine	11	Major structural component of HDL Ligand for HDL binding Activator of LCAT Reverse cholesterol transport
apo A-II	77	Liver	1	Structural component of HDL Activator of hepatic lipase
apo A-IV	377	Intestine Liver	11	Regulator of LPL activity Activator of LCAT Intestinal lipid absorption
apo B-48	2152	Intestine	2	Structural component of TRL Secretion of chylomicrons
apo B-100	4536	Liver	2	Structural
apo C-I	57	Liver Intestine	19	Activator of LCAT Inhibitor of the LRP
apo C-II	79	Liver Intestine	19	Activator of LPL
apo C-III	79	Liver Intestine	11	Inhibits LPL
apo D	169	Most tissues	3	Radical scavenger Reverse cholesterol transport Binding of haem-related compounds
apo E	299	Liver Macrophage	19	Ligand for the LDL receptor Ligand for the LRP Reverse cholesterol transport
apo(a)	Variable	Liver	6	?

allows the separation of several triacylglycerol-rich lipoproteins subfractions.

Lipoproteins containing apo A-I can be separated into two major species: those containing both apo A-I and apo A-II, known as LpAI:AII, and those containing apo A-I but not apo A-II (LpAI). Small numbers of particles containing apo A-II, but not apo A-I, have been detected in normal subjects; however, these particles could become predominant in the presence of rare genetic disorders associated with HDL deficiency. Another HDL species containing apo A-I and apo E is important in reverse cholesterol transport by transporting cholesterol from the cell membranes to the liver for elimination from the body.

Lipoproteins containing apo B consist of four lipoprotein families. Lipoproteins containing apo B only (Lp(B)) are cholesteryl ester-rich and are found primarily within the LDL density range, but they have also been detected within the VLDL range. Particles containing both apo B and apo C (LpB:C), apo B and apo E (LpB:E), and all three apolipoprotein groups (LpB:E:C), are triacylglycerol-rich and are found within the VLDL and IDL density range. The apo C and apo E content decreases as density increases.

More recently, the affinity for lectins of Lp(a), a lipoprotein containing apo B-100 as well as an antigenically unique apolipoprotein [apo(a)], has been used to develop a new technique to measure the levels of this lipoprotein in plasma.

Synthesis and Catabolism of Lipoproteins

Metabolism of Lipoproteins Carrying Exogenous Lipids

Dietary fats absorbed in the intestine are packaged into large, triacylglycerol-rich chylomicrons for delivery through the bloodstream to sites of lipid metabolism or storage. These lipoproteins interact with lipoprotein lipase (LPL) and undergo lipolysis, forming chylomicron remnants. The major sites of LPL activity are adipose tissue, skeletal muscle, the mammary gland, and the myocardium. In these sites, the fatty acids from the trcacylglycerols are used for storage, oxidation, or secretion back to the circulation. The triacylglycerol-depleted particles resulting from the lipolysis, known as chylomicron remnants, pick up apo E and cholesteryl ester from HDL and are rapidly taken up by the liver via a process mediated by the apo E receptor. This is a fast process and chylomicron particles are not usually present in the blood after a prolonged fasting period. The occurrence of chylomicronemia can be easily detected by the presence of a creamy supernatant floating on top of the plasma or serum kept several hours at 4 °C.

Transport of Endogenous Lipids

The liver cell secretes triacylglycerol-rich VLDL, which can be converted first to intermediate-density lipoprotein (IDL) and then to LDL through lipolysis by a mechanism similar to that described for chylomicrons. The excess surface components are usually transferred to HDL, and the triacylglycerol-depleted VLDL becomes an IDL. Some of these particles may be taken up by the liver via an apo E receptor, whereas others are further depleted of triacylglycerols, becoming cholesteryl ester-enriched particles known as LDL, which contain apo B as their only apolipoprotein. Consumption of fat-rich meals or glucose enhances VLDL production.

Some primary causes of elevated VLDL or IDL levels are familial endogenous hypertriglyceridemia (type IV according to Fredrickson's classification) and familial dysbetalipoproteinemia (type III hyperlipidemia). Genetic mutations at the apo E gene locus are responsible for the type III phenotype. Some secondary causes for elevated VLDL levels are obesity, diabetes mellitus, alcohol consumption, as well as the use of high doses of certain drugs (e.g., thiazide diuretics and estrogens). The presence of elevated levels of IDL has been associated with an increased atherosclerotic risk.

LDL particles are major carriers of cholesteryl ester in the blood. An LDL receptor that recognizes apo B-100 and apo E, but not apo B-48, allows the liver and other tissues to catabolize LDL. High-fat and high-cholesterol diets can decrease the activity of the LDL receptor, leading to increased levels of circulating LDL. These particles supply cholesterol to cells in the periphery for synthesis of cell membranes and steroid hormones. Modified or oxidized LDL can also be taken up by the scavenger receptor on macrophages in various tissues, including the arterial wall. This process is a potential initiator of foam cell formation and atherosclerosis.

Several LDL subclasses have been identified using gradient gel electrophoresis. Large, less dense LDL particles are commonly found in premenopausal women and men at low risk for CHD, whereas the small, more dense particles have been associated with a significant increased risk for myocardial infarction. The distribution of these particles appears to have a significant genetic component modulated by age and environmental factors.

Reverse Cholesterol Transport

HDL is synthesized by both the liver and the intestine. Its precursor form is discoidal in shape and matures in circulation as it picks up unesterified cholesterol from cell membranes and other lipids (phospholipid and triacylglycerol) and proteins (A-I, E, and C apolipoproteins) from triacylglycerol-rich lipoproteins (chylomicron and VLDL) as these particles undergo lipolysis. The cholesterol is esterified by the action of the lecithin–cholesterol acyltransferase (LCAT) and the small HDL_3 particle becomes a larger HDL_2 particle. The esterified cholesterol is either delivered to the liver or transferred by the action of cholesteryl ester transfer protein (CETP) to other lipoproteins (such as chylomicron, VLDL remnants, or LDL) in exchange for triacylglycerols. This cholesterol may then be taken up by the liver via receptors specific for these lipoproteins, or it can be delivered again to the peripheral tissues. The triacylglycerol received by HDL_2 is hydrolyzed by hepatic lipase and the particle is converted back to HDL_3, completing the HDL cycle in plasma. In the liver, cholesterol can be excreted directly into bile, converted to bile acids, or reutilized in lipoprotein production.

Several genetic disorders have been identified associated with low levels or total deficiency of HDL.

Effects of Dietary Fats and Cholesterol on Lipoprotein Metabolism

The cholesterolemic effects of dietary fatty acids have been extensively studied. The saturated fatty acids $C_{12:0}$, $C_{14:0}$, and $C_{16:0}$ have a hypercholesterolemic effect, whereas $C_{18:0}$ has been shown to have a neutral effect. Monounsaturated and polyunsaturated fatty acids in their most common *cis* configuration are hypocholesterolemic in comparison with saturated fatty acids. The effects of *trans* fatty acids on lipid levels are under active investigation. Our current knowledge shows that their effect is intermediate between saturated and unsaturated fats. The effect of dietary cholesterol on lipoprotein levels is highly controversial. This may be due in part to

the dramatic interindividual variation in response to this dietary component. Specific effects of dietary fats and cholesterol on each lipoprotein fraction are the focus of other articles and they are only briefly summarized below and in **Table 3**.

Effects of Diet on Chylomicron Metabolism

Diets very high in saturated fat have been associated with increased postprandial chylomicrons and chylomicron remnants compared with diets rich in n-6 polyunsaturated fats; however, human experiments carried out using moderate to high fat intake have not shown significant effects of different types of dietary fat or dietary cholesterol on postprandial lipoproteins.

The effects of dietary carbohydrates on postprandial lipoproteins have also been studied. Most protocols have used diets very high in simple carbohydrates. In general, high carbohydrate intake has been associated with increased levels of fasting triacylglycerols and increased postprandial levels of chylomicrons and chylomicron remnants.

Effects of Diet on VLDL Metabolism

It is well-known that diets high in simple carbohydrate increase hepatic secretion of VLDL. This carbohydrate induction of hypertriglyceridemia is the source of the current controversy regarding the optimal diet for subjects at high risk for cardiovascular disease. Some authors have demonstrated that the increased hepatic triacylglycerol secretion induced by high-carbohydrate diets was not accompanied by parallel increases in apo B-100 secretion. In other words, the consumption of low-fat, high-carbohydrate diets did not affect the number of particles but resulted in larger, more triacylglycerol-enriched VLDL particles.

Intake of saturated fat results in an increased secretion of the number of VLDL particles by the liver, whereas the opposite effect is observed with polyunsaturated fat. Of special note are the dramatic effects on VLDL production found following high intakes of n-3 fatty acids. These diets are associated with marked decreases in triacylglycerol secretion by mechanisms not fully understood. It

Table 3 Effects induced on the major lipoprotein fractions by different dietary components following isoenergetic replacement of saturated fatty acids

	MUFA	PUFA n-6	PUFA n-3	trans FA	Simple carbohydrate	Carbohydrate plus fiber
VLDL-C	≈	≈/↓	↓	↑	↑	≈
LDL-C	↓	↓	≈/↓	↑	↓	↓
HDL-C	≈/↑	≈/↓	↓	↓	↓	≈/↓

≈ equivalent effect; ↓ concentration reduced; ↑ concentration increased.

has been speculated that n-3 fatty acids may stimulate intracellular degradation of apo B in hepatocytes. Dietary cholesterol, within the physiological range, appears to play a minor role in hepatic VLDL production.

Effects of Diet on LDL Metabolism

The effects of dietary fat and cholesterol on LDL metabolism have been extensively studied. However, the effects of dietary cholesterol are still highly controversial. Whereas some studies have demonstrated increased LDL production and decreased catabolism associated with high cholesterol intakes, others have failed to find such associations.

Replacement of saturated by polyunsaturated fats has been associated with decreased LDL apo B production in some studies, whereas in other studies, increased ratios of polyunsaturated to saturated fats resulted in increased LDL apo B catabolism. Unlike the effects described for VLDL metabolism, intake of n-3 fatty acids appears to play a minor role on LDL metabolism.

Effects of Diet on HDL Metabolism

Diets high in simple carbohydrates reduce HDL cholesterol levels. This effect appears to be mediated by increases in the catabolism of apo A-I; however, one study has also demonstrated an additional decrease in apo A-I production.

Disorders of Lipoprotein Metabolism

For historical reasons the classification of disorders of lipoprotein metabolism will be presented according to the classical Fredrickson's classification (Table 4).

Type I or Familial Chylomicronemia

This disorder is characterized by greatly elevated levels of exogenous triacylglycerols and it is the result of impaired lipolysis of chylomicrons due to a deficiency of LPL or its activator, the apo C-II. Several genetic mutations at the structural genes for both LPL and apo C-II have been reported. These are autosomal recessive traits. In the heterozygous state, subjects have normal to slightly elevated plasma triglycerides, whereas homozygotes have triacylglycerol levels that may exceed $1000 \, \text{mg dl}^{-1}$ in the fasting state. The diagnosis of the homozygous state takes place during the first years of life from the presence of recurrent abdominal pain and pancreatitis. Eruptive xanthomas and lipemia retinalis may also occur.

The recommended treatment includes a diet low in simple carbohydrates and with a fat content below 20% of total energy. The use of medium-chain triglycerides (MCT) has also been reported to be efficacious. Body weight should be maintained within the normal limits and alcohol consumption should be avoided.

Other secondary causes leading to the presence of chylomicrons in the fasting state include uncontrolled diabetes mellitus, alcoholism, estrogen use, and hypothyroidism.

Fasting chylomicronemia has not been clearly associated with increased risk for atherosclerosis; however, there is considerable evidence supporting the atherogenic properties of chylomicron remnants.

Type II or Familial Hypercholesterolemia

Familial hypercholesterolemia (FH) is an autosomal dominant disorder characterized by elevation of plasma LDL cholesterol levels. Mutations at the LDL receptor gene locus on chromosome 19 are

Table 4 Classification of hyperlipidemias according to Fredrickson

Type	Plasma cholesterol	Plasma triacylglycerol	Lipoprotein fraction(s) affected	Atherosclerosis risk	Genetic disorder
I	Normal to elevated	Very elevated	Chylomicrons	No	Familial LPL deficiency Apo C-II deficiency
IIa	Elevated	Normal	LDL	High	Familial hypercholesterolemia Familial combined hyperlipidemia Polygenic hypercholesterolemia
IIb	Elevated	Elevated	LDL and VLDL	High	Familial hypercholesterolemia Familial combined hyperlipidemia
III	Elevated	Very elevated	IDL	High	Familial dysbetalipoproteinemia
IV	Normal or elevated	Elevated	VLDL	Moderate	Familial hypertriglyceridemia Familial combined hyperlipidemia
V	Normal or elevated	Very elevated	VLDL and chylomicrons	Moderate	Familial hypertriglyceridemia

responsible for this disorder. Multiple different mutations have been described at this locus resulting in the FH phenotype. In the heterozygous state, subjects develop tendinous xanthomas, corneal arcus, and CHD. Elevations of LDL can result from well-characterized genetic disorders such as FH or familial defective apo B-100.

The ranges of LDL cholesterol levels in plasma of FH subjects are 200–400 mg dl^{-1} in heterozygotes and above 450 mg dl^{-1} in homozygotes. The frequency of defects at the LDL receptor locus is about 1 in 500 for the heterozygous state and 1 in a million in the homozygous state.

Inhibitors of 3-hydroxy-3-methylglutaryl (HMG) coenzyme A are useful in the treatment of hypercholesterolemia. Most pharmacological therapies are ineffective in the homozygous state. FH homozygotes may be treated with LDL apheresis, liver transplantation, and portacaval shunt. More recently, encouraging results have been obtained using *ex vivo* gene therapy.

The genetic defect(s) associated with a common form of hypercholesterolemia present in most subjects with cholesterol levels between 250 and 300 mg dl^{-1} has not been elucidated. This disorder may be due to a combination of minor gene defects (i.e., presence of apo E-4 allele) that in combination with the environment (i.e., diet, lack of exercise) predispose individuals to moderately elevated LDL cholesterol levels. This disorder has been also named polygenic hypercholesterolemia.

Familial Defective apo B-100

Familial defective apo B-100 is an autosomal dominant genetic disorder that presents with a phenotype similar to FH. The frequency of this disorder may be similar to FH; however, it varies considerably depending on the ethnicity of the population studied. The specific mutation responsible for this disorder is a point mutation at amino acid 3500 of the mature apo B. The diagnosis of this disorder requires molecular biology techniques.

Type III or Familial Dysbetalipoproteinemia

In this disorder both plasma triacylglycerol and cholesterol are increased. Several mutations within the apo E gene locus have been found to be responsible for this disease; however, in most patients the complete expression of the clinical genotype needs additional interactions such as age, obesity, and diabetes. In addition to the accumulation in plasma of VLDL remnants and chylomicrons, other characteristics of this disorder are tuboeruptive xanthomas and in some cases also planar xanthomas. Therapies

include diet and hypolipidemic agents such as fibrates, statin, or nicotinic acid. In most cases, diagnosis can be carried out first by agarose gel electrophoresis, followed by molecular biology techniques to detect the presence of the apo E-2 allele.

Familial Type IV and Type V Hypertriglyceridemias

These two disorders may have overlapping phenotypes. In type IV or familial endogenous hypertriglyceridemia, triacylglycerol levels are increased and HDL is usually decreased. This disorder appears to be autosomal dominant and relatively frequent in populations consuming high-fat diets. The precise molecular defect has not been defined; however, the increase in triacylglycerol is associated with overproduction of triacylglycerol by the liver and often with consequent reduced clearance. Diet should be the first step in therapy, followed if necessary by pharmacotherapy using fibrates or nicotinic acid. Premature CHD has been seen in some but not all cases presenting with this phenotype.

Type V hyperlipidemia is a much more rare disorder. Usually the first signs of this abnormality are abdominal pain or pancreatitis. VLDL levels are high and chylomicrons are present in the fasting state. This abnormality has not been linked to any specific molecular defect. Besides the primary genetic defect, other secondary causes of type V hyperlipidemia are poorly controlled diabetes mellitus, nephrotic syndrome, hypothyroidism, glycogen storage disease, and pregnancy. Recent data indicate increased susceptibility to atherosclerosis.

Familial Dyslipidemia

Familial dyslipidemia may be a variant of the familial hypertriglyceridemias described previously. It is characterized by hypertriglyceridemia in combination with low HDL cholesterol. Patients are generally overweight, with male pattern obesity, insulin resistance, diabetes, and hypertension. These subjects have both increased hepatic triacylglycerol secretion and increased HDL apo A-I catabolism.

Familial Combined Hyperlipidemia

Familial combined hyperlipidemia (FCH) was initially described as the combination of hypercholesterolemia and hypertriglyceridemia within the same kindred, and with kindred members having one of these abnormalities or both. Moreover, most subjects with FCH have HDL cholesterol levels below the 10th percentile. Affected subjects have elevation in VLDL, LDL, or both. This disorder has a frequency of approximately 10% in survivors of premature myocardial infarction (less than 60 years of age) and about 14% in kindred with CHD.

It has been reported that affected subjects have overproduction of apo B-100. The precise molecular defect has not been elucidated, although there are already several candidate gene loci, including the LPL. The expression of this disorder may be triggered by other factors, such as overweight, hypertension, diabetes, and gout. The treatment should include diet and exercise and, if necessary, niacin, HMC CoA reductase inhibitors, or fibrates, depending on the major lipid present in excess.

Familial Hyperapobetalipoproteinemia

Familial hyperapobetalipoproteinemia is characterized by apo B values above the 90th percentile in the absence of other lipid abnormalities; it has been suggested to be a variant of FCH. This disorder is relatively common (~5%) in kindreds with premature CHD. The molecular defect is not known, but metabolic studies suggest overproduction of apo B-100.

Familial Hypoalphalipoproteinemia

Severe HDL deficiency, characterized by HDL cholesterol levels $<10\,\mathrm{mg\,dl}^{-1}$ is rare and may be due to Tangier disease, apo A-I deficiencies, LCAT deficiency, or fish-eye disease. The apo A-1 deficiency states are due to rare deletions, rearrangements, or point mutations within the apo A-I/C-III/A-IV gene complex. Familial hypoalphalipoproteinemia is relatively common and is characterized by HDL cholesterol levels below the 10th percentile of normal. These subjects have been reported to have either decreased HDL production or increased HDL apo A-I catabolism. This phenotype is present in about 4% of kindred with premature CHD.

The genetic defect or defects are not known; however, it has been suggested that familial combined hyperlipidemia, familial hyperapobetalipoproteinemia, familial dysbetalipoproteinemia, and familial hypoalphalipoproteinemia may be variants of a single disorder. This disorder is characterized by a genetic predisposition in subjects consuming high-fat, high-cholesterol diets to an increased secretion of apo B-containing lipoproteins and an increased catabolism of apo A-I-containing lipoproteins. The expression of the phenotype is usually enhanced by the presence of male pattern obesity.

Familial Lipoprotein (a) Excess

Lipoprotein (a) (Lp(a)) is an LDL particle with one molecule of apolipoprotein (a) attached to it. Elevated levels of Lp(a) (>35–40 mg dl^{-1} or 90th percentile) have been associated with premature CHD. This increased risk appears to result from two different mechanisms: cholesterol deposition in the arterial wall and inhibition of fibrinolysis.

Lp(a) concentrations are highly variable among individuals; however, they tend to remain constant during a person's lifetime. Between 80 and 90% of the variability appears to be of genetic origin, owing, for the most part, to variations at the structural apo(a) gene locus. Lp(a) concentrations are inversely associated with a size polymorphism of apo(a). This polymorphism is due to differences in the number of a multiple repeat of a protein domain highly homologous to the kringle 4 domain of plasminogen. Diets and medications used to lower LDL cholesterol levels do not appear to have a significant effect on Lp(a) concentrations; however, niacin has been reported to decrease Lp(a) levels. There have been reports suggesting that diets high in *trans* fatty acids have some raising effects on Lp(a) levels, whereas estrogen replacement lowers Lp(a) in postmenopausal women.

General Guidelines for the Treatment of Lipoprotein Abnormalities for CHD Prevention

There is a clear benefit from lowering LDL cholesterol with diet or drug therapy in patients with hyperlipidemia or CHD or both. Dietary therapy includes using diets that are restricted in total fat (<30% of calories), saturated fat (<7% of calories), and cholesterol (<200 mg day^{-1}). Pharmacological therapies include anion exchange resins, niacin, and HMG CoA reductase inhibitors. The latter agents have been demonstrated to also lower CHD mortality. It should be noted that dramatic interindividual variations have been demonstrated in response to diet and drug therapies. Consequently the efficacy of hypolipidemic therapies will vary from individual to individual. More information is needed about the benefits of HDL cholesterol raising in patients with low HDL cholesterol levels as well as the benefits of lowering triacylglycerol plasma concentrations, and more specifically the triacylglycerol carried in lipoprotein remnants. This is also true regarding the benefits of Lp(a) lowering using niacin in patients with elevated Lp(a) levels.

See also: **Body Composition**. **Cholesterol**: Sources, Absorption, Function and Metabolism; Factors Determining Blood Levels. **Coronary Heart Disease**: Hemostatic Factors; Lipid Theory; Prevention. **Fatty Acids**: Metabolism; Monounsaturated; Omega-3

Polyunsaturated; Omega-6 Polyunsaturated; Saturated; *Trans* Fatty Acids. **Fertility**.

Further Reading

Alaupovic P (1996) Significance of apolipoproteins for structure, function, and classification of plasma lipoproteins. In: Bradley WA, Gianturco SH, and Segrest JP (eds.) *Methods in Enzymology, Plasma Lipoproteins*, part C, vol. 263, pp. 32–60. San Diego: Academic Press.

Austin MA, Breslow JL, Henneckens CH *et al.* (1988) Low density lipoprotein subclass patterns and risk of myocardial infarction. *Journal of the American Medical Association*, **260**: 1917–1921.

Li Z, McNamara JR, Ordovas JM, and Schaefer EJ (1994) Analysis of high density lipoproteins by a modified gradient gel electrophoresis method. *Journal of Lipid Research* **35**: 1698–1711.

National Cholesterol Education Program (1994) Second Report of the Expert Panel on Detection, Evaluation and Treatment of High Blood Cholesterol in Adults (Adult Treatment Panel II). *Circulation* **89**: 1329–1445.

Ordovas JM (1991) Molecular biological approaches to the understanding of lipoprotein metabolism. In: Witiak DT, Newman HAI, and Feller DR (eds.) *Medical, Chemical and Biochemical Aspects of Antilipidemic Drugs*, pp. 97–121. Amsterdam: Elsevier.

Ordovas JM (1993) Metabolism of triglyceride-rich lipoproteins: Genetic mutations associated with its pathology. *Cardiovascular Risk Factors* 3: 1–8.

Ordovas JM (1994) Genetic and environmental factors: Effects on plasma lipoproteins. In: Serrano Rios (ed.) *Dairy Products in Human Health and Nutrition*, pp. 303–307. Rotterdam: Balkema.

Ordovas JM, Civeira F, Genest J, and Schaefer EJ (1990) Genetic high density lipoprotein deficiency states. In: Lenfant C, Albertini A, Paoletti R, and Catapano A (eds.) *Atherosclerosis Reviews. Biotechnology of Dyslipoproteinemias. Application in Diagnosis and Control*, vol. 20, pp. 261–274. New York: Raven Press.

Ordovas JM, Lopez-Miranda J, Mata P *et al.* (1995) Gene–dict interaction in determining plasma lipid response to dietary intervention. *Atherosclerosis* 118: S11–S27.

Schaefer EJ and Ordovas JM (1992) Diagnosis and management of HDL deficiency states. In: Miller NE and Tall AR (eds.) *High Density Lipoproteins and Atherosclerosis*, vol. III, pp. 235–251. Amsterdam: Elsevier.

Schaefer EJ, Genest Jr JJ, Ordovas JM, Salem DN, and Wilson PWF (1993) Familial lipoprotein disorders and premature coronary artery disease. *Current Opinion in Lipidology* 4: 288–298.

Schaefer EJ, Lichtenstein AH, Lamon-Fava S, McNamara JR, and Ordovas JM (1995) Lipoproteins, nutrition, aging, and atherosclerosis. *American Journal of Clinical Nutrition* 61(supplement): 726S–740S.

Zannis VI, Kardassis D, and Zanni EE (1993) Genetic mutations affecting human lipoproteins, their receptors, and their enzymes. *Advances in Human Genetics* 21: 145–319.

LIVER DISORDERS

J Hampsey and K B Schwarz, Johns Hopkins School of Medicine, Baltimore, MD, USA

This article covers the role of the liver in normal nutrition, including the important functions of bile salt production, macronutrient metabolism, and fat-soluble vitamin absorption, metabolism, and storage. Next, the pathogenesis of malnutrition in liver disease is discussed, starting with the mechanisms of malnutrition in both acute and chronic liver failure. Specific nutritional issues in liver failure are addressed, including metabolic disturbances of carbohydrates, protein, and fats. Nutritional disturbances in the major types of specific liver diseases are reviewed: hepatocellular, metabolic liver disease, and biliary tract disorders. Nutritional assessment and management of patients with acute, chronic liver disease and end stage liver disease are discussed.

Liver in Normal Nutrition

Bile Salts

A normal functioning liver will secrete 600–1200 ml of bile to the gall bladder on a daily basis. Bile is made up of bile salts, lecithin, conjugated bilirubin, phospholipids, cholesterol, electrolytes, and water. Bile salts, which are the predominant component of bile, are synthesized from cholesterol in the hepatocyte. The primary function of bile salts lies in their interaction with lipid digestion. Bile salts bind with large fat particles, which alone are insoluble in water, and act on them as an emulsifier, breaking down into smaller particles called micelles. Micelles, the product of the fat particle and bile salt structure, aid in the transport of fat to the mucosal membrane for absorption. Fat-soluble vitamins and cholesterol are also incorporated into mixed micelles for proper absorption.

Micellar solubilization is only required for long-chain fatty acids. Short-chain fatty acids (10 carbons or less) do not require micelle formation for absorption; instead, they enter the portal circulation directly, bound to albumin, and are transferred to the liver for oxidation. Approximately 94% of the micelle forming bile acids are reabsorbed in the ileum and shuttled via the portal hepatic vein bound to albumin back to the liver. Only 6% of bile acids are lost in excretion.

Macronutrient Metabolism

Carbohydrates The liver is responsible for maintaining normal blood glucose concentrations under various metabolic conditions. Among the several metabolic processes that allow this fine regulation are glycogenesis, gluconeogenesis, and glycolysis. The end product of carbohydrate digestion is 80% glucose, with the remaining 20% being fructose and galactose; the latter two are quickly converted into glucose in the liver. Once transported into the hepatocyte, the glucose molecule is phosphorylated (via glucokinase) and cannot leave the cell unless dephosphorylated with glucose phosphatase. Glucose is either used for immediate energy release or stored as glycogen.

Proteins The liver plays a major role in protein metabolism in the deamination of amino acids, urea formation for removal of ammonia, plasma protein synthesis, and in the interconversions among amino acids. Ingested protein is the sole source of the 10 essential amino acids and the primary source of nitrogen necessary for the synthesis of other amino acids. Protein is digested and broken down to amino acids that are absorbed into the circulation and taken to cells throughout the body, primarily the liver, and quickly become combined by peptide linkages. The plasma level of amino acids is tightly controlled and maintained near a constant level. Once the cellular limit of protein storage is met, excess amino acids are degraded and used for energy or stored as fat or glycogen. The liver is the primary site of all amino acid catabolism with the exception of branch-chained amino acid catabolism, which occurs in the muscle cells. The urea cycle, in which the toxic compound ammonia is converted to urea, occurs solely in the liver. The synthesis of the plasma proteins albumin, fibrinogen, and globulin also occurs in the liver.

Lipids The liver plays a role in fat metabolism in four key processes: fatty acid oxidation for energy, lipoprotein syntheses, the synthesis of cholesterol and phospholipids, and the conversion of carbohydrate to fat for storage. Digested fat is a major source of energy in which after splitting into fatty acids and glycerol, the fatty acid components further split via beta oxidation into acetyl-CoA. Two molecules of acetyl-CoA become paired together to form acetoacetic acid and are transported to other cells to provide energy in the citric acid cycle.

Fat-soluble vitamins The liver plays a key role in the absorption of the fat-soluble vitamins—A, D, E, and K—as they are only successfully absorbed in association with fat and sufficient quantities of bile salts. The liver is also the primary storage site for several vitamins, including A, E, K, and B^{12}. Vitamin A is stored in the largest quantity in a sufficient amount to prevent deficiency for 5–10 months. Vitamin D is stored in amounts sufficient for 2–4 months. Vitamin B_{12} is stored in amounts sufficient for at least 1 year. The liver is responsible for the hydroxylation of vitamin D to its storage form, 25-hydroxy vitamin D. It is released into circulation and thence delivered to the kidney where it is converted to its active form, 1, 25-dihydroxy vitamin D.

Specific Nutritional Issues

Carbohydrates As discussed earlier, the liver plays a major role in the maintenance of normal blood sugar levels and overall glucose metabolism. Not surprisingly, in the patient with liver disease, glucose intolerance and insulin resistance are common. Cirrhotic patients are prone to developing diabetes. Energy from carbohydrates plays an important role in protein sparing mechanisms, preventing the use of protein as energy.

Lipids In cholestatic liver disease there is malabsorption of dietary lipid and consequent malnutrition. There are experimental data from primates showing that chronic ethanol consumption results in a decrease of liver phospholipids and of phosphatidycholine (PC). Consequently, the total phospholipid content of the mitochondrial membranes is decreased; mitochondria are altered both structurally and functionally. There is diminished mitochondrial oxidation because of decreased cytochrome oxidase activity, which can be restored by administration of PC. The extent to which chronic liver disease of etiologies other than chronic ethanol consumption results in similar perturbations is unknown.

Protein Plasma proteins such as albumin and coagulation factors constitute approximately 50% of the proteins synthesized in the liver. In liver disease, decreased synthesis of these proteins has important clinical consequences, including ascites from hypoalbuminemia and coagulopathy from decreased synthesis of coagulation factors. In end stage liver disease, hypoglycemia can result from decreased hepatic gluconeogenesis from amino acids. Decreased activity of the urea cycle enzymes results in hyperammonemia and hepatic encephalopathy, the ultimate expression of which can be cerebral edema.

Fat-soluble vitamins Deficiencies of fat-soluble vitamins are common in liver disease associated with steatorrhea due to the concomitant malabsorption of fat. Vitamin A deficiency can result in anorexia, growth failure, decreased resistance to infections, and night blindness. Vitamin D deficiency results in osteopenia or osteoporosis as well as rickets. The prevalence of fractures is increased in women being treated for alcohol abuse and also following sobriety; deficiencies of vitamin D as well as calcium, phosphorus, and fluoride may play a role. The deficiency of vitamin E results in neuraxonal dystrophy, clinically manifesting as peripheral neuropathy and cerebellar disturbances. Vitamin K deficiency results in hemorrhage because of reduced synthesis of clotting factors.

Trace elements Zinc deficiency in cirrhotics may contribute to hypoalbuminemia and dermatitis as well as anorexia from hypogeusia. Deficiency of selenium can lead to decreased synthesis of important antioxidant selenoproteins such as glutathione peroxidase. Little is known about the effect of acute or chronic liver disease on other trace elements.

Liver in Specific Hepatobiliary Disorders

Hepatocellular Diseases

Alcoholic liver disease The term 'alcoholic liver disease' refers to a spectrum of types of hepatic injury associated with continuous alcohol ingestion, ranging from alcoholic fatty liver to alcoholic steatohepatitis, fibrosis, and cirrhosis. Nutritional disturbances in alcoholics are an important cause of morbidity and mortality; all classes of nutrients are affected. Anorexia leads to decreased food intake and subsequent protein-calorie malnutrition. Maldigestion and malabsorption can occur secondary to chronic alcohol injury to small intestinal mucosa. Alcohol consumption is often associated with chronic pancreatic insufficiency, which results in steatorrhea and decreased absorption of dietary protein, fat, and fat-soluble vitamins. Chronic alcohol ingestion also results in impaired hepatic amino acid uptake and protein synthesis.

In alcoholics, utilization of lipids and carbohydrates is markedly compromised due to an excess of reductive equivalents and impaired oxidation of triglycerides. Alcoholics are often resistant to insulin and exhibit impaired uptake of glucose into muscle cells. Insulin-dependent diabetes is common. Heavy alcohol consumption is frequently associated with deficiencies of a wide variety of micronutrients, including the fat- and water-soluble vitamins, particularly folate, pyridoxal-5′-phosphate, thiamine, and vitamin A.

Table 1 summarizes the five published controlled trials of the effect of oral or enteral nutritional supplements on patients with alcoholic hepatitis. In most, nitrogen balance and/or protein synthesis improved, although no effect on mortality was shown, perhaps because of the small number of patients studied and/or the duration of follow-up. In the largest study, at 1-year follow-up, the experimental group had a significantly better survival: 2/24 (8%) died compared to 10/27 (37%) of the controls. In general, the effects of parenteral nutrition in alcoholic liver disease are similar to those noted the studies of enteral nutritional supplements.

Many studies have examined the effect of oral or enteral nutritional supplementation in patients with alcoholic cirrhosis. Results are summarized in **Table 2**. Many studies are small and of short duration, so it is not surprising that results are inconclusive. Most studies demonstrated an improvement in nitrogen balance and protein synthesis; only one showed increased survival in the treated group. Taken together, these studies suggest that there are benefits to nutritional supplementation in this population.

A variety of international associations have made nutritional recommendations for patients with various types of alcoholic liver disease. The primary recommendation is of course abstinence, which may be all that is needed in patients with fatty liver. Patients with alcoholic hepatitis should take 40 kcal/kg, 1.5–2.0 g protein/kg, 4–5 g/kg of carbohydrates, and 1–2 g/kg of lipids per day. Those with cirrhosis without malnutrition should take 35 kcal/kg, 1.3–1.5 g protein/kg, and carbohydrates and lipids as recommended for patents with alcoholic hepatitis. Those with cirrhosis and malnutrition should take higher amounts of protein (1.5–2.0 g/kg) and lipids (2.0–2.5 g/kg) and lower amounts of carbohydrates (3–4 g/kg). Fluid should be restricted to 2–2.5 l/day and all eight B vitamins, including folate and thiamine, as well as vitamins C and K should be routinely supplemented. In addition, patients with cholestasis should take 50% of their dietary lipids as medium-chain triglycerides

Table 1 Studies on therapy of alcoholic hepatitis with oral or enteral nutritional supplements

Reference	Design	Patients (No.)	Duration (days)	Experimental treatment (EXP)	Control treatment (CTR)	Mortality	Secondary end points
Galambos et al. (1979)[a]	Open label	16	16–42	Oral (standard hospital diet) or intravenous supplement (51.6–77.4 g protein)	None	Not assessed	Nitrogen balance + albumin improved in EXP, CTR not assessed Improvement of albumin, transferrin, RBP
Mendenhall et al. (1985)[b]	Historical controls	57	30	Standard hospital diet (2500 kcal/day) + 2200 kcal/day BCAA	Standard hospital diet	NS	Positive nitrogen balance in EXP, delayed hypersensitivity improved
Calvey et al. (1985)[c]	Randomized, controlled	64	21	Standard diet (~2000 kcal/day) + 65 g standard AA or BCAA	Standard diet, 80 g protein/day	NS	Positive nitrogen balance in EXP, delayed hypersensitivity improved
Soberon et al. (1987)[d]	Crossover	14	6	Nasoduodenal tube, 35 kcal/kg/day, fat/carbohydrate/protein 45/40/15%	3 days standard hospital diet (35 kcal/kg/day)	0/6 controls 3/8 treatment	Nitrogen balance improved five-fold at 2 weeks
Cabre et al. (2000)[e]	Randomized, controlled	71	28	Nasogastric tube, 2000 kcal/day, 72 g protein/day, 31% BCAA	Standard diet (1 g protein/kg) + 40 mg/day prednisolone	11/35 TEN 9/36 PRED NS FU: 2/24 TEN 10/27 ($P = 0.04$)	No dropouts in PRED, 8 dropouts in TEN; equal improvements of albumin, Child score, Maddrey score; equal rate of infections

[a]Galambos JT, Hersh T, Fulenwider JT et al. (1979) Hyperalimentation in alcoholic hepatitis. *American Journal of Gastroenterology* **72**: 535–541.

[b]Mendenhall CL, Bongiovanni G, Goldberg S et al. (1985) VA cooperative study on alcoholic hepatitis. III: Changes in protein-calorie malnutrition associated with 30 days of hospitalization with and without enteral nutritional therapy. *Journal of Parenteral and Enteral Nutrition* **9**: 590–596.

[c]Calvey H, Davis M, and Williams R (1985) Controlled trial of nutritional supplementation, with and without branched chain amino acids enrichment, in treatment of acute alcoholic hepatitis. *Journal of Hepatology* **1**: 141–151.

[d]Soberon S, Pauley MP, Duplantier R et al. (1987) Metabolic effects of enteral formula feeding in alcoholic hepatitis. *Hepatology* **7**: 1204–1209.

[e]Cabre E, Rodriguez-Iglesias P, Caballeria J et al. (2000) Short-term and long-term outcome of severe alcohol-induced hepatitis treated with steroids or enteral nutrition: A multicenter randomized trial. *Hepatology* **32**: 36–42.

AA, amino acids; BCAA, branched-chain amino acid; FU, follow-up; NS, not significant; PRED, prednisolone group; TEN, total enteral nutrition group.

From Stickel F, Hoehn B, Schuppan D, and Seitz HK (2003) Review article: Nutritional therapy in alcoholic liver disease. *Alimentary Pharmacology & Therapeutics* **18**: 357–373.

Table 2 Studies on treating alcoholic cirrhosis with oral and enteral nutritional therapy[a]

Reference	Design	Patients (No.)	Duration (days)	Experimental treatment (EXP)	Control treatment (CTR)	Mortality	Secondary end points
Smith et al. (1982)[a]	Open label	10	10–60	Three different formulae: Oral 76–143 g protein, 2000–3716 kcal/day	None	None	Positive nitrogen balance, improved albumin, transferrin, creatinine/height, midarm muscle, fat areas
Keohane et al. (1983)[b]	Open label	10	3–23	Oral BCAA formula: 80 g protein/day through nasogastric tube	None	1 death (HRF)	Positive nitrogen balance, improved albumin
McGhee et al. (1983)[c]	Randomized, double-blind, crossover	4	11	20 g casein + 30 g BCAA formula	50 g casein/day	None	EXP equal to CTR, positive nitrogen balance
Christie et al. (1985)[d]	Randomized, double-blind, crossover	8	12	BCAA (50%) formula	Standard diet (18% BCAA)	1 death (infection)	EXP equal to CTR, positive nitrogen balance
Okita et al. (1985)[e]	Open label	10	4	40 g protein + 40 g BCAA formula/day	2100 kcal/day 80 g protein/day	None	EXP equal to CTR, positive nitrogen balance
Bunout et al. (1989)[f]	Randomized, controlled	36	28	50 kcal/kg, 1.5 g protein/day	Standard diet	EXP 2/17 CTR 5/19 (NS)	No differences
Cabre et al. (1990)[g]	Randomized, controlled	35 (23 alc.)	23–35	2115 kcal/day including 71 g BCAA formula	Standard diet	Improved ($p = 0.02$)	Child score improved, albumin improved
Marchesini et al. (1990)[h]	Randomized	64	90	Standard diet + BCAA supplement (0.24 g/kg)	Standard diet + casein supplement	None	Nitrogen balance improved in both, BCAA better than standard diet
Kerans et al. (1992)[i]	Randomized	31	28	Casein supplement (1.5 g protein/day, 40 kcal/day/kg/day)	Standard diet	NS	Both groups improved nitrogen balance and albumin
Hirsch et al. (1993)[j]	Randomized, controlled	51	12 (months)	Standard diet + casein supplement (1000 kcal/day, 34 g protein/day)	Standard diet	EXP 3/26 CTR 6/25 (NS)	Fewer hospitalizations, improved albumin and visceral protein
Nielsen et al. (1995)[k]	Open label	15	38	Increasing amounts of protein via standard diet (1.0–1.8 g/kg/day)	None	None	Increased protein retention through gradual or protein intake

Continued

Table 2 Continued

Reference	Design	Patients (No.)	Duration (days)	Experimental treatment (EXP)	Control treatment (CTR)	Mortality	Secondary end points
Campillo et al. (1995)[l]	Open label	26	30	Standard diet	None	None	Anthropometric ratios improved
Hirsch et al. (1992)[m]	Open label	31	6 (months)	Standard diet + casein supplement (1000 kcal/day, 34 g protein/day)	None	6 deaths/31	Increased albumin, improved cellular immunity

[a]Smith J, Horowitz J, Henderson JM et al. (1982) Enteral hyperalimentation in undernourished patients with cirrhosis and ascites. American Journal of Clinical Nutrition **2**: 1209–1218.

[b]Keohane PP, Attrill H, Brimble G et al. (1983) Enteral nutrition in malnourished patients with hepatic cirrhosis and acute encephalopathy. Journal of Parenteral and Enteral Nutrition **7**: 34–50.

[c]McGhee A, Henderson JM, Millikan WJ et al. (1983) Comparison of the effects of hepatic-aid and casein modular diet on encephalopathy, plasma amino acids, and nitrogen balance in cirrhotic patients. Annals of Surgery **197**: 288–293.

[d]Christie ML, Sack DM, Pomposelli J et al. (1985) Enriched branched-chain amino acid formula versus a casein-based supplement in the treatment of cirrhosis. Journal of Parenteral and Enteral Nutrition **9**: 671–678.

[e]Okita M, Watanabe A, and Nagashima H (1985) Nutritional treatment of liver cirrhosis by branched-chain amino acid-enriched nutrient mixture. Journal of Nutritional Science and Vitaminology **31**: 291–303.

[f]Bunout D, Alcardi V, Hirsch S et al. (1989) Nutritional support in hospitalized patients with alcoholic liver disease. European Journal of Clinical Nutrition **43**: 615–621.

[g]Cabre E, Gonzalez-Huix F, Abad-Lacruz A et al. (1990) Effect of total enteral nutrition on the short-term outcome of severely malnourished cirrhotics. A randomized controlled trial. Gastroenterology **98**: 715–720.

[h]Marchesini G, Dioguardi FS, Bianchi GP et al. (1990) Long term oral branched-chain amino acid treatment in chronic hepatic encephalopathy. A randomized double-blind casein-controlled trial. The Italian Multicenter Study Group. Journal of Hepatology **11**: 92–101.

[i]Kearns PJ, Young H, Garcia G et al. (1992) Accelerated improvement of alcoholic liver disease with enteral nutrition. Gastroenterology **102**: 200–205.

[j]Hirsch S, Bunout D, De la Maza MP et al. (1993) Controlled trial on nutritional supplementation in outpatients with symptomatic alcoholic cirrhosis. Journal of Parenteral and Enteral Nutrition **17**: 119–124.

[k]Nielsen K, Kondrup J, Martinsen I et al. (1995) Long-term oral refeeding of patients with cirrhosis of the liver. British Journal of Nutrition **74**: 557–567.

[l]Campillo B, Bories PN, Leluan M et al. (1995) Short-term changes in energy metabolism after 1 month of a regular oral diet in severely malnourished cirrhotic patients. Metabolism **44**: 765–770.

[m]Hirsch S, de la Maza MP, Gattas V et al. (1999) Nutritional support in alcoholic cirrhotic patients improves host defenses. Journal of the American College of Nutrition **18**: 434–414.

BCAA, branched-chain amino acid; HRF, hepatorenal failure; NS, not significant.

From Stickel F, Hoehn B, Schuppan D, Seitz HK (2003). Review article: Nutritional therapy in alcoholic liver disease. Alimentary Pharmacology & Therapeutics **18**: 357–373.

and should be supplemented with the fat-soluble vitamins—A, D, E, and K. The major strategy in the management of alcoholic cirrhotics with ascites and edema is to restrict fluids to 1–1.5 l/day and to restrict sodium as well.

Autoimmune liver disease The two major categories of autoimmune liver disease are primary biliary cirrhosis (PBC), a disease generally presenting in young female adults, and autoimmune hepatitis, which also most frequently presents in adults but can affect both sexes and present at any time from young childhood to mid-adulthood. PBC results in steatorrhea and malabsorption of the fat-soluble vitamins. Osteoporosis and osteopenia are common.

The nutritional consequences of autoimmune hepatitis, which can evolve into cirrhosis, are similar to those of alcoholic hepatitis and cirrhosis secondary to alcoholic liver disease, and thus the management is similar as well. Occasionally, autoimmune hepatitis can be accompanied by intestinal diseases such as inflammatory bowel disease or celiac disease, and the nutritional management should take both organ systems into account. Although mild liver function abnormalities are common in celiac disease, there are reports of celiac disease in patients with severe liver disease, all of whom demonstrated an improvement in their liver disease with introduction of a gluten-free diet.

Neonatal cholestasis The major differential diagnosis of conjugated hyperbilirubinemia in the first 30 days of life is extrahepatic biliary atresia and the neonatal hepatitis syndrome, for which a large number of specific genetic disorders have been identified. These include α-1 antitrypsin deficiency, inborn errors of bile salt synthesis or transport, cystic fibrosis/liver disease, Alagille syndrome, hypothyroidism, and panhypopituitarism. The nutritional consequences are similar for all: steatorrhea and malabsorption of the fat-soluble vitamins and failure to thrive. Nutritional management is also similar for all: use of an elemental formula rich in medium-chain triglycerides (MCTs) and supplementation with vitamins A, D, E, and K. Water-miscible vitamin E is poorly absorbed; administration of vitamin E solubilized in polyethylene glycol succinate is a more effective way to administer vitamin E to cholestatic infants.

Nonalcoholic fatty liver disease and nonalcoholic steatohepatitis Nonalcoholic fatty liver disease (NAFLD) and nonalcoholic steatohepatitis (NASH) have become very important causes of liver disease in both children and adults, particularly because obesity is being diagnosed in epidemic proportions in both age groups and both liver disorders are most commonly associated with obesity. Children with NAFLD may present before their fifth birthday. The disorder is more common in males. Hepatic fibrosis is common and may even evolve into cirrhosis during childhood. Treatment consists of weight reduction and aerobic exercise. Vitamin E may be beneficial.

In adults, NASH and NAFLD have been recognized for at least 25 years as chronic liver diseases associated with obesity (with or without non-insulin-dependent diabetes mellitus and with or without hyperlipidemia). NAFLD may account for as much as 80% of cases of elevated liver enzymes in the United States. Most adults with the disorders are 110–130% above ideal body weight. The prognosis of NAFLD is good if weight reduction is achieved. NASH is usually slowly progressive but can lead to cirrhosis and the need for liver transplantation in the minority of individuals affected.

In many patients, NAFLD is a component of the insulin-resistance syndrome known as the 'metabolic syndrome,' which is characterized by central obesity, hypertension, hypertriglyceridemia, low levels of high-density lipoprotein-cholesterol, and hyperglycemia. In patients with this syndrome, it is hypothesized that there is greater insulin resistance in muscles and adipose tissue than in liver. As shown in **Figure 1**, in adult patients with NAFLD, the body mass index class >30 kg/m^2 is associated with an increased prevalence of each of the five components of the metabolic syndrome.

As shown in **Table 3**, compared to controls, patients with NASH exhibited a higher intake of

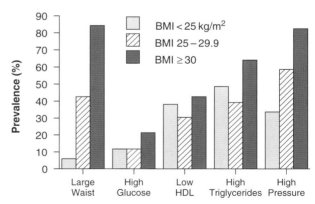

Figure 1 Prevalence of metabolic alterations fitting the criteria of the metabolic syndrome in patients with NAFLD according to classes of body mass index. (Reproduced with permission from Marchesini G, Buigianesi E, Forlani G *et al.* (2003) Nonalcoholic fatty liver, steatohepatitis, and the metabolic syndrome. *Hepatology* **37**: 917–923.)

Table 3 Daily intake of main dietary constituents in NASH patients and controls[a]

	NASH patients (n = 25)	Controls (n = 25)	p value
Total energy intake (kcal)	2638 ± 444	2570 ± 739	0.695
kcal/kg body weight	33 ± 5	32 ± 6	0.580
Dietary fat (g)	102.8 ± 31.6	92.1 ± 35.2	0.264
Dietary carbohydrate (g)	295.1 ± 53.7	315.2 ± 101.9	0.387
Dietary protein (g)	121.2 ± 25.2	107.2 ± 32.7	0.096
Alcohol (g)	13.3 ± 7.3	13.5 ± 8.9	0.705
Dietary fat (% kcal)	35.1 ± 7.1	32.3 ± 6.7	0.158
Dietary carbohydrate (% kcal)	44.7 ± 8.7	48.6 ± 9.1	0.128
Simple carbohydrate (% total carbohydrate)	30.3 ± 6.4	32.5 ± 5.1	0.185
Fiber (g)	12.9 ± 4.1	23.2 ± 7.8	0.000
Dietary protein (% kcal)	20.2 ± 3.7	16.7 ± 4.3	0.003
SFA (g)	40.2 ± 12.7	28.7 ± 11.1	0.001
MUFA (g)	52.1 ± 17.4	47.8 ± 16.7	0.377
PUFA (g)	103.9 ± 4.9	13.4 ± 4.1	0.019
Cholesterol (mg)	506 ± 108	405 ± 111	0.002
SFA (% total kcal)	13.7 ± 3.1	10.0 ± 2.1	0.000
MUFA (% total kcal)	17.7 ± 4.4	16.7 ± 5.1	0.462
PUFA (% total kcal)	3.5 ± 1.3	4.7 ± 2.0	0.015
SFA (% total fat)	39.1 ± 4.8	31.1 ± 5.2	0.000
MUFA (% total fat)	50.9 ± 6.5	51.9 ± 5.9	0.572
PUFA (% total fat)	10.0 ± 3.5	14.5 ± 4.0	0.000
(P:S ratio)	0.24 ± 0.10	0.46 ± 0.12	0.000
Vitamin A (μg)	582.6 ± 383.7	647.1 ± 507.3	0.614
Vitamin C (mg)	84.3 ± 43.1	144.2 ± 63.1	0.000
Vitamin E (mg)	5.4 ± 1.9	8.7 ± 2.9	0.000
Iron (mg)	12.1 ± 2.3	14.5 ± 3.9	0.011

[a]Data are presented as mean ± SD.
SFA, saturated fat intake; PUFA, polyunsaturated fat intake; MUFA, monounsaturated fat intake; P:S ratio, polyunsaturated to saturated fat.
From Musso R, Gambino R, DeMichiele F et al. (2003) Dietary habits and their relations to insulin resistance and postprandial lipemia in nonalcoholic steatohepatitis. Hepatology 37(4): 909–915.

saturated fatty acids, total fat, and cholesterol and a lower intake of polyunsaturated fat, fiber, and the antioxidant vitamins C and E. These findings provide a strong rationale for specific dietary modifications in NASH patients.

Pregnancy and liver disease Liver diseases that predominantly affect females, such as PBC and autoimmune hepatitis, decrease the chances of conception and demand that pregnant women with these disorders should be managed in high-risk obstetric facilities. Liver diseases that can evolve as a consequence of pregnancy include intrahepatic cholestasis of pregnancy, acute fatty liver of pregnancy, and HELLP (hemolysis, elevated liver enzymes, and low platelets syndrome). The latter has been associated with disorders of fatty acid oxidation in offspring. Successful pregnancies are the rule for women who have undergone liver transplantation, but preterm delivery and low-birth-weight infants are common. Careful attention to the nutritional management of the pregnant female with liver disease is necessary to ensure the best outcome for the fetus.

Total parenteral nutrition-associated liver disease Premature infants and children with short gut syndrome are particularly prone to develop this disorder, and in the pediatric age group total parenteral nutrition (TPN) liver disease is usually cholestatic. The cholestasis can be solely intrahepatic or can be associated with cholelithiasis. TPN liver disease can be seen at any age and with any disease etiology resulting in long-term dependence on parenteral nutrition; in older children and adults, steatosis is more common as an initial presentation rather than cholestasis. Potential pathogenetic mechanisms include the gastrointestinal dysfunction associated with the lack of enteral nutrients as well as components of the parenteral nutrition solutions as potential hepatotoxins, including amino acids, glucose, lipids (particularly peroxidizable lipids), and photo-exposed multivitamins. The most effective management is aggressive administration of enteral nutrients and a decrease and/or discontinuation of parenteral nutrition as early as possible.

Viral hepatitis Hepatitis A virus infection never results in chronic liver disease, so there are no specific nutritional recommendations for patients with this disorder. Hepatitis B virus infection evolves to chronic hepatitis in ~95% of neonates who acquire the infection perinatally but only ~5% of adults. Hepatitis C virus (HCV) infection has a much higher rate of chronicity in adults—up to 80% of those infected will develop chronic infection. Approximately 20–30% of those will progress to cirrhosis over 10–20 years and a smaller proportion of those will develop hepatocellular carcinoma. There is much less information about nutritional disturbances and nutritional management of patients with chronic viral hepatitis than there is for patients with alcoholic liver disease.

In general, the nutritional recommendations for management of alcoholic hepatitis, cirrhosis, or cholestasis detailed previously can be applied to patients with these various manifestations of chronic viral hepatitis. For example, it has been shown that thiamine deficiency is common in patients with cirrhosis secondary to either chronic alcohol consumption or chronic HCV and thiamine supplementation is indicated for patients with either type of liver disease.

Metabolic Disorders

Galactosemia Galactosemia is secondary to the deficiency of galactose-1-phosphate uridyl transferase. Galactose-1-phosphate is toxic and accumulates in liver and other organs, causing liver failure in early infancy. The usual presentation is hypoglycemia and encephalopathy in the first few days of life. Vomiting, diarrhea, jaundice, and failure to thrive are common. Treatment is by elimination of galactose (and, consequently, lactose) from the diet for life. Liver function improves by this maneuver, but long-term complications such as mental disability, speech defects, ovarian failure, and neurologic syndromes are common despite dietary restriction.

Glycogen storage disease Glycogen storage disease (GSD) I, II, and III are the most common glycogen storage diseases to present with hepatomegaly. Type IV (amylopectinosis) is the only one of these disorders to present with cirrhosis; however, most of the disorders originate from deficiency of a key hepatic enzyme of glycogenolysis. The main nutritional management strategy, most important for types I and III, is the prevention of hypoglycemia; night time administration of cornstarch is often effective. Since restricted diets are key to the management of most inborn errors of metabolism, patients with these disorders are at high risk for nutrient deficiencies.

Hemochromatosis This disorder is among the most common autosomal recessive diseases in the world, occurring as frequently as 1/300. Two mutant alleles of the HFE gene are responsible for essentially all cases. Hepatomegaly and hepatic dysfunction as manifested by elevation of serum aminotransferases are common. Pancreatic dysfunction and darkening of the skin may occur. Transferrin saturation, serum iron concentration, and ferritin levels are the usual tests for iron overload, but molecular testing is rapidly becoming the diagnostic modality of the future. Liver biopsy may still be necessary to determine the degree of hepatic iron overload; management is by dietary iron restriction and phlebotomy.

Hepatorenal tyrosinemia I This disorder, which is secondary to deficiency of fumarylacetoacetate hydrolase, is the most common and severe of the genetic defects of tyrosine metabolism. Initial management is with a phylalanine- and tyrosine-restricted diet. The current intervention with 2-(2-nitro-4-trifluoro-methylbenzoyl)-1,3 cyclohexenedione (NTBC) has improved the quality of life of patients suffering from this disorder because it decreases the frequency of episodes of acute liver failure and coagulopathy.

Hereditary fructose intolerance This disorder results from a deficiency of the enzyme fructose-1-phosphate aldolase, which results in the accumulation of fructose-1-phosphate in the liver. This substance is a competitive inhibitor of phosphorylase, which regulates the conversion of glycogen to glucose. With inhibition of this enzyme, hypoglycemia and lactic acidosis result. The clinical presentation is with vomiting, diarrhea, choelestasis, and hepatomegaly, usually in early infancy. Renal injury and growth retardation are common. Standard treatment is restriction of fructose (and sucrose) from the diet and early treatment results in an excellent clinical outcome.

Urea cycle disorders There are six of these disorders, all of which present with varying degrees of hyperammonemia. In the neonatal period, these disorders present dramatically with somnolence, poor feeding, vomiting, lethargy, seizures, and even hyperammonemic coma. In older children and adults, the presentation may be more subtle and begin with chronic vomiting, developmental delay, seizures, psychiatric illness, postpartum decompensation, and hyperammonemia associated with valproate therapy. Nutritional management includes restriction of upstream essential nutrients to prevent intoxication and supplementation of downstream nutrients to prevent secondary deficiency. In addition, alternative routes of disposal of precursor metabolites can be stimulated. For the severe deficiencies, including severe neonatal ornithine transcarbamylase deficiency and carbamyl phosphate synthetase deficiency, more aggressive strategies, such as liver transplantation and gene therapy, are being investigated.

Wilson's disease   Wilson's disease is an autosomal recessive disorder of copper accumulation secondary to mutations in ATP7B, a copper-binding ATPase primarily expressed in the liver. The clinical expression in children and adolescents is often dramatic subacute hepatic necrosis or fulminant liver failure accompanied by hemolysis. In adults, the hepatic presentation is more subtle—manifestations of portal hypertension and cirrhosis, such as fatigue and ascites, and neuropsychiatric manifestations are common. The management of severe liver disease is liver transplantation. However, in the absence of severe liver disease, treatment is with a copper-restricted diet and copper chelating agents.

Hepatobiliary Disorders

Biliary atresia   This disorder is the prototypic biliary tract disorder in infancy, accounting for ~50% of all liver transplants in the pediatric age group and ~10% of all liver transplants. It presents with cholestasis in early infancy; there is a palliative surgical procedure called the Kasai hepatic portoenterostomy that, if performed before 60 days of age, may at least delay disease progression. In ~20–25% of infants in whom the procedure is done in a timely fashion, liver transplantation may never be necessary. Severe steatorrhea and malnutrition are common and malabsorption of the fat-soluble vitamins is profound, sometimes requiring parenteral administration (particularly of vitamin K) to achieve sufficiency. Nutritional deficiency disorders such as osteoporosis are common.

Primary sclerosing cholangitis   This disorder most commonly presents in association with ulcerative colitis and less commonly with Crohn's disease or as an isolated entity. The nutritional management of the disorder is essentially like that of other cholestatic disorders; in patients with Crohn's disease of the small bowel, aggressive administration of an elemental diet rich in medium-chain triglycerides may be beneficial. It is accepted, however, that endoscopic interventions should be used as needed in the case of significant biliary obstruction. For prevention of severe osteoporosis, supplementation with vitamin D and calcium is needed. Vitamin K and alendronate may be beneficial in increasing bone mineral density. Serum levels of the fat-soluble vitamins should be monitored in high-risk patients and vitamins replaced as appropriate.

Nutritional Management

Acute Liver Failure

The nutritional status of someone with acute liver failure versus chronic liver failure can differ greatly. The primary goal of the nutritional management in acute liver failure is supportive. An increase in nausea, vomiting, and anorexia may be associated with acute liver disease, which may result in decreased oral intake. If normal nutritional status prior to the insult is assumed, the patient will have a much higher nutritional reserve than that of a patient in chronic liver failure. Energy needs can be met by providing the Dietary Reference Intakes for infants and children and approximately 30 kcal/kg for adults. The provision of adequate protein is crucial in fulminant hepatic failure and encephalopathy. Adequate protein must be provided to minimize catabolism, which may exacerbate any hyperammonemia present. Excessive protein intake should be avoided because it may increase ammonia levels.

Protein recommendations for adults and teenagers are 0.5–1.0 g/kg/day and for infants and children 1.2–1.5 g/kg/day. Additional protein restrictions or an increase in the intake of branched-chain amino acids intake may be beneficial. In health, the ratio of branched-chain amino acids/aromatic amino acids (leucine + isoleucine + valine/phenylalanine + tyrosine) = ~3:1, and in liver failure the ratio may decline to ~1, often in association with some degree of hepatic encephalopathy. There are data indicating that normalization of this ratio by administration of branched-chain amino acid formulae can improve hepatic encephalopathy.

Chronic Liver Disease

Chronic liver disease is often accompanied by nutritional deficiencies. The goals of nutritional management are to provide adequate energy and protein to prevent energy deficits and protein catabolism and to

Table 4 Management of chronic liver failure in children

Nutritional support
Energy intake, 120–150% (recommended daily amount)
Carbohydrate, 15–20 g/kg/day
Protein, 3–4 g/kg/day
Fat, 8 g/kg/day (50% medium-chain triglyceride)
Fat-soluble vitamins

Fluid balance
Avoid excess sodium (<2 mmol/kg)
Ascites: spironolactone (3 mg/kg), furoseimide (0.5–2 mg/kg),
    albumin infusion, paracentesis

Encephalopathy
Low protein (2 g/kg)
Lactulose (5–20 ml/day)

Coagulopathy
Vitamin K (2–10 mg/day)
Fresh frozen plasma, cryoprecipitate, platelets

From Kelly DA (2002) Managing liver failure. *Postgraduate Medical Journal* **78**: 660–667.

promote hepatic cell growth. Recommendations for nutritional management of children with chronic liver disease are presented in **Table 4**. The energy need for adults with chronic liver disease is 30–35 kcal/kg/day. Energy requirements are increased to compensate for the weight loss that often occurs in cirrhosis. Protein should be provided as 0.8–1 g/kg for adults; unnecessary protein restriction should be avoided because it may only worsen total body protein losses. Energy from fat is best delivered as MCTs due to malabsorption of long-chain fatty acids. Several infant, pediatric, and adult formulas are available with a large percentage of fat in the form of MCTs.

Supplementation with fat-soluble vitamins (A, D, E, and K) in water-miscible solutions is necessary due to the potential for deficiencies associated with fat malabsorption. Serum levels should be monitored regularly to ensure appropriate levels and prevent toxicity. Supplementation with zinc, selenium, iron, and calcium should be given as needed. Copper and manganese should not be supplemented because they are excreted via the bile and may build to toxic levels. Sodium and/or fluid restrictions may be necessary in cirrhosis characterized by ascites and edema. This can impose difficulty because this restriction decreases the palatability of the diet, further decreasing oral intake.

End Stage Liver Disease Pre- and Post-Liver Transplantation

Maintaining optimal nutritional status is important in the patient with end stage liver disease both pre- and post-transplant. However, nutritional assessment in end stage liver disease is particularly problematic. In the pretransplant setting, fluid retention, ascites, and hepatosplenomegaly make body weight an unreliable nutritional index. True decreases in body weight, due to loss of fat stores and lean body mass, may not be fully appreciated solely following weight trends. In the pediatric population, linear growth is often a better indicator of nutritional status. Chronic malnutrition is often present, as reflected in a decrease in linear growth velocity.

Although anthropometric measurements, 24-h creatinine, bioelectric impedance analysis, and indirect calorimetry have all been used, they are affected by ascites and peripheral edema. *In vivo* neutron activation analysis and isotope dilution techniques are more accurate ways of assessing body composition but are time-consuming and costly. For practical purposes, the indirect assessments of 24-h urinary creatinine excretion to determine body muscle mass and mid-arm muscle area can be used for patients without high volumes of extracellular fluid; in those with ascites, the creatinine–height index is a better way of assessing body muscle mass.

Visceral proteins, including albumin, transferrin, prealbumin, and retinol binding protein, are typically used in monitoring nutritional status due to the decrease seen in inadequate dietary protein intake. However, they should be used with caution in liver disease because the synthesis of these proteins is also decreased in end stage liver disease. Serum levels of fat-soluble vitamins should be monitored closely as well.

Improving nutritional status prior to transplant is imperative because malnutrition affects morbidity and mortality post-transplant. Although it may not be possible to reverse the degree of malnutrition, aggressive nutrition support should be implemented to prevent further worsening of the nutrition state and possibly reduce pre- and post-transplant infection and complications.

Post-transplant nutrition support should not be overlooked because the nutrition deficit is not cured merely by the transplant. Additionally, the surgery poses increased nutritional demand for post-surgery healing and support. Nutrition repletion may occur at a more rapid rate than pretransplant because the patient now has a functional liver in which metabolism and digestion of macro- and micronutrients will be improved.

See also: **Celiac Disease. Cystic Fibrosis. Obesity:** Definition, Etiology and Assessment; Fat Distribution; Complications; Prevention; Treatment. **Osteoporosis. Pregnancy:** Role of Placenta in Nutrient Transfer; Nutrient Requirements; Energy Requirements and Metabolic Adaptations; Weight Gain; Safe Diet for

Pregnancy; Prevention of Neural Tube Defects; Pre-eclampsia and Diet. **Vitamin A**: Biochemistry and Physiological Role; Deficiency and Interventions. **Vitamin D**: Physiology, Dietary Sources and Requirements; Rickets and Osteomalacia. **Vitamin E**: Metabolism and Requirements.

Further Reading

Guyton AC and Hall JE (1996) Digestion and absorption in the gastrointestinal tract. In *Textbook of Medical Physiology*. Philadelphia: WB Saunders.

Guyton AC and Hall JE (1996) The liver as an organ. In *Textbook of Medical Physiology*. Philadelphia: WB Saunders.

Hoffmann GF, Nyhan WL, Zschocke J, Kahler SG, and Mayatepek E (2002) *Inherited Metabolic Diseases*. Baltimore, MD: Lippincott Williams & Wilkins.

Lowell JA and Shaw BW (2001) Critical care of liver transplant recipients. In: Maddrey WC (ed.) *Transplantation of the Liver*. Philadelphia: Lippincott Williams & Wilkins.

Marchesini G, Buigianesi E, Forlani G *et al.* (2003) Nonalcoholic fatty liver, steatohepatitis, and the metabolic syndrome. *Hepatology* **37**: 917–923.

Mckiernan PJ (2002) Neonatal cholestasis. *Seminars in Neonatology* **7**: 153–165.

Musso G, Bambino R, De Michieli F *et al.* (2003) Dietary habits and their relations to insulin resistance and postprandial lipemia in nonalcoholic steatohepatitis. *Hepatology* **37**: 909–916.

Rigby SH and Schwarz KB (2001) Nutrition and liver disease. In *Nutrition in the Prevention and Treatment of Disease*. San Diego: Academic Press.

Roberts EA (2002) Steatohepatitis in children. *Best Practice and Research Clinical Gastroentrology* **16**: 749–765.

Sandhu BS and Sanyal AJ (2003) Pregnancy and liver disease. *Gastroenterology Clinics of North America* **32**(1): 407–436.

Stickel F, Hoehn B, Schuppan D, and Seitz HK (2003) Review article: Nutritional therapy in alcoholic liver disease. *Alimentary Pharmacology & Therapeutics* **18**: 357–373.

LOW BIRTHWEIGHT AND PRETERM INFANTS

Contents
Causes, Prevalence and Prevention
Nutritional Management

Causes, Prevalence and Prevention

M Merialdi and M de Onis, World Health Organization, Geneva, Switzerland

It is widely accepted that weight at birth is a key indicator of fetal and neonatal health, both for individuals and for populations. The strong association between low birthweight and perinatal mortality and morbidity is now well recognized by health care providers, as are the different determinants and health consequences of low birthweight. These epidemiological associations became progressively evident during the past century. In the United States, the practice of weighing infants at birth was introduced at the end of the nineteenth century when low birthweight infants were categorized as 'premature' and usually left unattended with minimal or no intervention attempted to prevent their deaths.

When information on birth weight and gestational age was introduced in the birth certificate in mid-twentieth century, it became apparent that prematurity was the most important cause of infant deaths at the national level.

With progressive awareness of the importance of low birthweight as a predictor of infant mortality, it appeared that being born small could be due either to a restriction of the normal process of fetal growth or to delivery before the term of gestation. Thus, the World Health Organization (WHO) made a distinction between the condition of low birthweight (birth weight less than 2500 g) and prematurity (delivery at less than 37 completed weeks, i.e., 259 days). A further development was the introduction of the concept of small for gestational age (SGA) that better describes infants affected by intrauterine growth restriction (IUGR). According to this classification, infants with birth weight below the 10th percentile of a reference population are considered SGA. Although these distinctions and definitions are commonly applied in developed countries, their use is more difficult in developing countries where information on gestational age is often nonexistent or unreliable. This is unfortunate because low birthweight conditions due to growth restriction or preterm birth have different determinants and prognosis, as well as different epidemiological distributions that vary by country and socioeconomic status. Thus, before discussing the causes, prevalence, and prevention of low birthweight, it is important to understand how its two components (gestational age and fetal growth) can be correctly identified and quantified for epidemiological purposes and what are the major limitations in doing so.

Assessment of Gestational Age and Fetal Growth: Methods and Limitations

Preterm birth is defined as delivery before 37 completed weeks (259 days). To accurately differentiate between preterm and term delivery it is crucial to have a reliable estimate of gestational age. Sonographic determination is the most accurate method to estimate gestational age. When ultrasonography is not available, gestational age can be determined by patient's recall of the time of last menstrual period, physical examination of the size of the uterus, and examination of the neonate. These methods can be used alone or in combination but are inaccurate.

Early pregnancy sonographic estimation of gestational age is crucial also for estimation of fetal growth *in utero*, which is assessed by evaluating the size of several fetal anatomical parameters and comparing those measurements with the normal ranges at specific gestational ages obtained from reference populations with growth that can be considered unaffected by pathological conditions. Alternatively, fetal growth can be assessed by the anthropometrical evaluation of the neonate. Several classification systems have been proposed for newborn birth weight. The simplest is categorizing newborns <2500 g as having a low birthweight, but this classification does not differentiate between infants born small for their gestational age and infants who are small because they are born preterm. Reference charts of birthweight at different gestational ages classify infants as SGA, a proxy for IUGR; adequate for gestational age; and large for gestational age. WHO defines SGA as a birth weight below the 10th percentile for a given gestational age based on the sex-specific reference by Williams *et al.* Because it is based on percentile distributions, this classification categorizes some normal, constitutionally small, newborns at the lower end of the normal fetal growth distribution as growth restricted. In addition, the interpretation of the reference data is complicated by inaccuracies in the estimation of gestational age at delivery and by the pathological processes that may affect the size of infants born early in gestation.

Causes

Recognizing that low birthweight may be due to either IUGR or preterm delivery, and, in some cases, a combination of the two, the scientific community has progressively started to consider that IUGR and preterm delivery are two conditions likely caused by various and possibly independent etiopathological factors.

Several complications of pregnancy, such as preeclampsia, fetal distress, fetal growth restriction, abruptio placenta, fetal death, placenta previa, and multiple gestations, are associated with preterm delivery, either spontaneous or induced. Importantly, developments in obstetric and neonatal care, and the consequent increase in obstetric interventions, are likely to be associated with the increase in rates of preterm delivery observed in recent years. Although several lifestyle factors and conditions have been implicated as possible causes, a definitive etiology has not been determined, making it difficult to identify women at risk and to implement preventive strategies. Poor nutrition, cigarette smoking, and alcohol and drug abuse have been indicated as possible risk factors, as well as young maternal age, poverty, short stature, occupational factors, and psychological stress. In addition, genetic factors are likely to be involved in the etiopathogenesis of preterm delivery, as suggested by the fact that the condition tends to recur in families and that prevalence varies across races. The possible role of infection in triggering preterm delivery has been suggested by several studies that have shown associations between delivery before term and amniotic fluid and chorioamniotic infection, bacterial vaginosis, genitourinary clamydial infection, and periodontal disease. Despite the biological plausibility of these associations, their causal relationship has not been definitely proved by unequivocal scientific and epidemiological evidence.

Several conditions have been associated with intrauterine growth restriction. However, present knowledge of the process of fetal growth is limited by the difficulty of differentiating between constitutional and environmental determinants of fetal growth. This limitation complicates the investigation of an important determinant of fetal growth such as maternal size. Small women tend to have smaller babies. There is evidence that intergenerational effects on birth weight are transmitted through the maternal line, thus suggesting a genetic effect. However, poor maternal nutrition and social deprivation have been related to impaired fetal growth and may also be related to small maternal size. Similarly, the relationship between fetal size and race may be mediated by genetic and environmental factors. Specifically designed studies are necessary to determine the contribution of genetic and environmental determinants to the process of fetal growth.

Other factors that have been associated with fetal growth restriction are fetal infections, congenital malformations, chromosomal abnormalities, chemical teratogens, vascular disease such as preeclampsia, chronic renal disease, chronic hypoxia, placental and cord abnormalities, and multiple fetuses.

Health Consequences

Low birthweight, due to either preterm delivery or IUGR, is associated with increased neonatal mortality. Mortality tends to increase with decreasing gestational age at delivery and birth weight (**Figures 1 and 2**). Preterm delivery is the most important obstetric complication in developed

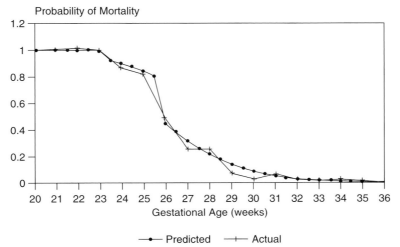

Figure 1 Probability of neonatal mortality as a function of gestational age at delivery in 3386 births between 20 and 37 weeks. The predicted mortality curve is smoothed using statistical methods. Reproduced with permission from Copper RL *et al.* (1993) A multi-centre study of preterm birth weight and gestational age-specific neonatal mortality. *American Journal of Obstetrics and Gynecology* **168**: 78–84.

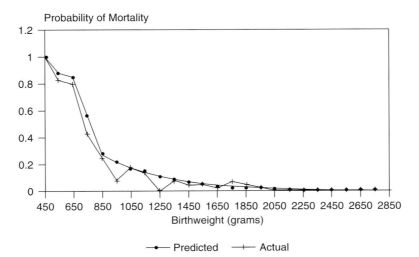

Figure 2 Probability of neonatal mortality as a function of birthweight in 3386 births between 20 and 37 weeks. The predicted mortality curve is smoothed using statistical methods. Reproduced with permission from Copper RL *et al.* (1993) A multicentre study of preterm birth weight and gestational age-specific neonatal mortality. *American Journal of Obstetrics and Gynecology* **168**: 78–84.

countries and, together with IUGR, a major cause of neonatal deaths both in developed and in developing countries. However, the burden of disease of preterm delivery and IUGR in terms of neonatal death is disproportionally heavier for developing countries. Ninety-eight percent of neonatal deaths occur in developing countries, and they account for 33% of all deaths of children younger than 5 years of age. Importantly, 50% of all neonatal deaths are due to being born underweight.

Morbidity is also increased in low birthweight newborns and the negative effects of preterm delivery and/or IUGR tend to persist in infancy as deficits in growth and neurological development. In addition, there is evidence that the negative effects of IUGR may persist long after infancy because low birthweight has been associated with the development of cardiovascular disease, high blood pressure, obstructive lung disease, diabetes, high cholesterol concentrations, and renal damage in adulthood.

Epidemiology

Table 1 shows estimates of prevalence of low birthweight, IUGR, and preterm delivery from three major multicountry studies: the WHO Antenatal Care Trial, the WHO Collaborative Study on Pregnancy Outcomes, and the WHO Misoprostol Trial. The data presented demonstrate that the distribution of low birthweight varies across populations, and the observed differences are due to the varying contribution of preterm delivery and IUGR to the total rates of low birthweight. Rates of low birthweight are higher in developing than in developed countries, as shown by the data presented in **Table 2**. Data from 11 developed areas and 25 developing ones indicate that rates of low birthweight steadily increase as the level of development decreases. The observed differences in low birthweight rates between geographical areas are enormous, with rates ranging from as low as 3.6% in Sweden to as high as 43% in Mumbai, India. Importantly, a global review of the magnitude of the problem demonstrates that many countries currently exceed the internationally recognized cutoff levels for triggering public health action (IUGR >20% and low birthweight (LBW) >15%). Most of low birthweight infants born in developed countries are the result of preterm delivery, whereas in developing countries they are more likely to be IUGR infants. In addition, differences in the distribution of low birthweight are observed at country level, as indicated by the higher prevalence of low birthweight (due mainly to preterm delivery) among African Americans compared to other ethnic groups in the United States.

Prevention

Results from clinical trials provide the most powerful scientific evidence to guide policy and programmatic public health strategies. Interventions aimed at preventing low birthweight either acting toward preterm delivery or IUGR have usually not proven to be effective by randomized clinical trials. The multicausal nature of these conditions is likely responsible for the fact that single interventions do not show an effect of enough magnitude to be detected by medium-sized clinical trials. Thus, appropriate combinations of interventions should be a priority for evaluation in the context of large, methodologically sound trials. Evidence shows that some interventions may be effective and their combined implementation may have a significant public health impact. Interventions likely to be beneficial in preventing IUGR are smoking cessation, antimalarial chemoprophylaxis in primigravide, and balanced protein energy supplementation. Treatment of urinary tract infection, placement of circumferential stitches on a structurally weak uterine cervix (cerclage), and treatment of bacterial vaginosis in high-risk women have been shown to be effective in preventing preterm birth. Unfortunately, these interventions are applicable only to a small number of high-risk women, and their overall effect in the general population is likely to be limited.

In the following sections, nutritional interventions to prevent preterm delivery and IUGR are reviewed with the aim of identifying potentially effective interventions and suggesting possible mechanisms that may link maternal nutritional status to low birthweight. The focus is on the review of randomized clinical trials that provide the most unbiased epidemiological evidence on the effectiveness of interventions. Clinical trials testing the same or similar interventions can be pooled together to estimate an overall effect by means of a systematic review of published and unpublished studies and the meta-analysis of the trials' results.

Nutritional Interventions to Prevent Preterm Delivery

Of the nutritional interventions conducted during pregnancy that have been tested by clinical trials to prevent preterm delivery, only calcium and fish oil supplementation appear promising. In addition, nutritional advice and magnesium supplementation are likely to be effective; however, methodological problems in the analysis of the trials' results prevent from drawing definitive conclusions. Most of the other

Table 1 Prevalence of LBW, IUGR, and preterm delivery in different countries

Country	Location	Years	Sample size	LBW (% of live births)	IUGR (% of live births)	Preterm (% of live births)	Data source
Argentina	City of Rosario	1996–1998	6,789	7.0	9.0	9.7	ANC
Argentina	City of Rosario	1984–1986	5,634	6.3	9.7	7.2	CSPO
Argentina	City of Rosario	1998–1999	2,709	4.0	6.0	6.3	MiT
China	Six subdistricts of Nanshi in Shanghai	1981–1982	4,753	4.2	9.4	7.5	CSPO
China	Shanghai	1998–1999	2,195	3.5	5.3	5.4	MiT
Colombia	City of Cali	1989	4,598	16.1	17.8	15.7	CSPO
Cuba	Havana	1996–1998	5,573	6.9	14.4	5.2	ANC
Cuba	Mixed urban and rural centres	1981	4,779	8.1	14.7	7.2	CSPO
Gambia	Keneba village	1976–1984	379	12.1	13.5	13.5	CSPO
Guatemala	Four highland rural villages	1969–1977	286	12.5	25.3	15.8	CSPO
India	Pune	1990	4,307	28.2	54.2	9.7	CSPO
Indonesia	City of Bogor and surrounding villages	1983	1,647	10.5	19.8	18.5	CSPO
Ireland	Dublin	1979–1980	6,424	5.6	6.9	6.2	CSPO
Ireland	Dublin	1998–1999	447	3.1	7.8	5.1	MiT
Malawi	Three rural communities	1986–1989	938	11.6	26.1	8.2	CSPO
Myanmar	Communities in rural and urban areas	1981–1982	3,542	17.8	30.4	24.6	CSPO
Nepal	Rural areas	1990	NA	14.3	36.3	15.8	CSPO
Saudi Arabia	Jeddah	1996–1998	3,923	7.5	17.1	7.9	ANC
Sri Lanka	Rural areas	1990	1,851	18.4	34.0	14.0	CSPO
Switzerland	Zurich	1998–1999	353	1.1	5.6	2.5	MiT
Thailand	Khon Kaen province	1996–1998	6,289	8.3	20.9	8.0	ANC
Thailand	Rural and urban centres	1979–1980	4,124	9.6	17.0	21.3	CSPO
Thailand	Khon Kaen province	1998–1999	1,816	5.5	13.3	7.5	MiT
United Kingdom	Aberdeen	1971–1976	4,803	6.2	12.3	4.6	CSPO
USA/CDC (Black)	17 states and District of Columbia	1989	4,614	10.6	11.2	16.6	CSPO
USA/CDC (Hispanic)	17 states and District of Columbia	1989	2,205	4.8	5.8	10.2	CSPO
USA/CDC (White)	17 states and District of Columbia	1989	16,481	6.0	6.9	9.3	CSPO
Vietnam	City of Hanoi and one rural district	1982–1984	4,428	5.2	18.2	13.6	CSPO
Vietnam	Ho Chi Min City	1998–1999	3,001	11.1	27.8	6.2	MiT

ANC, WHO Antenatal Care Trial; CSPO, WHO Collaborative Sudy on Pregnancy Outcomes; IUGR, intrauterine growth restriction; LBW, low birthweight; MiT, WHO Misoprostol Trial; NA, not available.

Table 2   Low birthweight rates in developed and developing areas

Location	Year	No. of newborn infants	Incidence of LBW ($\leq 2500\,g$)	Proportion of IUGR–LBW ($\leq 2500\,g$, $\geq 37\,weeks$) (%)	Source of gestational age other than LMP
Developed areas					
Sweden	1973	107,717	3.6	46	
Japan	1973	206,629	4.7	62	
Finland	1966	11,931	4.2	24	
Italy	1965	963,653	4.3	49	
New Zealand	1976	59,568	4.9	50	
Austria	1973	48,758	5.7	35	
Canada	1977	348,000	6.4	64	
United Kingdom	1970	16,815	6.9	57	
United States	1977	3,148,910	7.4	45	
Hungary	1973	152,996	10.8	28	
United States	1968–1974		6.0	30	
Developing areas					
Bogota, Colombia	1979	407	9.8	65	Early pregnancy detection[a]
Rosario, Argentina	1975	689	10.0	50	Neonatal examination[b]
Cuba	1973	208,503	10.1	38	
Tanga, Tanzania	1966	1,000	11.2	56	Neonatal examination
Nairobi, Kenya	1971	3,160	13.6	34	Neonatal examination
Eastern Guatemala	1977	1,276	16.0	73	Prospective amenorrhea detection[c]
Dominican Republic	1975–1976	304	17.8	68	
Nairobi, Kenya	1974	3,700	18.9	34	Neonatal examination
Johannesburg, South Africa	1971–1972	1,800	19.5	73	Neonatal examination
Colombo, Sri Lanka	1971	1,988	21.0	76	Neonatal examination
Vellore, India	1971–1972	2,626	22.1	76	Neonatal examination
Central Guatemala	1977	1,000	23.0	77	Neonatal examination
Jakarta, Indonesia	1967–1968	2,210	23.1	72	
New Delhi, India	1964–1966	2,273	24.1	79	
Tirupati, India	1968–1969	1,000	24.7	73	
Ibadan, Nigeria	1973–1974	1,290	24.9	43	Neonatal examination
Berhampur, India	1972	986	26.3	65	
New Delhi, India	1968–1969	4,100	30.0	78	
10 states, India	1969	10,739	30.5	77	
Rajasthan, India	1970	1,651	30.7	71	Neonatal examination
Tamil Nadu, India	1969–1975	4,420	31.8	77	Prospective amenorrhea detection
Hyderabad, India	1969	846	33.1	88	Neonatal examination
Pondicherry, India	1970–1971	1,279	34.0	66	Neonatal and amniotic fluid examination
Western Guatemala	1964–1972	415	41.6	83	Prospective amenorrhea detection
Mumbai, India	1966–1967	10,000	43.0	96	

[a]During the first trimester and follow-up during pregnancy to validate gestational age.
[b]The use of one or more recognized methods to measure neonatal maturation.
[c]Periodic home visits to detect the first lack of menstruation.
IUGR, intrauterine growth restriction; LBW, low birthweight.
From Villar J and Belizán JM (1982) The relative contribution of prematurity and fetal growth retardation to low birthweight in developing and developed societies. *American Journal of Obstetrics and Gynecology* **143**: 793–798.

interventions that have been hypothesized to have potential to prevent preterm delivery, such as protein and energy supplementation, protein and energy restriction, salt restriction, iron and/or folate supplementation, zinc supplementation, and vitamin A supplementation, have not been proved to be effective.

Nutritional Interventions to Prevent IUGR

Among the interventions that have been tested by randomized clinical trials to prevent IUGR, balanced energy protein supplementation has been shown to reduce the risk of SGA by approximately 30%. On the basis of these results, it has been proposed that universal balanced energy supplementation should be provided to women in areas with a high prevalence of maternal undernutrition to prevent impaired fetal growth. There is evidence that magnesium supplementation and calcium supplementation may be effective, even though for the latter it is not clear if the observed effect on low birthweight is due to a direct effect on fetal growth or mediated by a prolongation of gestational age at delivery. Other interventions, such as nutritional advice, energy protein restriction, salt restriction, iron and/or folate supplementation, fish oil supplementation, zinc supplementation, and vitamins E, C, and D supplementation, did not show any effect in preventing IUGR. Interestingly, high protein supplementation in women of low socioeconomic status in the United States has been associated with an increase in the rate of SGA infants, suggesting that nutritional supplementation may, in some cases, have potentially harmful effects.

Conclusion

Low birthweight, due to either preterm delivery or IUGR, represents a major public health problem for developing and developed countries. In developed countries, access to adequate obstetrics and neonatal care prevents most of the negative short- and long-term outcomes associated with low birthweight that are observed in developing countries in terms of both mortality and morbidity. Thus, public health efforts should be aimed at improving the level and accessibility of health care in developing countries. This is particularly important because most preventive strategies have been shown by clinical trials to be ineffective. Among nutritional interventions to prevent low birthweight, only balanced energy protein supplementation has been shown to be effective in reducing the risk of SGA and has been proposed to be provided to women in areas with a high prevalence of maternal undernutrition.

Research efforts should focus on the determination of the etiological factors responsible for preterm delivery and IUGR. Despite the considerable burden of disease related to these conditions, very little progress has been made in identifying their causes, thus limiting the possibility to implement effective preventive and primary care therapeutic interventions that would particularly benefit the populations of developing countries with limited access to secondary and tertiary health care.

See also: **Infants**: Nutritional Requirements; Feeding Problems. **Low Birthweight and Preterm Infants**: Nutritional Management. **Pregnancy**: Role of Placenta in Nutrient Transfer; Nutrient Requirements; Safe Diet for Pregnancy; Dietary Guidelines and Safe Supplement Use; Pre-eclampsia and Diet. **Supplementation**: Dietary Supplements.

Further Reading

Barker DJ (1992) *Fetal and Infant Origins of Adult Disease.* London: BMJ.

Battaglia FC and Lubchenco LO (1967) A practical classification of newborn infants by weight and gestational age. *Journal of Pediatrics* 71: 159–163.

Cunningham FG, Gant NF, Leveno KJ *et al.* (2001a) Preterm birth. In: *Williams Obstetrics*, 21st edn., pp. 689–727. New York: McGraw-Hill.

Cunningham FG, Gant NF, Leveno KJ *et al.* (2001b) Fetal growth disorders. In: *Williams Obstetrics*, 21st edn., pp. 743–764. New York: McGraw-Hill.

de Onis M, Blossner M, and Villar J (1998) Levels and patterns of intrauterine growth retardation in developing countries. *European Journal of Clinical Nutrition* 52(supplement 1): S5–S15.

Goldenberg RL and Rouse DJ (1998) Prevention of premature birth. *New England Journal of Medicine* 339: 313–320.

Gulmezoglu M, de Onis M, and Villar J (1997) Effectiveness of interventions to prevent or treat impaired fetal growth. *Obstetrical and Gynecological Survey* 52: 139–149.

Kramer MS and Victora CG (2001) low birthweight and perinatal mortality. In: Semba RD and Bloem MW (eds.) *Nutrition and Health in Developing Countries*, pp. 57–70. Totowa, NJ: Humana Press.

Merialdi M, Carroli G, Villar J *et al.* (2003) Nutritional interventions during pregnancy for the prevention or treatment of impaired fetal growth: An overview of randomized controlled trials. *Journal of Nutrition* 133: 1626S–1631S.

Villar J and Belizan JM (1982) The relative contribution of prematurity and fetal growth retardation to low birthweight in developing and developed societies. *American Journal of Obstetrics and Gynecology* 143: 793–798.

Villar J, Merialdi M, Gulmezoglu AM *et al.* (2003) Nutritional interventions during pregnancy for the prevention or treatment of maternal morbidity and preterm delivery: An overview of randomized controlled trials. *Journal of Nutrition* 133: 1606S–1625S.

World Health Organization (1961) *Public Health Aspects of Low Birth Weight. WHO Expert Committee on Maternal and Child Health.* Geneva: WHO.

World Health Organization (1995) The newborn infant. In *Physical Status: The Use and Interpretation of Anthropometry. WHO Expert Committee on Physical Status.* Geneva: WHO.

Nutritional Management

J M Cox, Johns Hopkins Hospital, Baltimore, MD, USA

Introduction

Thanks to advances in modern medicine and technology the outcome of preterm infants has improved dramatically. Many infants are now surviving who are born as young as 23 weeks' gestation and as small as 450 g. These infants enter life with their maternal nutrient supply abruptly disconnected and with only minimal nutrient stores. There is no other time in the life cycle when nutrition is more crucial. Additionally, nutrition in this early neonatal period may have an impact upon health throughout life.

These infants are vulnerable to poor growth and abnormal developmental outcome if not nourished appropriately. Since the preterm infant lacks the ability to voluntarily consume and process nutrients, all of the infant's needs must be provided through enteral and frequently parenteral nutrition. Preterm infants have numerous nutritional risk factors. Nutrient stores are accumulated during the third trimester; therefore, preterm infants have low energy reserves as well as minimal reserves of other nutrients. In fact, infants with birth weights less than 1000 g have energy reserves of less than 200 kcal kg^{-1} (836 kJ kg^{-1}). The metabolic rate of the preterm infant is elevated due to the predominance of metabolically active tissue and minimal fat stores. Protein, fat, and glucose needs are very high to provide adequate energy for metabolism, fat deposition, and growth. The preterm infant has excessive evaporative losses and increased urinary losses, which greatly increase fluid needs. The gastrointestinal tract of the preterm infant is very immature with minimal production of enzymes and growth factors, poor gastric emptying, and discoordinated peristalsis. To further complicate the provision of nutrients, preterm infants have episodes of metabolic instability including hypo- and hyperglycemia, poor lipid clearance, and electrolyte disturbances. The preterm infant also has high rates of stressful events including respiratory distress, hypoxemia, hypercarbia, and sepsis.

Usually, the goal is to provide sufficient nutrients to achieve the fetal growth rate. However, since the fetus and newborn differ in both physiology and metabolism this may not be an appropriate goal and in actuality this goal is rarely achieved both in regards to growth as well as body composition.

Most preterm and low-birth-weight infants show significant delays in growth due to the inability to provide adequate nutrients especially in the first few weeks following birth. Over the past several years, improvements in neonatal management and a more aggressive approach to nutrition have accelerated growth but it still lags behind the fetal growth rate. However, the growth potential of preterm infants may actually be greater than even that of the normal infant. Growth velocity in the infant is greatest between 25 and 30 weeks' gestation, greater than at 40 weeks. If the infant is undernourished during this key growth period, adequate catch-up growth may never be achieved. Protein and energy are the key nutrients for growth, but they must be provided in appropriate proportions for the optimal utilization of both. Vitamins, minerals, and electrolytes must also be supplied in adequate amounts and proportions to contribute to growth. During the first few weeks after birth most preterm infants are usually undernourished due to instability so that once stability is achieved an increased supply of nutrients may be necessary to achieve catch-up growth. Nutrients are usually supplied parenterally in the initial period, gradually transitioned to a combination of parenteral and enteral nutrition, and finally when stability has been achieved full enteral nutrition.

Energy Needs

Most estimates of energy expenditure in preterm infants have been done using indirect calorimetry in relatively healthy infants weighing greater than 1200 g. The energy needs of the smaller and more preterm infant may differ somewhat. Basically, energy needs of the preterm infant involve several energy-requiring functions. Resting metabolic rate accounts for the greatest percentage of energy needs. Resting metabolic rate is equivalent to basal metabolic rate plus some of the energy used for growth; estimates have ranged from 45 to 60 kcal kg^{-1} day^{-1}(188–251 kJ kg^{-1} day^{-1}). The energy cost of activity ranges between 2 and 12% of the total energy expenditure. The smaller more premature infants are probably at the lower end of the range while the larger less preterm infant has increased activity and therefore a higher expenditure. Although preterm infants are cared for in a thermoneutral environment, there is, nevertheless, energy lost to thermoregulation during nursing care and medical procedures. There may also be energy lost to thermoregulation in a stable growing infant during bathing, feeding, and when weaned to a bassinette. The energy cost of growth includes that needed for

Table 1 Energy needs of the growing preterm infant

Energy factor	$kcal\ kg^{-1}day^{-1}$	$kJ\ kg^{-1}day^{-1}$
Resting metabolic rate	45–60	188–250
Activity	10–15	42–63
Thermoregulation	10	42
Thermic effect of food	8	33
Fecal losses	12	50
Growth	25	105
Total	**110–130**	**460–545**

tissue synthesis as well as the energy stored in tissues. The estimates for growth needs vary widely probably depending on the composition of weight gain in the infant. For the enterally fed infant the thermic effect of food and fecal losses also contribute to total energy need. The total energy needs of the growing preterm infant are summarized in **Table 1**.

Parenteral Nutrition

Since the gastrointestinal tract of the preterm infant is immature, substantive enteral nutrition is not possible in the first 2–3 weeks after birth, especially in those infants whose birth weights are less than 1500 g; therefore, the preterm infant is dependent on intravenous fluid for the bulk of fluid needs. Parenteral nutrition (PN) is basically the infusion of a nutrient solution into the circulation. Its development has allowed for the provision of nutrients during the time that enteral nutrition cannot meet nutrient needs. The use of PN has reduced the catabolism that occurs until full enteral nutrition can be achieved. PN should definitely be considered in infants whose birth weights are <1500 g and/or gestational age <30 weeks. It may also be needed for the infant whose birth weight is between 1500 and 2000 g and/or gestational age 30–32 weeks especially if the initiation or progression of enteral feeding is likely to be prolonged.

Historically, parenteral nutrition was delayed for several days after birth, probably due to metabolic instability of the infant and concern for tolerance of the components in the solution. More recently, the early use of PN has been recommended within 24 h after birth. This practice minimizes the interruption of nutrient delivery and the catabolism that occurs when only dextrose solutions are infused.

Parenteral nutrition can be administered by two different routes. There are both risks and benefits associated with each route. In the early days of parenteral nutrition it was always infused via an indwelling, surgically placed catheter into a central vein. Since some of the complications with this method were related to the catheter, the use of peripheral veins for infusion became popular and is still employed today. The dextrose concentration of peripheral PN is limited to ~10%; thus, the nutrient intake by this route is somewhat limited without excessive fluid intake. Peripheral parenteral nutrition is usually recommended when its use will be of short duration. While peripheral lines are considered less risky complications can occur. If the intravenous line infiltrates some infants have experienced serious deep sloughing, sometimes requiring skin grafts. These lines require vigilance on the part of nursing to prevent infiltrates and some infants will have multiple intravenous attempts daily because the line needs to be replaced. The advent of the percutaneously inserted central catheter and its liberal use in the last few years has improved and stabilized the delivery of parenteral nutrition to the preterm infant. Central parenteral nutrition is recommended when it is anticipated that it will be used for >5–7 days, usually in infants weighing <1000–1250 g. If the infant tolerates glucose and clears lipids well it is possible to meet estimated nutrient needs using this route. Complications such as pneumothorax, pleural effusions, and increased risk of sepsis are associated with central lines (**Table 2**).

Components of Parenteral Nutrition

Parenteral nutrition solutions contain dextrose, amino acids, lipids, electrolytes, vitamins, and minerals.

Glucose Glucose, provided as a dextrose solution, is the predominant energy source in PN. It is the main energy substrate for the fetus as well as the

Table 2 Risks and benefits of parenteral nutrion routes

Peripheral	Central
Adequate for short-term use	Recommended when PN needed >7 days
Dextrose limited to 10–12.5%	Requires placement of central line/PICC line
Can provide 80–85 kcal kg^{-1} day^{-1} if adequate fluid available	Able to meet estimated needs if adequate fluid available
Possible complications	**Possible complications**
Intravenous line can infiltrate and cause deep skin sloughing	Sepsis
Requires nursing vigilance to care for intravenous line	Line complications (pleural effusions, pneumothorax)
Can require multiple intravenous attempts	

neonate after birth. Preterm infants often require more glucose than the term infant secondary to the higher brain to body weight ratio and the need for additional energy for central nervous system energy requirements. Measurements of glucose utilization in the preterm infant range from 6 to $10\,mg\,kg^{-1}\,min^{-1}$($0.033$–$0.055\,mmol\,kg^{-1}\,min^{-1}$). Glycogen stores are very limited in the preterm infant; therefore, it requires a large and continuous source of glucose. This should be initiated at a rate of $\sim6\,mg\,kg^{-1}\,min^{-1}$ ($0.033\,mmol\,kg^{-1}\,min^{-1}$) and can be advanced 1–$2\,mg\,kg^{-1}\,min^{-1}$ (0.0055–$0.011\,mmol\,kg^{-1}\,min^{-1}$) each day to an optimum of 12–$14\,mg\,kg^{-1}\,min^{-1}$ (0.066–$0.78\,mmol\,kg^{-1}\,min^{-1}$) as long as the infant does not become hyperglycemic. Above this rate, glucose is not used for energy but rather fat deposition. This is an inefficient process that can result in increased energy expenditure and carbon dioxide production.

Difficulties with glucose metabolism are a common problem in preterm infants. This may be due to decreased energy stores, increased gluconeogenesis secondary to stress, decreased insulin secretion, or insulin resistance. When hyperglycemia occurs the glucose infusion rate should be decreased, however the rate should not be decreased below 4–$6\,mg\,kg^{-1}\,min^{-1}$ (0.022–$0.33\,mmol\,kg^{-1}\,min^{-1}$) as this is the minimum supply rate necessary to provide adequate energy to the brain. Usually, the infusion of amino acids improves glucose tolerance by decreasing glucose production, stimulating insulin secretion, and enhancing insulin action. The use of continuous insulin infusions to treat hyperglycemia is controversial. If used, the insulin infusion should be initiated at a rate of $0.05\,U\,kg^{-1}\,h^{-1}$ and titrated to achieve and maintain a plasma glucose concentration between 80 and $120\,mg\,dl^{-1}$ (4.44–$6.66\,mmol\,l^{-1}$).

Protein   The early administration of protein in the form of crystalline amino acids to the preterm infant is one of the changes to have occurred over the last decade. Early studies of amino acid administration in preterm infants in the 1960s and 1970s raised the concern for protein toxicity because these infusions were associated with acidosis, azotemia, and hyperammonemia; this caused a delay in the routine administraton of protein. However, the above conditions were probably the result of the preparations being casein or fibrin hydrolysates and of suboptimal quality. Since the 1980s crystalline amino acid solutions have been used. In the late 1980s amino acid solutions specifically for use in infants were designed to produce a plasma amino

acid level comparable to that of a postprandial breast-fed infant.

The early administration of amino acids is crucial because studies have shown that the preterm infant suffers protein losses of between 0.8 and $1.2\,g\,kg^{-1}\,day^{-1}$. A number of studies have demonstrated that the infusion of amino acids along with glucose decreased protein catabolism. As little as 1–$1.5\,g\,kg^{-1}\,day^{-1}$ of amino acids have been shown to prevent negative nitrogen balance. Studies have also shown that the infusion of $3\,g\,kg^{-1}\,day^{-1}$ within the first 2 days of life resulted in increased protein synthesis, suppressed protein breakdown, and produced plasma aminograms similar to the breast-fed infant.

The provision of adequate energy is needed for protein metabolism and deposition. Most infants can achieve positive nitrogen balance at $2\,g\,kg^{-1}\,day^{-1}$ of protein intake when given 50–$60\,kcal\,kg^{-1}\,day^{-1}$ (209–$251\,kJ\,kg^{-1}\,day^{-1}$) of energy. Additionally, approximately $22\,kcal$ ($92\,kJ$) per g protein (15–20% of kcal) results in reasonable amino acid utilization.

Therefore, protein should be started if possible on the first day of life at 1.5–$2\,g\,kg^{-1}\,day^{-1}$ and advanced to 3.5–$4\,g\,kg^{-1}\,day^{-1}$ to achieve *in utero* accretion rates.

Cysteine   The amino acid cysteine is a conditionally essential nutrient in the preterm infant because they have low cystathionase activity. Cystathionase, an enzyme, is necessary to convert methionine to cysteine. However, this amino acid is unstable in liquid solutions so commercially available crystalline amino acid solutions do not contain cysteine. Plasma levels of cysteine are low in infants receiving cysteine-free PN. Cysteine hydrochloride however is soluble and is stable in aqueous solutions for a short period of time so $40\,mg\,g\,protein^{-1}$ is often added to PN solutions when prepared. The addition of cysteine may result in acidosis necessitating an increase in acetate. However, an additional advantage is that the addition of cysteine decreases the pH of the PN solution, which allows the addition of more calcium and phosphorous.

Lipids   Lipids are the most concentrated source of calories in the PN solution. They are available as lipid emulsions of soy bean and safflower oil; 20% emulsions are recommended for use because they contain less phospholipid than the 10% emulsion. Lipids are critical for central nervous system development. Additionally, when infused with the PN solution they may also prevent phlebitis. Lipids are usually infused to prevent essential fatty acid deficiency and as an energy source. Maximum lipid clearance occurs when lipids are infused over 24 h. Starting recommendations vary; but it is generally accepted to start with $0.5-1\,g\,kg^{-1}\,day^{-1}$ between 1–3 days of life. Lipids should be advanced to an optimum of $3\,g\,kg^{-1}\,day^{-1}$. Studies have shown that preterm infants have optimal protein retention when approximately 30–40% of calories are provided as lipids. Plasma triglycerides can be used to monitor lipid clearance. It is generally accepted that levels below $150-200\,mg\,dl^{-1}$ indicate adequate clearance. Lipoprotein lipase and hepatic lipase are the major enzymes for clearance of intravenous lipid. These activities are inducible by low-dose heparin, which is usually present in central PN solutions. Administration of heparin should be considered in those infants receiving peripheral PN showing poor lipid clearance. In infants with hypertriglyceridemia the provision of $0.5-1\,g\,kg^{-1}\,day^{-1}$ of lipid is adequate to prevent essential fatty acid deficiency and is a dose likely to be tolerated by most infants.

Carnitine Carnitine is necessary for the transport of free fatty acids into the inner mitochondrial membrane, the site of oxidation. Since the preterm infant has decreased carnitine synthesis capability and low plasma and tissue concentrations, carnitine may be an essential nutrient. Studies are conflicting as to whether there is benefit to adding it to parenteral nutrition. Its use should be considered in infants with birth weights $<1000\,g$, those receiving long-term parenteral nutrition without enteral feedings, and those with hypertriglyceridemia.

Electrolytes The electrolyte content of parenteral nutrition solutions is usually similar to that found in normal intravenous solutions: usually $3-4\,mmol\,kg^{-1}\,day^{-1}$ of sodium and $2-3\,mmol\,kg^{-1}\,day^{-1}$ of potassium. Very immature infants and those on diuretics may require additional amounts to maintain normal plasma concentrations. Chloride and acetate need to be dosed based on electrolyte levels. The very young preterm infant may need a higher proportion of acetate secondary to urinary bicarbonate losses. Later, when chronic diuretics are used a greater proportion of chloride may be needed.

Calcium, phosphorous, and magnesium Calcium and phosphorous are relatively insoluble in solution together. This makes it difficult to provide adequate levels of these minerals to meet the needs of the preterm infant. When parenteral nutrition solutions are advanced to 10% dextrose and 2 g protein per 100 ml usually 60–80 mg (1.5–2 mmol) calcium and 40–60 mg (1.3–1.9 mmol) phosphorous can

be added to the solution. Since the accretion rate of calcium in the fetus is normally $100\,mg\,kg^{-1}\,day^{-1}$ ($2.5\,mmol\,kg^{-1}\,day^{-1}$), infants on prolonged parenteral nutrition may develop osteopenia and fractures. The usual dose of magnesium is $0.3-0.5\,mEq\,kg^{-1}\,day^{-1}$ ($0.3-0.5\,mmol\,kg^{-1}\,day^{-1}$).

Trace minerals Zinc and copper deficiencies occurred in some preterm infants before these trace elements were routinely added to parenteral nutrition solutions. There is very little research that defines the parenteral requirements of trace minerals in preterm infants. The current recommendations for trace minerals are summarized in **Table 3**.

Vitamins Like trace minerals, the recommendations for intake of vitamins are not based on randomized trials but are based on the best information available. Infants receiving these parenteral intakes do not develop deficiencies or evidence of excessive intake (**Table 4**).

Table 3 Suggested parenteral intakes of trace minerals

Trace mineral	$\mu g\,kg^{-1}day^{-1}$
Zinc	400
Iron	200
Copper	15–20
Selenium	1.5–2
Manganese	1
Iodide	1
Molybdenum	0.25
Chromium	0.2

Table 4 Suggested parenteral intake of vitamins

Vitamin	Amount/per kg per day
Vitamin A (μg)	280–500
Vitamin E (mg)	2.8
Vitamin K (μg)	100
Vitamin D (μg)	4
Vitamin (IU)	160
Ascorbic acid (mg)	25
Thiamin (μg)	350
Riboflavin (μg)	150
Pyridoxine (μg)	180
Niacin (mg)	6.8
Pantothenate (mg)	2
Biotin (μg)	6
Folate (μg)	56
Vitamin B_{12}	0.3

Total dose should not exceed the amounts provided by 5 ml of reconstituted MVI Pediatric (Armor Pharmaceutical Co., Chicago, IL, USA): $700\,\mu g$ vitamin A, $7\,\mu g$ vitamin E, $200\,\mu g$ vitamin K, $10\,\mu g$ vitamin D, 80 mg ascorbic acid, 1.2 mg thiamin, 1.4 mg riboflavin, 1.0 mg pyridoxine, 17 mg niacin, 5 mg pantothenic acid, $20\,\mu g$ biotin, $140\,\mu g$ folic acid, $1\,\mu g$ vitamin B_{12}.

Table 5 Suggested initiation and advancement of parenteral nutrition for the preterm infant

Component	Initial	Advancement/day	Goal
Dextrose	6–8 m kg^{-1} min^{-1} (0.033–0.044 mmol kg^{-1} min^{-1})	1–2 mg kg^{-1} min^{-1} (0.0055–0.011 mmol kg^{-1} min^{-1})	12–14 mg kg^{-1} min^{-1} (0.066–0.077 mmol kg^{-1} min^{-1})
Protein	1.5–2 g kg^{-1}	1 g kg^{-1}	3.5
Lipids	0.5–1 g kg^{-1}	0.5–1 g kg^{-1}	3

Suggested initiation and advancement of parenteral nutrition in the preterm infant is shown in **Table 5**.

Enteral Nutrition

The provision of adequate enteral nutrition is the goal of those caring for the preterm infant. However, a fear of the development of necrotizing enterocolitis, a serious intestinal disease of preterm infants associated with enteral feedings, has influenced feeding practices. Necrotizing enterocolitis (NEC) is a major cause of morbidity and mortality in preterm infants. The incidence of this disease is estimated to be between 8 and 10% of preterm infants. The cause of NEC is considered multifactorial including enteral feeds, hypoxia, ischemia, patent ductus arteriosus, and infection. Approximately 90% of infants who develop NEC have been enterally fed and several studies have shown that the rapid advancement of enteral feedings is associated with NEC. With the advent of parenteral nutrition, the tendency was to delay enteral feeding for prolonged periods of time in order to prevent this disease and to use parenteral nutrition as the sole source of nutrition. However, it is known that delayed enteral feeding has a negative effect on gastrointestinal structure and function. Lack of enteral nutrition induces gastrointestinal atrophy, depresses gut hormone secretion, and delays the maturation of gastrointestinal motility. There are now numerous studies that demonstrate the benefits of early enteral feeding including the promotion of endocrine adaptation, the accelerated maturation of gut motility patterns, the provision of luminal nutrients, and possible benefits to the immune system. In fact, early enteral nutrition may enhance feeding tolerance and may actually decrease the incidence of NEC.

Trophic Feedings

Even though it is recognized that early enteral feeding is beneficial, there is still hesitation to begin feedings in the early days following birth. One of the strategies that has been extensively studied since the late 1980s is trophic feeding, also referred to as minimal enteral nutrition or gut priming. This method involves giving the infant small volumes of feedings, approximately 10–20 ml kg^{-1} day^{-1}, for a period of 10–14 days before advancing to full enteral feedings. The benefits found are greater energy intake, earlier attainment of full enteral feedings, improved growth, less PN-related complications, reduced risk of infection, and earlier hospital discharge. Furthermore, infants who received trophic feedings had no increased incidence of NEC. Many clinicians have adapted variations of this practice, some with a shortened period of trophic feeds, others reserving this practice for the smallest, most preterm infants while employing advancement of feeds in larger, more stable infants. Once minimal enteral nutrition has been established and the infant is stable enough to advance feedings, it is generally considered a safe practice to increase feedings by 20 ml kg^{-1} day^{-1} while using PN for the balance of intake until an adequate enteral intake has been established and tolerated. Although fast feeding advancement has been associated with NEC, one study has shown no increase in the incidence of NEC amongst preterm infants whose feeds were advanced by 35 ml kg^{-1} day^{-1}.

Feeding Route

Because preterm infants lack the ability to coordinate sucking, swallowing, and breathing, tube feedings must be used. Jejunal feeding was a popular method for feeding infants during the 1970s to early 1980s. It was felt that this method would minimize the risk of reflux and aspiration. This method is now generally reserved for infants in whom reflux and aspiration is complicating chronic lung disease or those who have poor gastric emptying. Now, most infants are fed using an orogastric or nasogastric tube; the former usually selected for the tiniest babies as the feeding tube may occlude one naris and impair nasal breathing.

Feeding Selection

Breast milk expressed by the infant's mother is the preferred type of feeding for most preterm infants. It is nutritionally superior to artificial formula in many respects. There is improved gastric emptying, more stool frequency, and improved fat absorption when breast milk is used. There are many trophic factors found in human milk that enhance the development of the gastrointestinal tract. Human milk contributes to host defense and reduces the risk of NEC. Preterm infants who have been fed expressed human milk also show a neurodevelopmental advantage but it is difficult to isolate this from the social variables also associated with mothers willing to express their milk. The use of expressed breast milk also enhances mother-infant bonding as this is one task that only the baby's mother is able to perform. However, there are also nutritional concerns related to the use of breast milk in infants born less than 33 weeks' gestation. Protein supplementation is necessary for optimal growth and maintenance of optimal protein status. Supplementation of calcium and phosphorous is also needed for adequate bone mineralization. There are multinutrient fortifiers available that can be added to breast milk to improve nutrient intake. The use of these fortifiers has been associated with improved intake of protein and minerals and growth and bone mineralization, and balance studies show improved nutrient retention.

If breast milk is not available, the feeding of choice becomes preterm infant formulas. These formulas have greater protein content and are cow's milk whey predominant. The carbohydrate is a mixture of lactose and glucose polymers, and the fat a mixture of both long-chain and medium-chain triglycerides for improved nutrient absorption. The concentration of minerals, electrolytes, and vitamins is increased to meet the estimated nutrient needs of the preterm infant when fed in an amount to provide $120\,kcal\,kg^{-1}\,day^{-1}$. Studies have shown that infants fed preterm infant formulas have improved growth over those fed term formula or even fortified breast milk.

Feeding Rate

The decision regarding how to feed must also be made: continuous versus bolus feeding. The preferred method is controversial. Some clinicians feel that continuous feedings are better tolerated while others feel that bolus feedings are more physiologic. In studies, bolus feedings have been associated with improved gastric emptying, and more mature intestinal motility patterns. It is difficult to compare feeding tolerance between continuous and bolus feeds due to differences in the criteria used. Comparison feeding studies have found fewer gastric residuals in those infants given bolus feedings than those fed continuously. A more recent study has found that

feeds given as a slow bolus, over 2 h, resulted in a normal duodenal motility pattern, suggesting that some infants may benefit from slow intermittent feedings. Regardless of the method chosen, if an infant does not tolerate one method it may be beneficial to try a different one.

Monitoring Feeding Tolerance

Feeding tolerance among preterm infants must be closely monitored since NEC is associated with enteral feedings. The presence of gastric residuals is one factor that is frequently used, but because preterm infants have poor gastric emptying amounts less than 50% of a previous feed should not be considered significant. Other indicators that should be used in conjunction with gastric residuals include the increase in abdominal girth, the absence of active bowel sounds, the presence of blood in the stool, a change in the number or quality of stools, and the presence of emesis. A careful exam is warranted if these symptoms are present.

Estimated calorie and protein intakes to achieve fetal weight gain are shown in **Table 6**.

Monitoring Nutritional Status

The nutritional status and growth of the preterm infant should be monitored throughout the hospitalization. The daily fluid and caloric intake should be monitored daily, body weight should be recorded daily, length and head circumference should be measured weekly, and all three measurements plotted on standardized growth charts. If growth is inadequate the volume or caloric density of feeds and or the protein content should be increased. Biochemical measurements should also be assessed periodically.

Preparation for Discharge

Approximately 1 week prior to discharge, preterm infants should be converted to the feeding regimen that will be used at home. Infants who have been fed expressed breast milk should demonstrate the ability to directly breast-feed and/or to feed supplemented breast milk or formula from the bottle as needed to gain adequate weight. The infant who weighs less than 2500 g at discharge, especially those infants born at less than 30 weeks' gestation, may require the supplementation of some breast-milk feedings with post discharge formula powder or the feeding of a concentrated post discharge formula for some of the daily feedings.

Table 6 Estimated calorie and protein intakes to achieve fetal weight gain

	Body weight (g)				
	500–700	700–900	900–1200	1200–1500	1500–1800
Protein (g)					
Parenteral	3.5	3.5	3.5	3.4	3.2
Enteral	4.0	4.0	4.0	3.9	3.6
Energy (kcal/(kJ) kg^{-1} day^{-1})					
Parenteral	89 (372)	92 (385)	101 (422)	108 (451)	109 (456)
Enteral	105 (440)	108 (451)	119 (500)	127 (530)	128 (535)
Protein/energy (g/100 kcal or 418 kJ)					
Parenteral	3.9	4.1	3.5	3.1	2.9
Enteral	3.8	3.7	3.4	3.1	2.8

Adapted from Ziegler EE, Thureen PJ, and Carlson SJ (2002) Aggressive nutrition of the very low birthweight infant. *Clinical Perinatology* **29**(2): 225–244.

For those infants who were fed preterm formula, conversion to a nutrient-enriched post discharge formula is recommended. These formulas contain additional protein, vitamins, and minerals compared to term formulas. Studies have shown that infants fed these formulas for the first 9–12 months of life have improved gains in weight, length, and head circumference.

If growth is inadequate with either feeding regimen then alteration in caloric density may be needed. Arrangements should be made for the nutritional status of these infants to be monitored after discharge.

Conclusions

Preterm infants have specialized nutritional needs and each infant must be carefully and continuously assessed to ensure that the best possible nutritional support is provided to promote optimal growth without causing additional morbidity and mortality.

Table 7 Periodic monitoring of nutritional status

Indicator	Frequency
Weight	Daily
Length	Weekly
Head circumference	Weekly
Electrolytes (PN)	Daily until stable then 2 times weekly
Electrolytes (enteral)	Weekly
Albumin	Weekly
Bili/transaminases (PN)	Weekly
Calcium, phosphorous, magnesium, alkaline phosphatase	Weekly
Hemoglobin/hematocrit	Weekly

See also: **Breast Feeding. Energy:** Requirements. **Growth and Development, Physiological Aspects. Growth Monitoring. Infants:** Nutritional Requirements; Feeding Problems. **Low Birthweight and Preterm Infants:** Causes, Prevalence and Prevention. **Nutritional Support:** Infants and Children, Parenteral.

Further Reading

Berseth CL (2001) Feeding methods for the preterm infant. *Seminars in Neonatology* **6**: 417–424.

Denne SC (2001) Protein and energy requirements in preterm infants. *Seminars in Neonatology* **6**: 377–382.

Embleton NE, Pang N, and Cooke RJ (2001) Postnatal malnutrition and growth retardation: an inevitable consequence of current recommendations in preterm infants? *Pediatrics* **107**(2): 270–273.

Griffinc IJ (2002) Postdischarge nutrition for high risk neonates. *Clinical Perinatology* **29**(2): 327–344.

Hay WW, Lucas A, Heird WC *et al.* (1999) Workshop summary: nutrition of the extremely low birth weight infant. *Pediatrics* **104**: 1360–1368.

Hay WW (1996) Assessing the effect of disease on nutrition of the preterm infant. *Clinical Biochemistry* **29**(5): 399–417.

Heird WC and Gomez MR (1996) Parenteral nutrition in low birthweight infants. *Annual Review of Nutrition* **16**: 47–99.

Heird WC (2002) Determination of nutritional requirements in preterm infants, with special reference to "catch-up" growth. *Seminars in Neonatology* **6**: 365–375.

Neu J and Koldovsky O (1996) Nutrient absorption in the preterm neonate. *Clinical Perinatology* **23**(2): 229–243.

Newell SJ (2000) Enteral feeding of the micropremie. *Clinical Perinatology* **27**(1): 221–234.

Thureen PJ and Hay WW (2000) Intravenous nutrition and postnatal growth of the micropremie. *Clinical Perinatology* **27**(1): 197–219.

Tyson JE and Kennedy KA (1997) Minimal enteral nutrition in parenterally fed neonates. www.nichd.nih.gov/cochraneneonatal.

Ziegler EE, Thureen PJ, and Carlson SJ (2002) Aggressive nutrition of the very low birthweight infant. *Clinical Perinatology* **29**(2): 225–244.

LUNG DISEASES

A MacDonald, The Children's Hospital, Birmingham, UK

Respiratory disease covers a wide range of disorders and interest has grown in the provision of its nutritional support. Epidemiological studies suggest that dietary habits influence lung function and the tendency to common lung diseases, such as asthma, chronic obstructive pulmonary disease (COPD), and lung cancer. Malnutrition and weight loss are commonly reported in patients with COPD, and intensive, specialist nutritional support is required. For cystic fibrosis (CF), nutritional therapy has been shown to improve the prognosis. Novel diet therapies, including exclusion of food allergens and reduction of salt intake, have been tried as possible treatments for asthma. This article outlines the rationale for and describes methods of nutritional support and therapy in the treatment of lung disease.

Chronic Obstructive Pulmonary Disease

COPD is a term used to describe a spectrum of disorders characterized by reduced maximal expiratory flow and slow forced emptying of the lungs (**Table 1**). It is associated with symptoms of obstructive lung diseases, such as cough, mucus production, breathlessness, airflow limitation, and wheezing. COPD can be present with or without substantial physical impairment or symptoms. The World Health Organisation states that it is the fourth leading cause of global mortality. In the United Kingdom, it is estimated that 18% of males and 14% of females aged 40–68 years may have developed features of COPD. Severe exacerbations remain the largest single cause of emergency admissions for respiratory disease, with a mean hospital stay of 10 days.

Table 1 Consequences of disease-related malnutrition in COPD

Reduced lung function and dyspnea
Reduced maximal O_2 consumption
Decreased peripheral muscle function
Decreased exercise performance
Decreased quality of life
Increased need for hospitalization
Increased postoperative complications during lung volume reduction surgery
Increased mortality

Adapted from Stratton et al. (2002).

The prevalence of COPD is greatest in socioeconomically deprived people. It is probably underdiagnosed partly because many people do not consult their general practitioners or do not reveal all their symptoms. In general, the major cause of COPD is smoking. Other causes include α_1-antitrypsin deficiency, cystic fibrosis, air pollution, occupational exposure, and bronchietasis.

Chronic bronchitis and emphysema are two of the major diseases grouped under COPD. Patients with COPD have features of both conditions, although one may be more prominent than the other.

Chronic Bronchitis

Definition and etiology Chronic bronchitis is defined by the presence of chronic bronchial secretions sufficient to cause expectoration occurring on most days for a minimum of 3 months for 2 consecutive years. It became recognized as a distinct disease in the late 1950s associated with the great British Smog. It develops in response to long-term irritants on the bronchial mucosa. Important irritants include cigarette smoke, dust, smoke, and fumes; other causes include respiratory infection, particularly in infancy, and exposure to dampness, sudden changes in temperature, and fog. In the United Kingdom, it affects 10% of older people, and it is more common in industrial countries. Chronic bronchitis is a slowly progressive disorder unless the precipitating factors are avoided and it is treated.

Clinical features Symptoms include productive cough and frequent and recurrent chest infections. The disease progresses over many years from a troublesome cough producing a little clear sputum to marked wheezing, severe breathlessness leading to poor exercise tolerance, and copious and purulent sputum. It may cause right heart failure (i.e., cor pulmonale), such as oedema and cyanosis.

Pathology There is hypertrophy of the mucus-secreting glands. The structural changes described in the airways include atrophy, focal squamous metaplasia, ciliary abnormalities, variable amounts of airway smooth muscle hyperplasia, inflammation, and bronchial wall thickening. The respiratory bronchioles display a mononuclear inflammatory process, lumen occlusion by mucus plugging, goblet cell metaplasia, smooth muscle hyperplasia, and distortion due to fibrosis. These changes combined with loss of supporting alveolar attachments cause airflow limitation by allowing airway walls to deform and narrow the airway lumen.

Emphysema

Diagnosis and etiology   Emphysema means 'inflation' in the sense of abnormal distension with air. It is a condition in which there is permanent destructive enlargement of the airspace distal to the terminal bronchioles without obvious fibrosis. In the general population, emphysema usually develops in older individuals with a long smoking history. However, other causes include exposure to heavy metals such as cadmium, and 5% of early presenting cases are caused by the autosomal recessive disorder α_1-antitrypsin deficiency. It affects almost 5% of older people, and it is more common in industrialised countries. The prognosis is variable. Progression is slow, provided it is treated.

Clinical features   Patients may be very thin with a barrel chest and have little or no cough expectoration. Symptoms include intense dyspnea with purse-lip breathing and overinflation of the chest. Breathing may be assisted by pursed lips and use of accessory respiratory muscles. The chest may be hyperresonant, and wheezing may be heard. Heart sounds are very distant and overall appearance is more like classic COPD exacerbation.

Chemical Pathology   There are three types of emphysema:

Panacinar emphysema: A generalized destruction of the alveolar walls. As a consequence, the elastic network of the normal lung is badly disorganized and the lung becomes floppy, leading to a severe degree of airways obstruction, particularly during expansion. It generally develops in patients with α_1-antitrypsin deficiency.
Centriacinar emphysema: Distension and damage affect the respiratory bronchioles; the more distal alveolar ducts and alveoli tend to be well preserved. This is very common and not necessarily associated with disability.
Paraseptal emphysema: The least common form, involving distal airway structures and alveolar ducts and sacs.

Nutritional Management in COPD

Malnutrition is an important clinical problem in a subpopulation of patients with COPD. Emaciation with emphysema was reported as early as 1898. Studies suggest malnutrition occurs in between 27 and 71% of all patients, increasing with the severity of airways obstruction. In one of the larger studies examining patients with stable COPD, one-fourth of 779 men were less than 90% of their ideal body weight. However, in patients who need hospital admission, malnutrition approaches or exceeds 50%. When acute respiratory failure complicates the clinical course, severe malnutrition is observed in 60% of cases.

Malnutrition has a considerable impact on both morbidity and mortality. Reduced respiratory muscle mass and function as well as increased susceptibility to infection are recognised as deleterious consequences of malnutrition in patients with or without lung disease. In a necropsy study, diaphragm muscle mass was reduced by 43% in malnourished patients whose weights were 71% of ideal body weight. Decreases in body weight, creatinine–height index, total lymphocyte count, serum transferrin, and retinol binding protein have been documented.

Nutritional depletion is an independent risk factor for mortality and hospitalization in patients with COPD. Studies have indicated a hospital stay of approximately 30 days for patients with a body mass index (BMI) of less than 20 compared with 18 days for those with a BMI of less than 30. If a patient with COPD begins to lose weight progressively, the average reported life expectancy is only 2.9 years, and it is considerably less in malnourished patients who have survived an episode of acute respiratory failure during an acute exacerbation of their disease. However, it is not certain whether this implies a casual relationship or whether low weight is a marker for more severely impaired lung function.

Reasons for Malnutrition

The cause of progressive weight loss in patients with COPD is not well understood but two factors have been implicated.

Increased resting energy expenditure   The relationship between resting energy expenditure (REE), lung function, oxygen cost of breathing, and malnutrition in COPD has been the focus of much attention in recent years. Results of studies on REE are conflicting. In two early studies on malnourished patients with COPD, Goldstein and coworkers described 10 patients whose REE was 113% of predicted, and Wilson and colleagues described 7 patients with a REE 115% of predicted. In contrast, two later studies found REE to be only 94 and 104% of predicted in stable fasted COPD patients, respectively. It has therefore been hypothesized that if patients with COPD are not hypermetabolic, malnutrition is related more to impaired gas exchange (as evidenced by a low diffusing capacity of carbon monoxide) than to airflow obstruction. The impaired gas exchange results from loss of the pulmonary capillary bed and may result in an inability to augment cardiac output in response to the stress of even minimal effort, leading to lack of oxygen delivery to the tissues and nutritional depletion. An alternative hypothesis is that malnutrition is precipitated by acute illnesses, leading to a combination of anorexia and hypercatabolism causing significant weight loss.

Reduced energy intake Many studies have examined the energy intake of malnourished COPD patients and have shown it to be either similar to that of well-nourished patients with COPD or higher than the respective dietary recommendations. Most of these studies were conducted on stable patients, but several factors may adversely affect energy and nutrient intake:

Hypoxia-related appetite suppression or anorexia due to acute exacerbation
Chronic sputum production and frequent coughing, which may alter desire for and taste of food
Fatigue, which can interfere with the ability to shop for food and prepare and eat meals
Depression
Side effects of medications, including nausea, vomiting, diarrhea, dry mouth, and gastric irritation, which may limit dietary intake
Raised plasma tumor necrosis factor-α levels
Arterial oxygen desaturation due to altered breathing pattern during chewing and swallowing

Nutritional Support

Several controlled studies have evaluated the effect of nutritional support in COPD in either outpatients or inpatients, and their outcome was related to the overall energy intake achieved. Weight gain was only achieved by substantially increasing energy intake by more than 30% above the usual intake, amounting to more than 45 kcal/kg per day. Moreover, improvement in muscle function or exercise tolerance occurred only with concomitant weight gain. In one of these controlled studies, oral supplementation was given for 3 months to ambulatory malnourished patients with chronic obstructive lung disease. Daily energy intake increased by 48% above the usual intake and corresponded to 47 kcal/kg on average. The authors reported a mean weight gain of 4.2 kg, an increase in maximal respiratory pressures and in handgrip and stemomastoid strength, and a decrease in stemomastoid muscle

fatigability; similar improvements were not observed in a control group. However, these improvements were not maintained when oral supplementation was discontinued. In another study, six malnourished patients received an additional 1000 kcal via a nasogastric tube for 16 days, whereas a control group of four received only an additional 100 kcal. A weight gain of 2.4 kg, and improvements in respiratory muscle strength and endurance were seen in the fed patients but not in the control group. Other studies have not demonstrated improvements in weight gain or muscle performance and have been less successful in increasing energy intake.

Type of Nutritional Support

If the patient with COPD is less than 90% ideal body weight for height, nutritional support should be considered. This can be difficult in COPD, but it can be provided on three levels.

Normal high-energy, high-protein diet For many patients with COPD, advising small, frequent nutrient-dense meals, regular snacks, and food fortification using high-energy and -protein foods, such as milk, yoghurt, butter, and cream, may provide adequate nutritional support. Foods of low nutritional value, such as tea, squash, and clear soup, should be discouraged. For some patients who lack vitality, use of readily prepared microwave dinners with a rest prior to mealtime is helpful. A daily multivitamin and minerals supplement may be indicated.

Use of high-energy, high-protein supplements These products can be used to augment a patient's dietary intake. They are available in the form of milk, sweet and savoury drinks, fortified fruit juices, milkshake powder, glucose polymer powders and liquids, and puddings. Patients and caregivers need to be given complete instructions regarding their use to optimise this form of nutritional supplementation. Unfortunately, many studies found that in COPD the use of these supplements led to a reduction in usual energy intake and caused symptoms such as bloating, nausea, and early satiety. Oral supplements are probably less effective in older patients with a systematic inflammatory response.

Tube feeding Overnight tube feeding should be considered in patients with COPD when oral methods of maintaining nutritional status have failed, although few studies have investigated this method. The composition of tube feeds for patients with COPD has received attention. Carbon dioxide production (VCO_2) is higher when carbohydrates are the main energy sources and lower when fat is mainly oxidised. However, patients with COPD who are in a stable clinical state usually appear to tolerate carbohydrates without difficulty. Respiratory failure has not been reported in studies of patients with COPD receiving nutritional support with enteral feeds and nutritional supplements containing up to 54% carbohydrate, but further work is needed to determine the optimal and safest feeding regimens for these patients.

Feeding Patients on Artificial Ventilation

The artificial ventilator may be used to control the breathing patterns of patients who have acute breathing problems (e.g., respiratory failure with worsening blood gases). If the patient can be enterally fed, the composition of feed has a profound effect on gas exchanges, especially CO_2 production, and therefore respiratory quotient. This is expressed as the ratio of CO_2 produced to oxygen consumed. Because CO_2 production is greater during carbohydrate metabolism, a diet high in carbohydrate requires increased ventilation to eliminate the excess CO_2, whereas high-fat feeds reduce CO_2 production and are therefore potentially beneficial. Overfeeding negates any beneficial response to high-fat feeds because the conversion of energy to fat involves a disproportionately large production of CO_2.

Cystic Fibrosis

Definition and Etiology

In CF, there is widespread dysfunction of exocrine glands that causes chronic pulmonary disease; pancreatic enzyme deficiency; intestinal obstruction in the neonate (distal intestinal obstruction syndrome); liver disease; infertility, especially in males; and abnormally high concentrations of electrolytes in sweat, resulting from the failure of salt reabsorption in the sweat gland ducts. This is the most common inherited disease in Caucasian populations. A gene located on chromosome 7, coding for the protein called cystic fibrosis transmembrane regulator (CFTR), is defective. CFTR acts as a cyclic-AMP-activated chloride channel blocker. More than 800 mutations of the gene have been identified, and they are categorized into five classes on the basis of CTFR alterations. The most predominant mutation, which accounts for approximately 70% of all the CTFR genes worldwide, is $\Delta 508$, but there is geographical variation and it is less common in non-white races.

Although previously this disease was considered lethal in childhood, the median survival for newborns in the 1990s is predicted to be 40 years. Survival is largely dependent on the severity and progression of lung disease, and more than 90% of mortality is due to chronic bronchial infections and their complications. Patients with pancreatic insufficiency have a worse prognosis in terms of growth, pulmonary function, and long-term survival. The mortality of females is generally greater than that of males.

Incidence

CF affects 1 in 2500 births in Caucasian populations, 1 in 20 000 in black populations, and 1 in 1 million in Oriental populations. It is extremely rare in Japan, China, and black Africa.

Clinical Features

Most children with CF present with malabsorption and failure to thrive accompanied by recurrent or persistent chest infections. In the lungs, viscid mucus in the smaller airways predisposes to chronic infection, particularly with *Staphylococcus aureus* and *Haemophilis influenzae*, and subsequently with *Pseudomonas* species. This leads to damage of the bronchial wall, bronchietasis, and abscess formation.

Approximately 90% of CF patients have pancreatic insufficiency, requiring pancreatic enzyme supplements. Untreated patients pass frequent, large, pale, offensive, greasy stools. Ten to 15% of infants present with a meconium ileus resulting from the blockage of the terminal ileum by highly proteinaceous meconium at birth. Distal intestinal obstruction syndrome may occur later in childhood or adult life. In addition to these symptoms, a number of other complications may occur in CF that are identified in **Table 2**.

Chemical Pathology

CTRF regulates the chloride channel in the cell at its luminal surface, and its absence or dysfunction results in an abnormally high concentration of sodium in sweat and in a low water content in the mucus produced by airways, pancreas, and intestine. In the lung, this leads to ciliary dysfunction and repeated infection and colonisation with bacteria, resulting in a vicious cycle of bacterial colonization, 'lung inflammation,' and scarring. These in turn result in severe bronchiectasis, which progressively destroys lung function.

Table 2 Complications of cystic fibrosis

Respiratory
Pneumothorax
Asthma/wheezing
Hemoptysis
Nasal polyps
Respiratory failure
Cor pulmonale
Allergic bronchopulmonary aspergillosis

Gastrointestinal
Meconium ileus
Rectal prolapse
Distal intestinal obstruction syndrome
Abdominal distension
Colonic strictures
Intussusception
Gastro-oesophageal reflux
Biliary cirrhosis
Hepatomegaly
Portal hypertension
Cholelithiasis
Cholecystitis
Obstructive jaundice
Pancreatitis

Other
Diabetes
Male infertility
Amyloidosis
Arthropathy
Salt depletion
Growth failure/weight loss/failure to thrive
Delayed puberty
Osteopenia

Nutritional Management

Nutritional intervention is associated with better growth and improvement or stabilization of pulmonary function and possibly may improve survival in CF. Malnutrition has several adverse effects, including poor growth, impaired muscle function, decreased exercise tolerance, increased susceptibility to infection, and decreased ventilatory drive. Studies indicate that BMI strongly correlates with lung function, but the exact mechanism of this relationship has not been fully determined. Achieving optimum nutrition and growth may minimize the progressive decline in pulmonary function commonly seen in CF. As early as the 1970s, the Toronto CF clinic was able to show that a high-fat diet promoted a normal growth pattern and improved survival.

Reasons for Malnutrition

A variety of complex organic and psychosocial factors contribute to malnutrition in CF.

Malabsorption Pancreatic exocrine secretions contain less enzymes and bicarbonate, have a lower pH, and are of a smaller volume, and the physical properties of proteins and mucus within the lumen are affected. This results in obstruction to the small ducts and secondary damage to pancreatic digestive enzyme secretions causing malabsorption. Other problems, such as gastric hypersecretion, reduced duodenal bicarbonate concentration and pH, disorders of bile salt metabolism, disordered intestinal motility and permeability, liver disease, and short bowel syndrome after intestinal resection in the neonatal period, may contribute to malabsorption. The severity of malabsorption is variable, and there can be significant malabsorption of protein and fat-soluble vitamins despite adequate use of enzyme supplements.

Increased energy expenditure Resting energy expenditure, an estimate of basal metabolic rate, is 10–20% greater than in healthy controls and may contribute to energy imbalance. Increased REE appears to be closely associated with declining pulmonary function and subclinical infection. Bronchial sepsis leads to local release of leukotrienes, free oxygen radicals, and cytokines, including tumour necrosis factor-α. Antibiotics have been shown to reduce energy requirements of moderately ill patients with chronic *Pseudomonas aeruginosa*.

Anorexia and low energy intake Inadequate energy intake is often the main reason for growth failure in CF. Factors associated with a reduced appetite include

Chronic respiratory infection and other complications of CF, such as distal ileal obstruction syndrome, abdominal pain, GOR resulting in oesophagitis, pain, and vomiting
Behavior feeding problems in preschool and school-age children
Media pressure to eat a healthy low-fat, low-sugar diet
Inappropriate concepts regarding body image
Depression
Eating disorders in teenagers
Poor use of dietary supplements
Dislike of high-energy foods

Nutritional Support

Nutritional requirements will vary according to the clinical state as well as the age, sex, and activity of the individual. Because of the heterogeneity of CF, it is impossible to give universal recommendations. Crude estimates suggest an energy intake of 120–150% of estimated average requirements; it is better to assess and monitor energy intake and equate this to the nutritional status of the patient. If weight gain or growth is poor, the usual energy intake is increased by an additional 20–30% of total intake. Likewise, exact protein requirements are unknown; but it is generally accepted that the protein intake should be increased to compensate for excessive loss of nitrogen in the feces and sputum and increased protein turnover in malnourished patients. Protein should provide 15% of the total energy intake.

High-energy/high-protein diet The encouragement of a high-calorie, high-protein diet will produce growth in the majority of children and adults with CF. A good variety of energy-rich foods should be encouraged, such as full cream milk, cheese, meat, full cream yoghurt, milk puddings, cakes, and biscuits. Extra butter or margarine can be added to bread, potatoes, and vegetables. Frying foods or basting in oil will increase energy density. Extra milk or cream can be added to soups, cereal, desserts, or mashed potatoes and used to top canned or fresh fruit. Regular snacks are important. Malnourished children achieve higher energy intake when more frequent meals are offered. Attention should be given to psychological, social, behavioral, and developmental aspects of feeding. A meta-analysis of differing treatment interventions to promote weight gain in CF demonstrated that a behavioural approach was as effective in promoting weight gain as evasive medical procedures.

Dietary supplements Although almost half of adult patients take dietary supplements, there are few published data to demonstrate their efficacy in CF. One study was unable to show any improvement in height and weight z scores when up to 30% of energy requirements were supplied by a supplement for 3 months. As a consequence, dietary supplements should be reserved for weight loss, any decline in height z score, if intake of a range of nutrients does not meet dietary reference values, or during acute chest infections. They should complement normal food intake and not replace food. In order to avoid reducing the intake of normal food, the recommended quantities are age dependent and are given in **Table 3**.

Enteral nutrition Enteral feeding is more commonly used in teenagers and adults, reflecting their deterioration in nutritional status. It is considered if the patient is less than 85% expected weight for height, the patient's weight has declined by two centile positions, the patient has failed to gain weight over a 6-month period, or the patient has a BMI less than 19. Enteral feeding is associated with

Table 3 Recommended dosage of dietary supplements in cystic fibrosis

Age (years)	Daily dosage (Kcal)
1–2	200
3–5	400
6–11	600
>12	800

Adapted from MacDonald A (2001). Cystic fibrosis. In: Shaw V and Lawson M (eds.) *Clinical Paediatric Dietetics*, pp. 137–157. Oxford: Blackwell Scientific.

improvements in body fat, height, lean body mass, muscle mass, increased total body nitrogen, improved strength, and development of secondary sexual characteristics. To produce lasting benefit, numerous studies have demonstrated that enteral feeding should be continued long term. The choice of route used is influenced by the duration of feeding and the preference of the patient and family, but gastrostomies, sited by endoscopic placement, are usually chosen for long-term feeding (**Table 4**).

It is common practice to give enteral feeding for 8–10 h overnight, with at least 40–50% of the estimated energy requirement given via the feed. Most patients tolerate an energy-dense polymeric feed providing at least 1.5 kcal/ml with additional pancreatic enzymes. However, there is some support for the use of chemically defined elemental or short-chain peptide feeds. These are generally low in fat and are administered without the use of pancreatic enzymes, although there is little evidence to support this practice and it is disputed by some. Monitoring for glucose intolerance is important. Patients receiving supplemental feeds who demonstrate repeated blood sugar levels higher than 11.1 mmol/l during the feed may benefit from insulin given before the feed.

Vitamin and mineral supplements Malabsorption of fat-soluble vitamins is likely in most pancreatic-insufficient patients with CF, and the United Kingdom recommends vitamin A, D, and E supplements. Low fat-soluble vitamin concentrations are associated with poorer clinical status and reduced lung function. Clinical features of vitamin A deficiency include night blindness, conjunctival and corneal xerosis, dry thickened skin, and abnormalities of bronchial mucosal epithelialisation. Vitamin A status is difficult to assess due to lack of a reliable marker and serum levels of retinol do not adequately mirror the concentration of vitamin A in the liver. Some researchers have found liver stores of vitamin A in CF to be 2.5 times higher than those in control subjects, despite lower serum levels of retinol and retinol binding protein.

Table 4 Advantages and disadvantages of enteral feeding routes

Method	Advantages	Disadvantages
Nasogastric	Short-term feeding	Tube reinsertion may be Distressing to patient/caregiver/nurse Easily removed Risk of aspiration Discomfort to nasopharynx Psychosocial implications
Nasojejunal	Less risk of aspiration Short-term feeding	Difficulty of insertion Radiographic check of position Easily removed Risk of perforation Abdominal pain and diarrhoea unless continuous infusion of feed Discomfort in nasopharynx Reflux of bile is facilitated
Gastrostomy	Cosmetically more acceptable Long-term feeding	Increase reflux if present Local skin irritation Infection Granulation tissue Leakage Gastric distension Stoma closes within a few hours if accidentally removed
Jejunostomy	Reduced risk of aspiration Long-term feeding	Surgical/radiology procedure Risk of perforation Must be constant infusion of feed Bacterial overgrowth Dumping syndrome can occur

Adapted from MacDonald A, Holden C, and Johnston T (2001) Paediatric enteral nutrition. In Payne-James J, Grimble G, and Silk D (eds.) *Artificial Nutrition Support in Clinical Practice*, pp. 347–366. London: Greenwich Medical Media.

Decreased bone mineral density and osteopenia associated with low 25-hydroxyvitamin D levels have been described in patients with CF but may be related to poor nutritional status and delayed puberty. Rickets is rarely seen. Possible contributory factors include low body mass index, disease severity, inadequate calcium intake, delayed puberty, or widespread use of systemic or inhaled steroids.

Blood levels of vitamin E are nearly always low unless supplements are given. In older patients, undetectable serum concentrations of vitamin E have been noted in association with neurological syndromes. Symptoms and signs include absent deep tendon reflexes, loss of position sense and vibration sense in lower limbs, dysarthria, tremor, ataxia, and decreased visual activity.

Some CF centres recommend routine salt supplements to all CF infants on normal infant formula, which is low in sodium, and CF patients during hot weather. Anorexia and poor growth may result from chronic salt depletion. Significant hyponatremia may be accompanied by vomiting.

Pancreatic Enzymes

Approximately 90% of patients with CF require pancreatic enzymes to reduce steatorrhea. They are based on animal pancreatic extracts; presented in powder; tablet, or capsule form; and contain a combination of lipase, protease, and amylase. In addition to enzyme content, many factors affect bioavailability of pancreatic enzymes, including enzyme source, manufacturing process, stability, enteric coating of acid-resistant tablets, formulation as either microspheres or microtablets, and particle size. The smallest dose of pancreatin to control steatorrhoea and achieve a normal pattern of growth and weight gain should be used. The Committee on Safety for Medicines recommends that patients with CF not exceed a daily dose of enzymes equivalent to 10 000 IU lipase/kg/day.

Asthma

Definition and Etiology

The word 'asthma' originates from an ancient Greek word meaning panting. It is a chronic obstructive disease characterized by tracheobronchial hyperreactivity leading to paroxysmal airway narrowing, which may reverse spontaneously or as a result of treatment. The smooth muscle surrounding the bronchi has an abnormally increased reaction to stimuli. Specific bronchial stimuli include inhaled allergens (e.g., house-dust mite, pollen, and moulds). Nonspecific bronchial stimuli include upper respiratory tract infections, cold air, exercise, cigarette smoke, excitement, emotional stress, and chemical irritants. Aspirin and other nonsteroidal antiinflammatory medications provoke asthma in some patients.

Prevalence

Since the 1980s there has been a worldwide increase in the prevalence of asthma in both children and adults. This escalating prevalence has led to significant increases in morbidity and mortality due to the disease. It is the most common chronic respiratory disorder, affecting 3–5% of adults and 10–15% of schoolchildren. Half of the people with asthma develop it before age 10, and most develop it before age 30. In childhood, it is twice as common in boys as in girls, but by adolescence equal numbers are affected. Asthma symptoms can decrease over time, especially in children. Many people with asthma have an individual and/or family history of allergies, such as hay fever (allergic rhinitis) or eczema. Others have no history of allergies or evidence of allergic problems.

It is responsible for 10–20% of all acute medical admissions in pediatric wards in children aged 1–16 years. There are 15–20 deaths from asthma in children each year in the United Kingdom. However, from 1979 to 1999, mortality rates of asthma have decreased in England and Wales in all age groups up to 65 years.

Clinical Features

Asthma is characterized clinically by wheezing, dyspnea, and cough. Coughing commonly produces small amounts of yellowish sputum or bronchial plugs. Some patients present with breathlessness. Most people with asthma have periodic wheezing attacks separated by symptom-free periods. Other asthmatics may have cough as their predominant symptom. Asthma attacks can last minutes to days.

Chemical Pathology

The development and phenotypic expression of allergic airway disease depend on a complex interaction between genetic and environmental factors. Exposure of the sensitized airway to a number of trigger factors results in bronchoconstriction, mucosal oedema, and excessive mucus production that in turn leads to airway narrowing and the clinical features of asthma. Airway inflammation is due to an immune-mediated process in which inflammatory cells and inflammatory mediators enter airway tissues to cause disease. Many cell-mediated immunologic factors participate in the inflammatory process of asthma. The most important inflammatory cells involved are eosinophils, mast cells, and T lymphocytes. The first months of life seem to be a particularly vulnerable period and there is evidence that sensitization is related to the level of allergen exposure during early life.

Dietary Management

There is an increasing interest in the relationship between nutrition and asthma. Associations have been reported between the intake of fruit and the antioxidant vitamins A, C, and E and selenium. Suboptimal nutrient intake may enhance asthmatic inflammation, consequently contributing to bronchial hyperreactivity. There is some suggestion that people who have a diet rich in fruit and vegetables have a lower risk of poor respiratory health, and this may be due to the antioxidant nutrients that food contains. Several issues need to be addressed before causality of these associations can be established. Nevertheless, it appears reasonable to issue dietary guidelines for the primary and secondary prevention of asthma that are in line with a healthy diet for the prevention of coronary heart disease and cancer.

Epidemiological studies also suggest that a diet high in marine fatty acids (fish oil) may have beneficial effects on asthma. However, a Cochrane review of nine randomized controlled trials conducted between 1986 and 2001 indicated there is little evidence to recommend that people with asthma supplement or modify their dietary intake of marine n-3 fatty acids (fish oil) in order to improve their asthma control. Equally, there is no evidence that they are at risk if they do so.

Food intolerance There is much controversy surrounding the role of food in the development and onset of asthma. Evidence suggests that atopic or asthmatic parents, whose children have a high risk of developing asthma, should be advised to avoid smoking during pregnancy; avoid cigarette smoke exposure after the child is born; undertake house dust mite control strategies; exclusively breast-feed their infants for 6 months; and subsequently provide their child with a nutritious, balanced diet. In contrast, there is little to suggest that a low allergen diet for high-risk women during pregnancy is likely to reduce the risk of having an atopic child.

Generally, the incidence of food intolerance in asthma is thought to be small, although there is evidence that intolerance to foods may act as a trigger for some cases of asthma. Common food allergens identified include milk, eggs, nuts, orange squash, wheat, and red wine. The additives sulfur dioxide, tartrazine, sodium benzoate, and salicylates have been implicated, although in the case of sulfur dioxide its ability to cause asthma depends on the nature of the food to which it is added, the level of residual sulfur dioxide in the food, and the sensitivity of the patient. Foods such as nuts, cola drinks, ice, and those cooked in oil have been found to cause symptoms more frequently in Asian children. Many of the studies that have identified certain foodstuffs as triggering asthma have had limitations or flaws in their design, leading to difficulties in interpreting and extrapolating their results.

Both immediate and delayed-onset symptoms have been reported in asthma. The use of diagnostic diets is difficult, partly because of the variability of asthma, delayed reactions, effect of other precipitating triggers, and dangers of inducing an asthma attack during food challenges. A simple exclusion diet excluding food(s) implicated on history is perhaps the most useful diagnostic diet. Because of the inherent problems with asthma, strict food diets are rarely used.

High-sodium diets Epidemiological studies have suggested that dietary salt may play a role in airway responsiveness and a high salt intake may act as a trigger for asthma. A correlation between regional mortality from asthma and purchase of table salt per person has been reported in England and Wales. Epidemiological studies have also suggested an association between a higher dietary sodium intake and a higher prevalence of self-reported wheeze in adults and children. However, not all of the evidence supports this hypothesis. At least three epidemiological surveys and two experimental studies found no evidence of an association between sodium intake and asthma.

See also: **Cancer**: Epidemiology of Lung Cancer. **Cystic Fibrosis**. **Food Intolerance**. **Malnutrition**: Primary, Causes Epidemiology and Prevention; Secondary, Diagnosis and Management. **Nutritional Support**: Adults, Enteral. **Sodium**: Physiology. **Supplementation**: Role of Micronutrient Supplementation.

Further Reading

Ardern KD and Ram FS (2001) Dietary salt reduction or exclusion for allergic asthma. *Cochrane Database of Systematic Reviews* 2001(4): CD000436.

Berry JK and Baum CL (2001) Malnutrition in chronic obstructive pulmonary disease: Adding insult to injury. *AACN Clinical Issues* 12: 210–219.

Couriel J (1997) Respiratory disorders. In: Lissauer T and Clayden G (eds.) *Illustrated Textbook of Paediatrics*, pp. 157–171. London: Mosby.

Felbinger TW, Suchner U, Peter K, and Askanazi J (2001) Nutrition support in respiratory disease. In: Payne-James J, Grimble G, and Silk D (eds.) *Artificial Nutrition Support in Clinical Practice*, pp. 537–552. London: Greenwich Medical Media.

Ferreira IM, Brooks D, Lacasse Y, Goldstein RS, and White J (2002) Nutritional supplementation for stable chronic obstructive pulmonary disease. *Cochrane Database of Systematic Reviews* 2002(1): CD000998.

Hind CRK and Walshaw MJ (1996) Chest disease. In: Axford J (ed.) *Medicine*. Oxford: Blackwell Science.

Hodge L, Yan KY, and Loblay RL (1996) Assessment of food chemical intolerance in adult asthmatic subjects. *Thorax* Sl: 805–809.

Kramer MS (2002) Maternal antigen avoidance during pregnancy for preventing atopic disease in infants of women at high risk. *Cochrane Database of Systematic Reviews* 2000(2): CD000133.

MacDonald A (2001) Cystic fibrosis. In: Shaw V and Lawson M (eds.) *Clinical Paediatric Dietetics*, pp. 137–157. Oxford: Blackwell Scientific.

MacDonald A, Holden C, and Johnston T (2001) Paediatric enteral nutrition. In: Payne-James J, Grimble G, and Silk D (eds.) *Artificial Nutrition Support in Clinical Practice*, pp. 347–366. London: Greenwich Medical Media.

Manaher S and Burke F (1996) Pulmonary disease. In: Morrison G and Hark L (eds.) *Medical Nutrition and Disease*, pp. 279–287. Oxford: Blackwell Science.

Mickleborough TD, Gotshall RW, Cordain L, and Lindley M (2001) Dietary salt alters pulmonary function during exercise in exercise-induced asthmatics. *Journal of Sports Science* 19(11): 865–873.

Price D and Duerden M (2003) Chronic obstructive pulmonary disease. *British Medical Journal* 326(7398): 1046–1047.

Stratton RJ, Green CJ, and Elia M (2003) *Disease-Related Malnutrition: An Evidence Based Approach to Treatment.* Cambridge, UK: CABI.

UK Cystic Fibrosis Trust Nutrition Working Group (2002) *Nutritional Management of Cystic Fibrosis.* London: Cystic Fibrosis Trust.

Woods RK, Thien FC, and Abramson MJ (2002) Dietary marine fatty acids (fish oil) for asthma in adults and children. *Cochrane Database of Systematic Reviews* 2002(3): CD001283.

LYCOPENES AND RELATED COMPOUNDS

C J Bates, MRC Human Nutrition Research, Cambridge, UK

Introduction

Lycopene, the most abundant pigment in ripe red tomatoes and in a few other fruits, is one of the major carotenoid pigments that is widely present in the diet of the human population in the world today. **Figure 1** illustrates the chemical formula of selected carotenoids that occur widely both in human diets and in the noncellular fraction of human blood in most regions of the world. Carotenoids are yellow-to-red in color, with lycopene being nearer the red end of the carotenoid series. However, unlike the carotenes and cryptoxanthins, it does not possess a beta-ionone ring structure at either end of the molecule, and this precludes it from becoming a precursor of vitamin A in humans and animals. Nevertheless, it is readily transformed from the all-*trans* form that is characteristic of most plants and plant foods for animals and humans, to a range of mono- and di-*cis* forms within the animal's body. In addition, oxidation to epoxides and hydroxylated derivatives occurs, although the control of these oxidation pathways and the nature of their products are not yet well understood or characterized.

In plant tissues, where it is synthesized, lycopene is thought to help protect vulnerable photosynthetic tissues from light- and oxygen-catalyzed damage. Its role in humans and other animals, which can only obtain the pigment from their diet, is less well understood. Indeed it remains unproven that there is an essential role for lycopene in animal tissues. Nevertheless, considerable research effort is currently being undertaken to test hypotheses that are attempting to link human dietary and tissue lycopene levels to the risk of degenerative diseases, such as vascular diseases, cancers, etc., especially in older people. As discussed in more detail below, this research is being performed in a wide range of tissue culture and animal model systems and human epidemiological studies.

In this article, some key aspects of the chemical and physical properties, the dietary sources, biochemical status indices, and biological significance of lycopene will be described.

Chemical and Physical Properties of Lycopene; its Food Sources and Enteral Absorption

Lycopene is the most commonly encountered of that subgroup of the naturally occurring carotenoids that have a straight-chain poly-isoprenoid molecule without any terminal β-ionone ring structures (**Figure 1**). The chain length and number of conjugated double bonds determine the absorption spectrum, which peaks at 472 nm with a molar extinction coefficient, $\varepsilon^{1\%}$ of 3450. It is one of the most nonpolar members of the carotenoids, and in organic solution it is also one of the most easily oxidized and thus is easily destroyed, which necessitates the use of rigorous precautions against its oxidative destruction during its extraction and analysis from plants, foods, animal tissues, and body fluids. Currently, such analytical determination is usually based on high-performance liquid chromatography (HPLC), using either its characteristic light absorption property, or its natural fluorescence, or its redox character, for detection and quantitation by absorbance or fluorometric or electrochemical detection. Another characteristic that greatly affects its stability and the problems of its storage and analysis is the phenomenon of *cis-trans* isomerization. Naturally occurring lycopene in tomatoes, the major human food source of this carotenoid, is nearly 100% all-*trans* (**Figure 1**), but during the processing of food, and then during the processes of absorption and accumulation in animal tissues, there is a progressive increase in the proportion of a variety of *cis*-forms. Most of these *cis*-forms contain a single *cis*-bond (mono-*cis*-lycopene), and the 5-, 9-, 13- and 15- mono-*cis*-lycopenes account for more than 50% of the total lycopene in human serum. Smaller quantities of di-*cis*-lycopenes are normally also present. Curiously, another food source of lycopene, red palm oil, has a much higher natural proportion of the *cis*-forms of the pigment. Isomerization is catalyzed by low pH; therefore, stomach acid is believed to be a major factor in the conversion of the all-*trans*-lycopene ingested from tomatoes and their products to a mixture of *cis*-forms in the digestive tract. There is also evidence that further isomerization occurs between the digestive tract and the portal lymphatic lipid micelles. The *cis*-isomers differ from the all-*trans* form in their absorption and intertissue transportation properties, and also in their functional characteristics; for instance, they are more soluble in lipophilic solvents and structures and

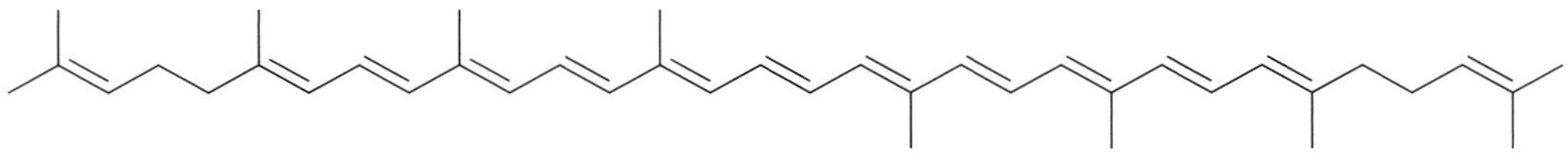

All-*trans* lycopene

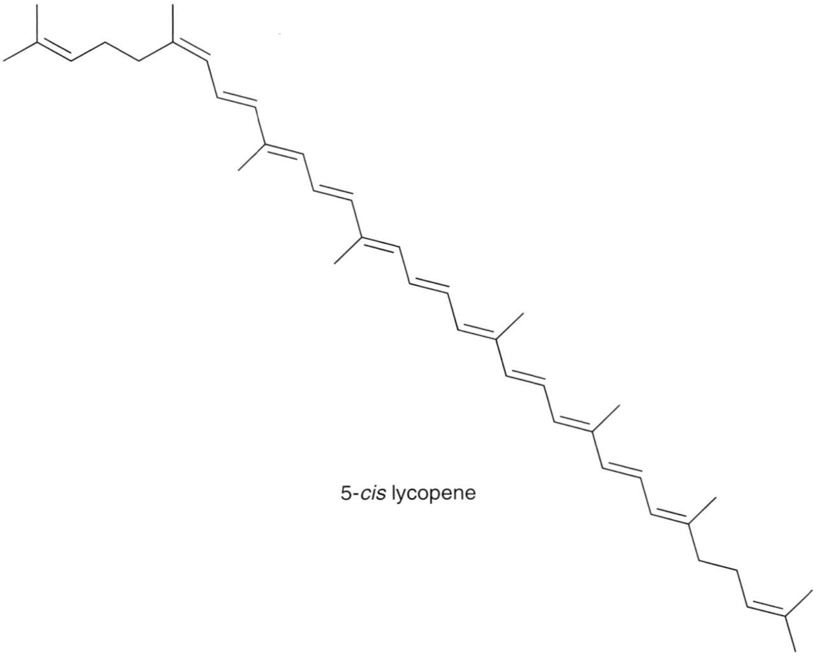

5-*cis* lycopene

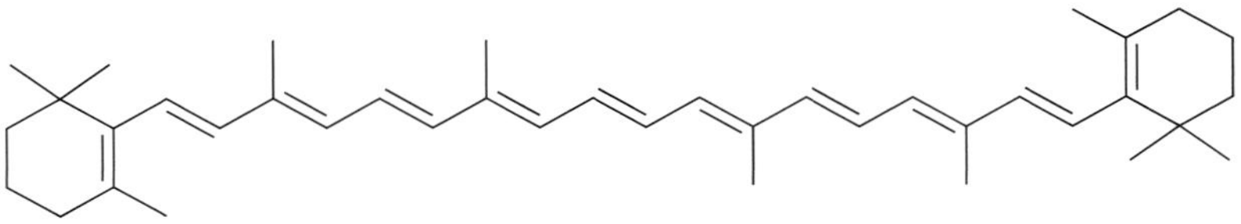

All-*trans* β-carotene

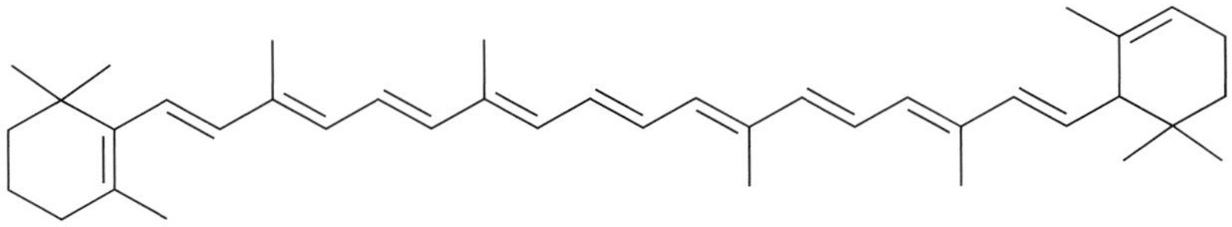

All-*trans* α-carotene

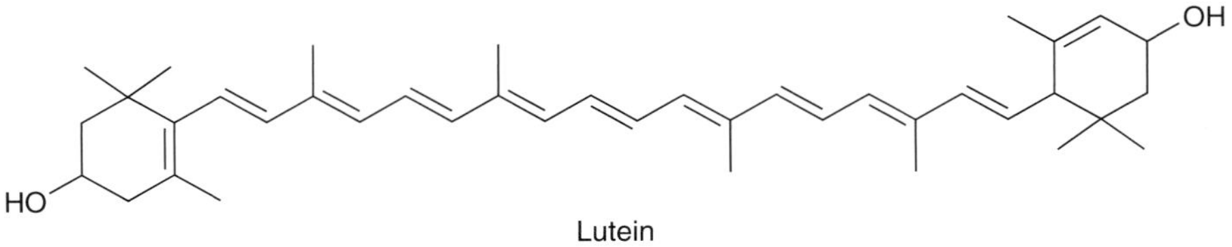

Lutein

Figure 1 Structures of lycopene and certain other carotenoids found in human blood and tissues.

are less likely to aggregate into crystalline forms. However, these physicochemical differences and their biological consequences have yet to be adequately explored and described.

Of all the most common naturally occurring carotenoids, lycopene is by far the most efficient in reacting with and quenching singlet oxygen, $^1O_2$, which is a non-free-radical excited and reactive

Table 1 Lycopene content of selected foods

Food category	Content as summarized by Clinton (1998) (mg per 100 g wet weight)
Fresh tomatoes	0.9–4.2
Canned tomatoes	
Tomato sauce	6.2
Tomato paste	5–150
Tomato juice	5–12
Tomato ketchup	10–13
Tomato soup	
Grapefruit	3.4
Guava	5.4
Papaya	2–5.3
Watermelon	2.3–7.2

Source: Clinton SK (1998) Lycopene: Chemistry, biology and implication for human health and disease. *Nutrition Reviews* **56**: 35–51.

form of oxygen. This form of oxygen reacts rapidly with lycopene to yield nonexcited triplet oxygen and excited triplet lycopene. The latter then dissipates its extra energy by solvent interactions, thus regenerating nonexcited lycopene and preserving its original structure by recycling. However, another of its chemical interactions with molecular oxygen appears to result in irreversible oxidation to yield one or more cyclic epoxides, which then probably undergo ring-opening. Nevertheless, there are many unresolved questions about the nature and importance of the many degradation and catabolic pathways that are believed to result in the irreversible destruction of lycopene both *in vitro* and *in vivo*.

Lycopene is an essential intermediate in the pathway for synthesis of the β-ionone ring-containing carotenoids such as β-carotene in plant tissues, and in most plant tissues it is present in only minor amounts. However, in a few, including tomato fruit, watermelon, and red grapefruit, this conversion to the β-ionone ring products by the enzyme lycopene cyclase is hindered, so that the intermediate carotenoid forms, lycopene, phytoene and phytofluene, accumulate instead.

In the US, tomato products provide more than 85% of the total quantity of lycopene consumed by the human population. Mean lycopene intakes in the US are considerably greater than they are in the UK, where the mean daily intake is thought to be less than one-third that in the US, while lycopene intakes in Far Eastern countries such as China and Thailand appear to be much lower still. Wild tomatoes originated in Central America and were introduced into Europe following the opening up of the New World,

and were later introduced back into North America from Europe. Because tomatoes are the major source of dietary lycopene in many human populations, some epidemiological studies have been designed on the simplistic assumption that tomato consumption can be used as a general proxy for lycopene consumption, and that any disease associations with tomato consumption can be attributed to the biological effects of lycopene. However, tomatoes also contain significant amounts of other carotenoids, vitamin C, bioflavonoids such as naringenin, and phenolic acids such as chlorogenic acid. Much of the existing epidemiological evidence for possible beneficial effects of lycopene (see below) cannot distinguish unequivocally between the biological effects of lycopene and those of the many other bioactive constituents present in tomatoes.

The bioavailability of lycopene from raw tomatoes is low, but it is greatly increased by cooking or by commercial processing such as conversion to soup, sauce, ketchup, etc., and its availability is also increased by increasing the fat content of the food. Interactions with other carotenoids are complex and have only partly been studied, for instance β-carotene in the same dish seems to increase the absorption of lycopene, but large doses of β-carotene given separately seem to decrease the lycopene content of serum lipoproteins. The contribution of several categories of tomato product to intakes in a recent survey of older people in Britain is shown in **Table 2**. The strength of the correlation between dietary lycopene intake and blood (serum or plasma) lycopene concentration varies greatly among studies

Table 2 Tomato products consumed by people aged 65 years and over in Britain

Categories of tomatoes and tomato products	Percentage of each category consumed
Raw tomatoes	36.2
Processed tomatoes	
Soups	8.8
Canned tomatoes	7.0
Grilled	5.4
Fried	3.2
Ketchup	0.4
Tomato-based products	
Canned food	29.5
Pizza	2.3
Other	7.1
Total	99.9

Source: Re R, Mishra GD, Thane CW, and Bates CJ (2003) Tomato consumption and plasma lycopene concentration in people aged 65 years and over in a British National Survey. *European Journal of Clinical Nutrition* **57**: 1545–1554. Reproduced with permission from Nature Publishing Group.

and clearly depends on many factors, one of which is the degree of sophistication of the food table values, since subtle differences in food sources and meal composition affect its bioavailability very considerably.

Tissue Contents and Kinetics of Lycopene Turnover

Once absorbed, passively from lipid micelles by the enterocyte, lycopene enters the portal lymphatics and thence the liver, from which it enters the peripheral bloodstream, mainly in association with the β-lipoproteins, in which it is transported to the peripheral tissues. Its half-life in plasma is of the order of 12–33 days; longer than that of β-carotene, which is less than 12 days. Clearly, many of these factors are interdependent, and there is a need for further clarification of the key independent determinants of lycopene status, and whether plasma levels can provide an adequate picture of tissue and whole body status.

Patients with alcoholic cirrhosis of the liver have greatly reduced hepatic lycopene concentrations; indeed, hepatic lycopene seems to offer a sensitive index of hepatic health. Studies of organ concentrations (**Table 3**), suggest a gradient from circulating levels in plasma to different ones in specific tissues. The different carotenoid ratios between organs (not shown) also indicate selective transport and accumulation. However, the mechanisms involved are poorly understood. No lycopene is detectable in the retina or lens of the eye, where lutein and zeaxanthin are found; however, lycopene is present in the ciliary body.

Table 3 Concentrations of lycopene reported in human tissues

Tissue	Range of mean or median lycopene concentrations (nmol per g wet weight)
Adrenal	1.9–21.6
Testis	4.3–21.4
Liver	0.6–5.7
Brain	2.5
Lung	0.2–0.6
Kidney	0.1–0.6
Stomach, colon	0.2–0.3
Breast, cervix	0.2–0.8
Skin	0.4
Adipose tissue	0.2–1.3
Prostate	0.1–0.6
Plasma	0.2–1.1

Values were gathered from 11 publications, all based on HPLC analyses.

Functional Properties and Tissue Health

The capacity for quenching of singlet oxygen has been mentioned above; the exceptionally high rate constant, $K = 3.1 \times 10^{10}\,mol^{-1}\,s^{-1}$, renders it one of the most efficient of known quenchers of this powerful oxidant. In the plant, it probably protects chlorophyll, which produces singlet oxygen as a by-product of photosynthesis. In experiments with lymphoid cells, lycopene provided better protection against singlet oxygen damage than several other carotenoids tested. In skin exposed to UV light, lycopene disappears much more rapidly than β-carotene. Lycopene is also able, in model systems, to inhibit the peroxidation of polyunsaturated lipids and the oxidation of DNA bases to products such as 8-hydroxydeoxyguanosine (8-OHdG). It can react directly with hydrogen peroxide and nitrogen dioxide.

Several studies in cell culture have shown a reduction in the formation of oxidation damage products such as malondialdehyde, and have found less injury to cells exposed to oxidants such as carbon tetrachloride, if lycopene (or other carotenoids) are present.

Another characteristic of lycopene and other carotenoids that may be relevant to inhibition of cancer cell growth is the modulation of gap junction cell–cell communication processes. In particular, carotenoids including lycopene have been shown to enhance the efficacy of the protein, connexin43, which helps to ensure the maintenance of the differentiated state of cells and to reduce the probability of unregulated cell division, and which is deficient in many tumors. They may also interact with and enhance the synthesis of binding proteins that downregulate the receptor for the growth-promoting hormone insulin-like growth factor-1 (IGF-1).

In certain circumstances, lycopene can reduce LDL-cholesterol levels, possibly by inhibiting hydroxymethylglutaryl CoA reductase (HMGCoA reductase), the rate-limiting enzyme for cholesterol synthesis (see below). Lycopene was shown to have modest hypocholesterolemic properties in one small clinical trial.

Health, Research Models and Epidemiological Evidence

Table 4 summarizes the various types of evidence that have been used to test the hypothesis that lycopene may have health-promoting or protective properties in man. The ultimate proof of efficacy, which would be long-term controlled intervention studies with clinical diseases and or mortality as the end points, are extremely difficult,

Table 4 Types of evidence being sought, that a nutrient such as lycopene may protect against oxidation-induced or other disease processes

1. Model *in vitro* systems, e.g., oxygen-derived free-radical trapping in pure chemical mixtures.
2. Tissue (cell and organ) cultures, e.g., reduction of optical opacity development in cultured eye lenses; reduced growth rates or apoptosis in tumor cell cultures.
3. Animal studies demonstrating a reduction of oxidation-induced damage or disease with lycopene supplements or with lycopene-rich foods such as tomatoes or tomato products.
4. Human observation studies using intermediate biochemical markers: e.g., inverse relationships between lycopene intakes or its blood levels and biochemical markers, such as lipid or DNA oxidation products.
5. Studies using pathology-related intermediate markers, e.g., arterial thickening or reduced arterial elasticity; precancerous polyposis, etc.
6. Relationships (without intervention) between tomato intakes or estimated lycopene intakes or lycopene contents of serum, plasma, or tissues (e.g., fat biopsies) and actual disease prevalence or incidence in human cross-sectional, case-control, or prospective epidemiological studies.
7. Intervention studies: lycopene supplements producing a reduction in biochemical markers of oxidation damage or in functional markers, or, eventually, in actual human disease incidence or progression.

expensive, and time-consuming to obtain, and cannot address all possible benefits in a single intervention trial.

The two disease categories that have so far received most attention for possible long-term benefits of lycopene have been the amelioration of cancers and of heart disease. Both benefits are plausible in view of the physicochemical and biological properties of lycopene outlined above, because both categories of disease are characterized by tissue damage, which is thought to be induced or exacerbated by reactive oxygen species in the environment or those generated within the body.

Evidence for Possible Anticancer Protection by Lycopene

Most of the indications with respect to cancer comes from human studies linking tomato intake, total estimated lycopene intake, and serum or plasma lycopene concentrations to the subsequent development of cancers (**Table 5**). There is a small amount of evidence from experimental animal studies, for instance, rat and mouse dimethylbenzanthracene-induced mammary tumor studies have supported

the hypothesis, as has a model of spontaneous mammary tumor formation in one strain of mice, but many of the animal models of tumor promotion have been criticized as being too dissimilar from the likely processes of spontaneous tumorigenesis in humans.

Partly for historical reasons, there has been a particular interest in prostate cancer (**Table 5**). A large and early trial in the US (US Health Professionals Follow-up Study) reported an impressive difference between groups with high and low intakes of tomatoes and hence of lycopene for subsequent prostate cancer development, which was not shared with other carotenoids. Plausibility was enhanced by the fact that although human prostate lycopene concentrations are not especially high on an absolute basis (**Table 3**), they are higher than those of other carotenoids in this tissue. Subsequent studies have had variable outcomes. A small pilot study reported that tomato oleoresin supplements given for a short period to prostate cancer sufferers who were due for radical prostatectomy resulted in smaller tumor size and other apparent benefits, but this trial now needs to be repeated on a larger scale.

Table 5 Summary evidence for possible lycopene protection against prostate cancer

No. of studies	Locations	Total no. of participants	Types of trial	Outcome conclusion
2	Greece, Canada	937	Case–control (intake of tomato or lycopene, or blood level)	Significant association
7	USA, UK, Canada, New Zealand	3824	As above	No significant association
3	USA	954	Prospective studies based on dietary estimates	Significant association
1	Netherlands		As above	No association
3	USA	723	Prospective studies based on serum or plasma lycopene	Inconclusive; one study found a marginal ($P = 0.05$) benefit vs. aggressive cancer

Table 6 Summary evidence of association of relatively high serum or plasma lycopene with lowered risk of cardiovascular disease (CVD)

Study	Location	Sex (total participants)	Types of trial and outcome measures	Outcome conclusion
Euramic	Europe, multicenter	M (1379)	C-C, MI	Significant association with protection[a]
ARIC	USA	M + F (462)	C-C, IMT	NS
Street	USA	M + F (369)	NC-C, MI in smokers	NS
Rotterdam	Netherlands	M + F (216)	C-C, PC	Significant association with protection
Bruneck	Italy	M + F (392)	CS + PFU, PC	NS
Linkoping –Vinus	Sweden and Lithuania	M (210)	CS, mortality from heart disease	NS
Kuopio (KHID)	Finland	M (725)	PFU, acute coronary event or stroke	Significant association with protection
Kuopio (ASP)	Finland	M + F (520)	IMT	Males significant; females not significant.

[a]No association with plasma β-carotene in this study.

C-C, case–control study; NC-C, nested case–control study; CS, cross-sectional study; PFU, prospective follow-up study; MI, myocardial infarct; IMT, intima-media thickness estimate; PC, plaque count. NS, no significant evidence for protection.Significance generally after appropriate adjustment for other known CVD risk factors.

Several studies have provided evidence for protection of certain regions of the digestive tract against tumor occurrence or growth. Two studies, one in Iran and another in Italy, found an inverse relationship between esophageal cancer and tomato consumption. Two Italian and one Japanese study reported evidence for protection against gastric cancer, and two studies claimed a reduction in pancreatic cancer. Results with others cancer have been mixed and inconclusive.

Lycopene and Cardiovascular Disease

Table 6 summarizes the evidence. The European Multicentre Euramic Study, which reported that risk of developing myocardial infarct was inversely related to lycopene intake, after appropriate adjustment for other cardiovascular risk factors. Some Scandinavian studies have subsequently supported this claim; moreover, lycopene is capable of reducing LDL-cholesterol levels, possibly by inhibiting hydroxymethylglutaryl CoA reductase (HMGCoA reductase), the rate-limiting enzyme for cholesterol synthesis.

Other Disease-Related Investigations

In an organ culture model, some evidence for protection of rat lenses against induction of cataractogenesis has been reported. There is good reason to believe that carotenoids in general may play a role in the protection of ocular tissues against the damaging effects of UV light and of reactive oxygen substances, whose exposure to light carries some analogy with the known functions of carotenoids in plant tissues. A possible protective role in the ciliary body and iris has been proposed, but not yet tested.

Conclusions

Clearly lycopene possesses chemical and biological properties, which make it a very attractive candidate for tissue protection and reduction of disease, especially degenerative diseases. Lycopene probably interacts more efficiently with one particular reactive oxygen species, singlet oxygen, than any other commonly occurring nutrient. It appears to share with several other carotenoids the capacity to reduce lipid peroxidation and DNA oxidative damage, and to enhance cell–cell gap junction communication and to protect normal IGF-1 function. It may reduce cholesterol formation and its tissue accumulation in some circumstances. Studies related to cancers and cardiovascular disease are ongoing and are attracting increased research interest.

See also: **Alcohol**: Disease Risk and Beneficial Effects. **Antioxidants**: Diet and Antioxidant Defense; Observational Studies; Intervention Studies. **Ascorbic Acid**: Physiology, Dietary Sources and Requirements. **Carotenoids**: Chemistry, Sources and Physiology; Epidemiology of Health Effects. **Fruits and Vegetables**. **Vitamin A**: Biochemistry and Physiological Role; Deficiency and Interventions.

Further Reading

Arab L and Steck S (2000) Lycopene and cardiovascular disease. *American Journal of Clinical Nutrition* **71**(supplement): 1691S–1695S.

Arab L, Steck-Scott S, and Bowen P (2001) Participation of lycopene and beta-carotene in carcinogenesis: Defenders, aggressors or passive bystanders? *Epidemiologic Reviews* **23**: 211–230.

Britton G (1995) Structure and properties of carotenoids in relation to function. *FASEB J* **9**: 1551–1558.

Clinton SK (1998) Lycopene: chemistry, biology, and implications for human health and disease. *Nutrition Reviews* **56**: 35–51.

Gerster H (1997) The potential of lycopene for human health. *Journal of the American College of Nutrition* **16**: 109–126.

Giovanucci E (1999) Tomatoes, tomato-based products, lycopene, and cancer: review of the epidemiologic literature. *Journal of the National Cancer Institute* **91**: 317–331.

International Symposium on the Role of Tomato Products and Carotenoids in Disease Prevention (2002) 14 review articles by different authors, plus 17 symposium abstracts. *Experimental Biology and Medicine* **227**: 843–937.

Nguyen ML and Schwartz SJ (1999) Lycopene: chemical and biological properties. *Food Technology* **53**: 38–45.

Rao AV and Agarwal S (1999) Role of lycopene as antioxidant carotenoid in the prevention of chronic diseases: A review. *Nutrition Research* **19**: 305–323.

Stahl W and Sies H (1996) Lycopene: a biologically important carotenoid for humans? *Archives of Biochemistry and Biophysics* **336**: 1–9.

Weisburger J (1998) International symposium on lycopene and tomato products in disease prevention. *Proceedings of the Society for Experimental Biology and Medicine* **218**: 93–143.

MAGNESIUM

C Feillet-Coudray and Y Rayssiguier, National
Institute for Agricultural Research, Clermont-Ferrand,
France

Magnesium (Mg), the second intracellular cation after
sodium, is a essential mineral. It is a critical cofactor in
more than 300 enzymatic reactions. It may be required
for substrate formation (Mg-ATP) and enzyme activation. It is critical for a great number of cellular functions, including oxidative phosphorylation, glycolysis,
DNA transcription, and protein synthesis. It is
involved in ion currents and membrane stabilization.
Mg deficiency may be implicated in various metabolic
disorders, including cardiovascular diseases, immune
dysfunction and free radical damage.

Magnesium Metabolism

Distribution of Mg within the Body

The normal adult body contains approximately 25 g
of Mg, with more than 60% in bone tissue
(**Table 1**). Only a fraction of bone Mg (at the
surface of the bone crystal) is exchangeable with
extracellular Mg. The muscle contains 25% of
total body Mg, and extracellular Mg accounts for
only 1%. Plasma Mg is approximately 0.8 mmol/l,
half of which is ionised and active in physiological
reactions half bound to proteins or complexed to
anions. In cells, Mg is associated with various
structures, such as the nucleus and intracellular
organelles, and free Mg accounts for 1–5% of total
cellular Mg. Intracellular free Mg is maintained at a
relatively constant level, even if extracellular Mg
level varies. This phenomenon is due to the limited
permeability of the plasma membrane to Mg and the
existence of specific Mg transport systems that regulate the rates at which Mg is taken up by cells or
extruded from cells. Mechanisms by which Mg is
taken up by cells have not been completely
elucidated, and Mg efflux particularly requires the
antiport Na^+/Mg^{2+}. Various hormonal and
pharmacological factors influence Mg transport,
and it can be assumed that recent developments in
molecular genetics will lead to the identification of
proteins implicated in Mg transport.

Intestinal Absorption

Net Mg absorption results from dietary Mg
absorption and Mg secretion into the intestinal
tract via bile and gastric and pancreatic juice.
In healthy adults, 30–50% of dietary Mg is absorbed.
The secreted Mg is efficiently reabsorbed and endogenous fecal losses are only 20–50 mg/day. Mg
absorption occurs along the entire intestinal tract,
but the distal small intestine (jejunum and ileum) is
the primary site. It is essentially a passive intercellular process by electrochemical gradient and solvent
drag. The active transport occurs only for extremely
low dietary Mg intake and its regulation is
unknown. Mg uptake in the brush border may be
mediated by a Mg/anion complex, and Mg
efflux across the basolateral membrane may involve
Na^+/Mg^{2+} antiport systems. A gene implicated in
Mg deficit in humans has been identified. It is
expressed in intestine and kidney and appears to
encode for a protein that combines Ca- and Mg-
permeable channel properties with protein kinase
activity. This gene may be implicated in Mg absorption. Because of the importance of the passive process, the quantity of Mg in the digestive tract is the
major factor controlling the amount of Mg
absorbed.

The possibility of an adaptative increase in the
fraction of Mg absorbed as Mg intake is lowered is
controversial. In fact, experimental studies indicate
that fractional intestinal absorption of Mg is
directly proportional to dietary Mg intake. Because
only soluble Mg is absorbed, all the factors increasing Mg solubility increase its absorption while formation of insoluble complexes in the intestine may
decrease Mg absorption. Most well-controlled studies indicate that high calcium intake does not
affect intestinal Mg absorption in humans. In contrast, dietary phytate in excess impairs Mg

Table 1 Magnesium in human tissues

	% distribution	Concentration
Bone	60–65	0.5% of bone ash
Muscle	27	6–10 mmol/kg wet weight
Other cells	6–7	6–10 mmol/kg wet weight
Extracellular	<1	
Erythrocytes		2.5 mmol/l
Serum		0.7–1.1 mol/l
Free	55	
Complexed	13	
Bound	32	
Mononuclear blood cells		2.3–3.5 fmol/cell
Cerebrospinal fluid		1.25 mmol/l
Free	55	
Complexed	45	
Sweat		0.3 mmol/l (in hot environment)
Secretions		0.3–0.7 mmol/l

From *Molecular Aspects of Medicine*, vol. 24, Vormann J: Magnesium: nutrition and metabolism, pp. 27–37, Copyright 2003, with permission from Elsevier.

absorption by formation of insoluble complexes in the intestinal tract. Negative effects of a high intake of dietary fiber have often been reported, but these actions have certainly been overestimated. In fact, only the impact of purified fiber was considered, but fiber-rich diets are a major source of Mg and roles of the intestinal fermentation and the large bowel in mineral absorption were neglected. It was demonstrated in animal models that fermentable carbohydrates (oligosaccharides and resistant starch) enhance Mg absorption in the large bowel and that a similar effect exists in humans. Other nutrients may influence Mg absorption but these effects are important only at low dietary Mg intake.

Urinary Excretion

Magnesium homeostasis is essentially regulated by a process of filtration–reabsorption in the kidney. Urinary Mg excretion increases when Mg intake is in excess, whereas the kidney conserves Mg in the case of Mg deprivation. Usually, 1000 mmol/24 h of Mg is filtered and only 3 mmol/24 h is excreted in urine.

A total of 10–15% of the filtered Mg is reabsorbed in the proximal tubule by a passive process. The majority of filtered Mg (65%) is reabsorbed in the thick ascending loop of Henle. The reabsorption in this segment is mediated by a paracellular mechanism involving paracellin-1. It is also related to sodium transport by a dependence on the transepithelial potential generated by NaCl absorption. Thus, factors that impair NaCl reabsorption in the thick ascending loop of Henle, such as osmotic diuretics,

loop diuretics, and extracellular fluid volume expansion, increase Mg excretion. At least 10–15% of the filtered Mg is reabsorbed in the distal tubule. The reabsorption occurs via an active transcellular mechanism and is under the control of special divalent cation-sensing receptors. Thus, elevated plasma Mg concentrations inhibit reabsorption of Mg from the distal tubule, leading to an increased magnesuria. Other active transport may also exist since some hormones (parathyroid hormone, glucagon, calcitonin, and insulin) may increase Mg reabsorption. Other factors may also influence Mg reabsorption, such as hypercalciuria or hypophosphatemia, which inhibit the tubular reabsorption of Mg. Metabolic alkalosis leads to renal Mg conservation, whereas metabolic acidosis is associated with urinary Mg wasting. Thus, the chronic low-grade metabolic acidosis in humans eating Western diets may contribute to decreased Mg status.

Dietary Sources of Magnesium

Mg is present in all foods, but the Mg content varies substantially (**Table 2**). Cereals and nuts have high Mg content. Vegetables are moderately rich in Mg, and meat, eggs, and milk are poor in Mg. A substantial amount of Mg may be lost during food processing, and refined foods generally have a low Mg content. In addition to Mg content, it is important to consider the Mg density of food (i.e., the quantity of Mg per unit of energy). Vegetables, legumes, and cereals thus contribute efficiently to daily Mg intake, whereas fat- and/or sugar-rich products have a minor contribution. Some water can also be a substantial source of Mg, but it depends on the area from which the water derives.

Table 2 Mg density of foods

Food	Magnesium density (mg/MJ)
Vegetables (lettuce, broccoli)	211
Legumes (bean)	113
Whole cereal (wheat)	104
Nuts (almond)	105
Fruits (apple)	30
Fish (cod)	75
Meat (roast beef)	40
Whole milk	38
Cheese (camembert)	15
Eggs	18
Dessert	
Biscuit	10
Chocolate	52

From *Répertoire Général des Aliments* (1996).

Requirements

Assessment of Mg Status

Several potential markers for estimating daily Mg requirement have been suggested. Plasma Mg concentration is the most commonly used marker to assess Mg status. In healthy populations, the plasma Mg value is 0.86 mmol/l and the reference value is 0.75–0.96 mmol/l. A low plasma Mg value reflects Mg depletion, but a normal plasma Mg level may coexist with low intracellular Mg. Thus, despite its interest, plasma Mg is not a good marker of Mg status.

Ion-specific electrodes have become available for determining ionized Mg in plasma, and this measurement may be a better marker of Mg status than total plasma Mg. However, further investigation is necessary to achieve a standardized procedure and to validate its use as an appropriate marker of Mg status.

Erythrocyte Mg level is also commonly used to assess Mg status, and the normal value is 2.06–2.54 mmol/l. However, erythrocyte Mg level is under genetic control, and numerous studies have shown no correlation between erythrocyte Mg and other tissue Mg.

The total Mg content of white blood cells has been proposed to be an index of Mg status. However, lymphocytes, polymorphonuclear blood cells, and platelets may have protective mechanisms against intracellular Mg deficiency, and the determination of total Mg content in leukocytes and platelets to assess Mg status is of questionable usefulness.

Mg excretion determination is helpful for the diagnosis of Mg deficit when there is an hypomagnesemia. In healthy populations, the urinary Mg value is 4.32 mmol/day and the reference value is 1.3–8.2 mmol/day. In the presence of hypomagnesemia, normal or high urinary Mg excretion is suggestive of renal wasting. On the contrary, Mg urinary excretion lower than normal values is convincing evidence of Mg deficiency.

The parenteral loading test is probably the best available marker for the diagnosis of Mg deficiency. The Mg retention after parenteral administration of Mg seems to reflect the general intracellular Mg content, and a Mg retention more than 20% of the administered Mg suggests Mg deficiency. However, this test is not valid in the case of abnormal urinary Mg excretion and is contraindicated in renal failure.

Determination of exchangeable Mg pools using Mg stable isotopes is an interesting approach to evaluate Mg status. In fact, Mg exchangeable pool sizes vary with dietary Mg in animals. However, more studies are necessary to better appreciate the relationship between Mg status and exchangeable Mg pool size in humans.

Magnesium Deficit

Two types of Mg deficit must be differentiated. Dietary Mg deficiency results from an insufficient intake of Mg. Secondary Mg deficiency is related to dysregulation of the control mechanisms of Mg metabolism.

Dietary Mg Deficiency

Severe Mg deficiency is very rare, whereas marginal Mg deficiency is common in industrialized countries. Low dietary Mg intake may result from a low energy intake (reduction of energy output necessary for physical activity and thermoregulation, and thus of energy input) and/or from low Mg density of the diet (i.e., refined and/or processed foods). Moreover, in industrialized countries, diets are rich in animal source foods and low in vegetable foods. This leads to a dietary net acid load and thus a negative effect on Mg balance. In fact, animal source foods provide predominantly acid precursors (sulphur-containing amino acids), whereas fruits and vegetables have substantial amounts of base precursor (organic acids plus potassium salts). Acidosis increases Mg urinary excretion by decreasing Mg reabsorption in the loop of Henle and the distal tubule, and potassium depletion impairs Mg reabsorption. Mg deficiency treatment simply requires oral nutritional physiological Mg supplementation.

Secondary Mg Deficiency

Failure of the mechanisms that ensure Mg homeostasis, or endogenous or iatrogenic perturbing factors of Mg status, leads to secondary Mg deficit. Secondary Mg deficiency requires a more or less specific correction of its causal dysregulation.

Intestinal Mg absorption decreases in the case of malabsorption syndromes, such as chronic diarrhoea, inflammatory enteropathy, intestinal resection, and biliary and intestinal fistulas.

Hypermagnesuria is encountered in the case of metabolic and iatrogenic disorders, such as primary and secondary hyperaldosteronism (extracellular volume expansion), hypercalcemia (competition Ca/Mg at the thick ascending loop of Henle), hyperparathyroidism, and phosphate or potassium depletion. Hypermagnesuria may also result from tubulopathy, as the selective defect of the Mg tubular reabsorption (chromosome 11q23), Bartter's syndrome (thick ascending loop of Henle), or Gitelman's syndrome (distal convoluted tubule).

Administration of medications can be a causal factor in the development of secondary Mg deficiency. Administration of diuretics is the main cause of iatrogenic deficit because it decreases NaCl reabsorption in the thick ascending loop of Henle and thus increases the fractional excretion of Mg.

Causes of Mg Deficit

Complex relations exist between Mg and carbohydrate metabolism. Diabetes is frequently associated with Mg deficit and insulin may play an important role in the regulation of intracellular Mg content by stimulating cellular Mg uptake. Hypomagnesemia is the most common ionic abnormality in alcoholism because of poor nutritional status and Mg malabsorption, alcoholic ketoacidosis, hypophosphatemia, and hyperaldosteronism secondary to liver disease.

Stress can contribute to Mg deficit by stimulating the production of hormones and thus increasing urinary Mg excretion and by impairing neurohormonal mechanisms that spare Mg.

Consequences of Mg Deficit and Implications in Various Metabolic Diseases

Mg deficit causes neuromuscular manifestations, including positive Chvostek and Trousseau signs, muscular fasciculations, tremor, tetany, nausea, and vomiting. The pathogenesis of the neuromuscular irritability is complex, and it implicates the central and peripheral nervous system, the neuromuscular junction, and muscle cells.

Mg deficit perturbs Ca homeostasis and hypocalcemia is a common manifestation of severe Mg deficit. Impaired release of parathyroid hormone (PTH) and skeletal end organ resistance to PTH appear to be the major factors implicated, probably by a decrease in adenylcyclase activity.

Perturbations in the action and/or metabolism of vitamin D may also occur in Mg deficit. Because Mg plays a key role in skeletal metabolism, Mg deficit may be a possible risk factor for osteoporosis. However, epidemiologic studies relating Mg intake to bone mass or rate of bone loss have been conflicting, and further investigation is necessary to clarify the role of Mg in bone metabolism and osteoporosis.

Hypokalemia is frequently encountered in Mg deficit. This is due to an inhibition of Na,K-ATPase activity that impairs K and Na transport in and out of the cell and to stimulation of renin and aldosterone secretion that increases K urinary excretion.

There is increasing evidence that Mg deficiency may be involved in the development of various pathologies. Mg deficit is frequent in diabetes and can be a factor in insulin resistance. It can modify insulin sensitivity, probably by influencing intracellular signaling and processing. Mg deficit has also been implicated in the development or progression of micro- and macroangiopathy and neuropathy.

Mg deficit appears to act as a cardiovascular risk factor. Experimental, clinical, and epidemiological evidence points to an important role of Mg in blood pressure regulation. Mg deficit can lead to cardiac arrhythmias and to increased sensitivity to cardiac glucosides. Mg deficit may also play a role in the development of atherosclerosis. In experimental animal models, dietary Mg deficiency results in dyslipidemia, increased sensitivity to oxidative stress, and a marked proinflammatory effect, thus accelerating atherogenosis. Macrophages and polynuclear neutrophils are activated and synthesize a variety of biological substances, some of which are powerful inducers of inflammatory events (cytokines, free radicals, and eicosanoids). The effect of Mg depletion or Mg supplementation may result in the ability of Mg to modulate intracellular calcium. Pharmacological doses of Mg may reduce morbidity and mortality in the period following infarction. The beneficial effect of Mg may result from calcium-antagonist action, decreased platelet aggregation, and decreased free radical damage.

Magnesium Excess

Magnesium overload can occur in individuals with impaired renal function or during massive intravenous administration of Mg. It is most often iatrogenic. Clinical symptoms such as drowsiness and hyporeflexia develop when plasma Mg is 2- or 3-fold higher than the normal value.

Recommended Dietary Allowances

The Estimated Average Requirement (EAR) is the nutrient intake value that is estimated to meet the requirement of 50% of individuals in a life stage and a gender group. Balance studies and data on stable isotopes suggest an EAR of 5 mg/kg/day for males and females. This value is greater during growth in adolescents and is estimated to be 5.3 mg/kg/day. The Mg requirement is also higher during pregnancy because of Mg transfer to the fetus in the last 3 months; therefore, an additional 35 mg/day is recommended.

In infants, the determination of the Adequate Intake (AI) is based on the Mg content of mother's milk and the progressive consumption of solid food.

Table 3 Recommended dietary allowances of Mg

Age	RDA (mg/day)		AI (mg/day)	
	Male	Female	Male	Female
0–6 months			30	30
6–12 months			75	75
1–3 years	80	80		
4–8 years	130	130		
9–13 years	240	240		
14–18 years	410	360		
19–30 years	400	310		
31–50 years	420	320		
51–70 years	420	320		
<70 years	420	320		
Pregnancy		+40		
Lactation		+0		

From the Institute of Medicine (1997).

Thus, the AI is 30 mg/day during the first 6 months of life and 75 mg/day the second 6 months of life.

The Recommended Dietary Allowance (RDA) is the average daily dietary intake that is sufficient to meet the nutrient requirement of 97.5% of individuals and is set at 20% above the EAR $+2$ CVs where the CV is 10%. During recent years, dietary reference intakes have been revised by the US Institute of Medicine. The recommended intakes of Mg are given in **Table 3**. It is not known whether decreased urinary Mg and increased maternal bone resorption provide sufficient amounts of Mg to meet increased needs during lactation. Thus, the French Society for Nutrition suggests adding 30 mg/day to intake for lactation.

The intake of Mg has been determined in various populations. Evidence suggests that the occidental diet is relatively deficient in Mg, whereas the vegetarian diet is rich in Mg. For instance, the mean Mg intake of the subjects in the French Supplementation with Antioxidant Vitamins and Minerals Study was estimated to be 369 mg/day in men and 280 mg/day in women. Thus, 77% of women and 72% of men had dietary Mg intakes lower than the RDA, and 23% of women and 18% of men consumed less than two-thirds of the RDA.

Conclusion

Based on evidence of low Mg intake in industrialized countries, intervention studies to improve Mg status and to assess its impact on specific health outcomes are required.

See also: **Calcium**. **Cereal Grains**. **Electrolytes**: Water–Electrolyte Balance. **Fruits and Vegetables**. **Malabsorption Syndromes**. **Vitamin D**: Rickets and Osteomalacia.

Further Reading

Coudray C, Demigné C, and Rayssiguier Y (2003) Effects of dietary fibers on magnesium absorption in animals and humans. *Journal of Nutrition* 133: 1–4.

Durlach J (1988) *Magnesium in Clinical Practice* London: John Libbey.

Elin RJ (1989) Assessment of magnesium status. In: Itokawa Y and Durlach I (eds.) *Magnesium in Health and Disease*, pp. 137–146. London: John Libbey.

Feillet-Coudray C, Coudray C, Gueux E, Mazur A, and Rayssiguier Y (2002) A new approach to evaluate magnesium status: Determination of exchangeable Mg pool masses using Mg stable isotope. *Magnesium Research* 15: 191–198.

Galan P, Preziosi P, Durlach V et al. (1997) Dietary magnesium intake in a French adult population. *Magnesium Research* 10: 321–328.

Institute of Medicine (1997) *Dietary Reference Intakes for Calcium, Phosphorus, Magnesium, Vitamin D and Fluoride*. Washington, DC: National Academy Press.

Rayssiguier Y, Mazur A, and Durlach J (2001) *Advances in Magnesium Research, Nutrition and Health* London: John Libbey.

Répertoire général des aliments (1996) *Table de Composition Minérale*. Paris: Tec & Doc, Lavoisier.

Rude RK (1998) Magnesium deficiency: A cause of heterogeneous disease in humans. *Journal of Bone Mineral Research* 13(4): 749–758.

Shils ME (1994) Magnesium. In: Shils ME, Olson JA, and Shike M (eds.) *Modern Nutrition in Health and Disease*, 8th ed, pp. 164–184. Philadelphia, PA: Lea & Febiger.

Vormann J (2003) Magnesium: Nutrition and metabolism. *Molecular Aspects of Medicine* 24: 27–37.

Wilkinson SR, Welch RM, Mayland HF, and Grunes DL (1990) Magnesium in plants: Uptake, distribution, function and utilization by man and animals. In: Sigel H and Sigel A (eds.) *Compendium of Magnesium and Its Role in Biology, Nutrition and Physiology*, pp. 33–56. New York: Marcel Dekker.

MALABSORPTION SYNDROMES

P M Tsai and C Duggan, Harvard Medical School, Boston, MA, USA

The human gastrointestinal tract has an impressive capacity for water, electrolyte, and nutrient absorption. In some disease states, however, this excess capacity is outpaced by either intestinal secretion or inadequate absorption. Malabsorption is defined as the inability of the gastrointestinal tract to adequately absorb nutrients. Although strictly speaking, malabsorption is distinct and contrasted with maldigestion (inadequate breakdown of nutrients in the intestinal lumen), the therapeutic implications of these two conditions are often similar. Multiple causes of malabsorption exist (e.g., inflammatory bowel disease, cystic fibrosis, and short bowel syndrome). We review the pathophysiology, symptoms, and nutritional therapies for common malabsorption syndromes.

Pathophysiology and Symptoms

Malabsorption can occur when any of the several steps in nutrient digestion, absorption, and/or assimilation are interrupted; see **Table 1** for a list of congenital defects in nutrient assimilation. Carbohydrate malabsorption can occur, for instance, when intestinal disaccharidases are reduced in concentration at the enterocyte. The brush border membrane produces four disaccharidases that are important in carbohydrate digestion. These enzymes are sucrase–isomaltase, maltase–glucoamylase, trehalase, and lactase–phlorizin hydrolase. Worldwide, lactase deficiency is the most common type of acquired disaccharidase deficiency since much of the world's population exhibits a noticeable reduction in intestinal lactase concentration after the age of 2 years. In addition, infants and children with diarrheal disease may suffer from acquired lactase deficiency due to intestinal villous damage that is often temporary. With either congenital or acquired lactase deficiency, malabsorbed carbohydrate remains in the intestinal lumen and exerts an osmotic pull on fluids and electrolytes, leading to abdominal cramping and loose stools. Malabsorbed carbohydrate can be metabolized by gastrointestinal tract bacteria, and the fermented gas produced is associated with flatulence and bloating. Bacterial overgrowth of the small intestine, as seen with short bowel syndrome, can also be associated with carbohydrate malabsorption.

Steatorrhea, excessive fat in the stools, results from fat malabsorption and can have several causes, most notably pancreatic insufficiency due to cystic fibrosis, chronic pancreatitis, Shwachman–Diamond syndrome, and Johanson–Blizzard syndrome. Failure of pancreatic secretion of lipase, amylase, and other digestive enzymes leads to persistence of dietary fat in the intestinal lumen, causing bloating, abdominal pain, and bulky, foul-smelling, oily stools. The stools often float due to a high gas content and test positive for fat. Patients also complain of blunted appetite and nausea. Other causes of fat malabsorption include hepatobiliary disease with inadequate bile salt circulation, severe mucosal disease, and short bowel syndrome.

The most common cause of protein malabsorption is so-called protein-losing enteropathy. Etiologies include diffuse mucosal disease such as celiac disease or Crohn's disease, elevated right heart pressure with resultant dilatation of lymphatics and leakage of lymph into the lumen, and colitides such as *Shigella* or *Salmonella* infections. Since protein is a relatively minor component of dietary energy compared with carbohydrate and fat, symptoms of protein malabsorption can sometimes be minimal. However, infectious colitis or exacerbations of inflammatory bowel disease often present with frequent loose stools, which may be bloody. Rare, congenital etiologies of protein malabsorption include enterokinase and trypsinogen deficiencies (**Table 1**).

Finally, the malabsorption of various micronutrients can occur in conjunction with or separate from the macronutrient malabsorption syndromes noted previously. For instance, steatorrhea can be accompanied by excessive fecal losses of the fat-soluble vitamins A, D, E, and K as well as calcium and other minerals. Alternatively, atrophic gastritis or surgical resection of the terminal ileum can lead to vitamin B_{12} malabsorption in the absence of any symptoms of diarrhea. Proximal bowel resection can result in iron, zinc, and calcium malabsorption. A rare cause of micronutrient inadequacy is abetalipoproteinemia, in which fat-soluble nutrients are normally digested and absorbed by the intestine but are not delivered to the circulation due to defective transepithelial transport. Other rare causes of micronutrient malabsorption are noted in **Table 1**.

Table 1 Congenital defects in nutrient assimilation[a]

Disorder	Enzyme/protein affected	Symptoms
Carbohydrate digestion		
Congenital lactase deficiency	Lactase	Lactose-induced diarrhea
Hypolactasia	Lactase	Lactose-induced diarrhea
Congenital sucrase–isomaltase deficiency	Sucrase–isomaltase	Sucrose-induced diarrhea
Glucoamylase deficiency	Glucoamylase	Starch-induced diarrhea
Trehalase deficiency	Trehalase	Trehalose-induced diarrhea
Carbohydrate absorption		
Glucose–galactose malabsorption	Sodium–glucose cotransport (SGLT1)	Glucose-induced diarrhea
Fructose malabsorption	Facilitative fructose transport (GLUT5)	Fructose-induced diarrhea
Fanconi–Bickel syndrome	Facilitative glucose transport (GLUT2)	Diarrhea and nephropathy
Protein digestion		
Enterokinase deficiency	Enterokinase	Diarrhea and edema
Trypsinogen deficiency	Trypsinogen	Diarrhea and edema
Fat digestion		
Pancreatic lipase deficiency	Pancreatic lipase	Steatorrhea
Fat assimilation		
Abetalipoproteinemia	Microsomal triglyceride transfer protein	Steatorrhea
Hypobetalipoproteinemia	Apolipoprotein B	Steatorrhea
Chylomicron retention disease	Sar1-ADP-ribosylation factor family GTPases	Steatorrhea
Primary bile acid malabsorption	Sodium–bile acid transporter	Steatorrhea, bile acid diarrhea
Tangier disease	ATP binding cassette transporter 1	Hepatosplenomegaly
Sitosterolemia	ATP binding cassette subfamily G, member 8	Atherosclerosis
Ion and metal absorption		
Congenital sodium diarrhea	Defective Na^+/H^+ exchange	Secretory diarrhea
Congenital chloride diarrhea	Defective $Cl^-/HCO3^-$ exchange	Secretory diarrhea
Cystic fibrosis	CFTR	Pancreatic insufficiency, meconium ileus
Acrodermatitis enteropathica	Zinc and iron-regulated transport proteins (ZIP4)	Diarrhea and dermatitis
Menkes disease	Copper transporter	Developmental delay
Wilson's disease	Copper transporter	Cirrhosis
Primary hypomagnesemia	Paracellin	Seizures, deafness and polyuria
Hemachromatosis	Hepcidin, others	Cirrhosis, cardiomyopathy, diabetes
Vitamin absorption		
Folate malabsorption	?	Macrocytic anemia, diarrhea, developmental delay
Congenital pernicious anemia	Intrinsic factor	Macrocytic anemia, developmental delay
Imerslund–Graesbeck syndrome	Cubilin, amnionless	Macrocytic anemia, proteinuria
Congenital deficit of transcobalamin II	transcobalamin II	Macrocytic anemia, diarrhea, developmental delay
Thiamine-responsive megaloblastic anemia	Thiamine transport protein	Anemia, diabetes, cranial nerve defects
Familial retinol binding protein (RBP) deficiency	RBP-4	Vitamin A deficiency
Selective vitamin E deficiency	α-Tocopheral transport protein	Vitamin E deficiency

[a]Included are congenital defects that are associated with gastrointestinal symptoms and/or nutritional deficiencies. Congenital defects not included here include multiple defects in amino acid absorption.
Adapted from Martin M and Wright EM (2004) Congenital intestinal transport defects. In: Walker WA, Goulet O, Kleinman RE et al. (eds.) Pediatric Gastrointestinal Disease: Pathophysiology, Diagnosis, Management, 4th edn. Hamilton, Ontario: BC Decker.

General Nutritional Management of Malabsorption

As with all nutritional disorders, a thorough nutritional assessment is needed to plan rational therapy of malabsorption. Important historical points to review include duration of symptoms, underlying etiology of malabsorption, ability to meet nutritional needs by mouth, the presence of food allergies, and concurrent medical and surgical problems. The patient's nutritional status (weight, height, body mass index, and their respective percentiles) should be determined. Tests of body composition such as arm anthropometrics, bioelectrical impedance, or DXA studies should be considered. If the underlying cause of malabsorption is not known, diagnostic gastrointestinal endoscopy, laboratory studies, and/or imaging studies are indicated.

Specific Nutritional Management of Malabsorption

Fluids and Electrolytes

Diarrhea is usually the most distressing problem for patients with malabsorption and may cause dehydration. Care should be taken to correct fluid losses with appropriately designed oral rehydration solutions. Even in the setting of massive secretory diarrhea, such as seen with cholera infections, oral rehydration solutions are effective at treating dehydration. Data support the safety and efficacy of oral rehydration solutions of reduced osmolarity in children with dehydration from acute diarrhea. An oral rehydration solution composed of glucose 75 mmol/L, sodium 75 mmol/L, potassium 20 mmol/L, base 30 mEq/L, and osmolality 245 mOsm/L is well suited for the rehydration and maintenance therapy during dehydration due to diarrhea.

In some cases of severe diarrhea, parenteral hydration is the mainstay of therapy. Examples include glucose–galactose malabsorption, congenital chloride diarrhea, microvillous inclusion disease, and tufting enteropathy. These cases, as well as other severe causes of more common malabsorptive syndromes, also frequently require the use of parenteral nutrition therapy.

Carbohydrate Malabsorption

Lactose intolerance   Lactose intolerance is defined by the occurrence of symptoms due to the inability to digest lactose, the main carbohydrate in milk. These symptoms may include abdominal pain, bloating, diarrhea, or flatulence. Lactose malabsorption is attributed to a relative deficiency of the disaccharidase lactase. Primary lactase deficiency is a condition in which lactase activity declines after weaning. Secondary lactose intolerance is usually due to mucosal injury associated with a condition or disease such as infectious diarrhea, Crohn's disease, or short bowel syndrome.

Although people of Northern European ancestry commonly maintain the ability to digest lactose into adulthood, the majority of the world's population produces less lactase after weaning. In addition to the presence or absence of the lactase enzyme, other factors determine whether a person will have symptoms of lactose malabsorption, including the amount of lactose in the diet, the mixture of lactose with other foods, gastric emptying rate, colonic scavenge of malabsorbed carbohydrate, ethnic origin, and age. Primary lactose intolerance is prevalent in African American, Hispanic, Native American, and Asian populations.

Nutritional management of lactose intolerance consists largely of the removal of lactose from the diet. Lactose is a common ingredient in many foods, including breads, crackers, soups, cereals, cookies, and baked goods. Eliminating or reducing lactose-containing ingredients from one's diet is usually adequate to relieve symptoms. Individuals with primary lactose intolerance may require a permanent dietary change. Individuals with secondary lactose intolerance should eliminate all lactose from their diets for a short period of time ranging from 2 to 6 weeks. If symptoms resolve, lactose may be reintroduced slowly as tolerated by the individual. The amount of lactose that an individual can tolerate is highly variable. Many children can tolerate small amounts of lactose, particularly yogurt, hard cheese, or ice cream, without discomfort. Many adults who consider themselves lactose-intolerant can actually tolerate moderate amounts of milk.

For individuals who choose to restrict lactose in their diets, a variety of lactose-free and low-lactose food choices are available. Lactose-reduced products, containing 70–100% less lactose than standard foods, are available commercially. Individuals may also choose to consume dairy products with concomitant administration of lactase enzyme tablets or drops.

Frequent consumption of milk and other dairy foods has been associated with better bone health in some studies, and a strict lactose-free diet may not contain adequate amounts of calcium and vitamin D. **Table 2** provides a list of some commercially available lactose-free calcium supplements.

Table 2   Commercial calcium supplements

Product	Manufacturer	mg Calcium/ tablet	IU vitamin D
Citracal + D	Mission Pharmacal	315	200
OsCal 500 + D	Marion Lab	500	200
Tums	Smith-Kline Beecham	200	0
Calcium Milk Free (2)	Nature's Plus	500	100
Cal-citrate + D	Freeda	250	100

From DiSanto C and Duggan C (2004) Gastrointestinal diseases. In: Hendricks KM and Duggan C (eds.) *Manual of Pediatric Nutrition*, 4th edn. Hamilton, Ontario: BC Decker.

Sucrose Congenital sucrase–isomaltase deficiency (SID) is the most common congenital disaccharidase deficiency. Patients with this disorder lack functional sucrase, although isomaltase deficiency may be normal or absent. Symptoms of SID can include diarrhea, abdominal pain, and poor weight gain. Dietary avoidance of sucrose or table sugar helps relieve symptoms and can sometimes help with the diagnosis. Sucraid, a sacrosidase produced from *Saccharomyces cerevisiae*, is an enzyme that can be given with meals and allows increased tolerance to sucrose.

Fat Malabsorption: Fat and Fat-Soluble Nutrients

Patients with pancreatic insufficiency are unable to produce and secrete enough enzymes to aid with the breakdown of fats in the intestinal lumen. Studies of normal adults and those with pancreatic insufficiency have demonstrated that pancreatic enzyme secretion needs to be less than 15% of normal levels before significant steatorrhea is seen (**Figure 1**). Once clinically significant steatorrhea is determined, recovery of pancreatic function is unlikely.

Historically, patients with pancreatic insufficiency due to cystic fibrosis (CF) were told to minimize symptoms of steatorrhea by limiting dietary fat. However, epidemiologic studies confirmed that this advice led to negative energy balance, undernutrition, and higher mortality rates compared to communities in which CF patients were treated with high-energy, high-fat diets. The introduction of effective pancreatic replacement therapy has been heralded as one of the

most significant breakthroughs in the nutritional management of CF, responsible in part for the substantial increase in life span enjoyed by recent generations of CF patients. In fact, the finding of a lower incidence of growth failure in CF patients diagnosed and treated with aggressive nutritional therapy early in infancy has been used as justification for neonatal screening of this condition.

Judicious use of pancreatic replacement enzymes is the hallmark of nutritional therapy of CF and other disorders of pancreatic insufficiency. Multiple commercial preparations of porcine pancreatic enzymes are available, most of which contain lipase, amylase, and protease enzymes. The dose is usually titrated to the amount of steatorrhea. If meals take more than 30 min, the dose may be divided, with half given before the meal and half given during the meal. Patients who cannot swallow pills may open the capsules and sprinkle the enzymes into acidic foods.

Another critical aspect of the nutritional management of fat malabsorption is routine supplementation with the fat-soluble vitamins A, D, E, and K. Multiple studies have confirmed that patients with CF, Crohn's disease, and other malabsorptive disorders are prone to micronutrient deficiencies, and some literature suggests that dietary needs for these and other antioxidant nutrients may be increased in settings of infectious and catabolic stress often suffered by these patients. The contribution of fat malabsorption to other important mineral malabsorption, as in the case of calcium or zinc, should also be recognized.

Routine supplementation of fat-soluble vitamins is indicated in patients with fat malabsorption. In addition, serial measurement of fat-soluble vitamin biochemical status is recommended. Since blood nutrient concentrations of these and other nutrients can vary with the concentration of transport proteins, correction for these can aid the interpretation of these lab findings. For instance, vitamin A toxicity should be suspected if the molar ratio of vitamin A:retinol binding protein exceeds 1. Vitamin E concentrations should be corrected for circulating lipids. **Table 3** lists recommendations for therapy of fat-soluble vitamin deficiencies.

Some patients with pancreatic malabsorption may benefit from a diet enriched with medium-chain triglycerides (MCTs). MCTs are absorbed directly into the portal circulation and therefore bypass the steps of intraluminal digestion, reesterification, and enterocyte uptake. Thus, MCTs may be a dietary source of fats more easily absorbed in settings of fat malabsorption due to either pancreatic insufficiency or mucosal disease. However, MCT oils are less energy dense than long-chain fats, more expensive, and do

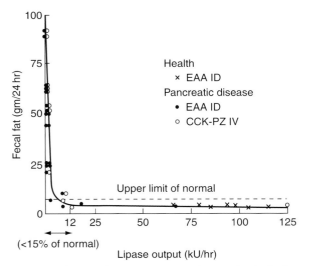

Figure 1 Pancreatic enzyme secretion and steatorrhea. Significant steatorrhea ensues when pancreatic function is less than 15% of normal. (Reproduced with permission from DiMagno EP, Go VLW, and Sumerskill WHJ (1973) Relations between pancreatic enzyme output and malabsorption in severe pancreatic insufficiency. *New England Journal of Medicine* **288**: 814).

Table 3 Assessment and treatment of fat-soluble vitamin deficiencies

Vitamin assessment	Therapy if deficiency	Considerations
A		
Normal: >20 µg/dl	Severe deficiency with xerophthalmia	Serum level is not a good indicator of liver stores.
Marginal stores: 10–19 µg/dl	<6 months old: 50 000 IU PO QD ×2 days, then again at 2 weeks	Low in chronic infection, liver disease, or during an acute phase response.
Deficient: <10 µg/dl	6–12 months: 100 000 IU PO QD ×2 days, then again at 2 weeks	Check retinol binding protein (RBP) circulation in plasma. Assess toxicity by using molar ratio of retinol to RBP:
	>12 months: 200 000 IU PO QD ×2 days, then again at 2 weeks	Retinol(µg/dl) × 0.0349 = µmol/l
	1–8 years: 5000 IU/kg/day ×5 days PO, then 5000–10 000 units/day ×2 months	RBP(mg/dl) × 0.476 = µmol/l
	>8 years and adults: 500 000 IU QD ×3 days, then 50 000 units/day ×14 days, then 10 000–20 000 units/day ×2 months	Molar ratio should be between 0.8 and 1.0. Ratios >1.0 suggest increased levels of free retinol and possible toxicity.
D		
25-OHD:	Vitamin D$_2$ (Ergocalciferol)	Low in dietary deficiency, decreased absorption, UV light deficiency, prematurity, liver disease, and with certain drugs (anticonvulsants). Higher in summer.
Normal: 9–75 ng/ml	Oral (Drisdol) liquid or capsule	
	Children with malabsorption 10 000–25 000 USP units PO/day until normal	
	Children with normal absorption 1000–5000 units PO ×6–12 weeks	Watch for hypercalcemia and hypercalciuria and other signs of toxicity.
	IM (Calciferol)—100 000 units/ml	
	10 000–100 000 units IM once. Larger single IM doses may be given.	
	Follow calcium, PTH, 25-OHD concentrations.	
E		
Deficiency if	1 unit/kg/day of water-miscible form plus usual vitamin E supplementation until normal blood levels	Carried exclusively on plasma lipoproteins; thus, vitamin E:total lipid ratio or vitamin E:chol + tryglycerides (TG) is a better indicator of stores than serum levels.
Plasma level <5 mg/L		
Vitamin E:total lipid ratio <0.6–0.8 mg/g in adults	1 unit = 1 mg dl-α-tocopherol acetate	Conversions
Vitamin E:chol + TG <1.59 µmol/mmol		Total lipids = cholesterol + TG + phospholipids
Erythrocyte hemolysis >10%		Chol (mg/dl) × 0.0259 = chol (mmol/l)
		TG (mg/dl) × 0.0113 = TG (mmol/l)
		Vitamin E (mg/l) × 2.32 = vitamin E (µmol/l)
		Do not give with medications that interfere with vitamin E absorption (vitamin A, cholestyramine, and antacids).
K		
Prothrombin time (PT) deficiency if >13.5 s	Infants and children 1–2 mg single IM, SC, or IV dose	Deficiency in malabsorption, long-term antibiotic therapy.
PIVKA-II deficiency if <3.0 ng/ml	Adults 10 mg single IM, SC, or IV dose	

From Corrales K (2005) Cystic fibrosis. In: Hendricks KM and Duggan C (eds.) *Manual of Pediatric Nutrition*, 4th edn. Hamilton, ON: BC Decker.

not contain the fatty acids linoleic and linolenic acid, which are essential to humans.

Protein Malabsorption

Protein-losing enteropathy (PLE) can also be treated with a variety of nutritional interventions. PLE due to dilated lymphatics, as with right heart failure, results in leakage of lymphocytes, proteins, and fats into the intestinal lumen. As with fat malabsorption, MCT-supplemented foods and formulas are indicated to allow improved fat absorption in PLE. Fat-soluble vitamin supplementation is indicated. In congenital protein malabsorption syndromes, peptide- or amino acid-based formulas are often helpful.

Mucosal disorders, including inflammatory bowel disease, allergic diseases, and celiac disease, are additional examples of disorders causing protein malabsorption. Once intestinal inflammation is reduced with appropriate medical or nutritional therapy, absorption of protein is usually improved. In Shigella infections, some studies have demonstrated improved nutritional outcomes with a high-protein diet during recovery from the acute symptoms of diarrhea.

Route of Nutrition in Malabsorption

Several factors need to be considered when recommending whether oral, enteral, or parenteral nutrition should be used to provide nutrition to the patient with malabsorption, including etiology of malabsorption, severity of gastrointestinal disease, and underlying nutritional and medical condition. Oral nutrition using modified diets as noted previously is the most customary and desirable by physician and patient alike. In cases of mild lactose malabsorption, modification of a regular, healthy diet to avoid foods high in lactose should be sufficient. In cases in which widespread gastrointestinal disease is leading to severe malabsorption, enteral or 'tube' feeding is helpful for two main reasons: (i) Use of proprietary formulas specially designed for malabsorption is often indicated, and these formulas may be unpalatable, and (ii) enteral feedings, especially slow continuous 'drip' feedings, make efficient use of nutrient transport kinetics, thereby maximizing residual gastrointestinal absorptive function. In severe cases of malabsorption in which tube feedings are unable to achieve adequate nutritional intake, parenteral nutrition may be indicated.

Selection of Enteral Formulas for Malabsorption

A number of commercially available formulas are designed for patients with malabsorption, and these differ with regard to energy density, macronutrient composition, and indicated age. Since infant formulas are often handled in a separate regulatory manner by governments, infant formulas are usually considered separately from formulas designed for older children and adults. In addition, formulas are also conventionally categorized by the extent of the hydrolysis of their protein source. Categories include intact protein formulas, protein hydrolysate formulas, and amino acid-based formulas. Protein hydrolysate formulas are also sometimes referred to as 'semielemental' formulas, and amino acid formulas are sometimes called 'elemental' formulas. However, these terms suffer from vagueness and inaccuracies since not all of their macronutrients are semi- or completely elemental. Marketing strategies often compound the confusion with misleading formula names. These terms should be discouraged, and the terms that refer to the composition and/or biochemical processing should be used instead.

Patients who have carbohydrate malabsorption from lactose intolerance should use lactose-free formula. Fat malabsorption calls for MCT-enriched formula. In cases of protein malabsorption or severe enteropathy, a formula that is a protein hydrolysate or amino acid-based would be most appropriate. Since many malabsorption syndromes overlap in terms of the macronutrient affected, as in cases of severe mucosal disease, some formulas are designed for fat, protein, and carbohydrate malabsorption. For example, all formulas designed for use in adults are lactose-free, and several formulas contain both hydrolyzed proteins and MCT oils.

Clinical Management of Malabsorption

Two of the most clinically challenging scenarios for the management of malabsorption are inflammatory bowel disease (especially Crohn's disease) and short bowel syndrome.

Inflammatory Bowel Disease

Patients with Crohn's disease have widespread and intermittent gastrointestinal inflammation. Some patients with inflammatory bowel disease may require complete bowel rest for several days or even a few weeks to allow time for mucosal healing. In order to provide nutrition during this period, parenteral nutrition may be needed.

Numerous studies have shown that patients with Crohn's disease may safely and effectively achieve clinical remission with primary nutritional therapy. Early literature in the field highlighted the use of protein hydrolysate formulas that, due to unpalatability, often required supplementation with a nasogastric or gastrostomy tube. Recent data have confirmed that intact protein formulas, termed 'polymeric' formulas when describing formulas designed for adults, may work as well as protein hydrolysates, and these formulas can feasibly be given by mouth.

As patients are recovering from an exacerbation and begin advancing their diet, they should temporarily minimize the amount of fiber ingested to decrease trauma to healing mucosa. Patients whose disease affects the small intestine often benefit from temporary avoidance of lactose products as the mucosa heals and brush border membrane enzyme production is restored.

Micronutrients are also needed in the nutritional management of inflammatory bowel disease. Iron supplementation is recommended for anemia that may be secondary to acute or chronic blood loss. Treatment of inflammatory bowel disease frequently requires the use of steroids, which affects bone density. Calcium and vitamin D supplementation is commonly needed to minimize the osteopenic effects of steroid therapy and/or the effects of malabsorption and chronic inflammation.

Short Bowel Syndrome

Patients who have suffered acquired or congenital loss of small intestinal surface area that makes them dependent on specialized enteral or parenteral support are said to have short bowel syndrome (SBS). Patients with SBS often malabsorb carbohydrates, proteins, fat, as well as numerous micronutrients, depending on the extent and location of bowel resection as well as the presence of mucosal disease in the nonresected bowel.

Special attention should be given to the part of the intestine that remains as well as the length of the intestine. Some patients may have the terminal ileum removed and are unable to absorb vitamin B_{12} and bile acids. Removal of the ileocecal valve increases the risk of bacterial overgrowth. Reduced length also means reduced surface area for the absorption of nutrients and decreased intestinal transit time.

In the immediate postoperative period, parenteral nutrition and gut rest should be used because significant stool output is the norm. Output should be quantified, and electrolytes must be carefully monitored in order to determine appropriate replacement fluids to make up for excess urine, stool, and ostomy losses. Replacement fluids should generally be given separately from standard parenteral nutrition so that they can be adjusted as needed to rapid shifts in fluid and electrolyte status.

As patients recover from surgery, every attempt should be made to feed them enterally as soon as is feasible. Enteral feeds facilitate growth and adaptation of the remaining bowel to allow partial compensation for the missing portion, and several studies have correlated early feeding with better long-term outcome. Attaining independence from parenteral nutrition may take weeks, months, or years. **Table 4** outlines an approach to determining feeding advancement. Whereas some patients are able to grow well or maintain their body weight with enteral feeds, many are dependent on parenteral nutrition. Some patients with SBS also have oral feeding aversion due to prematurity, prolonged mechanical ventilation, and/or prolonged orogastric or nasogastric feeding. Gastrostomy tubes are particularly helpful in this regard.

In infants, breast milk should be used if available. The breast milk may need to be fortified to increase calories, protein, or fat. For older patients or infants who are not receiving breast milk, protein hydrolysates or amino acid-based formulas may be better tolerated since the residual bowel more easily absorbs these nutrients. Lactose-free and MCT-containing formulas are often used as well. Formulas may need to be supplemented with oral rehydration solutions if electrolyte abnormalities persist, particularly with sodium losses through persistent high stool or ostomy output.

Since many patients with SBS are dependent on parenteral nutrition for prolonged periods of time,

Table 4 Feeding advancement in short bowel syndrome

Stool output

If <10 g/kg/day or <10 stools/day	→ Advance rate by 10–20 ml/kg/day
If 10–20 g/kg/day or 10–12 stools/day	→ No change
If >20 g/kg/day or >12 stools/day	→ Reduce rate or hold feeds[a]

Ileostomy output

If <2 g/kg/h	→ Advance rate by 10–20 ml/kg/day
If 2–3 g/kg/h	→ No change
If >3 g/kg/h	→ Reduce rate or hold feeds[a]

Stool reducing substances

If <1%	→ Advance feeds per stool or ostomy output
If = 1%	→ No change
If >1%	→ Reduce rate or hold feeds[a]

Signs of dehydration

If absent	→ Advance feeds per stool or ostomy output
If present	→ Reduce rate or hold feeds[a]

Gastric aspirates

<Four times previous hour's infusion	→ Advance feeds
>Four times previous hour's infusion	→ Reduce rate or hold feeds[a]

[a]Feeds should generally be held for 8 h and then restarted at three-fourths of the previous rate.
Adapted from Utter SL and Duggan C (2004) Short bowel syndrome. In: Hendricks KM and Duggan C (eds.) *Manual of Pediatric Nutrition*, 4th edn. Hamilton, Ontario: BC Decker.

selenium, carnitine, copper, and zinc blood concentrations should be checked periodically and supplemented if needed. Parenteral nutrition should be cycled off for a few hours each day to help simulate more natural cyclic fluctuations of gastrointestinal hormones. These patients also often have poor absorption of calcium and need calcium supplements to prevent osteopenia, which increases the risk of fractures. Iron may also be needed in patients with anemia from decreased absorption secondary to resection of the duodenum or jejunum. Ultimately, weaning from parenteral and enteral nutrition remains the goal of treatment, although lifelong dietary therapy is often needed.

Summary

Malabsorption can involve any of the macronutrients or micronutrients, and these disorders may be congenital or acquired. Determining the type of malabsorption and root cause is essential to providing appropriate nutritional therapy. Multiple formulas, supplements, and dietary regimens exist to target specific defects in the digestion, absorption, and assimilation of nutrients. In addition, many new nutrients are undergoing investigation that may become a standard part of care in the future, including probiotics, prebiotics, and various amino acids.

See also: **Celiac Disease**. **Colon**: Disorders; Nutritional Management of Disorders. **Cystic Fibrosis**. **Diarrheal Diseases**. **Lactose Intolerance**. **Microbiota of the Intestine**: Prebiotics; Probiotics. **Nutritional Support**: Adults, Enteral.

Further Reading

Basu TK and Donaldson D (2003) Intestinal absorption in health and disease: Micronutrients. *Best Practice and Research: Clinical Gastroenterology* 17(6): 957–979.

Borowitz D, Baker RD, and Stallings V (2002) Consensus report on nutrition for pediatric patients with cystic fibrosis. *Journal of Pediatric Gastroenterology and Nutrition* 35(3): 246–259.

Duggan C, Gannon J, and Walker WA (2002) Protective nutrients and functional foods for the gastrointestinal tract. *American Journal of Clinical Nutrition* 75: 789–808.

Heuschkel RB, Menache CC, Megerian JT *et al.* (2000) Enteral nutrition and corticosteroids in the treatment of acute Crohn's disease in children. *Journal of Pediatric Gastroenterology and Nutrition* 31: 8–15.

Holt PR (2001) Diarrhea and malabsorption in the elderly. *Gastroenterology Clinics of North America* 30(2): 427–444.

Schmitz J (2004) Maldigestion and malabsorption. In: Walker WA, Goulet O, Kleinman RE *et al.* (eds.) *Pediatric Gastrointestinal Disease: Pathophysiology, Diagnosis, Management*, 4th edn. Hamilton, Ontario: BC Decker.

Treem WR, McAdams L, Stanford L *et al.* (1999) Sacrosidase therapy for congenital sucrase-isomaltase deficiency. *Journal of Pediatric Gastroenterology and Nutrition* 28(2): 137–142.

Vanderhoof JA and Young RJ (2003) Enteral and parenteral nutrition in the care of patients with short-bowel syndrome. *Best Practice and Research: Clinical Gastroenterology* 17(6): 997–1015.

MALNUTRITION

Contents

Primary, Causes Epidemiology and Prevention

A Briend, Institut de Recherche pour le Développement, Paris, France
P Nestel, International Food Policy Research Institute, Washington, DC, USA

Undernutrition is a condition of poor health resulting from an inadequate intake of energy and/or essential nutrients. It can also be caused by an imbalance between energy and nutrient intakes and requirements due to infection that results in malabsorption, anorexia, or excessive losses.

Causes

The determinants of undernutrition can be categorized as being immediate, underlying, or basic (**Figure 1**). The immediate causes include dependence on a diet that is inadequate in quantity and/or quality. This can be due to low food availability or anorexia from recurrent infections and also poor health status that can result in a vicious cycle of ill health and undernutrition. The underlying determinants are food insecurity, inadequate care for mothers and children, and poor sanitation. The basic determinants influence the underlying determinants and include the environmental, technological, and human resources available to a country or community. Access to and use of resources are influenced by both the political and the economic structures as well as cultural and social factors that affect how resources are used to maintain and improve food security, the provision of care, and sanitation. The following discussion is limited to the immediate causes of undernutrition.

Undernutrition is intergenerational, and a cycle of ill health and growth failure frequently occurs in which undernutrition in childhood leads to small body size in adulthood (**Figure 2**). Genetic and environmental influences also affect both maternal height and prepregnancy weight, both of which are important determinants of birth size and, to a lesser extent, later growth and size.

Food Availability and Diet Quality

Poor access to and an inadequate intake of a good quality diet is the major cause of undernutrition in

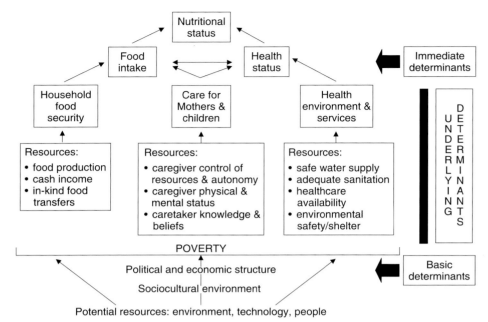

Figure 1 Determinants of undernutrition (Reproduced with permission from Smith LC and Haddad L (2000) *Overcoming Child Malnutrition in Developing Countries: Past Achievements and Future Choices*, Food, Agriculture, and the Environment Discussion Paper No. 30. Washington, DC: International Food Policy Research Institute.)

developing countries. Children are particularly at risk of becoming undernourished due to their high energy and nutrient requirements. Diet diversity, including the intrahousehold distribution of animal source foods, feeding patterns, and child growth are all related to household socioeconomic status.

Low energy intake is associated with growth retardation and often related to a poor quality diet.

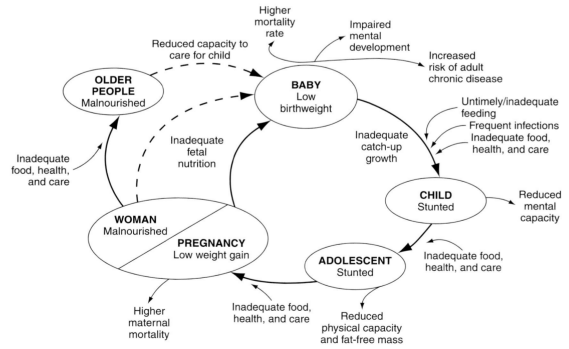

Figure 2 Nutrition throughout the life cycle. (Reproduced with permission from ACC/SCN (2000) *Fourth Report on the World Nutrition Situation*. Geneva: ACC/SCN (in collaboration with the International Food Policy Research Institute).)

Moreover, children can become anorectic when fed monotonous diets, and this can be compounded when superimposed on frequent and repeated bouts of infections. A high-carbohydrate, low-fat diet with a low energy density also precipitates undernutrition in children. Protein deficiency per se is not the major cause of growth retardation, but little is known about the specific effects of essential fatty acid deficiencies on growth. Micronutrient deficiencies, particularly zinc deficiency, cause growth retardation. Zinc supplementation can increase body weight and length/height, but the effect is modest compared with the growth deficit usually observed in growth-faltered children. Children in poor communities are likely to have multiple micronutrient deficiencies, and the combined effect of these coupled with inadequate fat and energy intake will affect growth patterns.

Low income is associated with a low intake of the more expensive animal source foods (meat, fish, dairy, and eggs). The mainly vegetarian diets eaten by children in poor families are frequently associated with growth retardation. Children in developed countries who for cultural reasons eat a diet that lacks any animal products have growth patterns similar to those observed in developing countries.

Women of reproductive age and adolescent girls are also susceptible to micronutrient deficiencies, especially iron, due to their increased physiological requirements for nutrients that can rarely be met from a diet low in animal source foods. In addition, food availability for women is often compounded by sociocultural practices that discriminate against women, and this can start in early childhood and continue throughout the life span.

Infections

Longitudinal studies have shown that infections, especially diarrheal diseases, are associated with growth faltering due to anorexia and/or malabsorption. However, the effect of acute infections on growth is transient, at least in children older than 6 months of age, and no longer apparent after a few weeks. The lack of a long-term effect on growth can be explained by the lower proportion of energy and nutrients needed for growth after 6 months of age, which facilitates catch-up growth after an acute disease. However, chronic infections, even if asymptotic, may lead to anorexia and malabsorption. The frequently observed inverse correlation between markers of chronic infection—such as elevated white blood cell, lymphocyte and platelet counts, C-reactive protein, and gut permeability—and growth supports this hypothesis. A similar mechanism may also explain the delayed growth observed in children

infested with worms and the undernutrition observed in adults with chronic diseases, such as HIV infection and tuberculosis.

The edematous form of severe malnutrition, kwashiorkor, has been hypothesized to be due to oxidative stress resulting from insufficient intake of antioxidant nutrients, including selenium, vitamins E, C, and B_2, niacin, and sulfur amino acids. This suggests that infections, leading to an increased production of free radicals, can be one cause of this form of severe undernutrition.

Epidemiology: Assessing the Prevalence of Undernutrition

Food Balance Sheets

The Food and Agriculture Organization (FAO) uses national-level data on the production, export, and import of food in food balance sheets to calculate the average daily per capita energy supply. This value, combined with a measure of the inequality in food distribution, is used to calculate the proportion of undernourished individuals in a population. Globally, 840 million people are undernourished: 11 million in developed countries, 30 million in countries in transition, and 799 million in the developing world. The total number of undernourished people has increased during the past decade, despite the increase in per caput food availability, because of population growth. The proportion of undernourished individuals is highest in Africa, particularly in sub-Saharan Africa, but the greatest number of undernourished people is in Asia (**Figure 3**).

The precision of the FAO estimate for the number of undernourished individuals is dependent on the accuracy and reliability of agricultural statistics in developing countries, many of which include a large sector that produces food for subsistence and not the market economy. FAO is refining its method to adjust for the latter by including data collected at the household level. The food balance method, however, only deals with estimating the deficit in energy but not nutrient intakes. The latter can be obtained from detailed household or individual-level food consumption surveys, although nationally representative dietary intake surveys are rare in developing countries.

Anthropometric Surveys

When energy intake is insufficient to meet requirements, energy is derived by metabolizing fat and lean tissues, mainly muscle. Children first stop gaining height/length and then lose weight, whereas adults lose weight. Weight loss is more rapid in children

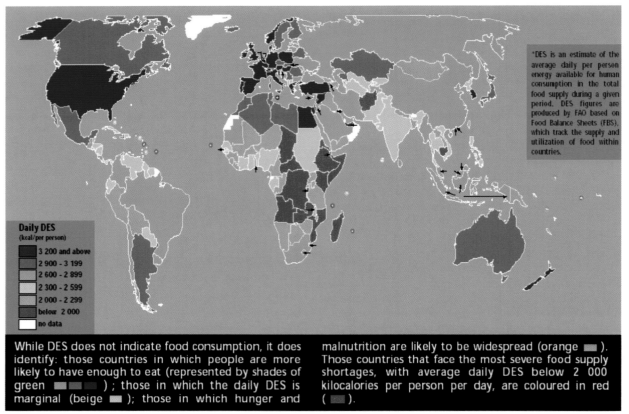

While DES does not indicate food consumption, it does identify: those countries in which people are more likely to have enough to eat (represented by shades of green ■■■); those in which the daily DES is marginal (beige ■); those in which hunger and malnutrition are likely to be widespread (orange ■). Those countries that face the most severe food supply shortages, with average daily DES below 2 000 kilocalories per person per day, are coloured in red (■).

Figure 3 Dietary energy supply (DES), 1994–1996. (Reproduced with permission from the Food and Agriculture Organization (2000) Undernourishment around the world. Counting the hungry: Latest estimates. In: *The State of Food Insecurity in the World.* Rome: FAO.)

than in adults because of their higher energy requirements per kilogram body weight, mainly due to a different body composition. Population-level measurements of body weight and height/length in children indirectly assess the adequacy of food intake on the assumption that a low average body weight and height/length compared with a growth reference reflects an inadequate diet. WHO recommends that the following be used to compare undernutrition in children in different areas of the world:

- Underweight is defined as the proportion of children whose weight in relation to their age is below -2 standard deviations (-2 z scores) of the median of the National Center for Health Statistics (NCHS) reference.
- Wasting is the proportion of children whose weight in relation to their height is below -2 z scores of the median of the NCHS reference.
- Stunting is the proportion of children whose height in relation to their age is below -2 z scores of the median of the NCHS reference.

The previous calculations underestimate the true prevalence of undernutrition because a child can be below his or her optimal weight or height/length yet remain above the -2 z score cutoff point. Wasting is often described as acute malnutrition because it reflects relatively recent weight loss, and stunting is described as chronic malnutrition. Growth retardation is often described as protein–energy malnutrition, which is a misnomer because there is increasing evidence that other nutritional deficiencies besides protein–energy, such as zinc, can lead to growth faltering. Severe undernutrition is defined by a weight in relation to height below -3 z scores of the NCHS reference (marasmus) and/or by the presence of nutritional edema (kwashiorkor or marasmus kwashiorkor), and it is associated with a high risk of dying. WHO and UNICEF maintain a global database on the prevalence of undernutrition among children. Stunting is more prevalent than underweight (**Table 1**) and is often used to monitor long-term trends in undernutrition.

In emergency situations, rapid assessment surveys are often carried out using the mid-upper arm circumference as a proximate indicator of nutritional status in children and, increasingly, adults. This approach is less reliable than methods based on

Table 1 Prevalence of undernutrition by region

UNICEF region	Under-5 population, 2000[a]	Wasting prevalence (%)		Underweight prevalence (%)		Stunting prevalence (%)	
		Moderate and severe	Severe	Moderate and severe	Severe	Moderate and severe	Severe
Sub-Saharan Africa	106 394	10	3	30	9	41	20
Middle East and North Africa	44 478	7	2	15	4	23	9
South Asia	166 566	15	2	46	16	45	22
East Asia and Pacific	159 454	4	—	17	—	21	—
Latin America and Caribbean	54 809	2	0	8	1	16	5
CEE/CIS and Baltic states	30 020	4	1	7	2	16	7
Industrialized countries	50 655	—	—	—	—	—	—
Developing countries	546 471	9	2	28	10	32	17
Least developed countries	110 458	10	2	37	11	43	20

[a]In thousands.
Sources: http://childinfo.org/eddb/malnutrition/database1.htm (underweight), http://childinfo.org/eddb/malnutrition/database2.htm (stunting), and http://childinfo.org/eddb/malnutrition/database3.htm (wasting).

weight and height for epidemiological assessment of undernutrition. Measures of mid-upper arm circumference, however, are useful for screening to quickly identify the severely undernourished, especially children, who are at high risk of dying and need urgent case management.

Anthropometry is also used to assess undernutrition in adults, usually as the body mass index (weight/height^2). A body mass index of less than 18.5 defines chronic energy deficiency, and that less than 16.0 defines severe chronic energy deficiency. A global database on maternal nutrition is not available.

Anthropometric surveys do not give information on the causes (dietary, infectious, or other) of the weight and height deficits they measure. Genetic factors are unlikely to determine child growth at a population level because growth is very similar among well-off children from different countries. Breast-feeding patterns, however, may affect growth patterns, and WHO is developing new growth references based on a longitudinal study of infants from diverse geographic sites who are exclusively or predominantly breast fed for at least 4 months with continued breast feeding throughout the first year and on a cross-sectional study of infants and young children age 18–71 months.

Approximately 55% of all child deaths in developing countries are associated with undernutrition (**Figure 4**), of which at least three-fourths are related to moderate or mild undernutrition rather than severe undernutrition. Some nutritional deficiencies,

such as vitamin A, can result in higher mortality without a clear effect on growth. Hence, studies examining the association between undernutrition and mortality, using anthropometry as proxy for undernutrition, are likely to underestimate the strength of this relationship.

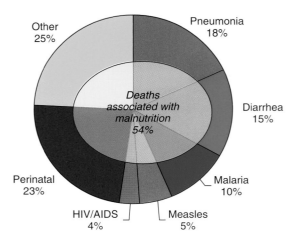

Figure 4 Association between malnutrition assessed by anthropometry and cause-specific mortality in children younger than 5 years of age. (Reproduced with permission from the WHO Department of Child and Adolescent Health and Development (2002) Available at www.who.int/child-adolescent-health/OVERVIEW/CHILD_HEALTH/map_02_world.jpg. Sources: for cause-specific mortality, EIP/WHO; for malnutrition, Pelletier DL, Frongillo EA Jr, and Habicht JP (1993) Epidemiological evidence for a potentiating effect of malnutrition on child mortality. *American Journal of Public Health* **83**: 1130–1133.)

Biochemical Surveys

Because of the interest and focus on controlling iodine, vitamin A, and iron deficiencies, national-level surveys for these micronutrients are conducted in developing countries. Urinary iodine level is a good marker of iodine deficiency, which can cause retarded physical development. However, the biochemical markers of vitamin A and iron are acute phase proteins, which are altered during infection, even subclinical infection. Serum retinol declines during infection, overestimating the prevalence of vitamin A deficiency, whereas serum ferritin rises and overestimates adequate iron stores. Hemoglobin, which is often used as a proxy for iron deficiency, is also affected by the prevalence of infection (as is serum zinc). For these reasons, biochemical surveys need to include markers of infection, which adds to their complexity and cost; thus, they are rarely done.

Prevention

Increasing both the purchasing power of poor families and women's access to and control of household resources can prevent undernutrition. Improving the social and economic status of women and households, however, is insufficient to eliminate undernutrition and interventions that affect each stage of the life cycle and are necessary to break the intergenerational cycle of undernutrition (**Table 2**).

Table 2 Intervention points in the life cycle continuum

Nutritional risks	Interventions to improve nutritional status and growth
Infancy and early childhood (<6 months)	
Suboptional breast feeding	Feeding colostrum
	Exclusive breast feeding for 6 months
Complementary feeding period (6–24 months)	
Suboptional breast-feeding	Breast feeding
Inadequate and low-quality diet	Nutrition education
Micronutrient deficiencies	Infection control
Frequent infections and parasites	Food supplements
Gender discrimination in food and health care	Micronutrient supplements
Childhood (2–9 years)	
Inadequate and low-quality diet	Nutrition education
Micronutrient deficiencies	Infection control
Frequent infections and parasites	Micronutrient supplements
Gender discrimination in food and health care	School feeding
Adolescence (10–19 years)	
Inadequate and low-quality diet	Iron supplementation (schools)
Rapid growth	Deworming through schools (endemic areas)
Anemia with onset of menstruation	Nutrition and health education (schools)
Infections (including STDs) and parasites	Prevention and management of STDs and other infections
Early pregnancy and lactation	School meals
Gender discrimination in food and health care	Income-earning skill training
Adult women of reproductive age (20–49 years)	
Food insecurity	Income generation
Micronutrient deficiencies	Family planning/birth spacing
Infections and parasites	Prevention and management of STDs
Gender inequities	Agricultural/gardening
STDs and AIDS	Improved technologies
	Adult literacy
Pregnant women	
Inadequate food intake to meet increased demands for fetal growth	Increase intake of bioavailable nutrients and energy
Micronutrient deficiencies	Malaria chemoprophylaxis (endemic areas)
Maternal mortality	Deworming (endemic areas)
Low birth weight	Iron/folic acid supplementation
Birth defects	Postpartum vitamin A
Lactating women	
Decreased quantity of vitamins in breast milk	Increase intake of bioavailable nutrients and energy
Micronutrient deficiencies	Iron/folic acid supplementation
Weight loss	
Post-reproductive age (49+ years)	
Undernutrition	Food security

Early Infancy (<6 Months)

All newborns should be fed colostrum immediately after delivery. Because breast milk is the best food for infants, exclusive breast feeding is the best way to prevent undernutrition in this age group. Exclusive breast feeding also reduces the risk of diarrhea and other infections that can reduce appetite and absorption or increase nutrient losses.

The advantages of breast feeding should be balanced with the risk of HIV transmission if the mother is known to be HIV positive. In early infancy, breast milk may not easily be replaced, and risks should be carefully assessed by program managers before recommending breast milk substitutes.

Beyond exclusive breast feeding, there is a role for micronutrient supplementation for some high-risk children. For example, low birthweight infants can benefit from zinc, iron, and vitamin A supplementation. Where there is a risk of rickets, such as in areas where young infants do not get any exposure to sunlight or calcium intake is very low, vitamin D supplementation is recommended.

Complementary Feeding Period (6–24 Months)

Undernutrition, especially wasting and micronutrient deficiencies, is most prevalent during the complementary feeding period. Linear growth retardation is usually well established during this stage of the life cycle. This age group is particularly vulnerable because of its high nutrient requirements that cannot be supplied through breast milk alone. A variety of nutrition interventions have been proposed to prevent undernutrition, and the use of multiple approaches is likely to be most successful.

Breast feeding promotion   Beyond 6 months of age, breast milk alone is not sufficient to sustain optimal growth and its contribution to energy and nutrient intake progressively declines. After the age of 12 months, breast fed children are not better nourished than non-breast fed children. However, prolonged breast feeding is very important and needs to be promoted because it improves child survival. The poor nutritional status of breast fed children older than 6 months of age is due to late introduction of an appropriately balanced diet. Family planning is an important intervention for promoting prolonged breast feeding because a new pregnancy can be a frequent cause of breast feeding cessation.

Nutrition education   Undernutrition among children is often ascribed to ignorance, and nutrition education programs are often proposed to resolve

this. However, choosing and recommending foods that are appropriate for promoting child growth at low cost is not easy. Moreover, micronutrient requirements in this age group are high, and it is usually not possible to provide a balanced diet without large quantities of animal source foods or fortified foods that are generally not readily available to the poor.

In theory, advising mothers to use nutrient-dense foods when they are available might improve child nutrition. Some nutrition education programs have be shown to be efficacious in pilot studies, but their effectiveness when scaled up has been disappointing.

Infection control   Acute infections have a transient effect on the growth of young children. However, controlling chronic infections, including parasitic and other subclinical infections, can have a positive effect on growth. A general improvement in environmental hygiene and sanitation may be more effective in removing this cause of undernutrition than medical interventions per se, with the possible exception of regular deworming.

Food supplements   Food supplements are designed to provide nutrients missing from the diet. They are usually made from a cereal flour mixed with a lysine-rich flour, generally soy flour, or milk powder to improve the amino acid balance (e.g., corn–soy blend). The fat content is usually low because fat mixed with flour is rapidly oxidized and cannot be added to food without costly packaging. Nowadays, such food supplements are usually fortified with micronutrients that are likely to be missing in childrens' diet, especially iron, zinc, retinol, and riboflavin.

The efficacy of food supplements has been tested in pilot programs, and most randomized trials that compared the growth of children receiving food supplements with that of children receiving the usual family diet failed to show a major effect on growth, especially height. The reasons for this are not clear. Biological factors may be involved. For example, most trials tested a low-cost supplement that had a high phytate content, which would limit the bioavailability of minerals such as zinc (known to be important for growth) and iron. Moreover, the food supplements were low in fat, which may be a limiting nutrient for children who usually have a very low fat intake. Finally, even in carefully controlled trials the food supplement may be shared within the family, especially if it requires special preparation, which would dilute its effect.

Besides the pilot trials, the use of donated food supplements has been usually limited to food crises, such as wars and environmental catastrophes. Food supplements are also available in the commercial market, but their price often precludes their use by those most in need of them.

Micronutrient supplements Vitamin A is routinely distributed through immunization programs and is a standard health package delivered in under-5 clinics to improve child survival. In very few countries, prophylactic liquid iron is given to older infants. Routine iron supplementation to children is not without controversy in malarial areas. Most micronutrient supplementation trials have been carried out using syrups, which are expensive to use on a large scale, or tablets/capsules, which are difficult to administer to young children. New formulations, such as multiple micronutrient sprinkles or water-dispersible tablets, are being tested. Highly fortified spreads that can provide fat along with micronutrients are also being tested.

Childhood (2–9 Years)

The nutritional problems of 2- to 5-year-old children are similar to those of younger children. The critical factors being that these children do not eat enough food and they are still susceptible to repeated bouts of infection. Because there is no obvious contact point with these children (e.g., measles immunization), it is difficult to deliver programs that reach them.

Children 6–9 years old can be reached through school feeding programs. School health programs increasingly include deworming, malaria chemoprophylaxis, and iron supplementation to improve student nutrition and health. Where institutional feeding is provided, the potential exists to provide fortified food in a meal or as a snack food. In situations in which institutional feeding is not provided, community mobilization activities in primary education can incorporate messages to support student health and nutrition.

Adolescents (10–19 Years)

Adolescent girls are at special nutritional risk, especially for iron deficiency anemia, with menstruation taking place while growth is still not complete. Few intervention studies have been done on adolescent girls, and those that have focused on anemia prevention. Well-supervised intermittent iron supplementation to adolescent girls in schools or the workplace can reduce their prevalence of anemia. Although iron supplements have been shown to be important for correcting iron deficiency anemia in adolescent girls, there is only a modest improvement in storage iron status in early pregnancy following supplementation in adolescence if the time between the end of supplementation and conception is more than a few months. Iron supplementation in adolescence cannot build sufficient stores to substitute for the need for iron supplements in pregnancy.

Secondary schools are the easiest way to reach adolescents, although in many countries relatively few girls go to school compared to boys. Supplementary food can also be provided through school meals to induce growth and maximize the pubertal growth spurt, increase school attendance, and serve as an excellent opportunity for nutrition and health education relevant to the age group. Such interventions are likely to be effective because of the potential for good supervision. However, any credible intervention program will have to reach the girls who do not attend school. Currently, the few activities targeted to this age group center around HIV/AIDS awareness and education, including the prevention and management of sexually transmitted diseases. These children, especially girls, are particularly vulnerable and often have no voice in the community.

Women of Reproductive Age (20–49 Years)

Many programs designed to improve food security include adult women of reproductive age, who may not be pregnant or lactating. Managers of these programs recognize that the nutritional benefits are not necessarily direct, and it is not easy to measure or attribute any change in nutritional status to the intervention. Such projects, which invariably strive to empower women, include income-generation or credit schemes, home gardening and agriculture, improved technologies, and adult literacy, alone or in combination.

Health-based interventions, such as family planning and longer birth spacing, are assumed to have a more direct effect on women's nutritional status, but the inputs and outcomes rarely, if ever, include issues related to improving the nutritional status of women. However, the potential is there to change this.

The role of iron/folic acid supplements remains equivocal, except where severe deficiency exists. Insufficient data are available to justify the provision of free multiple micronutrient supplements through the public health system, although there is some rationale to improve micronutrient status before these women become pregnant so that they are in the best nutritional state possible. The demand side issues for supplementation need to be addressed concurrently; otherwise, it is unlikely that these programs can be successful.

In urban areas, adult women of reproductive age may be reached through the workplace, social/community groups, religious centers, etc., where the possibility exists of getting institutional support for health-related activities that include nutrition. Similar groups could be used in rural areas where they exist, and activities that support or strengthen group 'cohesion' should be seen as a component of an add-on nutrition/health activity. As with the other groups of the life cycle framework, it is important to put nutrition in the context of perceived priorities.

Pregnancy

Prenatal programs focus on identifying and counseling pregnant women on appropriate care and nutrition, including breast-feeding, tetanus toxoid immunization, iron/folic acid supplementation, and referral of high-risk pregnancies. Malaria chemoprophylaxis, especially among primigravidae, and deworming need to be encouraged to prevent anemia in areas where these parasites are public health problems. The provision of postpartum vitamin A supplementation is increasing and needs to be further expanded.

Some programs provide and target supplementary food to at-risk and undernourished women. These programs are effective in increasing weight gain during pregnancy, but they have a significant beneficial effect on birth weight only in women who are genuinely at risk of an inadequate diet, such as rural African women who continue to perform difficult manual work during the hungry season. In other settings, the effect is less clear.

Despite the research evidence that iron supplementation is efficacious, this relatively simple program has not been effective in reducing the prevalence of anemia among women. Most iron/folic acid supplement programs suffer from serious operational constraints related to supply and distribution systems, access to health care services, motivation of health care providers, and compliance. Lack of good quality, low-cost, generic iron supplements, suitable compounds and dispensing mechanisms, and potential side effects are unsolved problems that affect compliance.

Although there is little evidence that an iron supplement program works, it remains one of the few options available to improve iron status of the population, and it is the only program that has the potential to meet the high iron requirements of pregnancy. Operation research has shown that intermittent supplementation is less appropriate for pregnant women and daily iron supplementation should be continued as the intervention of choice.

Lactation

Except under extreme famine-like conditions, undernourished women produce sufficient breast milk, but its micronutrient quality can vary depending on the nutritional status of the mother.

Postnatal programs cover the lactation period and include counseling on nutrition (including breast-feeding) and family planning, although these two programs are not usually integrated. Where the prevalence of anemia is higher than 40%, iron/folic acid supplementation should be extended through the first 3 months of lactation. Clinical signs of vitamin A deficiency are known to exist in lactating women, and postpartum supplementation within 6–8 weeks of giving birth has been shown to be beneficial and safe for both the mother and the newborn.

Some programs include provision of a protein and energy supplement during lactation. Controlled trials have failed to show an effect on milk production, but increased weight gain and a sensation of well-being among mothers are potential positive outcomes.

Post-reproductive Age (49+ Years)

There are no reports on nutrition interventions for older people in developing countries, successful or otherwise. At best, they are covered in food security projects targeted at the household level, although the focus is generally on maternal and child nutrition. This age group deserves more attention, especially in areas with a high prevalence of HIV, where older people often play a key role in sustaining the household.

See also: **Adolescents**: Nutritional Problems. **Anemia**: Iron-Deficiency Anemia. **Breast Feeding**. **Children**: Nutritional Problems. **Dietary Surveys**. **Infants**: Feeding Problems. **Infection**: Nutritional Interactions; Nutritional Management in Adults. **Lactation**: Dietary Requirements. **Malnutrition**: Secondary, Diagnosis and Management. **Nutritional Assessment**: Anthropometry; Biochemical Indices; Clinical Examination. **Older People**: Nutrition-Related Problems. **Pregnancy**: Nutrient Requirements. **Supplementation**: Role of Micronutrient Supplementation; Developing

Countries; Developed Countries. **United Nations Children's Fund**. **Vegetarian Diets**. **World Health Organization**. **Zinc**: Deficiency in Developing Countries, Intervention Studies.

Further Reading

Allen LH and Gillespie SR (2001) *ACC/SCN. What Works? A Review of the Efficacy and Effectiveness of Nutrition Interventions*. Geneva: ACC/SCN (in collaboration with the Asian Development Bank, Manila). Available at www.adb.org/documents/books/nutrition/what_works/default.asp.

Awasthi S, Bundy DA, and Savioli L (2003) Helminthic infections. *British Medical Journal* **327**: 431–433.

Brown KH, Peerson JM, Rivera J, and Allen LH (2002) Effect of supplemental zinc on the growth and serum zinc concentrations of prepubertal children: A meta-analysis of randomized controlled trials. *American Journal of Clinical Nutrition* **75**: 1062–1071.

Checkley W, Epstein LD, Gilman RH, Cabrera L, and Black RE (2003) Effects of acute diarrhea on linear growth in Peruvian children. *American Journal of Epidemiology* **157**: 166–175.

Davidsson L and Nestel P (2003) *Efficacy and Effectiveness of Interventions to Control Iron Deficiency and Iron Deficiency Anemia*. Washington, DC: International Nutritional Anemia Consultative Group. Available at http://inacg.ilsi.org/file/efficacyscreen.pdf.

Food and Agriculture Organization (2002) Undernourishment around the world. Counting the hungry: Latest estimates In: *The State of Food Insecurity in the World*. Rome: FAO. Available at http://ftp.fao.org/docrep/fao/005/y7352e/y7352e01.pdf.

Gera T and Sachdev HP (2002) Effect of iron supplementation on incidence of infectious illness in children: Systematic review. *British Medical Journal* **325**: 1142–1152.

International Vitamin A Consultative Group (2002) *IVACG Statement on Maternal Night Blindness: A New Indicator of Vitamin A Deficiency*. Washington, DC: IVAGC. Available at http://ivacg.ilsi.org/file/Nightblindness.pdf.

Merialdi M, Carroli G, Villar J *et al.* (2003) Nutritional interventions during pregnancy for the prevention or treatment of impaired fetal growth: An overview of randomized controlled trials. *Journal of Nutrition* **133**(5 supplement 2): 1626S–1631S.

Sazawal S, Black RE, Menon VP *et al.* (2001) Zinc supplementation in infants born small for gestational age reduces mortality: A prospective, randomized, controlled trial. *Pediatrics* **108**: 1280–1286.

Steketee RW (2003) Pregnancy, nutrition and parasitic diseases. *Journal of Nutrition* **133**(5 supplement 2): 1661S–1667S.

Tomkins A (2003) Assessing micronutrient status in the presence of inflammation. *Journal of Nutrition* **133**(5 supplement 2): 1649S–1655S.

UNICEF (2003) *UNICEF statistics: Malnutrition*. Available at http://childinfo.org/eddb/malnutrition/index.htm.

World Health Organization (2003) *HIV and Infant Feeding: Framework for Priority Action*. Available at www.who.int/child-adolescent-health/publications/NUTRITION/HIV_IF_Framework.htm.

World Health Organization (2003) *Department of Nutrition for Health and Development. Global Data Base on Child Growth and Malnutrition*. Available at www.who.int/nutgrowthdb/.

Secondary, Diagnosis and Management

N Solomons, Center for Studies of Sensory Impairment, Aging and Metabolism (CeSSIAM), Guatemala City, Guatemala

Definitional Considerations

In its broadest context, malnutrition is a state of having an inappropriate nutritional status with respect to one or more macronutrient (water, electrolyte, protein, or fat) or micronutrient (vitamin or mineral) constituent of the body. This imbalance can be a deficit, leading to an insufficient supply or content of the nutrient (undernutrition), or an excess, leading to an excessive content or overloading of the organism with a nutrient (overnutrition).

Victor Herbert enumerated six possible causes for all nutrient deficiencies as: decreased intake; impaired absorption; increased wastage; impaired utilization; increased destruction; and elevated requirements. Correspondingly, with the exception of any utilization defect, overnutrition and excesses can result from the reciprocal defects, that is: hyperphagia; hyperabsorption; increased retention; decreased destruction; and decreased requirements.

As discussed in the previous chapter, the term 'primary' malnutrition relates almost exclusively to the first of these mechanisms, that of the ingestion of nutrients from the diet. It is about food consumption and intake. Secondary malnutrition, by contrast, concerns the disturbed and disordered handling of nutrients. When diseases or abnormal physiological conditions interfere with the normal disposition of nutrients ingested from the diet, this is the basis of a situation of 'secondary' malnutrition. A representative, but not exhaustive, list of diseases and conditions producing secondary undernutrition is provided in **Table 1**. The roster of causes of secondary overnutrition is provided in **Table 2**.

The basis for suspecting the presence of secondary undernutrition emerges when there is evidence of malnutrition (deficiency or excess) but food and nutrients are presumably being consumed with in abundance. Once the suspicion emerges, three distinct diagnostic principles need to be addressed: (1) the confirmation of dietary intake, and estimation of its adequacy; (2) the diagnosis and classification of abnormal nutritional status; and (3) the diagnosis of the functional, physiological, or pathological origins of disordered nutrient disposition. To emphasize the

Table 1 Diseases and conditions associated with secondary macronutrient or micronutrient undernutrition

Decreased nutrient absorption
Gastric atrophy
Pernicious anemia
Celiac disease
Inflammatory bowel disease
Intestinal cryptosporidiasis
Pancreatic insufficiency
Biliary obstruction
Cystic fibrosis
Radiation enteritis
Chronic intestinal pseudoobstruction

Increased nutrient excretion
Hepatic cirrhosis
Laxative abuse
Peptic ulcer
Gastrointestinal fistula
Gastric adenoma
Colonic adenoma
Amebiasis
Hookworm
Schistosomiasis
Diabetes mellitus
Fanconi syndrome
Hypoaldosteronism
Hemodialysis; peritoneal dialysis

Increased destruction or internal consumption nutrients
Hyperthyroidism
Cardiac cachexia
HIV/AIDS
Cancer cachexia
Cystic fibrosis
Bone marrow transplants
Pulmonary tuberculosis

Decreased utilization of nutrients
Lead poisoning
Menkes' copper storage disease

point, one must remain attuned to the nutritional status of patients, clients, or populations, and sensitive to the possibility of a nonprimary origin of any under- or overnutrition.

Table 2 Diseases and conditions associated with secondary macronutrient or micronutrient excess (overnutrition)

Increased nutrition absorption
Wilson's disease
Hemochromatosis

Increased nutrition retention
Prader–Willi syndrome
Hypercorticosterism
Hyperpituitarism
Acute tubular necrosis
Chronic renal failure

Decreased destruction of nutrients
Hypothyroidism

Coexistence of Primary and Secondary Malnutrition

It is important to recognize the potential for the simultaneous coexistence of primary and secondary malnutrition in the same individual. Primary malnutrition in the free-living populations can be associated with famine conditions (crop failure, conflict, natural disaster, refugee crisis), in which sufficient food is simply not available. Alternatively, it can arise from the poverty of landlessness or urban margination, where food is not accessible within the household income. A large number of communicable diseases with consequences for nutrient absorption, retention or utilization, such as parasitoses, tuberculosis or HIV/AIDS, are common in these situations of deprivation and misery.

To the extent that a disease process produces anorexia or dysphagia, or even psychic depression, the net effect is to reduce total intake of dietary energy and nutrients. Whatever, malabsorptive or nutrient-wasting components of the underlying disorders will further compromise the nutritional state.

The Reverse Paradigm: Underlying Pathology Revealed by Detection of Abnormal Nutrition

In clinical medicine, a type of 'reversal of roles' often occurs. Rather than primarily recognizing the presentation of the underlying pathology, recognition of an abnormal nutritional status without a suitable dietary cause leads to the diagnosis of the underlying disorder before any specific (pathognomonic) sign or symptom has yet occurred. For instance, the Prader-Willi syndrome of pathological obesity would initially present as common obesity. Similarly, in hypercorticosteroidism (Cushing's syndrome), abnormal fat deposition and weight gain can be the changes that lead to the recognition of the underlying pituitary or adrenal dysfunction.

Classically, in type 2 diabetes, unexplained weight loss is a presenting complaint when polyuria is mild or absent. Moreover, with common forms of childhood gastrointestinal disorders, such as celiac sprue or Crohn's disease, arrested linear growth is often the first clue that something is clinically awry. It provokes the diagnostic inquiry that leads to the recognition of the bowel lesions. In milder presentations of cystic fibrosis, a similar growth failure occurring in infancy, can indicate an underlying pathological disorder.

In fact, the entire roster of conditions listed in **Table 1** and **Table 2**, as well as others of a similar nature, are subject to being diagnosed as the result

Table 3 Three-level diagnostic principles related to secondary malnutrition

Assessment of dietary and nutrient intake: A quantitative and qualitative evaluation of usual dietary intake by a nutritionally trained practitioner or clinical dietician serves to exclude the possibility that the situation is not primary (low intake) in nature and suggests the secondary basis of the nutritional problem. Caveat: In certain situations, a **combination** of reduced intakes **and** nutritional stress at absorption, retention, or utilization may coexist.

Assessment of nutritional status: This includes the measures of anthropometry and body composition, hematological status, biological indices, and functional indicators, as well as clinical (physical) evaluation.

Diagnosis of underlying cause(s) of secondary nutritional imbalance: It is important, where possible, to identify the underlying entitie(s) that are causing the nutritional problem, to enable (where possible) a direct remedial approach to the cause of malnutrition and to orient management based on any pathophysiological knowledge about the underlying disease.

of a secondary change in nutritional status. The practical message is that the nutritional specialist, physician, or nonphysician may be the first person to whom the secondarily malnourished patient is referred and the acumen of recognising a secondary causation will guide the case to an appropriate clinical diagnostic program to uncover (and hopefully address and remedy) the underlying medical or surgical problems. Overarching guideline principles for uncovering secondary malnutrition states are provided in **Table 3**.

Diagnosis of Secondary Malnutrition

In general terms, a common set of principles applies for assessment of nutrient status whether the bases are primary, secondary, or a combination of both. These principles include: body composition measures, hematological and biochemical findings, functional variables, and clinical signs and symptoms. It is more productive to focus here on the nuances, caveats, and distinctions for the detection of altered nutrition due to background conditions beyond spontaneous food intake.

Caveats for the Diagnosis of Secondary Excess Nutriture

The conditions that cause increased retention of energy and hypometabolism are listed in **Table 2**. When it comes to overweight and obesity, the absence of clear-cut overeating combined with other characteristic signs of the different entities should raise suspicion. Excesses of vitamins and minerals may not easily be detected because the homeostatic control of circulating concentrations confounds biochemical diagnosis. Excessive urinary excretion rates of the nutrients or their metabolites often provide better indications than blood levels when micronutrient overload is the issue.

Caveats for the Diagnosis of Secondary Undernutrition

Undernutrition due to disease and dysfunction obviously requires establishment of the following: (1) the existence of deficiencies; and (2) that factors other than underconsumption are influencing the deficiency states. The body composition standard is a body mass index (BMI) of $<18.5 \, \mathrm{kg \, m^{-2}}$. With the worldwide pandemic of overweight, recent weight loss of 10% or more of usual body weight may be a more sensitive and reliable indicator of an incipient undernutrition problem. Weight problems diagnosed in this manner would certainly be detectable well before the BMI will have fallen to the aforementioned criterion.

Ill patients with adequate or excessive body mass indices can manifest metabolic substrate metabolism reminiscent of the severe malnutrition syndromes of adult kwashiorkor or marasmus (inanition). Moreover, fluctuations in weight under acute or semiacute situations often reflect changes in fluid balance. This is also the situation in patients with end-stage renal failure undergoing chronic dialysis. Methods such as bioelectrical impedance, dual X-ray absorbance, or isotope dilution in association with indirect calorimetry can assess true lean- and fat-mass status and macronutrient metabolism in patients of apparently normal body mass.

Hematological evaluation is important in nutritional assessment. A low hemoglobin, hematocrit, or red cell count signifies anemia, but in individuals with associated diseases, anemia can have a series of origins (hemolytic, hypoproliferative) that are nonnutritional and will not respond to nutritional therapy.

Biochemical evaluation for nutrient deficiency status in patients with associated disease is fraught with caveats and limitations. Michael Golden has defined two classes of nutritional deficiency: in type 1 deficiencies, nutritional desaturation of tissue stores occurs, and circulating levels of nutrients reflect the total body nutrient status; in type 2 deficiency, there is homeostatic conservation of tissue and circulating concentrations of nutrients, such that blood concentrations remain virtually unaltered in the face of depletion. Deficiencies of zinc and magnesium, among others, fall into this second category. Inflammation and infection are stimuli that directly alter the circulating concentrations of nutrient indicators. Ferritin and circulating copper are elevated whereas zinc, iron, and vitamin A concentrations are depressed with activation of the acute-phase response to injury. In liver disease, depressed production of binding proteins can alter the usual indicators of nutritional status as a consequence of hepatic pathophysiology itself, rather than preexisting secondary malnutrition. Finally, it almost goes without saying that attempting biochemical nutrient evaluations from blood samples taken during concurrent infusion of micronutrient solutions in parenteral nutrition regimens – and without a period of distribution and equilibration – will not reflect the tissue stores and total body reserves of the respective nutrients of interest.

Functional indicators of nutritional status have been applied to the assessment of secondary malnutrition and have been plagued by pitfalls. This applies to tests of nitrogen status, immune function, and hepatic protein secretion. Tests such as creatinine excretion, white blood cell counts, and cutaneous delayed hypersensitivity anergy, as well as decreased serum albumin, transferrin, transthyronein (prealbumin), and retinal-binding protein concentrations are sensitive to alteration by stress and injury. Failure to recognize distortion from stress underlies an early fallacy in surgical nutrition, in which low values for albumin, lymphocyte counts, and pre-albumin, together with anergy, predicted poor postoperative outcomes. This misconception justified aggressive preoperative parenteral nutrition and albumin infusions, with little impact on predicted outcomes. In these situations, it was the stress and injury of the underlying disease, rather than nutritional status, that was producing the abnormal values for the biomarkers. Recently, insulin-like growth factor has been advanced as a sensitive indicator of protein status in older patients, but whether it is confounded by nonnutritional features of disease remains to be clarified.

Management of Secondary Malnutrition

Secondary malnutrition has many faces and facets. It may have to be addressed both in a public health sense, for communicable diseases, such as parasitoses or HIV/AIDS, and in a medical care context, for disorders that are particular and clinical in nature, such as hereditary or degenerative diseases.

Principles of Management

The first principle is to identify the underlying functional, physiological, or pathological cause of the malnourished state. If the condition is curable, then the management issues are simplified. For instance, if a person is dehydrated because of hyperglycemic diuresis in uncontrolled diabetes mellitus, the short-term management involves administration of exogenous intravenous fluids to restore normal hydration; however, restoring adequate diabetic control to the patient would be the long-term and definitive solution. The undernutrition and growth failure due to undetected celiac disease is easily eliminated by institution of a gluten-free diet. With deficient nutrition in cystic fibrosis, adequate management of pulmonary problems and digestive-enzyme should allow patients to recover and maintain normal nutrition on a balanced oral diet. Thus, medical or surgical address of the underlying disorder, where possible, is the primary tool for management of secondary undernutrition.

Public Health Approaches

The management of the secondary nutritional deficiency attributable to hookworm or schistosomiasis, i.e., iron deficiency, can be achieved both by anthelmintic medications or by supplemental iron to compensate for parasite-induced losses. In countries where HIV/AIDS is rampant efforts for its prevention are fundamental. A food-security crisis grips the whole society in AIDS endemic areas, and this must be relieved with food and economic assistance. The wasting syndromes produced by tuberculosis are best addressed proactively by prevention of transmission and early detection. However, when primary prevention fails, as in the aforementioned infections, efforts to enhance the enteral intake of infected members of the community are particularly essential for their comfort and well being.

Dietary Management of Secondary Overnutrition

The dietary management of secondary overnutrition would logically be to restrict the intake of the nutrients accruing in excess. This is not always facile or feasible, however, due to the intrinsic complexity of foods and beverages, where most are sources of multiple essential micronutrients. Marked reduction in total energy intake can jeopardize the intake of proteins and essential fats. For the metal-storage afflictions such as Wilson's disease and hemochromatosis, removing copper and iron from the diet, respectively, are the fundamental elements of management. Some additional benefits can be gained by blocking the metals' absorption, as with high doses of zinc in Wilson's disease or with strong black tea (tannins) in hemochromatosis. Fundamentally, however, the management of metal-storage diseases requires some interventions to selectively remove the overload by chelating agents in Wilson's disease and recurrent phlebotomy in hemochromatosis. In a related variant condition, African hemosiderosis, common among Bantu in southern Africa, removing concentrated iron sources from the diet, specifically the iron-loaded native beers, provides effective long-term control.

Dietary and Nutritional Management of Secondary Undernutrition

The syllogism for dietary and nutritional management is to get enough nutrients into the body to restore nutritional adequacy and balance, taking any chronic barriers to uptake and retention into consideration. The blend of nutrients must be tailored to the specific absorptive or utilization problems, e.g., compensatory fat-soluble vitamins in water-miscible forms with severe fat malabsorption, and extra doses of highly available iron with chronic blood loss. These can be delivered within a dietary context with supplements and fortified vehicles in nonacute conditions. Even nondietary routes have been devised as in the treatment of vitamin D deficiency due to Crohn's disease with tanning bed ultraviolet B radiation.

When accumulated undernutrition is dangerously advanced, absorptive barriers are especially severe, or nutrient losses are excessive more concerted nutritional intervention is required. Intensive therapy can be delivered by three routes: orally, with special diets supplemented by liquid formulas; enterally, with liquid formulas perfused by intragastric or intraintestinal feeding tubes; and parenterally, with intravenous formulas infused into peripheral or central veins. Up to 50% of patients on dialysis have protein-energy malnutrition, which may continue undetected. For end-stage renal patients, intra-dialytic alimentation (adding nutrients to the dialysis fluids) has been used to reduce nutrient loss. Each approach has its distinct costs, special potential, and limitations and risks, and has been explored and refined in the context of age, physiological status, and specific disease states or surgical indications.

Tailoring of nutrient delivery is required with both enteral and parenteral nutrition, depending upon the pathophysiology of the underlying conditions. Both hypo- and hypermetabolic states can occur; indirect calorimetry with metabolic carts is in vogue for prescribing energy delivery in intensive care. When pulmonary compromise is present, the balance among macronutrients is important to minimize carbon dioxide formation in metabolism.

Maintaining abundant amino acid supply promotes protein-sparing and prevents loss of lean tissue in catabolic states. Enrichment of enteral or parenteral regimens with branched-chain amino acids or keto-analog amino acids has been devised to compensate for the metabolic defects of nitrogen handling in hepatic or renal failure states. The objective of nutritional support in patients with liver failure is to provide adequate macronutrients to ensure the specific substrates for energy and protein synthesis and integrity of normal hepatic tissue function, without inducing or accentuating encephalopathy or otherwise aggravating hepatic insufficiency.

In juvenile cholestasis, large amounts of fat-soluble vitamin supplements and medium-chain triglycerides are usually required for optimum growth. With protracted secretory diarrheal diatheses, fluid and electrolyte balance may be the primary concern, followed by macro- and micronutrient nutriture, invoking the institution of parenteral feeding. Cancer cachexia is a major secondary consequence of disseminated neoplasms. It is tempting to prescribe aggressive nutritional support, but a caveat is that certain nutrients acting with certain neoplasms favor the tumor's growth and dissemination. To the extent that various forms of cachexia are partly driven by catabolic responses mediated by proinflammatory cytokines, antagonists directed at countering their action hold promise for retarding the nutrient-wasting in various forms of cachexia.

With intensive nutrition, there are risks and adverse consequences intertwined with the benefits. A variation of the refeeding syndrome, that is hyper-alimentation complications from excessive energy substrate perfusion or infusion, can produce hypophosphatemic and hypokalemic episodes. Improper formulation of fluids or liquids with micronutrients can cause deficiency or toxicity states in chronic nutritional support. The hazards of indwelling catheters are multiple, from phlebitis of the veins to sudden dislocation or migration. Fluid overload and sepsis are the most troubling complications of intravenous parenteral nutrition.

For tube-feeding enteral alimentation, tube placement is the crucial element. With nasal placement of the tube, there is a finite risk of respiratory tract inflammation and infection from aspiration of formula and secretions. In hospital, enteral nutrition is a risk factor for nosocomial pneumonia. An alternative site for long-term administration of tube-feeds is percutaneous placement of an intragastric feeding tube under endoscopic control.

Aggressive nutritional support, with its attendant expense and potential morbidity, in critically ill patients remains controversial. In terms of cost–benefit analysis, the use of the intensive formats of enteral artificial nutrition seems to be cost effective to reduce post-hip-fracture hospital stay in underweight women and for preoperative nutritional support, if carried out at home. Preoperative parenteral nutrition has been judged as prohibitively expensive for the small reduction in postoperative morbidity that it produces.

Conclusions

Dietary intake is the most important determinant of over- or undernutrition, but it is not the only influence on an individual's nutritional status. A series of extrinsic environmental factors or intrinsic clinical or physiological disorders can alter the absorption, retention, utilization, and integrity of nutrients. These give origin to secondary malnutrition states. Primary (dietary origin) and secondary (environmental, pathological) factors often combine within the same individuals. From a public health perspective, the goal is to implement broad policies and programs that increase the availability of specific nutrients imperiled by the local environmental problems, e.g., iron in hookworm infested areas, while addressing the primary diseases. In the clinical setting, management requires diagnosing and managing the underlying pathological states interfering with nutritional health while providing compensatory measures to correct secondary nutritional imbalances.

See also: **Cystic Fibrosis**. **Diabetes Mellitus**: Etiology and Epidemiology. **Handicap**: Prader–Willi Syndrome. **Liver Disorders**. **Malnutrition**: Primary, Causes Epidemiology and Prevention. **Nutritional Support**: Adults, Enteral; Adults, Parenteral; Infants and Children, Parenteral. **Zinc**: Deficiency in Developing Countries, Intervention Studies.

Further Reading

Brooks MJ and Melnik G (1995) The refeeding syndrome: an approach to understanding its complications and preventing its occurrence. *Pharmacotherapy* **15**: 713–726.

Dudrick SJ, Maharaj AR, and McKelvey AA (1999) Artificial nutritional support in patients with gastrointestinal fistulas. *World Journal of Surgery* **23**: 570–576.

Herbert V (1973) The five possible causes of all nutrient deficiencies: Illustrated by deficiencies of vitamin B12 and folic acid. *American Journal of Clinical Nutrition* **26**: 77–88.

McKenzie C, Vicca N, Ward JE, and Coles SJ (2000) Prevalence of malnutrition on admission to four hospitals in England. The Malnutrition Prevalence Group. *Clinical Nutrition* **19**: 191–195.

Murray MJ, Marsh HM, Wochos DN, Moxness KE, Offord KP, and Callaway CW (1988) Nutritional assessment of intensive-care unit patients. *Mayo Clinic Proceedings* **63**: 1106–1115.

Ofman J and Koretz RL (1997) Clinical economics review: nutritional support. *Alimention and Pharmacological Therapy* **11**: 453–471.

Paccagnella A, Calo MA, Caenaro G, Salandin V, Jus P, Simini G, and Heymsfield SB (1994) Cardiac cachexia: preoperative and postoperative nutrition management. *Journal of Parenteral and Enteral Nutrition* **18**: 409–416.

Phang PT and Aeberhardt LE (1996) Effect of nutritional support on routine nutrition assessment parameters and body composition in intensive care unit patients. *Canadian Journal of Surgery* **39**: 212–219.

Solomons NW (1993) Pathways to impairment of nutritional status by gastrointestinal pathogens, with emphasis on protozoal and helminthic parasites. *Parasitology* **107**(supplement): S19–S35.

Solomons NW and Keusch GT (1999) Clinical issues: Childhood illnesses, vaccinations and nutritional status. In: Gershwin ME, German JB, and Keen CL (eds.) *Nutrition and Immunology: Principles and Practice*, pp. 469–474. Totowa, NJ: Humana Press.

Thapa BR (1994) Intractable diarrhoea of infancy and its management: modified cost effective treatment. *Journal of Tropical Pediatrics* **40**: 157–161.

Von Roenn JH, Roth EL, and Craig R (1992) HIV-related cachexia: potential mechanisms and treatment. *Oncology* **49**(supplement 2): 50–54.

Zipf WB (2004) Prader–Willi syndrome: the care and treatment of infants, children, and adults. *Advances in Pediatrics* **51**: 409–434.

MANGANESE

C L Keen, J L Ensunsa, B Lönnerdal and S Zidenberg-Cherr, University of California at Davis, Davis, CA, USA

The essentiality of manganese was established in 1931, when it was demonstrated that a deficit of it resulted in poor growth and impaired reproduction in rodents. Manganese deficiency can be a practical problem in the swine and poultry industries, and it may be a problem in some human populations. Conversely, manganese toxicity can be a significant human health concern. Here, literature related to manganese nutrition, metabolism, and metabolic function is reviewed.

Chemical and Physical Properties

Manganese is the 12th most abundant element in the Earth's crust and constitutes approximately 0.1% of it. Chemical forms of manganese in their natural deposits include oxides, sulfides, carbonates, and silicates. Anthropogenic sources of manganese are predominantly from the manufacturing of steel, alloys, and iron products. Manganese is widely used as an oxidizing agent, as a component of fertilizers and fungicides, and in dry cell batteries. Methylcyclopentadienyl manganese tricarbonyl (MMT) improves combustion in boilers and motors and can substitute for lead in gasoline as an antiknock agent. Concentrations of manganese in groundwater normally range between 1 and $100 \mu g \, l^{-1}$, with most values being below $10 \mu g \, l^{-1}$. Typical airborne levels of manganese (in the absence of excessive pollution) range from 10 to $70 \, ng \, m^{-3}$.

Manganese is a transition element located in group VIIA of the periodic table. It occurs in 11 oxidation states ranging from -3 to $+7$, with the physiologically most important valences being $+2$ and $+3$. The $+2$ valence is the predominant form in biological systems and is the form that is thought to be maximally absorbed. The $+3$ valence is the form in which manganese is primarily transported in biological systems.

The solution chemistry of manganese is relatively simple. The aquo-ion is resistant to oxidation in acidic or neutral solutions. It does not begin to hydrolyze until pH 10, and therefore free Mn^{2+} can be present in neutral solutions at relatively high concentrations. Divalent manganese is a $3d^5$ ion and typically forms high-spin complexes lacking crystal field stabilization energies. The previous properties, as well as a large ionic radius and small charge-to-radius ratio, result in manganese tending to form weak complexes compared with other first-row divalent ions, such as Ni^{2+} and Cu^{2+}. Free Mn^{2+} has a strong isotropic electron paramagnetic resonance (EPR) signal that can be used to determine its concentration in the low micromolar range. Mn^{3+} is also critical in biological systems. For example, Mn^{3+} is the oxidative state of manganese in superoxide dismutase, is the form in which transferrin binds manganese, and is probably the form of manganese that interacts with Fe^{3+}. Given its smaller ionic radius, the chelation of Mn^{3+} in biological systems would be predicted to be more avid than that of Mn^{2+}. Cycling between Mn^{3+} and Mn^{2+} has been suggested to be deleterious to biological systems because it can generate free radicals. However, at low concentrations Mn^{2+} can provide protection against free radicals, and it appears to be associated with their clearance rather than their production.

Dietary Sources

Manganese concentrations in typical food products range from $0.4 \mu g \, g^{-1}$ (meat, poultry, and fish) to $20 \mu g \, g^{-1}$ (nuts, cereals, and dried fruit). Breast milk is exceptionally low in manganese, containing only $0.004 \mu g \, g^{-1}$, whereas infant formula can contain up to $0.4 \mu g \, g^{-1}$. Teas can be particularly rich in manganese, containing up to $900 \mu g \, g^{-1}$ of the element. An important consideration with respect to food sources of manganese is the extent to which the manganese is available for absorption. For example, although tea contains high amounts of the element, the tannin in tea can bind a significant amount of manganese, reducing its absorption from the gastrointestinal tract. Similarly, the high content of phytates and fiber constituents in cereal grains may limit the absorption of manganese. Conversely, although meat products contain low concentrations of manganese, absorption and retention of manganese from them is relatively high. Based on studies utilizing whole body retention curves after dosing with ^{54}Mn, the estimated percentage absorption of 1 mg of manganese from a test meal was 1.35%, whereas that from green leafy vegetables (lettuce and spinach) was closer to 5%. Absorption from wheat and sunflower seed kernels was somewhat lower than that from the leafy greens at 1 or 2%, presumably due to a higher fiber content or to higher amounts of phytates and similar compounds in the wheat and sunflower seeds. The dephytinization of soy formula increased manganese absorption 2.3-fold from 0.7 to 1.6%.

Analysis

Although manganese is widely distributed in the biosphere, it occurs in only trace amounts in animal tissues. Serum concentrations can be as low as 20 nM and typical tissue concentrations are less than $4 \mu mol \, g^{-1}$ wet weight; tissue concentrations of $4–8 \mu mol \, g^{-1}$ wet weight are considered high. Because of the high environmental levels of manganese relative to its concentration in animal tissues, considerable effort must be made to minimize contamination of samples during their collection and handling.

The most common analytical methods that can sensitively measure manganese include neutron activation analysis, X-ray fluorescence, proton-induced X-ray emission, inductively coupled plasma emission, EPR, and flameless atomic absorption spectrophotometry (AAS). Currently, the most common method employed is flameless AAS. All of these methods, with the exception of EPR, measure the total concentration of manganese in the samples. EPR allows selective measurement of bound versus free manganese.

Physiological Role

Tissue Concentrations

The average human body contains between 200 and 400 μmol of manganese, which is fairly uniform in distribution throughout the body. There is relatively little variation among species with regard to tissue manganese concentrations. Manganese tends to be highest in tissues rich in mitochondria; its concentration in mitochondria is higher than in cytoplasm or other cell organelles. Hair can accumulate high concentrations of manganese, and it has been suggested that hair manganese concentrations may reflect manganese status. High concentrations of manganese are normally found in pigmented structures, such as retina, dark skin, and melanin granules. Bone, liver, pancreas, and kidney tend to have higher concentrations of manganese ($20–50\,\mathrm{nmol\,g^{-1}}$) than do other tissues. Concentrations of manganese in brain, heart, lung, and muscle are typically $<20\,\mathrm{nmol\,g^{-1}}$; blood and serum concentrations are approximately 200 and $20\,\mathrm{nmol\,l^{-1}}$, respectively. Typical concentrations in cow milk are on the order of $800\,\mathrm{nmol\,l^{-1}}$, whereas human milk contains $80\,\mathrm{nmol\,l^{-1}}$. Bone can account for up to 25% of total body manganese because of its mass. Bone manganese concentrations can be raised or lowered by substantially varying dietary manganese intake over long periods of time, but bone manganese is not thought to be a readily mobilizable pool. The fetus does not accumulate liver manganese before birth, and fetal concentrations are significantly less than adult concentrations. This lack of fetal storage can be attributed to the apparent lack of storage proteins and the low prenatal expression of most manganese enzymes.

Absorption, Transport, and Storage

Absorption of manganese is thought to occur throughout the small intestine. Manganese absorption is not thought to be under homeostatic control. For adult humans, manganese absorption has been reported to range from 2 to 15% when ^{54}Mn-labeled test meals are used and to be 25% when balance studies are conducted; given the technical problems associated with balance studies, the ^{54}Mn data are probably more reflective of true absorption values. Data from balance studies indicate that manganese retention is very high during infancy, suggesting that neonates may be particularly susceptible to manganese toxicosis.

The higher retention of manganese in young animals relative to adults in part reflects an immaturity of manganese excretory pathways, particularly that of bile secretion, which is very limited in early life.

The avid retention of the small amount of manganese from milk and the postnatal changes in its excretory pattern underscore the considerable changes in manganese metabolism that occur during the neonatal period.

In experimental animals, high amounts of dietary calcium, phosphorus, fiber, and phytate increase the requirements for manganese; such interactions presumably occur via the formation of insoluble manganese complexes in the intestinal tract with a concomitant decrease in the soluble fraction available for absorption. The significance of these dietary factors with regard to human manganese requirements remains to be clarified. Studies in avian species have demonstrated that high dietary phosphorus intakes decrease manganese deposition in bone by approximately 50%. Given that the diet of many individuals may be marginal in manganese ($\leq 2\,\mathrm{mg}$ per day intake) while high in phosphorus ($\geq 2000\,\mathrm{mg}$ per day intake), this antagonism may have important implications for human health. For example, the low fractional absorption of manganese from soy formula has been related to its relatively high phytate content. The mechanism underlying this effect of soy protein on manganese absorption/retention has not been fully delineated. However, dephytinization of soy formula with microbial phytase can markedly enhance manganese absorption.

An interaction between iron and manganese has been demonstrated in experimental animals and humans. Manganese absorption increases under conditions of iron deficiency, whereas high amounts of dietary iron can accelerate the development of manganese deficiency. The chronic consumption of high levels of iron supplements ($>60\,\mathrm{mg\,Fe}$ per day) can have a negative effect on manganese balance in adult women. The mechanisms underlying the interactions between iron and manganese have not been fully elucidated; however, they likely involve competition for either a transport site or a ligand. Both iron and manganese can utilize divalent metal transporter 1 (DMT1); however, the expression of DMT1 is regulated by iron status via the IRE/IRP system. Thus, during iron deficiency, DMT1 is upregulated causing an increase in manganese absorption. Rats fed iron-deficient diets accumulate manganese in several brain regions compared to rats fed control diets; the involvement of DMT1 in this accumulation of manganese is an area of active study. It should be noted that the interaction between manganese and iron can also affect the functions of some enzymes. For example, manganese can replace iron in the iron–sulfur center of cytosolic aconitase (IRP-1), resulting in an inhibition of the enzyme and an increase in iron regulatory protein (IRP) binding activity. Given the central role of IRPs in cellular iron metabolism, elevated cellular manganese concentration could in theory disrupt numerous translational events dependent on IRPs. That this in fact occurs is illustrated by the observation that following the addition of manganese to cells in culture, there can be sharp reductions in ferritin protein abundance, whereas there are increases in transferrin receptor abundance. This results in changes in intracellular iron metabolism, as reflected by decreases in mitochondrial aconitase (m-aconitase) abundance.

Manganese entering the portal blood from the gastrointestinal tract may remain free or become associated with α_2-macroglobulin, which is subsequently taken up by the liver. A small fraction enters the systemic circulation, where it may become oxidized to Mn^{3+} and bound to transferrin. Studies *in vivo* suggest that the Mn^{3+} complex forms very quickly in blood, in contrast to the slow oxidation of the Mn^{2+}–transferrin complex *in vitro*. Manganese uptake by the liver has been reported to occur by a unidirectional, saturable process with the properties of passive mediated transport. After entering the liver, manganese enters one of at least five metabolic pools. One pool represents manganese taken up by the lysosomes, from which it is transferred subsequently to the bile canaliculus. The regulation of manganese is maintained in part through biliary excretion of the element; up to 50% of manganese injected intravenously can be recovered in the feces within 24 h. A second pool of manganese is associated with the mitochondria. Mitochondria have a large capacity for manganese uptake, and the mitochondrial uptake and release of manganese and calcium are thought to be related. A third pool of manganese is found in the nuclear fraction of the cell; the roles of nuclear manganese have not been fully delineated, but one function may be to contribute to the stability of nucleosome structure. A fourth manganese pool is incorporated into newly synthesized manganese proteins; biological half-lives for these proteins have not been agreed upon. The fifth identified intracellular pool of manganese is free Mn^{2+}. Fluctuations in the free manganese pool may be an important regulator of cellular metabolic control in a manner analogous to those for free Ca^{2+} and Mg^{2+}. Consistent with this concept, in pancreatic islets manganese blocks glucose-induced insulin release by altering cellular calcium fluxes, and manganese directly augments contractions in smooth muscle by a mechanism comparable to that of calcium.

The mechanisms by which manganese is transported to, and taken up by, extrahepatic tissues have not been identified. Transferrin is the major manganese binding protein in plasma; however, it is not known to what extent transferrin facilitates the uptake of manganese by extrahepatic tissue. The concentration of manganese citrate in blood can be fairly high, and this complex may be important for manganese movement across the blood–brain barrier. DMT1 may be involved in manganese transport because it is expressed in discrete areas of the brain. Manganese uptake by extrahepatic tissue does not seem to be increased under conditions of manganese deficiency, suggesting that manganese, in marked contrast to iron, does not play a role in the induction (or suppression) of manganese transport proteins.

There is limited information concerning the hormonal regulation of manganese metabolism. Fluxes in the concentrations of adrenal, pancreatic, and pituitary–gonadal axis hormones affect tissue manganese concentrations; however, it is not clear to what extent hormone-induced changes in tissue manganese concentrations are due to alterations in cellular uptake of manganese-activated enzymes or metalloenzymes.

Metabolic Function and Essentiality

Manganese functions as a constituent of metalloenzymes and as an enzyme activator. Manganese-containing enzymes include arginase (EC 3.5.3.1), pyruvate carboxylase (EC 6.4.1.1), and manganese–superoxide dismutase (MnSOD) (EC 1.15.1.1). Arginase, the cytosolic enzyme responsible for urea formation, contains 4 mol Mn^{2+} per mole of enzyme. Reductions in arginase activity resulting from manganese deficiency result in elevated plasma concentrations of ammonia and lowered plasma concentrations of urea. Reductions in arginase activity due to manganese deficiency may affect flux of arginine through the nitric oxide synthase (NOS) pathway, resulting in alterations in NO production. It has been suggested that arginase plays a regulatory role in NO production by competing with NOS for the same substrate, arginine. Rats fed manganese-deficient diets have shown effects indicative of increased NO production, such as increases in plasma and urinary nitrates plus nitrites and decreased blood pressure; however, neither NOS activity nor NO production have been measured directly. In addition, manganese binding by arginase is critical for the pH-sensing function of this enzyme in the ornithine cycle, suggesting that manganese plays a role in the regulation of body pH. With experimental diabetes, liver and kidney manganese concentrations and arginase activity can be markedly elevated.

This manganese effect on arginase has been suggested to be due to an effect of Mn^{2+} on the conformational properties of the enzyme with a resultant modification of arginase activity. Whether this finding implies an increased manganese requirement for people with diabetes has not been determined.

Pyruvate carboxylase, the enzyme that catalyses the first step of carbohydrate synthesis from pyruvate, also contains $4\,mol\ Mn^{2+}$ per mole enzyme. Although the activity of this enzyme can be lower in manganese-deficient animals than in controls, gluconeogenesis has not been shown to be markedly inhibited in manganese-deficient animals.

MnSOD catalyzes the disproportionation of O_2^- to H_2O_2 and O_2. The essential role of MnSOD in the normal biological function of tissues has been clearly demonstrated by the homozygous inactivation of the *SOD2* gene for MnSOD in mice. Mice with this phenotype die within the first 10 days of life with a dilated cardiomyopathy, accumulation of lipid in liver and skeletal muscle, and metabolic acidosis. The activity of MnSOD in tissues of manganese-deficient rats can be significantly lower than in controls due to downregulation of MnSOD at the (pre)transcriptional level. That this reduction is functionally significant is suggested by the observation of higher than normal levels of hepatic mitochondrial lipid peroxidation in manganese-deficient rats. Tissue MnSOD activity can be increased by several diverse stressors, including alcohol, ozone, irradiation, interleukin-1, and tumor necrosis factor-α, presumably as a consequence of stressor-associated increases in cellular free radical (or oxidized target(s)) concentrations. Stressor-induced increases in MnSOD activity can be attenuated in manganese-deficient animals, potentially increasing their sensitivity to these insults. Transgenic mice have also been produced that overexpress MnSOD; a decreased severity of reperfusion injury has been noted in these animals, further supporting its physiological significance.

Considerable research is focused on the introduction of the human MnSOD gene into research animals utilizing viral vectors or plasmid/liposome delivery. This gene therapy has been shown to decrease radiation-induced injury, extend pancreatic islet transplant function, and slow the growth of malignant tumors in animal models via overexpression of the MnSOD protein. Another field of research that is rapidly advancing utilizes MnSOD mimetics for treatment of a variety of diseases in which the native SOD enzyme has been found to be effective. These mimetics are small manganese-containing synthetic molecules that have catalytic activity equivalent or superior to the native enzyme. They possess the additional beneficial properties of being nonimmunogenic because they are nonpeptides, able to penetrate cells, selective for superoxide (they do not interact with biologically important molecules), stable *in vivo*, and not deactivated by the destructive free radical peroxynitrite, which is capable of deactivating native MnSOD via nitration of tyrosine. These mimetic compounds have been found to be protective in animal models of acute and chronic inflammation, reperfusion injury, shock, and radiation-induced injury. Both of these therapies, MnSOD gene delivery and MnSOD mimetics, hold promise for future treatments in human chronic and acute conditions.

Finally, further evidence for the biological and research relevance of MnSOD is that experiments have been undertaken on the International Space Station to improve three-dimensional growth of MnSOD crystals in order to develop a better understanding of the role of structure in the reaction mechanism of this enzyme.

In contrast to the relatively few manganese metalloenzymes, there are a large number of manganese-activated enzymes, including hydrolases, kinases, decarboxylases, and transferases. Manganese activation of these enzymes can occur as a direct consequence of the metal binding to the protein, causing a subsequent conformation change, or by binding to the substrate, such as ATP. Many of these metal activations are nonspecific in that other metal ions, particularly Mg^{2+}, can replace Mn^{2+}. An exception is the manganese-specific activation of glycosyltransferases. Several manganese deficiency-induced pathologies have been attributed to a low activity of this enzyme class. A second example of an enzyme that may be specifically activated by manganese is phosphoenolpyruvate carboxykinase (PEPCK; EC 4.1.1.49), the enzyme that catalyzes the conversion of oxaloacetate to phosphoenolpyruvate, GDP, and CO_2. Although low activities of PEPCK can occur in manganese-deficient animals, the functional significance of this reduction is not clear.

A third example of a manganese-activated enzyme is glutamine synthetase (EC 6.3.1.2). This enzyme, found in high concentrations in the brain, catalyzes the reaction $NH_3 + glutamate + ATP \rightarrow glutamine + ADP + P_i$. Brain glutamine synthetase activity can be normal even in severely manganese-deficient animals, suggesting that the enzyme either has a high priority for this element or magnesium can act as a substitute when manganese is lacking. It should be noted that this enzyme can be inactivated by oxygen radicals; therefore, a manganese deficiency-induced reduction in MnSOD activity theoretically could act to depress further the activity of glutamine synthetase.

Manganese Deficiency

Manganese deficiency has been demonstrated in several species, including rats, mice, pigs, and cattle. Signs of manganese deficiency include impaired growth, skeletal abnormalities, impaired reproductive performance, ataxia, and defects in lipid and carbohydrate metabolism.

The effects of manganese deficiency on bone development have been studied extensively. In most species, manganese deficiency can result in shortened and thickened limbs, curvature of the spine, and swollen and enlarged joints. The basic biochemical defect underlying the development of these bone defects is a reduction in the activities of glycosyltransferases; these enzymes are necessary for the synthesis of the chondroitin sulfate side chains of proteoglycan molecules. In addition, manganese deficiency in adult rats can result in an inhibition of both osteoblast and osteoclast activity. This observation is particularly noteworthy, given the reports that women with osteoporosis tend to have low blood manganese concentrations and that the provision of manganese supplements might be associated with an improvement in bone health in postmenopausal women.

One of the most striking effects of manganese deficiency occurs during pregnancy. When pregnant animals (rats, mice, guinea pigs, and mink) are deficient in manganese, their offspring exhibit a congenital, irreversible ataxia characterized by incoordination, lack of equilibrium, and retraction of the head. This condition is the result of impaired development of the otoliths, the calcified structures in the inner ear responsible for normal body-righting reflexes. The block in otolith development is secondary to depressed proteoglycan synthesis due to low activity of manganese-requiring glycosyltransferases.

Defects in carbohydrate metabolism, in addition to those described previously, have been shown in manganese-deficient rats and guinea pigs. In the guinea pig, perinatal manganese deficiency results in pancreatic pathology, with animals exhibiting aplasia or marked hypoplasia of all cellular components. Manganese-deficient guinea pigs and rats given a glucose challenge often respond with a diabetic-type glucose tolerance curve. In addition to its effect on pancreatic tissue integrity, manganese deficiency can directly impair pancreatic insulin synthesis and secretion as well as enhance intracellular insulin degradation. The mechanism(s) underlying the effects of manganese deficiency on pancreatic insulin metabolism have not been fully delineated, but they are thought to be multifactorial. For example, the flux of islet cell manganese from the cell surface to an intracellular pool may be a critical signal for insulin release. It is also known that insulin mRNA levels are reduced in manganese-deficient animals, which is consistent with their depressed insulin synthesis. In addition, insulin sensitivity of adipose tissue is reduced in manganese-deficient rats, a phenomenon that may be related to fewer insulin receptors per adipose cell. Manganese deficiency may also affect glucose metabolism by means of a reduction in the number of glucose transporters in adipose tissue by an unidentified mechanism. Finally, the effect of manganese deficiency on insulin production may also be due to the destruction of pancreatic J3 cells. It is worth noting that constitutive pancreatic MnSOD activity is lower than in most tissues; this, coupled with the observation that most diabetogenic agents function via the production of free radicals with subsequent tissue damage, suggests that an additional mechanism underlying pancreatic dysfunction in manganese-deficient animals may be free radical mediated.

In addition to its effect on endocrine function, manganese deficiency can affect pancreatic exocrine function. For example, manganese-deficient rats can be characterized by an increase in pancreatic amylase content. The mechanism underlying this effect of manganese deficiency has not been delineated; however, it is thought to involve a shift in amylase synthesis or degradation because secretagogue-stimulated acinar secretion is comparable in control and manganese-deficient rats.

Although the majority of studies concerning the influence of manganese deficiency on carbohydrate metabolism have been conducted with experimental animals, there is one report in the literature of an insulin-resistant diabetic patient who responded to oral doses of manganese (doses ranged from 5 to 10 mg) with decreasing blood glucose concentrations. Although this is an intriguing case report, others have reported a lack of an effect of oral manganese supplements (up to 30 mg) in diabetic subjects, and low blood manganese concentrations have not been found to be a characteristic of diabetics.

Abnormal lipid metabolism is also characteristic of manganese deficiency: Specifically, a lipotrophic effect of manganese has been suggested in the literature. Severely manganese-deficient animals can be characterized by high liver fat, hypocholesterolemia, and low high-density lipoprotein (HDL) concentrations. Deficient animals can also be characterized by a shift to smaller plasma HDL particles, lower HDL apolipoprotein (apoE) concentrations, and higher apoC concentrations. As stated previously, tissue lipid peroxidation rates can be increased in manganese-deficient animals, possibly as a result of low tissue MnSOD activity.

There is considerable debate as to the extent to which manganese deficiency affects humans under free-living conditions. Manganese deficiency can be induced in humans under highly controlled experimental conditions. In one study, manganese deficiency was induced in adult male subjects by feeding a manganese-deficient diet (0.1 mg Mn per day) for 39 days. The subjects developed temporary dermatitis, as well as increased serum calcium and phosphorus concentrations and increased alkaline phosphatase activity, suggestive of bone resorption. Since the late 1980s, several diseases have been reported to be characterized, in part, by low blood manganese concentrations. These diseases include epilepsy, Mseleni disease, maple syrup urine disease and phenylketonuria, Down's syndrome, osteoporosis, and Perthes' disease. The finding of low blood manganese levels in subsets of individuals with the previously mentioned diseases is significant since blood manganese levels can reflect soft tissue manganese concentrations. The reports of low blood manganese concentrations in individuals with epilepsy are particularly intriguing, given the observations that manganese-deficient animals can show an increased susceptibility to drug and electroshock-induced seizures and a genetic model for epilepsy in rats (the GEPR rat) is characterized by low blood manganese concentrations. It is evident that a deficiency of manganese may contribute to the pathology of epilepsy at multiple points, given that Mn^{2+} is implicated in activation of glutamine synthetase, a Mn^{2+}-specific brain ATPase; production of cyclic AMP; altered synaptosomal uptake of noradrenalin and serotonin; glutamate, GABA, and choline metabolism; and biosynthesis of acetylcholine receptors.

Evidence of widespread manganese deficiency in human populations is lacking. Typically, manganese intakes approximate the 2001 US Institute of Medicine's suggested adequate intakes as follows: 3 µg/day for infants 0–6 months old, 0.6 mg/day for infants 7–12 months old, 1.2–1.9 mg/day for children 1–13 years old, 1.6–2.2 mg/day for older children, and 1.8–2.6 mg/day for adults. The Tolerable Upper Intake Level (UL) is the highest level of a daily nutrient intake that is likely to pose no risk of adverse health effects in almost all individuals. The Institute of Medicine's recommended intakes for manganese set ULs at 2, 3, and 6 mg/day for children 1–3, 4–8, and 9–13 years old, respectively. Values were set at 9 mg/day for adolescents 14–18 years old and at 11 mg/day for adults.

Manganese Toxicity

In domestic animals, the major reported lesion associated with chronic manganese toxicity is iron deficiency, resulting from an inhibitory effect of manganese on iron absorption. Additional signs of manganese toxicity in domestic animals include depressed growth, depressed appetite, and altered brain function.

In humans, manganese toxicity represents a serious health hazard, resulting in severe pathologies of the central nervous system. In its most severe form, the toxicosis is manifested by a permanent crippling neurological disorder of the extrapyramidal system, which is similar to Parkinson's disease. In its milder form, the toxicity is expressed by hyperirritability, violent acts, hallucinations, disturbances of libido, and incoordination. The previous symptoms, once established, can persist even after the manganese body burden returns to normal. Although the majority of reported cases of manganese toxicity occur in individuals exposed to high concentrations of airborne manganese ($>5\,mg\,m^{-3}$), subtle signs of manganese toxicity, including delayed reaction time, impaired motor coordination, and impaired memory, have been observed in workers exposed to airborne manganese concentrations less than $1\,mg\,m^{-3}$. Therefore, an inhalation reference concentration range for manganese has been established by the US Environmental Protection Agency to be between 0.09 and $0.2\,\mu g\,m^{-3}$. Manganese toxicity has been reported in individuals who have consumed water containing high levels ($\geq10\,mg\,Mn\,l^{-1}$) of manganese for long periods of time. Recently, there has been concern that the risk for manganese toxicity may be increasing in some areas because of the use of MMT in gasoline as an antiknock agent, although there is little evidence that air, water, or food manganese concentrations have increased where this fuel is used.

In addition to neural damage, reproductive and immune system dysfunction, nephritis, testicular damage, pancreatitis, lung disease, and hepatic damage can occur with manganese toxicity, but the frequency of these disorders is unknown. Although there is a limited body of epidemiological data that suggests that high levels of manganese can result in an increased risk for colorectal and digestive tract cancers, most investigators do not consider manganese to be a carcinogen. In contrast, both divalent ($MnCl_2$) and heptavalent forms ($KMnO_4$) of manganese are recognized to be strong clastogens both *in vitro* and *in vivo*; exposure to high concentrations of either form results in chromosomal breaks, fragments, and exchanges. High concentrations of manganese can also induce forward and point mutations in mammalian cells. High levels of dietary manganese have not been reported to be teratogenic in the absence of overt signs of maternal toxicity. However, there are reports that exposure to high levels of manganese during prenatal development can result in behavioral abnormalities. High levels of brain manganese have been reported in subjects with amyotrophic lateral sclerosis, and it has been suggested that this increase may contribute to the progression of the disease. Similar to the cases in humans, chronic manganese toxicity in rhesus monkeys is characterized by muscular weakness, rigidity of the lower limbs, and neuron damage in the substantia nigra. Findings from a recent study suggest that iron and aluminum, which accumulate in the globus pallidus and the substantia nigra of these animals, induce tissue oxidation that may contribute to the damage associated with manganese toxicity. Neural toxicity is a consistent finding in rats exposed to chronic manganese toxicity. Significant manganese accumulation was accompanied by an increase in cholesterol content in the hippocampal region of manganese-treated rats, which was associated with impaired learning; this impairment was corrected by an inhibitor of cholesterol synthesis. The development of manganese toxicity in individuals with compromised liver function, or compromised biliary pathways, is well documented. Significantly, these individuals can have abnormal magnetic resonance imaging (MRI) patterns, which improve following the alleviation of the manganese toxicity. For example, in some cases improvements in brain function have been achieved after liver transplant. The mechanisms underlying the toxicity of manganese have not been agreed upon but may involve multiple etiologies, including endocrinological dysfunction, excessive tissue oxidative damage, manganese-mediated disruptions in intracellular calcium and iron metabolism, and mitochondrial dysfunction caused by manganese inhibition of some pathways of the mitochondrial respiratory chain.

Severe cases of manganese toxicity in humans have been reported for adults, as well as isolated cases in other groups of individuals who are vulnerable, including children on long-term parenteral nutrition and parenteral nutrition patients who have cholestasis or other hepatic disease. In many cases, the previously mentioned groups of individuals have been reported to be characterized by high brain manganese concentrations based on MRI. Although no known cases have been reported, infants may be at a high risk for manganese toxicity due to a high absorptive capacity for the element and/or an immature excretory pathway for it. If manganese is taken up by extrahepatic

tissues via the manganese–transferrin complex, the developing brain may be particularly sensitive to manganese toxicity due to the high number of transferrin receptors elaborated by neuronal cells during development, coupled with the putative need by neural cells for transferrin for their differentiation and proliferation. Newborn rats given daily doses of dietary manganese at a level equivalent to that of soy formula exhibited significant neurodevelopmental delays as assessed by several behavioral tests. It should be noted that the concentration of manganese in soy formula is relatively modest but approximately 60–100 times higher than that of breast milk. Brain manganese concentration was increased and striatal dopamine concentrations were significantly decreased even 45 days after the supplementation ended, suggesting that the impact of manganese on the brain and behavior was irreversible. Thus, dietary exposure to high levels of manganese during infancy can be neurotoxic to rat pups and result in developmental deficits. Further studies on human infants fed diets with different levels of manganese are needed to assess whether there are any long-term consequences of early manganese exposure of newborns.

Another group of neuropathological conditions that has been associated with elevated levels of brain manganese is transmissible spongiform encephalopathies. These diseases found in animals and humans are also referred to as prion diseases. There is strong evidence that in their native state, prions are normal brain glycoproteins that bind copper and have an antioxidant function. However, it has been suggested that in the disease process an abnormal isoform of the protein is generated in which manganese is substituted for copper. This isoform is proteinase resistant, no longer has antioxidant activity, and may play a role in the etiology of these diseases. Indeed, elevated levels of brain manganese, along with lower than normal levels of brain copper, have been measured in patients with the prion disease, Creutzfeld–Jakob disease. Whether the elevated levels of brain manganese observed in these patients as well as in animal models of these diseases play an important role in their pathogenesis or are secondary to other factors remains to be determined.

Assessment of Manganese Status

Reliable biomarkers for the assessment of manganese status have not been identified. Whole blood manganese concentrations are reflective of soft tissue manganese levels in rats; however, it is not known whether a similar relationship holds for humans. Plasma manganese concentrations decrease in individuals fed manganese-deficient diets and are slightly higher than normal in individuals consuming manganese supplements. Lymphocyte MnSOD activity and blood arginase activity are increased in individuals who consume manganese supplements; however, their value as biomarkers for manganese status may be complicated due to the number of cytokines and disease states that may also increase their expression. Urinary manganese excretion has not been found to be sensitive to dietary manganese intake. With respect to the diagnosis of manganese toxicosis, the use of MRI appears to be promising because the images associated with manganese toxicity are relatively specific. Whole blood manganese concentrations can be correlated with MRI intensity and Ti values in the globus pallidus even in the absence of symptoms of neurological damage. Thus, although it is relatively expensive, MRI may be particularly useful as a means of identifying susceptible individuals in, or around, manganese-emitting factories. In addition, the method may be useful in the evaluation of patients with liver failure.

See also: **Carbohydrates**: Regulation of Metabolism. **Cofactors**: Inorganic. **Iron**.

Further Reading

Brown DR (2002) Metal toxicity and therapeutic intervention. *Biochemical Society* **30**: 742–745.

Crossgrove JS, Allen DD, Bukaveckas BL, Rhineheimer SS, and Yokel RA (2003) Manganese distribution across the blood–brain barrier. I. Evidence for carrier-mediated influx of manganese citrate as well as manganese and manganese transferrin. *Neurotoxicology* **24**: 3–13.

Davey CA and Richmond TJ (2002) DNA-dependent divalent cation binding in the nucleosome core particle. *Proceedings of the National Academy of Sciences of the United States of America* **99**: 11169–11174.

Garrick MD, Dolan KG, Horbinski C et al. (2003) DMT1: A mammalian transporter for multiple metals. *BioMetals* **16**: 41–54.

Gerber GB, Léonard A, and Hantson PH (2002) Carcinogenicity, mutagenicity and teratogenicity of manganese compounds. *Critical Reviews in Oncology/Hematology* **42**: 25–34.

Guo H, Seixas-Silva JA, Epperly MW et al. (2003) Prevention of radiation-induced oral cavity mucositis by plasmid/liposome delivery of the human manganese superoxide dismutase (SOD2) transgene. *Radiation Research* **159**: 361–370.

Kwik-Uribe CL, Reaney S, Zhu Z, and Smith D (2003) Alterations in cellular IRP-dependent iron regulation by *in vitro* manganese exposure in undifferentiated PC12 cells. *Brain Research* **973**: 1–15.

Normandin L and Hazell AS (2002) Manganese neurotoxicity: An update of pathophysiologic mechanisms. *Metabolic Brain Disease* **17**: 375–387.

Sabbatini M, Pisani A, Uccello F et al. (2003) Arginase inhibition slows the progression of renal failure in rats with renal ablation. *American Journal of Renal Physiology* **284**: F680–F687.

Salvemini D, Muscoli C, Riley DP, and Cuzzocrea S (2002) Superoxide dismutase mimetics. *Pulmonary Pharmacology and Therapeutics* **15**: 439–447.

Takagi Y, Okada A, Sando K et al. (2002) Evaluation of indexes of *in vivo* manganese status and the optimal intravenous dose for adult patients undergoing home parenteral nutrition. *American Journal of Clinical Nutrition* **75**: 112–118.

Takeda A (2003) Manganese action in brain function. *Brain Research Reviews* **41**: 79–87.

Tran T, Chowanadisai W, Crinella FM, Chicz-DeMet A, and Lönnerdal B (2002) Effect of high dietary manganese intake of neonatal rats on tissue mineral accumulation, striatal dopamine levels, and neurodevelopmental status. *Neurotoxicology* **158**: 1–9.

Vahedi-Faridi A, Porta J, and Borgstahl GEO (2002) Improved three-dimensional growth of manganese superoxide dismutase crystals on the International Space Station. *Biological Crystallography* **59**: 385–388.

Yokel RA, Crossgrove JS, and Bukaveckas BL (2003) Manganese distribution across the blood–brain barrier. II. Manganese efflux from the brain does not appear to be carrier mediated. *Neurotoxicology* **24**: 15–22.

MEAL SIZE AND FREQUENCY

F E Leahy, University of Auckland, Auckland, New Zealand

Man's eating habits are changing. Terms such as 'super-sizing,' 'portion distortion,' and 'grazing' have appeared in the contemporary vernacular. Therefore, a better understanding of meal size and frequency is particularly important, especially considering the potential role that these new eating patterns may be playing in the dramatic increase in the incidence of illnesses such as obesity, diabetes, and cardiovascular disease in society.

The principal consequences that changes in meal size and frequency have on the body relate to the absorption and metabolism of food. Several factors in addition to meal size and frequency influence absorption and metabolism, such as the physical characteristics of the food, its macronutrient composition, the energy density of the diet, and the physical volume of the meal. However, the particular contribution that changes in meal size and frequency have made to the dramatic change in society's eating patterns makes them worthy of special attention.

Effect of Meal Size on Absorption

When a meal of mixed macronutrient composition is consumed, the rate at which the carbohydrate, protein, and fat in that meal is absorbed differs. Carbohydrate in the form of glucose and protein in the form of amino acids enter the portal vein within 30 minutes of meal ingestion and later appear in the general circulation. As the glucose concentration in the portal vein increases, there is an increase in the uptake of glucose into the hepatocytes. Pancreatic islet cells react to the increase in blood glucose and secrete insulin, among other hormones, into the circulation. As a result, there is a decline in the release of nonesterified fatty acids from the adipose tissue. Fatty acid oxidation in the skeletal muscle tissue decreases, and as glucose uptake takes place, the muscle cells increase the rate at which glucose is oxidized. Glycogen synthesis in the muscle and liver cells is increased and the uptake of amino acids by muscle tissue may also occur. Up to 4 h after ingestion of the meal, fat in the form of chylomicron triacylglycerol enters the circulation via the lymphatic system. The action of the hormone lipoprotein lipase in the adipose tissue has by now increased, which promotes the storage of fatty acids as triacylglycerol in adipocytes. This synopsis indicates that following the ingestion of a meal, there is a marked increase in glucose oxidation with a corresponding decrease in fat utilization resulting in the storage of fat.

The larger the meal consumed, the more pronounced are the responses described previously. After a large meal is eaten, the plasma glucose concentration will remain elevated for up to 4 h following ingestion. Conversely, the smaller the meal, the more subtle the effect. This indicates that meal size does indeed influence absorption. However, in order for the relationship between meal size and absorption to be fully understood, the role that absorption plays in determining meal size needs to be considered. The following section focuses on the process of absorption and the systems that control the amount of food eaten.

Regulation of Meal Size by Satiety Peptides and Adiposity Signals

Peptides in the gastrointestinal tract and brain are believed to play an important role in the body's decision to commence and conclude meal consumption. When a meal is being consumed, these peptides are secreted by the gut to indicate the level of satiety. Some of this information can be used by the brain to determine the feeling of fullness, in turn influencing the decision to cease consumption. Cholecystokinin (CCK), a polypeptide located in the peripheral and central nervous systems, is one such satiety signal. It is released in proportion to the amount of food being consumed and helps to determine the amount consumed. Following a meal, CCK is secreted from mucosal epithelial cells in the first segment of the duodenum and stimulates the delivery of digestive enzymes from the pancreas, as well as bile from the gallbladder, into the small intestine. In addition, CCK is produced by neurons in the enteric nervous system and is widely distributed in the brain. The exogenous administration of CCK (and CCK-8, its synthetic analogue) has been shown to influence the amount of food consumed in proportion to the dose given. Although CCK (and other satiety signals) acts to limit meal size, it is important to note that it has little effect on body fat stores, meaning that it does not take into consideration the existing adiposity of the individual when signaling the onset of satiety. Therefore, adiposity signals must be considered in parallel because they also play a part in the process of determining meal size.

Adiposity signals such as leptin act in conjunction with satiety signals in the brain during digestion and their concentration is determined in relation to the degree of adiposity. Like CCK, the effect on meal consumption and body weight of their exogenous administration is dose dependent. Leptin is a peptide hormone produced predominantly by adipocytes, and it is also secreted by the epithelial cells of the stomach. The definitive role of leptin in digestive physiology is still being determined, but it is thought to play a part in limiting food intake in conjunction with CCK. It is when the adiposity signals interact with, and influence, the satiety signals originating from the gut that an attempt at controlling energy intake and meal size is made.

Effect of Meal Size on Metabolism

Energy homeostasis, or the state of balance, achieved by matching energy intake with energy expenditure, is partially dependent on the regulation of meal size consumed. In order for meal size to have an effect on energy metabolism, it must affect either or both components involved in the regulation of energy balance, namely energy intake and energy expenditure. Energy balance is the difference between energy ingested and energy expended over a given period of time. Consequently, energy storage is equal to intake minus expenditure. The following sections examine the effect of meal size on the two components of the energy balance equation.

Effect of Meal Size on Energy Intake

Meal portion sizes have been increasing steadily since the 1970s, in parallel with the increasing prevalence of obesity in society. It is known that portion and meal sizes vary depending on the food source and location of consumption. Not surprisingly, the largest portions consumed are generally those obtained at fast-food restaurants, although the portion sizes of home-cooked meals have been increasing steadily as well. Meal size may thus be contributing to the problem of obesity by leading to a daily total energy intake that is greater than the daily total energy expenditure, resulting in a positive energy balance.

Effect of Meal Size on Energy Expenditure

Total energy expenditure (EE) can generally be divided into three major components: basal metabolic rate (BMR), thermogenesis, and physical activity (Table 1). In order for meal size to have an effect on the EE side of the energy balance equation, it must have an effect on one or more of these components. There is no evidence that meal size has an effect on BMR, which refers to the energy expended to maintain the body on a day-to-day basis. Thermogenesis broadly refers to the body's production of heat, which is divided into three categories: dietary, thermoregulatory, and adaptive. It is the dietary category, commonly known as dietary-induced thermogenesis (DIT), that is of greatest relevance to the discussion of the effect of meal size on energy expenditure. It refers to the heat lost by the body as a result of the absorption and metabolism of a recently ingested meal. DIT represents approximately 10% of energy intake, and therefore the energy expended on DIT increases and decreases in relation to the size of the

meal and, more important, the energy value of the meal consumed. The larger the meal, the more energy will be expended to absorb, transport, and metabolize the nutrients consumed during that meal. For example, in the case of a meal containing 2000 kJ (478 kcal) of energy, approximately 200 kJ (48 kcal) will be expended on DIT alone. It is in the physical activity component of energy expenditure that the greatest variation between individuals is observed because physical activity levels (and therefore the energy expended on activity) are contingent on lifestyle choices such as employment and leisure time activities. The effect that meal size may have on physical activity is somewhat difficult to quantify. Meal size is perhaps more important to elite athletes, whose energy expenditure is two or three times greater than that of untrained weight-matched athletes with up to 40% of their energy expenditure being the cost of training.

Effect of Meal Frequency on Absorption

The perceived health advantages of increased meal frequency (as opposed to eating larger, infrequent meals) have been of interest to researchers since the 1930s. In particular, the benefits of this approach were made apparent by the discovery that insulin requirements in diabetics could be decreased in a frequent meal regime. In a series of case reports on patients taking high insulin doses, it was demonstrated that improved glycemic control and decreased insulin requirements can be achieved when glucose is sipped at hourly intervals throughout the day. Similarly, in healthy individuals a diet composed of many small meals compared with an isoenergetic diet composed of larger meals results in decreased insulin and glucose fluctuations.

Meal frequency not only affects insulin and glucose levels but also influences an individual's circulating lipids. An inverse relationship exists between meal frequency and lipid levels, suggesting that infrequent feeding leads to an increased risk of cardiovascular disease due to large fluctuations in circulating lipids. Increased meal frequency, on the other hand, is associated with several benefits, such as decreased serum cholesterol levels, decreased total:high-density lipoprotein cholesterol ratio, decreased esterified fatty acids, and decreased enzyme levels in adipose tissue associated with fatty acid storage. Paradoxically, individuals who report that they eat more frequently not only have lower total and low-density lipoprotein cholesterol (LDL-C) but also have a greater intake of energy, total fat, and saturated fatty acids. Considering that some of these results were found in a free-living

Table 1 Major components of energy expenditure

Component	Total energy expenditure (%)	Represents
BMR	60–75	Day-to-day running costs of an individual (e.g., circulation)
Thermogenesis	10–20	Heat produced by the body through dietary, adaptive, and thermoregulatory processes
Physical activity	100 − (BMR + thermogenesis)	The sum of work carried out by an individual

BMR, basal metabolic rate.

population, it is possible that dietary misreporting, a common occurrence in overweight populations, may be the cause of this inconsistency.

Mechanisms Underlying the Metabolic Effect of Meal Frequency

The mechanisms underlying beneficial responses to frequent feeding as opposed to an infrequent meal pattern are not fully understood. Frequent feeding has been shown to elicit lower plasma glucose fluctuations than does a more infrequent eating pattern. The absolute amount of carbohydrate eaten at each episode of ingestion in a frequent feeding pattern is simply not great enough to elevate glucose to the same extent as more infrequent eating. Small elevations in plasma insulin seen with frequent feeding are most likely in response to minimal fluctuations in glucose. The mechanisms responsible for the effect of an increased frequency of meal eating on lipid metabolism are not as clear-cut. The lower serum cholesterol levels observed during frequent feeding may be related to lower serum insulin levels. Insulin appears to have a key role in enhancing the hepatic synthesis of cholesterol through its ability to stimulate hydroxymethylglutaryl-coenzyme A reductase (HMG-CoA), the rate-limiting enzyme in hepatic cholesterologenesis. Exogenous insulin quickly increases HMG-CoA reductase activity in rats with diabetes and raises levels of the enzyme in animals without the disorder. It is possible that the reduction of serum cholesterol during a diet of habitual frequent feeding in normal healthy individuals may result from a reduction in hepatic cholesterol synthesis, secondary to the maintenance of euglycemia at lower serum insulin levels. A reduction in cholesterol synthesis would result in an increase in LDL receptors, further lowering total and LDL-C levels.

Alternatively, or in addition, the benefits associated with an increased feeding regimen may reflect unintentional or uncontrolled changes in dietary energy and fat intake that may occur when an individual's meal frequency is altered. It is not clear whether a diet of frequent eating results in any adaptational responses of enzymes or hormones that in turn may be providing additional benefit to the individual.

Much of the research that found these benefits is difficult to interpret due to the variety of methods used, the lack of information available regarding the foods consumed, and the exact nature of the dietary intervention. The majority of measurements are made on fasted blood samples, when in fact most individuals are in a postprandial state for the greater part of every 24-h period. The results of such research must be interpreted with caution for a number of reasons, such as the small sample size used and the interactions with other factors that may prolong absorption time (e.g., soluble fiber, low-glycemic index foods, and the administration of α-glycosides).

As discussed previously, frequent feeding has been demonstrated to lower circulating plasma glucose, insulin, and lipids in both healthy and diabetic subjects in the short term. In addition to the lack of clarity on the mechanisms involved, further research is needed to investigate any medium- and long-term benefits of frequent feeding. It is important that, if deemed desirable in terms of metabolic control, increasing the number of periods of feeding encourages the desired dietary pattern and mix of macro- and micronutrients and is not offset by the failure to decrease meal size.

Effect of Meal Frequency on Metabolism

The maxim that was applied earlier to the study of meal size, namely that it can only influence energy metabolism if it affects energy intake and/or energy expenditure, is applicable to meal frequency. The following sections focus on energy intake and energy expenditure, respectively.

Effect of Meal Frequency on Energy Intake

It has long been argued that the frequency of meal intake may have an effect on body weight regulation. It has been suggested that there is an inverse association between meal frequency and body weight. However, there are a number of flaws in the design of many of the studies from which these data have been derived, and caution is required in the interpretation of the results. Design flaws include (i) dietary underreporting, especially of snacking occasions; (ii) reverse causality, which refers to the possibility that people abstain from eating meals when they become overweight in an attempt to lose weight or to prevent further weight gain; (iii) lack of measurement of physical activity or energy expenditure; and (iv) inclusion of people in a diseased state. These important confounding factors may help to resolve the contradictory results of many research trials. Erroneous conclusions have been drawn from the misinterpretation of such results because these studies are extremely vulnerable to methodological errors that may generate spurious relationships that may not actually exist.

There appears to be very little direct empirical evidence in humans to suggest that frequent feeding per se affects appetite and energy intake. Individuals who eat frequently seem to exhibit a greater capacity to compensate for changes in the energy content of specific meals relative to individuals who derive most of their energy intake from fewer larger meals. Over very short periods, and under highly controlled experimental conditions, frequent feeding can decrease energy intake at a subsequent meal, which may in turn have an effect on appetite regulation. It remains to be seen, however, whether the same would occur in free-living conditions.

Mechanisms by which meal frequency may influence energy intake   Although the evidence is inconclusive, feeding frequency may have an impact on appetite and hence affect energy intake. The control of appetite is very complex and is determined by a number of factors. However, the question remains as to whether the frequency of feeding elicits effects on any of these factors, in turn affecting appetite and possibly body weight.

Frequency of feeding may potentially affect the release of neuroendocrine hormones such as neuropeptide Y, galanin, orexin, and melanocortins from the hypothalamus. The release of such hormones may be either stimulated or suppressed during frequent feeding, leading to either higher or lower than normal hormone levels, which may in turn have knock-on effects on energy intake and/or expenditure. Because it is not feasible to investigate such effects in humans, no studies have been carried out to determine this. The release of gut hormones such as CCK, glucagon-like peptide (GLP), and glucose-dependent insulotropic polypeptide (GIP) may be altered in relation to feeding frequency. In rats, the infusion of the sulfated octapeptide of cholecystokinin (CCK-8) causes a significant reduction in meal size as previously mentioned, whereas meal frequency is increased to compensate for the small meals. However, little is known about the effects of meal pattern on CCK in animals or humans. It is possible that frequent feeding may affect CCK release in one of two ways: It may cause the regular release of the hormone in response to each feed, persistently alerting the brain that the individual is satiated, or CCK may be released into the circulation in such small amounts in response to frequent feeding that it is not recognized by the brain and the individual continues to eat. Similar effects may occur with GLP and GIP.

Effect of Meal Frequency on Total Energy Expenditure

As discussed earlier, the three components of energy expenditure are BMR, thermogenesis, and physical activity. For meal frequency to have an influence on energy expenditure, it must affect one or more of these components. BMR (which represents 60–75% of energy expenditure in sedentary individuals) is not known to be influenced by meal frequency. Much the same can be said for thermogenesis, for which extensive research has failed to demonstrate a link between feeding frequency and DIT. It is reasonable and logical to expect that any difference between frequent and infrequent meal-eating patterns would be seen most clearly during the postprandial period when food has just been eaten, where the rate of ingestion of nutrients may alter EE and fuel storage.

Although much research has been carried out on the effects of meal frequency on total energy expenditure, few studies have isolated the physical activity component per se. Greater attention has been paid to the relationship between meal frequency and physical activity with regard to the performance of elite athletes because the manipulation of the meal pattern can potentially be used as a tool to achieve optimal performance. Because carbohydrate requirements in elite athletes are high and endogenous glycogen reserves are limited, athletes undertaking prolonged strenuous exercise seek to maximize carbohydrate availability at all times.

Irrespective of the above, the key determinant of feeding frequency's overall effect on energy balance is whether it has an impact on 24-h energy expenditure, where energy intake is fixed in content and composition and physical activity is kept constant. Numerous studies have been carried out to investigate this, and all have found that no relationship exists. The majority of these studies used either direct or indirect calorimetry or doubly labeled water in their measurements, both of which are highly reliable energy expenditure measurement techniques.

Conclusion

The contemporary terminology referring to the tendency to increase the amount of food eaten at a meal and the greater frequency at which food is eaten demonstrates the importance of a clear understanding of the consequences of meal size and frequency on health. Satiety peptides and adiposity hormones attempt to control the size of a meal eaten, and increased meal frequency, within the constraints of energy balance, has been found to have beneficial effects attenuating circulating substrates. However, to elucidate the influence that meal size and frequency have on absorption and metabolism, and to clarify whether the increase in the volume of food eaten at a meal and the greater frequency at which food is eaten have a direct affect on health, further research on the free-living population is required.

See also: **Appetite**: Physiological and Neurobiological Aspects; Psychobiological and Behavioral Aspects. **Energy**: Metabolism; Balance; Requirements. **Energy Expenditure**: Indirect Calorimetry. **Weight Management**: Approaches; Weight Maintenance; Weight Cycling.

Further Reading

Bellisle F, McDevitt R, and Prentice AM (1997) Meal frequency and energy balance. *British Journal of Nutrition* **77**: S57–S70.

Blevins JE, Schwartz MW, and Baskin DG (2002) Peptide signals regulating food intake and energy homeostasis. *Canadian Journal of Physiology & Pharmacology* **80**: 396–406.

Blundell JE and King NA (1996) Overconsumption as a cause of weight gain: Behavioral–physiological interactions in the control of food intake (appetite). *Ciba Foundation Symposium* **201**: 138–154; discussion 154–158, 188–193.

Drummond S, Crombie N, and Kirk T (1996) A critique of the effects of snacking on body weight status. *European Journal of Clinical Nutrition* **50**: 779–783.

Frayn KN (1997) In: Keith Snell (ed.) *Metabolic Regulation, A Human Perspective*, 2nd edn. Oxford: Portland Press.

Jenkins DJA (1997) Carbohydrate tolerance and food frequency. *British Journal of Nutrition* **77**: S71–S81.

Mann J (1997) Meal frequency and plasma lipids and lipoproteins. *British Journal of Nutrition* **77**: S83–S90.

Moran TH, Ladenheim EE, and Schwartz GJ (2001) Within-meal gut feedback signalling. *International Journal of Obesity and Related Metabolic Disorders* **25**: S39–S41.

Wilding JP (2002) Neuropeptides and appetite control. *Diabetic Medicine* **19**: 619–627.

Woods SC and Seeley RJ (2000) Adiposity signals and the control of energy homeostasis. *Nutrition* **16**: 894–902.

MEAT, POULTRY AND MEAT PRODUCTS

P A Lofgren, Oak Park, IL, USA

Animal source foods are major contributors to the nutrients in the food supply in many countries. Of these foods, animal muscle (or meat) foods and products are excellent examples of nutrient-dense, or naturally nutrient-rich, foods that provide a relatively large amount of many nutrients per the amount of calories provided in a typical serving. For purposes of this article, discussion is limited to the muscle foods: beef, pork, lamb, veal, poultry, and some of the processed products made from these muscle species.

For meat and meat products there are extensive and comprehensive nutrient databases available for reference for particular products of interest. Thus, this article will provide a sampling of the data available for representative meats and meat products.

One of the best and most comprehensive listings of the nutrient values of all meat, poultry, and other meat products is the nutrient database developed and maintained by the US Department of Agriculture. In this database, complete nutrient profiles are listed for more than 700 beef, 200 pork, 195 lamb, 85 veal, 140 poultry, and 130 turkey products. This database can be accessed and searched on-line at the Web site www.nal.usda.gov/fnic/foodcomp. This database is updated as new data become available for various food products. The most recent version of this database is the *USDA National Nutrient Database for Standard Reference*, Release 17, published in 2004.

For another extensive listing of the nutrient values of many meat and meat products, including some by brand name, the reader is referred to the publication *Bowes & Church's Food Values of Portions Commonly Used* (18th edn.). This reference, although not as extensive in terms of products listed, provides data directly in common serving sizes and provides available data on some additional nutrient and nutrient-related components of meat products (e.g., values for ω-3 and *trans* fatty acids, glutathione, vitamin D activity, and other vitamin-like compounds).

Nutritional Value

The nutritional value of foods, including meat and meat products, can be defined in a number of different ways, from simply listing the quantities of various nutrients contained in the foods to consideration of biological factors that affect the utilization of these nutrients by the body. Some foods may contain nutrients in forms that the body cannot readily utilize. Thus, nutrient bioavailability, or availability, becomes important.

The nutritional value of meat and meat products is related to the quantity and utilization of nutrients and the potential for these products to either enhance or restrict nutrient utilization by the body. There are five major classes of nutrients: protein, lipid, carbohydrate, vitamins, and minerals.

The nutrient content of meat (muscle foods) is fairly similar among the various mammals, birds, and fish. However, differences in the levels of the various nutrients may result from differences in the carcass composition among species and within species as a result of different fat-to-muscle ratios in the edible portion. As fat percentage increases, nutrient concentration of the muscle portion decreases. Also, to a certain extent, the fat profile/composition and other nutrient content levels may be modified or affected by the animal's diet and/or genetic makeup.

In general, cooking or heat processing has only minimal effects on the nutritional value of muscle foods. In most cases, cooking usually decreases moisture content and concentrates other nutrients, including fat content, especially in lower fat products. This is due to moisture loss. However, in some intensely heated meat products, fat content may also be reduced significantly with negligible loss of other nutrients.

Classes of Nutrients and Meat Products

Protein

Proteins comprise the structural unit of all muscle cells and connective tissue. As such, meat and meat products (muscle foods) are major protein sources. Furthermore, muscle foods, as a group, are excellent sources of high-quality protein that supplies all the essential amino acids in desirable proportions for human consumption. Amino acids are the building blocks of protein, and those provided by meat match or exceed the profile required by humans.

The protein content of most muscle foods, on a wet basis, is between 15 and 35%. This percentage will change due to the moisture and lipid content of the specific product. On a raw weight basis as purchased at a store, the protein content is generally less than 20%. However, people do not eat muscle foods raw, and visible fat in red meat products and skin in poultry products are usually trimmed away. Therefore, muscle foods, as consumed, have a much higher protein content, in the range of 30%.

Lipids

The lipid component of meat and meat products includes a diverse group of substances, such as glycerides (glycerol with fatty acids attached), phospholipids, and sterols. The basic component of most meat lipids is the fatty acids, which can be saturated, monounsaturated, or polyunsaturated.

The relative amount of lipid in muscle foods is probably the most variable aspect of the nutritional profile. Within the lipid component, the relative amount of the different forms of fatty acids present is another variable among meat products. Despite the common reference to animal fats (and especially meat and meat products) as 'saturated,' less than half of all the fatty acids of meats are saturated.

The largest proportions of fatty acids in meats are monounsaturated, followed by saturated and then polyunsaturated fatty acids. Among meat products, poultry has a higher proportion of polyunsaturated fatty acids and slightly less saturated fatty acids compared to other meat sources.

The fat in meat products provides much of the flavor associated with these foods and also contributes to the palatability and overall acceptability by consumers.

In addition, the fats in meat and meat products also contain several essential fatty acids (linoleic and linolenic acid), and they contain the fat-soluble vitamins A, D, E, and K.

Carbohydrates

Meat and meat products are not significant sources of dietary carbohydrates. Almost all dietary carbohydrates come from plant sources. The only naturally occurring carbohydrate in muscle foods is glycogen. In some processed meat products, such as those that are 'sugar-cured,' there may be additional sucrose or glucose added.

Vitamins

Meat and meat products are especially good sources of most of the water-soluble vitamins. In general, meat is the major dietary source of vitamin B_{12} and is an excellent source of many of the other B vitamins, such as pyridoxine (B_6), biotin, niacin, pantothenic acid, riboflavin, and thiamin. For vitamin B_{12}, red meat products such as beef and lamb are especially good sources. Pork products are one of the very best sources of thiamin. Although present in muscle foods, the fat-soluble vitamins are less abundant than in plant foods. Vitamins E and K are present, but at lower levels.

Vitamin D activity may be present in some meat products, but at extremely low levels. This is reflected in the USDA nutrient database, in which vitamin D activity is not listed for beef, pork, lamb, veal, and chicken/turkey products; however, it is listed for some processed meat products. In recent years, there has been production research on beef, pork, and lamb to determine if added vitamin D_3 or its metabolites, fed to the animal for a brief period of time prior to slaughter, can result in improved meat tenderness. Although the results are inconsistent, and commercial application is premature, there is some indication that tenderness may be improved with relatively low levels of vitamin D supplementation, which seems to leave very little residual vitamin D_3 or its metabolites in the muscle. Research in Denmark notes that the more biologically active 25-OHD is present at low levels in meat; however, there is no consensus on the conversion factor for 25-OHD to calculate vitamin D activity. Also, there are very few data on the vitamin D and 25-OHD levels in most meat products. This represents a potential future area of research regarding the nutrient composition of meat.

Minerals

Meat and meat products are good to excellent sources of most minerals. Among the macrominerals, calcium is not high in muscle foods, although phosphorus and potassium are prominent. In natural meat products, sodium is present but not a significant contributor to the diet. However, processed meat products may contain significantly higher levels of sodium (added as part of curing, preserving, or flavor-enhancing ingredients). Some of the microminerals (trace elements) are especially abundant in meat and meat products. Iron is of greatest significance from meat sources because it is present in the 'heme' form, which is more bioavailable than the non-heme form. Of meat products, beef is an especially rich source of iron in this bioavailable form.

Muscle tissue is a very rich source of minerals, such as phosphorus, potassium, magnesium, iron, copper, zinc, and selenium. For instance, pork, poultry, and beef are especially good sources of selenium.

Bioavailability of Nutrients

Muscle foods have been shown to contain 'intrinsic' factors that improve the bioavailability of a variety of nutrients. Moreover, the bioavailability of these nutrients from muscle foods is high, often exceeding the availability for the same nutrients in foods derived from plants. Heme iron is one example. Zinc and copper have been shown to be more available from meat sources than from plant sources. Several of the B vitamins may also be more bioavailable from meat sources than from plant sources.

Another interesting aspect of meat products is their ability to promote the bioavailability of nutrients in nonmuscle foods when the two are eaten together. This has been referred to as the 'meat factor.' Perhaps the best example of this is the positive effect of meat in the diet on non-heme iron sources, also in the diet.

Nutrient Density of Meat and Meat Products

The nutrient density of meat is high. Muscle foods have high levels of essential nutrients per unit of weight and per amount of calories provided. Meat and meat products (muscle foods) provide significant amounts of essential nutrients at levels/concentrations higher than those of most other foods relative to the caloric content provided. The US Food and Drug Administration food labeling guidelines allow a food to be designated a 'good' source of a nutrient if it contributes 10% or more of the Daily Value (DV) and an 'excellent' source if it contributes 20% or more of the DV, for that nutrient, per 3-oz. serving. Most meat products are good or excellent sources of many nutrients. It is generally recognized that in diets that lack muscle foods, greater care is required in diet/menu selection to ensure that adequate levels of essential nutrients are present and bioavailable.

Meat Sources and Nutritional Values

Beef

Beef is an excellent source of high-quality protein, and provides significant contributions of many B vitamins and minerals. In macronutrient terms, the lean-to-fat ratio of the particular beef product influences the calorie and nutrient composition. In general, as the fat content decreases, the concentration of other nutrients (especially protein, B vitamins, and minerals) in beef tends to increase. Most beef products available to the consumer are much leaner than they were 20 or 30 years ago. This is a result of changes in feeding and genetics, producing leaner animals, and also due to closer trim levels on the products that consumers see in the meat case. Whereas in the past, beef cuts with 1/4 in. of fat trim were common, now the same products have only 1/8 in. fat trim or, in some cases, even 0 in. fat trim. In the case of ground beef products, 10 or 20 years ago 17% fat ground beef was considered as 'extra lean.' Today, ground beef is commonly available at fat levels as low as 5 or 10%. Other common fat levels for ground beef are 15, 20, and 25%; however, a large proportion of current ground beef sales are in the 5–15% fat level range.

The fat content of beef contains a varied fatty acid profile, with the largest proportion being contributed by monounsaturated fat, followed by saturated fat and polyunsaturated fatty acids. In addition, because it is a ruminant product, beef is an excellent source of the naturally occurring fatty acid conjugated linoleic acid (CLA), which has been demonstrated to provide anticarcinogenic properties among other health benefits.

Table 1 provides the energy, protein, and lipid profile of beef along with other meat sources. For a comparison of the mineral composition of beef products versus that of other common meat sources, see **Table 2**. For a comparison of the vitamin composition of beef products versus that of other common meat sources, see **Table 3**.

Table 1 Energy, protein, and lipid profile of meats and meat products[a]

Meat species/cut	Serving size (g)	Energy (kcal/kJ)	Total protein (g)	Total fat (g)	Total SFA (g)	Total MUFA (g)	Total PUFA (g)	Total cholesterol (mg)
Beef								
Composite, Ln 0 in., ckd, all grades	85	179/751	25.4	7.9	3.01	3.32	0.27	73
Top round, Ln 0 in., brld, all grades	85	158/662	27.0	4.8	1.67	2.02	0.18	65
Top loin, Ln 0 in., brld, all grades	85	155/649	24.9	5.4	2.06	2.16	0.20	54
Arm pot roast, Ln 0 in., brsd, all grades	85	173/722	28.4	5.7	2.17	2.44	0.20	57
95% Ln ground beef, brld	85	151/633	22.4	6.2	2.53	2.31	0.28	65
Pork								
Composite, fresh, Ln, ckd	85	180/754	24.9	8.2	2.90	3.70	0.64	73
Tenderloin, fresh, Ln, rstd	85	139/583	23.9	4.1	1.41	1.64	0.35	67
Center loin chop, fresh, Ln, pan-fried	85	197/825	27.4	8.9	3.09	3.78	1.14	78
Shoulder, blade steak, fresh, Ln, brld	85	193/808	22.7	10.7	3.78	4.79	0.92	80
Ham, fresh, Ln, rstd	85	179/751	25.0	8.0	2.80	3.78	0.72	80
Lamb								
Composite, Australian, Ln 1/8 in., ckd	85	171/715	22.7	8.2	3.44	3.28	0.36	74
Loin, Australian, Ln 1/8 in., brld	85	163/683	22.6	7.4	3.13	2.97	0.31	69
Leg, Australian, Ln 1/8 in., rstd	85	162/676	23.2	6.9	2.80	2.81	0.32	76
Foreshank, Australian, Ln 1/8 in., brsd	85	140/586	23.4	4.4	1.60	1.99	0.25	78
Composite, New Zealand, Ln, ckd	85	175/733	25.2	7.5	3.28	2.96	0.44	93
Composite, US domestic, Ln 1/4 in., ckd	85	175/733	24.0	8.1	2.89	3.54	0.53	78
Veal								
Composite, Ln, ckd	85	167/697	27.1	5.6	1.56	2.00	0.50	100
Cutlet, leg top round, Ln, pan-fried	85	156/651	28.2	3.9	1.10	1.40	0.35	91
Loin chops, Ln, rstd	85	149/622	22.4	5.9	2.19	2.12	0.48	90
Shoulder, blade, Ln, brsd	85	168/704	27.8	5.5	1.54	1.96	0.49	134
Chicken/turkey								
Broilers, meat only, rstd	85	162/676	24.6	6.3	1.73	2.26	1.44	76
Broilers, Lt meat only, rstd	85	147/615	26.3	3.8	1.08	1.31	0.83	72
Broilers, Dk meat only, rstd	85	174/729	23.3	8.3	2.26	3.03	1.92	79
Turkey, all classes, meat only, rstd	85	145/604	24.9	4.2	1.39	0.88	1.22	65
Turkey, all classes, Lt meat only, rstd	85	133/558	25.4	2.7	0.88	0.48	0.73	59
Turkey, all classes, Dk meat only, rstd	85	159/665	24.3	6.1	2.06	1.39	1.84	72
Processed meats								
Bacon, pork, cured, pan-fried, 1 slice	7.9	42/176	3.0	3.2	1.05	1.42	0.35	9
Sausage, pork, fresh, ckd, 2 links	48	163/680	9.3	13.6	4.38	5.94	1.79	40
Bologna, beef & pork, low fat, 1 slice	28	64/269	3.2	5.4	2.05	2.56	0.46	11
Salami, beef, ckd, 1 slice	26	67/280	3.3	5.8	2.56	2.77	0.27	18

[a]Amount per 3 oz./85 g, lean only, cooked, except as noted.

Ln, lean and trim level; ckd, cooked; brld, broiled; rstd, roasted; brsd, braised; Lt, light; Dk, dark.

Data from USDA, ARS (2004) *USDA National Nutrient Database for Standard Reference*, Release 17. Nutrient Data Laboratory Web site: www.nal.usda.gov/fnic/foodcomp.

Table 2 Mineral composition of meats and meat products[a]

Meat species/cut	Serving size (g)	Ca (mg)	Fe (mg)	Mg (mg)	P (mg)	K (mg)	Na (mg)	Zn (mg)	Cu (mg)	Mn (mg)	Se (μg)
Beef											
Composite, Ln 0 in., ckd, all grades	85	7	2.54	22	196	302	56	5.76	0.11	0.02	18.1
Top round, Ln 0 in., brld, all grades	85	6	2.28	18	172	223	36	4.67	0.07	0.01	30.8
Top loin, Ln 0 in., brld, all grades	85	16	1.56	21	195	314	51	4.56	0.07	0.01	28.6
Arm pot roast, Ln 0 in., brsd, all grades	85	14	2.38	19	173	225	46	6.76	0.10	0.01	28.7
95% Ln ground beef, brld	85	6	2.41	19	175	296	55	5.47	0.08	0.01	18.4
Pork											
Composite, fresh, Ln, ckd	85	18	0.94	22	201	319	50	2.52	0.05	0.02	38.2
Tenderloin, fresh, Ln, rstd	85	5	1.25	24	220	371	48	2.24	0.04	0.03	40.9
Center loin chop, fresh, Ln, pan-fried	85	20	0.83	27	230	382	73	2.07	0.07	0.01	40.6
Shoulder, blade steak, fresh, Ln, brld	85	28	1.33	20	187	292	63	4.27	0.05	0.01	33.4
Ham, fresh, Ln, rstd	85	6	0.95	21	239	317	54	2.77	0.09	0.03	42.4
Lamb											
Composite, Australian, Ln 1/8 in., ckd	85	14	1.74	20	176	270	68	4.37	0.13	0.01	9.3
Loin, Australian, Ln 1/8 in., brld	85	18	1.85	22	187	289	68	2.96	0.13	0.01	8.8
Leg, Australian, Ln 1/8 in., rstd	85	8	1.83	21	182	277	61	4.11	0.13	0.01	5.0
Foreshank, Australian, Ln 1/8 in., brsd	85	12	1.62	19	150	217	85	6.74	0.11	0.01	7.7
Composite, New Zealand, Ln, ckd	85	11	2.00	19	209	160	42	3.65	0.10	0.03	1.7
Composite, US domestic, Ln 1/4 in., ckd	85	13	1.74	22	178	292	65	4.48	0.11	0.02	22.2
Veal											
Composite, Ln, ckd	85	20	0.99	24	212	287	76	4.33	0.10	0.03	11.1
Cutlet, leg top round, Ln, pan-fried	85	6	0.74	27	246	376	65	2.87	0.05	0.03	8.8
Loin chops, Ln, rstd	85	18	0.72	22	189	289	82	2.75	0.10	0.03	9.9
Shoulder, blade, Ln, brsd	85	34	1.25	24	214	259	86	6.28	0.15	0.03	12.3
Chicken/turkey											
Broilers, meat only, rstd	85	13	1.03	21	166	207	73	1.78	0.06	0.02	18.7
Broilers, Lt meat only, rstd	85	13	0.90	23	184	210	65	1.05	0.04	0.01	20.7
Broilers, Dk meat only, rstd	85	13	1.13	20	152	204	79	2.38	0.07	0.02	15.3
Turkey, all classes, meat only, rstd	85	21	1.51	22	181	253	60	2.63	0.08	0.02	31.3
Turkey, all classes, Lt meat only, rstd	85	16	1.15	24	186	259	54	1.73	0.04	0.02	27.3
Turkey, all classes, Dk meat only, rstd	85	27	1.98	20	173	247	67	3.79	0.14	0.02	34.8
Processed meats											
Bacon, pork, cured, pan-fried, 1 slice	7.9	1	0.11	3	44	47	192	0.29	0.01	0.00	5.1
Sausage, pork, fresh, ckd, 2 links	48	6	0.65	8	78	141	360	1.00	0.04	0.00	0.0
Bologna, beef & pork, low fat, 1 slice	28	3	0.18	3	51	44	310	0.42	0.02	0.00	3.1
Salami, beef, ckd, 1 slice	26	2	0.57	3	53	49	296	0.46	0.05	0.01	3.8

[a]Amount per 3 oz./85 g, lean only, cooked, except as noted.

Ln, lean and trim level; ckd, cooked; brld, broiled; rstd, roasted; brsd, braised; Lt, light; Dk, dark.

Data from USDA, ARS (2004) *USDA National Nutrient Database for Standard Reference*, Release 17. Nutrient Data Laboratory Web site: www.nal.usda.gov/fnic/foodcomp.

Table 3 Vitamin composition of meats and meat products[a]

Meat species/cut	Serving size (g)	Thiamin (mg)	Riboflavin (mg)	Niacin (mg)	Pantothenic acid (mg)	Vitamin B_6 (mg)	Folate (μg)	Vitamin B_{12} (μg)	Vitamin E (mg)	Vitamin K (μg)
Beef										
Composite, Ln 0 in., ckd, all grades	85	0.08	0.20	3.40	0.33	0.30	7	2.64	0.14	1.50
Top round, Ln 0 in., brld, all grades	85	0.06	0.15	4.84	0.53	0.36	9	1.49	0.34	1.30
Top loin, Ln 0 in., brld, all grades	85	0.07	0.13	7.12	0.49	0.53	8	1.39	0.32	1.20
Arm pot roast, Ln 0 in., brsd, all grades	85	0.06	0.18	4.13	0.56	0.27	9	2.07	0.37	1.30
95% Ln ground beef, brld	85	0.04	0.15	5.05	0.55	0.35	6	2.10	0.59	1.10
Pork										
Composite, fresh, Ln, ckd	85	0.72	0.29	4.40	0.58	0.37	1	0.64	0.15	0.00
Tenderloin, fresh, Ln, rstd	85	0.80	0.33	4.00	0.58	0.36	5	0.47	0.17	0.00
Center loin chop, fresh, Ln, pan-fried	85	1.06	0.28	5.10	0.85	0.44	5	0.65	0.19	0.00
Shoulder, blade steak, fresh, Ln, brld	85	0.64	0.37	3.66	0.69	0.26	4	0.96	0.23	0.00
Ham, fresh, Ln, rstd	85	0.59	0.30	4.20	0.57	0.38	10	0.61	0.22	0.00
Lamb										
Composite, Australian, Ln 1/8 in., ckd	85	0.11	0.31	4.94	0.75	0.34	b	2.56	b	b
Loin, Australian, Ln 1/8 in., brld	85	0.15	0.28	6.93	0.71	0.44	b	1.71	b	b
Leg, Australian, Ln 1/8 in., rstd	85	0.12	0.36	4.87	0.84	0.39	b	2.71	b	b
Foreshank, Australian, Ln 1/8 in., brsd	85	0.08	0.24	4.58	0.56	0.22	b	2.72	b	b
Composite, New Zealand, Ln, ckd	85	0.11	0.43	6.53	0.49	0.12	0	2.51	0.16	b
Composite, US domestic, Ln 1/4 in., ckd	85	0.09	0.24	5.37	0.59	0.14	20	2.22	0.16	b
Veal										
Composite, Ln, ckd	85	0.05	0.29	7.16	1.13	0.28	14	1.40	0.36	5.60
Cutlet, leg top round, Ln, pan-fried	85	0.06	0.32	10.74	1.04	0.43	14	1.28	0.36	4.20
Loin chops, Ln, rstd	85	0.05	0.26	8.04	1.08	0.32	14	1.11	0.42	4.70
Shoulder, blade, Ln, brsd	85	0.05	0.31	4.83	1.35	0.21	13	1.71	0.38	5.80
Chicken/turkey										
Broilers, meat only, rstd	85	0.06	0.15	7.80	0.94	0.40	5	0.28	0.23	2.00
Broilers, Lt meat only, rstd	85	0.06	0.10	10.56	0.83	0.51	3	0.29	0.23	0.30
Broilers, Dk meat only, rstd	85	0.06	0.19	5.57	1.03	0.31	7	0.27	0.23	3.30
Turkey, all classes, meat only, rstd	85	0.05	0.16	4.63	0.80	0.39	6	0.31	0.28	3.10
Turkey, all classes, Lt meat only, rstd	85	0.05	0.11	5.81	0.58	0.46	5	0.31	0.08	0.00
Turkey, all classes, Dk meat only, rstd	85	0.05	0.21	3.10	1.09	0.31	8	0.31	0.54	3.30
Processed meats										
Bacon, pork, cured, pan-fried, 1 slice	7.9	0.04	0.02	0.91	0.10	0.03	0	0.10	0.02	0.00
Sausage, pork, fresh, ckd, 2 links	48	0.14	0.10	3.00	0.35	0.16	1	0.57	0.26	0.20
Bologna, beef & pork, low fat, 1 slice	28	0.05	0.04	0.71		0.05	1	0.37	0.06	0.10
Salami, beef, ckd, 1 slice	26	0.03	0.05	0.84	0.25	0.05	1	0.80	0.05	0.30

[a]Amount per 3 oz./85 g, lean only, cooked, except as noted.

[b]Comparable data not available.

Ln, lean and trim level; ckd, cooked; brld, broiled; rstd, roasted; brsd, braised; Lt, light; Dk, dark.

USDA, ARS (2004) *USDA National Nutrient Database for Standard Reference*, Release 17. Nutrient Data Laboratory Web site: www.nal.usda.gov/fnic/foodcomp.

Pork

Pork, like beef, is an excellent source of high-quality protein and contributes significant amounts of many B vitamins and minerals. As for other muscle foods, pork's nutrient composition is greatly affected by its fat and water content. As fat percentage decreases, the concentration of other nutrients increases. In addition, as pork is cooked and moisture is removed, the concentration of nutrients also increases. Pork is an excellent source of minerals, such as selenium, iron, zinc, phosphorus, and potassium. Compared to other muscle foods, the contribution of pork to selenium in the food supply is especially significant.

Pork is an excellent source of the B vitamins. Pork is an especially good source of thiamin (vitamin B_1), being the single best source of this vitamin among commonly eaten foods. The fat profile of pork can be influenced by feeding regimes such that it is more or less saturated or firm. However, overall the fatty acid profile of pork is largely monounsaturated, followed by saturated and then polyunsaturated fatty acids.

Lamb

Although it represents a smaller portion of overall muscle food consumption, lamb still provides a nutrient profile with significant benefits for the human diet. In addition to being a source of high-quality protein, lamb is also a good source of many minerals and B vitamins. Vitamin B_{12} is especially abundant in lamb. It is also a good source of the minerals iron and zinc.

In addition, as a ruminant, lamb is another naturally occurring dietary source of CLA, a unique fatty acid with anticarcinogenic and other health benefits (from animal model studies).

Veal

Although representing a smaller proportion of overall meat consumption, veal still provides a nutrient profile that is very beneficial. As with all meat sources, veal provides high-quality protein in a product that may be slightly leaner (in terms of fat) than other red meat sources. Compared to other meat sources, veal has a lower iron content.

Poultry

The nutrient composition of poultry (chicken and turkey) is similar to that of red meat animals with a few exceptions. Poultry is lower in iron content, and thus heme iron, than beef. Turkey is slightly higher in several minerals (Ca, Fe, P, K, Zn, and Cu) than chicken. As in red meats, there are significant amounts of several B vitamins (e.g., niacin, B_6, and pantothenic acid) compared to other meat sources, and these are not significantly reduced during cooking.

The fat content of poultry is predominantly monounsaturated fat, followed by saturated fat and polyunsaturated fat. Poultry fat, like pork fat, is somewhat more unsaturated than beef fat. Poultry is significantly higher in polyunsaturated fat compared to beef, pork, lamb, and veal.

Processed Meats

Processed meats represent a diverse array of products that have undergone additional treatment from the fresh meat form to the point of consumption, including curing with other ingredients added and the addition of salt or other flavor or preservative mixtures. Also, these products often represent combined meat sources.

Summary

Muscle foods provide significant amounts of essential nutrients at levels/concentrations higher than those of most other foods relative to the caloric content provided. Almost all of the essential nutrients are present in muscle foods at some level. Furthermore, muscle foods provide nutrients in a form that enhances the bioavailability of nutrients from both the meat and other dietary sources. It is generally recognized that in diets that lack muscle foods, greater care is required in diet/menu selection to ensure that adequate levels of essential nutrients are present and bioavailable.

See also: **Amino Acids**: Chemistry and Classification; Metabolism; Specific Functions. **Bioavailability**. **Biotin**. **Carbohydrates**: Chemistry and Classification; Regulation of Metabolism; Requirements and Dietary Importance; Resistant Starch and Oligosaccharides. **Cholesterol**: Sources, Absorption, Function and Metabolism; Factors Determining Blood Levels. **Copper**. **Dairy Products**. **Dietary Surveys**. **Eggs**. **Energy**: Balance; Requirements; Adaptation. **Fats and Oils**. **Fatty Acids**: Metabolism; Monounsaturated; Omega-3 Polyunsaturated; Omega-6 Polyunsaturated; Saturated; *Trans* Fatty Acids. **Fish**. **Folic Acid**. **Food Composition Data**. **Fruits and Vegetables**. **Iron**. **Lipids**: Chemistry and Classification; Composition and Role of Phospholipids. **Magnesium**. **Manganese**. **Niacin**. **Nuts and Seeds**. **Pantothenic Acid**. **Phosphorus**. **Potassium**. **Protein**: Synthesis and Turnover; Requirements and Role in Diet; Digestion and Bioavailability; Quality and Sources; Deficiency.

Riboflavin. **Selenium**. **Sodium**: Physiology. **Thiamin**: Physiology. **Ultratrace Elements**. **Vegetarian Diets**. **Vitamin A**: Biochemistry and Physiological Role. **Vitamin B₆**. **Vitamin E**: Metabolism and Requirements. **Vitamin K**. **Zinc**: Physiology.

Further Reading

Council for Agricultural Science and Technology (1997) *Contribution of Animal Products to Healthful Diets*, Task Force Report No. 131. Ames, IA: CAST.

Council for Agricultural Science and Technology (1999) *Animal Agriculture and Global Food Supply*, Task Force Report No. 135. Ames, IA: CAST.

Foote MR, Horst RL, Huff-Lonergan EJ *et al.* (2004) The use of vitamin D₃ and its metabolites to improve beef tenderness. *Journal of Animal Science* 82(1): 242–249.

Godber JS (1994) Nutritional value of muscle foods. In: Kinsman DM, Kotula AW, and Breidenstein BC (eds.) *Muscle Foods—Meat, Poultry and Seafood Technology*, pp. 430–455. New York: Chapman & Hall.

Ovesen L, Brot C, and Jakobsen J (2003) Food contents and biological activity of 25-hydroxyvitamin D: A vitamin D metabolite to be reckoned with? *Annals of Nutrition and Metabolism* 47(3–4): 107–113.

Pennington JAT and Douglass JS (2004) *Bowes & Church's Food Values of Portions Commonly Used*, 18th ed. Baltimore: Lippincott Williams & Wilkins.

US Department of Agriculture, Agricultural Research Service (2004) *USDA National Nutrient Database for Standard Reference*, Release 17. Nutrient Data Laboratory Web site: http://www.nal.usda.gov/fnic/foodcomp.

Menkes Syndrome *see* **Copper**

MICROBIOTA OF THE INTESTINE

Contents
Prebiotics
Probiotics

Prebiotics

J M Saavedra and N Moore, John Hopkins School of Medicine, Baltimore, MD, USA

Introduction

The gastrointestinal (GI) system in humans comprises the largest surface area of any organ in the body. The complexity of this system and its functions provides us with the ability to take in nutrition, selectively process it, assist in maintaining fluid and electrolyte balance, and offers a vehicle for excretion of waste while at the same time offering the first line of defense against toxins, pathogens, and other noxious agents. The indigenous gut microflora make up the complex ecosystem that inhabits the GI lumen, which mediates part of the interaction between the external environment and the host.

The basic development and makeup of the human intestinal microflora, and the metabolic, immune, and functional effects of the host are discussed below. The importance of maintaining a balance in this ecosystem, and the recent use of nutrition for providing beneficial microflora and the clinical effect this offers will be presented.

Normal Microflora

The intestinal microflora of healthy humans is comprised of more than 400 species of bacteria with a population of 10^{12}–10^{14} colony-forming units (CFU) per gram, of which more than 98% are resident in the colon. This bacterial population nearly exceeds the population of cells in the human body. The microflora is composed of both aerobic and predominantly anaerobic microorganisms that when equilibrium within an individual is maintained confer nutritional and immune benefits. A prime example of the importance of microorganisms in the GI tract was the study of gnotobiotic (germ-free) mice, which suffered persistent enteritis and severe infections with poor survival rate. Through the interaction of the mucosal surface with the GI tract microflora an important system of immune defense is established.

The presence of microorganisms in different segments of the GI tract varies both qualitatively and quantitatively. Bacteria from the mouth are predominantly anaerobes including streptococci, *Bacteroides*, *Lactobacillus*, and some yeasts; these wash down to the stomach with the intake of food and function of swallowing. In the stomach the acid environment destroys most of the oral and food-ingested microorganisms. The microflora of the stomach is comprised of mostly Gram-positive and aerobic microflora at very low levels (10^3 CFU ml^{-1}). *Peptostreptococcus*, *Fusobacterium*, and *Bacteroides* species are present in low numbers while *Clostridium* is uncommon.

The volume of microflora increases exponentially from the small intestine, which is sparsely colonized, to the richly populated colon. The concentrations of bacteria found in the small intestine are between 10^3 and 10^4 CFU ml^{-1}, again both facultative anaerobes and aerobic bacteria with almost complete absence of coliforms and *Bacteriodes*.

The microflora of the colon dramatically increases to a concentration of 10^{11}–10^{12} CFU gm^{-1}. This bacterial load accounts for up to 50% of the volume of colonic content. Although the colonic microflora comprises more than 400 different species it is predominantly anaerobic including *Bacteroides*, *Fusobacterium*, *Bifidobacterium*, *Lactobacillus*, *Enterobacter* and coliforms, and other facultative anaerobes (*Staphlococcus* and *Candida* species).

Development of Microflora

The GI tract is essentially sterile at the time of birth and bacterial colonization begins upon exposure to the environment. Progression of colonization is initially fast, followed by a gradual process of modification over the first few years of life. As the baby passes through the birth canal bifidobacteria and lactobacilli are typically acquired and rapid colonization of mainly enterobacteria occurs. The hospital environment, type of feeding, and type of delivery affect the early colonization of the intestine after birth. Normal vaginal birth permits the transfer of bacteria of the mother as the infant passes through

the birth canal. However, with Cesarean delivery this transfer is absent and the hospital or other immediate environment can have a more significant effect on colonization. In these infants, colonization with anaerobic bacteria, especially *Bacteroides*, occurs later than with vaginally delivered infants.

Within the first few days and with introduction of feeding, the newborn intestine (through oxidation–reduction) promotes the establishment of aerobic bacteria, predominantly enterobacteria, *Enterococcus* and staphylococci, and anaerobic bacteria, bifidobacteria, *Bacteroides* and *Clostridia*. As the aerobic bacteria consume oxygen the intestinal milieu becomes more amenable to anaerobic bacteria and aerobic bacteria in turn decline. In breast fed infants bifidobacteria counts increase dramatically and account for 80–90% of the total fecal flora. Lactobacilli and *Bacteroides* also increase but to a lesser extent, while enterobacteria decrease. In formula fed babies *Enterococcus* is the predominant bacteria present with significantly less bifidobacteria and *Bacteroides* than the breast-fed infant. It is the difference in microflora, especially in the greater presence of bifidobacteria, and the presence of oligosaccharide and other bifido-genic factors in breast milk that likely confer a protective effect to the infant against infection, particularly against diarrheal disease.

With the introduction of weaning foods the fecal flora of babies begins to change resembling that of adults by 1 year of age. Concentrations of aerobes decrease and anaerobes (streptococci, *Enterobacter*, *Escherichia coli*, *Bacteroides*, and *Lactobacillus*) increase and predominate by 1–2 years of age. Bifidobacteria concentration also decreases but is generally maintained throughout adulthood (**Figure 1**).

Once well established the microflora is unique to each individual and maintained fairly undisturbed throughout adult life. Changes in general health

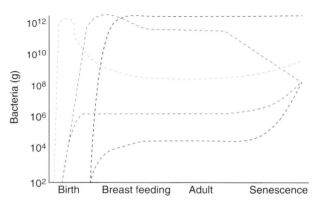

Figure 1 The intestinal flora and its relation to age. (purple), *Bacteroides*, Eubacteriae, Peptococcaceae; (red), Bifidobacteriae; (orange), *E. coli*, streptococci; (blue), lactobacilli; (green), Clostridiae.

and wellbeing, exposure to toxins in the food supply, and utilization of medications, particularly antibiotics, all transiently alter the colonic flora, often profoundly. When the equilibrium of this complex system occurs the host is potentially compromised. However, recovery to the original state of colonization usually occurs upon removal of the altering factors.

Metabolic Activity of Microflora

The structure and function of the gastrointestinal tract is influenced greatly by the presence and make-up of indigenous microflora. In the germ-free murine model, lack of microflora leads to a thinner, less cellular intestinal wall; the villi are thinner, crypts shallower and mucosal surface area is decreased, thus interfering with the gut immune system and nutrient handling processes. The intestinal flora is responsible for production of some micronutrients, particularly vitamins (biotin, folate, and vitamin K), and also fermentation of carbohydrates, which results in the production of short-chain fatty acids (acetate, proprionate, and butyrate). These end products are known to be active in the regeneration and health of the mucosal cellular make up. Glycosylation of complex carbohydrates on the microvillus membrane are specifically related to anaerobic bacteria in the gut lumen. Additionally, the microflora modulates the release of peptides and some proteins from the endocrine cells in the mucosa of the GI tract.

Innate bacteria induce many beneficial responses of the gut immune system. Bacterial interaction with the epithelial cells can enhance local immunity and deter response to antigens. Gram-negative bacteria cause the production of proinflammatory cytokines including interleukin-6 and tumor necrosis factor alpha (TNF-α).

Gut Barrier Effect

Health of intestinal mucosa and the equilibrium of the microflora are essential for the immune response of the GI tract to both ingested and systemic invaders. The colonic microflora plays a key role in maintaining mucosal integrity and the deterrence of pathogenic/toxic bacteria. To maintain the bacterial equilibrium the indigenous bacteria appear to compete with pathogenic bacteria predominantly in the colon for enterocyte receptors, as well as for luminal nutrient. Additionally, the production of short-chain fatty acids from bacterial fermentation of carbohydrates and the transformation of proteins to sterols and bile acids destroy potential mutagens of ingested foods. Dietary antigens are prevented through this system of barrier protection. Alterations will produce an immunoinflammatory response; ultimately entrance of antigens into the body can occur, inducing a systemic allergic response.

Flora-Nutrient Interactions

There is a complex interaction between food and microflora in a feedback-like system. Different types of diets can lead to changes in fecal flora, and its resultant metabolic activity can be altered. When individuals consuming a vegetarian diet were compared to those on a typical Western diet, the latter had microflora that showed greater hydrolyzing ability leading to a more effective metabolism of bile acids and subsequently reduced cholesterol. Similar studies in mice have shown differences with high-fat diets versus low-fat diets.

Disaccharides are broken down in the proximal small intestine by enzymes in the brush border and microvilli of the intestinal epithelium. Glucose, sucrose, lactose, and maltose are the predominant disaccharides hydrolyzed and these rarely reach the colon. When the brush border is unable to produces the enzymes needed for metabolism, the disaccharides are not absorbed in the small bowel and ultimately reach the colon where they interact with the abundant colonic bacteria. Subsequent fermentation causes an osmotic imbalance pulling water into the lumen and causing diarrhea. Significant and rapid production of short-chain fatty acids causes changes in the fecal pH and can irritate the colonic mucosa.

Complex carbohydrates, such as dietary fibers, are predominantly fermented in the colon by colonic bacteria, mostly anaerobic flora. Short-chain fatty acids, acetate, propionate, and butyrate are the predominant by-products and in lesser amounts carbon dioxide, hydrogen, methane, and water. Slow and regular production of short-chain fatty acids provides an energy source that helps the regeneration of colonic mucosa. Fatty acids are also used for hepatic very low density lipoprotein synthesis, which has been reported to have influence in cardiovascular disease.

Dietary protein is only partially digested in the small intestine producing amino acid (NH_2) and carboxyl groups ($COOH$). These amines enter the colon and are hydrolyzed by enzymes of colonic bacteria. Amines and short-chain fatty acids will enter the systemic system through absorption by the colonic mucosa and portal vein into the bloodstream where they will be appropriately utilized by tissues. These substances then return to the liver through the portal circulation and are excreted as urea in the urine.

Primary bile acids originating from the liver are excreted into the small intestine and conjugate with amino acids, particularly taurine and glycine. Conjugated compounds in general are not well absorbed and cannot re-enter the hepatic circulation without further breakdown. Bacterial action hydrolyzes the conjugated amines, releasing free bile acids 7α- and 7β-dehydroxylation of the bile acid nucleus, and hydroxyl groups C_{-3}, C_{-6}, and C_{-7}. *Bacteroides, Bifidobacterium, Fusobacterium, Clostridium, Lactobacillus*, and *Streptococcus* are the main bacteria that assist in this hydrolysis. These free bile acids can recirculate through the enterohepatic circulation. Bile acids assist in digestion of fats in the intestine. Colonic microflora also transform excess cholesterol found in the large intestine to coprostanol thus reducing available cholesterol and increasing cholesterol to be excreted in stool.

Bacterial microflora of both the small and large bowel synthesizes a number of essential vitamins. Most importantly vitamin K production by the liver is dependent on the metabolic activity of bacteria in the ileum. Prothrombin, a blood-clotting factor, is synthesized in the liver. Glycoprotein arising from the prothrombin complex cannot be synthesized unless the liver contains menaquione. Bacteria in the intestine synthesize menaquione at the terminal ileum where it can be absorbed and reach the liver to promote clotting factors.

Vitamin B_{12} is completely synthesized from microflora in animals. Meats and dairy products from these animals is a primary source of B_{12} for humans, but it is also synthesized in the large bowel. However, the small bowel is the site of optimal absorption of B_{12} so synthesized B_{12} is not well absorbed. Additionally, biotin and other B complex vitamins (folic acid and thiamine) are synthesized by GI microflora.

Microflora and Host Interactions

The immune response within the GI tract is both innate and adaptive. The innate immune system is a pre-existing system that begins to eliminate invading pathogenic microorganisms immediately upon exposure. Natural barriers of the mucosal epithelium begin this immune response. Rapid induction of an immune response occurs with initial inflammation through phagocytosis. Neutrophils and macrophages engulf bacteria in an effort to get rid of them before insult to the epithelium occurs. Phagocytes also release important chemokines and cytokines that increase the inflammatory response activating the adaptive immune mechanisms when necessary.

The adaptive immune mechanisms are able to differentiate indigenous microflora and mount a response to pathogenic microbes. This process involves cells of the gut-associated lymphoid tissue (GALT) resulting in production of IgA. The adaptive branch of the GI immune system is antigen specific allowing a 'memory' of such and responding specifically to re-exposure to offensive bacteria or toxins. It is through this delicate interplay between innate and adaptive immune mechanisms that an adequate immunologic defense response can be maintained while the adaptive immune system is activated in the hope of averting a harmful systemic reaction.

Mucus/Mucin Glycoproteins

Mucus is continuously produced by goblet cells to lubricate and protect the GI epithelium. The primary gene identified that is located in the goblet cell and predominantly responsible for the production and secretion of mucus and its resulting sugar, mucin, is the MUC_2 gene. This is through an elaborate process of encoding a peptide modified by *o*-glycosidic bonds to a variety of carbohydrate residues to amino acids serine or threonine resulting in a glycoprotein with high carbohydrate content that provides the potential to bind sites for both indigenous and pathogenic bacteria. Mucin, the resulting glycoprotein, forms a viscous gel that coats the epithelial surface of the intestine protecting it from chemical and mechanical stress. Coating of the epithelia thus denies pathogenic bacteria the opportunity to adhere preventing an inflammatory response. This is the first line of defense of the intestine against pathogenic microbes. Indigenous bacteria also utilize the carbohydrate component of mucins as fuel, encouraging the growth of health-promoting bacteria (particularly anaerobes).

Colonization Resistance

Varying levels of bacteria throughout the GI tract have inherent benefit to the function of each portion of the GI tract. Thus, selective discouragement of colonization is necessary. For example, the low number of bacteria in the small bowel allows the function of nutrient breakdown and absorption. Intrinsically, the small bowel limits the levels of bacteria through antegrade peristalsis, and bactericidal action of the gastric acid and biliary enzymes of the liver. The ileocecal valve at the terminal end of the small bowel functions as a gate deterring the entrance of colonic bacteria into the small bowel. Presence of higher concentrations of colonic bacteria causes mucosal inflammation and villous atrophy ultimately interfering in its function.

Bacterial overgrowth syndrome is due to anatomical and physiologic alterations of the small bowel causing proliferation of bacteria in the upper GI tract. Conditions causing hypochlorhydria (decreased secretion of hydrochloric acid) such as gastritis, drug therapy, and dysmotility contribute to bacterial overgrowth. Surgical or anatomical malformations resulting in ineffective peristalsis or absence of the ileocecal valve also contribute to this syndrome. Impaired micelle formation causes fat malabsorption and steatorrhea. Higher levels of free bile acids in the proximal portion of the small bowel bind with vitamin B_{12} thus preventing absorption in the terminal end. Additionally, amino acid and carbohydrate malabsorption occurs leading to increased fecal nitrogen, lower serum proteins, and ultimately protein calorie malnutrition.

The Gut-Associated Lymphoid Tissue (GALT)

The complex function of the gut-associated lymphoid tissue (GALT) is the critical protective immune system in the GI tract. Peyer's patches are cells found in the mucosa and submucosa of the small intestine and contain CD4, CD8 T cells and B cells. M cells that overlay the epithelium transport antigens to the Peyer's patches that initiate the adaptive immune response. Production of secretory IgA occurs and other immune cells then enter systemically through the Peyer's patches and into the mesenteric lymph system. IgA cells prevent pathogens from adhering to the intestinal surface thus preventing gut cell damage.

Altering Gut Flora

The concept of manipulating microflora to enhance the positive aspects of the GI tract has become a more focused endeavor. However, this concept is not new. The early recognition of fermented foods offering health benefits dates back to the early 1900s. Eli Metchnikoff was the first to recognize this benefit when he observed the long lives and good health of Bulgarian peasants and associated this with the large amounts of milk soured with lactic acid bacteria (LAB) they consumed.

Since then much study of the health benefits from introduction of orally supplemented beneficial bacteria has taken place. This concept has been termed probiotics and is defined as the consumption of microbes that confer a positive effect on the host in prevention and treatment of specific pathologic conditions. Bifidobacteria, *Lactobacillus*, and *Streptococcus thermophilus* have been the most recognized and studied probiotics because of their ability to survive the upper GI tract and proliferate, although transiently, in the colon. The purported health benefits of these and other probiotics include

prevention and treatment of diarrhea (particularly rotaviral and antibiotic associated), improved lactose digestion, enhanced gut immune function, and, most recently, prevention and treatment of food allergy and its systemic effects (atopic dermatitis and possibly gastrointestinal allergic disease). Use of probiotics to beneficially alter flora composition and its effects will be elaborated on in a separate chapter.

The effects of probiotics on the host are transient and without regular consumption of these products the colon cannot maintain the level of beneficial colonization that connfers the health benefits. Therefore, a key to the probiotic effect and possible enhancement of native colonic flora would be a substrate for gut bacterial growth through fermentation. Certain dietary carbohydrates and fibers that escape digestion in the upper GI tract are ideal for this action. This recent concept involving such carbohydrates is termed prebiotics.

Prebiotics: Definition and Uses

Definition

A prebiotic is generally accepted as a nondigestible food ingredient that selectively stimulates the growth and/or activity of native bacteria in the colon to beneficially affect the host. This generally, but not always, implies:

- a 'natural' food component;
- ability to by-pass the upper GI tract (not digested);
- ability to be selectively fermented by 'beneficial,' nonpathogenic colonic bacteria;
- ability to modify the established microflora; and
- ability to confer an advantageous physiologic activity to the host.

Classifications

Various food components have been recognized to have prebiotic activity, including various fermentable carbohydrates (lactulose, gums, lactilol, soyoligosaccharides, galacto-oligosaccharides Xylo-oligosaccharides. However, the best studied of these have been those classified as dietary fructans. Dietary fructans can either be derived from naturally occurring oligosaccharides or can be artificially synthesized. These carbohydrates contain one or more fructosyl-fructose links that make up the majority of osidic bonds. They are linear or branched fructose (oligo)polymers with either β-2-1 linked inulins or β-2-6 linked levans. These oligosaccharides exist naturally in many plants including onions, garlic, the roots of Jerusalem artichoke, asparagus root, chicory root, and wheat (**Table 1**). Inulin is extractable from root plants particularly Jerusalem artichoke and chicory, while fructooligosaccharide is hydrolyzed from inulin yielding a shorter chain sugar. It is the degree of polymerization (DP) that distinguishes the fructans. Fructooligosaccharides are β-D-fructans with DP between 2 and 10 while inulin has DP 10–60. Essentially, they are sucrose molecules with 1–3 fructose units linked by a β-(2,1)-glycosidic bond. Most oligosaccharides are synthesized from sucrose and therefore usually have a terminal glucose end. Inulin, derived from chicory, is broken down using an inulase enzyme making a smaller (2–10) chain with lower DP (4). Oligofructose is a form synthesized from sucrose by β-fructofuranosidase linking fructose monomers to sucrose.

Both inulin-derived and synthesized fructooligosaccharides have been shown to resist digestion in the upper GI tract. Ninety per cent of consumed inulin and fructooligosaccharide was excreted at the terminal ileum of adult ileostomy patients. Furthermore, the undigested oligosaccharides are

Table 1 Fructo-oligosaccharide (FOS) content of common fruits, vegetables, and grains

Food type	FOS concentration (mg gm^{-1})
Fruits	
Apples	0.1
Banana	0.1
Banana, ripe	2.0
Blackberry	0.2
Orange, navel	0.3
Peach	0.4
Raspberry, red	0.2
Vegetables	
Acorn squash	0.4
Artichoke, globe	2.4
Artichoke, Jerusalem	58.4
Chicory root, raw	3.9
Garlic	3.9
Onion, red	1.4
Onion, white	3.1
Onion powder	45.0
Peas, snap	1.1
Peas, snow	0.6
Shallot	8.5
Grains	
Barley	1.7
Oats	0.3
Rye	3.8
Wheat	1.3
Wheat bran	3.5
Wheat germ	4.2

Adapted from Campbell J, Bauer L, Fahey G, Hogarth AJCL, Wolf B, and Hunter D (1997) *Journal of Agricultural and Food Chemistry* **45**: 3076–3082.

not recovered in the fecal mass indicating they are completely fermented in the colon. In many ways, prebiotics behave as a form of dietary fiber that has specific effects on colonic flora.

The mother's milk is a key factor in the early establishment of the infant's colonic environment. Up to 10% of the carbohydrates in human milk are not lactose, and human milk contains high concentrations of other carbohydrates and glycoconjugates that fall under the general category of prebiotic food substances. The monosaccharides of breast milk include D-glucose, D-glactose, sialic acid, L-fructose, and N-acetylglucosamine. Chain lengths range from three to ten with the majority having a lactose end. Combinations of these monosaccharides result in more than 130 varieties of oligosaccharides in human milk. These galacto-oligosaccharides in breast milk have lactose as their reducing end. Many human milk oligosaccharides elongate by enzymatic attachment of N-acetylglucosamine linked to a galactose residue. Several of these carbohydrates, including N-acetylglucosamine, are considered 'bifidus factors' or 'bifidogenic,' increasing the growth and establishment of bifidobacteria in the intestine of the breast fed infant. Human milk oligosaccharides also appear to prevent attachment of pathogenic microorganisms by competing with epithelial ligands for bacterial binding sites. Several types of human milk oligosaccharides appear to be bacteria specific. For example, sialyated oligosaccharides inhibit attachment of *Pneumococci* and influenza viruses, while galacto-oligosaccharides and fructosylated oligosaccharides can inhibit *E.coli* attachment. The bifidogenic effects, as well as those of direct interaction with the intestinal mucosa, are considered to be some of the mechanisms by which these agents confer a protective effect on the lactating infant.

Oligosaccharide content of the breast milk varies among individuals and within an individual. Levels are highest in the newborn period peaking after 5 days and slowly declining through the first 3 months. The levels of oligosaccharide in the breast milk also are dependent on time of feeding and generally are higher at the beginning of the feed.

Other, less well-studied oligosaccharides including maltose, soya, and xylose-oligosaccharides have some effect on increasing microbe colonization; however, they are weak prebiotics because of the lack of specificity of their fermentation.

Clinical Effects of Prebiotics

Average consumption of dietary fructans as part of a normal diet has been estimated to be 1–4 g day^{-1} in the US. Europeans tend to have a higher intake ranging from 3 to $10\,\mathrm{g\,day^{-1}}$. Many products worldwide are produced with supplemental oligosaccharides. Owing to the nondigestible nature of dietary fructans, the nutritional value in terms of calories and energy is negligible. The actual energy produced by these carbohydrates relates to the by-products of fermentation, specifically short-chain fatty acids (SCFA) and lactate.

Effect in the Upper GI Tract

From the dietary point of view, oligosaccharides meet the criteria to be considered a dietary fiber. Fibers are categorized as soluble, insoluble, or mixed. Definition of dietary fiber has focused on biochemical attributes and physiologic effects. Insoluble fibers (nonfermentable) decrease colonic transit time and increase fecal volume thus acting as a bulking agent.

Oligosaccharides because of their fermentable nature are considered a soluble fiber. Their effect on the upper GI tract is to slow down gastric and small bowel transit time, thereby altering glucose metabolism and increasing sensitivity to insulin. Altered fat metabolism by the binding of bile acids thus decreasing serum cholesterol and triglyceride levels has been reported with oligosaccharide supplementation in hypercholestrolemic patients.

There is a strong link between oligosaccharide consumption and the integrity of the GI mucosa. A trophic effect of the mucosa and hyperplasia of the epithelial cells occurs from a hormonal response to dietary fructans although the mechanism it not clear. Adequate or improved trophism of the intestinal wall may increase the absorption capacity for such minerals as calcium, magnesium, iron, copper, and zinc. Of particular interest is the effect of oligosaccharides on calcium absorption. Recent studies have demonstrated increased calcium absorption in teenage girls consuming a prebiotic mixture. Although there are not enough studies as yet to determine what compounds and at what doses connfer this health benefit, it is proposed that the short-chain fatty acids produced from fermentation lower fecal pH and increase colonic absorption of calcium.

Effects in the Colon

The main effect of inulin and fructooligosaccharide in the colon is directly related to fermentation. The process of fermentation from innate bacteria produces short-chain fatty acids and lactate. Increase in biomass contributes to the bulking effect that oligosaccharides have on stool. Additionally, fecal pH is decreased due to suppression of the production of putrefactive substances.

Carbon dioxide and hydrogen are produced in this process contributing to disagreeable side effects when given in high doses. Abdominal cramping, increased flatulence, and bloating have been shown to occur significantly more in studies where adults received $15\,\mathrm{g\,day^{-1}}$ or more of fructooligosaccharide and inulin as compared to a placebo group. However, in a limited number of controlled pediatric studies these symptoms were not seen at doses of up to $3\,\mathrm{g\,day^{-1}}$.

The greatest value of inulin and fructooligosaccharide is their role in stimulating the growth of innate microbes in the colon. Inulin and fructooligosaccharide selectively promote proliferation of bifidobacteria and *Bacteriodes*. In adult studies fructooligosaccharide and inulin given in doses of $10\,\mathrm{g\,day^{-1}}$ resulted in increased levels of bifidobacteria and decreased levels of enterobacteria and enterococci without GI side effects. In establishing a predominant microbial environment of bifidobacteria, epithelial adherence of pathogenic bacteria is deterred.

It is generally assumed that the immunologic effects seen with probiotic consumption (bifidobacteria, lactobacilli) would apply with the altered microbial balance with prebiotics. However, there is a lack of well-designed trials to support this. Limited animal studies of prebiotics have shown increased lymphocytes in the GALT and peripheral blood, although any impact on the host has not been addressed.

Conclusion

It is clear that the intestinal ecosystem of organisms in humans play a critical role in the development and health maintenance of the human intestine. The intestinal flora can be modified in a positive way via dietary means. Further studies should help define future dietary recommendations in support of improvement in gastrointestinal and immunologic function.

See also: **Biotin**. **Breast Feeding**. **Carbohydrates**: Requirements and Dietary Importance; Resistant Starch and Oligosaccharides. **Colon**: Structure and Function; Disorders. **Dietary Fiber**: Potential Role in Etiology of Disease. **Folic Acid**. **Lactose Intolerance**. **Microbiota of the Intestine**: Probiotics. **Thiamin**: Physiology. **Vitamin K**.

Further Reading

Campbell JM, Bauer LL, Fahey GC Jr, Hogarth AJCI, Wolf BW, and Hunter DE (1997) Selected fructooligosaccharide (1-kestose, nystose and 1 ^{F}-β-Fructofuranosylnystose) composition of foods and feeds. *Journal of Agricultural and Food Chemistry* **45**: 3076–3082.

Day A and Sherman PM (1998) Normal intestinal flora: pathobiology and clinical relevance. *International Seminars in Pediatric Gastroenterology and Nutrition* 7(3): 2–7.

Gibson GR (1999) Dietary modulation of the human gut microflora using the prebiotics oligofructose and inulin. *Journal of Nutrition* **129**: 1438S–1441S.

Goldin BR, Lichtenstein AH, and Gorbach SL (1994) Nutritional and metabolic roles of intestinal flora. In: Shills ME, Olson JA, and Shike M (eds.) *Modern Nutrition in Health and Disease*, 8th edn. Malvern, PA: Lea & Febiger.

Hentges D (ed.) (1983) *Human Intestinal Microflora in Health and Disease*. New York: Academic Press.

Kunz C, Rudloff S, Baier W, Klein N, and Strobel S (2000) Oligosaccharides in human milk: structural, functional, and metabolic aspects. *Annual Review of Nutrition* **20**: 699–722.

Mahida YR (ed.) (2001) *Immunological Aspects of Gastroenterology*. Dordrecht: Kluwer Academic Publishers.

Roberfroid MB (1997) Health benefits of non-digestible oligosaccharides. In Kritchevsky D and Bonfield (eds.) *Dietary Fiber in Health and Disease*. New York: Plenum Press.

Roberfroid MB and Delzenne NM (1998) Dietary fructans. *Annual Review of Nutrition* **18**: 117–143.

Simon GL and Gorbach SL (1984) Intestinal flora in health and disease. *Gastroenterology* **86**(1): 174–193.

Probiotics

M Gueimonde and S Salminen, University of Turku, Turku, Finland

Introduction

The human gastrointestinal (GI) tract harbors a complex collection of microorganisms. The individual digestive system contains about 1.5 kg of viable (live) bacteria, made up of more than 500 different identified microbial species. Indeed, the total number of bacteria in the gut amounts for more than 10 times that of eukaryotic cells in the human body, and this bacterial biomass can constitute up to 60% of fecal weight. This complex microbiological community is called the intestinal microflora. While most people are familiar with the side-effects of some members of it (e.g., diarrhea), the beneficial effects in stabilizing gut well-being and general health are less well known. These so-called 'friendly' bacteria are naturally present in the GI tract as part of the normal healthy intestinal microflora and ensure the balance that creates a healthy individual. Such beneficial microbes and a healthy intestinal microflora also constitute the main source of probiotics used to improve intestinal and host health.

Fermented products containing living microorganisms have been used for centuries to restore gut health. Such utilization of live microorganisms to improve host health forms the basis of the probiotic concept.

Usually probiotics are taken in the form of dairy products, drinks, or supplements, but in African countries they have traditionally also been ingested in fermented cereal and in fermented vegetables in Asian countries. The claimed benefits of traditional fermented foods range from treatment of diarrheal diseases to alleviation of the side-effects of antibiotics to the prevention of a number of other health problems. In some countries fermented foods have even been associated with benefits to the skin.

Definition of Probiotics

Probiotics have been defined as 'bacterial preparations that impart clinically verified beneficial effects on the health of the host when consumed orally.' According to this definition the safety and efficacy of probiotics must be scientifically demonstrated. However, as different probiotics may interact with the host in different manners, their properties and characteristics should be well defined. It is understood that probiotic strains, independent of genera and species, are unique and that the properties and human health effects of each strain must be assessed in a case-by-case manner. Most probiotics are currently either lactic acid bacteria or bifidobacteria, but new species and genera are being assessed for future use. The probiotic bacteria in current use have been isolated from the intestinal microflora of healthy human subjects of long-standing good health and thus most of them are also members of the healthy intestinal microflora.

It has been demonstrated that probiotics have specific properties and targets in the human intestinal tract and that they are able to modulate the intestinal microflora.

Intestinal Microflora

Composition of the Intestinal Microflora

The human GI tract hosts a rich and complex microflora that is specific for each person depending on environmental and genetic factors. Different bacterial groups and levels are found throughout the GI tract, as corresponds with the different ecological niches present from mouth to colon. The stomach and the upper bowel are sparsely populated regions (10^3–10^4 CFU per g contents) while the colon is heavily populated (10^{11}–10^{12} CFU g contents). In the small intestine genera such as *Lactobacillus* and *Bacteriodes* are usually found, whereas those considered predominant in the large bowel include *Bacteriodes*, *Bifidobacterium*, *Eubacterium*, *Clostridium*, *Fusobacterium*, and *Ruminococcus* among others. Several health-promoting properties have been attributed to defined members of the intestinal microflora such as lactobacilli and bifidobacteria. A balanced microflora provides a barrier against harmful food components and pathogenic bacteria and has a direct impact on the morphology of the gut. Hence, the intestinal microflora constitutes an important factor for the health and well-being of the human host and a healthy stable microflora affords a potential source of future probiotics.

Development and Succession of Microflora during Life-Time

The human fetus is sterile and the maternal vaginal microflora comprises the first inoculum of microbes. The indigenous intestinal microflora develops over time, determined by an interplay between genetic factors, mode of delivery, contact with the initial surrounding environment, diet, and disease. As a result, every individual has a unique characteristic microflora. The human intestinal microbiota does not exist as a defined entity; this population comprises a dynamic mixture of microbes in each individual.

The establishment of the gut microflora, a process commencing immediately upon birth, provides an early and massive source of microbial stimuli, and may consequently be a good candidate 'infection.' This step-wise succession begins with facultative anaerobes such as the enterobacteria, coliforms, and lactobacilli first colonizing the intestine, rapidly succeeded by bifidobacteria and lactic acid bacteria. The indigenous gut microflora plays an important role in the generation of an immunophysiological regulation of the gut, providing key signals for the development of the immune system in infancy and also interfering with and actively controlling the gut-associated immunological homeostasis later in life. A healthy microflora can thus be defined as the normal individual microflora of a child that both preserves and promotes well-being and absence of disease, especially in the GI tract, but also beyond it. It provides the first step in long-term well-being for later life and the basis for this development lies in early infancy. Failure in the establishment of a healthy microflora has been linked to the risk of infectious, inflammatory, and allergic diseases later in life. Demonstration of this has stimulated researchers to elucidate the composition and function of the intestinal microflora.

Microflora Research

In spite of the recent development of DNA based methods, microbiota development and characterization in the human host still rests largely on the culture-based assessment pioneered by Japanese researchers. The identification of different microbial species and strains has been dependent on microbial characterization, which is usually based on limited phenotypic properties and the metabolic activity of the microbes, for example, sugar fermentation profiles. There are several bacteria, however, that cannot be cultured and isolated or identified by the traditional methods. The culture technique as used in microbial assessments of feces is also hindered by the fact that microbes in the feces will mainly represent the microflora in the lumen of the sigmoid colon, while the composition of the intestinal microflora differs both along the GI tract and between the lumen and the mucosa. For more accurate information on the population elsewhere in the intestine, samples should be taken by endoscopy or during surgery. Most of our current data on microflora are derived from results obtained from fecal samples and culturing. These data indicate that there are several successive phases in microflora development related to age (**Figure 1**). In early infancy the microflora is scant and simple consisting mainly of bifidobacteria. During breast-feeding it remains so, but following weaning its complexity increases, reaching the state observed in adults where the microflora is specific to each person. Aging is related to further changes and the diversity is again decreased. The microflora becomes more unstable and vulnerable to diseases, for example, diarrheal diseases caused by intestinal pathogens.

Current research efforts focus on revealing genomic data on both probiotic microorganisms and certain important intestinal commensals. This has

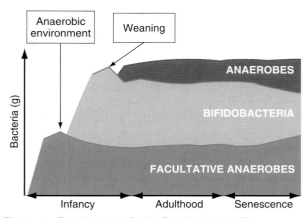

Figure 1 Development of microflora throughout life.

provided information indicating that gut commensals not only derive food and other benefits from the intestinal contents but also have a role in influencing the human host by providing maturational signals for the developing infant and child and providing later signals for alteration to gut barrier mechanisms.

The genomic data on, for instance, *Bifidobacterium longum* and *Bacteroides thetaiotaomicron*, both important members of the human intestinal microflora, give an indication as to how specific bacteria are adapted to the development of the gut by specific genes enabling the use of intestinal mucins and breast milk oligosaccharides as main sources or nutrients.

Genomic information on *B. longum* also gives insight into the adhesive mechanisms that comprise a basis both for populating the infant gut and for communicating developmental signals to specific areas and sites of the gut mucosa. Furthermore, a large part (>8.5%) of the *B. longum* genome is devoted to carbohydrate transport and metabolism, indicating a versatile metabolism well adapted to life in the intestine and making it very different from, for instance, *Lactobacillus johnsonii*.

Bacteroides thetaiotaomicron has also been shown to modulate glycosylation of the intestinal mucus and to induce expression of angiogenins, revealing proposed mechanisms whereby intestinal microbes may influence the gut microecology and shape the immune system. Incorporating such information with host gene expression data from the exposed mucosal sites and beyond them will enable us to understand the role of both microbial transfer and succession and microbe–microbe and host–microbe interactions. Recent information demonstrates that the vast community of indigenous microbes colonizing the human gut also shapes our development and biology.

Role of Microflora in Health and Disease

Major dysfunctions of the GI tract are thought to be related to disturbances or aberrationss of the intestinal microflora. Recent findings confirm that aberrations can be documented and related to disease risk. The microorganisms present in our GI tract thus have a significant influence on our health and well-being.

The development of the intestinal microbiota needs to be characterized to define the composition that helps us to remain healthy. Specific aberrations in the intestinal microflora may predispose to disease. Such aberrations have been identified in allergic disease, including decreased numbers of

bifidobacteria and an atypical composition of bifidobacterial microflora. Also, aberrations in *Clostridium* content and composition have been reported to be important. Similar predisposing factors may also exist in the case of microflora and both inflammatory gut diseases and rotavirus diarrhea. Microflora aberrations have also been reported in rheumatoid arthritis, juvenile chronic arthritis, ankylosing spondylitis, and irritable bowel syndrome patients. A thorough knowledge of the intestinal microflora composition will offer a basis for future probiotic development and the search for new strains for human use. Many diseases and their prevention can be linked to the microflora in the gut.

Modulation by Probiotics

In general, probiotic bacteria do not colonize the human intestinal tract permanently, but specific strains are able to transiently colonize or persist for some time in the intestine and may modulate the indigenous microflora. The rationale for modulating the gut microflora by means of probiotics derives from the demonstration that this microflora is important to the health of the host. Specific probiotics have been shown to colonize temporarily the human intestinal tract, thereby modulating the intestinal microflora both locally and at the commensal level. Such modification has not been reported to be permanent; rather it is related to a balancing of aberrant or disturbed microflora to assist it to return to normal metabolic and physiological activities. Such modulation and restoration of the normal state of the microflora activity is a key target for probiotic action. However, the state of the microflora should be well characterized to enable the selection of specific probiotics to counteract the aberration or disturbance in question.

Specific probiotic bacteria can modulate both the intestinal microflora and local and systemic immune responses. Activation of immunological cells and tissues requires close contact of the probiotic with the immune cells and tissue on the intestinal surface. Interestingly, both lactobacilli and bifidobacteria, which colonize mainly the small and large intestine respectively, when given as probiotic supplements were able to modify immunological reactions related to allergic inflammation, whereas lactobacilli were ineffective in protection against cows' milk allergy. In this respect, preferential binding of probiotics on the specific antigen-processing cells (macrophages, dendritic, and epithelial cells) may be even more important than the location of adhesion. It is also known that the cytokine stimulation profiles of different *Bifidobacterium* strains vary and that strains isolated from healthy infants stimulate mainly noninflammatory cytokines.

Results of an increasing number of clinical and experimental studies demonstrate the importance of constituents within the intestinal lumen, in particular the resident microflora, in regulating inflammatory responses. Probiotic bacteria may counteract inflammatory processes by stabilizing the disturbed gut microbial environment, forming a stable healthy microflora and thus improving the intestine's permeability barrier. Another mode of action comprises enhancing the degradation of enteral antigens and altering their immunogenicity. Yet another mechanism for the gut-stabilizing effect could be improvement of the intestine's immunological barrier, particularly intestinal IgA responses. Probiotic effects may also be mediated via control of the balance between pro- and anti-inflammatory cytokines. Such effects may be mediated through changes in the intestinal microflora, especially by modulation of the bifidobacteria microflora.

Importance of Understanding Intestinal Microflora

It is obvious that an understanding of the cross-talk that occurs between the intestinal microflora and its host promises to expand our conceptions of the relationship between the intestinal microflora and health. There is also an increasing amount of information indicating that specific aberrations in the intestinal microflora may render us more vulnerable to intestinal inflammatory diseases and other diseases beyond the intestinal environment. It is likely that some aberrations may even predispose us to specific diseases. Unfortunately, however, we are still far from knowing the qualitative and quantitative composition of the intestinal microflora and the factors governing its composition in an individual.

Probiotic Effects

Living microorganisms have long been used as supplements to restore gut health at times of dysfunction. It is clear that different strains from a given microbial group may possess different properties. It is thus important to establish which specific microbial strain may have a beneficial effect on the host; even closely related strains can have significantly different or even counteracting effects. Their properties and characteristics should thus be well defined; studies using closely related strains cannot be extrapolated to support each other.

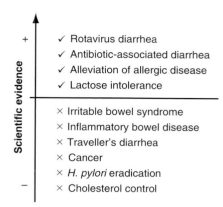

Figure 2 Health benefits of probiotics.

Working hypotheses can be supported by studies carried out *in vitro* using cell culture models or *in vivo* using animal models. However, the studies most important for efficacy assessment are carefully planned and monitored clinical studies in humans.

In summary, well-designed human studies are required to demonstrate health benefits. Using the criteria thus obtained it can be concluded that certain specific probiotics have scientifically proven benefits that can be attributed to specific products (see below). Other reported probiotic health-related effects are only partially established (**Figure 2**), and require more data from larger double-blind placebo controlled studies before firm conclusions can be reached.

Scientifically Documented Effects

Diarrhea The mechanisms by which probiotics prevent or ameliorate diarrhea may involve stimulation of the immune system, competition for binding sites on intestinal epithelial cells (**Figure 3**), or the elaboration of bacteriocins or binding of virus particles in the gut contents. These and other mechanisms are thought to be dependent on the

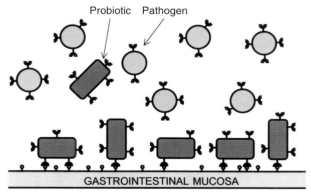

Figure 3 Probiotic adhesion and replacement of pathogenic bacteria.

type of diarrhea being investigated, and may therefore differ between viral diarrhea, antibiotic-associated diarrhea, or traveller's diarrhea.

Viral diarrhea Shortening of the duration of rotavirus diarrhea using *Lactobacillus* GG (LGG) is perhaps the best-documented probiotic effect. A reduction in the duration of diarrhea was first shown in several studies around the world and also in a recent multicenter European study on the use of LGG in acute diarrhea. Other investigators demonstrated that supplementation with a combination of *Bifidobacterium bifidum* and *Streptococcus thermophilus* reduces the incidence of diarrhea and shortens the duration of rotavirus shedding in chronically hospitalized children. On average, the duration of diarrhea was shortened by 1 day in both hospitalized children and those treated at home.

Other investigators have studied the immune modulating effects of probiotics as a means of reducing diarrhea, suggesting that the humoral immune system plays a significant role in the probiotics' effect.

From these numerous studies it is clear that probiotics do indeed play a therapeutic role in viral diarrhea. Even meta-analyses have been conducted in this area, showing that probiotic therapy shortens the duration of acute diarrhea in children. However, the exact mechanism of action involved is not clear and is very likely multifactorial.

Antibiotic-associated diarrhea The incidence of antibiotic-associated diarrhea is between 5 and 30%. The success of probiotics in reducing or preventing this form of diarrhea has been convincing, and includes a number of probiotics as well as various antibiotics.

LGG has been shown to prevent antibiotic-associated diarrhea when consumed in both yogurt form or as a freeze-dried product. Also, *Saccharomyces boulardii* has been found to be effective in preventing antibiotic-associated diarrhea. Other microorganisms such as *Enterococcus faecium* or a combination of *L. acidophilus* and *L. bulgaricus* have also been reported to be effective.

Alleviation of symptoms of allergic disease It has been shown that changes in intestinal microflora composition precede the development of some allergic diseases, indicating a potential area for probiotic application. LGG given prenatally to mothers and during the first months to infants with a high risk of atopic disease has reduced the prevalence of atopic eczema to about half in the infants receiving the strain. Furthermore, extensively hydrolyzed whey formula supplemented with LGG or *Bifidobacterium lactis* Bb12 is more effective than unsupplemented formula in eczema alleviation in infants with atopic eczema.

These results indicate a high potential for probiotic application in the treatment and reduction of risk of allergic diseases.

Lactose intolerance Several studies have shown that lactose-intolerant individuals suffer fewer symptoms if milk in the diet is replaced with fermented dairy products. The mechanisms of action of lactic acid bacteria and fermented dairy products include the following: lower lactose concentration in the fermented product due to lactose hydrolysis during fermentation; high lactase activity of bacterial preparations used in production; and increased active lactase enzyme entering the small intestine with the fermented product or within the viable bacteria.

The bacterial enzyme beta-galactosidase, which can be detected in the duodenum and terminal ileum after consumption of viable yogurt, is thought to be the major factor improving digestibility by the hydrolysis of lactose, mainly in the terminal ileum. Another factor suggested to influence lactose digestion is the slower gastric emptying of semisolid milk products such as yogurt.

In conclusion, there is good scientific evidence to demonstrate the alleviation of lactose intolerance symptoms by specific probiotic lactic acid bacteria. However, the strain-specific lactase activities may vary from nil to very high values. Thus, different products may have varying lactose contents and individual strains, when released into the duodenum, vary in their lactase activity.

Potential Effects Requiring Further Clinical Work

Intestinal microecology and cancer A number of studies have focused on the impact of probiotics on intestinal microecology and cancer. *Lactobacillus acidophilus*, *L. casei* Shirota strain, and LGG have been shown to have inhibitory effects on chemically induced tumors in animals. Some specific strains of probiotic bacteria are able to bind carcinogens and to downregulate some microbial carcinogenic enzymatic activities. This phenomenon may then reduce carcinogen production and exert a beneficial effect in the colon, the urinary tract, and the bladder.

The most interesting documentation is that concerning *L. casei* Shirota. There have been several mechanistic studies on the effects of the strain reporting decreased mutagen excretion, and some human clinical studies have been conducted using this strain. In clinical and multicenter studies carried out in Japan, prophylactic effects of oral administration of *L. casei* Shirota on the recurrence of superficial bladder cancer have been reported. Recently, a large Japanese case control study has been conducted on the habitual intake of lactic acid bacteria and risk reduction of bladder cancer. Results suggested that the habitual intake of fermented milk with the strain reduces the risk of bladder cancer in the Japanese population. More studies, and especially human studies in other countries, are needed prior to the establishment of firm conclusions.

Irritable bowel syndrome There is a rationale for investigating the effect of probiotics in the treatment of this common disorder where intestinal motility and dysfunctions in the intestinal microflora are important factors to consider. In a recent study using *L. plantarum* 299v, a reduction of symptoms was reported. *Enterococcus faecium* preparations have also been evaluated for the treatment of patients with irritable bowel syndrome, and although patient-recorded symptoms did not show significant differences, the physician's subjective clinical evaluation revealed an improvement.

Inflammatory bowel disease Inflammatory bowel disease (IBD) comprises a heterogeneous group of diseases of unknown etiology (Crohn's, ulcerative colitis, and pouchitis), but here also factors related to the intestinal microflora seem to be involved, providing a rationale for the application of probiotics. From reviewing studies on the use of probiotics in IBD it can be concluded that, although there are some promising preliminary findings, more well-planned long-term studies are needed before any firm conclusions can be drawn.

Traveller's diarrhea There are a few studies on the prevention of traveller's diarrhea using probiotics and these show a positive outcome for LGG and a combination of *L. acidophilus* LA5 with *B. lactis* Bb-12. The results offer some indication of beneficial effects, even though some studies yielded no reported effects, but information from good and extensive human studies using defined strains for traveller's diarrhea is still largely lacking. The current data on traveller's diarrhea show no scientifically proven effects for any of the strains used. More studies are required for efficacy assessment.

Helicobacter pylori eradication Specific strains of lactic acid bacteria have been reported to inhibit a wide range of intestinal pathogens including *Helicobacter pylori*, which is involved in the process

of gastric ulcer development. Lactic acid bacteria are often able to survive acidic gastric conditions and it has therefore been proposed that they may have a beneficial influence during the eradication of *H. pylori*. It has been reported that both the inhibitory substances produced and the specific strains may influence the survival of *Helicobacter*, and studies have been conducted, particularly with a *L. johnsonii* strain. It has been shown that there is good *in vitro* inhibition and that fermented milk containing the strain has a positive effect when consumed during *Helicobacter* eradication therapy. However, more controlled human studies in different populations need be conducted to verify this effect.

Cholesterol control The cholesterol-lowering effects of probiotics have been the subject of two recent reviews with contradictory results. The first, which focused on short-term intervention studies with one yogurt type, reported a 4% decrease in total cholesterol and a 5% decrease in LDL. Contrary to this, the second review concluded that no proven effects could be found. In this context, it is clear that long-term studies are required before the establishment of any conclusion.

Safety

Safety assessment is an essential phase in the development of any new food. Although few probiotic strains or prebiotic compounds have been specifically tested for safety, the long history of safe consumption of some probiotic strains could be considered the best proof of their safety. Although some lactobacilli and bifidobacteria have been associated with rare cases of bacteremia, usually in patients with severe underlying diseases, the safety of members of these genera is generally recognized due to their long history of safe use and their lack of toxicity. Furthermore, the low incidence of infections attributable to these microorganisms, together with a recent study showing that there is no increase in the incidence of bacteremia due to lactobacilli in Finland despite the increased consumption of probiotic lactobacilli, supports this hypothesis. With regard to other bacteria such as enterococci, *S. boulardii*, *Clostridium butyricum*, or some members of the genus *Bacillus* the situation is more complicated, even though they have been used as probiotics for some time.

In addition to the possibility of infection there are other risks that must be taken into account (**Table 1**). These include those risks associated with the metabolic properties of the strain (capacity for deconjugation/dehydroxylation of bile salts,

Table 1 Probiotic action: potential benefits and risks

Action mechanisms	Potential risks
Improvement of gut barrier (immunologic, nonimmunologic)	Proinflammatory effects
Modulation of aberrant gut microbiota	Adverse effects on innate immunity
Modulation of inflammatory response	Infection
Degradation of antigens	Production of harmful substances
Binding/inhibition of carcinogens	Antibiotic resistance (Specific risks related to host, strain characteristics, or interactions)

production of enzymes favoring the invasion/translocation through the epithelium, etc.), with the presence of active substances in the probiotic or product (immunoactive substances, toxic compounds, etc.), or with antibiotic resistance. It is clear that strains harboring transferable antibiotic resistance genes should not be used. In this context the specific risks related to each probiotic strain must be carefully identified.

Guidelines are needed to test the safety of probiotics. However, taking into account the great diversity of probiotic microorganisms, it is necessary to identify the specific risks associated with the respective strains, as well as the risk factors associated with the host and the possible interactions between probiotic–host–food components in order to assess the safety of these products. Additional epidemiological surveillance and follow-up of novel strains should be conducted. In this context, the specific risks related to each probiotic strain must be carefully identified. With regard to this, knowledge of mechanisms involved is a key factor not only for the assessment of health effects but also for the safety aspects of probiotics.

Future Challenges

Some of the claimed beneficial effects of probiotics are backed by good clinical studies. However, other possible effects call for further investigation in new, well-planned, long-term human clinical studies prior to any firm conclusions being made. Protocols for human studies need to be developed for probiotics. In some cases, even postmarketing surveillance studies on intakes and long-term effects are useful; such studies have in fact already been used for the safety assessment of current probiotics.

The assessment of potential probiotic strains must be based on a valid scientific hypothesis with realistic studies supporting it. In this respect, knowledge of mechanisms of action is a key factor for hypothesis formulation and for the selection of biomarkers appropriate to the specific state of health and well-being or reduction of risk of disease. It is thus important to improve our knowledge of the mechanisms involved and take into account the fact that probiotic mechanisms of action are multifactorial and that each probiotic may have specific functions affecting the host.

It is also of key interest to increase our knowledge of intestinal microflora composition and to understand its role in health and disease, identifying those microorganisms related to the health status of the host, in order to select probiotic strains able to modulate the intestinal microflora in a beneficial manner.

Knowledge accrued regarding the intestinal microflora, nutrition, immunity, mechanisms of action and specific diseases should be carefully combined with genomic data to allow the development of a second generation of probiotics; strains for both site- and disease-specific action.

See also: **Breast Feeding**. **Cancer**: Epidemiology of Gastrointestinal Cancers Other Than Colorectal Cancers. **Cholesterol**: Sources, Absorption, Function and Metabolism. **Colon**: Disorders. **Diarrheal Diseases**. **Food Allergies**: Etiology; Diagnosis and Management. **Lactose Intolerance**. **Microbiota of the Intestine**: Prebiotics.

Further Reading

Benno Y and Mitsuoka T (1986) Development of intestinal microflora in humans and animals. *Bifidobacteria Microflora* 5: 13–25.

Dai D and Walker WA (1999) Protective nutrients and bacterial colonization in the immature human gut. *Advances in Pediatrics* 46: 353–382.

De Roos N and Katan M (2000) Effects of probiotic bacteria on diarrhea, lipid metabolism, and carcinogenesis: a review of papers published between 1988 and 1998. *American Journal of Clinical Nutrition* 71: 405–411.

Falk PG, Hooper LV, Midvedt T, and Gordon JI (1998) Creating and maintaining the gastrointestinal ecosystem: What we know and need to know from gnotobiology. *Microbiology and Molecular Biology Reviews* 62: 1157–1170.

Guandalini S, Pensabene L, Zikri M, Dias J, Casali L, Hoekstra H, Kolacek S, Massar K, Micetic-Turk D *et al.* (2000) *Lactobacillus* GG administered in an oral rehydration solution to children with acute diarrhea: a multicenter European trial. *Journal of Pediatric Gastroenterology and Nutrition* 30: 54–60.

Guarner F and Malagelada JR (2003) Gut flora in health and disease. *Lancet* 381: 512–519.

Gueimonde M, Ouwehand AC, and Salminen S (2004) Safety of probiotics. *Scandinavian Journal of Nutrition* 48: 42–48.

He F, Morita H, Hashimoto H, Hosoda M, Kurisaki J, Ouwehand AC, Isolauri E, Benno Y, and Salminen S (2002) Intestinal Bifidobacterium species induce varying cytokine production. *Journal of Allergy and Clinical Immunology* 109: 1035–1036.

Isolauri E, Kirjavainen PV, and Salminen S (2002) Probiotics: a role in the treatment of intestinal infection and inflammation? *Gut* 50(Suppl. 3): iii54–iii59.

Isolauri E, Salminen S, and Ouwehand AC (2004) Probiotics. *Best Practice and Research Clinical Gastroenterology* 18: 299–313.

Jonkers D and Stockbrügger R (2003) Probiotics and inflammatory bowel disease. *Journal of the Royal Society of Medicine* 96: 167–171.

Kalliomäki M, Kirjavainen P, Eerola E, Kero P, Salminen S, and Isolauri E (2001) Distinct patterns of neonatal gut microflora in infants developing or not developing atopy. *Journal of Allergy and Clinical Immunology* 107: 129–134.

Kalliomäki M, Salminen S, Arvilommi H, Kero P, Koskinen P, and Isolauri E (2001) Probiotics in the prevention of atopic diseases: a randomised placebo-controlled trial. *Lancet* 357: 1076–1079.

Ohashi Y, Nakai S, Tsukamoto T, Masumori N, Akaza H, Miyanaga N *et al.* (2002) Habitual intake of lactic acid bacteria and risk reduction of bladder cancer. *Urology International* 68: 273–280.

Pridmore RD, Berger B, Desiere F, Vilanova D, Barretto C, Pittet A-C, Zwahlen M-C, Rouvet M, Altermann E, Barrangou R, Mollet B, Mercenier A, Klaenhammer T, Arigoni F, and Schell MA (2004) The genome sequence of the probiotic intestinal bacterium Lactobacillus johnsonii NCC 533. *Proceedings of the National Academy of Sciences of the United States of America* 101: 2512–2517.

Salminen S, Bouley MC, Boutron-Rualt MC, Cummings J, Franck A, Gibson G, Isolauri E, Moreau M-C, Roberfroid M, and Rowland I (1998) Functional food science and gastrointestinal physiology and function. *British Journal of Nutrition* Suppl 1: 147–171.

Salminen SJ, von Wright AJ, Ouwehand AC, and Holzapfel WH (2001) Safety assessment of probiotics and starters. In: Adams MR and Nout MJR (eds.) *Fermentation and Food Safety*, 1st edn, pp. 239–251. Gaithersburg: Aspen Publishers, Inc.

Schell MA, Karmirantzou M, Snel B, Vilanova D, Berger B, Pessi G, Zwahlen M-C, Desiere F, Bork P *et al.* (2002) The genome sequence of *Bifidobacterium longum* reflects its adaptation to the human gastrointestinal tract. *Proceedings of the National Academy of Sciences of the United States of America* 99: 14422–14427.

Schiffrin EJ, Brassart D, Servin AL, Rochat F, and Donnet-Hughes A (1997) Immune modulation of blood leukocytes in humans by lactic acid bacteria: criteria for strain selection. *American Journal of Clinical Nutrition* 66: 515S–520S.

Shanahan F (2002) Crohn's disease. *Lancet* 359: 62–69.

Sudo N, Sawamura S, Tanaka K, Aiba Y, Kubo C, and Koga Y (1997) The requirement of intestinal bacterial flora for the development of an IgE production system fully susceptible to oral tolerance induction. *Journal of Immunology* 159: 1739–1745.

Tannock GW (2003) Probiotics: time for a dose of realism. *Current Issues in Intestinal Microbiology* 4: 33–42.

Van Niel CW, Fewudtner C, Garrison MM, and Christakis DA (2002) Lactobacillus therapy for acute infectious diarrhea in children: a meta-analysis. *Pediatrics* 109: 678–684.

Vaughan E, de Vries M, Zoentendal E, Ben-Amor K, Akkermans A, and de Vos W (2002) The intestinal LABs. *Antonie Van Leeuwenhoek* 82: 341–352.

Xu J, Chiang HC, Bjursell MK, and Gordon JI (2004) Message from a human gut symbiont: sensitivity is a prerequisite for sharing. *Trends in Microbiology* 12: 21–28.

Milk *see* **Dairy Products**

Minerals *see* **Calcium. Magnesium. Phosphorus. Potassium. Sodium**: Physiology

---

Molybdenum *see* **Ultratrace Elements**

Monosaturated Fat *see* **Fatty Acids**: Monounsaturated

Mycotoxins *see* **Food Safety**: Mycotoxins

N

NIACIN

C J Bates, MRC Human Nutrition Research, Cambridge, UK

This article is reproduced from the previous edition, pp. 1290–1297, © 1999, Elsevier Ltd.

Absorption, Transport, and Storage

Niacin is a B vitamin that is essential for health in humans and also in most other mammals that have been investigated. Niacin is associated with a characteristic deficiency disease in humans known as pellagra. Pellagra has been described and identified in various communities, notably in Spain and North America, in the last century and the early years of this century. It has persisted in Yugoslavia, Egypt, Mexico, and some African countries. Pellagra is characteristically associated with maize-based diets. The skin lesions found in pellagra are most severe during the summer months because of the effects of the exacerbating sun exposure. However, some countries with a maize diet (e.g., Guatemala) avoid pellagra by means of the niacin present in roasted coffee (**Table 1**). Others avoid it by lime treatment, e.g., in the preparation of tortillas.

Preformed niacin occurs in foods either as nicotinamide (niacinamide) or as the pyridine nucleotide coenzymes derived from it, or as nicotinic acid, without the amide nitrogen, which is the form known as 'niacin' in North America. Both nicotinamide and nicotinic acid are equally effective as the vitamin, but in large doses they exert markedly different pharmacological effects, so it is important, at least in that context, to make and maintain the distinction. In addition to the preformed vitamin, an important *in vivo* precursor is the amino acid L-tryptophan, obtained from dietary protein. Because the human total niacin supply, and hence niacin status, depends on the dietary tryptophan supply as well as on the amount of preformed dietary niacin and its bioavailability, it has become the accepted practice to express niacin intakes as 'niacin equivalents,' which is a combination of mg preformed dietary niacin and mg niacin which can become available by conversion from tryptophan within the body. As discussed later, this calculation involves several assumptions, and is therefore only an approximation to the actual supply to the body for any particular individual; however, it is considered adequate for most practical purposes.

It appears likely that the most important ultimate sources of preformed niacin in most foods, particularly those of animal foods, are the pyridine nucleotides: $NAD(H_2)$ and $NADP(H_2)$. Hydrolases and pyrophosphatases present in biological tissues convert these coenzymes to partly degraded products, which are then available as sources of the vitamin. NAD glycohydrolase and pyrophosphatase enzymes are present in the gut mucosa to assist hydrolysis and absorption of the hydrolyzed products, and these are likely to include both nicotinamide and nicotinamide ribonucleotide, the latter being further degraded to the riboside. Absorption of nicotinamide or nicotinic acid by the mammalian intestine has been shown to consist of a saturable transport component, dominant at low intakes, which is dependent on sodium, energy and pH, and a nonsaturable component, which becomes dominant at high doses or intake levels. Absorption is efficient even at such high discrete doses as 3 g or more: as much as 85% of such a dose is subsequently excreted into the urine. Absorption of test niacin doses introduced directly into the human upper ileum is rapid, with peak levels appearing in blood plasma within 5–10 min.

Transport of niacin between the liver and the intestine can occur *in vivo*, as indicated by radioactive probes in animals, and the liver appears to be a major site of conversion of niacin to its ultimate functional products: the nicotinamide nucleotide coenzymes. Nicotinamide can pass readily between the cerebrospinal fluid and the plasma, thus ensuring a supply also to the brain and spinal cord. Liver contains greater niacin coenzyme concentrations than most other tissues, but all metabolically active tissues contain these essential

Table 1 Niacin equivalents in selected foods[a]

	Niacin equivalents from preformed niacin[b] (mg per 100 g, wet)	Niacin equivalents from tryptophan[c] (mg per 100 g, wet)	Total niacin equivalents (mg per 100 g, wet)
Milk	0.1	0.8	0.9
Raw beef	5.0	4.7	9.7
Raw white fish	2.4	3.4	5.8
Raw eggs	0.1	3.7	3.8
Raw potatoes	0.6	0.5	1.1
Raw peas	2.5	1.1	3.6
Raw peanuts	13.8	5.5	19.3
White bread	0.8	1.7	2.5
Polished rice	0.2	1.5	1.7
Maize	0.1	0.9	1.0
Cornflakes (fortified)	16.0	0.9	16.9
Coffee[d]	24.1	2.9	27.0

[a]Data adapted from: Paul AA (1969) The calculation of nicotinic acid equivalents and retinol equivalents in the British diet. *Nutrition* (*London*) **23**: 131–136,[a] and supplements to *McCance and Widdowson's The Composition of Foods* (Holland B, Welch AA, Unwin ID, Buss DH, Paul AA, and Southgate DAT (1991), The Royal Society of Chemistry and MAFF),[a] and from Bressani R *et al.* (1961) Effect of processing method and variety on niacin and ether extract content of green and roasted coffee. *Food Technology* **15**: 306–308.
[b]Amount available for absorption. In the case of bread, rice, and maize, the total amounts present are 1.7, 1.5, and 1.2 mg per 100 g, but apart from the niacin added in the fortification of white flour, 90% of this is unavailable for utilization by humans.
[c]Assuming that 60 mg tryptophan yields 1 mg niacin equivalent.
[d]Niacin is released from trigonelline in coffee beans by the roasting process.

metabolic components. Both facilitated diffusion (which is sodium- and energy-dependent and saturable), and passive diffusion (which is nonsaturable) contribute to tissue uptake from the bloodstream. With the exception of muscle, brain and testis, within the body nicotinic acid is a better precursor of the coenzyme form than is nicotinamide. The liver appears to be the most important site of conversion of tryptophan to the nicotinamide coenzymes.

Of the two pyridine nucleotide coenzymes, NAD is present mainly as the oxidized form in the tissues, whereas NADP is principally present in the reduced form, $NADPH_2$. There are important homeostatic regulation mechanisms which ensure and maintain an appropriate ratio of these coenzymes in their respective oxidized or reduced forms in healthy tissues. Once converted to coenzymes within the cells, the niacin therein is effectively trapped, and can only diffuse out again after degradation to smaller molecules. This implies, of course, that the synthesis of the essential coenzyme nucleotides must occur within each tissue and cell type, each of which must possess the enzymatic apparatus for their synthesis from the precursor niacin. Loss of nicotinamide and nicotinic acid into the urine is minimized (except when the intake exceeds requirements) by means of an efficient reabsorption from the glomerular filtrate.

Metabolism and Excretion

The conversion of tryptophan to nicotinic acid *in vivo* is depicted in **Figure 1**. The rate of conversion of tryptophan to niacin and the pyridine nucleotides is controlled by the activities of tryptophan dioxygenase (known alternatively as tryptophan pyrrolase), kynurenine hydroxylase, and kynureninase. These enzymes are, in turn, dependent on factors such as other B vitamins, glucagon, glucocorticoid hormones, and estrogen metabolites, and there are various competing pathways which also affect the rate of conversion. For these reasons, a variety of nutrient deficiencies, toxins, genetic and metabolic abnormalities, etc. can influence niacin status and requirements.

For practical purposes, on the basis of studies performed in the 1950s, 60 mg tryptophan is deemed to give rise to 1 mg nicotinic acid; hence 60 mg tryptophan contributes 1 mg niacin equivalent, for dietary intake calculations and food tables (see **Table 1**).

The two pyridine nucleotide coenzymes, formerly known as 'coenzymes I and II,' then for a period as 'DPN and TPN,' and known nowadays as 'NAD' and 'NADP' (nicotinamide adenine dinucleotide and nicotinamide adenine dinucleotide phosphate), are involved in hundreds of enzyme-catalyzed redox reactions *in vivo*. Although a minority of these

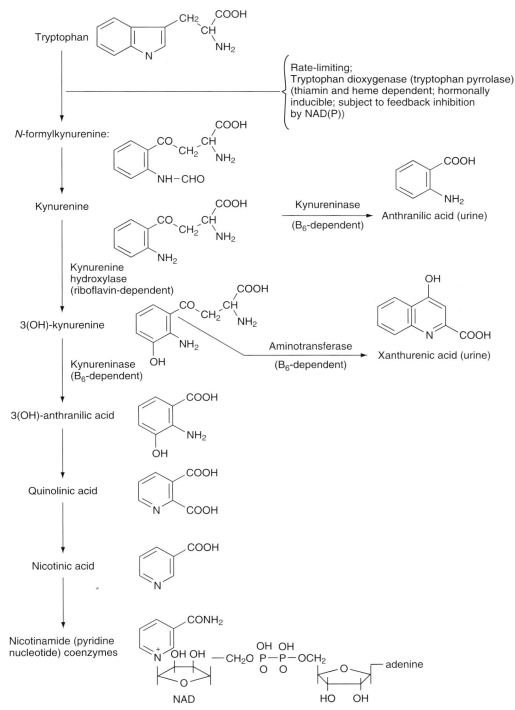

Figure 1 *In vivo* conversion of tryptophan to nicotinic acid and NAD.

diverse reactions can use either of the two niacin-derived cofactors, most are highly specific for one or the other.

Catabolism of the pyridine nucleotide coenzymes *in vivo* is achieved by four classes of enzymes: NAD glycohydrolase, ADP ribosyl transferase, and poly (ADP ribose) synthetase, (all of which liberate nicotinamide), and NAD pyrophosphatase (which liberates nicotinamide mononucleotide which is then further hydrolyzed to nicotinamide). Turnover of nicotinamide then results in the formation of 1-methylnicotinamide (usually described as

N^1-methyl nicotinamide or NMN), an excretory product which is excreted in the kidney and appears in the urine, together with some further oxidation products, typically the 1-methyl-2-pyridone-5-carboxamide and 1-methyl-4-pyridone-3-carboxamide (usually referred to as '2-pyridone' and '4-pyridone', respectively). These excretory turnover products can be used as indicators of whole body niacin status (see below). At high intakes of niacin, as much as 85% of the intake may be excreted unchanged; however the excretion of nicotinamide always predominates over that of nicotinic acid.

Hydrolysis of hepatic NAD to yield nicotinamide allows the release of niacin for utilization by other tissues. Relative protection of the pyridine nucleotide within certain key enzymes such as glyceraldehyde 3-phosphate dehydrogenase confers a protection on certain key metabolic pathways, thus ensuring good homeostatic control. By contrast, there is evidence that the enzymes which catalyze pyridine nucleotide turnover may be hyperactivated within cells that have been damaged by carcinogens, including mycotoxins, thus starving these damaged cells of essential cofactors and causing their death, presumably to protect the rest of the organism. This effect may help to explain the otherwise puzzling observation that moldy grain in the diet can increase the risk of pellagra when niacin and tryptophan intakes are marginal. In normal, healthy cells, the compartmentalization of hydrolytic enzymes prevents unwanted coenzyme turnover, and this compartmentalization seems to become breached in damaged or dying cells.

Other urinary excretion products of niacin include nicotinuric acid (nicotinoyl glycine); nicotinamide N-oxide, and trigonelline (N^1-methyl nicotinic acid); the latter may arise from bacterial action in the gut or from the absorption of this substance from foods. The pattern of the different turnover metabolites varies between species, between diets (depending partly on the ratio of nicotinamide to nicotinic acid in the diet), and partly with niacin status; thus there are complex regulatory mechanisms to be considered.

Metabolic Function and Essentiality

The best-known functions of niacin are derived from the functions of its coenzymes: NAD and NADP in the hydrogen/electron transfer redox reactions in living cells. Like most B vitamins, niacin is not extensively stored in forms or in depots that are usually metabolically inactive, but rather those that can become available during dietary deficiency. However, some 'storage' of the coenzymes NAD and NADP in the liver is thought to occur. An inadequate dietary intake leads rapidly to significant tissue depletion within 1–2 months, and then successively to biochemical abnormalities, followed by clinical signs of deficiency, and eventually to death. As with the other B vitamins, rates of turnover and hence the rates of excretion of coenzyme breakdown products decline progressively as dietary deficiency becomes more severe and prolonged, so that the tissue levels are relatively protected and spared. In adult humans a severe deficiency may take many months to develop before it results in the clinical signs of pellagra.

Some of the most important and characteristic functions of NAD manifest in the principal cellular catabolic pathways, responsible for liberation of energy during the oxidation of energy-producing fuels. NADP, however, functions mainly in the reductive reactions of lipid biosynthesis, and the reduced form of this coenzyme is generated via the pentose phosphate cycle. NAD is essential for the synthesis and repair of DNA. NAD has, in addition, a role in supplying ADP ribose moieties to lysine, arginine, and asparagine residues in proteins such as histones, DNA lyase II, and DNA-dependent RNA polymerase, and to polypeptides such as the bacterial diphtheria and cholera toxins. In the nucleus, poly (ADP ribose) synthetase is activated by binding to DNA breakage points and is involved in DNA repair. It is also concerned with condensation and expansion of chromatin during the cell cycle and in DNA replication. Niacin status affects the level of ADP ribolysation of proteins. A high level of poly (ADP ribose) synthetase activity, which is found in some tumors, can result in low levels of NAD. A chromium dinicotinate complex found in yeast extracts may function as a glucose tolerance factor or in detoxification, but this has not yet been proven.

Because the electron transport functions of NAD frequently involve flavin coenzymes, and because both flavin coenzymes and vitamin B_6 coenzymes are involved in the conversion of tryptophan to niacin *in vivo*, there are important metabolic interactions between these B vitamins. A similarity of clinical deficiency signs, making it difficult to distinguish between them, may be encountered in population studies of deficiency.

Because the body's need for niacin can be met completely by dietary tryptophan, it is not, strictly speaking, an essential vitamin. In this respect it resembles carnitine, which can be synthesized entirely from lysine, but for which in some circumstances a dietary requirement exists. Traditionally, however, niacin is classified as an essential vitamin, because some human diets have tended to be lacking in niacin and its precursor, tryptophan. Some animals such as sheep and cattle appear to be able to synthesize sufficient niacin for their needs from tryptophan, and do not therefore need preformed niacin in their diets.

Assessment of Niacin Status

Whereas the measurement of B vitamin status has, in recent years, tended to focus on blood analysis, perhaps mainly because of the convenience of sample collection, the development of blood-based status analysis for niacin has lagged behind that of the other components of the B complex. Some studies have indeed suggested that the erythrocyte concentration of the niacin-derived coenzyme NAD may provide useful information about the niacin status of human subjects; that a reduction in the ratio of NAD to NADP to below 1.0 in red cells may provide evidence of niacin deficiency; and that a decline in plasma tryptophan levels may indicate a more severe deficiency than a decline in red cell NAD levels. These claims now need to be tested in naturally deficient human populations. The niacin coenzymes can be quantitated either by enzyme-linked reactions or by making use of their natural fluorescence in alkaline solution.

At present, niacin status is most commonly assessed by the assay of some of the breakdown products of niacin coenzymes in the urine. Of these, N^1-methyl nicotinamide (NMN) is the easiest to measure, because of a convenient conversion *in vitro* to a fluorescent product, which can then be quantitated without the need for separation. However, more definitive and reliable information can be obtained by the measurement of urinary NMN in conjunction with one or more of the urinary pyridone turnover products (N^1-methyl-2-pyridone-5-carboxamide and N^1-methyl-4-pyridone-3-carboxamide), which can be detected and quantitated by UV absorption following high-pressure liquid chromatography. The Interdepartmental Committee on Nutrition for National Defense (USA) selected the criterion of niacin deficiency in humans as an NMN excretion rate of $<5.8\,\mu mol$ (0.8 mg) NMN per day in 24 h urine samples.

Requirements and Signs of Deficiency

As for most other micronutrients, the requirement of niacin to prevent or reverse the clinical deficiency signs is not known very precisely, and probably depends on ancillary dietary deficiencies or other insults occurring in natural human populations. For the purpose of estimating niacin requirements

for dietary reference values, the criterion of restoration of urinary excretion of NMN during controlled human depletion–repletion studies has been selected, and on this basis, the average adult requirement has been estimated as 5.5 mg (45 μmol) of niacin equivalents per 1000 kcal (4200 kJ). Adding a 20% allowance for individual variation this needs to be increased to 6.6 mg (54 μmol) per 1000 kcal, (4200 kJ), which is the current reference nutrient intake (UK). Niacin requirements were, by convention, expressed as a ratio to energy expenditure. For subjects with very low energy intakes, the daily intake of niacin equivalents should not fall below 13 mg, however. If dietary protein levels and quality are high, it is possible for tryptophan alone to provide the daily requirement for niacin equivalents. Dietary niacin deficiency is now rare in most Western countries.

The appearance of severe niacin deficiency as endemic pellagra, especially in North America in the nineteenth and early twentieth centuries, has been ascribed to the very poor availability of bound forms of niacin (in niacytin, a polysaccharide/glycopeptide/polypeptide-bound form, which is 90% indigestible), together with the relatively low content of tryptophan occurring in grains (see **Table 1**). However, the lack of available niacin and tryptophan may not have been the whole story, since coexisting deficiencies or imbalances of other nutrients, including riboflavin, may also have contributed to this endemic disease. It appears also that the choice of cooking methods may have been critical, since the Mexican custom of cooking maize with lime in the preparation of tortillas helps to release the bound niacin from its carbohydrate complex and to increase the bioavailability of tryptophan-containing proteins, and thus to reduce the prevalence of clinical deficiency disease. In parts of India, pellagra has been encountered in communities whose main staple is a form of millet known as 'jowar', which is rich in leucine. It was proposed, and evidence was obtained from animal and *in vitro* studies, that high intakes of leucine can increase the requirements for niacin. However, other evidence is conflicting (this interaction is not fully understood). In parts of South Africa, iron overload has been reported to complicate the metabolic effects of low niacin intakes.

The average content of niacin in human breast milk is 8 mg (65.6 μmol) per 1000 kcal (4200 kJ), and this is the basis for the recommendations (and dietary reference values) for infants up to 6 months. In the UK, the Reference Nutrient Intake niacin increment during pregnancy is nil, and during lactation it is 2 mg per day.

The most characteristic clinical signs of severe niacin deficiency in humans are dermatosis (hyperpigmentation, hyperkeratosis, desquamation – especially where exposed to the sun), anorexia, achlorhydria, diarrhea, angular stomatitis, cheilosis, magenta tongue, anemia, and neuropathy (headache, dizziness, tremor, neurosis, apathy). In addition to the pellagra caused by dietary deficiency or imbalance, there are also reports of disturbed niacin metabolism associated with phenylketonuria, acute intermittent porphyria, diabetes mellitus, some types of cancer (carcinoid syndrome), thyrotoxicosis, fever, stress, tissue repair, renal disease, iron overload, etc. The picture in other species is not radically different; however, deficient dogs and cats typically exhibit 'black tongue' (pustules in the mouth, excessive salivation) and bloody diarrhea, pigs exhibit neurological lesions affecting the ganglion cells, rats exhibit damage to the peripheral nerves (cells and axons), and fowl exhibit inflammation of the upper gastrointestinal tract, dermatitis, diarrhea, and damage to the feathers. All species exhibit reduction of appetite and loss of weight; however, it is of interest that the skin lesions seen in humans are rare in most other species.

Dietary Sources, High Intakes, and Antimetabolites

As can be seen from **Table 1**, different types of foods differ considerably, not only in their total contribution to nicotinic acid equivalents, but also in the ratio of the contribution from preformed niacin and from tryptophan. In a typical Western diet, it has been calculated that if the 60 mg tryptophan = 1 mg niacin formula is applied, then preformed niacin provides about 50% of the niacin supply in the diet. In practice it seems possible for all of the niacin requirement to be provided by dietary tryptophan in Western diets. As is the case for the other B vitamins, meat, poultry, and fish are excellent sources of niacin equivalents, followed by dairy and grain products, but as noted above, certain grains such as maize, and whole highly polished rice, can be very poor sources and may be associated with clinical deficiency if the diets are otherwise poor and monotonous.

In recent years, both nicotinamide and nicotinic acid have been proposed and tested for possibly useful pharmacological properties at high intake levels. This new phase of interest in the vitamin has, in turn, raised concerns about the possible side effects of high intakes, and the definition of maximum safe intakes.

The greatest interest, in pharmacological terms, has been centered around nicotinic acid, which has been shown to have marked antihyperlipidemic properties at daily doses of 2–6 g. Nicotinamide does not share this particular pharmacological activity. Large doses of nicotinic acid reduce the mobilization of fatty acids from adipose tissue by inhibiting the breakdown of triacylglycerols through lipolysis. They also inhibit hepatic triacylglycerol synthesis, thus limiting the assembly and secretion of very low-density lipoproteins from the liver and reducing serum cholesterol levels. Large doses of nicotinic acid ameliorate certain risk factors for cardiovascular disease: for instance they increase circulating high-density lipoprotein levels. The ratio of HDL_2 to HDL_3 is increased by nicotinic acid; there is a reduced rate of synthesis of apolipoprotein A-II and a transfer of some apolipoprotein A-I from HDL_3 to HDL_2. These changes are all considered potentially beneficial in reducing the risk of cardiovascular disease. If given intravenously, large doses of nicotinic acid can, however, produce side effects such as temporary vasodilatation and hypotension. Other side effects can include nausea, vomiting, diarrhea and general gastrointestinal disturbance, headache, fatigue, difficulty in focusing, skin discoloration, dry hair, sore throat, etc. A large trial for secondary prevention of myocardial infarction, with a 15 year period of follow-up, produced convincing evidence for moderate but significant protection against mortality, which was attributed either to the cholesterol-lowering effect or an early effect on nonfatal reinfarction, or both. Nicotinic acid is still the treatment of choice for some classes of high-risk hyperlipidemic patients, although newer drugs may have fewer side effects and therefore be preferred.

The potential benefits of the lipid-lowering effects of nicotinic acid have to be considered in the light of possibly toxic effects, particularly for the liver. These may manifest as jaundice, changes in liver function tests, changes in carbohydrate tolerance, and changes in uric acid metabolism including hyper-uricemia. There may also be accompanying ultrastructural changes. Hyperuricemia may result from effects on intestinal bacteria and enzymes, and from effects on renal tubular function. Such toxic effects are especially severe if sustained release preparations of nicotinic acid are used.

Nicotinamide does not share with nicotinic acid these effects on lipid metabolism or the associated toxicity. However, it has been shown to be an inhibitor of poly (ADP ribose) synthetase in pancreatic β cells in animal studies. A high-risk group of children aged 5–8 years in New Zealand given large doses of nicotinamide daily for up to 4.2 years had only half the predicted incidence of insulin-dependent diabetes.

Other claims for megadoses of nicotinic acid or nicotinamide, such as the claim that abnormalities associated with schizophrenia, Down's syndrome, hyperactivity in children, etc. can be reduced, have so far failed to win general acceptance. Clearly niacin deficiency or dependency can exacerbate some types of mental illness such as depression or dementia. There have been a number of attempts to treat depression with tryptophan or niacin, or both, on the basis that the correction of depressed brain levels of serotonin would be advantageous. However, these have met with only limited success. Schizophrenics have been treated with nicotinic acid on the basis that their synthesis of NAD is impaired in some parts of the brain, and that the formation of hallucinogenic substances such as methylated indoles may be controlled.

There are various medical conditions and drug interactions that can increase the requirement for niacin. Examples are: Hartnup disease, in which tryptophan transport in the intestine and kidney is impaired; carcinoid syndrome, in which tryptophan turnover is increased; and isoniazid treatment, which causes B_6 depletion and hence interference with niacin formation from tryptophan. Hartnup disease (the name of the first patient being Hartnup) is a rare genetic disease in which the conversion of tryptophan to niacin is reduced, partly as a result of impaired tryptophan absorption. Affected subjects exhibit the classical skin and neurological lesions of pellagra, which can be alleviated by prolonged treatment with niacin. Another genetic disease which may respond to niacin supplements is Fredrikson type I familial hypercholesterolemia; nicotinic acid is effective in reducing the raised blood cholesterol levels associated with this abnormality.

There are several analogs and antimetabolites of niacin that are of potential use or metabolic interest. The closely related isoniazid is commonly used for treatment of tuberculosis; indeed, nicotinamide itself has been used for that purpose. Nicotinic acid diethylamide ('nikethamide') is used as a stimulant in cases of central nervous system depression after poisoning, trauma or collapse. Possible antineoplastic analogs include 6-dimethylaminonicotinamide and 6-aminonicotinamide; however, the latter is also highly teratogenic. These latter compounds inhibit several key enzymes whose substrates are NAD or NADP, by being converted *in vivo* to analogs of these coenzymes. The compound 3-acetyl pyridine, which also forms an analog of NAD, can have either antagonistic or niacin-replacing properties, depending on the dose used. Commonly used drugs such as metronidazole are also niacin antagonists.

See also: **Bioavailability. Energy**: Metabolism. **Hyperlipidemia**: Overview; Nutritional Management. **Riboflavin. Vitamin B$_6$**.

Further Reading

Bender DA (1992) Niacin. In: *Nutritional Biochemistry of the Vitamins*, ch. 8, pp. 184–222. Cambridge: Cambridge University Press.

Carpenter KJ (ed.) (1981) *Pellagra: Benchmark Papers in the History of Biochemistry/II*. Stroudsburg, Pennsylvania: Dowden, Hutchinson & Ross Publ. Co.

Di Palma JR and Thayer WS (1991) Use of niacin as a drug. *Annual Review of Nutrition* 2: 169–187.

Fu CS, Swendseid ME, Jacob RA, and McKee RW (1989) Biochemical markers for assessment of niacin status in young men: levels of erythrocyte niacin coenzymes and plasma tryptophan. *Journal of Nutrition* 119: 1949–1955.

Hankes LV (1984) Nicotinic acid and nicotinamide. In: Machlin LJ (ed.) *Handbook of Vitamins*, ch. 8, pp. 329–377. New York: Marcel Dekker Inc.

Henderson LM (1983) Niacin. *Annual Review of Biochemistry* 3: 289–307.

Horwitt MK, Harvey CC, Rothwell WS, Cutler JL, and Haffron D (1956) Tryptophan–niacin relationship in man. *Journal of Nutrition* 60(supplement 1): 1–43.

Jacob RA, Swendseid ME, McKee RW, Fu CS, and Clemens RA (1989) Biochemical markers for assessment of niacin status in young men: urinary and blood levels of niacin metabolites. *Journal of Nutrition* 119: 591–598.

Sauberlich HE, Dowdy RP, and Skala JH (1974) *Laboratory Tests for the Assessment of Nutritional Status*, pp. 70–74. Boca Raton: CRC Press.

Swendseid ME and Jacob RA (1984) Niacin. In: Shils ME and Young VR (eds.) *Modern Nutrition in Health and Disease*, 7th edn., ch. 22, pp. 376–382. Philadelphia: Lea & Febiger.

Nitrogen *see* **Amino Acids**: Chemistry and Classification; Metabolism. **Protein**: Digestion and Bioavailability; Quality and Sources; Requirements and Role in Diet; Deficiency

NUCLEIC ACIDS

E A Carrey, Institute of Child Health, London, UK
H A Simmonds, Guy's Hospital, London, UK

The nucleic acids, vital constituents of all living cells, were discovered by Miescher in 1868 and isolated from the nuclei of pus cells and spermatozoa of Rhine salmon. The major constituents of nucleic acids were shown to be sugars, phosphate groups, and the characteristic purine and pyrimidine bases, now considered to be some of the first chemicals to emerge from the 'primordial soup' before life began on Earth. Emil Fischer and colleagues established the chemical structure of the purine bases, including uric acid—the end (waste) product of purine metabolism in humans—at the end of the nineteenth century.

This article outlines the biosynthesis of nucleic acids and gives a brief overview of the physiological functions of nucleosides, nucleotides, and nucleic acids. It describes the toxicity that may arise from degradation of both endogenous and dietary (exogenous) nucleic acids in humans and provides a summary of the nucleic acid content of foods.

Physiology

Structure

The nucleic acids are fundamental to genetics and to metabolism. Deoxyribonucleic acid (DNA) is found in the chromosomes within the nucleus and the mitochondria, and it contains the genetic information. Ribonucleic acid (RNA) is found both in the nucleus and in the surrounding cytoplasm, and its various forms fulfill several tasks associated with the transfer of the genetic message and its eventual translation into proteins.

Each nucleic acid is a linear polymer of nucleotides (**Figure 1A**). Nucleosides, the related small molecules, consist of a pentose sugar bound to the N-9 atom of a purine or to the N-1 of the

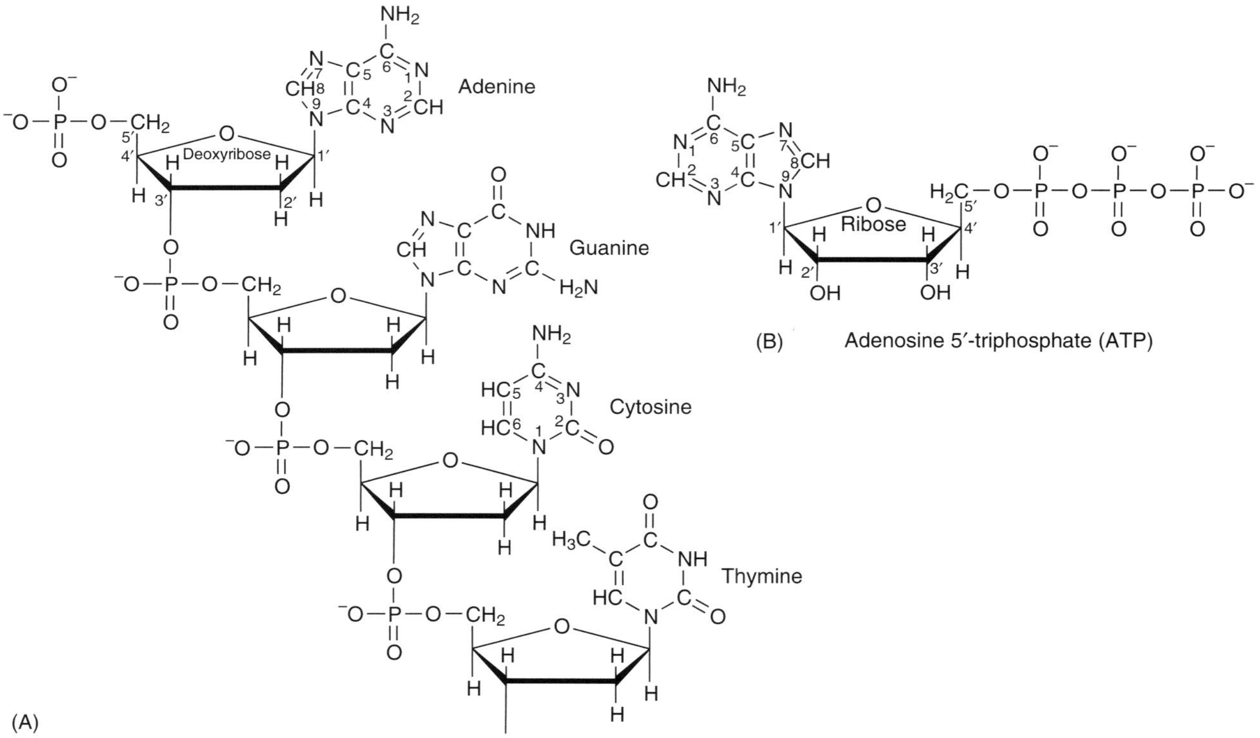

Figure 1 (A) Schematic representation of part of a DNA strand showing the structural formulas of the four constituent bases, adenine, guanine, cytosine, and thymine, linked via the 3′-OH group of the deoxyribose moiety to the 5′-phosphate group of the next nucleotide. Also shown is the numbering of the atoms in the deoxyribose, as well as the pyrimidine and purine rings. The latter consist of a six-membered pyrimidine ring fused to a five-membered imidazole ring. (B) Structural formula of ATP indicating that the ribose, as distinct from deoxyribose, has an OH group at the 2′ position on the pentose ring.

pyrimidine ring: With one or more phosphate groups at the 5′ position of the sugar, the molecule is a nucleotide (**Figure 1B**). When nucleoside triphosphates (NTP) are linked through the 5′ phosphate groups to the 3′ position of the previous residue on the growing chain, the chemical energy for the polymerization is provided by the removal of the second and third phosphate groups.

In DNA the pentose is 2′-deoxyribose (**Figure 1A**) and the bases are adenine (A), guanine (G), cytosine (C), and thymine (T). Two strands are wound in opposing chemical directions in the well-defined double-helix structure of DNA, with each nucleotide of one strand linked by hydrogen bonding to a complementary nucleotide on the other (A-T and G-C). The deoxyribose and phosphate groups form the outer sides of the 'ladder.'

The RNA molecule is chemically single stranded, but double-helical regions arise when stretches of complementary sequences allow hairpin loops to form. In addition, the base uracil (U) is found instead of thymine, and the pentose is ribose.

Nucleic Acid Biosynthesis in Humans

The first step in the synthesis of DNA and RNA in humans involves the formation of the purine and pyrimidine ribonucleotides. They are derived endogenously by two routes: the energetically expensive multistep *de novo* route (**Figure 2**), using small

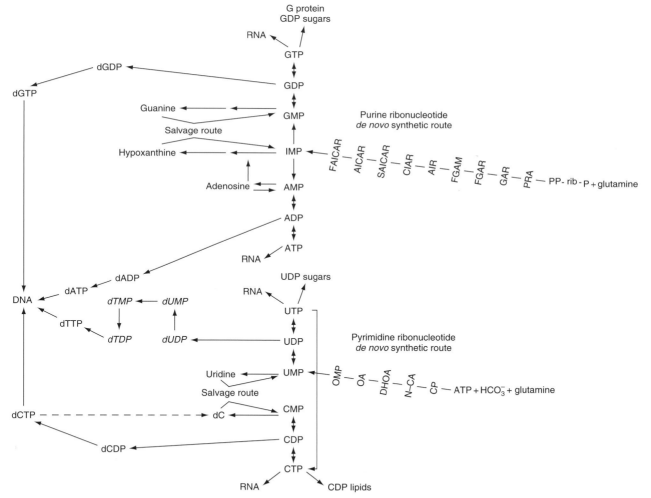

Figure 2 Metabolic pathways for the synthesis of DNA and RNA from their purine and pyrimidine ribo- and deoxyribonucleotide precursors. The dotted line from dCTP indicates the route of breakdown to deoxycytidine (dC), which can be salvaged by dC kinase and incorporated into dCDP lipids or DNA. HCO_3^-, bicarbonate; CP, carbamoyl phosphate; N-CA, carbamoyl aspartate; DHOA, dihydroorotic acid; OA, orotic acid; OMP, orotidylic acid; PP-rib-P, 5-phosphoribosyl-1-pyrophosphate; PRA, 5-phosphoribosylamine; GAR, glycinamide ribotide; FGAR, *N*-formyl glycinamide ribotide; FGAM, *N*-formylglycinamidine ribotide; AIR, 5-aminoimidazole ribotide; CAIR, 5-aminoimidazole-4-carboxy ribotide; SAICAR, *N*-succino-5-aminoimidazole-4-carboxamide ribotide; AICAR, 5-aminoimidazole-4-carboxamide ribotide; FAICAR, 5-formamidoimidazole-4-carboxamide ribotide.

molecules such as carbon dioxide, amino acids, and ribose sugars as precursors; and the energetically less expensive 'salvage' pathway. Purine bases and pyrimidine nucleosides from the breakdown of nucleic acids and nucleotide cofactors are salvaged within the cells, generating nucleotides that can be incorporated into nucleic acids. In most cells in the body, salvage processes are more important than *de novo* synthesis, and the ribonucleotides recycled in this way exert feedback control on the *de novo* routes.

The ribonucleoside 5′-monophosphates generated from either pathway are rapidly phosphorylated within the cell to the triphosphate form for immediate use in the synthesis of RNA or in a variety of cellular processes. The most abundant ribonucleotide in the body is adenosine 5′-triphosphate (ATP), which is the universal energy carrier of all living organisms (**Figure 1B**). In addition, ATP molecules are part of the coenzymes (NAD, NADP, FAD, etc.), which assist in many reactions including the conversion of food into energy. Adenosine and guanosine nucleotides within cells have roles in the transduction of external signals into cellular responses and in the translation and synthesis of proteins. Pyrimidines, present at much lower concentrations in cells, also fulfill diverse functions. UDP-glucose and CDP–lipids are active intermediates in the synthesis of glycogen and membranes, respectively, and sugars linked to UDP or GDP are used in the glycosylation of proteins, many of which are exposed on the outer surface of cells. UDP-glucuronic acid is an essential component of the pathways in liver, gut, and kidney that convert foreign molecules and steroids into soluble forms for disposal from the body.

To make DNA, the ribonucleoside diphosphates (rNDP) are reduced to the corresponding 2′-deoxyribonucleoside diphosphates (dNDP) in a reaction catalyzed by ribonucleotide reductase. This reaction produces dADP, dGDP, and dCDP, which are phosphorylated to the triphosphate form; dUDP is converted via dUMP to dTMP, providing the four substrates essential for DNA synthesis. The DNA polymerase enzymes form double-stranded DNA by sequential addition of monomers complementary to the bases on the opposite strand. Crucially, a 'proofreading' activity in the enzyme ensures the accuracy of the process, and hence double-stranded DNA provides a stable format for genetic information.

Nucleic Acids in the Storage and Transmission of Genetic Information

The role of DNA and RNA in the storage and transmission of genetic information is well established and can be found in standard textbooks. The hereditary material in the nucleus of human cells is packed into 23 chromosomes, and additional DNA is found in the mitochondria. The human genome is known to contain approximately 30 000 coding sequences, or genes, and a substantial proportion of DNA has a regulatory role in transcription of the genes. The sequence of the four bases and the capacity of DNA to be copied into two complementary strands underlie the genetic information of all living organisms. Interactions between DNA and the transcription factors determine the time and place in the body where genes are transcribed, causing development and metabolism to occur.

RNA molecules are synthesized initially on a DNA template by a DNA-dependent RNA polymerase in a process called transcription, in which ribonucleotides complementary to the bases of one strand of DNA are joined by 3′–5′ phosphodiester bonds.

Cells contain three types of RNA, each of which is chemically modified after transcription from the DNA template. The three kinds of RNA together are important in the translation of the genetic message to synthesize proteins in the cell. Most RNA is in the cytoplasm, principally in the form of ribosomal RNA (80% of the total), which performs structural and catalytic roles in ribosomes, the site of the growing polypeptide chain in protein synthesis, whereas messenger RNA (5%) provides the template for protein synthesis. The amino acids are brought to the assembly site covalently bonded to transfer RNA (15%), with their order in the growing protein being specified by the order of the bases in mRNA.

Synthesis of nucleic acids and their precursors in different human cells is related to cellular function
Synthesis of both DNA and RNA is prominent in cells and tissues with a high rate of turnover or metabolism (e.g., liver, gut epithelium, skin, dividing lymphocytes, bone marrow, and hair follicles). In most tissues in the adult, cells differentiate to perform specialized tasks and therefore cell division is used only to replace cells that have been lost. Different complements of enzymes are expressed in each cell type, and therefore tissues have characteristic profiles of internal metabolites, including nucleotides and nucleosides.

For example, in cells that do not continuously divide, such as heart and muscle, nucleotide profiles are relatively simple, relating to the major requirement to sustain levels of cofactors and ATP. In contrast, rapidly dividing cells in liver and intestine show a complex nucleotide pattern, supporting these organs as major sites of nucleic acid metabolism. The gut is particularly important in this respect. The rate of cell turnover in the luminal villi is high, and it has been calculated in rat that approximately 30 mg of endogenous nucleic acid from dead cells enters the gut lumen daily. This means that the rate of nucleic acid synthesis in liver and intestine is much higher than in tissues such as muscle.

Metabolism of Endogenous Nucleic Acids and Excretion of End Products

There is a considerable turnover of endogenous nucleic acids and ribonucleotides daily during muscle work, wound healing, erythrocyte senescence, mounting an immune response, etc. However, only a small fraction of these vital endogenous compounds are actually degraded and lost from the body. The contents of dead cells are normally used by nearby cells, and degraded RNA or cofactors are recycled within living cells using active 'salvage' routes.

Salvage of the polynucleotides DNA and RNA begins when the molecules are degraded by enzymes—ribonucleases for RNA and deoxyribonucleases for DNA—to liberate nucleotides. The next step, degradation by specific 5′-nucleotidases (removing the phosphate groups) to nucleosides or deoxynucleosides, is essentially irreversible. In turn, removal of amino groups and the sugar residue will give the purine bases hypoxanthine and xanthine or the pyrimidine bases uracil and thymine.

Any pyrimidine nucleosides that are not salvaged are converted first to the bases uracil and thymine, which are further catabolized in a series of steps to β amino acids. All are soluble and readily excreted. There is thus normally no measurable pyrimidine end product and therefore no toxicity from endogenous or dietary pyrimidines.

In contrast, the purine bases are converted to xanthine (an insoluble metabolite) by the enzyme xanthine dehydrogenase (XDH) and then to the equally insoluble end product uric acid. This compound can normally be disposed of in the urine, but high concentrations can lead to the formation of kidney stones or deposits in the joints and under the skin. Some rare genetic disorders of purine biosynthesis can remove feedback regulation, or excessive breakdown of cells may overload the salvage system, resulting in very high endogenous levels of uric acid.

Metabolism of Dietary Nucleic Acids in Humans

The normal human diet is rich in both DNA and RNA since food is derived from once-living organisms. The metabolism of these exogenous nucleic acids follows a similar pattern to the intracellular process described previously, but the bacterial flora of the intestine are the first point of attack. This digestion is rapid. Studies in pigs (confirmed by later studies in humans) demonstrated that up to 50% of radiolabeled dietary purine was degraded and lost as carbon dioxide gas within 30 min, with the remaining 43% being recovered in the urine and 5% in the feces (**Figure 3**). It has been shown that dietary pyrimidine nucleotides, but not purines, are incorporated into RNA.

Humans thus have no apparent requirement for purines from the diet, and the intestinal mucosa provides an effective barrier to their uptake through a battery of enzymes that rapidly degrade purine nucleotides, nucleosides, and bases to the metabolic waste product, uric acid. This phenomenon may represent an important evolutionary development to protect the integrity of the cellular DNA or to ensure that levels of ATP do not fluctuate in concert with the dietary intake of purines.

The potential toxicity of dietary nucleic acids to humans usually arises not from the nucleic acids but

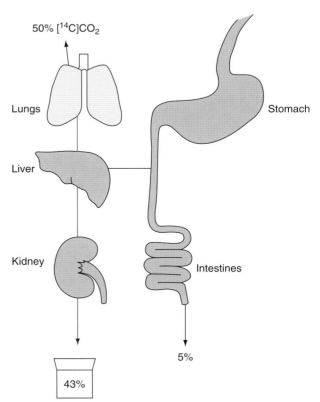

Figure 3 Diagram showing the fate of ^{14}C-labeled exogenous purine (guanine) in an animal model (pig). Radiolabel was recovered only in carbon dioxide gas, urine, or feces. No incorporation into any tissues was found.

from their metabolic end products (principally uric acid). Many investigators have shown that the fate of the dietary purine moiety depends on whether it is administered in the form of DNA, RNA, mononucleotides, nucleosides, or bases, with some being catabolised more readily than others. When normal subjects are fed RNA, the increase in the excretion of uric acid is dramatic alongside a modest increase in plasma urate concentrations. The effect of RNA is also twice that of DNA when the increase in purines in the plasma is measured.

On the other hand, pyrimidine mononucleotides and uridine, but not the base uracil, are absorbed readily from the intestine and utilised for nucleic acid synthesis. This has been demonstrated by studies of humans with hereditary oroticaciduria, a rare defect in *de novo* pyrimidine synthesis at the fourth step involving conversion of orotic acid to UMP. Such patients have a severe megaloblastic anemia that does not respond to the usual forms of treatment. They have been sustained for more than 40 years on oral uridine, indicating that the dietary pyrimidine is absorbed intact and can compensate totally for lack of *de novo* synthesis in humans. Studies using radiolabelled purines and pyrimidines in mice have provided further evidence for the incorporation of dietary pyrimidine nucleosides, but not purine nucleosides, into hepatic RNA.

Nucleosides and Nucleotides in the Diet

In healthy adults, the normal diet is a good source of nucleic acids, nucleotides, and nucleosides, and no supplementation is necessary.

Pharmacological uses for nucleosides and nucleotides Oral uridine, as described earlier, can be used where *de novo* biosynthesis of pyrimidines is defective, and it may be useful in reversing some effects of mitochondrial dysfunction and to minimize the toxic effect of the antitumor drug 5-fluorouracil. Uridine is also a precursor for UDP-glucose, essential for the deposition of glycogen in the liver. Enzymes in the liver, however, rapidly degrade much of each oral dose of uridine. Oral administration of a new prodrug, PN401, inhibits the degradative processes and delivers more uridine into circulation than oral uridine.

Oral CDP–choline is rapidly converted to its components, CDP (which can be recycled to uridine) and choline, an essential component of lipid membranes. Each molecule can then cross the blood–brain barrier, where CDP–choline is used in regeneration of membranes within and around nerve cells. Research in rats and early studies in humans suggest that its

pharmacological effects may extend to protection against dementia, memory loss, visual degeneration, and recovery from ischemic strokes.

Beneficial effects of dietary nucleosides and nucleotides There is substantial evidence (principally from research in animal models) that the presence of nucleotides or nucleosides in the diet helps cellular proliferation in the gut, in postoperative trauma, and in the development of the immune response. Although dietary purines are not taken into circulation from the gut, purine nucleotides influence the transcription of several genes in intestinal cells. Nucleotides based on both adenosine and uridine can activate the purinergic receptors on a wide range of cell types. In lymphocytes and other cells, synthesis of nucleotides *de novo* is expanded dramatically when a signal for proliferation is received; the rate of pyrimidine biosynthesis increases more than that of purine biosynthesis. Thus, nucleotides are considered to be 'conditionally essential' since their provision in the diet will provide help through the salvage system where cells are dividing rapidly or where other nutrients, used as precursors, are scarce.

Human milk contains maternal cells, providing nucleic acids, and also nucleosides (particularly cytidine and uridine), and nucleotides equivalent to 10–20 mg/day. Cow's milk contains the *de novo* intermediate orotic acid, which can be taken up by erythrocytes and converted to UMP. Dietary nucleotides have been shown to promote the incorporation of essential fatty acids into membrane lipids in healthy newborn infants and to enhance the integrity and maturation of the intestine and of the immune system. Thus, these components may contribute to the improved immunity seen in breast-fed infants. Many infant formulas are now supplemented with nucleotides/nucleosides, but usually in lower concentrations than in human milk.

Purine ribonucleotides as flavor-enhancing additives The purine 5′-nucleotide monophosphates IMP and GMP, derived from degradation of RNA, have received much attention as the taste-active components in a variety of seafoods and meat. Both IMP and GMP enhance the *umami* flavor generated by monosodium glutamate (MSG). This flavor was generated only by the purine 5′-nucleotides, and not by the pyrimidine nucleotides CMP and UMP, by interaction with receptors on the specific *umami* tastebuds in the mouth. Since ATP is the major free nucleotide in muscle cells, its breakdown into the flavor-enhancing IMP provides a scientific rationale for the improved palatability of meat or game birds that have been hung for several days after slaughter. Similarly, the distinctive flavors of several cheeses are related to the metabolism, by bacteria, of the characteristic range of nucleotides present in the original milk.

Toxicology

Pathophysiology of Genetic Metabolic Disorders in Nucleotide Metabolism

The important physiological roles played by the nucleic acid precursor rNTP and dNTP molecules in humans has become apparent since the 1970s by the recognition of 28 different inborn errors of purine and pyrimidine metabolism. The spectrum of clinical manifestations ranges from fatal immunodeficiency syndromes to muscle weakness, severe neurological deficits, anemia, renal failure, gout, and urolithiasis (uric acid kidney stones).

Patients in whom the gene encoding a crucial enzyme is absent or defective harbor an 'experiment of nature,' equivalent to the artificial 'knockout' of individual genes in animals. The metabolic consequences of the disorders have highlighted the importance of individual steps in the nucleotide pathways to a particular cell or tissue, particularly the need for intact pathways for nucleic acid synthesis as well as for metabolism, degradation, and recycling of nucleotides.

It is evident from two genetic disorders associated with immunodeficiency that rapid turnover of DNA from cells of the immune system normally produces significant amounts of free deoxyribonucleotides in the bone marrow, which must be degraded to the corresponding base or nucleoside for recycling. The absence of either of two enzymes critical to this pathway, adenosine deaminase and purine nucleoside phosphorylase, results in the accumulation of dATP or dGTP, respectively. Each of these nucleotides inhibits ribonucleotide reductase and may also lead to misincorporation during DNA synthesis. The lymphocytes are particularly sensitive, resulting in a potentially fatal immunodeficiency syndrome with a clinical course similar to that in AIDS. Other rapidly dividing cells, such as those of the skin or the gut, are also affected. These disorders highlight the sensitivity of lymphocytes to the efficient removal of waste from DNA catabolism and, in fact, have provided the basis for development of novel immunosuppressant drugs based on inhibitors of these enzyme activities.

Role of Nucleotide Analogs as Cytotoxic and Antiviral Drugs

DNA in the chromosomes is normally protected by active repair systems against damage by a variety of chemical and physical agents, including ionizing radiation and ultraviolet light. Proofreading activities guard against the incorporation of mismatched nucleotides during DNA replication or transcription. In contrast, the use of certain nucleotide analogs as drugs depends on their incorporation into DNA—the chemical must be recognized and used by the replication enzymes but must prohibit further elongation of the nucleic acid chain. Analogs used in HIV therapy are incorporated by the reverse transcriptase of the virus and bring the reaction to a halt. Toxicity associated with several analogs is known to arise from erroneous incorporation into the patient's mitochondrial DNA because of less stringent proofreading by the mitochondrial DNA polymerase enzyme. Azidothymidine remains one of the most effective and least toxic drugs for AIDS, albeit it is now usually taken in triple therapy.

Nucleotide analogs have been used to inhibit the *de novo* pathways for the synthesis of the precursor nucleosides and nucleotides, leading to depletion of metabolites and imbalance of dNTPs, and hence to misincorporation of nucleotides in RNA or DNA, respectively. Malaria and other parasites rely exclusively on *de novo* pyrimidine biosynthesis; thus, they may be susceptible at drug doses that do not affect the host because the human body can obtain nucleotides from the salvage pathway. Similarly, because of the increased requirement for nucleotides in rapidly proliferating cells, almost all the enzyme reactions (**Figure 2**) have been investigated as potential targets for treatment of cancer, inflammation, or to prevent rejection of transplanted organs. Again, combinations of drugs with different modes of action have often proved most effective.

Toxicity of Exogenous Nucleic Acids to Humans

Dietary nucleic acids are digested fully to their component nucleosides and bases, so nucleic acids are not absorbed *per se* into the body. The potential toxicity to humans of dietary purine bases arises principally because primates lack expression of the gene for the hepatic enzyme uricase. Excess purines are therefore converted to uric acid rather than to the extremely soluble allantoin, as in most other mammalian species. In reptiles, snakes, spiders, and birds, uric acid is the end product of the metabolism of all nitrogenous compounds, analogous to urea in mammals. The main advantage to using this insoluble end product is that there is no obligatory water loss for its excretion, as there is for urea. Consequently, uric acid can be excreted as a slurry by these animals—an evolutionary adaptation enabling survival in arid environments. In contrast, in humans, excess uric acid may accumulate in the tubules of the kidney as uric acid stones or as crystals in the interstitium, resulting in renal disease. Likewise, crystals can accumulate in the joints or subcutaneously, giving rise to gout symptoms. The most common and effective treatment for gout is the well-known drug allopurinol, which prevents conversion of xanthine to uric acid. The uricase enzyme may be prescribed as short-term therapy to avoid tumor lysis syndrome (the release of massive amounts of nucleic acids when cancerous cells are destroyed by chemotherapy or radiotherapy).

Although the uricase gene appears to be present in human cells, the promoter is not activated, so no enzyme activity is detected in the liver. The biological value of the normal circulating concentration of urate has been debated, but urate ions may provide more than half the antioxidant activity in the plasma of primates.

Not only is uric acid a relatively insoluble form of metabolic waste but also plasma concentrations are kept high because the renal proximal tubule reabsorbs approximately 90% of the filtered uric acid (**Figure 4**) before it can be excreted in the urine. Net reabsorption is higher in healthy males (92%) than in females (88%) and is lower in children of either sex (80–85%). This difference explains the higher plasma uric acid in adult males and means that uric acid is circulating in their plasma at concentrations close to its solubility limit. Reabsorption is much

higher (95%) in middleaged males with 'primary gout'—and increasingly in men and elderly women who are treated with thiazide diuretics for high blood pressure. Poor excretion of uric acid is also seen in a familial renal disease associated with gout symptoms in children and young adults of both sexes. Without treatment to lower the uric acid accumulation, the kidney function may be seriously diminished.

Origin of the Body Uric Acid Pool in Humans

The body pool of urate, and hence the plasma urate concentration, is the result of a balance between production, ingestion, and excretion. The main causes of high plasma uric acid concentrations are high intake of exogenous nucleic acid in the diet and overproduction of endogenous purine. Eating less meat, seafood, and other high-purine foods (**Tables 1** and **2**) leads to a lower dietary intake of nucleic acids. In contrast, subjects with genetic defects that remove the usual controls on purine biosynthesis may have overwhelmingly high endogenous levels of the waste product, uric acid.

The contribution of the two sources can be assessed by placing the subject on a purine-free diet for 1 week and measuring the urinary uric acid. In this way, fewer than 5% of patients with gout have been found to excrete abnormally large amounts of urate (>3 mmol/day) derived from endogenous

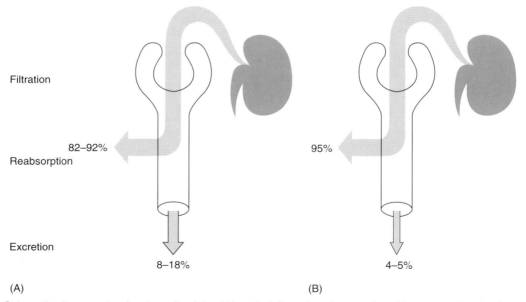

Filtration

Reabsorption 82–92%

95%

Excretion 8–18%

4–5%

(A)   (B)

Figure 4 Schematic diagram showing the role of the kidney in influencing plasma uric acid concentration. In the brush border membrane of the proximal tubule, reabsorption by the urate anion exchanger and secretion via a voltage-sensitive pathway both occur. This results in a mean fractional urinary excretion of only 8–18% of the filtered load in healthy subjects and 5% or less in 'primary' gout. The net uric acid reabsorption is (A) higher in healthy men (92%) than in women (88%) and lower in children of either sex (82%), and (B) much higher in middle-aged males with primary gout (95%).

Table 1 Reference guide to the purine content of foods

Foods and beverages rich in nucleic acids/purines
Offal: sweetbreads, liver, kidney, heart, and paté
Wild or farmed game meats (venison, pheasant, rabbit, hare)
Seafoods: sardines, sprats, herring, bloaters, anchovies, fish roe, caviar, taramasalata, trout or salmon, lobster, crab, prawns
Vegetables: asparagus, avocado pears, peas, spinach, mushrooms, broad beans, cauliflower
Pulses and grains: legumes, pulses and soya products such as bean curd, tofu, Quorn
Cereals: all bran, oat, rye, or wheat cereals and products; whole meal, rye, and brown breads
Other: beer and yeast extracts/tablets (Barmene, Tastex); meat or vegetable extracts (Marmite, Vegemite, Bovril, Oxo)

Foods that are moderate or low sources of purine
Beef, lamb, pork (steak or chops), bacon, ham, sausages, some poultry, tongue (all should be eaten in moderation)
Carrots, parsnip, potatoes, lettuce, leeks, cabbage, sprouts, marrow, courgettes
Peanuts, cashew nuts
White bread or flour, cakes, scones, biscuits, cereals
Some fish (see **Table 2**)

Foods and beverages that are purine-free
Milk, cheese, eggs, butter, margarine, cream, ice cream
Sugar, jam, marmalade, honey, sweets
Cucumber, tomato, onions, pumpkin
Fresh, cooked or tinned fruits, nuts
Puddings, custards, yogurt
Fruit juices, soft drinks

Table 2 Concentrations of purines in some common foods and beverages[a]

Food	Purine (mg/100 g)	Protein (mg/100 g)
Meat		
Beef liver	333	19.7
Beef kidney	285	15.4
Beef heart	285	16.8
Beef tongue	167	16.4
Beef steak	151	19.5
Calf liver	348	19
Sweetbreads	1212	19.6
Veal cutlet	152	19.2
Sheep kidney	312	16.8
Lamb chop	196	14.9
Pork liver	289	22
Pork cutlet	164	16.4
Bacon	85	9.1
Ham	136	19.5
Sausage (beef)	79	13.8
Sausage (pork)	66	11.5
Rabbit	118	20.4
Venison	156	20
Vegetables		
Asparagus	32	2.1
Cauliflower	32	2.1
Celery	20	1.1
Kohlrabi	44	2.1
Mushrooms	72	3.5
Peas	72	6.7
Spinach	96	2.2
Dried legumes		
Split peas	195	21
Red bean	162	20
Lentils	222	28
Haricot beans	230	22
Lima bean	149	21
Other		
Bovril	340	18
Marmite	356	2
Oxo cubes	236	10
Yeast extracts	2257	46
Poultry		
Chicken flesh	181	20.6
Chicken liver	372	22.1
Chicken heart	223	18
Duck	181	16
Goose	177	16.4
Turkey	239	20.1
Fish, seafoods		
Anchovies	411	20
Bass	73	19.5
Bloaters	133	22.6
Bream	72	19.7
Cod	62	18
Crab	61	19.2
Clams	136	17
Eel	108	18.6
Fish cakes	36	12.1
Herring	378	17
Kippers	91	21.2
Lobster	100	20
Lemon sole	54	19.9
Mackerel	246	29
Plaice	53	18.1
Salmon	250	23
Sardines	345	23
Scallops	117	22.3
Sprats	250	25.1
Squid	135	15
Trout	92	19.2
Canned seafoods		
Anchovies	321	30
Herring	378	17
Mackerel	246	26
Oysters	116	6
Salmon	88	26
Sardines	399	24
Shrimp	231	22
Tuna	142	29

[a]Results are recorded relative to 100 g of food for purine and for protein, although serving size for each ingredient may be larger or smaller than 100 g.

purines. In these cases, overproduction of purine nucleotides leading to excess uric acid can be traced to a genetic defect. Two such sex-linked disorders are hypoxanthine–guanine phosphoribosyltransferase (HPRT) deficiency and phosphoribosyltransferase superactivity (PRPS). Boys presenting in infancy usually have severe and eventually fatal neurological deficits. Neurological problems are milder or absent, and only gout may be evident, in those presenting as adolescents. It is important for clinicians to be aware of these disorders, especially when encountering a young patient with gout or an older male with a history dating back to adolescence. In some families, siblings are also affected, and although the gout symptoms can be alleviated, other aspects are less amenable to treatment and genetic counselling should be given.

Gout

Gout is a painful, acute form of arthritis caused by the accumulation of crystals of uric acid in the joints (typically the great toe is the first site to be affected). The pain may be relieved by antiinflammatory drugs or by colchicine, and the accumulation of urate is halted by the drug allopurinol, which inhibits xanthine dehydrogenase. Nevertheless, adopting a low-purine diet has an important role in alleviating the effects of gout.

Historically, 'primary' gout—affecting predominantly middle-aged males—has long been associated with excessive consumption of 'rich' food and drink (**Tables 1** and **2**). Until World War I, affluent European gentlemen habitually consumed vast nucleic acid-rich meals including many different courses and meats. Alcoholic drinks also played their part, with beer being particularly rich in purines derived from yeast RNA and port a potential cause of lead poisoning from glass bottles and decanters.

Both hyperuricemia and gout are relatively common in Polynesians due to a genetic defect in excretion of urate and in Australasians, traditionally high consumers of nucleic acid-rich seafood, meat, and beer. In such countries, the prevalence of gout is as high as 10% compared with 1–4% in Europe. In Europe, the prevalence is higher in countries such as France where the consumption of seafoods and paté is high. The role of diet in the etiology of primary gout is confirmed by the fact that during and immediately after the two world wars this type of gout was virtually unknown. Gout, a hitherto little known disease, is now more common worldwide where affluence or the consumption of meat have increased.

Urolithiasis (Kidney Stones)

Although modest overindulgence in purine-rich food by normal subjects does not precipitate gout, it can predispose to uric acid lithiasis. Uric acid stones are relatively common in countries where the consumption of nucleic acid-rich beverages and food is high and in hot climates if insufficient fluids are consumed. Health foods such as yeast tablets, Spirulina,

or supplements containing nucleotides also contribute to uric acid lithiasis.

A number of compounds, such as vitamin C, increase uric acid clearance and thus can precipitate urolithiasis. Perhaps not so well recognized is the uricosuric effect of a high-protein diet and the fact that purine-rich foods also predispose to renal calcium stones. This may be because many purine-rich foods, such as spinach, are equally rich in calcium oxalate. Approximately 25% of vitamin C intake is also excreted as oxalate, which can compound the problem.

The solubility of uric acid is very sensitive to the pH of the urine, which in turn may be altered by components of the diet. The solubility of uric acid in urine at pH 5.0 is low (approximately $1 \, \text{mmol} \, l^{-1}$), but it can be increased 12-fold at pH 8.0 by alkalinising regimens, such as sodium bicarbonate or potassium citrate.

Exacerbation of kidney stone formation by dietary nucleic acids in inherited purine disorders Excess uric acid from dietary purines can also precipitate symptoms that may draw attention to milder forms in adults of HPRT deficiency or PRPS superactivity. A third genetic defect raises levels of adenine, which is converted by XDH to the even more insoluble uric acid analog, 2,8-dihydroxyadenine (2,8-DHA). Undiagnosed, such subjects have progressed to renal failure and even death. One child presenting in coma had a diet of pulses and grains, which have a particularly high adenine content. Since the accumulation of 2,8-DHA is treatable with allopurinol, such nephropathy can be avoided if the defect is recognized and the consumption of nucleic acid-rich foods reduced to a minimum.

Dietary Sources

Nucleic Acid Content of Foods

The nucleic acid content of different foods is expressed generally in terms of purine equivalents, with the data derived from the hydrolysis of nucleic acids and free nucleotides to the constituent bases. Careful analysis by Robert McCance, Elsie Widdowson, and colleagues since the 1930s forms the basis of tables of the composition of foodstuffs.

Foods may be classified into three groups: high, low, or essentially purine free (**Table 1**). As a general rule, growing organisms such as yeast, or rapidly metabolizing tissues such as liver, will be rich in both DNA and RNA. Seeds, grain, and fish eggs are good sources of the genetic material, DNA. Muscle tissue is an excellent source of nucleotides, such as the energy source ATP. Extracts of meat and yeast have very high purine contents but are usually eaten in small quantities. Some vegetables may provoke gout attacks by virtue of their oxalic acid content rather than that of purines, but legumes, fast-growing parts of brassicas, and asparagus tips may also have significant nucleic acid content. Fats, white flour, sugar, and fruit juices have been separated from the 'living' part of the food and so they are poor sources of nucleic acids.

Table 2 provides data for specific foodstuffs, obtained from the Documenta Geigy Chemical Composition of Foodstuffs tables. The ideal diet for subjects at risk of gout or of uric acid lithiasis is no more than one meat meal per day, using only the low-purine meat and vegetables indicated.

See also: **Ascorbic Acid**: Physiology, Dietary Sources and Requirements. **Choline and Phosphatidylcholine**. **Gout**.

Further Reading

Becker MA (2001) Purines and pyrimidines. In: Scriver CR, Beaudet AL, Sly WS, and Valle D (eds.) *The Metabolic and Molecular Basis of Inherited Disease*, 8th edn., pp. 2513–2537. New York: McGraw-Hill.

Carver JD (2003) Advances in nutritional modifications of infant formulas. *American Journal of Clinical Nutrition* **77**(supplement): 1550S–1554S.

Christopherson RI, Lyons SD, and Wilson PK (2002) Inhibitors of de novo nucleotide biosynthesis as drugs. *Accounts of Chemical Research* **35**: 961–971.

Diem K and Lentner C (eds.) (1970) *Scientific Tables—Chemical Composition of Foodstuffs*, 7th edn., pp. 230–243. Basel: Geigy.

Fuke S and Konosu S (1991) Taste-active components in some foods: A review of Japanese research. *Physiology and Behaviour* **49**: 863–868.

Grahame R, Simmonds HA, and Carrey EA (2003) *Gout: The 'At Your Fingertips' Guide* London: Class Publishing.

Lee H, Hanes J, and Johnson KA (2003) Toxicity of nucleoside analogues used to treat AIDS and the selectivity of the mitochondrial DNA polymerase. *Biochemistry* **42**: 14711–14719.

Rolls ET (2000) The representation of umami taste in the taste cortex. *Journal of Nutrition* **130**: 960S–965S.

Secades JJ and Frontera G (1995) CDP-choline: Pharmacological and clinical review. *Methods and Findings in Experimental and Clinical Pharmacology* **17**(supplement B): 1–54.

Uauy R (1989) Dietary nucleotides and requirements in early life. In: Lebenthal E (ed.) *Textbook of Gastroenterology and Nutrition in Infancy*, pp. 265–280. New York: Raven Press.

Zöllner N and Gresser U (eds.) (1991) *Urate Deposition in Man and Its Clinical Consequences*. Berlin: Springer-Verlag.

NUTRIENT–GENE INTERACTIONS

Contents
Molecular Aspects
Health Implications

Molecular Aspects

C D Berdanier, University of Georgia, Athens, GA, USA
H C Freake, University of Connecticut, Storrs, CT, USA

The completion of the sequencing of the human genome has resulted in a broadening of focus to include the investigation of the complex environment in which these genes operate. Although the term 'gene' refers to a specific sequence of DNA, the biological effects of that gene are manifest through its expression as a protein or peptide product. Nutrients affect the expression of genes in a variety of ways. Nutrients are required for the synthesis and packaging of DNA. Some have specific effects on the synthesis of messenger RNA (i.e., either suppress or enhance transcription). Others affect the synthesis of the pyrimidine and purine bases used for DNA and RNA synthesis. Some nutrients have an overall effect on protein synthesis, whereas others influence the translation of the messenger RNA into protein or the post-translational modification of the newly synthesized protein. Still others can affect the outcome of gene expression by influencing the environment in which the gene product functions. This article outlines the process of gene expression, focusing on the ways in which it is influenced and regulated by particular nutrients.

DNA Characteristics

The characteristics of every living creature are dictated by the genetic material, DNA. Nuclear DNA is organized into units called chromosomes, of which there are 46 in the human. The chromosomes are found in pairs and contain the individual units called genes. DNA is a double-stranded helix composed of four bases, two pyrimidines (cytosine and thymine) and two purines (adenine and guanine), that are joined together by ribose and phosphate groups (**Figure 1**). DNA is formed when the bases are joined through phosphodiester bonds using ribose as the common linkage. The phosphodiester linkage is between the 5′ phosphate group of one nucleotide and the 3′ OH group of the adjacent nucleotide. This provides a direction (5′ to 3′) to the chain. The bases are hydrophobic and contain charged polar groups. These features are responsible for the helical shape of the nuclear DNA chain. A double helix forms when the bases of each chain interact through hydrogen bonding.

The DNA base sequence is unique for every protein and peptide that synthesized in the body. The sequence of these bases determines the genotype of the individual for each gene product. Although only four different bases are used for the DNA, it is the sequence of these bases that determines the product being produced. Each gene product is uniquely derived from a specific gene. Although all cells contain the same DNA, not all genes are expressed in every cell; some are particular to specific cell types. Thus, the function of DNA is to determine not only the particular characteristics of the individual but also the properties of each cell through the provision of a multitude of genes, each coding for a particular protein found in that cell. Therefore, it functions to transmit genetic information from one generation to the next in a given species and ensures the identity of specific cell types.

The Human Genome Project has detailed the specific base sequence of nuclear and mitochondrial DNA in the human cell. The identification of each gene and its corresponding controls of expression have not been completely elucidated. Although the nuclear genome has been sequenced, it has not been completely mapped; that is, the location, within the DNA, of each gene (and its promoter region) and the identification of the protein or peptide it encodes

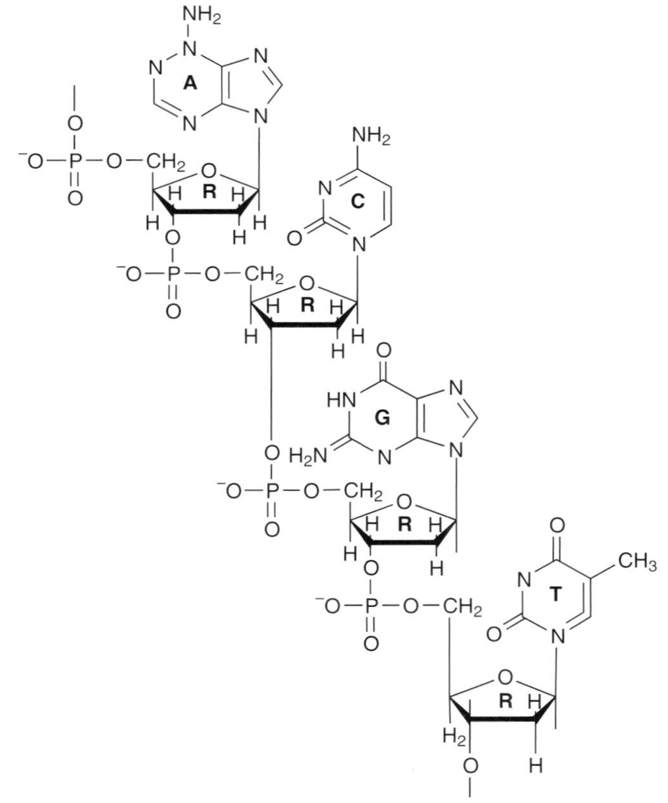

Figure 1 Representation of a segment of DNA showing the phosphodiester bond that uses ribose as the common link between the bases. A, adenine; C, cytosine; G, guanine; T, thymine; R, ribose.

have not been fully determined. In addition, we do not know all the details of the regulation of gene expression. Some genes have been intensely studied, whereas others have yet to be identified. In contrast, the genome in the mitochondria has been completely sequenced and mapped. It is a very small genome encoding only 13 gene products (components of the mitochondrial respiratory chain) under the control of a single promoter sequence, the D-loop. Despite its small size and apparent simplicity, however, we know even less about the regulation of its expression than we know about some of the nuclear-encoded genes.

DNA Synthesis

In the adult, some cell types are extremely long-lived (e.g., neuronal cells), whereas others last only a few days and therefore need constant replacement (epithelial cells, e.g., intestine and skin). This synthesis requires a number of micronutrients, protein, and energy. Should any of these be in short supply, symptoms of malnutrition will be observed, especially in those cell types that have very short half-lives. Typical of niacin deficiency (pellagra), for example, are skin lesions. As epithelial cells die and must be replaced, niacin is needed for this replacement. All the components of the new cells including DNA must be synthesized. The purines and pyrimidines that comprise DNA must be synthesized and this requires energy as well as micronutrients (niacin, riboflavin, pyridoxine, folic acid, vitamin B_{12}, copper, iron, sulfur, zinc, magnesium, and phosphorus). Anemia is another characteristic of malnutrition. Not only must new blood cells be made but also the essential ingredient of these cells, hemoglobin, must be synthesized. Among the nutrients needed for red blood cell synthesis are iron, copper, magnesium, folic acid, vitamin B_{12}, vitamin B_6, and, of course, energy and protein sufficient to support this synthesis.

The nutritional requirements for new cell synthesis are much greater in growing individuals than in adults because growth and cell division are much greater. Thus, energy and protein deficiency can be particularly detrimental. In addition, an adequate supply of specific micronutrients is crucial. For example, zinc deficiency was first described in teenage boys who were stunted and also sexually undeveloped. This report showed that zinc was required for both growth in general and the development of specific organ systems. Folic acid is required for DNA synthesis. Meeting this requirement is crucial during embryonic development. Inadequate folate intake by prepregnant and pregnant women can result in neural tube defects due to insufficient cell division during this time period. Not all women are so affected; there may be genetic differences in the need for folate that in turn determine whether the embryo is affected.

Transcription

Messenger RNA (mRNA) synthesis using DNA as the template is called transcription. The mRNA carries genetic information from the DNA of the chromosomes in the nucleus to the surface of the ribosomes in the cytosol. It is synthesized as a single strand. Chemically, RNA is similar to DNA. It is an unbranched linear polymer in which the monomeric subunits are the ribonucleoside $5'$ monophosphates. The bases are the purines (adenine and guanine) and the pyrimidines (uracil and cytosine). Thymine is not used in mRNA. Instead, uracil is used. This base is not present in DNA. Messenger RNA is much smaller than DNA and is far less stable. It has a very short half-life (from seconds to minutes or hours) compared to that of nuclear DNA (years). Because it has a short half-life, the purine and pyrimidine bases that are used to make mRNA must be continually resynthesized. This requires the same array of nutrients noted previously for DNA synthesis.

The synthesis of mRNA from DNA occurs in several stages: initiation, elongation, editing (processing), and termination. Initiation of transcription (the synthesis of mRNA) occurs when factors that serve to stabilize nuclear DNA are perturbed. Perturbation signals pass in to the nucleus and stimulate transcription. A small portion of the DNA (~17,000 bases) is exposed and used as the template for mRNA synthesis. The exposed portion also contains one or more sequences that have control properties with respect to the initiation of transcription. This region is called the promoter region and represents a key site for nutrient interaction. The promoter region precedes the start site of the structural gene and is said to be upstream of the structural gene. Those bases following the start site are downstream. The exposed DNA contains groups of bases called exons and introns. The introns are noncoding and are removed by editing prior to the movement of the mRNA from the nucleus to the cytosol.

Transcription is highly regulated. The DNA in all cell types is identical. However, not all of this DNA is transcribed in all cells all the time. Only certain genes are activated and transcribed into mRNA and subsequently translated into protein or peptides. As mentioned previously, these gene products give the individual cell type its identity. Central to this regulation are protein:DNA interactions and protein:nutrient interactions. At initiation, basal transcription factors recognize and bind to the start site of the structural gene. They form a complex with RNA polymerase II, an enzyme that catalyzes the formation of mRNA. Transcription factors bind to particular base sequences, called response elements, in the promoter region of the DNA that are upstream of the transcription start site (**Figure 2**). Each gene promoter contains a characteristic array of response elements, and these will determine to which signals the particular gene responds. Transcription factors also bind nutrients, and it is here that some nutrients have their effects on gene expression.

The regulation of transcription often occurs through the regulation of transcription factors. These factors can be regulated by the rates of their synthesis or degradation, by phosphorylation or dephosphorylation, by ligand binding, by cleavage of a pro-transcription factor, or by release of an inhibitor. One class of transcription factors important for nutrition is the nuclear hormone receptor superfamily that is regulated by ligand binding. Ligands for these transcription factors include retinoic acid (the gene active form of vitamin A), fatty acids, vitamin D, thyroid hormone, and steroid hormones. These receptors are proteins with a series of domains. The retinoic acid receptor can serve as an example. Its ligand-binding domain recognizes and binds with high affinity the nutrient signal, retinoic acid. The DNA-binding domain gives

gene specificity. It binds to a segment of the gene promoter that contains its corresponding response element, the retinoic acid response element (RARE). A transactivation domain then signals the effective occupation of this response element to the gene as a whole, including RNA polymerase II and its associated proteins. There are additional factors responsible for mediating this interaction between nutrient receptor and the transcription process. They include coactivating proteins, which stimulate transcription, and corepressor proteins, which can cause inhibition of transcription from a particular protein. In general, nutrients can signal the activation of transcription of some genes while at the same time turning off the transcription of others.

An interesting additional feature of this superfamily of nuclear hormone receptors is that they contain two zinc atoms in their DNA-binding domains. Each zinc is bound by four cysteine residues and causes the folding of the protein in a finger-like shape that binds DNA. The zinc ion plays an important role in gene expression because of its central use in the zinc finger of a wide variety of DNA binding proteins. In the case of the receptor superfamily, although zinc is required for receptor function, there is no evidence that it plays a regulatory role. However, there are other transcription factors in which it does play a role. MTF-1 (metal response element (MRE)-binding transcription factor-1) responds to increasing zinc concentrations within the cell by translocating to the nucleus and activating the transcription of genes containing MREs in their promoter region. These genes include

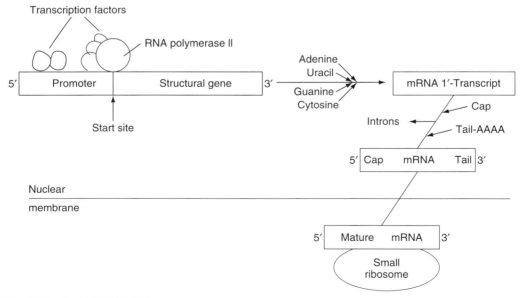

Figure 2 Schematic view of transcription.

metallothionein, which binds zinc and may play a key role in zinc homeostasis.

The direct binding of a nutrient signal to a transcription factor is perhaps one of the simpler ways in which nutrients impact gene transcription. There are other less direct but equally important mechanisms. Genes involved in cholesterol homeostasis are characterized by a sterol response element (SRE) in their promoter regions, which interacts with a sterol response element binding protein (SREBP). This protein is synthesized as a large precursor, incorporated into endoplasmic reticulum membranes, and is unavailable to function in gene regulation until it is cleaved and released. Limited cholesterol availability results in the cleavage and release of SREBP from the membrane compartment and its translocation to the nucleus. There it can perform its gene regulatory function by activating the transcription of genes for cholesterol synthesis as well as the LDL receptor gene. The LDL receptor facilitates cholesterol uptake by the liver. When it is abnormal due to a mutation in its gene, hypercholesterolemia results. The liver is unable to remove cholesterol from the blood and continues to synthesize it since SREBP remains active.

The metabolism and availability of macronutrients also influence gene transcription. Promoter elements have been described that allow a response to glucose (the carbohydrate response element (CHORE)). Although the specifics are unclear, the activity of the protein that binds this element responds to the metabolism of glucose and then stimulates the transcription of relevant genes—for example, those required for glucose metabolism (pyruvate kinase) and fatty acid synthesis (acetyl-coA carboxylase and fatty acid synthase). Fatty acids also influence gene expression. They can affect transcription by binding directly to their own transcription factor (the peroxisome proliferator activated receptor) and also indirectly by reducing the availability of SREBP within the nucleus. The latter mechanism provides a means for linking cholesterol and fatty acid metabolism with the cell.

Nutrients can also affect gene expression indirectly by regulating the release of hormones into the blood. Thus, glucose, in addition to having its own effects on gene expression through the CHORE, also stimulates insulin secretion from the pancreas. Insulin has its own transcriptional effects, often on the same genes that are regulated by glucose. In the postabsorptive state, insulin drops and glucagon is released. This hormone activates an intracellular signaling pathway that results in inhibition of genes involved in glucose metabolism and fatty

acid synthesis and stimulation of genes involved in gluconeogenesis (e.g., phosphenolpyruvate carboxykinase). Taken as a whole, macronutrient availability regulates the expression of the complex set of genes responsible for macronutrient metabolism by an aggregate of direct and endocrine-mediated pathways.

Nuclear Processing of mRNA

Once the bases are joined together in the nucleus to form mRNA, it is edited with a reduction in size. Through editing and processing, less than 10% of the original mRNA actually leaves the nucleus. Editing and processing are needed because immature RNA contains all those bases corresponding to the DNA introns. The removal of these introns is a cut-and-splice process whereby the intron is cut at its 5′ end, pulled out of the way, and cut again at its 3′ end. After this group of bases is excised, the bases corresponding to the DNA exons are joined. This cut-and-splice routine is continued until all the introns are removed and the exons joined. Some genes can give rise to multiple protein products since not all exons are necessarily retained in the mature mRNA. Some editing of the RNA also occurs with base substitutions made as appropriate. The mRNA is capped at the 5′ end in a process that adds a guanine base and some methyl groups. Finally, a 3′-terminal poly A tail is added and the mature mRNA is ready to leave the nucleus and move to the cytoplasm for translation. The nucleotides that have been removed during editing and processing are either reused or degraded. Some mRNA is totally degraded, never leaving the nuclear compartment. This serves to control the amount of mRNA. Regulation of the amount of mRNA that leaves the nucleus is a key step in metabolic control.

mRNA Stability

The stability of mRNA can also be regulated within the cytoplasm. Some mRNA have very short half-life (seconds to minutes), whereas others have longer half-lives (hours). This is important because some gene products (i.e., hormones and cell signals) must be short-lived and the body needs to control/counterbalance their synthesis and action. A nutritionally important example of regulation of mRNA stability involves iron and the transferrin receptor. The transferrin receptor is the protein responsible for the uptake of iron into cells. The expression of the transferrin receptor is downregulated by iron in order to limit uptake and potential toxicity of the mineral at times of high availability. This regulation is achieved through an iron regulatory protein. When iron is limited, this protein is bound to the 3′ untranslated region of the transferrin receptor mRNA. This serves to protect the mRNA from degradative attack and permits its continued translation into active protein. As iron concentrations rise, the binding protein becomes occupied with iron, which results in its dissociation from the transferrin receptor mRNA. The mRNA is then degraded more quickly, concentrations fall, and protein production is limited.

Translation

Following transcription is translation. Translation is the synthesis of the protein or peptide, the gene product. Translation occurs on the ribosomes; some ribosomes are located on the membrane of the endoplasmic reticulum and some are free in the cell matrix. Ribosomes consist of RNA and protein. Ribosomal RNA makes up a large fraction of total cellular RNA. Ribosomal RNA is synthesized via RNA polymerase I in the cell nucleus as a large molecule; there, this RNA molecule is split and leaves the nucleus as a large and a small subunit. The large ribosomal unit serves as the 'docking' point for the activated amino acids bound to the transfer RNA (tRNA). The mRNA is bound to the small ribosomal unit. The two ribosomal units reassociate in the cytosol for the translation step. tRNA is used to bring an amino acid to the large ribosome, the site of protein synthesis. Each amino acid has a specific tRNA. Each tRNA molecule is thought to have a cloverleaf arrangement of nucleotides. This arrangement allows the formation of the maximum number of hydrogen bonds between base pairs. Hydrogen bonding stabilizes the tRNA. tRNA also contains a triplet of bases that pair to a corresponding triplet found in the mRNA. This triplet is not identical to the mRNA triplet and is called the anticodon. The bases pair in a preordained manner: adenine to thymine, guanine to uracil, guanine to guanine, uracil to cytosine, inosine to adenine, and so forth. The amino acid carried by tRNA is identified by the codon of mRNA through its anticodon; the amino acid is not involved in this identification.

Translation takes place in four stages, as illustrated in **Figure 3**. Each stage requires specific cofactors and enzymes. The first stage involves the esterification of the amino acids to specific tRNAs. Each of these esterification reactions requires a molecule of ATP. Here again is an explanation of why the provision of energy is crucial to protein synthesis. If a protein contains several hundred

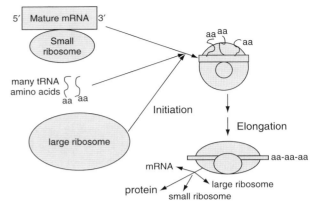

Figure 3 Schematic view of translation.

amino acids, this step in translation will require several hundred molecules of ATP. Energy-deficient diets result in a shortfall in ATP and so protein synthesis is compromised.

During the second stage of translation, polypeptide chain synthesis begins. mRNA binds to the small ribosome and an initiation complex is formed. The complex consists of the mRNA cap and the first activated amino acid–tRNA. The ribosome finds the correct reading frame on the mRNA by 'scanning' for an AUG codon. This is the so-called start codon. The large ribosomal unit then attaches and forms a functional ribosome. A number of specific protein initiation factors are involved in this step.

In the third stage of translation, the peptide chain is elongated by the sequential addition of amino acids from the amino acid–tRNA complexes. The amino acid is recognized by base pairing of the codon of mRNA to the bases found in the anticodon of tRNA, and a peptide bond is formed between the peptide chain and the newly arrived amino acid. The ribosome then moves along the mRNA; this brings the next codon into the proper position for attachment to the anticodon of the next activated amino acid–tRNA complex. The mRNA and nascent polypeptide appear to 'track' through a groove between the two ribosomal subunits. This protects the protein being synthesized from attack by enzymes in the surrounding environment.

The final stage of translation is the termination and release of the amino acid chain. The mRNA contains a stop codon that signals termination at the carboxy terminus. The carboxy-terminal amino acid, although attached to the peptide chain, is also esterified to its cognate tRNA–ribosome. A protein release factor promotes the hydrolysis of the ester link between the tRNA and the amino acid. Now the polypeptide is released from the ribosome and is free to assume its characteristic three-dimensional structure.

Translation is influenced by nutritional status as well as by specific nutrients. Protein synthesis is dependent on the simultaneous presence of all the amino acids necessary for the protein being synthesized and on the provision of energy. If there is an insufficient supply of either, protein biosynthesis will not proceed at its normal pace. This is an example of the consequences of malnutrition with respect to gene expression. Malnourished individuals will not be able to support the full range of *de novo* synthesis of body proteins because their diets are energy poor and/or contain proteins of poor quality. This condition is known as protein-energy malnutrition. It is commonly found in children but may also be observed in adults under severe food deprivation.

An example of an effect of a nutrient on translation of a specific mRNA is that of iron in the synthesis of ferritin. Iron storage in cells occurs through chelation to a protein called ferritin. Ferritin synthesis is highly regulated by iron intake. In iron deficiency, the mRNA start site for ferritin translation is obstructed by an iron regulatory protein. This protein binds to the $5'$ untranslated region and inhibits the movement of the 40s ribosome from the cap to the translation start site. When the diet contains sufficient iron and iron status is improved, the iron regulatory protein dissociates from the ferritin mRNA and translation proceeds. When iron availability is limited, the same iron regulatory protein binds to ferritin mRNA (to inhibit its translation) and to the transferrin receptor mRNA, as described previously (to prevent its degradation and ensure its translation). These exquisite mechanisms serve to maintain iron homeostasis.

Post-translational Protein Modification

After translation, the primary amino acid sequence is complete. The secondary and tertiary structure of the protein evolves via numerous interactions between amino acids via hydrogen bonding, disulfide bridges, and ionic bonds. The newly synthesized proteins can be further modified via post-translation reactions. Post-translational protein modification includes the association of various subunits of an enzyme or a carrier or a cell component. For example, the association of the four subunits that make up hemoglobin occurs after the initial synthesis of each of the subunits has occurred. Again, specific nutrients can influence the process. Another example is the post-translational carboxylation of the proteins osteocalcin and prothrombin. Osteocalcin and prothrombin each have glutamic acid-rich regions that, when carboxylated, allow the protein to bind significant amounts of calcium. Calcium binding is an essential feature of the functions of each of these proteins. The post-translational carboxylation of osteocalcin and prothrombin requires vitamin K. Should vitamin K be in short supply, this carboxylation will not occur (or will occur in only a limited way) and these proteins will not be able to bind calcium. Both must bind calcium in order to function. Hence, vitamin K deficiency is characterized by prolonged blood clotting times (inadequate calcium binding by prothrombin) and poorly mineralized bone (inadequate calcium binding by osteocalcin).

Some protein modifications occur in a nutritionally dependent reversible manner. The means whereby macronutrients influence their own metabolism at the level of transcription was outlined previously. In addition, the nutritionally regulated hormones insulin and glucagon influence enzyme activity by phosphorylation/dephosphorylation

Table 1 Examples of nutrient effects on gene expression

Nutrient	Intermediary protein	Gene/gene product	Effect
Cholesterol	Sterol response element binding protein	LDL receptor	Suppresses transcription
Fatty acids	Sterol response element binding protein	Fatty acid synthase	Suppresses transcription in liver
	Peroxisome proliferator activated receptor	Fatty acid binding protein	Increases transcription
Glucose	Carbohydrate responsive factor	Pyruvate kinase, acetyl-coA carboxylase	Increases transcription in liver
Iron	Iron regulatory protein	Ferritin	Increases translation
		Transferrin receptor	Destabilizes mRNA
Vitamin A	Retinoic acid receptor	Retinoic acid receptor	Increases transcription
		Collagenase	Decreases transcription
Vitamin D	Vitamin D receptor	Calcium binding proteins	Increases transcription
Vitamin K		Prothrombin, osteocalcin	Serves as cosubstrate for the post-translational carboxylation of glutamic acid-rich regions of these proteins
Zinc	MTF-1	Metallothionein	Increases transcription

mechanisms. This allows metabolic flux to respond to nutrient availability much more rapidly than would be possible with mechanisms dependent on new protein synthesis.

There are numerous examples of specific nutrients' effects on gene expression. Some of these effects concern the transcription of genes that encode enzymes or receptors or carriers that are important to the use of that nutrient. Examples are listed in **Table 1**. Many nutrients serve more than one function with respect to gene expression. Some influence both transcription and translation, whereas others serve to enhance the transcription of one gene while suppressing the transcription of another. Nutrient–gene interactions can result in either an increase or a decrease in specific mRNA, but there may be no increase in gene product or a measurable increase in gene product function. This speaks to the complicated nature of metabolic control. Simply synthesizing more message units or more enzyme protein does not automatically result in an increase in enzyme activity, an increase in a metabolic pathway, or an increase in a metabolic product. The processes of gene expression and metabolic regulation comprise a complex web of interactions in which nutrients are major and diverse players.

See also: **Carbohydrates**: Regulation of Metabolism. **Cholesterol**: Factors Determining Blood Levels. **Fatty Acids**: Metabolism. **Folic Acid**. **Iron**. **Nutrient–Gene Interactions**: Health Implications. **Vitamin A**: Biochemistry and Physiological Role. **Vitamin K**. **Zinc**: Physiology.

Further Reading

Berdanier CD (1998) In *Advanced Nutrition: Micronutrients*. Boca Raton, FL: CRC Press.

Berdanier CD (2000) *Advanced Nutrition: Macronutrients*, 2nd edn. Boca Raton, FL: CRC Press.

Eisenstein R (2000) Iron regulatory proteins and the molecular control of mammalian iron metabolism. *Annual Review of Nutrition* 20: 627–662.

Horton JD, Goldstein JL, and Brown MS (2002) SREBPs: Activators of the complete program of cholesterol and fatty acid synthesis in the liver. *Journal of Clinical Investigation* 109: 1125–1131.

Jump DB and Clark SD (1997) Regulation of gene expression by dietary fat. *Annual Review of Nutrition* 19: 63–90.

Mangelsdorf DJ, Thummel C, Beato M *et al.* (1995) The nuclear receptor superfamily: The second decade. *Cell* 83: 835–839.

Matthews JM and Sunde M (2002) Zinc fingers—Folds for many occasions. *IUMBM Life* 6: 351–355.

Moustaid-Moussa N and Berdanier CD (eds.) (2001) *Nutrient–Gene Interactions in Health and Disease*. Boca Raton, FL: CRC Press.

Health Implications

C D Berdanier, University of Georgia, Athens GA, USA
H C Freake, University of Connecticut, Storrs, CT, USA

Food, and the nutrients it contains, has long been known to influence the health and well-being of humans. Included in the list of nutrition-related diseases that afflict humankind are the specific nutrient deficiency diseases and several of the chronic diseases, including some of the most common ones. Each of these conditions has both a nutrition component and a genetic component. With respect to the nutrient deficiency diseases, there is considerable variation in nutrient requirements since the genetics of the consumer dictates how much of each essential nutrient is needed. If the individual's requirement is met, the deficiency disease is prevented. **Table 1** lists the essential nutrients and the symptoms of the deficient state caused by inadequate intake of the nutrients. Some symptoms (i.e., anemia) characterize several different nutrient deficiency states.

In addition to the diseases that are clearly nutritionally related, many of the chronic diseases have a nutritional component. They are also influenced by genetics, and often these two factors interact so that when certain dietary behaviors are found with a susceptible genotype, the disease results. A third kind of nutrient gene interaction relevant to health occurs when dietary constituents either promote or protect against changes in DNA that result in aging or disease. Nutrients that affect the redox balance within the cell are important in this case.

Some disease states result from alterations in a single gene. Function of the gene product is compromised and the specific pathology develops. Acrodermatitis enteropathica is an example of this, in which the affected individual has impaired zinc absorption due to a mutation in the gene encoding a zinc transporter. Menkes' disease is another example; copper absorption is impaired due to an X-linked mutation in the protein needed to release absorbed copper from the enterocyte into the circulation. People with this disorder develop symptoms of copper deficiency. Single gene mutations have been identified that affect the use of a single nutrient. However, in many genetically determined instances of nutrient malabsorption or abnormal use, the situation is more complex and the disease state may develop as a result of small changes in several genes. These situations may be more common than individual

Table 1 Nutrient deficiency disorders[a]

Nutrient	Disease: signs of inadequate intake
Ascorbic acid	**Scurvy**: hyperkeratosis, congestion of the hair follicles, skin hemorrhages, conjunctival lesions, gum swelling and bleeding, peripheral neuropathy with hemorrhages into the nerve sheaths, painful joints, deformed chests in children
Thiamin	**Beriberi**: muscle tenderness and peripheral neuropathy, edema, fast pulse, high blood pressure, decreased urine volume, disorientation, memory loss, ataxia, jerky movements of the eyes
Riboflavin	Ill-defined symptoms that are not necessarily related to inadequate intake: poor growth, poor appetite, cracks in the corners of the mouth, dermatitis of the scrotum
Niacin	**Pellagra**: black, roughened skin especially in areas exposed to sunlight; insomnia; loss of appetite; sores in mouth and tongue; indigestion; diarrhea; mental confusion; nervousness; headache; apprehension; forgetfulness
Vitamin B_6	Ill-defined symptoms: poor growth, muscular weakness, fatty liver, convulsions, anemia, reproductive impairment, edema, neural degeneration, enlarged adrenal glands
Folic acid	**Anemia**; macrocytic anemia. Neural tube defects in infants are associated with inadequate folic acid intakes of the mother during the first trimester of pregnancy
Vitamin B_{12}	**Pernicious anemia**; macrocytic anemia. Also loss of peripheral nerve function
Vitamin A	**Night blindness**, poor growth and reproduction, roughened skin (keratomalacia); **xerophthalmia**, leading to blindness, anemia, reduced immune function
Vitamin D	**Rickets**; inadequate calcification of bones resulting in bone deformities
Vitamin K	Poor blood clotting
Vitamin E	Red cell fragility, increase in blood peroxides
Phosphorus	Anorexia, muscle weakness, rickets, impaired growth, bone pain
Magnesium	Muscle spasms, twitching, tremor, anorexia, nausea
Iron	**Anemia**; microcytic anemia due to low hemoglobin, fatigue, inability to concentrate
Zinc	Growth failure, hypogonadism, impaired immune function, enlarged liver and spleen, mental lethargy
Copper	**Anemia**, poor wound healing
Selenium	**Keshan disease**: fragile red blood cells, enlarged heart, cardiomyopathy, growth retardation, skeletal muscle degeneration, cataract formation
Iodine	**Goiter**: enlarged thyroid gland, poor growth, reduced metabolic rate, mental retardation if deficiency occurs in the perinatal period

[a]Some nutrients have no defined deficiency syndromes.

gene mutations. They are also much more complex and more difficult to identify.

Before discussing the different kinds of nutrient–gene interactions in detail, an outline of the kind of variability found within the human genome is presented.

DNA Variability

The DNA in the nucleus is very stable with respect to the base sequence and content. Humans are more similar than different. Variations in DNA sequence have occurred and continue to occur. DNA replication is not 100% faithful nor is DNA repair 100% accurate. Changes in the sequence of bases that comprise the individual genes and their promoter sequences occur as base substitutions, deletions, or rearrangements. Chemicals that generate free radicals can cause DNA strand breaks and a possible loss of a base. Replacement of that base can occur and the strand can be repaired. However, in some instances, the base used for the repair might not be identical to the one lost, and a base substitution will be made. If any of these changes affect the amino acid sequence of the gene product and this substitution is in a critical area that affects function, then a mutation is said to have occurred. Otherwise, the difference in base sequence is referred to as a polymorphism rather than a mutation.

The significance of a deletion or substitution of bases in the DNA of a particular gene will depend on where it occurs and what change it engenders. It may occur in a noncoding region of the DNA or be a base substitution that does not affect the amino acid sequence of the gene product. Some amino acids have more than one base triplet (codon) that dictate its use in the gene product. If the change results in a substitution of a relatively similar amino acid, the function of the protein may be conserved. Some amino acids can be replaced without affecting the secondary, tertiary, or quaternary structures of the protein (and hence its chemical and physical properties), particularly if the base substitution occurs in an area that encodes a nonactive portion of the gene product. If any of these occur there will be little discernable effect on the gene product. The resultant gene product retains its premutation function but has a slightly different amino acid sequence. Polymorphisms in DNA, particularly mitochondrial DNA, are useful tools because they allow scientists to genetically identify individuals and their relatives and also allow population geneticists to track mutation and evolutionary events through related family members. Particularly useful in this respect are the polymorphisms in mitochondrial DNA. Anthropologists use this information to track population shifts that have occurred over time.

The amino acid sequence within a given species for a given protein is usually similar. However, some individual variation does occur. Examples of 'acceptable' amino acid substitutions are those that account for the species differences in the amino acid sequence of the hormone insulin. As a hormone, it serves a variety of important functions in the regulation of carbohydrate, lipid, and protein metabolism. However, even though there are species differences in the amino acid sequence of this protein, insulin from one species can be given to another species and be functionally active. Obviously, the species differences in the amino acid sequence of this protein are not at locations in the insulin molecule that determine its biological function in promoting glucose use.

Whether the substitution of one amino acid for another affects the functionality of the protein being generated depends entirely on the amino acid in question. An example of potentially important changes in sequence involves three related proteins important to energy balance regulation—the uncoupling proteins (UCPs) 1, 2, and 3. The UCPs function to uncouple the synthesis of ATP from the synthesis of water in the mitochondrial compartment. If UCPs are present, the cell makes less ATP and releases more energy as heat (thermogenesis), thereby decreasing energetic efficiency. If one or more UCPs are absent or nonfunctional due to a mutation(s) in the codes for these proteins, the reverse occurs. More energy is trapped in the high-energy bond of ATP, and this energy is subsequently transferred to synthetic reactions that produce storage energy products: fats and glycogen. With a decrease in energy wastage by the mitochondria, excess fat accumulates. For whatever reason, the individual is unable to produce or release one or more of the UCPs, and fuel metabolism and energy balance are adversely affected. The individual may not be able to rapidly adjust to changes in the environment, such as a dramatic decrease in environmental temperature. This is an example of a nutrient–gene interaction that is part of a disease process, in this case obesity. However, it is not a single nutrient but all energy-containing nutrients—carbohydrates, fats, and proteins—that play a role in obesity development. If the individual does not have access to a plentiful food supply, the obesity phenotype may not be apparent.

Genetics Affects Nutrient Requirements

There are many examples of nutrient requirements being influenced by genetic background. For example, in the early years of determining the human need for vitamin C, human studies showed that there could be large individual differences in the need for this essential vitamin. In addition to genetic variability, vitamin C need was increased in smokers versus nonsmokers and in people with diabetes compared to people without this disease. Similar observations have been reported for vitamin A. A rare but quite profound example of genetically determined differences in nutrient need is that of vitamin D-resistant rickets. Vitamin D constitutes part of an endocrine system within the body that allows calcium absorption to be adjusted to need. Among other actions, it is responsible for stimulating calcium uptake in the small intestine. It works through a protein, the vitamin D receptor (VDR), that, in association with the activated form of the vitamin, stimulates the transcription of genes associated with calcium transport. The VDR gene is subject to mutation, like all other genes. These can affect function, but since there are two alleles for each gene, one inherited from each parent, even those carrying a mutated gene can usually maintain calcium homeostasis using half the complement of receptors. However, if both parents carry an allele for the mutation, their child may inherit two copies of the mutated VDR genes and vitamin D would not therefore stimulate the transcription of the calcium transport proteins. These children would develop a severe form of rickets that would be vitamin D resistant. This is a rare event. These children can be treated with calcium, but they have a requirement for vitamin D that can never be satisfied.

There is another genetic condition, vitamin D-dependent rickets, in which the affected gene is not the VDR but rather an enzyme required for the activation of vitamin D. The receptor is fully functional, but affected individuals are unable to metabolize vitamin D to its active form. In this case, treatment with vitamin D is possible, giving the active form of the vitamin rather than the precursor form normally found in food. Both kinds of rickets are rare but provide a clear example of the influence of genetic background on nutrient function.

A more common example may be found with folate. Folate deficiency in some prepregnant and pregnant women can result in an infant with a condition known as spina bifida. Hydrocephaly can also result. This is a neural tube defect in which the bony covering of the spinal column is incomplete. The defect occurs early in embryonic development when the cells are differentiating into specific cell types. Folate plays an important role in this differentiation, and in some women (not all) an insufficient intake of folate just before pregnancy and in the early weeks of pregnancy can result in these neural tube defects. It was estimated that 2500 infants per year were born with this problem. As a prevention measure, foods are now fortified with the vitamin. However, many women with very low intakes of folate give birth to healthy infants. It appears likely that some women have an enhanced requirement for folate, and it is the infants of these women who are at risk. Although the specific gene mutations are not clear, a number of candidate genes involved in folate metabolism and transport have been identified.

Another example is hemochromatosis (HH). This is a disorder resulting from unregulated absorption of iron. Usually, iron absorption is downregulated when stores are adequate, but this does not occur with HH and toxic levels build up. The condition is caused by a mutation in the *HFE* gene. Although mutation of both alleles of the gene is rare, it has been estimated that 10% of some population groups may be heterozygous carriers. This is important because enhanced iron absorption is found in heterozygotes and results in liver disease, diabetes, and other chronic conditions. For many individuals and populations, a lack of dietary iron and its association with a host of iron deficiency disorders are concerns. However, individuals with HH need to limit iron intake; thus, information about genotype is clearly useful.

It is interesting to note that for some genes involved in nutrient function, no clinical syndromes linked to their mutation or deletion have been described. A possible explanation for this comes from experimental work with mice, in which gene function is typically investigated using gene deletion studies. MTF-1 is a transcription factor that regulates genes in response to zinc availability. Knock-out of the *MTF-1* gene is embryonically lethal (i.e., no offspring develop in the absence of this gene). Thus, mutations or deletions of genes that play a key role in embryonic development will not be seen in adults.

The examples given previously demonstrate a general principle that holds true for all nutrients: There is a variation in requirement that depends on genetic background. This may result from alterations in a single gene, but perhaps more likely it is due to the aggregate effect of differences in many genes that encode products relevant to that nutrient's function. As the human genome becomes better annotated and the significance of sequence differences better understood, it will be possible to make more precise recommendations for nutrient intakes for both individuals and populations.

Nutrient–Gene Interactions in Chronic Disease

A further refinement for recommended nutrient intakes is to include consideration of the relationship of one or more nutrients to the development of chronic disease. Many chronic diseases are the result of an interaction between the genetic heritage or genotype of the individual and the lifestyle choices that individual makes. Conditions such as heart disease, diabetes mellitus, and obesity are in this category. There are also a number of genetic conditions that can be managed by diet. One of the most common of these is lactose intolerance. Approximately 75–80% of the adult population in the world today is lactose intolerant. That is, they cannot consume quantities of milk and some milk products without experiencing gastrointestinal distress. **Table 2** lists some genetic disorders that are amenable to dietary management. There are also some relatively rare genetic diseases that affect genes involved in key nutritionally relevant biological processes. For example, mutations in the gene encoding the low-density lipoprotein receptor can impair the ability of the liver to clear cholesterol from the circulation. If cholesterol in the circulation cannot be removed by the liver, it can accumulate in the blood and perhaps lead to cardiovascular disease.

Many of the major chronic diseases (i.e., heart disease, cancer, stroke, diabetes, and obesity) have identifiable genetic linkages that are nutritionally responsive. That is, if an individual carries one or more gene messages that predispose that individual to one of these diseases, nutrient intake can affect the time course and appearance of the disease. For example, more than 150 mutations have been identified that associate with the development of

Table 2 Genetic disorders amenable to dietary management

Disorder	Nutrition strategy
Acrodermatitis enteropathica	Increase zinc intake
Fructosemia	Avoid fructose-containing foods
Galactosemia	Avoid lactose-containing foods
Hereditary hemochromatosis	Limit iron intake
Lactase deficiency	Avoid lactose-containing foods (milk and milk products)
Methylmalonuria	Vitamin B_{12} injections
Obesity (some forms)	Consume only enough energy to meet energy need; increase energy output (exercise)
Phenylketonuria	Control phenylalanine intake such that the need for this amino acid is met but that no surplus is consumed
Sucrase deficiency	Avoid sucrose-containing foods

diabetes. The phenotypic expression (the development of diabetes) of some of these genotypes can be influenced by diet. Numerous mutations, especially in the genes for the lipid-carrying proteins, have been identified as being associated with heart disease. These too may be nutrient responsive, but the details of this responsiveness are not known. Still other mutations have been found that associate with the development of obesity or with one or more of the diseases generically referred to as cancer. Again, the details of nutrient–gene expression in these diseases are lacking.

Although many genetic signatures have been associated with specific diseases, not all people who have these genetic characteristics develop the associated disease. This suggests that not only must one have the genetic characteristic but also one must provide the environment for the disease to flourish. An example of this was reported in the early 1960s. Newly arrived Yemenite Jews and Yemenite Jews who had resided in Israel for at least 20 years were compared with respect to diet, lifestyle, and the prevalence of type 2 diabetes. The newly arrived immigrants had very little diabetes, whereas the established Yemenite Jews had as much diabetes in their population as in the Israeli Jewish populations from other areas of the world. The diets and lifestyles of these population groups were compared to a matched group of Arabs living in the same locations in Israel. The diets were not greatly different among the groups, but the disease was far more prevalent in the Jews than in the Arabs. Studies of the diet consumed by the Jews in Yemen versus that in Israel revealed that there were very few differences with one exception: In Yemen very little refined carbohydrate was consumed. Sugar was not readily available, and what was available was very expensive. Once the Yemenites settled in Israel and adopted the Israeli diet with its abundance of refined carbohydrates, type 2 diabetes began to appear. It was suggested that the change in diabetes prevalence in the Yemenite group was due to an interaction between their genetic heritage and their increased consumption of refined carbohydrate. This report was the first to suggest such an interaction.

As mentioned previously, more than 150 mutations associate with diabetes mellitus, but the presence of one or more of these mutations does not necessarily mean that the person will become a diabetic. Diabetologists have acknowledged that there are far more people with a diabetes genotype than with a diabetes phenotype. That many of the diabetes phenotypes take so many years to develop suggests that given the appropriate lifestyle choices, the phenotype may never develop; however, it may

develop very rapidly if poor lifestyle choices are made. In support of this argument, one has only to examine the numbers of new cases of diabetes in times of abundant food supplies and in times of food restriction. During World War II when food was rationed (as was gasoline for automobiles), people ate less and were more active. During this period, the number of new cases of type 2 diabetes declined. The number of new cases of type 1 diabetes (autoimmune diabetes or insulin-dependent diabetes) remained fairly constant. Because food was rationed and activity was increased, fewer people had excess fat stores, and this was probably a contributing factor to the decrease in diabetes development. When food became abundant after the war, food intake again was unrestricted, and over time the prevalence of both diabetes and obesity increased.

Some forms of diabetes and obesity share a genotype that phenotypes as obesity/diabetes, called 'diabesity.' As with the group of diseases called diabetes, obesity has a number of mutations that associate with it. The expression of these genotypes depends largely on whether sufficient food is available and consumed to make possible the phenotypic expression of the obesity genotype. Several of these mutations affect food intake regulation and thus energy balance. If the brain does not receive an appropriate appetite-suppressing signal, then excess energy is consumed, with the result of excess body fat stores. Excess fat stores, particularly in the adipocyte, interfere with the action of insulin in facilitating the entry of glucose into the fat cell. When this occurs, abnormal glucose metabolism (type 2 diabetes) develops. Individuals with excess fat stores can normalize their glucose metabolism if these stores are significantly reduced through food intake restriction and increased physical activity. However, not all instances of diabesity can be resolved in this way.

Technological developments have made it easier to routinely determine the presence of polymorphisms in genes associated with the development of diseases. Given the significance of cardiovascular disease and its association with lipoprotein metabolism, much effort has been focused on this area. Currently, dietary recommendations on fat intake are made for the whole population, but it appears reasonable to suppose that individual responses to a diet designed to lower plasma lipid concentrations will depend on genotype. Evidence for this comes from a G/A polymorphism in the promoter region of the gene encoding the ApoA1 lipoprotein, a major constituent of the high-density lipoprotein (HDL). The A polymorphism is less common and some studies have found an association with the possession of this form of the gene and higher HDL concentrations.

HDL is thought to be protective against heart disease. However, the association between the A polymorphism and elevated HDL is quite inconsistent. This is explained by considering diet. Women with the A polymorphism who consumed >6% of energy as polyunsaturated fatty acids (PUFA) had higher HDL cholesterol concentrations than women consuming <6% dietary PUFA. In women lacking this polymorphism, no such effect of diet was seen. Thus, although women with the A polymorphism would clearly benefit from the standard recommendation for increasing dietary PUFA, those who lack it may not, at least with respect to HDL.

The extent to which individual polymorphisms determine disease risk is likely to be limited. These chronic diseases are complex and outcome is likely to depend on polymorphisms in a number of genes and their interactions with dietary as well as other lifestyle factors. However, as technology improves and more polymorphisms are identified, an aggregate picture of risk will develop that will allow much more refined and specific dietary recommendations to be made. Knowing that these conditions are influenced by lifestyle choices, the identification of susceptible individuals should enable the design of effective strategies to delay disease development. It may not be possible to eliminate the problem, but it may be possible to appreciably delay its onset.

Nutrition Influences Mutation Risk

Although parents largely determine one's genotype, DNA is always subject to mutation. A few or many bases can be destroyed by free radicals, for example, leaving the cell unable to produce a given protein. In turn, this affects the function of the cell. It should be noted that a single affected cell does not represent a lethal event, except for that particular cell. It becomes a problem when many cells have their DNA damaged in the same way and the loss of cell function is significant. In most instances, DNA repair will occur so well that there is little noticeable effect of the initial insult. However, over time, mismatch repair or cumulative assaults on the DNA can have cumulative effects on DNA and cellular function. This cumulative effect of assault has been suggested to explain aging. Aging as a result of cumulative effects of free radical attack on DNA as well as on the vulnerable membranes within and around the cell has been used to explain the gradual loss in cellular function that occurs with age.

Nutrients that protect cells against free radical attack are additional examples of nutrient–gene interactions in health and disease. Such nutrients as vitamin E, ascorbic acid, carotene (vitamin A),

Table 3 Nutrients that have a role in free radical protection

Nutrient	Role
Vitamin E	Quenches free radicals as they form via the conversion of tocopherol to tocopheroxyl radical, which is then converted to a quinone
Vitamin K	Serves as a H^+/e^- donor/acceptor
Carotene	Serves as a H^+/e^- donor acceptor (precursor of vitamin A)
Ascorbic acid	Serves as a H^+/e^- donor acceptor; copper is used as well
Selenium	Incorporated as selenocysteine into glutathione peroxidase
Copper, zinc	Essential cofactors for cytosolic superoxide dismutase
Manganese	Essential cofactor for mitochondrial superoxide dismutase

selenium, and others serve to suppress free radical formation or to promote the synthesis of enzymes that function in the free radical suppression system. **Table 3** lists nutrients and their roles in free radical protection.

Whereas the nucleus has a very efficient DNA repair process, the mitochondrion does not. However, there is only one nucleus in each cell, whereas there are many mitochondria in that same cell. If one or two are damaged, there are many in the cell to compensate. Disease develops only when damage occurs to a large majority of the mitochondria. A certain threshold of damage must be reached for such damage to have a physiological effect. Again, nutrients that function as free radical suppressants or that enhance the synthesis of enzymes of the free radical suppression system function to protect mitochondria from free radical damage. In the nucleus, the DNA is protected from free radical attack by histone and nonhistone proteins. Histones are highly basic proteins varying in molecular weight from ~11 000 to ~21 000. The histones keep the DNA in a very compact form. In contrast, the mitochondrial DNA does not have this protective histone coat. It is 'naked' and much more vulnerable to damage. In addition, ~90% of oxygen free radicals are generated in the mitochondria, providing the means for such damage should the enzyme superoxide dismutase, a manganese-dependent enzyme found in this compartment, not suppress these radicals. The damage can be quite severe, but because each mitochondrion contains 8–10 copies of its genome and there are many mitochondria in each cell (up to 2000), the effects of this damage may not be apparent. There is another superoxide dismutase found in the cytosol that has a similar function. It is a copper/zinc-dependent enzyme. Again, note the dependence of function on particular nutrients (manganese, zinc, and copper) that in turn have effects on gene expression in health and disease.

Another way that changing DNA in a single cell can profoundly affect the health of the whole organism involves cancer. In this case, the DNA changes occur in particular genes related to the growth regulatory properties of the cell. Normal homeostatic mechanisms fail and the individual cell multiplies rapidly and therefore has a widespread influence. Nutrition interacts with cancer in a number of ways. It can promote or prevent the initiating mutation. It also will influence the progression of cancer by providing the nutrients required for its growth. The cancer often ultimately influences nutrition by limiting food intake. Another level of complexity is added with chemo- and radiotherapies and their interactions with nutrition.

Throughout this article, examples have been given that illustrate the interactions that occur between nutrients and genes. The ultimate goal of understanding such interactions is to use our knowledge to enhance the expression of genes that sustain good health while suppressing the expression of genes associated with disease. Although it is currently not possible to identify individuals with genetic dispositions to chronic diseases, there is no doubt that such screening tests will be developed and will be used as a basis for recommending nutrient (food) intakes. Optimizing health, after all, is the ultimate goal of good nutrition.

See also: **Aging**. **Antioxidants**: Diet and Antioxidant Defense. **Cancer**: Epidemiology and Associations Between Diet and Cancer; Effects of Nutritional Status. **Children**: Nutritional Problems. **Coronary Heart Disease**: Hemostatic Factors; Lipid Theory; Prevention. **Diabetes Mellitus**: Etiology and Epidemiology.

Folic Acid. **Hyperlipidemia**: Overview. **Inborn Errors of Metabolism**: Classification and Biochemical Aspects. **Iron**. **Lactose Intolerance**. **Nutrient–Gene Interactions**: Molecular Aspects. **Obesity**: Definition, Etiology and Assessment. **Vitamin D**: Rickets and Osteomalacia. **Zinc**: Physiology; Deficiency in Developing Countries, Intervention Studies.

Further Reading

Acworth IN and Bailey B (1995) *Handbook of Oxidative Metabolism*. Chelmsford, MA: ESA.

Berdanier CD (1998) *Advanced Nutrition: Micronutrients*. Boca Raton, FL: CRC Press.

Krauss RM (2001) Dietary and genetic effects on low-density lipoprotein heterogeneity. *Annual Review of Nutrition* 21: 283–295.

Malloy PJ and Feldman D (1999) Vitamin D resistance. *American Journal of Medicine* 106: 355–370.

Moustaid-Moussa N and Berdanier CD (eds.) (2001) *Nutrient–Gene Interactions in Health and Disease*. Boca Raton, FL: CRC Press.

Moyers S and Bailey LB (2001) Fetal malformations and folate metabolism: Review of recent evidence. *Nutrition Reviews* 59(7): 215–224.

Ordovas JM (2002) Gene–diet interaction and plasma lipid responses to dietary intervention. *Biochemical Society Transactions* 30: 68–73.

Pietrangelo A (2002) Physiology of iron transport and the hemochromatosis gene. *American Journal of Physiology: Gastrointestinal and Liver Physiology* 282: G403–G414.

Strachen T and Read AP (1996) *Human Molecular Genetics*. New York: Wiley–Liss.

Tolstoi LG (2000) Adult-type lactase deficiency. *Nutrition Today* 35: 134–141.

Wei Y-H and Lee H-C (2002) Oxidative stress, mitochondrial DNA mutation, and impairment of antioxidant enzymes in aging. *Experimental Biology and Medicine* 227: 671–682.

Zeisel SH, Allen LH, Coburn SP *et al.* (2001) Nutrition: A reservoir for integrative science. *Journal of Nutrition* 131: 1319–1321.

NUTRIENT REQUIREMENTS, INTERNATIONAL PERSPECTIVES

A A Yates, ENVIRON Health Sciences, Arlington, VA, USA

Determining human requirements for nutrients has been a major activity for nutritionists, biochemists, and physiologists for the past 100 years since the advent of methods that have allowed for their isolation, quantification in food, and determination of their function in cell and whole body metabolism. Whereas initial efforts focused on identifying constituents in food required to maintain life and promote growth and thus were considered essential or indispensable, research during the past 60 years has become increasingly focused on elucidating the specific roles each nutrient plays in health and quantifying, through experimentation and study of healthy populations, the amounts needed on a daily basis to provide for optimal health and prevent disease. This process of estimating requirements for an individual with any level of precision is still in the early stages of development. Nevertheless, many facets of maintaining and improving the health of the public hinge on knowing how much is needed of which nutrients or chemical components of food, and how this differs at different stages of growth and development.

Multiple terms have been adopted to define nutrient requirements, allowances, or standards (**Table 1**). They have been established or adopted by various countries and then used for the major functions of planning food programs or assessing diets for adequacy or excess (**Figure 1**). Major efforts during the past two decades by nutrition scientists throughout the world have resulted in a shift from establishing and periodically revising nutrient allowances or recommendations based on general consensus of adequate levels (e.g., the Recommended Dietary Allowances (RDAs) of the Food and Nutrition Board in the United States, the Recommended Nutrient Intakes (RNIs) of Canada, or the Safe Levels of Intake derived by the expert groups convened by the World Health Organization and Food and Agriculture Organization of the United Nations) to more definitively anchoring the reference values to specific, well-described scientific studies so that when new information becomes available from research, it is clear that new evaluations need to be undertaken. For example, in the past, the RDAs in the United States have been used as the reference values in many situations, from setting the standards for nutrient content in programs that provide single meals, such as in school lunch programs, to the basis for government reimbursement for costs of care in skilled nursing homes (**Table 2**). It is not surprising that one reference value or number, even when adjusted for age or body size and based on scientific studies, is at times not appropriate for the situation in which it is used.

What Is a Nutrient?

The traditional approach to establishing the human essentiality of a nutrient is to show that it can be chemically isolated from foods and can improve or remove a deficiency sign resulting from its lack in the diet. The number of required nutrients defined in this way has increased over the years (**Table 3**).

During the past two decades, as a result of scientific inquiry and experimentation, the line between nutrients that might be considered essential versus nonessential has blurred. There are few new chemicals in foods or food components that, when identified, have been shown to cause severe dysfunction or death when removed from the diet in a similar manner to many of those listed in **Table 3**. However, many chemical constituents of food do contribute to health; current controversy focuses on whether such substances should be considered nutrients. The major difference with the use of modern scientific techniques is the ability now to detect finer gradations of inadequacy so that with some newer constituents the end result is not necessarily death or severe organ dysfunction but decline in health status or ability to function optimally. It could be said that there is merely a longer latency period than with typical nutrient deficiencies or excesses before the effect becomes manifest; such a situation may well characterize the typical diet-related chronic disease. An example of this is the role of vitamin E in decreasing onset of cardiovascular disease: Demonstrated to be effective in animal studies, large-scale studies in humans have so far not documented the expected positive effects on primary prevention of the specific chronic disease.

Groups throughout the world have come to define health as not just the absence of overt disease, such as nutrient deficiency diseases like pellagra (inadequate vitamin B_6) or goiter (inadequate iodine), but also a level of reserve to protect against stress, either environmental or self-induced, and preventive in nature rather than therapeutic. In 1946, the World Health Organization defined health as follows: "Health is a state of complete physical, mental, and social well-being and not merely the absence of disease or infirmity."

Scientific Basis for Establishing Recommended Intakes

Since the initial development of quantitative recommended intakes of nutrients in the 1930s and 1940s, new approaches have provided a stronger science base to the reference values so established. Early development of recommended intakes usually involved convening a group of scientists who considered the available literature and, based on their expert judgment, developed quantitative estimates of requirements for specific subpopulation groups, including by age and gender. Newer statistically supported methods allow for a more science-based approach to such deliberations and consensus.

Table 1 Definitions of reference nutrient values used by selected countries and groups

AI: Adequate Intake

Canada and the United States (1997–present): A value based on experimentally derived intake levels or approximations of observed mean nutrient intakes by a group (or groups) of healthy people. The AI for children and adults is expected to meet or exceed the amount needed to maintain a defined nutrition state or criterion of adequacy in essentially all members of a specific apparently healthy population.

The Netherlands (2000–present): An amount of the nutrient that provides for the needs of almost all those in the group.

DRI: Dietary Reference Intake

United States and Canada: A set of nutrient-based reference values, each of which has special uses.

DRV: Dietary Reference Value

United Kingdom: A term used to cover LRNI, EAR, RNI, and safe intake.

EAR: Estimated Average Requirement

United Kingdom: The required intake of a group of people for energy, protein, a vitamin, or a mineral. About half will usually need more than the EAR and half less.

United States: The daily intake value that is estimated to meet the requirement, as defined by the specified indicator or criterion of adequacy, of half of the apparently healthy individuals in a life stage or gender group.

LRNI: Lower Reference Nutrient Intake

United Kingdom: An amount of the nutrient that is enough for only the few people in a group who have low needs.

RDNI: Recommended Daily Nutrient Intake

Nordic countries: The average nutrient intake that meets the requirement needs of 50% of a group. The remaining 50% of the group will have requirements above the RDNI.

RNI: Recommended Nutrient Intake (formerly in Canada); Reference Nutrient Intake (United Kingdom)

Canada (prior to 1997): The recommended intakes of essential nutrients.

United Kingdom: An amount of the nutrient that is enough, or more than enough, for about 97% of people in a group. If average intake of a group is at the RNI, then the risk of deficiency in the group is small.

PRI: Population Reference Intake

Belgium and European Community: The intake that is enough for virtually all healthy people within a group.

RDA: Recommended Dietary Allowance

United States (prior to 1997): The intake that meets the nutrient needs of 97 to 98% of a group.

Canada and the United States (1997–present): The average daily dietary intake level that is sufficient to meet the nutrient requirements of nearly all (97–98%) healthy individuals in a particular life stage and gender group.

The Netherlands (since 2000): The mean requirement plus twice the standard deviation of the requirement (defined as the smallest intake of a nutrient that both prevents symptoms of deficiency and at which, at the same time, the risk of chronic diseases—to the extent that this is influenced by the nutrient concerned—is minimal, and is thus sufficient for almost all people in a group).

SUL: Safe Upper Level

United Kingdom: An intake level that can be consumed daily over a lifetime without significant risk to health on the basis of available evidence.

UL: Tolerable Upper Intake Level

Canada and the United States (1997–present): Highest level of daily nutrient intake that is likely to pose no risk of adverse health effects for almost all apparently healthy individuals in the specified life stage group. As intake increases above the UL, the potential risk of adverse effects may increase.

European Community (2000–present): The maximum level of total chronic intake of a nutrient (from all sources) judged to be unlikely to pose a risk of adverse health effects to humans.

The Netherlands (2000–present): Intake level above which there is a risk of adverse effects.

Sources: Committee on Medical Aspects of Food Policy (1991) *Dietary Reference Values for Food Energy and Nutrients in the United Kingdom*, Report on Health and Social Subjects No. 41. London: HMSO.

Food Standards Agency, Expert Group on Vitamins and Minerals (2003) *Safe Upper Levels for Vitamins and Minerals*. London: HMSO.

Health Council of the Netherlands (2001) *Health Council of the Netherlands; Reports 2000*, Publication No. A2001/01, pp. 53–54. The Hague: Health Council of the Netherlands.

Institute of Medicine, Standing Committee on the Scientific Evaluation of Dietary Reference Intakes, Food and Nutrition Board (1997) *Dietary Reference Intakes for Calcium, Phosphorus, Magnesium, Vitamin D, and Fluoride*. Washington, DC: National Academy Press.

Institute of Medicine, Subcommittee on Upper Reference Levels of Nutrients and the Standing Committee on the Scientific Evaluation of Dietary Reference Intakes, Food and Nutrition Board (1998) *Dietary Reference Intakes: A Risk Assessment Model for Establishing Upper Intake Levels for Nutrients*. Washington, DC: National Academy Press.

Institute of Medicine, Subcommittee on Interpretation and Uses of Dietary Reference Intakes and the Standing Committee on the Scientific Evaluation of Dietary Reference Intakes, Food and Nutrition Board (2003) *Dietary Reference Intakes: Applications in Dietary Planning*. Washington, DC: National Academies Press.

European Commission, Scientific Committee on Food, Health and Consumer Protection Directorate-General (2000) *Guidelines of the Scientific Committee on Food for the Development of Tolerable Upper Intake Levels for Vitamins and Minerals*, SCF/CS/NUT/UPPLEV/11 Final, 28 November.

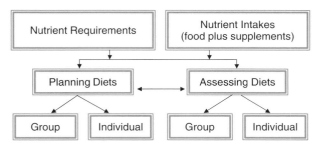

Figure 1 Uses of reference intakes in planning and assessing diets.

Table 2 Pre-1997 uses of RDAs in the United States

Planning for feeding groups of healthy people (school lunch, elderly feeding programs)

Nutrient goals for healthy individuals

Basics for foods provided in supplemental feeding programs (e.g., WIC)

Procurement of and purchasing food supplies for groups of healthy people

Reference point for evaluating the dietary intake of population subgroups

Nutrient intake targets in intervention programs

Basis of food groups in food and nutrition education programs

Reference point for the nutrition labeling of food and dietary supplements

Basis for fortification of food products

Basis for formulating dietary supplements and special dietary foods

Standards for menu planning for hospitals, correctional facilities, military operations, and other institutional feeding settings

Table 3 Nutrients for which RDAs and recommended intakes or ranges (in parentheses) have been established since 1941

Nutrient	1941	1989	1997–2004
Calories	X	X	X
Protein	X	X	X
Calcium	X	X	X
Iron	X	X	X
Vitamin A	X	X	X
Thiamin	X	X	X
Riboflavin	X	X	X
Niacin	X	X	X
Vitamin C	X	X	X
Vitamin D	X	X	X
Vitamin E		X	X
Vitamin K		X	X
Vitamin B_6		X	X
Vitamin B_1		X	X
Folate		X	X
Pantothenic acid		(X)	X
Biotin		(X)	X
Choline			X
Chromium		(X)	X
Copper		(X)	X
Fluoride		(X)	X
Iodine		X	X
Magnesium		X	X
Manganese		(X)	X
Molybdenum		(X)	X
Phosphorus		X	X
Selenium		X	X
Zinc		X	X
Potassium		(X)	X
Sodium			X
Chloride			X
Total water			X
Carbohydrate			X
Total fiber			X
Linoleic acid (n-6)			X
α-Linolenic acid (n-3)			X

From the Food and Nutrition Board, US National Research Council, Institute of Medicine.

A number of factors must be present before quantitative requirements for nutrients can be made most useful to those who use such estimates for program planning and evaluation:

- There must be some understanding of the chemical. For example, in early work on vitamins, an isolated fraction of cod liver oil was determined to be required for normal eye growth and bone development and was named 'vitamin A.' Subsequent isolation and characterization allowed the isolated mixture to be further separated into what was called the fat-soluble factor for bone growth compared to another required for sight. Thus, vitamin A was differentiated from vitamin D in the lipid-soluble fraction.

- There must be data on how much is present in the diet. In order to obtain these data, the content of the nutrient or food component in multiple typical foods must be analyzed, which thus allows the data to be used to estimate intake or exposure.

- There should be some idea of intake among the population groups of interest. Studies in which known amounts of a nutrient are consumed at varying levels and evidence of inadequacy

detected should be conducted. This is typically done first with animal models, followed by human clinical trials or metabolic studies, which include at least one level of intake at which effects of inadequacy are observed and can be linked directly to the nutrient under study. Frequently, it is not possible to remove or add some nutrients to a diet without altering the content of other nutrients; this is particularly true for energy-yielding nutrients, such as omega-3 fatty acids, or substances such as fiber. This makes the interpretation of the resulting data less clear.

Adequate for What?

Usually, once these data are known or have been estimated, it becomes possible to establish an intake recommendation, initially based on observations of how much appears to prevent the deficiency and how much is in the diet of those not demonstrating the symptoms or signs (indicators) of inadequacy. Many of the earlier recommended intakes were established on this basis, which is why, in many cases, the values may vary greatly across expert groups and countries. As additional data derived from experiments, observations of intake, and consequences of inadequacy of a nutrient in the diet are generated, there is a need for periodic updates of nutrient requirements and recommended intakes (**Table 4**). Changing recommendations may result in the need to make changes in programs and activities, such as food labeling, and thus frequently represent new costs. Of great importance from a scientific perspective is an overt statement of the goal of the derived reference value: Will the reference value provide guidance for minimizing overt deficiencies, usually by providing enough to prevent a known deficiency sign or symptom, or is it set at a dietary level required to maintain a blood concentration or function that might represent storage or a reserve and thus be available in times of stress?

For example, the prevention of scorbutic gums, one of the signs of overt vitamin C deficiency, requires far less vitamin C on a daily basis than the amount needed to maintain 70% saturation of white blood cell ascorbate (vitamin C) levels to counteract potential oxidative stress and damage at the cellular level. Generally, for a nutrient there exists a growing list of possible indicators or outcomes that could be used to estimate requirements (**Table 5**), and for each, a different amount may be needed daily for the specific indicator to meet the body's need and thus demonstrate adequacy.

There is usually a continuum of benefits that occur as the level of intake increases. It becomes very important to define what the criterion(ia) is that has been used to establish the quantitative level of intake recommended. **Figure 2** shows data relating iron intake to three possible criteria or indicators that could be used to determine adequate intakes for women in a national survey in The Netherlands and analyzed by George Beaton. The data show that as the level of iron intake decreases, the number of individuals (or percentage of the population group of women in this age group) who would have their needs met as documented by a given indicator of adequacy decreases. Thus, if prevention of anemia is used as the criterion (in this case, hemoglobin value $<110\,g/l$), an individual whose intake averaged 6 mg/day would have a 40% probability that she would be inadequate (i.e., her hemoglobin value would be below the cutoff). However, if a biochemical marker of function of iron (e.g., total iron binding capacity) were used, the level of intake needed for a 40% probability of being inadequate using that criterion would be approximately 9 mg/day. Finally, if the goal were to maintain a level of storage, such as ferritin concentration, the dietary level would need to approximate 18 or 19 mg/day. Thus, when comparing recommended

Table 4 Changing US recommendations for nutrients: RDAs for vitamins (adult males, moderately active)

Vitamin	1941	1943	1945	1948	1953	1958	1968	1976	1980	1989	1997–2001
Vitamin A (mg RE)	1000	1000	1000	1000	1000	1000	1000	1000	1000	1000	900[c,d]
Vitamin D	400 IU[a]	400 IU[a]	[b]	[b]	[b]	[b]	400 IU	400 IU	5 μg	5 μg	5 μg[d]
Vitamin E							30 IU	15 IU	10 IU	10 mg	15 mg[e]
Vitamin K (μg)										80	120[d]
Vitamin C (mg)	75	75	75	75	75	75	60	45	60	60	90
Thiamin (mg)	1.8	1.8	1.5	1.5	1.5	1.6	1.3	1.4	1.4	1.5	1.2
Riboflavin (mg)	2.7	2.7	2.0	1.8	1.6	1.8	1.7	1.6	1.6	1.7	1.3
Niacin (mg)	18	18	15	15	15	21	17	18	18	19	16
Vitamin B_6 (mg)							1–2[f]	2.0	2.0	2.2	2.0	1.3
Pantothenic acid (mg)										4–7[f]	5[d]
Biotin (mg)										0.03–0.1[f]	0.03[d]
Folate (μg)						500[f]	400	400	400	200	400[g]
Vitamin B_{12} (μg)							3.0	3.0	5.0	2.0	2.4

[a]When not exposed to sunshine (400 IU ≈ 10 μg).
[b]Small amount needed when not exposed to sunshine.
[c]Unit changed from RE (Retinol Equivalent) to RAE (Retinol Activity Equivalent).
[d]Adequate Intake (AI), not RDA.
[e]As α-tocopherol only.
[f]Estimate or range, no recommendation made.
[g]As Dietary Folate Equivalents (DFE).
From the Food and Nutrition Board, US National Research Council/Institute of Medicine.

Table 5 Possible indicators or criteria to evaluate adequacy of iron intakes

Erythrocyte indexes
Erythrocyte protoporphyrin levels
Factorial modeling
Hemoglobin concentration and hematocrit
Iron balance studies[a]
Plasma total iron binding capacity
Serum ferritin concentration
Soluble serum transferrin receptor levels
Serum transferrin saturation

[a]Balance studies measure or estimate total excretion of a nutrient at different levels of intake and determine the lowest level of intake at which intake = excretion.

intakes, it is critical to know specifically the criterion or criteria used in setting the recommended intake and evaluating adequacy.

Role of Estimates of Average (Median) Requirements

For many of the uses given for reference values, it becomes important statistically to not depend on an allowance that would cover the needs of everyone and thus might include a safety factor added to some adequate level of intake but, rather, to apply estimates of the average requirement for the group of interest. For most nutrients, with iron a notable exception, it can be assumed that nutrient requirements are symmetrically distributed in a population of similar people (**Figure 3**), which means that some will have higher requirements than other similar individuals due to genetics and other factors, and that a median requirement intake level can be determined, such that consumption of a nutrient at that level would be adequate for half of the individuals in the group but inadequate for the other half. If this

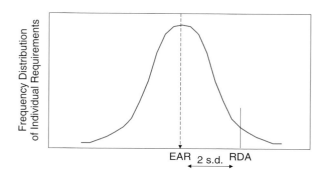

Figure 3 Probability distribution of individual nutrient requirements.

distribution of requirements is symmetrical, then the median and the mean requirement are the same.

Why have an Estimated Average Requirement? There are two main reasons to have an Estimated Average Requirement (EAR): to use as the basis for establishing the recommended intake for an individual and to assess the adequacy of intakes of similar population groups. The concept of establishing an average requirement, and assuming that the requirements of individuals in a population of similar people are symmetrically (or normally) distributed, is not new. Conceptually, it has served as the ideal basis for recommended intakes during the past few decades. However, it was rigorously used on only rare occasions. The RDA has been conceptually defined in the United States during the past few decades as the lowest amount of a nutrient that, in the judgment of the Food and Nutrition Board, meets the known nutritional needs of almost all of the population (subgroup), and it was also more mathematically defined as the mean requirement plus two standard deviations (SD), which would equal an amount required by 97 or 98% of the population to whom it is applied.

The Dietary Reference Intake (DRI) process—a joint effort of the United States and Canada—retained the term RDA, limiting its use to serving as the goal for intake when planning diets for individuals and standardizing the method by which it is established. It is defined as follows: $RDA = EAR + 2SD_{EAR}$. When data on variation in requirements of a specific nutrient are lacking, it is assumed that the standard deviation (variation) in requirements is approximately 10%. This variation in requirements is derived from the variation seen in basal metabolic rate in individuals and the variation seen in protein requirements, with protein being the nutrient whose variability has been most studied.

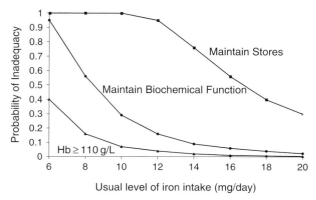

Figure 2 Probability that specified usual iron intake would be inadequate to meet the needs of a randomly selected menstruating woman. (Used with permission, G. Beaton, 1994)

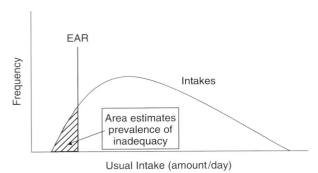

Figure 4 Using the EAR to estimate the prevalence of inadequacy in a population from the distribution of nutrient intakes.

It has been demonstrated statistically that the prevalence of inadequacy in a population whose requirements are symmetrically distributed can be estimated by comparing its intake to the EAR for that nutrient in the same (or a similar) population (**Figure 4**). Thus, in the DRI process, when evaluating vitamin C requirements, experimental data from a clinical study indicated that the average intake for men needed to achieve 70% white blood cell ascorbate saturation (the chosen indicator) was ∼75 mg/day, and the EAR was set at 75 mg/day. This is a value that can be applied to the intakes of other similar populations of men who have similar characteristics to determine the percentage of the population who may be inadequate based on this criterion of adequacy (**Figure 5**).

To use this method to assess adequacy of population groups, there are other basic statistical assumptions that should be met. First, an individual's requirement for a nutrient must be statistically independent of the intake for that nutrient (this does not hold for nutrients such as total energy or water—

people eat or drink because they know they need energy or water). Second, the amount of variation (the distribution) in the nutrient intake levels in the population group must be greater than the variation in the group of the requirements for the nutrient (this is almost always the case, except when everyone in the group consumes the same food in the same amounts—thus, there is little variability in intake). If these two assumptions are met, along with the symmetry mentioned previously, then the EAR can be used as the cut point for adequacy in other similar populations (as shown in **Figure 4**). This is called the EAR cut point method.

Because the RDA has been misused as a tool to assess adequacy of intakes of groups in the past by policymakers and scientists alike, it has been argued by some that it is better for scientific panels of experts not to provide, in addition to EARs, any recommended intakes since their only use is to provide guidance to the individual, and health professionals can easily develop recommended intakes from reference values that are average requirements. However, the concept of RDAs in the United States and RNIs in Canada has been accepted in the general population to the extent that to not provide RDAs (and, as an extension, recommended intakes such as Adequate Intakes (AIs) where data are lacking) would result in more misguided actions than would result from providing them along with instructions for their specific and only use: to plan diets for the individual.

Adequate Intake: Used when an EAR cannot be determined Whereas for many nutrients enough data exist to be able to establish levels of nutrient intake at which half of the individuals in a group would be inadequate based on the criterion chosen, for some nutrients the necessary data may be conflicting or lacking. In order to give some guidance to users of nutrient reference values, it is still necessary to provide quantitative numbers. To further differentiate the appropriate uses of the RDA, the DRI framework provides an additional category of a recommended intake for use with individuals to plan diets—termed the AI. This is a level that is considered adequate for all members of the group and thus may overestimate the needs of many, if not all. Statistically, it cannot be used as if it were an EAR to assess adequacy. It does, however, provide guidance for how much an individual should consume. In some cases, it is derived from the average intake of a population in which inadequacy appears to be nonexistent based on review of available indicators or criteria (such as is the case for vitamin K).

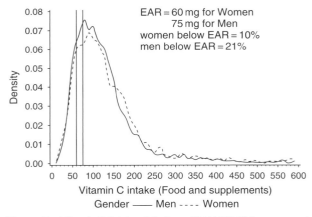

Figure 5 Vitamin C intake data from NHANES III for men and women; using the EAR to determine the expected prevalence of inadequacy.

Reference Values: Which to Use and When

As mentioned previously, there are two main uses of reference values: to assess diets for adequacy or excess and to plan diets (**Figure 1**). Although these may seem to be the same, in many ways the best reference values to use in these situations may be quite different from each other on a quantitative basis. In addition, each of these major functions is frequently applied in two different situations: to a group's intake (i.e., the intake of a population or subpopulation) or to an individual's intake.

Using DRIs to plan diets If the goal is to plan a diet or menu for a specific group so that the nutrient intake of all but a small number (e.g., 2 or 3%) in the group will have their needs met, it is not necessary for each person to consume at least the RDA; this actually overstates the need of almost all individuals. It is only necessary that the nutrient be consumed such that the intake of only 2 or 3% would be below the EAR. Thus, the goal would be to have a very low percentage of intakes below the EAR (**Figure 4**).

On the other hand, if one is planning a diet for the individual, and there is little knowledge about the individual other than his or her gender and age, then one would want to provide what is thought to be adequate for almost everyone in the group, which is the RDA—by definition set at 2 SD above the median or average requirement (EAR)—or the AI.

Using DRIs to assess diets Frequently, such as when considering whether to fortify the food supply with a specific nutrient or when evaluating the nutritional status of a subgroup in the population, it is necessary to assess the diets of groups through surveys of food intake and from such surveys determine which nutrients may be consumed at inadequate levels. If data on intakes for the group of interest are available, and the group possesses similar characteristics to the individuals studied when deriving the EARs, it is possible to estimate the prevalence of inadequacy in the group of interest from their intake data without information on their requirements or variation in intake.

This is a key reason for establishing EARs for nutrients, and it replaces the questionable past practice of comparing intakes to the RDA. Frequently when this was done, a group might appear to be at low risk of inadequacy because the mean intake of the group as a whole for a nutrient might be at or above the RDA, despite a sizable portion of the group being below their individual requirements, if they had been determined (**Figure 6**).

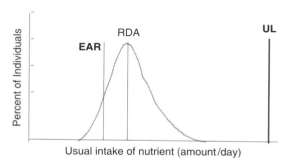

Figure 6 Example of assuming that when the mean intake of a population group is equal to the RDA, there will be a low prevalence of inadequacy. As shown, there may still be a substantial proportion of the population with intakes below the EAR, which would be a better estimate of the prevalence of inadequacy.

Whether this occurred or not would depend on whether the RDA was based on the mean intake of a population in which no one was inadequate or whether the RDA came from data for which some members of the population had inadequate intakes and thus demonstrated one or more possible criteria of inadequacy, which are usually not possible to determine. By using the EAR as the cutoff to determine the prevalence of inadequacy (this applies to those nutrients for which requirements are symmetrically or normally distributed), it is possible to set an acceptable level of inadequacy in situations of scarce resources in which it is not possible to assume that all have an adequate intake.

DRIs for Other Nutrients and Food Constituents

As indicated previously, assumptions regarding variability and independence are involved in using EARs to estimate adequacy and to plan diets. When these cannot be followed, the Food and Nutrition Board's DRI framework included other categories of reference values to provide guidance for program planning and nutrition policy: the AI, including the Estimated Energy Requirement (EER) and the Acceptable Macronutrient Distribution Range (AMDR). In the United Kingdom, population averages along with minima and maxima for some energy-yielding nutrients have been established.

The EERs for use in the United States and Canada are derived from regression equations for adults and for children based on pooled data obtained from a group of international investigators. They represent the first time that energy recommendations have been based on quantitative estimates of energy expenditure (made by the technique of measuring doubly labeled water metabolism) directly in individuals over 2 or 3 weeks for a large number of people rather than estimating the amount of time spent in various energy-requiring activities over a 24-h period and then multiplying each type of activity by indirect estimates of energy expended.

Reference values for macronutrients such as starch, fiber, and other carbohydrates, various fatty acids, and other lipids such as cholesterol are primarily related to the role that each macronutrient plays in chronic disease development and risk factor reduction. As such, the data that support such reference values are usually less definitive, and definitely more complex, than those for single nutrients that can be easily isolated and manipulated in the diet. This additional set of reference values is given as ranges to provide guidance to federal agencies and others related to nutrient intakes. The ability to identify and quantitate the relationship of accepted risk factors for diseases is also important in reviewing literature to develop macronutrient ranges compatible with low risk of disease and maintenance of health.

Finally, physical activity has been included in the recent DRI series to highlight the very important role it plays in decreasing risk of chronic disease in terms of both maintaining sufficient energy expenditure to allow for maintenance of body weight and maintaining cardiovascular fitness to decrease the risk of heart disease.

Application of Risk Assessment Methodology to Nutrients

One of the many needs for reference values is to provide guidance about when intake of a nutrient may be too much, where the level of intake has the potential for an increased risk through excess consumption. In the past, this was rarely a concern because it was difficult to consume, on a chronic basis, large enough amounts of a specific nutrient from foods to result in serious adverse effects.

Most adverse effects of overconsumption are self-limiting because they usually involve gastrointestinal disturbances (as is the case for dietary fiber) or involve objectionable and readily reversible effects (e.g., turning orange when consuming very high amounts of carotenoids from carotene-rich foods). However, instances of serious adverse effects have been reported in the past few decades due to over-ingestion of isolated nutrients or food constituents, typically in pill form and given in therapeutic doses, or through mistakes in fortification and enrichment of the food supply, but rarely from overconsumption of foods in their natural state.

Recent increases in demand for nutrients as a result of consumer interest in self-management of health, and provocative findings relating specific dietary constituents to possible health benefits, have provided incentives for industry to increase the availability and use of nutrients and food components in dietary supplements and for the voluntary fortification of foods. Thus, the need for science-based reviews of data on the potential for increased risk of serious adverse effects that may result from chronic consumption of individual nutrients in higher amounts than typically encountered with foods has grown in importance. Such reviews have been conducted by Canadian and US scientists through the Food and Nutrition Board, by the United Kingdom's Expert Group on Vitamins and Minerals, and by the Scientific Committee on Food of the European Commission, among others. Each has worked on developing approaches to evaluating reports of adverse effects and establishing, if possible, upper levels of intake for which little concern about risks of serious adverse effects may be expected. Although somewhat differing in the review of specific studies and in defining what might be considered serious, these efforts are all aimed at incorporating the basic components of toxicological risk assessment (**Figure 7**) in the review of nutrients, primarily from a qualitative perspective and on an individual (nutrient-by-nutrient) basis. In all cases, attempts are made to quantitate no-observed-adverse-effect levels as well as lowest-observed-adverse-effect levels of exposure and then divide by an uncertainty factor to obtain the upper reference level or limit (**Figure 8**).

Issues in Establishing Reference Intakes

Extrapolating Data to Other Life-Stage and Gender Groups

Invariably, there is not enough information on studied populations to establish reference values directly for each subgroup. Knowledge of nutritional needs as well as response to higher levels of intake and exposure for such groups, such as during pregnancy or preadolescence, would be very useful. In order to provide adequate guidance when data are lacking, reference intakes are routinely provided by extrapolating the available primary data to these important age or life-stage groups from those subgroups for whom data are available. Consensus on the best methods to use for extrapolation when data are lacking, with modeling and consideration of more sophisticated approaches than just body size or caloric expenditure, is needed to enhance the utility of the derived reference values.

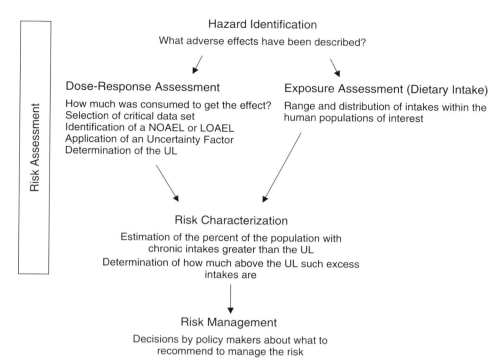

Figure 7 Steps in a model of risk assessment for nutrients.

Role of Nutrient Intake Surveys and Food Composition Databases

Surveys such as the National Health and Nutrition Examination Surveys and the What We Eat in America Survey in the United States, the Dutch National Food Consumption Survey in The Netherlands, and the National Diet and Nutrition Surveys in the United Kingdom serve as the underpinning for tracking changes in consumption and eating behavior of specific vulnerable population groups, such as young children or the elderly, in order to evaluate the potential for targeted intervention programs, either through programs aimed at changing eating behavior (e.g., the 5 A Day Program to enhance fruit and vegetable consumption in the United States) or through fortification of specific foods (e.g., calcium with bread in Canada) or changes in food product formulation (e.g., decreasing *trans* fat in high-fat

processed foods). The absence of surveys that link intake with health or quantifiable and validated disease indicators makes it almost impossible to determine risk of inadequacy as well as risk of excess, particularly in vulnerable groups, without very expensive laboratory tests and clinical observation.

Lack of data or nutrient content in a variety of foodstuffs, as well as lack of valid intake data, decreases the utility of subsequent estimates of inadequacy or exposure. An issue that continues to hamper reliable estimates of intake is selective underreporting and overreporting of intakes of specific foods or portion sizes by responders in surveys, usually related to foods known to be associated with causation of disease in the first case (underreporting) or considered more healthy in the second (overreporting). Although conducting large-scale surveys is costly and highly labor-intensive, poor collection of intake data and lack of replicate food composition information available to estimate intakes continue to hamper attempts to improve accuracy of the estimates. Much work is currently under way to increase the ability for such surveys to estimate intakes.

Approaches to Evaluating Bioactive Food Components

As new technologies, such as metabolomics, develop that allow better understanding of cell

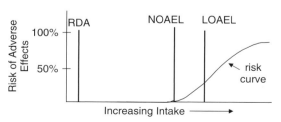

Figure 8 Identifying the hazard: dose–response.

metabolism and interaction among nutrients within cell systems, food constituents that have previously gone unnoticed are gaining recognition for their potential roles in maintaining health and decreasing risk of chronic disease. Some food components appear to work in concert with other nutrients and chemicals and are highly active at nanogram concentration levels in cellular systems involved in decreasing inflammatory responses or cell death. These bioactive substances may be difficult to analyze in food stuffs when they rapidly convert or oxidize into other less active compounds, making traditional methods of determining potential roles in health very difficult to apply. However, such new technologies offer the opportunity to study not pathways but, integrated circuits of multiple systems and bioactive food components simultaneously, modeling from multiple perspectives rather than the typical linear relationships diagrammed in the metabolic pathways identified by the mid-twentieth century. Using these tools, the integrated nature and role of known and unknown chemical constituents of foods will form the basis for evaluating human nutritional requirements in the future.

Steps Toward International Consensus

An issue that is obvious in any consideration of how best to approach estimating human requirements is the need to achieve consensus on the best science-based approaches to determine them. Internationally, the diversity of requirement estimates might mislead one to assume there was significant variability in nutrient needs based on geographic location or genetic makeup. As more information regarding the role that genetic factors play in disease becomes available, the variability seen in actual requirements will diminish. There will continue to be a need to recognize and use information about nutrient bioavailability, which may well be different for diets based on different foods and staples and thus require different reference values for such varied situations, but human physiology is remarkably similar.

Harmonizing approaches to reviewing data and achieving consensus among scientists is an important first step to deriving truly borderless reference values that represent differences that are physiologically and genotypically related rather than culturally related.

Efforts to harmonize are ongoing in a number of settings. Germanic language countries now have joint reference values; Australia and New Zealand are working on joint reference intakes, as are nutritionists in Southeast Asia; countries in the European Union have plans for increasing such joint deliberations beyond the activities involved in developing upper levels; and the United Nations, through the coordinating efforts of the United Nations University, is initiating extragovernmental discussion of basic issues involved in evaluating the human data that serve as the basis for establishing requirements and reference values. All these activities are in the beginning stages. With the enhanced level of communication due to computers and the Internet, such efforts are feasible as well as critical to undertake.

See also: **Antioxidants**: Diet and Antioxidant Defense. **Bioavailability. Dietary Guidelines, International Perspectives. Dietary Intake Measurement**: Methodology; Validation. **Dietary Surveys. Energy**: Balance; Requirements; Adaptation. **Food Composition Data. Food Fortification**: Developed Countries. **Functional Foods**: Regulatory Aspects. **Nutritional Surveillance**: Developed Countries; Developing Countries. **Phytochemicals**: Epidemiological Factors. **World Health Organization**.

Further Reading

Institute of Medicine (1997) Dietary Reference Intakes. In *Dietary Reference Intakes for Calcium, Phosphorus, Magnesium, Vitamin D, and Fluoride*, pp. 21–37. Washington, DC: National Academy Press.

Institute of Medicine (1998) *Dietary Reference Intakes: A Risk Assessment Model for Establishing Upper Intake Levels for Nutrients*. Washington, DC: National Academy Press.

Institute of Medicine (2000) Using the estimated average requirement for nutrient assessment of groups. In *Dietary Reference Intakes: Applications in Dietary Assessment*, pp. 73–105. Washington, DC: National Academy Press.

Trumbo P, Schlicker S, Yates A, and Poos M (2002) Dietary Reference Intakes for energy, carbohydrate, fiber, fat, fatty acids, cholesterol, protein, and amino acids. *Journal of the American Dietetic Association* **102**: 1621–1630.

NUTRITION POLICIES IN DEVELOPING AND DEVELOPED COUNTRIES

C Geissler, Kings College London, London, UK

This article reviews the definition of nutrition policy and aspects specific to developing and developed countries; components of typical policies; government structures for their formulation and implementation; the types of programs used to implement policy; historical trends of emphasis; the international promotion of nutrition policies; constraints imposed by major development organisations; the effectiveness and characteristics of successful policies and programs; and emerging issues.

What Is a Nutrition Policy?

Nutrition is the process whereby living organisms use food for maintenance of life, growth, the normal functioning of organs and tissues, and the production of energy. Human nutrition therefore encompasses food composition, food consumption, food habits, the nutritive value of foods, nutritional requirements, the relationship between diet and health, and research in all these fields. Diet in this context means the total solid and liquid foods consumed by an individual or a population group. Nutrition is therefore at the center of a web of a number of disciplines and so policy affecting nutrition involves many government sectors.

In the process of national policy formulation, various ministries and departments of the government (sectors) prepare programs for implementation during a specific plan period. Those aspects of the national policy that are specifically designed to improve the state of nutrition in a country are together defined as 'nutrition policy' or 'food and nutrition policy.'

In developing countries, national policies are published for each sector in periodic national development plans, usually every 5 years. In developed countries, they are formulated at irregular intervals within the term of office of the elected government. Nutrition does not usually constitute a separate sector and so aspects of nutrition policy appear under the policies of specific sectors, such as agricultural, food, health, education, and social welfare. These aspects are by no means comprehensive and during the stage of implementation are generally not coordinated through any official mechanism.

Policy Differences in Developing Countries

Nutrition policy preparation and implementation in developing countries differs from that in developed countries in two main aspects, as discussed in the following sections.

Types of Nutrition Problems Addressed

In developing countries, these are mainly undernutrition, labeled as protein energy malnutrition, and specific deficiency conditions, most commonly vitamin A, anemia, and goiter. Although the so-called 'diseases of affluence' often affect the richer urban sections of the population, they have not been policy priorities, but they have recently become so in some Asian and Latin American and other developing countries. However, countries such as China that are in nutritional transition between the predominance of diseases of poverty and of affluence have to consider how to reduce remaining nutritional deficiencies but avoid the nutrition-related problems afflicting developed countries. In developed countries, chronic diseases related to poor nutrition, such as obesity, coronary heart disease, diabetes, and osteoporosis (sometimes referred to as 'overnutrition'), are the main problems addressed because most micronutrient deficiencies have been contained, although anemia remains prevalent, as does goitre in some areas, and pockets of undernutrition also exist in developed countries.

Influence of External Aid Agencies

In many developing countries, governments are assisted in the formulation of nutrition policies by agencies such as the World Bank, the United Nations Children's Fund (UNICEF), the World Health Organisation (WHO), and the United Nations Food and Agricultural Organisation (FAO), and specific projects are often resourced by external funding, technical assistance, and food aid.

National Nutrition Policies and Government Structures

Since the 1970s, nutrition has been recognized as an important objective of national development and an indicator of such development. In developing countries, this objective determines the goals that form the major ingredients of a national nutrition policy. In both developed and developing countries, a typical policy would aim to ensure a biologically safe and physically clean food supply sufficient to amply meet people's physiological, social, and cultural requirements of a variety of foodstuffs at commonly affordable prices. The specific programs to implement such policies usually include a mixture of analyses of the situation and individual interventions of the types outlined in the following section. Analyses for the purpose of monitoring the nutritional situation and providing public information and recommendations may include the periodic assessment of consumption patterns and energy and nutrient intakes, the identification of populations at risk of deprivation and excessive or imbalanced food consumption through specific studies and surveys, analyzing and composing dietary patterns in terms of food groups and nutrients, and defining minimum and desirable standards of the requirement of food energy and nutrients for various age groups and specific groups of the population with special needs.

Because nutrition is generally not a sector *per se*, it usually does not have a direct budget and in many countries the ministry of health is charged with improving the state of nutrition of the people, whereas aspects of food come under the ministry of agriculture. In most developing countries, implementation of the nutrition policy is carried out by these ministries or a ministry of planning through autonomous or semiautonomous councils, commissions, or committees, which may or may not be intersectoral in their compositions. These may report to the relevant ministry, cabinet, or, rarely, directly to the president. In some countries, nutrition units also exist in the provinces to provide regional planning information and actions. Some nutrition planning bodies receive advice from ad hoc technical committees as needs arise. The weakness or strength of such bodies can be judged from the change in nutritional status of the people since their establishment.

In developed countries, the ministries or departments of health and agriculture also share the main responsibility for nutrition. However, there is often conflict between the interests of producers and consumers within ministries of agriculture. Many of the nutrition and health policies in both types of countries incorporate aspects such as education and modifying activity levels, and so other ministries become involved to provide the facilities for these.

Types of Programs and Interventions

The types of interventions that form part of national nutrition policies in both developing and developed countries tend to be limited to palliative measures such as vitamin supplementation, nutrition education, and child feeding programs because many of the underlying factors that lead to malnutrition, such as unemployment, low wages, and land tenure arrangements, involve fundamental economic and political interests that are much more difficult and contentious to address. In developed countries, which are by definition richer, the governments generally provide economic safety nets for the unemployed, disabled, and other disadvantaged sections of the population. These people have to be cared for by extended family or other means in developing countries. The pattern of programs is therefore different between developed and developing countries because of differences in the nutritional problems and the wealth of the population and government. However, the types of programs are similar. The types of interventions that affect nutrition can be divided into general categories summarized in **Table 1**.

Historical Trends

There have been changes in emphasis in the type of programs advocated throughout the decades to improve nutrition as knowledge of nutrition has grown and as governments and development agencies have experienced success or failure in various approaches.

During World War II and the postwar period of the 1940s, the emphasis in developed countries was on institutional feeding, such as school meals, school milk, and the distribution of concentrated vitamin sources to children and mothers. These approaches were continued in developing countries by international agencies, such as FAO and WHO, after their establishment postwar.

As decolonization progressed, a growing interest in the process of economic development and nutrition led to the recognition that individual interventions had little impact on malnutrition and that a more integrated approach was needed to improve the use of available resources. In the 1950s, the international agencies therefore promoted 'applied nutrition programs,' which are village-based

Table 1 Types of nutrition programs

Explicitly nutritional

Programs directly related to food, including those aiming to improve food availability, accessibility, quality, safety, consumption, and knowledge.

  Nutrition-oriented food policies
    Agricultural production, kitchen gardens, marketing, storage, processing, safety
    Food price and distribution control, food price subsidies, taxation, food stamps, rationing
  Feeding programs
    Mother and child: nutrition rehabilitation centres; on site, take home
    Schools: lunch, breakfast, snack, milk
    Workers: canteens, Food for Work
    Elderly: community center; Meals on Wheels
  Weaning foods
    Formulated, fermented, amylase rich
  Fortification, supplementation
    Iron, B vitamins, iodine, vitamin A, iron, vitamin D, vitamin C, amino acids
  Nutrition education

Implicitly nutritional

Programs with indirect nutritional impact through improvement of effective food demand, food utilization, and energy balance

  Health
    Primary health care: immunization, antiparasites, rehydration, basic medicines, prenatal care, health education, first aid
    Sanitation: water supply, water treatment, water storage, waste disposal, drainage and spraying, hygiene education
  Economic
    Income generation
    Income maintenance: welfare benefits, unemployment benefits, child allowances, etc.
    Income substitution by subsidized basic needs
  Activity moderation
    Cereal mills, water storage and transport, child care crèches
    Sports facilities, cycle paths, etc.

Integrated

Combining explicit and implicit nutritional interventions; For example, targeted 'applied nutrition programs', and 'community development programs'

---

programmes with components addressing several of the multiple factors of malnutrition, such as income generation activities, horticulture, health care, and nutrition education.

During the 1960s, attention focused on the world food supply and concern that the population could outstrip production. Thus, food and nutrition programs were centered around the production and dissemination of high-yielding varieties of cereals, wheat, rice, and maize—the 'green revolution' package. In the same decade, the idea developed that a specific 'protein gap' existed between the amount of protein available in national food supplies and population needs. A second focus was therefore on means to increase the production and consumption of protein from a variety of novel sources. During this same period, in the United States awareness increased that pockets of food poverty still existed in this affluent country. The resulting concern about 'Hunger in America' led to new welfare programs, such as the Women, Infants, and Children program.

By the 1970s, after 25 years of experience in nutrition interventions within economic development strategies in developing countries, it was recognized that increased national wealth did not always result in improved welfare and nutrition as predicted by the 'trickle-down' theory of development. Nutrition was therefore proposed as a specific goal for national development because a better nourished population would achieve more effective development. Government nutrition policy should be integrated and coordinated by a nutrition planning unit in an umbrella organization such as a ministry of planning or a prime minister's office so that the underlying causes would be simultaneously addressed by the appropriate government sector. This approach was fostered by development agencies such as FAO and the US Agency for International Development and was adopted by several countries, particularly after it was endorsed at the World Food Conference in 1974.

In developed countries, an increased interest in nutrition policy emerged as it was realized that existing legislation, based on food purity and the prevention of adulteration, and also the control of deficiencies, was not adequate to deal with the changing nature of nutrition problems of chronic nutrition-related diseases. Several government advisory, professional, and consumer bodies in the United States, United Kingdom, and other countries recommended appropriate dietary goals with the common theme of reducing fat, sugar, and salt intake and increasing the intake of dietary fiber, fruit, and vegetables. The recommendation to reduce the intake of certain nutrients appeared to be a threat to some sectors of the food industry, resulting in considerable opposition to the recommendation and arguments about the validity of the evidence on which the recommendation was based. Other constraints to updating food and nutrition policy included legislation designed to prevent adulteration and maintain quality as previously perceived, such as minimum fat levels in milk and premiums on animals with high fat content. However, the proposals were gradually accepted and incorporated into government policies, while industry recognized new opportunities in the production of high-fiber, low-fat, low-salt and -sugar food products. Norway was the first developed country to have an integrated food and nutrition policy in 1975. Other developed countries subsequently formulated food and nutrition policies within their health and agriculture sectors.

By the 1980s, attempts in developing countries to apply the rational procedures advocated by the national nutrition planning approach for the selection of appropriate interventions had demonstrated the paucity of data on which to decide nutritional priorities and the effectiveness of various interventions, the difficulties of placing a policy priority on nutrition, and the problems of effective intersectoral coordination. This approach was subsequently abandoned by the development agencies. These hurdles, however, led to better evaluation of interventions and to measurements of the functional impact of malnutrition. In the 1980s, the promotion of intersectoral planning gave way to ensuring that existing sectoral interventions such as agricultural development programs included nutrition considerations. The other main theme was the targeting of nutrition interventions to those most in need and the involvement of local communities in self-sustaining development programs. This was brought about by the structural adjustment programs described later.

The 1980s also saw greater recognition of the role that women play in child nutrition through their economic as well as reproductive roles; the income that they control empowers them to make decisions beneficial to their own health and that of their children. There was also a renewed recognition of the role of diet quality in the promotion of nutrition status by the understanding that micronutrients have a function in child survival beyond deficiency

diseases. This led to the promotion in developing countries of small-scale home gardening, capsule distribution, and fortification programs. Such programs had been in use for several decades in developed countries, providing land for kitchen garden allotments, the provision of supplements to children and mothers during the world wars, and the fortification of white flour with vitamins and minerals from that period to the present day as well as later compulsory fortification of margarine with vitamins A and D.

The main theme of the 1990s in developing countries was subsequently micronutrient intervention, including particularly vitamin A, iron, iodine, and, to a lesser extent, folic acid. There developed a research interest in population trials with several micronutrients that may lead to changes in nutrition policy and interventions. For example, the importance of vitamin A was investigated not only for eye lesions and blindness but also for resistance to respiratory and diarrheal infections; antioxidants began to be tested for their possible role in protection against cancer, heart disease, and other conditions; and zinc and other micronutrients were explored as a means to address the issue of restricted growth, which is widespread in developing countries.

In the 1990s, more developed countries produced explicit nutrition policies and also integrated measures to increase physical activity. For example, in the United Kingdom explicit nutritional goals were set for the first time in the 1992 government health policy, *The Health of the Nation*, which focused on five key areas for action—coronary heart disease and stroke, cancers, mental illness, HIV/AIDS and sexual health, and accidents—the first two of which are diet related. The diet and nutrition targets were as follows:

Reduce the average percentage food energy from saturated fats by at least 35% (to no more than 11% food energy)

Reduce the average percentage food energy from total fat by at least 12% (to no more than approximately 35% food energy)

Reduce the percentage of men and women aged 16–64 years who are obese by at least 25 and 35%, respectively (to no more than 6% of men and 8% of women)

Reduce the percentage of men drinking more than 21 units of alcohol per week and women drinking more than 14 units per week by 30% (to 18% of men and 7% of women)

By concentrating on these targets, it was expected that the associated dietary changes and reduction in obesity would have beneficial consequences on such diseases as cancer, osteoarthritis, diabetes, etc. A nutrition task force was set up to oversee implementation and a physical activity task force was also set up to develop physical activity targets and detailed strategies. On a regional basis, the WHO European Region prepared the First Action Plan for Food and Nutrition Policy 2000–2005, which includes a food and nutrition task force. Food-based dietary guidelines were produced in the United States and subsequently in other countries and by FAO/WHO.

Food safety became a major concern in the 1990s, particularly in the developed countries. European consumers in particular lost faith in the science establishment due to initial assurances that BSE (mad cow disease) was no danger to human health, and they became extremely cautious about the safety of the food they purchased. In the United Kingdom, this distrust also led to a revision in government structure via the Food Standards Act 1999 so that agricultural and consumer food interests that had been combined within the Ministry of Agriculture Food and Fisheries were separated into the Food Standards Agency to champion consumer interests and the Department for the Environment, Food and Rural Affairs to oversee agriculture. A similar body was established within the European Union, the European Food Safety Authority, in 2002. In the United States, food and nutrition are regulated by the Food and Drug Administration, whereas other aspects of food and nutrition policy are regulated by the US Department of Agriculture. Due to the increased requirements to adhere to the new food safety expectations, it is more difficult for developing country exporters to gain market share in the developed world, affecting their own food security through constrained export opportunities. Along with these new food safety considerations have been concerns about genetically modified (GM) foods.

Also in the 1990s, there was increased awareness that pockets of food poverty still existed in developed countries, following the increased economic inequality that occurred in the 1980s in both developed and developing countries, partly due to government cutbacks in welfare programs (see International Constraints). This led to actions to relieve the constraints of the poor. This echoed a similar period in the United States in the 1960s involving 'Hunger in America,' which resulted in new welfare programs.

In the twenty-first century, many of the interventions emphasized in previous decades continue to form the tools of nutrition policy, and community trials continue. The experiences of these efforts in developing countries have been drawn together in a United Nations Administrative Committee on Coordination/Standing Committee on Nutrition review of 'what works.' No such review has been carried out on the effectiveness of various interventions in reducing the chronic nutrition-related diseases, possibly because the history of interventions is shorter. However, some systematic reviews on interventions for specific diseases have been conducted.

The main new emerging intervention is the development of genetic modification to provide crops with higher levels of the micronutrients that are commonly deficient in developing countries, such as iron and vitamin A, and with resistance to poor environmental conditions, such as drought and soil salinity. To date, GM foods have realized benefits largely for producers in developed countries in terms of higher productivity and lower costs. Despite no obvious benefits to consumers other than perhaps lower prices, GM soybean products have been consumed in the United States since the 1990s. However, European consumers and many in the United States are concerned that the food safety and environmental safety issues related to GM foods have not been adequately researched. The mandatory labelling of foods as 'containing GM organisms' is proposed as one solution, allowing consumers to make informed choices, but this has been opposed by GM producers as being too expensive to keep the GM and non-GM crops separate throughout the food distribution chain. The public sector has a role to play, and some new institutional arrangements, including the Global Alliance for Improved Nutrition concerning food fortification, are seeking to create incentives for the private sector to develop fortified foods for the benefit of the poor.

International Context

International Promotion

Hunger and malnutrition were put on the international agenda by the League of Nations in the 1930s, and the first conference of the United Nations in 1943 was devoted to food and agriculture. It remained an important focus of the United Nations technical agencies, FAO, WHO, and UNICEF, which were created immediately after World War II. Other international organizations have since been established, including the World Food Programme, World Food Council, International Fund for Agriculture Development, United Nations Fund for Population Activities, the World Bank, and the Consultative Group on International Agriculture. All these organizations and other international supporting bodies have explicit objectives to eradicate human suffering due to hunger and malnutrition and to promote well-being and sound standards of health for all peoples of the world. The focus of these groups has been mainly on developing countries, but developed countries have recently been considered. These organizations have played an important role in relation to nutrition policies in developing countries by (i) providing technical assistance in the formulation and implementation of policies, programs, and activities; (ii) providing program and project funding; (iii) collecting and disseminating data, such as the World Food Surveys conducted by FAO every decade since 1946, which have greatly influenced the ideas of nutritionists and development policymakers in estimating the extent and defining the causes of malnutrition and have shaped the technical assistance deemed to be appropriate; (iv) organizing fora for debate on topics relevant to food and nutrition policy, such as the World Food Conference (1974); Alma Ata Conference of Primary Health Care (1978); World Conference on Agrarian Reform and Rural Development (1979); Convention on the Elimination of All Forms of Discrimination Against Women (1979); Fourth UN Development Decade (1990); World Summit for Children (1990); Innocente Declaration on Protection, Promotion and Support of Breast-Feeding (1990); Montreal Policy Conference on Micronutrient Malnutrition (1991); Rio Declaration on Environment and Development (1992); and International Conference on Nutrition (1992). The World Food Summit convened in November 1996, two decades after the influential World Food Conference of 1974, with the objective "to renew the commitment of the world leaders at the highest level to the eradication of hunger and malnutrition and the achievement of lasting food security for all." The UN Millennium Summit in 2000 produced the Millennium Development Goals, espoused by each of the UN agencies. These were to (i) eradicate extreme poverty and hunger; (ii) achieve universal primary education; (iii) promote gender equality and empower women; (iv) reduce child mortality; (v) improve maternal health; (vi) combat HIV/AIDS, malaria, and other diseases; (vii) ensure environmental sustainability; and (viii) develop global partnership for development. The agencies have set specific targets for each of these goals.

Some of the resolutions of these fora are very broad and clearly unachievable, such as the nutrition goals of the Fourth United Nations Development Decade (1990s), which were to (i) eliminate starvation and death caused by famine, (ii) reduce malnutrition and mortality among children substantially, (iii) reduce chronic hunger tangibly, and (iv) eliminate major nutritional diseases.

The more specific targets of the World Summit for Children (1990) to be reached by the year 2000, included (i) reduction in severe as well as moderate malnutrition among children younger than 5 years old by half of 1990 levels, (ii) reduction in the rate of low birth weights (2.5 kg or less) to less than 10%, (iii) reduction of iron deficiency anemia in women by one-third of the 1990 level, (iv) virtual elimination of iodine deficiency disorders, and (v) virtual elimination of vitamin A deficiency and its consequences, including blindness. These have clearly not been reached, and the setting of such unobtainable targets has been criticized on the grounds that they divert the attention of nutrition planners away from local priorities to global issues.

International Constraints

In the early 1980s, many developing countries experienced severe economic crises and had to implement a variety of 'structural adjustment policies,' enforced by the international finance agencies, the International Monetary Fund and the World Bank, to reduce government spending and improve balance of payments. Reduced spending resulted in cutting a variety of welfare programs that had been effective in controlling malnutrition, such as food price subsidies. Structural adjustment conditions have been rigidly imposed by the agencies for countries to obtain new financial loans. These institutions are funded by quotas from members who have voting rights in proportion to their contribution, assessed according to economic status, so that decisions are effectively in the hands of the major industrialized countries, especially the United States. This banking structure means that the policies of borrowing countries are dictated by the richer industrialized nations.

Structural adjustment has frequently resulted in changes of particular concern to the poor, such as increased food prices and decreased expenditure on social programs. The effects of these policies on health care, food consumption, incomes, and prices appear to have led to a serious deterioration in indicators of nutrition, health status, and school achievement in several countries, although it is difficult to distinguish policy effects from those of general economic decline. Efforts were subsequently made by UNICEF and other bodies to buffer vulnerable groups from these effects. During the same period, there were also cutbacks in welfare programs in developed countries, such as the provision of school meals.

International Trends in Malnutrition

To what extent have nutrition policies in developing and developed countries been effective in reducing malnutrition? During the 20 years between the World Food Conference in 1974 and the International Nutrition Conference in 1992, there have been considerable changes in the extent of malnutrition. The percentage of underweight children has declined in all areas of the world except sub-Saharan Africa and South America, but the numbers have declined only in China and have increased markedly in Southeast Asia and sub-Saharan Africa. Most data on nutritional status relate to preschool children because these are considered the most vulnerable, but other age groups are certainly not immune to malnutrition. Since 1992, international assessments of nutritional status have included women, but no information is available on trends. On the other hand, the prevalence of obesity and associated diseases has increased alarmingly in developed countries and also in several developing countries. Since the 1990s, international nutrition reports have moved from an almost exclusive focus on developing countries to include the nutrition concerns of developed countries.

What Is the Secret of Success?

Although undernutrition is clearly related to poverty, some countries are better nourished than others at similar levels of national wealth. Some countries are much better than others with a similar gross national product (GNP) in terms of indicators of nutrition and health, such as food available for consumption and infant mortality. Countries that have done best to improve undernutrition in recent years are those in which there is greater equity or in which policies have concentrated on ensuring the satisfaction of basic needs, including adequate food. Their political ideologies range from communist China to capitalist South Korea and Taiwan. China is the classic example of a country that is still poor but has largely dominated malnutrition and famine through effective organization of food production and distribution. Other examples are Costa Rica, Chile, Cuba, Kerala state in India, Sri Lanka, and Thailand, which have better nutrition conditions than other counties with similar GNPs. In contrast, some countries have extensive chronic malnutrition despite massive aid (e.g., Bangladesh) and rapid economic growth (e.g., Brazil).

These improvements cannot all be ascribed to specific nutrition policies. What are the lessons that can be learned about the effectiveness of the nutrition interventions commonly used to implement nutrition policies? This is not an easy question to answer because the evaluation of effectiveness of specific interventions is theoretically simple but practically difficult since evaluation has to take into account general economic change. An important function of international development and research agencies such as the World Bank, the International Food Policy Research Institute, FAO, UNICEF, and WHO since the 1970s has been to draw together research on the impact of policies and programs on the economic, health, and nutritional status of beneficiaries to distinguish the characteristics of success. Most of these have concentrated on developing countries. Several features of successful large-scale nutrition interventions in relation to undernutrition have been extracted and are summarized next.

The objectives must be based on a careful analysis of the real problem and be achievable in a timescale set within the program design. Community and local nongovernment organization involvement is essential in the design and implementation so that there is a sense of joint ownership for self-sustaining success. The overall effectiveness depends on coverage, and if interventions are targeted at specific groups there has to be a trade-off between the cost-effectiveness of targeting and wider coverage of the population. Charismatic leadership and good management are essential, and the appropriate mix of components must be accompanied by effective administration with a balance between bottom-up and top-down actions. Most successful programs include strong training and supervision. Effective implementation is helped by setting clear targets and by monitoring and evaluating the process, with flexibility to modify the program where necessary. The attitude of the workers is crucial in determining the potential for scaling up from a pilot project with selected staff to a large-scale operational program that has to use existing staff. Awareness of the consequences and causes of malnutrition and a political commitment at all levels are important. These common characteristics are a useful basis for the planning of future programs to maximize their success.

Emerging Issues in the Twenty-First Century

Some of the main emerging and reemerging nutrition issues of the new millennium for developing countries are those that reflect changing economic, demographic, and disease patterns and include HIV/ AIDS, the nutrition transition, refugees, adolescents, and aging.

In developed countries, aging is also one of the main emerging issues, along with the continued increase in obesity in both adults and children, with concomitant increases in related diseases such as diabetes. It has been recognised that this cannot be dealt with only on the nutrition front, and nutrition policies and recommendations are now including measures to increase activity in the population. Research continues to refine the association of various food factors with aspects of health and so determines policy. For example, the United States has already undertaken folic acid fortification of flour and the United Kingdom is considering doing so.

Millions have died of AIDS, especially in sub-Saharan Africa, with devastating effects on people's livelihoods. For the individual, the disease raises nutrient requirements and reduces the immune system, increasing vulnerability to other diseases. A major issue is the transmission of HIV from mother to child during pregnancy, at birth, or with breast-feeding. For the household, HIV/AIDS reduces the capacity to care for young children and infected household members and to work to ensure food security, resulting in deteriorating nutritional status. Women feel the impact most severely. Nutrition policy has to relate to prevention and nutritional care, which can significantly postpone illness and prolong life.

More developing countries will have to modify their nutrition policies to address the shift from problems of nutritional deficiency and infectious diseases to problems of chronic diet-related diseases, including obesity, diabetes, cardiovascular disease, hypertension, and various forms of cancer. These shifts are associated with changes in diet and life-style patterns that accompany industrialization, urbanization, economic development, and market globalization and that result in the increased consumption of energy-dense diets and sedentary work and leisure occupations.

National and international conflict has resulted in millions of refugees and internally displaced persons, estimated by the United Nations to be 35 million, of which 80% are women and children, and acute malnutrition is frequently reported. Nutritional support of these displaced populations is a concern for national governments and international agencies.

Most attention in the past has been focused on the nutrition of young children and on pregnant and lactating women, and other groups have been relatively neglected. Recently, the special needs of adolescents have begun to be addressed. Adolescents comprise approximately 20% of the world's population, and adolescence is a period of intense physical, psychosocial, and cognitive development, during which they gain up to 50% of their adult weight, height, and skeletal mass, caloric requirements are maximal, and poor eating habits and pregnancy are additional concerns. More attention will be paid to this group and to ways to avoid the consequences of poor nutrition during this period.

Another neglected group is the elderly. Currently, there are 580 million people older than 60 years (61% in developing countries), and this number is projected to increase to 1 billion by 2020 (71% in developing countries). The majority are women because they live longer than men. Special problems associated with nutrition include osteoporosis and fractures, vulnerability to malnutrition, and degenerative diseases.

Conclusions

A nutrition policy is easy to draw up on paper but is useless unless implemented. Many countries have adopted nutrition policies that were ineffective because they were not or could not be implemented. Some policies could not be implemented even if the political will existed because they were too complex, such as National Nutrition Planning, or could not be scaled up successfully from pilot projects to operational programs because they did not have funding for an equivalent level of training and supervision, such as the Applied Nutrition Program. Successful implementation depends on many economic and technical factors but most important on political will. Success in improving nutrition has been achieved in countries with a wide range of political ideologies but with a common theme of government commitment to promoting equity and to satisfying basic needs. Some types of specific interventions can be successful without such commitment, such as nutrient supplement programmes, but the criteria of success have to be clearly defined in terms of population coverage, sustainability, and to what extent the program addresses the main nutritional problems.

See also: **Dietary Guidelines, International Perspectives**. **Food Fortification**: Developing Countries. **Malnutrition**: Primary, Causes Epidemiology and Prevention. **Nutrient Requirements, International Perspectives**. **Nutritional Surveillance**: Developing Countries. **United Nations Children's Fund**. **World Health Organization**.

Further Reading

de Onis M, Frongillo EA, and Blossner M (2000) Is malnutrition declining? An analysis of changes in levels of child malnutrition since 1980. *Bulletin of the World Health Organisation* 78(10): 1222–1233.

FAO/WHO (2003) *Diet, Nutrition and the Prevention of Chronic Diseases. Report of the Joint FAO/WHO Expert Consultation*, Technical Report Series No. 916. Geneva: FAO/WHO.

Flores R and Gillespie S (eds.) (2001) *Health and Nutrition: Emerging and Re-emerging Issues in Developing Countries*, 2020 Focus 5. Washington, DC: International Food Policy Research Institute.

Geissler C (1995) Nutrition intervention. In: Ulijaszek SJ (ed.) *Health Intervention in Less Developed Countries*. Oxford: Oxford University Press.

Grantham-McGregor SM, Pollit E, Wachs TD, Meisels SJ, and Scott KG (1999) Summary of the scientific evidence on the nature and determinants of child development and their implications for programmatic interventions with young children. *Food and Nutrition Bulletin* 20(1): 4–6.

Heaver R (2002) *Improving Nutrition: Issues in Management and Capacity Development. Health, Nutrition and Population Discussion Paper, Human Development Network*. Washington, DC: World Bank.

Jolly R and Cornia GA (eds.) (1984) *The Impact of World Recession on Children. UNICEF Report*. New York: Pergamon Press.

Kennedy E (1999) Public policy in nutrition: The US nutrition safety net—Past, present and future. *Food Policy* 24: 325–333.

Khush GS (2002) The promise of biotechnology in addressing current nutritional problems in developing countries. *Food and Nutrition Bulletin* 23(4): 354–357.

Pinstrup-Andersen P (ed.) (1993) *The Political Economy of Food and Nutrition Policies*. Baltimore: Johns Hopkins University Press.

Popkin BM, Horton S, and Kim S (2001) The nutrition transition and prevention of diet-related chronic diseases in Asia and the Pacific. *Food and Nutrition Bulletin (United Nations University)* 22(4 supplement).

Riches G (ed.) (1997) *First World Hunger: Food Security and Welfare Politics*. Basingstoke, UK: Macmillan.

Standing Committee on Nutrition (2002) *Nutrition in the Context of Conflict and Crisis*, SCN News No. 24. Geneva: ACC/SCN.

United Nations Administrative Committee on Coordination, Standing Committee on Nutrition (2000) *Fourth Report on the World Nutrition Situation*. Geneva: ACC/SCN and IFPRI.

NUTRITION TRANSITION, DIET CHANGE AND ITS IMPLICATIONS

B M Popkin, University of North Carolina, Chapel Hill, NC, USA

The world is experiencing rapid shifts in structures of diet and body composition with resultant important changes in health profiles. In many ways, these shifts are a continuation of large-scale changes that have occurred repeatedly over time; however, the changes facing low- and moderate-income countries appear to be very rapid. Broad shifts continue to occur throughout the world in population size and age composition, disease patterns, and dietary and physical activity patterns. The former two sets of dynamic shifts are termed the demographic and epidemiological transitions. The latter, whose changes are reflected in nutritional outcomes, such as changes in average stature and body composition, is termed the nutrition transition. These three relationships are presented in **Figure 1**.

Human diet and activity patterns, and nutritional status, have undergone a sequence of major shifts, defined as broad patterns of food use and their corresponding nutrition-related diseases. During the past three centuries, the pace of dietary and activity change appears to have accelerated to varying degrees in different regions of the world. Furthermore, dietary and activity changes are paralleled by major changes in health status as well as by major demographic and socioeconomic changes. Obesity emerges early in these shifting conditions, as does the level and age composition of morbidity and mortality. Although there are five broad nutrition patterns dating back to the origins of modern man, the focus of this article is on the three most recent periods (**Figure 2**). For convenience, the patterns are outlined as historical developments; however, 'earlier' patterns are not restricted to the periods in which they first arose but, rather, they continue to characterize certain geographic and socioeconomic subpopulations. The first two patterns relate to earlier periods in the evolution of man—the first pattern of collecting food and the second

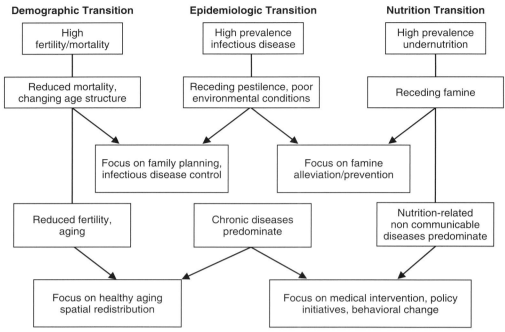

Figure 1 Stages of health, nutritional, and demographic change. (From Popkin BM (2002) The shift in stages of the nutrition transition in the developing world differs from past experiences! *Public Health Nutrition* **5**(1A): 205–214.)

pattern of famine. The following are the three later periods:

Pattern 3: Receding famine: The consumption of starchy staples had predominated and continues to do so, but these items become less important in this low-fat diet as limited amounts of fruits, vegetables, and animal protein are increasingly added to the low-fat and high-fiber diet. Many earlier civilizations made great progress in reducing chronic hunger and famines, but only in the last third of the past millennium have these

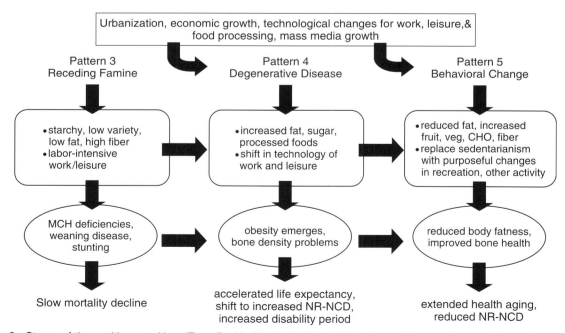

Figure 2 Stages of the nutrition transition. (From Popkin BM (2002) The shift in stages of the nutrition transition in the developing world differs from past experiences! *Public Health Nutrition* **5**(1A): 205–214.)

changes become widespread, leading to marked shifts in diet. However, famines continued well into the eighteenth century in portions of Europe and remain common in some regions of the world. Activity patterns start to shift and inactivity and leisure become a part of the lives of more people.

Pattern 4: Nutrition-related noncommunicable disease (NR-NCD): A diet high in total fat, cholesterol, sugar, and other refined carbohydrates, low in polyunsaturated fatty acids and fiber, and often accompanied by an increasingly sedentary life is characteristic of most high-income societies (and increasing proportions of the population in low-income societies), resulting in increased prevalence of obesity and contributing to the degenerative diseases that characterize the final epidemiologic transition stage.

Pattern 5: Behavioral change: A new dietary pattern appears to be emerging, evidently associated with the desire to prevent or delay degenerative diseases and prolong health. Whether these dietary changes, instituted in some countries by consumers and in others also prodded by government policy, will create a large-scale transition in dietary structure and body composition remains to be seen.

Our focus is increasingly on patterns 3–5, particularly the rapid shift in much of the world's low- and moderate-income countries from the stage of receding famine to NR-NCD. **Figure 2** presents this focus. The concern about this period is so great for many that the term 'nutrition transition' is synonymous with this shift from pattern 3 to 4.

Shifts in Dietary and Activity Patterns and Body Composition Seem to Be Occurring More Rapidly

The pace of the rapid nutrition transition shifts in diet and activity patterns from the period termed the receding famine pattern to one dominated by NR-NCDs seems to be accelerating in the lower and middle-income transitional countries. We use the word 'nutrition' rather than 'diet' so that the term NR-NCDs incorporates the effects of diet, physical activity, and body composition rather than solely focusing on dietary patterns and their effects. This is based partially on incomplete information that seems to indicate that the prevalence of obesity and a number of NR-NCDs is increasing more rapidly in the lower and middle-income world than it has in the West. Another element is that the rapid changes in urban populations are much greater than those experienced a century ago or less in the West; yet

another is the shift in occupation structure and the rapid introduction of the modern mass media. Underlying such changes is a general concern for rapid globalization as the root cause.

Clearly, there are quantitative and qualitative dimensions to these changes. On the one hand, changes toward a high-density diet, reduced complex carbohydrates, increased added sugar and other caloric sweeteners, and inactivity may be proceeding faster than in the past. The shift from labor-intensive occupations and leisure activities toward more capital-intensive, less strenuous work and leisure is also occurring faster. On the other hand, qualitative dimensions related to multidimensional aspects of the diet, activity, body composition, and disease shifts may exist. The social and economic stresses that people face and feel as these changes occur may also be included.

Scholars often note that the pace and complexity of life, reflected in all aspects of work and play, are increasing exponentially. There are also unanticipated developments, new technologies, and the impact of a very modern, high-powered communications system. It is this sense of rapid change that makes it so important to understand what is happening and anticipate the way in which changes in patterns of diet, activity, and body composition are occurring. Although the penetration and influence of modern communications, technology, and economic systems related to 'globalization' have been a dominant theme of the past few decades, there seem to be some unique issues that have led to a rapid increase in globalization and its impact.

Stating that globalization is the cause results in a focus on broad and vaguely measured sets of forces; this ignores the need to be focused and specific, which would allow us to develop potentially viable policy options. It is difficult to measure each element of this globalization equation and its impact. These processes certainly have been expanded, as indicated by enhanced free trade, a push toward reduction of trade barriers in the developing world, and the increasing penetration of international corporations into the commerce in each country (measured by share of gross national product (GNP) or manufacturing). Similarly, other economic issues related to enhanced value given to market forces and international capital markets are important. Equally, the increasing access to Western media, the removal of communication barriers enhanced by the World Wide Web, cable TV, mobile telephone systems, etc. are important. The accelerated introduction of Western technology into manufacturing and the basic sectors of agriculture, mining, and services is also a key element.

Another way to understand the types of changes the developing world is facing is to consider an urban squatter's life and a rural villager's life in China approximately 20 years ago and today. During the 1970s, food supply concerns still existed; there was no television, limited bus and mass transportation, little food trade, minimal processed food, and most rural and urban occupations were very labor intensive. Today, work and life activities have changed: Small gas-powered tractors are available, modern industrial techniques are multiplying, offices are automated, soft drinks and many processed foods are found everywhere, TVs are in approximately 89% of households (at least one-fifth of which are linked to Hong Kong Star and Western advertizing and programing), younger children do not ride bicycles, and mass transit has become heavily used. Considering that such changes are also occurring in much of Asia, North Africa, the Middle East, Latin America, and many areas (particularly cities) in sub-Saharan Africa, it is evident that the shift from a subsistence economy to a modern, industrialized one occurred in a span of 10–20 years, whereas in Europe and other industrialized high-income societies, this occurred over many decades or centuries.

To truly measure and examine these issues, we would need to compare changes in the 1980–2000 period for countries that are low and middle income to changes that occurred a half century earlier for the developing world. However, data on diet and activity patterns are not available, and there are only minimal data on NR-NCDs and obesity.

The elements of the nutrition transition known to be negatively linked with NR-NCDs are obesity, adverse dietary changes (e.g., shifts in the structure of diet toward a greater role for higher fat and added caloric sweeteners in food, reduced fruit and vegetable intake, reduced fiber intake, greater energy density, and greater saturated fat intake), and reduced physical activity in work and leisure. The causes of these elements of the nutrition transition are not as well understood as the trends in each of them. In fact, few studies have attempted to research the causes of such changes, and there are only a few data sets equipped to allow such crucial policy analyses to be undertaken.

Obesity Trends

The most commonly measured health outcome of the shifts in the structure of diet is obesity. The shifts in adult overweight and obesity in the developing world in the past 10–30 years are far faster than in the higher income countries. We examined the shifts in body composition among Chinese adults aged 20–45 years during an 8-year period. Not only did mean body mass index (BMI) increase but also the shape of the BMI distribution curve changed during the 8-year period. From 1989 to 1997, the proportion of underweight men and women declined considerably and the prevalence of both overweight and obesity increased greatly. In fact, the proportion of overweight or obese men more than doubled from 6.4.0 to 14.5% and the proportion of overweight or obese women increased 50%, from 11.5 to 16.2%.

China is not unique; here, data from a few low- and middle-income countries are presented to compare their increase in the annual prevalence of overweight and obese adults with that of the United States. **Figure 3** presents the annualized increase in the percentage points of prevalence for data from high-income countries with comparable data. **Figure 4** shows how quickly overweight and obesity have emerged in Mexico as a major public health problem. Compared to the United States and European countries, where the annual prevalence increase in overweight and obesity is approximately 0.25 each, the rates of change are very high in Latin America. Cuba's data only represent Havana. Similar shifts in the prevalence of obesity are presented for North Africa and the Middle East and Asia in **Figures 5** and **6**, respectively.

What is important to note is that the increase in the proportion of the adult population that is overweight is far greater in all the lower income countries than in the United States or most European countries. Only Spain, with its large shift in overweight in the past decade, is close to the speed of change of these countries.

Dietary Changes: Shift in the Overall Structure over Time

The diets of the developing world are shifting equally rapidly. There are no good data for most countries on total energy intake, but there are reasonable data to examine shifts in the structure of the diet. Food balance data were used to examine the shift over time in the proportion of energy from fat.

The dramatic changes in the aggregate income–fat relationship from 1962 to 1990 are displayed in **Figure 7** by the estimated regression lines based on cubic polynomial regressions. Most significantly, even the poor nations had access to a relatively high-fat diet by 1990, when a diet deriving 20% of energy (kcal) from fat was associated with countries having a GNP of only $750 *per capita*,

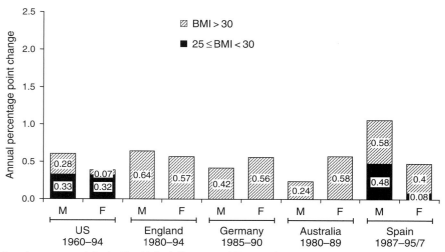

Figure 3 Obesity trends among adults in the United States and Europe (the annual percentage point increase in prevalence). BMI, body mass index; F, female; M, male. (Popkin BM (2002) The shift in stages of the nutrition transition in the developing world differs from past experiences! *Public Health Nutrition* 5(1A): 205–214.)

whereas in 1962 the same energy diet (20% from fat) was associated with countries having a GNP of $1475 (both GNP values in 1993 dollars). This dramatic change arose from a major increase (10–13%) in the consumption of vegetable fats by poor and rich nations; similar increases (3–6%) also occurred in mid- and high-income nations.

At the same time, there were decreases in the consumption of fat from animal sources for all except the low-income countries. The availability of animal fats continued to be linked to income,

though less strongly in 1990 than in 1962. These decreases, combined with the increase in vegetable fat intake for all income countries, resulted in an overall decrease in fat intake for moderate-income countries of approximately 3% but an increase of approximately 4 or 5% for low- and high-income countries. **Figure 7** shows these substantial shifts in the relationships between GNP and the composition of diets over time.

Vegetable fats in 1990 accounted for a greater proportion of dietary energy than animal fats for

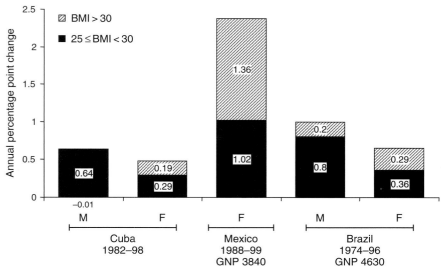

Figure 4 Obesity trends among adults in Latin America (the annual percentage point increase in prevalence). BMI, body mass index; F, female; GNP, gross national product; M, male. (Data from Rodriguez-Ojea A, Jimenez, Berdasco A and Esquivel M. (2002) The nutrition transition in Cuba in the nineties: an overview. *Public Health Nutrition* 5(1A): 129–33. Rivera (2002) Reference: Rivera JA, Barquera S, Campirano F, Campos I, Safdie M and Tovar V. (2002) Epidemiological and nutritional transition in Mexico: rapid increase of non-communicable chronic diseases and obesity. *Public Health Nutrition* 5(1A): 113–22.)

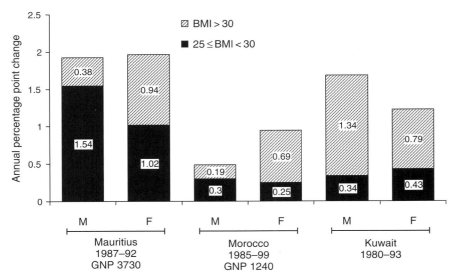

Figure 5 Obesity trends among adults in North Africa/Middle East (the annual percentage point increase in prevalence). BMI, body mass index; F, female; GNP, gross national product; M, male. (Data from Benjelloun S. (2002) Nutrition transition in Morocco. *Publlic Health Nutrition* **5**(1A): 135–40. Hodge (1996) Reference: Hodge AM, Dowse GK, Gareeboo H, Tuomilehto J, Alberti KG, Zimmet PZ. (1996) Incidence, increasing prevalence, and predictors of change in obesity and fat distribution over 5 years in the rapidly developing population of Mauritius. *International Journal of Obesity* **20**: 137–46. Al-Isa (1995,1997) References: 1-Isa AN. (1995) Prevalance of obesity among adult Kuwaitis: a cross-sectional study. *International Journal of Obesity and Related Metabolic Disorders*. **19**(6):431–3. A1-Isa AN. (1997) Changes in bidy mass index (BMI) and prevalance of obesity among Kuwaitis 1980–1994. *International Journal of Obesity* **21**: 1093–9.)

countries in the lowest 75% of countries (all of which have incomes less than $5800 per capita) of the per capita income distribution. The absolute level of vegetable fat consumption increased, but there remained at most a weak association between GNP and vegetable fat intake in these aggregate data. The change in edible vegetable fat prices, supply, and consumption is unique because it equally affected rich and poor countries, but the net impact is relatively much greater on low-

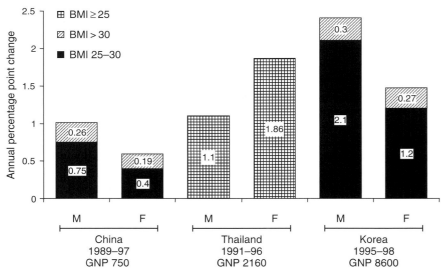

Figure 6 Obesity trends among adults in Asia (the annual percentage point increase in prevalence). BMI, body mass index; F, female; GNP, gross national product; M, male. (Data from Kosulwat V. (2002) The nutrition and health transition in Thailand. *Public Health Nutrition* **5**(1A): 183–89. Du (2002) Reference: Du S,Lu B, Zhai F and Popkin BM. (2002) A new stage of the nutrition in China. *Public Health Nutrition* **5**(1A): 169–74. Lee (2002) Reference: Lee M-J, Popkin BM and Kim S. (2002) The unique aspects of the nutritioin transition in South Korea: the retention of healthful elements in their traditional diet. *Public Health Nutrition* **5**(1A): 197–203.)

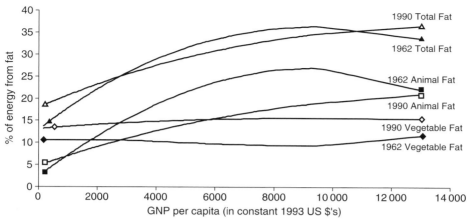

Figure 7 Relationship between the percentage of energy from fat and gross national product (GNP) *per capita*, 1962 and 1990. (Source: Nonparametric regressions run with food balance data from FAOUN and GNP data from the World Bank for 134 countries; Guo X, Mroz TA, Popkin BM and Zhai F (2000) Structural changes in the impact of income on food consumption in China, 1989–93. *Econoomic Development and Cultural Change* **48**: 737–60.)

income countries. Recent analysis in China shows that the pace of change for increased energy density and animal source foods in the diet has accelerated.

There is also an equally large and important shift in the proportion of energy from added caloric sweeteners in the diets of lower income countries. In fact, an additional 100–200 kcal per day was available for daily consumption from added caloric sweeteners in the diet in 2000 compared to 1962 in the developing world. In the United States, this added caloric sweetener increase derives mainly from soft drinks and fruit drinks, but in many other countries the source of this increase is other foods, even basic processed foods that have sweeteners added to them. Increasingly, high-fructose corn syrup is used as the sweetener of choice. This is unfortunate because there are mechanisms by which glucose may limit intake, but not fructose.

When we specifically examine the combined effect of these various shifts in the structure of rural and urban Chinese diets, we find an upward shift in the energy density of the foods consumed. In this study, the kilocalories of energy intake from foods and alcohol per 100 grams of food in both urban and rural Chinese adult diets increased by more than 10% (to 2.42) between 1989 and 1997. These are very rapid shifts in energy density. It is important to note that the value of 2.42 is not comparable with the normal measure of energy density of the diet. The normal method includes full measures of all beverages, whereas the Chinese Food Composition Table, from which this data was extracted, measures only a few beverages (milk,

coconut juice, sugarcane juice, spirits, beer, wine, champagne, and brandy) and excludes many beverages, particularly tea and coffee. A number of clinical investigations have varied the energy density of the diet in ad libitum studies. Each study shows that increases in energy density, often as small as from 1 to 1.3 kcal/g, can increase total energy intake. For these reasons, energy density changes in China, and most likely in other developing countries, are critical components of dietary change to be monitored.

Rapid Social Change Is Important: Urbanization, Rapid Demographic Change, and Other Behavioral Changes Are Occurring Simultaneously

Diets have shifted in urban areas in a far more dramatic fashion than in rural areas. We do not focus on many of the complex issues related to the type of urban change that has occurred. Nevertheless, critical sociodemographic issues include the following:

- Rapid reductions in fertility have enhanced the shift in the age distribution.
- Urbanization continues unabated in Asia and Africa. More poor will reside in urban than rural areas in future decades.
- Economic changes, particularly increased income and income inequality, appear to define changes in many regions of the developing world.
- Globalization of mass media is occurring at an earlier stage of economic development than occurred in higher income countries in the past.

Urbanization

In other published work, we have shown how the structure of diet has shifted markedly as populations have urbanized. This relationship will, by itself, shift the structure of diet significantly at the national level as urbanization continues and as the proportion of the population in urban areas grows.

Structural Shifts in Income–Diet Relationships Are Occurring

Changes in dietary behavior can be caused either by shifts in the composition of society regarding the plurality of the educated, rich, or urban residents or by changes in actual behavior of those with specific characteristics. This latter type can include a change in consumption behavior such that for the same level of education or income, a person would buy different amounts or types of commodities at different points in time. Research conducted in China shows that there have been profound behavioral shifts of this type during the past decade (i.e., for each extra dollar of income, additional high-fat foods are purchased vs. what would have been purchased in previous years for the equivalent extra dollar). Economists speak of this effect as one that shows how the decision-making demand pattern for food has changed, so for the same income level the patterns of demand have changed significantly from earlier periods. The explosion in access and exposure to mass media may very well have created this situation.

Mass Media

There is no doubt that access to modern mass media has increased very rapidly, particularly in the past decade. Elsewhere, we have shown worldwide trends. It is most useful to examine the proportion of households in a country that have TV sets to gain insight into this topic. Again, we use China Health and Nutrition Survey (CHNS) data to demonstrate the types of changes in one setting. Overall, 88.5% of Chinese households in the CHNS sample had TVs in 1997. It is important to note that not only the proportion of people with access to TV was shifting but also the types of programs and access to Western influences were shifting. In the 1980s, cable systems in China did not provide outside programming, but by 1997 approximately one-fourth of Chinese provinces provided access to Phoenix Star TV, a Hong Kong TV system that relies heavily on US and British programming and provides modern TV advertising.

Again, although there are no extensive data on the proportions of Chinese households with access to mass media 30–70 years ago, it is certain that the penetration into Chinese households in 1997 was far greater than it was into US households 50 years ago, when TV was in its infancy.

Health Effects: Is the Biology Different? Rather, Do We Have Different Social Structures and Body Composition Patterns That Affect BMI–Disease Relationships? Are There Genetic Variants That Are Important?

There are a number of different ways these questions could be answered in the affirmative. One is if the body composition and other unmeasured race/ethnic factors affect susceptibility to NR-NCDs. Another might be if previous disease patterns (e.g., the presence of malaria or other tropical diseases) led to disease patterns that predisposed the population to certain problems. One component of this may be the fetal insult syndrome developed and popularized by Barker.

There is a growing body of research that shows the international standards, used to delineate who is overweight and obese, are not appropriate for many large subpopulations in the world. For instance, a BMI of 25 in an Asian adult appears to have a far greater adverse metabolic effect than in a Caucasian adult. In fact, the World Health Organization and the International Obesity Task Force formed a group of scientists and agencies in Asia to review this topic. This group held international meetings and has proposed a lower BMI cutoff for Asians of 23 for overweight and 25 for obesity. In one paper comparing China, the Philippines, and US Hispanics, blacks, and whites, the odds of being hypertensive were higher for Chinese men and women compared to other subpopulation groups at lower BMIs in the 23–25 range. Ethnic differences in the strength of the association between BMI and disease outcomes warrant further consideration.

Zimmet and others who have focused on this issue as it relates to lower income countries believe that the highest genetic susceptibility for adult-onset diabetes is for Pacific Islanders, American Indians, Mexican Americans and other Hispanics, and Asian Indians. Those with modest genetic susceptibility include Africans, Japanese, and Chinese. The age of onset (usually after age 50 years) of non-insulin-dependent diabetes mellitus is much lower for these susceptible populations, and it appears that the prevalence is higher for a given level of obesity and waist:hip ratio. Zimmet summarizes a large selection of literature that has explored these issues relating to diabetes among susceptible populations.

It is not clear how much of this difference between subpopulations regarding BMI–diabetes or other BMI–morbidity relationships is a function of differences of body composition, metabolic or genetic factors, or social causes. We have shown that part of the apparent race–hypertension relationship may also be explained by socioeconomic status.

Another dimension relates to the issue of inflammatory burden. Evidence that inflammation plays a central role in cardiovascular disease (CVD), particularly at all stages of atherosclerosis, is persuasive. This position is supported by basic science and epidemiology. As reviewed in a meta-analysis, the magnitude of the associations between CVD outcomes and levels of inflammatory factors, such as C-reactive protein, albumin, white blood cell count, and fibrinogen, is surprisingly consistent across studies, despite differing designs, populations, duration of follow-up, and case definitions.

There is another pathway related to the role of previous health problems for which there is less understanding and no real documentation of its impact (e.g., malnutrition that caused a virus to mutate, parasitic infections that affected long-term absorption patterns, or a parasite that is linked to an unknown genotype—comparable to sickle cell anemia and its evolutionary linkage with malaria). We have no basis for speculation about this potential pathway.

However, the final pathway—the effect of fetal and infant insults on subsequent metabolic function—appears to be a critical area. If the rapid shifts toward positive energy imbalance are occurring concurrently with higher levels of low birth weight in a population, then this becomes a much more salient aspect of this argument. For the developing world, where intrauterine malnutrition rates are high and there is a high prevalence of nutrition insults during infancy, the work of Barker and many others portends important potential effects on the prevalence of NR-NCDs in the coming decades. Not only is there an emerging consensus that fetal insults, particularly with regard to thin, low-birth-weight infants who subsequently face a shift in the stage of the transition and become overweight, are linked with increased risk of NR-NCDs but also infancy may equally be a period of high vulnerability. Three studies by Hoffman suggest that fat metabolism of stunted infants is impaired to the extent that this may lead to increased obesity and other metabolic shifts. Other work on the role of stunting on obesity suggested such an effect, but Hoffman's work

suggests the mechanism and fits with the correlational work.

The CVD Epidemic Is Beginning

Evidence from many developing countries shows that nutrition-related chronic diseases prematurely disable and kill a large proportion of economically productive people, a preventable loss of precious human capital. This includes countries in which HIV/AIDS is a dominant problem. Four out of five deaths from nutrition-related chronic diseases occur in middle- and low-income countries. Reddy reviewed these data and noted that

> the current high burden of NCDs is highlighted by the estimates for 1998 that indicate these disorders contributed to 58.8% of global mortality and 43% of the global burden of disease, measured as disability adjusted life-years lost. The contribution of low- and middle-income countries to this burden is large; about 77% of the total mortality and 85% of the total burden of disease attributable to NCDs arises from these countries. (page 231)

The burden of cardiovascular disease alone is now far greater in India, and also in China, than in all economically developed countries in the world combined. Low-income communities are especially vulnerable to nutrition-related chronic diseases, which are not just diseases of affluence. CVD, cancer, diabetes, neuropsychiatric ailments, and other chronic diseases are becoming major contributors to the burden of disease, even as infections and nutritional deficiencies are receding as leading contributors to death and disability.

Furthermore, CVD in the developing world emerges at an earlier age. As Reddy notes,

> Thus in 1990, 46.7% of CVD-related deaths in developing countries occurred below the age of 70 years, in contrast to only 22.8% in the high-income industrial countries. The Global Burden of Disease Study projected 6.4 million deaths would occur due to CVD in the developing countries in 2020, in the age group of 30–69 years. (page 233)

A World Health Report updates this analysis and focuses on the important role of obesity and CVD and cancer deaths in the developing world.

There are major differences in the profiles of the CVD epidemic across the developing world. For instance, hypertension and stroke are more likely to emerge in east Asia, whereas diabetes occurs earlier in south Asia.

As would be expected from the dietary and obesity data noted previously, CVD levels are far greater in urban areas of the developing world, but often the opposite is true in the developed higher income countries.

Social Burden of Changes in Diet, Body Composition, and Health

In higher income countries, increasingly higher income groups follow a more healthful lifestyle, whereas the poor do not. Thus, higher income Americans consume a more healthful diet pattern, exercise more, and smoke less, and similar patterns are found in other high-income countries. In contrast, the prevailing opinion has been that the opposite is found in the developing world, namely that the poor are less likely to have a heavy burden of NR-NCDs compared to the rich. This is changing rapidly. It has been shown that obesity has declined among the better educated and increased among the lower educated in southeastern Brazil. It has also been shown that not only are less healthful dietary patterns consumed by higher income Chinese but also other dimensions of lifestyle (inactivity, smoking, and drinking) are poorer among the higher socioeconomic status (SES) Chinese. In other research, scholars of China have shown a rapid shift in food consumption patterns among different income groups in China that seems to indicate a shift in the burden of poor diets toward the poor in China. It has been shown that for countries with a GNP per capita of more than $2500, the likelihood is very great that there will be more obesity among the lower SES groups compared to higher SES groups.

The Future

Consuming a more tasteful and richer diet is a goal of most of the world's population. As shown here, dietary change is universal. In particular, rapid change is seen in the poorest areas of the world. The challenge is to learn how to continue to improve the palatability and quality of our diet while doing so in a more healthful manner.

See also: **Diabetes Mellitus**: Etiology and Epidemiology. **Dietary Intake Measurement**: Methodology; Validation. **Famine. Fats and Oils. Nutrient Requirements,**

International Perspectives. **Obesity**: Definition, Etiology and Assessment.

Further Reading

Adair LS, Kuzawa CW, and Borja J (2001) Maternal energy stores and diet composition during pregnancy program adolescent blood pressure. *Circulation* 104: 1034–1039.

Barker DJP (2001) *Fetal Origins of Cardiovascular and Lung Disease* New York: Marcel Dekker.

Bell AC, Adair LS, and Popkin BM (2002) Ethnic differences in the association between body mass index and hypertension. *American Journal of Epidemiology* 155: 346–353.

Bell C, Ge K, and Popkin BM (2001) Weight gain and its predictors in Chinese adults. *International Journal of Obesity* 25: 1079–1086.

Bell EA, Castellanos VH, Pelkman CL *et al.* (1998) Energy density of foods affects energy intake in normal-weight women. *American Journal of Clinical Nutrition* 67: 412–420.

Bray GA, Nielsen SJ, and Popkin BM (2004) Consumption of high-fructose corn syrup in beverages may play a role in the epidemic of obesity. *American Journal of Clinical Nutrition* 79: 537.

Drewnowski A and Popkin BM (1997) The nutrition transition: New trends in the global diet. *Nutrition Reviews* 55: 31–43.

Eaton SB and Konner M (1985) Paleolithic nutrition: A consideration on its nature and current implications. *New England Journal of Medicine* 312: 283–289.

Hoffman DJ, Sawaya AL, Coward WA *et al.* (2000) Energy expenditure of stunted and nonstunted boys and girls living in the shantytowns of Sao Paulo, Brazil. *American Journal of Clinical Nutrition* 72: 1025–1031.

International Diabetes Institute (2000) *The Asia-Pacific Perspective: Redefining Obesity and Its Treatment.* Victoria Australia: Health Communications Australia.

Monteiro CA, Conde WL, and Popkin BM (2002) Is obesity replacing or adding to undernutrition? Evidence from different social classes in Brazil. *Public Health Nutrition* 5(1A): 105–112.

Omran AR (1971) The epidemiologic transition: A theory of the epidemiology of population change. *Milbank Quarterly* 49: 509–538.

Popkin BM (2002) The shift in stages of the nutrition transition in the developing world differs from past experiences! *Public Health Nutrition* 5(1A): 205–214

Popkin BM and Nielsen SJ (2003) The sweetening of the world's diet. *Obesity Research* 11: 1325–1332.

Reddy KS (2002) Cardiovascular disease in the developing countries: dimensions, determinants, dynamics and directions for public health action. *Public Health Nutrition* 5(1A): 231–237.

Zimmet PZ, McCarty DJ, and de Courten MP (1997) The global epidemiology of non-insulin-dependent diabetes mellitus and the metabolic syndrome. *Journal of Diabetes Complications* 11(2): 60–68.

NUTRITIONAL ASSESSMENT

Contents
Anthropometry
Biochemical Indices
Clinical Examination

Anthropometry

J Eaton–Evans, University of Ulster, Coleraine, UK

This article is reproduced from the first edition, pp. 1357–1363, © 1999, Elsevier Ltd. with revisions made by the Editor.

Anthropometric measurements include weight, height, length, selected skinfold thicknesses, and head, waist, hip, and arm circumferences. When compared with reference values, these measurements or combinations of these measurements can provide information on body size and the proportion and distribution of body fat and lean body mass in adults; they can also be used to assess growth in children. Anthropometric measurements indirectly indicate present or past nutrition and may be markers of future ill-health.

This article reviews the uses, advantages, and limitations of anthropometric measurements; discusses the technical errors of the measurements; describes the most frequently used measurements, derived nutritional indices, and reference values; and summarizes the laboratory methods that may validate the assessments.

Uses of Anthropometric Measurements

In adults and children, anthropometric measurements can be used to estimate body fat and lean body mass and assess their distribution and change over time. Body fat includes storage fat, found inter- and intra-muscularly, around the organs and gastro-intestinal tract and subcutaneously, as well as lipids in bone marrow, central nervous tissue, mammary glands, and other organs. Normal-weight men and women have about 10 and 20% body fat, respectively. Lean body or fat-free mass is mostly water and protein with relatively small amounts of glycogen and minerals. Inadequate diets are associated with low body fat stores and reduced lean body mass in adults and growth failure of children. Consumption of food greater than requirements results in excessive body fat stores in adults and children. Body fat stores that are too low or too high are associated with increased risk of morbidity and mortality. The proportion and distribution of fat and fat-free mass varies with age, sex, genetics, disease, some hormones, and some drug treatments. Extensive physical exercise may be associated with increased muscle mass.

Different anthropometric measurements and combinations of measurements provide information on body composition and fat distribution and, therefore, nutritional status. The choice of measurements depends on the purpose of the assessment, the equipment available, the subjects being measured, and the skills of the observer making the measurements. Measurements can be made in laboratories, clinics, and hospitals using fixed, precision equipment with a high degree of accuracy, or in the field, including peoples' homes or rural centers, with lighter, robust, and portable equipment.

Advantages and Limitations of Anthropometric Measurements

Anthropometric measurements are noninvasive. Compared with other methods of assessing nutritional status, the measurements are quick and easy to make using relatively cheap and simple equipment. They can be made by relatively unskilled people.

Anthropometric measurements cannot identify protein and micronutrient deficiencies, detect small disturbances in nutritional status, nor identify small changes in the proportions of body fat to lean body mass. Some anthropometric measurements may not be socially or culturally acceptable, such as the measurement by men of womens' subscapular and supra-iliac skinfold thicknesses; some measurements may be impractical to make, such as the height in people who are unable to stand straight. Observers with limited literacy skills may not be able to read and therefore record some measurements. A single anthropometric measurement, such as weight, does not normally in itself assess growth and/or body composition and, therefore, indicate nutritional status. To interpret anthropometric measurements, single measurements or combinations of measurements must be compared with reference values, by age and sex. Such reference values are not available for all population groups nor for all ages.

Errors of Anthropometric Measurements

All anthropometric measurements should be made as accurately as possible. Measurement errors may result in the misclassification of subjects' nutritional status or may lead to changes in nutritional status over time being over- or underestimated. Very precise and accurate measurements are needed for nutrition research and in some clinical situations. The same degree of precision may not be possible in nutritional screening and surveillance programs in field studies. Errors in making measurements arise from the equipment, the physical state and age of the subjects, the time of day when the measurements are made, misreading of measurements by the observer, and as a result of rounding up or down to the nearest half or whole integer. These technical errors of measurement (TEM) vary with the age of the subjects, the measurements being made, and between (inter-) and within (intra-) observers. Values for a particular anthropometric measurement of a group of people by age and sex can be considered accurate if the inter- and intraobserver error is close to a reference value for TEM in a series of repeated measurements and if there are no biases in the measurement. For measurements of subjects outside the age range, the coefficient of variability (R) can be calculated as $R = 1 - [(TEM)^2/(SD)^2]$, where SD is the total intersubject variance including measurement error. It has been recommended that an R of 0.90, that is a measurement 90% error-free, is an acceptable lower limit of accuracy, although an intraobserver R of 0.95 might be more realistic in some circumstances.

TEM can be minimized by careful training of all observers and by making measurements using appropriate equipment in triplicate and then calculating the mean. If measurements for a research study are to be made by more than one person, the interobserver measurements made must be comparable. R can be calculated for interobserver variability by making a series of measurements.

Anthropometric Measurements

Height

Height, or stature, is measured in adults and children over the age of 2 years using a stadiometer, a portable anthropometer, or a moveable headboard on a vertical measuring rod. The measuring device should be checked for accuracy using a standard 2-m steel tape. Subjects should be measured to the nearest 0.1 cm. Subjects, in minimal clothing with bare heads and feet, should stand straight, arms hanging loosely to the side, feet together and with heels, buttocks and shoulder blades in contact with the vertical surface of the stadiometer. Errors occur if subjects do not stand straight, do not keep heels on the ground, or overstretch. Diurnal variation results in people being 0.5–1 cm shorter in the evening than in the morning.

Height cannot be measured accurately in adults with severe kyphosis of the spine and in those who are bed- or chair-ridden. Since knee height is highly correlated with stature, height in such adults can be estimated from the measurement of knee height, using a sliding calliper. The regression equations, derived from a nonrandom sample of American people over the age of 60 years, are:

$$Height\ (cm)\ for\ men = (2.02 \times knee\ height, cm) \\ - (0.04 \times age, years) \\ + 64.19$$

$$Height\ (cm)\ for\ women = (1.83 \times knee\ height, cm) \\ - (0.24 \times age, years) \\ + 84.88$$

Variations in the proportion of limb length to trunk length can lead to a standard error in the estimate (SEE) of height from knee height of ±8 cm. Demi-span, which is the distance between the sternal notch of the right collar bone and the left finger root of the middle and ring finger when the subject's arm is horizontal and in line with the shoulders, can also be used to estimate height.

Length, rather than height, is measured in infants and children under the age of 3 years. Length is measured by laying a child face upwards on a measuring board with the head against the fixed headboard, and moving another board up to and resting against the child's heels with the legs straight (**Figure 1**). Small changes in length (±0.5 cm) may not be significant as it is a difficult measurement to make. Children wriggle and will not stretch out their legs. Length measurements are 1–2 cm longer than height.

Height (stature) or length indicates attained size or growth of adults and children. Long periods of inadequate food intake or increased morbidity result in a slowing of skeletal growth and individuals being short for their age, or stunted. Consecutive measurements of height every 3–6 months can be used to assess growth velocity in children and to indicate the timing of the adolescent growth spurt.

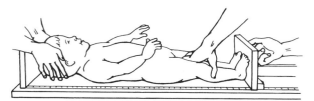

Figure 1 Measurement of recumbent length in children younger than 3 years of age. The head should be in contact with the fixed headboard, with child facing straight up. With legs fully extended, the mobile footboard should be placed firmly against the infant's heels. (Reproduced with permission from Frisancho AR (1990) *Anthropometric Standards for the Assessment of Growth and Nutritional Status.* Ann Arbor: University of Michigan Press.)

Weight

Weight is measured with digital weighing scales, using a pan, basket, sling, standing platform or chair, depending on the age and mobility of the people being measured. Weighing scales must be set on a hard, level, and even surface. Scales should be accurate, sensitive, and robust. They must be carefully maintained, calibrated, regularly checked for accuracy using known weights, and always set at zero before use. Weight is usually measured to the nearest 0.1 kg for adults and 0.01 kg for infants.

Weight measures total body mass but does not provide information on the proportions of fat, water, protein, and minerals. Weight and fat are only synonymous in very heavy people. Adults can be heavy for height if very muscular, overfat, and/or big framed. With accurate scales, small changes in weight are detectable but may not necessarily reflect change in body fat or lean body mass. In healthy persons, day-to-day variation in body weight is usually small (± 0.5 kg). Consecutive measurements of weight can be used to monitor the effects of treatment such as weight loss on reduction diets or weight gain with nutritional interventions and supplementation. Weight changes are assumed to reflect changes in the amount of body fat. However, changes in body weight may also result from differences in hydration, oedema, tumour growth, and trauma, as well as from factors such as the amount of food in the gastrointestinal tract and the fullness of the bladder. Weight may remain constant if the loss of muscle mass is masked by increased fat as seen in sarcopenia, the age-related loss of muscle, or by increased fluid retention.

Weight-for-height (or length) can be used to indicate body composition in adults and is an age-independent measure of body composition in children. Growth can be measured in children by consecutive measurements of weight over time (growth velocity) or by weight-for-age if the children's ages are known.

Head Circumference

Head circumference is measured in infants and young children, to the nearest 0.1 cm, with a narrow flexible nonstretch tape laid over the supraorbital ridges and the part of the occiput which gives the maximum circumference. The head circumference of infants increases rapidly in the first 2 years of life. Increase in head circumference in the first 2 years of life is affected by nutritional status and nonnutritional problems, including some diseases, genetic variation, and cultural practices.

Mid-Upper Arm Circumference

Mid-upper arm circumference (MUAC) is measured in adults and children, to the nearest 0.1 cm, using a flexible nonstretch tape laid at the midpoint between the acromion and olecranon processes on the shoulder blade and the ulna, respectively, of the arm (**Figure 2**). MUAC is a measure of the sum of the muscle and subcutaneous fat in the upper arm. In severe malnutrition both fat and muscle are reduced in the upper arm. Oedema may increase a limb's circumference but it is not usually a problem of the upper arm. MUAC can be used as a indicator of body composition in adults and children. Since MUAC increases little between the age of 6 months and 5 years, it can be used in preschool children as

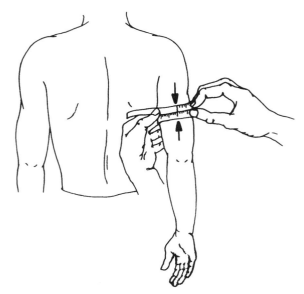

Figure 2 Measurement of upper arm circumference at the mid-point of the upper arm. (Reproduced with permission from Frisancho AR (1990) *Anthropometric Standards for the Assessment of Growth and Nutritional Status.* Ann Arbor: University of Michigan Press.)

an age-independent screening tool for severe malnutrition. A MUAC less than 12.5 cm suggests malnutrition. A MUAC greater than 13.5 cm is normal.

Skinfold Thickness

Precision skinfold thickness callipers are used to measure the double fold of skin and subcutaneous fat to the nearest millimeter. The usual sites of measurement are at the triceps (TSFT), the midpoint of the back of the upper arm (**Figure 3**); the biceps (BSFT) at the same level as the TSFT but to the front of the upper left arm; the subscapular (SSFT) just below and laterally to the left shoulder blade (**Figure 4**); and the suprailiac (SISFT) obliquely just above the left iliac crest. Skinfold thicknesses can also be measured at the mid-thigh, mid-calf, and abdomen.

Skinfold thicknesses are difficult measurements to make with precision and accuracy: It is difficult to pick up a consistent fold of skin and subcutaneous fat; in the very obese, the skinfold may be bigger than the callipers can measure; the fold of skin and fat compresses with repeated measurements; and the careless use of the callipers causes pain, bruising, and skin damage to subjects. There is, therefore, likely to be considerable inter- and intraobserver error in the measurements.

Skinfold thicknesses measure subcutaneous body fat and, therefore, indicate body composition. TSFT

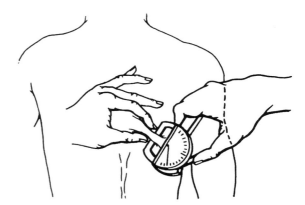

Figure 4 Measurement of subscapular skinfold using a Lange caliper. With subject's arm and shoulder relaxed, a horizontal skinfold is picked approximately 1 cm below the tip of the scapula with thumb and index fingers. The caliper is applied 1 cm from fingers. (Reproduced with permission from Frisancho AR (1990) *Anthropometric Standards for the Assessment of Growth and Nutritional Status*. Ann Arbor: University of Michigan Press.)

and SSFT indicate subcutaneous fat on the limbs and body trunk, respectively. Skinfold thickness measurements mistakenly assume that subcutaneous fat, measured at one or more selected sites, measures total body fat stores. However, subcutaneous fat at one site may not reflect fat stores at another site, and may not be positively correlated with the amount of visceral fat deposited around the internal organs of the body. Subcutaneous fat, and therefore skinfold thicknesses at the different sites, changes at varying rates with age, weight change, with diseases such as diabetes, and in women during pregnancy, postpartum, and at the menopause. Skinfold thicknesses are not useful for monitoring short-term change in fat stores. If only one skinfold thickness measurement is made, TSFT is most commonly selected. TSFT correlates with estimates of total body fat in women and children. SSFT is better than TSFT as an indicator of total body fat in men. SSFT has been shown to be a predictor of blood pressure in adults independently of age and racial group.

Waist and Hip Circumferences

Waist and hip circumferences are measured to the nearest 0.1 cm using a flexible narrow nonstretch tape in adults wearing minimal clothing, standing straight but not pulling in their stomachs. Waist circumference is measured halfway between the lower ribs and the iliac crest, while hip circumference is measured at the largest circumference around the buttocks. Measurement error occurs if the tape is pulled too tight or loose, or if subjects wear clothes with belts and/or full pockets.

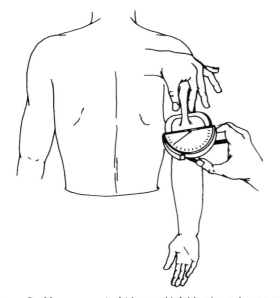

Figure 3 Measurement of triceps skinfold using a Lange caliper. With the subject's arm in a relaxed position, the skinfold is picked with thumb and index fingers at the mid-point of the arm. (Reproduced with permission from Frisancho AR (1990) *Anthropometric Standards for the Assessment of Growth and Nutritional Status*. Ann Arbor: University of Michigan Press.)

With increase in waist circumference there is an increase in insulin sensitivity, while a waist circumference greater than 94 cm in men and 80 cm in women has been associated with increased risk factors for cardiovascular disease.

Elbow Width

Elbow width is the width of the epicondyles of the humerus with the elbow flexed at 90°. Sliding callipers are used to measure elbow width in adults to the nearest 0.1 cm. Elbow width is a measure of bone size. Frame size can be determined by comparison with reference values either by age or by height and sex.

Nutritional Indices

Most single anthropometric measurements do not in themselves assess nutritional status. Nutritional indices are derived either by combining two or more anthropometric measurements, shown in laboratory studies to be predictive of body composition, or by comparison of the anthropometric measurements with reference values of healthy, well-fed populations. A combination of these methods can also be used.

Body Mass Index

Body mass index relates weight (kg) with height (m) by a simple calculation to indicate body composition (BMI = weight/height^2). It is the most commonly used screening measurement for both obesity and underweight as very low and high BMI are associated with increased mortality and morbidity. BMI classifies adults as underweight, normal, overweight, or obese (**Table 1**). BMI and percentage body fat is only highly correlated at extremes of the distribution. BMI cannot distinguish between adults who are heavy because of fat or heavy because of muscle, takes no account of frame size, and provides no information on body fat distribution. These limitations may result in heavy, muscled sports people being classified as overweight or obese.

Table 1 Classifications of nutritional status as a percentage of ideal body weight and body mass index

% of ideal body weight for height	Body mass index	Nutritional status
>120	>30	Obese
110–120	25–29.9	Overweight
90–109	20–24.9	Normal
<90	<20	Underweight

In children, BMI is age-dependent. BMI increases rapidly in the first year of life and then more slowly. Children, at extremes of the distribution of reference values by age and sex, can be identified as being abnormally thin or fat for height. The BMI classification used for adults should not be used for children.

Weight-for-Height

Weight-for-height is an indicator of body composition in adults. Reference values by age, sex, and frame size can be used to estimate desirable body weights (%desirable body weight = (actual weight ÷ ideal body weight) × 100), which are categorized by cutoff points (**Table 1**).

Weight-for-height by sex is a sensitive indicator of body composition in children. It appears to be relatively independent of ethnic group in children aged 1–5 years and age-independent in children aged 1–10 years. Children with weights less than 85% of the median reference weight-for-height are considered wasted. It is a useful screening tool for current malnutrition, especially if used with height-for-age. Oedema and obesity, however, may confound the index.

Weight-for-Age

Weight-for-age can be used to monitor growth in children of known age when a series of measurements are made and compared with reference values by sex. A single measurement of weight-for-age does not discriminate between a child who is light for age because of stunting and/or wasting owing to malnutrition, and one who is small for age but healthy and well fed. Children should gain weight as a percentile of the reference values. Failure to gain weight as expected or a weight loss indicates an inadequate diet, infection, and/or lack of care and should be investigated. Maintenance of weight or weight gain may mask the loss of lean body fat and the increased oedema of kwashiorkor.

Growth Velocity

Growth velocity, or change in weight or height over time, can be used to assess growth in children when compared with reference values by age and sex. Growth rates decline in the first few years of life and then increase with the pubertal growth spurt. Premature and small-for-dates children and those recovering from malnutrition and severe infections tend to have higher growth velocities (catch-up growth). Growth velocities are useful to monitor growth and assess the response to therapy including nutritional supplementation.

Head Circumference-for-Age

Head circumference-for-age by sex is used by paediatricians to identify children up to 2 years of age with severe chronic malnutrition pre- and postpartum and the need for further medical investigations. It is not a good indicator of children's nutritional status.

Mid-Upper Arm Circumference-for-Age

Mid-upper arm circumference (MUAC)-for-age indicates body composition (upper arm fat and muscle) in adults and children when used with measurements of weight and height. MUAC measurements are compared with reference values by age and sex. Since the rate of change of arm circumference is slow, it cannot be used to assess growth or monitor the response to therapy.

Mid-Upper Arm Circumference-for-Height

Mid-upper arm circumference-for-height (the QUAC stick) is a cheap, quick, age-independent screening tool for children with malnutrition. It is a vertical stick on which are inscribed the 80 and 85% median reference values for MUAC and height, respectively. A child is considered malnourished if the MUAC is less than 80% of the MUAC expected for height.

Skinfold Thickness-for-Age

Skinfold thickness-for-age and sex indicates subcutaneous body fat stores in adults and children. Reference values for TSFT, SSFT, and the sum of the TSFT and SSFT are available by age and sex.

Measurement of BMI with skinfold thicknesses can identify people who are heavy owing to excess fat or muscle mass. A high BMI and low TSFT and/or SSFT indicate a large muscle mass; a high BMI and high TSFT and/or SSFT indicate a high subcutaneous body fat.

Mid-Upper Arm Muscle Circumference and Upper Arm Muscle Area

Mid-upper arm muscle circumference (MUAMC) and upper arm muscle area (AMA) are estimates of upper arm muscle and, therefore, body composition. They can be used as indicators of muscle mass and protein stores. Both MUAMC and AMA are calculated from measurements of MUAC and TSFT on the mistaken assumption that the arm is cylindrical, the subcutaneous fat is equally distributed, the bone atrophies in proportion to muscle wastage in malnutrition, and the cross-sections of neurovascular tissue and bone are small. The formula, with MUAC and TSFT in mm, is:

$$MUAMC = MUAC - (\pi \times TSFT)$$

AMA can be calculated from revised formulae which take account of errors resulting from the noncircular nature of muscle and the inclusion of nonskeletal muscle with MUAC and TSFT in cm:

$$\text{For men: } AMA = \left[\frac{MUAC - (\pi \times TSFT)}{4\pi}\right]^2 - 10.0$$

$$\text{For women: } AMA = \left[\frac{MUAC - (\pi \times TSFT)}{4\pi}\right]^2 - 6.5$$

MUAMC and AMA can be compared with reference values by age and sex. AMA cannot be used to monitor change in muscle stores because of the problems in making this measurement. The ratio of AMA to total body muscle mass changes with age and certain diseases.

Arm Fat Area

Arm fat area (AFA) can be derived from measurements of MUAC and TSFT. AMA is a better indicator of total body fat but not percentage body fat, than TSFT alone. The formula used to calculate AFA (with MUAC and TSFT in mm) is:

$$AMA = \frac{TSFT \times MUAC}{2} - \frac{\pi \times (TSFT)^2}{4}$$

AMA can be compared with reference values by age and sex. Theoretically, limb fat area can be calculated for other limbs and the body trunk, but there are no reference values available.

Total Body Fat

Total body fat can be estimated as a percentage of body fat by comparing the sum of TSFT, BSFT, SSFT, and SISFT with reference values derived from laboratory studies by age and sex, or via the estimation of body density from regression equations with skinfold thickness measurements. There are no specific empirical equations which can be used for specific population groups. Lean body mass is calculated by difference. These calculations may overestimate body fat in lean individuals and underestimate body fat in fat adults. They should not be used in undernourished individuals or in those with diseases where the total body water content may be markedly increased.

Waist-to-Hip Ratio

The waist-to-hip ratio (WHR) in adults discriminates between those with upper body or intraabdominal obesity (WHR greater than 1 in men and 0.8 in women) and those with lower body or peripheral obesity. Genetics, sex, and age partly determine body fat distribution. A high WHR is associated with an increased risk of premature mortality and morbidity.

Reference Values

Anthropometric assessments are interpreted by comparison with reference values by age and sex. Ideally, reference values should represent the range of 'optimum' measurements for health and longevity of a population of the same ethnic origin. Individuals should be considered at nutritional risk when above or below predetermined reference limits or cutoff points, based on functional impairment, clinical signs of deficiency, or increased risk of mortality and morbidity.

In practice, reference values are derived from large sets of cross-sectional anthropometric measurements of representative samples of populations of the same ethnic origin, who are assumed to be well nourished and free from infection, parasitic disease, and any other environmental factors which may affect growth and nutritional status. These data can be supplemented by data derived from direct laboratory studies of body composition. International reference values are used if local reference data are too difficult, time-consuming, and expensive to obtain.

Normal, healthy, well-fed people vary in size. Therefore, reference values are usually presented as percentiles, with values less than the 5th centile or greater than the 95th centile considered outside the normal range. If international reference values are used, it may be necessary to modify the cutoff points used for identifying those at risk for particular populations. Since the rate of growth of children is age-dependent, growth charts of the most commonly used anthropometric measurements and derived indices have been constructed. Children's growth is best monitored by plotting their sequential measurements on growth charts. A well-nourished healthy child should progress along a centile between the 5th and 95th centile for each measurement. When a child's measurements cross centiles of the growth charts, whether owing to growth faltering, failure-to-thrive, or excessive growth, the cause needs to be investigated. In this way anthropometric measurements can indicate the adequacy of a child's diet, the timing of the introduction of weaning foods, the impact of illness, and the response to treatment. To use growth charts such as weight-for-age, height-for-age, and head circumference-for-age, it is essential to know the age of a child accurately. A child's age cannot be estimated

accurately by examination. A malnourished child is smaller and looks younger and less mature than a well-fed, healthy child.

To analyse data for screening, surveillance, or research programmes, measurements can be compared with the median (50th centile) of the reference data and expressed as either a percentage of the median value or a modified statistical z-score transformation, where

$$SD\ score = \frac{\substack{individuals'\ measurement \\ -\ median\ value\ of\ reference\ value}}{standard\ deviation\ value\ of\ reference\ value}$$

SD scores are appropriate for use in areas with a high incidence of malnutrition. A high proportion of the population have measurements less than the 5th centile of reference values in these areas. A child with a SD score less than -2, irrespective of the nutritional indices used, is considered malnourished. A SD score greater than 2 suggests obesity.

The most commonly internationally used anthropometric reference values for noninstitutionalized adults aged 25–74 years have been derived from the American NHANES I and NHANES II studies, which were undertaken during 1971–74 and 1976–80, respectively. Reference values by sex, height, and frame size for desirable weights-for-height have also been derived from data on the longevity of holders of life insurance policies. These reference values are not taken from a random sample of the population, as only the more affluent in society are likely to hold life insurance; in addition, these values take no account of body composition and make no reference to the incidence of disease.

Many countries have developed their own reference standards for weight and height of children and adolescents. In the United States, the Centers for Disease Control and Prevention (CDC) published in the year 2000 growth charts for children 0–20 years of age, which for the first time included age-adjusted BMI data. The CDC dataset excluded anthropometric information from the most recent surveys fro certain age groups because of the marked secular trend to higher body weights in the US population.

The United Kingdom, France, and several other countries have developed reference growth curves based on national datasets. The World Health Organization is also leading an international effort to develop a truly global reference standard for growth, including reference values that reflect growth rates of exclusively breast-fed infants, who are known to grow at lower rates than formula-fed infants during the first year of life. Although growth rates differ across countries, there is general consensus that in healthy populations these differences are encompassed within the boundaries of acceptable percentile ranges, usually the 5th and 95th. Furthermore, environmental rather than genetic factors appear to be the main determinants of differences in growth across populations since migration of individuals from a poor to an adequate nutritional environment is usually accompanied by marked gains in height after only a few generations.

Children's growth is influenced by many factors, including sex, ethnic group, breast or bottle milk feeding, their birth order, gestational age of premature children, as well as the size (height) of their parents. Growth charts do not allow for these factors. With the secular changes in height and weight, growth charts derived from anthropometric measurements of children made over 30 years ago may no longer be appropriate to monitor growth of all children today. However, they may still be relevant to disadvantaged groups in the population. Similarly, growth charts of children derived from reference data of today may not be relevant to the children of the future.

A new reference data set, derived from mostly cross-sectional studies undertaken between 1978 and 1990 of 23 000 British children aged 0–20 years, has been developed by the Human Measurements Anthropometry and Growth Research Group. Growth charts from these data have been produced by sex for weight-for-age, height-for-age, length-for-age, head circumference-for-age, and BMI-for-age.

See also: **Dietary Intake Measurement**: Methodology; Validation. **Growth Monitoring**. **World Health Organization**.

Further Reading

Centers for Disease Control and Prevention (2005) *Growth Charts Dataset*. Available at www.cdc.gov/nchs/about/major/nhanes/growthcharts/datafiles.htm.

Frisancho AR (1990) *Anthropometric Standards for the Assessment of Growth and Nutritional Status*. Ann Arbor: University of Michigan Press.

Gibson RS (1990) *Principles of Nutritional Assessment*. New York: Oxford University Press.

Jelliffe DB (1966) *The Assessment of the Nutritional Status of the Community*. Geneva: World Health Organization.

World Health Organization (1995) *Physical Status: The Use and Interpretation of Anthropometry*, WHO Technical Report Series No. 854. Geneva: World Health Organization.

Biochemical Indices

F Fidanza, University of Rome Tor Vergata, Rome, Italy

Biochemical methods are considered to be the most objective measures for the assessment of nutritional status of the individual. The method employed should cover a range of cutoff points specific and sensitive to depletion of the nutrient body pool or tissue store.

The evolution of deficiency for most nutrients, particularly vitamins, progresses in successive stages. The first stage of deficiency is when nutrient body stores begin to be depleted; in this stage, nutrient urine excretion decreases, whereas homeostatic regulation ensures that the level of nutrient in the blood does not change. In the next stage, depletion is more marked; nutrient urinary excretion continues to decrease and its blood and other tissue concentrations are reduced.

A lowering of nutrient metabolites and/or dependent enzymes often characterizes the following stage. Sometimes, lower hormone concentrations and some physiological alterations are observed. In the last stages, morphological and/or functional disturbances are present; at first they are reversible, and then they become irreversible. Nonspecific signs and symptoms can be present; without therapeutic intervention, death can be expected.

Within the framework of the evolution of nutrient deficiencies, the biochemical static and functional tests most commonly used in nutritional status assessment in humans are discussed here.

Static Biochemical Tests

Static tests measure chemically the content of nutrients, their active or inactive metabolites, or other related components in tissues and urine. The choice of tissue or fluid depends on the information required (short-term or long-term status, body pool or tissue store) and on the condition of the subject.

Various confounding factors affect static biochemical tests. Some are of a general kind, such as age, sex, ethnic group, physiological and hormonal status, seasonality, elevation, and thus cannot be eliminated; others are of a technical nature and can be reduced or eliminated by standardization; and others are biological or environmental (e.g., alcohol intake, smoking habits, and use of medicines). The most relevant confounding factors are considered for each method; those that occur during infection are examined separately.

Protein Nutritional Status

Total serum protein determination is very seldom used because it is no longer considered a sensitive index of status.

Plasma proteins are albumin, transport proteins (transthyretin (TTR) involved in thyroid hormone transport and formerly called prealbumin, retinol binding protein (RBP), and transferrin (TF)) and fibronectin (FB; an apsonic glycoprotein). Serum albumin, measured by an automated dye-binding method, has a rather large body pool and a long half-life and so it is a less sensitive index of immediate nutritional status. TTR, complexed with RBP in the carriage of vitamin A, TF, and FB have a smaller pool size and a shorter half-life than serum albumin and so their concentrations can change more rapidly. Therefore, they are immediate indicators of protein status. Plasma transport proteins are usually measured on radial immunodiffusion plates or alternatively with laser nephelometry. Useful commercial kits are available. Plasma fibronectin is measured only with laser nephelometry. Albumin and transport proteins are negative acute phase reactants. Other confounding effects of protein-losing diseases, such as reduced protein synthesis diseases, conditions involving an increase in plasma volume, or hemodilution and zinc depletion, have been reported. In addition, RBP is sensitive to deficiencies of vitamin A, and TF is affected by iron status. Insulin has also been demonstrated to interfere with plasma transport protein levels.

Urinary creatinine, usually measured with a colorimetric method (also automated), is used as a biochemical marker of muscle mass. In fact, urinary creatinine is a nonenzymatic product of creatine and cannot be reutilized. Various assumptions are required for correct urinary creatinine determination, and various confounding effects are reported (age, diet, intensive exercise, pregnancy, injury, fever, and renal diseases with impaired creatinine clearance). In a clinical setting, the creatinine/height index is preferred, but because of some limitations, it is not very useful.

Urinary 3-methyl-histidine (3-MH) can be measured by ion exchange chromatography or high-performance liquid chromatography (HPLC). 3-MH is present in myofibrillar proteins, and during breakdown it is excreted quantitatively because it cannot be reused or oxidized. Accordingly, it is used as an indicator of muscle protein turnover.

Various confounding effects are reported (sex, age, diet, intensive exercise, stress, hormonal and catabolic states, etc.) and so the use of the urinary 3-MH test is considered to be rather problematic.

Insulin-like growth factor-1 (IGF-1), or somatomedin C, is a regulator of anabolic properties. It has been proposed as a sensitive indicator of protein deficiency. It is assayed in serum by a radioimmunoassay method available also in a kit. IGF-1 can also be used as a nutritional marker in adults receiving total parenteral nutrition. Confounding effects of stress, some hormonal diseases, and obesity have been reported.

Plasma amino acid levels have been used in the past to diagnose protein–energy malnutrition. The ratio of free nonessential amino acid levels (glycine, serine, glutamine, and taurine) to the essential amino acid levels (leucine, isoleucine, valine, and methionine) was proposed for the diagnosis of kwashiorkor. In children with this disease, this ratio can be much higher than the normal value of 2. Plasma amino acids were previously assessed by paper chromatographic methods; automated ion exchange or HPLC techniques are now preferred. However, in recent years there has been much less interest in this test.

Essential Fatty Acid Status

A number of measures can be used to assess deficiency of essential fatty acids. In serum cholesterol esters, fatty acids determination is related to recent intake, in erythrocyte membranes it is related to intake during the previous 2 or 3 months, and in subcutaneous fat tissue it is related to intake of fatty acids for more than 1 year. Essential fatty acids are measured by gas–liquid chromatography.

Vitamin Nutritional Status

Vitamin A (retinol) status can be assessed in the liver and plasma/serum. The best method is determination in the liver, but hepatic biopsy is very invasive and unsuitable in population studies. Plasma retinol is usually measured by HPLC after separation from its carrier (RBP), but its marginal values do not always reflect status because of homeostatic control and confounding effects (e.g., protein–energy malnutrition, infection, parasitic diseases, zinc deficiency, liver disorders, and chronic alcoholism). In the case of inflammation, the degree of depression of serum retinol can be quantified by assessing the concentration of certain acute phase proteins (CRP and AGP).

Because serum retinol is closely correlated with serum RBP, the measurement of this transport protein by the immunodiffusion technique or a portable apparatus has been proposed to assess vitamin A status.

The RBP:TTR molar ratio has been introduced to detect vitamin A deficiency (VAD) in the presence of inflammation. This test was based on the observation that VAD and inflammation were independent causes of low plasma RBP, whereas plasma TTR concentration was reduced only by inflammation. Nonsatisfactory results were reported from two African population groups.

The deuterated-retinol-dilution (DRD) technique is used to indirectly assess total body vitamin A reserves. A dose of deuterium-labeled retinyl acetate is given orally. After allowing time to reach equilibration (3–20 days), deuterated and nondeuterated retinol is measured by gas chromatography-mass spectrometry. A mathematical formula is used to estimate total body stores of vitamin A. Because of a set of assumptions and technical difficulties, this method is used mostly in research projects. In inflammation, the release of RBP is inhibited, so the test is probably unreliable.

In connection with vitamin A, its provitamins and non-provitamins, the carotenoids, need some consideration. β-Carotene and a few other carotenoids play an independent and specific role in preventing oxidation, genotoxicity, and malignancy. The serum level of carotenoids is correlated with vegetable and fruit intake. Lutein is the best indicator of green leafy vegetable consumption. Lycopene is a good measure of tomato-based product consumption. α-Carotene in industrialized countries is probably a biomarker of carrot consumption and in West Africa a good marker of red palm oil consumption. The plasma level of carotenoids is measured by the HPLC system. However, there are difficulties with peak identification and quantification. Confounding effects of diet and season, sex and age, infection, smoking, and drinking habits are reported. With an appropriate HPLC system, it is possible to measure in a single assay vitamins A and E and individual carotenoids.

Vitamin D status is generally assessed by measurement of serum 25-hydroxyvitamin D (25-OHD) and in some circumstances 1,25-dihydroxyvitamin D (1,25(OH)$_2$D). The current test for 25-OHD and 1,25(OH)$_2$D determination in serum is by radioimmunoassay, also available as commercial kits. The HPLC method with ultraviolet detection can be used as an alternative. Confounding effects of seasons, age, sex, drugs, and liver and renal diseases are reported.

Vitamin E status can be assessed in plasma, erythrocytes, platelets, and adipose tissue. The most common and practical measure is α-tocopherol in plasma by HPLC. Because α-tocopherol is bound to lipoproteins, it is preferred to express plasma α-tocopherol relative to serum cholesterol. The determination of α-tocopherol in adipose tissue biopsy provides information on long-term nutritional status, but this test is too invasive. Confounding effects of chronic enteropathies, protein–energy malnutrition, hemolitic anemia, cholestatic liver disease, and some drugs and heavy metals are reported.

Vitamin K status requires a multiple approach including a functional test. Plasma phylloquinone is measured by reversed-phase HPLC using postcolumn chemical reduction followed by fluorometric detection. Determination of the serum undercarboxylated form of prothrombin (PIVKA-II) by enzyme-linked immunosorbent assay (ELISA) and urinary γ-carboxyglutamic acid by HPLC with fluorometric detection has been proposed. Confounding effects of age, sex, season, malfunction of gastrointestinal tract, osteoporosis, liver diseases, antibiotics, and other drugs are reported.

Thiamin status can be assessed by urinary excretion and erythrocyte thiamin pyrophosphate (TPP) tests. Thiamin urinary excretion is indicative of recent dietary intake; thiamin is detected fluorometrically after conversion to thiochrome. If 24-h urine cannot be collected, thiamin should be determined in the fasting morning urine and expressed in relation to creatinine concentration. Erythrocyte TPP is indicative of long-term nutritional status and is assessed by HPLC using fluorometric detection after precolomn derivatization to thiochrome pyrophosphate. The only limitation is TPP instability, and determination should be carried out within 2 h of blood drawing. Erythrocyte TPP levels present large interindividual variation probably as a results of confounding factors (age and sex, alcohol intake, smoking habits, physical activity, and drugs).

Riboflavin status can be assessed by urinary excretion and whole blood flavinadeninedinucleotide (FAD) tests. Riboflavin urinary excretion is indicative of recent dietary intake; riboflavin is measured by HPLC using fluorometric detection. As for thiamin, if fasting morning urine is collected, riboflavin value is expressed in relation to millimoles of creatinine. Confounding effects of physical activity, bed rest, chronic alcoholism, antibiotics, and other drugs are reported. Whole blood FAD is considered a reliable indicator of long-term nutritional status and is assessed by reversed-phase HPLC using fluorometric detection. This test presents some advantages over the functional test erythrocyte glutathion reductase activation coefficient (EGR-AC).

Vitamin B_6 status is generally assessed by urinary 4-pyridoxic acid (4-PA) and whole blood or plasma pyridoxal-5'-phosphate (PLP) tests. The 4-PA test is indicative of recent intake but also of a deep compartment with slow elimination rate. 4-PA is measured by reversed-phase HPLC using fluorescence detection. When the completeness of 24-h collection is impossible, 4-PA is expressed in relation to millimoles of creatinine. PLP in whole blood or plasma is considered to be an indicator of depletion of vitamin B_6 reserves. In whole blood, PLP can be measured by reversed-phase HPLC using fluorometric detection. A HPLC system with fluorescence detector for determination of vitamin B_6 vitamers and pyridoxic acid in plasma is available. Plasma PLP can also be measured by radioenzymatic assay using tyrosine decarboxylase apoenzyme, which is more sensitive than other methods of analysis. Confounding effects of age and sex, acute phase status, tissue injury, catabolic state, smoking habits, alcoholism, pregnancy, drugs, physical exercise, organic diseases, and some inborn errors of metabolism are reported.

Niacin status can be assessed by measuring the two end products N'-methylnicotinamide ($N'MN$) and N'-methyl-2-pyridone-5-carboxamine (2-Py) in urine by HPLC. The ratio of these two urinary products is considered to be the best index of niacin nutritional status. With a single HPLC assay, the previously mentioned two nicotinamide metabolites and N^1-methyl-4-pyridone-3-carboxamide (4-Py) can be measured. The ratio $(2\text{-Py} + 4\text{-Py})/N'MN$ is proposed; it has a diurnal variation and decreases with cold. However, for nutritional status assessment further investigation is needed.

Folate status can be assessed by serum/plasma folate, which provides information on recent intake, and erythrocyte folate, indicative of body folate stores and long-term nutritional status. Folate is measured by radioassay kits, sometimes simultaneously with vitamin B_{12}. Less practical, although more accurate, are microbiological assays. In a EC-Flair programme intercomparison study, it was observed that radioassay tends to overestimate serum folate and presents considerable between-kit variability; improved standardization of diagnostic kits and the provision of suitable reference material are still of paramount importance. HPLC, liquid chromatography–mass spectrometry (LC–MS), and LC–MSMS methods are now available. Confounding effects of starvation, dietary folate intake and alcohol abuse, pregnancy, smoking habits, and drugs are reported for serum folate; iron deficiency, age,

and other disease states are reported for erythrocyte folate.

Vitamin B_{12} status can be assessed by measuring serum or plasma total cobalamins and serum holo-transcobalamin II. Serum or plasma cobalamins are determined by competitive protein-binding assay. Kits are available to measure folate simultaneously. Microbiological assays tend to give lower results. Confounding effects of age, sex, impaired absorption by some diseases or drugs, myeloproliferative disorders, worm infestations, and severe liver disease are reported. Holotranscobalamin II is the transport protein of absorbed cobalamin and has been considered as an early indicator of vitamin B_{12} deficiency and possibly a marker of cobalamin malabsorption. Plasma holotranscobalamina II is measured by microparticle enzyme intrinsic factor assay (together with total vitamin B_{12}) or by indirect immunoadsorption method.

Biotin status can be assessed in whole blood by microbiological assay. Radioimmunoassay tests are also available not only for plasma but also for urine. These tests give slightly higher values than microbiological assay.

Vitamin C status can be assessed by ascorbic acid in plasma, buffy-coat, and leucocytes. Ascorbic acid in plasma is considered an index of the circulating vitamin available to tissues, in buffy-coat it is indicative of the intracellular content, and in leucocytes (particularly polymorphonuclear) it is believed to be a good indicator of tissue stores. Whole blood and erythrocyte ascorbic acid determinations are considered of lesser value than plasma for ascorbic acid status assessment. Ascorbic acid in the previously mentioned blood components is measured with a dinitrophenylhydrazine assay and with a more practical HPLC method coupled with electrochemical or amperometric detectors. Also, a HPLC with fluorometric detection method is available. Confounding effects of acute stress, infection, surgery, smoking habits, chronic alcoholism, sex, and drugs are reported. The urinary excretion of ascorbic acid is an index of recent intake; because of instability of the collected sample, the determination is limited to special cases.

Essential Mineral and Trace Element Nutritional Status

Sodium and potassium in plasma/serum have little meaning in nutritional terms; total body Na or K are measured by radioisotope dilution.

Calcium status can be assessed measuring serum or plasma ionized calcium or indirectly by measuring bone mass and bone density. Plasma ionized calcium provides information on physiological function and is measured by a calcium-selective electrode; bone calcium content is an index of body calcium stores and is measured by neutron activation analysis or dual-photon absorptiometry. Confounding effects of venous stasis, cardiac arrest, large volumes of citrated blood infusion, and high or low pH are reported for plasma ionized calcium.

Magnesium status can be assessed by measuring magnesium in serum, erythrocyte, leucocyte, and urine. Serum magnesium is the method most commonly used. Confounding effects of haemolysis, energetic exercise, and pregnancy are reported. Erythrocyte magnesium is considered indicative of a long-term status. Confounding effects of age, thyroid disease, and premenstrual tension are reported. Leucocyte magnesium is considered indicative of intracellular status. Urinary magnesium is used as an indicator of magnesium deficiency after a load test. Some precautions are necessary for this test. Magnesium is measured by flame atomic absorption spectroscopy (AAS) or automated colorimetric methods. The serum/plasma free ionized magnesium determination by selective electrode has been considered a better indicator of status. Further studies are required.

Iron status is assessed in relation to three stages of development of iron-deficiency anemia. In the first stage, to evaluate the size of body iron stores, serum or plasma ferritin can be measured by radiometric methods or using ELISA. Commercial kits are available. Confounding effects of infection, liver and malignant diseases, acute leukemia, Hodgkin's disease, rheumatoid arthritis, thalassemia major, alcohol consumption, age, and sex are reported. In the second stage, to determine the adequacy of iron supply to the erythroid marrow, serum iron (measured by the colorimetric method, available as commercial kits; AAS is not recommended because it gives higher values), plasma or serum total iron binding capacity (TIBC; by colorimetric or radioactive methods available as commercial kits), erythrocyte protoporphyrin (by specific hematofluorometer), and serum transferrin receptor (by ELISA using developed monoclonal antibodies) are measured. The percentage of transferrin saturation is computed as follows: serum iron/TIBC $\times$ 100. Confounding effects of infection, chronic alcoholism, folate and vitamins B_6, B_{12}, and C deficiencies, acute viral hepatitis, malignancy, shock, physical trauma, pregnancy, and altitude are reported for serum iron; infection, protein–energy malnutrition, alcoholic cirrhosis,

malignancy, nephrotic syndromes, entheropathy, pregnancy, viral hepatitis, and oral contraceptive intake are reported for TIBC; and infection, lead poisoning, and porphyrin disorders are reported for erythrocyte protoporphyrin. In the third stage, as indicators of iron-deficiency anemia, hemoglobin (by spectrophotometry or automatically with an electronic counter), hematocrit or packed cell volume (by specially designed centrifuge or an electronic counter), and red cell indices (mean cell volume and mean corpuscolar hemoglobin, both by electronic counter) are measured. Confounding effects of chronic infection, deficiencies of folate and vitamin B_{12}, chronic diseases, hemoglobinopathies, parasitosis, sex, altitude, and smoking habits are reported. All tests of the third stage present low sensitivity and, for the confounding factors, low specificity. The measure of serum transferrin receptor seems to be a promising technique for the evaluation of iron deficiency or toxicity because it is not influenced by infection, inflammation, and chronic diseases. The assessment of serum ferritin and transferrin receptors is considered valuable in screening iron deficiency. Because the measurement of only one variable is not sufficient for the assessment of mild iron deficiency, and also to avoid other limitations, it is recommended to combine two or more independent variables.

Zinc status can be assessed by using AAS to measure zinc in plasma or serum, leucocyte and leucocyte subsets, urine, hair, nails, and saliva. Plasma or serum zinc is the method most commonly used. Many precautions are required during sample collection to avoid the influence of time of day, proximity of meal, stress, hemolysis, and contamination. There are also many pathophysiological conditions that can negatively influence specificity and sensitivity of serum zinc (e.g., infection, stress, chronic disease, exercise, oral contraceptive use, pregnancy, hypoalbuminemia, diabetes, starvation, severe malnutrition, and other catabolic conditions). Therefore, plasma zinc levels are generally considered a poor measure of marginal zinc deficiency. Leucocyte subset zinc, particularly monocyte zinc, is considered a useful indicator of zinc deficiency, but monocyte separation is difficult and a large blood sample must be collected. Zinc in other fluids or tissues is not considered a useful or reliable indicator of zinc deficiency.

Copper status is most frequently assessed in serum or plasma by AAS, even though this measure is of low sensitivity or specificity in the general population. Levels of copper in other tissues or fluids are difficult to assess or are not considered valid indices of copper status. Confounding effects of infection, inflammation, pregnancy, leukemia, Hodgkin's disease, some anemias, myocardial infarction, malabsorption, ulcerative colitis, Wilson's disease, hepatitis, high-level physical activity, cigarette smoking, age, and sex are reported.

Selenium status is usually assessed measuring plasma or serum selenium by AAS with a Zeeman background correction and also by the fluorometric technique. Although plasma Se determination provides information on short-term Se status, the determination in whole blood or erythrocytes is indicative of long-term status. Confounding effects of some inborn errors of metabolism, congestive cardiomyopathy, age, and some physiological conditions are reported.

The determination of Se in urine presents some limitations and Se levels in hair and nails display some drawbacks.

Iodine status is generally assessed by measuring urinary iodine using the colorimetric method, which reflects iodine intake within the past few days. If 24-h urine cannot be collected, iodine excretion can be expressed per gram of creatinine but only in areas with very low inter-and intraindividual variation in urinary creatinine. In clinical settings, the measurement of uptake of radioactive iodine is used.

Functional Tests

Functional tests are defined by Solomons and Allen as tests that measure behavioral, physiological, or biochemical functions of the organism dependent on the adequate availability of a nutrient or responses to the regularity process to maintain body stores and harmonic internal distribution for those many nutrients that are homeostatically regulated by the organism.

There are few reliable and specific functional tests; other simpler tests, not commonly used, lack specificity. Further studies are required on these tests because they are important for a correct assessment of nutritional status in humans. Some of the confounding factors reported for static biochemical tests also apply to functional tests.

Vitamin Nutritional Status

Vitamin A functional tests are the relative dose–response (RDR) and the modified relative dose–response (MRDR). The RDR test can provide information on liver store and is indicative of marginal status of vitamin A. It consists of the determination of plasma retinol level at baseline (A0), administration of a small dose of retinyl acetate or retinyl palmitate, and a second determination of plasma retinol 5 h later (A5). The response is related to the release from the liver of holo-RBP, and in deficient subjects the plasma retinol will increase after 5 h. RDR is calculated as follows:

$$RDR = (A5 - A0) \times 100/A5$$

The MRDR uses a metabolite of vitamin A (3,4-didehydroretinol (DR)). After a test dose, DR binds to RBP and after 5 h appears in the serum if vitamin A reserves are low. Serum retinol (SR) and DR (SDR) are measured by HPLC. The ratio is calculated as follows:

$$MRDR = SDR/SR$$

This ratio is abnormal when greater than 0.06. Confounding effects of protein–energy malnutrition, malabsorption, inflammation (due to inhibition of release of RBP), and liver disease are reported for both tests.

The vitamin D functional test can be the measure of serum alkaline phosphatase activity. For determination of serum alkaline phosphatase, automated procedures and commercial kits are available. The specificity is not very high and confounding factors are age, sex, pregnancy, and unrelated pathologies.

Vitamin E functional tests consist of the following assays: erythrocyte hemolysis, erythrocyte malondialdehyde, breath pentane, susceptibility of low-density lipoprotein to oxidation, and diene conjugate second derivatives. For the first two assays, there are methodological limitations; for the other assays, further experimentation is needed.

A vitamin K functional test that has been recently proposed is the determination of serum underdecarboxylated osteocalcin by radioimmunoassay. This test is well correlated with static indices. Commercial kits are available, as is a semiautomated bead-based enzyme immunoassay that is less time-consuming.

A thiamin functional test that is commonly used is the erythrocyte transketolase activation coefficient (ETK-AC) test. Transketolase is a thiamin-dependent enzyme with a specific role in the glucose oxidative pathway. Transketolase activity in haemolysed erythrocytes (ETK) is measured either by the disappearance of pentose or by the appearance of hexose by spectrophotometry. In the case of thiamin deficiency, the quantity of hexose is reduced. When TPP is added to the reaction mixture, the enzyme activity is enhanced in thiamin-deficient hemolysates only. The activation coefficient is given by the ratio of enhanced (with TPP addition) to basal (without TPP addition) activity.

Because of limitations, to obtain a correct thiamin nutritional status, basal activity should be carried out together with the activation test. Automation of this test is available. Confounding effects of chronic ethanol exposure, conditions that reduce thiamin intake or absorption, uncontrolled diabetes, hyperparathyroidism, age, stress, and infections are reported. Because various methods of measurement have been proposed, in order to obtain a better interpretation and comparison of results, the standardization of the procedure and the use of quality control samples at various time points have been recommended.

A riboflavin functional test that is commonly used is the erythrocyte glutathione reductase activation coefficient (EGR-AC) test. Glutathione reductase is a flavoenzyme with FAD as a prosthetic group. By measuring the EGR activity by spectrophotometry in erythrocyte hemolysate without FAD addition (basal) and with FAD addition (stimulated), the activation coefficient (the ratio of stimulated to basal activity) can be calculated. The higher the coefficient, the lower the coenzyme content. Automation of this test is available. Confounding effects of glucose-6-phosphate dehydrogenase deficiency, severe uremia, liver cirrhosis, biliary disorders, diabetes, thyroid diseases, congenital heart disease, chronic alcoholism, pyridoxine deficiency, stress, and drugs are reported.

Vitamin B_6 functional tests are the erythrocyte aspartate aminotransferase activation coefficient test and the tryptophan load test. Erythrocyte aspartate aminotransferase activity is measured spectrophotometrically in erythrocyte hemolysate without PLP addition (basal) and with PLP addition (stimulated). The activation coefficient is given by the ratio of stimulated to basal activity. Automation of this test is available. Confounding effects of renal and liver diseases, cancer, celiac disease, high protein diet, thiamin status, alcohol intake, stress, and drugs are reported. The tryptophan load test was used in the past because vitamin B_6-dependent enzymes are involved in the conversion of tryptophan to niacin. After an appropriate loading dose of tryptophan and under controlled conditions, vitamin B_6-deficient subjects excrete tryptophan metabolites (kynurenine, kynurenic acid, and xanturenic acid) in urine measured spectrophotometrically after thin-layer or ion exchange chromatography separation. Confounding effects of protein intake, exercise, pregnancy, some hormones, and acute phase status in young people are reported. Plasma total homocysteine (tHcy) in the absence of folate and vitamin B_{12} deficiencies can be considered indicative of vitamin B_6 status. For its determination, see the following discussion of folate functional tests.

Folate functional tests are the plasma homocysteine, urinary formiminoglutamic acid (FIGLU), lymphocyte deoxyuridine (dU) suppression, and hypersegmentation of neutrophilic granulocytes assays. Folate and, to a lesser extent, vitamins B_{12} and B_6 are involved in tHcy metabolism. Plasma homocysteine concentration, in the absence of vitamin B_{12} and B_6 deficiencies, is considered a test of folate status. Because an elevated plasma tHcy concentration is associated with an increased risk of cardiovascular diseases, the determination of this amino acid in plasma has become very common. Various methods are available for tHcy determination. The most commonly used is the HPLC method with fluorescence or ultraviolet (UV) detection, which presents some problems for standardization. Capillary electrophoresis methods with laser fluorescent or UV detection have several advantages. Immunoassay methods are all automated, not time-consuming, and easy to use because of the availability of commercial kits. The chromatographic method coupled to mass spectrometry and with isotopic dilution is considered a reference method due to its high level of accuracy and precision. In a Dutch population study, it was observed that after adjustment for confounders (age, intake of other B vitamins and methionine, smoking, and alcohol consumption) folate was independently inversely associated with plasma tHcy concentration. Other confounding factors are renal failure, inborn errors affecting enzymes involved in lowering tHcy level, lack of exercise, hypothyroidism, psoriasis, and a few drugs. FIGLU acid is eliminated due to the inhibition of the conversion of histidine to glutamic acid in folate deficiency. However, the specificity of this test is low and its use limited. The other two tests are too complex, not very specific, and require further investigation.

Vitamin B_{12} functional tests are the urinary/serum methylmalonic acid (MMA), plasma/serum tHcy, and dU suppression assays. MMA increases in vitamin B_{12} deficiency; the loading with valine or isoleucine produces a marked increase in both urine and serum. MMA is measured by gas chromatography–mass spectrometry. In vitamin B_{12} deficiency in the absence of folate and vitamin B_6 deficiencies, tHcy in plasma increases and decreases with B_{12} administration. For tHcy determination, see the discussion of folate functional tests. The dU suppression test is rather complex and not specific for assessment of vitamin B_{12} status.

Vitamin C functional tests are the lingual vitamin C and intradermal 2,6-dichlorphenolindophenol solution assays. The time to decolorize this solution is inversely correlated with plasma vitamin C levels. However, in humans both methods have low precision.

Zinc functional tests are serum or plasma alkaline phosphatase, erythrocyte metallothionein (MT), monocyte metallothionein mRNA (MTmRNA), and serum thymulin assays. Alkaline phosphatase is a zinc metalloenzyme; rather than being indicative of zinc deficiency, it is considered to be of value after zinc supplementation but with contrasting results. A commercial kits is available for plasma alkaline phosphatase determination. Alkaline phosphatase activity has low specificity and is subject to pathophysiological conditions. Erythrocyte MT decreases in moderate and severe zinc depletion and changes in response to elevated dietary zinc intake. Erythrocyte MT is measured by sandwich ELISA assay. MTmRNA is a new approach to zinc status assessment. It responds more rapidly to zinc supplements than erythrocyte MT. MTmRNA is measured in monocytes by competitive reserve transcriptase-polymerase chain reaction. An improvement of the this method is the determination of MTmRNA on blood samples spotted onto filter paper. Confounding effects are limited to infection. MT and MTmRNA assays are very promising; further studies are needed because of the difficulty in their determination. Serum thymulin activity is decreased in zinc deficiency because it requires zinc to maintain its structure. This test needs further investigation.

Copper functional tests are serum caeruloplasmin, erythrocyte superoxide dismutase (SOD), and leucocyte/platelet cytochrome c oxidase assays. Serum caeruloplasmin, an acute phase reactant protein, can be measured for its oxidase activity on various substrates or by radial immunodiffusion (a commercial kit is available). Serum ceruloplasmin levels are increased with exercise, stress, pregnancy, trauma, cigarette smoking, infection, and malignancy and decreased with nephrosis, advanced liver disease, malnutrition, protein-losing enteropathies, and drugs. Cu, Zn SOD is a cytosolic metalloprotein that catalyzes the reduction of superoxide to hydrogen peroxide and oxygen. It is considered to be a better indicator of reduced copper status than serum copper or caeruloplasmin. The major disadvantage of this test is the lack of a standard assay. Reference values depend on the analytical method. For determination, commercial kits are available. Confounding effects of Down's syndrome, uraemia, various anaemias, Duchenne muscular dystrophy, glutathione reductase deficiency, and porphyria are reported. Tests on cytochrome c oxidase seem to

be more reliable than erythrocyte SOD as indicators of copper stores. They are not affected by sex and hormone use, but the enzyme is rather labile and presents large intersubject variations. For technical improvement, further studies are warranted.

Selenium functional tests are plasma, erythrocyte, and platelet glutathione peroxidase activity (GSF-px) assays. The plasma GSH-px is a useful index only in populations with low Se intake; it responds rapidly to supplementation. Erythrocyte GSH-px presents a plateau at $1.77\,\mu mol\,l^{-1}$, above which it is independent of Se status. In addition, erythrocyte GSH-px responds slowly to depletion and supplementation. Platelet GSH-px responds rapidly to Se dietary changes and presents the maximum activity at Se levels of $1.25{-}1.45\,\mu mol\,l^{-1}$. Accordingly, it is considered to be a sensitive indicator of changing Se status. GSH-px can be measured with coupled enzyme assay or ELISA; commercial kits are available. Confounding effects of age and sex, physical activity, essential fatty acid deficiency, vitamin B_{12}, and iron deficiencies, and stress from antioxidants are reported.

Iodine functional tests are the determination of the thyroid hormones, thyroxine (T_4) and 3,5,3'-triiodothyroxine (T_3), and pituitary thyroid-stimulating hormone (TSH) in serum by specific competitive radioimmunoassay methods (available in kits).

Choice of Laboratory Tests

The choice of laboratory tests depends on the type of study to be carried out. In field nutritional epidemiology studies, particularly in developing countries, the number of tests will be limited by the sample size, the suspected prevalence of deficiencies, the local laboratory conditions, and the availability of skilled personnel and economic resources. In general, the following common tests can be suggested: hemoglobin, hematocrit, serum iron, TIBC, serum ferritin, blood protoporphyrin, serum albumin, plasma transport proteins, and serum zinc. In specific cases, serum retinol, other vitamins in blood or urine, and some hormones (thyroxine and TSH) and minerals (urinary iodine) can be added.

In population studies to be carried out in developed countries with high-level laboratory facilities, the selection of laboratory tests depends on the purpose of the study, sample size, and financial resources. The assessment of protein status is in general limited to plasma transport proteins, unless there are other specific reasons for using other variables. Essential fatty acid status is assessed in lipid pattern studies; the choice of test is determined by

Table 1 Summary of Flair Concerted Action No. 10 recommended methods

Micronutrient	Recommended method	'Best available' method	Additional methods of use in some circumstances
Vitamin A		Serum retinol	RDR test
			MRDR test
			Isotope dilution technique
			RBP:TTR ratio
Carotenoids		Serum carotenoid profile	Serum lutein
			Serum lycopene
			Serum α-carotene
Vitamin E	Lipid standardized serum α-tocopherol		
Vitamin D	Serum 25-OH vitamin D		Serum 1,25-dihydroxyvitamin D
			Serum calcium
			Serum phosphate
			Serum alkaline phosphatase
Thiamin	ETK stimulation test		RBC TPP
Riboflavin	EGR stimulation test		
Vitamin B$_6$	Plasma PLP		EAST stimulation test
Vitamin B$_{12}$	Serum cobalamins		Serum MMA
Folate	RBC folate		Serum folate
Vitamin C	Plasma vitamin C		
	Leucocyte ascorbate		
Selenium		Plasma selenium	RBC GSHPx
Iron	Serum ferritin	Transferrin receptors	
Copper		Serum copper (?)	RBC SOD
Zinc		Serum zinc	RBC metallothionein

RDR, relative dose–response; MRDR, modified relative dose–response; RBP, retinol binding protein; TTR, transthyretin; ETK, erythrocyte transketolase; RBC, red blood cell; TPP, thiamin pyrophosphate; EGR, erythrocyte glutathione reductase; PLP, pyridoxal-5'-phosphate; EAST, erythrocyte aspartate aminotransferase; MMA, methylmalonic acid; GSHPx, platelet glutathione peroxidase; SOD, superoxide dismutase.Adapted with permission from van den Berg H, Heseker H, Lamand M, Sandstrom B and Thurnham D (1993) Flair Concerted Action No 10 Status Papers—Introduction, Conclusions and Recommandations. *International Journal for Vitamin and Nutrition Research* **63**: 247–251, with changes suggested by D. Thurnham (personal communication).

the interest in recent intake or long-term status. In association with this test, serum cholesterol and triacylglycerols and also lipoprotein fractions are measured. The selection of micronutrient tests can be determined by the suspected deficiencies from previous dietary surveys; in the absence of dietary data, several tests should be measured because preclinical deficiencies are common in developed societies. A sensible selection can be found in **Table 1**. In the US Third Nutritional Health and Nutrition Examination Survey, most of the recommended and best available methods were used. This is also the case for vitamin status analysis in the recent UK government diet and nutrition surveys of specific population groups.

In a hospital setting, the selection of laboratory tests depends on the clinical conditions of patients on admission and during the subsequent course of injury or illness. Because protein–energy malnutrition can be present in some cases, protein status should be assessed using laboratory tests for serum albumin, plasma transport proteins, and urinary creatinine and 3-methylhistidine, and also for acute phase proteins. Using some of the previous values associated with other variables (immunological functions and anthropometric measurements), indices relating nutritional status to clinical outcome can be computed. Among hospital patients, vitamin and trace element deficiencies are also common; the determination of deficient variables suspected on the basis of history and physical examination is suggested.

Because on various occasions major differences in interlaboratory comparisons and ring tests have been observed, it is essential in the selection of laboratory tests to favor definitive reference methods or, in their absence, standardized and validated methods for which careful collection and handling of samples is compulsory and also appropriate quality control. Commercial-quality control samples or external quality assurance schemes are available only in some cases. For quality control of in-house samples, it is suggested to prepare one sample with low or deficient content and one with normal or high content. Interlaboratory cross-comparison is highly recommended.

Evaluation of Laboratory Indices

In general, reference values are population specific; accordingly, each major laboratory in homogeneous areas has to derive them from a clinically healthy reference population selected with very specific criteria. These values should preferably be given in percentiles.

In general, cutoff points for an appropriate interpretation of results have been derived statistically from reference values. A current procedure for constructing cutoff point consists of determining the biochemical values that correspond to the earliest determinable physiological, metabolic, functional, and morphological alterations. Such an approach has been followed only in a very few cases, and consequently most available cutoff points should be considered as tentative.

For albumin, the guidelines for interpretation suggested in 1974 are still in use. For children and adults, values $<28 \, \text{g} \, \text{l}^{-1}$ are indicative of a deficient (high-risk) status, and for pregnant women this value is $<30 \, \text{g} \, \text{l}^{-1}$. A marginal (moderate-risk) status is indicated by the following values: infants, $<25 \, \text{g} \, \text{l}^{-1}$; children 1–5 years, $<30 \, \text{g} \, \text{l}^{-1}$; children 6–17 years, $<35 \, \text{g} \, \text{l}^{-1}$; adults, $28–34 \, \text{g} \, \text{l}^{-1}$; pregnant women at first trimester, $30–39 \, \text{g/l}^{-1}$; and pregnant women at second and third trimester, $30–34 \, \text{g} \, \text{l}^{-1}$. All values above the moderate risk are indicative of an acceptable (low-risk) status.

Reference values for transport proteins are provided by plate producers. Tentatively, $0.10 \, \text{g} \, \text{l}^{-1}$ for prealbumin and $25 \, \text{mg} \, \text{l}^{-1}$ for retinol binding protein are considered indicative of protein deficiency. For transferrin, values less than $1 \, \text{g} \, \text{l}^{-1}$ are considered indicative of severe protein depletion; marginal status values are between 1 and $2 \, \text{g} \, \text{l}^{-1}$.

For the interpretation of serum phospholipid essential fatty acid values, the ratio triene–tetraene (C 20:3 n-9/C 20:4 n-6) above 0.2 was considered by Holman to be the upper limit of normalcy. The ratio C 22:5 n-6/C 22:6 n-3 can be a sensitive index of n-3 fatty acid deficiency.

The cutoff points for the most widely used micronutrient tests in adults are reported in **Table 2**. Cutoff points are different for children, pregnant and lactating women, and the elderly. These values can be found in reference texts. For antioxidant vitamins and provitamins to prevent chronic diseases, the following optimal plasma levels have been proposed: retinol, $>2.5 \, \mu\text{mol} \, \text{l}^{-1}$; β-carotene, $>0.40 \, \mu\text{mol} \, \text{l}^{-1}$; α-tocopherol, $>30 \, \mu\text{mol} \, \text{l}^{-1}$; and ascorbic acid, $>50 \, \mu\text{mol} \, \text{l}^{-1}$.

Confounding Effects of Infection on Laboratory Assessment

As already indicated, many confounding effects of infection have been observed in many laboratory tests for nutritional status. For protein status, confounding effects of infection are reported for almost all laboratory tests, excluding that for total serum protein. In particular, serum albumin, plasma transport protein, and fibronectin levels decrease because of the increase of acute phase proteins.

For vitamin A, severe systemic infections (e.g., pneumonia, bronchitis, diarrhoea, septicaemia, rheumatic and scarlet fever, malaria, and measles) cause a marked decrease in serum retinol level. This decrease may be due to various factors (e.g., increased retinol excretion in urine and reduced liver release of retinol and RBP to plasma). A reduction of vitamin A liver reserves assessed by the RDR test has been observed in children with chickenpox.

Plasma vitamin E is reduced in malaria-infected patients. This influence is retained via the lipoproteins and not directly. Tests for thiamin status can be confounded by infections that prevent normal absorption (diarrhea and dysentery) or increase the requirement (fever).

For vitamin B_{12}, fish tapeworm or hookworm infestations give a low level of serum vitamin B_{12} because of their preferential consumption of this vitamin. For vitamin C, acute and chronic infections can depress markedly the serum ascorbic acid level due to a decrease in vitamin C reserves.

For iron status tests, infection induces an increase in serum ferritin and blood protoporphyrin levels and a decrease in serum iron binding capacity, serum iron, and hemoglobin. Zinc status tests are influenced by acute and chronic infections. A decrease in plasma zinc has been reported, due initially to redistribution of zinc within the body tissues and then to a negative body balance. This is due to anorexia, which reduces dietary intake, and also to increased losses via the faeces (diarrhea), sweat, and urine.

Regarding copper status tests, infection results in an increase in serum copper level because the leucocytic endogenous mediator induces an increase in serum ceruloplasmin. Iodine status can be influenced by infection because the synthesis of TTR is markedly suppressed.

In nutrition surveys, to correct misclassification of laboratory values due to positive acute phase proteins, the concurrent serum determination of these proteins has been suggested.

Table 2 Tentative cutoff points for interpretation of results of micronutrient tests in adults

	Severe deficiency	Marginal deficiency	Physiological level or range
Lv retinol (μmol g^{-1})	<0.07		
P retinol (μmol l^{-1})	<0.35	0.35–1.05	>1.05
RBP:TTR ratio	≤0.37		
Relative dose response (%)		>20	<20
S 25-OHD (nmol l^{-1})	<12.5	12.5–25.0	>25
P/S α-tocopherol (μmol l^{-1})	<11.6	11.6–16.2	>16.2
P α-tocopherol (μmol l^{-1})	<9.25	9.25–13.9	>13.9
E TPP (nmol l^{-1})	<120	120–150	>150
U thiamin (μg/24 h)	<27	27–65	>66
ETK-AC[a]	>1.25	1.15–1.25	1.00–1.15
E FAD (nmol l^{-1})	<200		
U riboflavin (μg/g creatinine)	<27	27–79	>80
EGR-AC[a]	>1.4	1.2–1.4	<1.2
EGR-AC[b]	>1.30	1.20–1.30	<1.20
P PLP (nmol l^{-1})	<20		20–86
U 4-PA (nmol/nmol creatinine)			128–680
EAST-AC[a,b]	>1.80	1.70–1.80	<1.70
P vitamin B$_{12}$ (pmol l^{-1})[b]	<258		>260
S TCII (pmol l^{-1})	<15		
S methylmalonic acid (μmol l^{-1})		0.5–1.0	<0.5
P homocysteine (μmol l^{-1})	>100	100–12	<12
P folate (nmol l^{-1})	>7.0		
P folate (nmol l^{-1})[b]	<5.7	5.7–11.4	>11.4
RBC folate (nmol l^{-1})	<317	317–354	>354
L lobe average	>3.6	3.6–3.2	<3.2
P biotin (nmol l^{-1})[b]	<0.5	0.5–1.0	>1.0
P ascorbic acid (μmol l^{-1})	<11.4	11.4–17	>17
B ascorbic acid (μmol l^{-1})	<17	17–27	>28
L ascorbic acid (nmol/10^8 cells)		53–95	114–301
S/P ferritin (μg)	<12	20	100
S iron (μmol l^{-1})	<10.7	20	
S TIBC (μmol l^{-1})	<71.6		
Transferrin saturation (%)	<15%		
E PP (μmol l^{-1})	<1.24		
Haemoglobin (g l^{-1})	M <130 F <120		
Haematocrit (%)	M <40 F <36		
MCV	<80		
P Zn (μmol l^{-1})	<10.7		
S caeruloplasmin (μmol l^{-1})			2–4
P Se (μmol l^{-1})	<0.38	0.38–0.76	0.76–1.52
E Se (μmol l^{-1})	~0.45		1.13–2.41

[a]The percentage stimulation is now very seldom used. It can be calculated as follows: $(AC \times 100) - 100$.

[b]From Benton D, Haller J and Fordy J (1997) The vitamin status of young british adults. *International Journal for Vitamin and Nutrition Research* 67: 34–40, with permission.

Lv, liver; P, plasma; S, serum; E, erythrocyte; U, urine; L, leucocytes; B, whole blood; RBP, retinol binding protein; TTR, transthyretin; TPP, thiamin pyrophosphate; ETK-AC, erythrocyte transketolase activation coefficient; FAD, flavinadeninedinucleotide; EGR-AC, erythrocyte glutathione reductase activation coefficient; PLP, pyridoxal-5'-phosphate; 4-PA, 4-pyroxic acid; EAST-AC, erythrocyte aspartate aminotransferase activation coefficient; TCII, transcobalamin II, RBC, red blood cell; TIBC, total iron-binding capacity; PP, protoporphyrin; MCV, mean cell volume.

Adapted with permission from Flair Concerted Action No. 10 Status Papers (1993) *International Journal for Vitamin and Nutrition Research* **63**: 252–316, with changes suggested by C.J. Bates (personal communication).

See also: **Ascorbic Acid**: Physiology, Dietary Sources and Requirements. **Carotenoids**: Chemistry, Sources and Physiology. **Cobalamins. Copper. Fatty Acids**: Omega-3 Polyunsaturated; Omega-6 Polyunsaturated. **Folic Acid. Iron. Magnesium. Niacin. Nutritional Assessment**: Anthropometry; Clinical Examination. **Potassium. Riboflavin. Selenium. Sodium**: Physiology. **Thiamin**: Physiology. **Vitamin A**: Physiology. **Vitamin B$_6$. Vitamin E**: Metabolism and Requirements. **Vitamin K. Zinc**: Physiology.

Further Reading

Bates CJ (1997) Vitamin analysis. *Annals of Clinical Biochemistry* 34: 599–626.

Bates CJ (1999) Diagnosis and detection of vitamin deficiencies. *British Medical Bulletin* 55: 643–655.

Brody T (1999) *Nutritional Biochemistry*, 2nd edn. San Diego: Academic Press.

De Leenheer AP, Lambert WE, and Van Boexlaer JF (2000) In *Modern chromatographic analysis of vitamins*. New York: Decker.

Fidanza F (1991) *Nutritional Status Assessment—A Manual for Population Studies*. London: Chapman & Hall.

Gibson RS (1990) *Principles of Nutritional Assessment*. New York: Oxford University Press.

Gregory J, Foster K, Tyler H, and Wiseman M (1990) *The Dietary and Nutritional Survey of British Adults (Office of Population Censuses and Surveys, Social Survey Division)*. London: HMSO.

Gunter EW, Lewis BG, and Koncikowski SM (1996) *Laboratory Procedures Used for the Third National Health and Nutrition Examination Survey*. Atlanta: Centers for Disease Control and Prevention.

Iyengar GV (1989) *Elemental Analysis of Biological System*. Boca Raton, FL: CRC Press.

Jelliffe DB and Jelliffe EFP (1989) *Community Nutritional Assessment—With Special Reference to Less Technically Developed Countries*. Oxford: Oxford University Press.

McLaren DS and Frigg M (2001) *Sight and Life Manual on Vitamin A Deficiency Disorder (VADD)*, 2nd edn. Basel: Task Force SIGHT AND LIFE.

Report of the International Nutritional Anemia Consultative Group (1985) *Measurements of Iron Status*. Washington, DC: Nutrition Foundation.

Sauberlich HE (1999) *Laboratory Tests for the Assessment of Nutritional Status*, 2nd edn. Boca Raton, FL: CRC Press.

van den Berg H, Heseker H, Lamand M, Sandstrom B, and Thurnham D (1993) Flair Concerted Action No. 10 Status Papers. *International Journal for Vitamin and Nutrition Research* 63: 247–316.

Wright R and Heymsfield S (1984) In *Nutritional Assessment*. Boston: Blackwell Scientific.

Clinical Examination

B Caballero, Johns Hopkins Bloomberg School of Public Health and Johns Hopkins University, Baltimore, MD, USA

The clinical evaluation of nutritional status is a fundamental component of health assessment at any age. Along with anthropometry, dietary assessment, and laboratory tests, the physical examination is one of the key tools to evaluate nutritional status.

The two most common settings for a clinical examination are the hospital (inpatient or outpatient) and the field health care unit. In the first situation, the physician or examiner may have access to resources that are usually not available in the field. Because of this and other constraints, the assessment of nutritional status in the field is frequently more narrowly aimed at identifying a specific clinical condition or set of signs and symptoms. In either case, it is essential that information on history and physical findings be collected in a standardized manner in terms of both format and procedures. The former is usually best achieved by the use of preprinted or computerized forms. Electronic forms can be programmed to perform immediate range checking as values are entered, thus alerting the operator when values out of range are entered. Procedures for examination must be clearly defined in writing, and any health worker should be able to follow the instructions and perform an acceptable measurement. Although many components of the examination are subjective, it is important to standardize as much as possible terms such as 'minor,' 'average,' and 'large' within the group of examining persons, attributing a numeric value whenever possible. If data entry requires selecting from a numeric scale, they should be also standardized by cross-validation with experienced personnel or by means of photographs or models.

The two components of the clinical assessment are the medical history and the physical examination (**Table 1**).

Table 1 Major components of a nutrition-oriented medical history

Medical history
History of weight loss or gain
Gastrointestinal symptoms (nausea, diarrhea, flatulence, pain, etc.)
History of changes in color or texture of skin, hair, conjunctiva, buccal mucosa
Use of medications
Physical activity level (work-related, leisure)
History of fatigue, shortness of breath, muscle cramps
Other lifestyle practices
Places of residence, travel (exposure to toxins, sunlight, food contaminants)
In children and adolescents
– Growth history
– Neurodevelopmental history
– General school performance
– Parental and siblings' body size (body mass index)
– Pubertal stage
– Food preferences, fads

Dietary history
Habitual dietary intake and preferences
Past diet history
Alcohol consumption
Food allergies and intolerances
Assessment of dietary intake
– 24-hr recall
– Food frequency questionnaire

Medical History

The medical history for nutritional assessment is no different from a general medical history, in which familial and past and present environmental factors and their possible association with specific diseases or disease risk are considered. For the purpose of nutritional assessment, this information will be used to determine if any nutritional finding or complaint may be caused by an underlying medical condition, particularly one that remains unrecognized at the time of the examination. Additionally, specific medical conditions and their current status are important factors altering nutrient requirements and dietary prescriptions.

One specific focus of medical history in a nutritional assessment context is the exploration of gastrointestinal function. Conditions such as chronic diarrhea, gastroesophageal reflux, and colonic disorders may be associated with reduced nutrient absorption or food avoidance that result in impaired nutritional status. Past history of gastrointestinal problems and/or surgery may also point to current alterations in nutrient digestion or absorption. Other important components of the medical history are history of weight loss or gain, past and present use of medications, use of special foods or formulas, changes in taste or smell, and food allergies and intolerances.

In children and adolescents, the medical history must also obtain information on neurodevelopmental stages, history of behavioral problems, and overall school performance. Food preferences must be noted, particularly in adolescence, when adoption of unconventional dietary practices is more likely to occur.

Physical Examination

As noted previously, anthropometric measurements are a key component of the physical examination. Measurement of weight and height is perhaps one of the most frequently performed nutritional measurements. Although its value is limited with regard to identifying specific nutrient deficiencies, it is invaluable to evaluate growth and adequacy of past and present diet in infants, children, and adolescents and to identify undernutrition and obesity in adults. Measurements should be done by trained personnel and following standard protocols. In addition to anthropometry, the physical examination focuses on signs of nutrient deficiency or excess. These signs usually appear only when the deficiency is advanced and are not to be expected in marginal

deficiencies. Furthermore, the time that it takes for a deficient intake of a given nutrient to cause clinical manifestation of deficiency varies considerably, depending on whether the nutrient is stored in the body and on the initial status of the reserves. Typical signs for selected nutritional deficiencies are presented in **Table 2**. Virtually none of these signs, with the exception of Bitot's spots, are pathognomonic for one specific deficiency. However, they are useful in indicating a specific nutrient impairment and prompting further evaluation.

The physical examination should start with a general visual assessment of the patient. In children, state of alertness, willingness to engage in play, or

Table 2 Typical clinical signs of selected nutritional deficiencies

Deficiency	Signs
Protein–energy malnutrition	Hair: depigmentation, thinning, pluckability
	Edema in lower extremities (generalized in severe cases)
	Muscle wasting
	Decreased subcutaneous fat
	Skin: diffuse depigmentation, flaky dermatosis
	Liver enlargement
Vitamin A	Bitot's spot
	Conjunctival xerosis
	Corneal xerosis
	Keratomalacia
	Night blindness
Riboflavin	Angular stomatitis
	Cheilosis
	Scrotal (vulvar) dermatosis
	Red tongue
	Corneal vascularization
Thiamin	Edema
	Hyporeflexia
	Muscle tenderness
	Cardiac enlargement
	Tachycardia
Niacin	Pellagroid dermatosis
	Scarlet, raw, fissured tongue
	Malar and supraorbital pigmentation
Vitamin C	Bleeding, spongy gums
	Petechiae
	Ecchymoses
	Epiphyseal enlargement
	Atrophy of lingual papillae
	Follicular hyperkeratosis
Vitamin D	Active rickets: rib beading, epiphyseal enlargement, persistently open fontanelle, craniotabes, hypotonia
	Residual rickets: frontal or parietal bossing, bowlegs, knock-knees, thorax deformities
Iron	Pale conjunctiva
	Atrophy of lingual papillae
	Koilonychia
Folic acid, B_{12}	Usually associated with pallor of anemia
	Peripheral neuropathy (B_{12})
Iodine	Thyroid enlargement

resisting examination are important clues to energy level and physical strength. A generalized loss of fat depots, or excess adiposity as in the obese, is readily identifiable in most circumstances. A general overview can also identify pallor, loss of muscle mass, and skin changes.

Numerous signs of nutritional deficiencies can be identified in the skin and hair. Because skin exhibits a relatively rapid turnover, impairments in protein synthesis can result in fragile, flaky, and discolored skin. Vitamin A deficiency typically causes a dry, hyperkeratotic skin. The dermatitis of pellagra consists of patchy areas of hypo- or hyperpigmentations, usually in sun-exposed body regions, eventually progressing to hardened, broken surfaces. In protein–energy malnutrition, hair may become brittle, thin, and easily pluckable. Fluctuations in the rate of synthesis of hair protein may result in band discoloration, where pale and normal colors alternate, resulting in the 'banner sign,' typical of kwashiorkor. Petechiae or hematomas may result from protein–energy malnutrition or vitamin K or vitamin E (in the newborn) deficiencies.

One of the most specific signs of nutritional deficiency can be identified in the eye. Vitamin A deficiency produces a series of alterations in the conjunctiva and the cornea that not only indicate a deficiency of this nutrient but also help grade its severity. The most commonly used classification of vitamin A deficiency is primarily based on eye findings, from Bitot's spots to perforated keratomalacia. Conjunctival pallor has been a classic sign of anemia, but its sensitivity varies substantially depending on ethnicity, ambient lighting, and experience of the observer.

The mouth and tongue are also areas where typical manifestations of deficiency can be detected. A red tongue is a classic sign of riboflavin deficiency but has also been associated with niacin deficiency; the latter may also include fissures. Conversely, a pale tongue may indicate iron deficiency. Glossitis, with or without color changes, has been linked to pyridoxine deficiency. A similar condition, including pain and intense red color, has been associated with biotin deficiency. Angular stomatitis and ulcerations and other lip lesions are associated with riboflavin or ascorbic acid deficiencies. In the latter, extensive involvement of the gums (swelling and bleeding) is also typical. Atrophy of the papillae occurs in vitamin B_{12}, niacin, and folate deficiencies. Excess vitamin A intake may result in discoloration of the gingival mucosa.

Rib beading (also known as rickets rosary) is a typical sign of vitamin D deficiency in children, but a similar manifestation may appear in vitamin C deficiency (scurvy). Ephyphiseal enlargement and bowlegs are other classic signs of rickets. A distended abdomen is characteristic of protein–energy malnutrition in children. In the lower limbs, inspection must ascertain the presence of edema, which is also associated with protein-energy malnutrition.

Peripheral neuropathies such as those associated with beriberi or vitamin B_{12} deficiencies may result in visible impairment of limb movements, such as the 'foot drop' of dry beriberi.

In preadolescents and adolescents, assessment of sexual maturation (usually following the Tanner staging) is an important component of the physical examination, although it is not always feasible due to cultural and practical reasons. Alternatively, more limited information may be obtained in girls by self-reported menarcheal status. Self-assessment of Tanner stage by comparison with photographs is another useful alternative, but use of these photographs with children may not be acceptable in some communities.

In order to obtain a unified rating of a person's nutritional status, it is desirable to integrate clinical, laboratory, and functional data into a single scoring system. Several approaches to achieve this have been proposed, and their use will depend primarily on the target population and the intended use of the score. The Subjective Global Assessment is an approach that relies primarily on data from the physical examination and thus can be readily performed after this examination has been completed. Other scoring systems, such as the Prognostic Nutritional Index or the Instant Nutritional Index, rely to variable degrees on combinations of clinical and laboratory data.

See also: **Dietary Intake Measurement**: Methodology; Validation. **Energy Expenditure**: Indirect Calorimetry; Doubly Labeled Water. **Nutritional Assessment**: Anthropometry; Biochemical Indices.

Further Reading

McLaren DS (1992) *A Colour Atlas and Text of Diet-Related Disorders*. London: Wolfe.

Morrison G and Hark L (1996) *Medical Nutrition* Cambridge, MA: Blackwell Science.

Newton JM and Halsted CH (1998) Clinical and functional assessment of adults. In: *Modern Nutrition in Health and Disease*, 9th edn., pp. 895–902. Philadelphia: Lippincott.

Sardesai VM (2003) *Introduction to Clinical Nutrition*, 2nd edn. New York: Marcel Dekker.

Stallings VA and Fung EB (1998) Clinical nutrition assessment of infants and children. In: *Modern Nutrition in Health and Disease*, 9th edn., pp. 885–893. Philadelphia: Lippincott.

NUTRITIONAL SUPPORT

Contents
In the Home Setting
Adults, Enteral
Adults, Parenteral
Infants and Children, Parenteral

In the Home Setting

M Elia and R J Stratton, University of Southampton, Southampton, UK

The prevalence of nutritional problems in developed societies is a cause of growing concern. At one end of the nutritional spectrum, the obesity 'epidemic' is spreading at an alarming rate. At the other end of the spectrum, protein–energy malnutrition and nutrient deficiencies are also common, especially in the elderly and in those with disease. **Table 1** shows the frequency of specific vitamin deficiencies and underweight (body mass index <20 kg/m^2) in people aged 65 years or older resident in the United Kingdom. Complimentary information on protein–energy status can be obtained by considering simple criteria, such as those used by the 'Malnutrition Universal Screening Tool' (MUST) (**Figure 1**). This tool, which depends on weight loss and body mass index (and an acute disease effect, which does not normally apply to community patients), has been used to estimate that 10–15% of older people in the United Kingdom are at medium to high risk of malnutrition. The prevalence of malnutrition increases with age, and it is more common in the presence of disease and in institutions, where about one in five people are at risk. With the growing number of older people, especially those living in nursing homes and alternative care facilities, the overall prevalence of malnutrition may increase. It is disturbing that malnutrition is underrecognized and undertreated, despite its adverse effects on the individual and society.

The first important step in the management of malnutrition is identifying it using one of a number of validated nutritional screening tools. MUST was developed specifically for all types of patients in all health care settings. The potentially broad application of the same tool encourages consistency of thought and continuity of care through different health care settings. The care plan linked to this tool varies from dietary restriction in the case of obesity to supplementation and other forms of nutritional support in the case of malnutrition. For special situations, enteral tube feeding (e.g., in some patients with swallowing problems) and parenteral (intravenous) nutrition are required.

This article focuses on the treatment of malnutrition (rather than obesity) in the home setting. This treatment includes dietary counselling and fortification, oral nutritional supplementation (mixed macro- and micronutrient supplements), and artificial nutritional support (enteral tube feeding (ETF) and parenteral

Table 1 Proportion of subjects 65 years or older with selected vitamin deficiencies and body mass index <20 kg/m^2

	Free living (%)	Institutions (%)[a]	Criteria	
Vitamin deficiencies				
Folate deficiency	29	35	Red blood cell concentration	<345 μmol/l
– Severe deficiency	8	16		<230 μmol/l
Thiamine deficiency	9	14	Erythrocyte transketolase activation coefficient (ratio)	>1.25
Vitamin B$_{12}$ deficiency	6	9	Plasma concentration	<118 pmol/l
Vitamin D deficiency	1–2	1–5		<12 μmol/l
Vitamin C deficiency	14	40	Plasma concentration	<11 μmol/l
– Severe deficiency	5	16		<5 μmol/l
Underweight	3	16	Body mass index	<20 kg/m^2

[a]Registered residential homes (57%), nursing homes (30%), dual-registration homes (9%), and other facilities (4%)
Based on the National Dietary and Nutrition Survey (1998) in the United Kingdom.

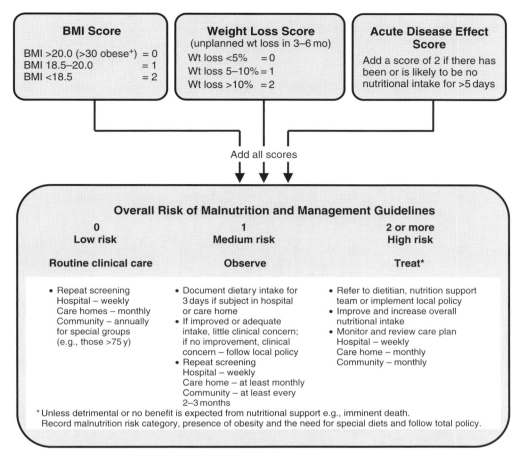

BMI Score

BMI >20.0 (>30 obese⁺) = 0
BMI 18.5–20.0 = 1
BMI <18.5 = 2

Weight Loss Score
(unplanned wt loss in 3–6 mo)
Wt loss <5% = 0
Wt loss 5–10% = 1
Wt loss >10% = 2

Acute Disease Effect Score
Add a score of 2 if there has been or is likely to be no nutritional intake for >5 days

Add all scores

Overall Risk of Malnutrition and Management Guidelines

0	1	2 or more
Low risk	**Medium risk**	**High risk**
Routine clinical care	**Observe**	**Treat***

- Repeat screening
  Hospital – weekly
  Care homes – monthly
  Community – annually
  for special groups
  (e.g., those >75 y)

- Document dietary intake for 3 days if subject in hospital or care home
- If improved or adequate intake, little clinical concern; if no improvement, clinical concern – follow local policy
- Repeat screening
  Hospital – weekly
  Care home – at least monthly
  Community – at least every 2–3 months

- Refer to dietitian, nutrition support team or implement local policy
- Improve and increase overall nutritional intake
- Monitor and review care plan
  Hospital – weekly
  Care home – monthly
  Community – monthly

* Unless detrimental or no benefit is expected from nutritional support e.g., imminent death.
Record malnutrition risk category, presence of obesity and the need for special diets and follow total policy.

Figure 1 'Malnutrition Universal Screening Tool' (MUST). A copy of MUST and further details on taking alternative measurements, special circumstances, and subjective criteria can be downloaded at www.bapen.org.uk.

nutrition (PN)). The simplest and most commonly used treatment involves oral nutritional support, which is considered before home enteral tube feeding (HETF) and home parenteral nutrition (HPN).

Oral Nutritional Support

Dietary Counselling and Fortification

Dietary counselling, usually provided by a dietitian, is an integral part of oral nutritional support. It includes advice on dietary fortification, which is often the first-line treatment of malnutrition in the home and other care settings. Counselling may involve advice on eating patterns (e.g., eating certain types of snacks at particular times of day) or addition of energy- and protein-rich food ingredients (e.g., cream, milk, oil, butter, sugar, and skimmed milk powder) to meals. Commercial energy- and protein-containing supplements can also be used to improve intake without substantially altering the taste of food and drink. The use of nutritionally

fortified food snacks as part of the diet may improve both the intake and the status of micronutrients. However, the success of these dietary strategies is limited in patients with severe anorexia, those living in poverty and due to other social factors, and in those with inadequate motivation. Thus, patients may find it difficult to purchase, manipulate, or prepare their meals. Financial or other forms of social support, such as help with shopping, cooking (or provision of 'meals on wheels'), and help with eating, may do much to improve intake in some individuals. Although dietary counselling, with or without dietary fortification, is widely used in clinical practice, there is little research supporting its clinical efficacy in patients at risk of malnutrition in developed countries.

Oral Nutritional Supplements

Mixed macro- and micronutrient liquid sip feeds and other oral nutritional supplements (bars, powders, and puddings) are widely used in the treatment

Table 2 Summary of significant functional and clinical outcome improvements following oral nutritional supplementation in community patients from randomised controlled trials

Patient group	Functional/clinical outcome
Chronic obstructive pulmonary disease	Respiratory muscle function Hand grip strength Walking distances
Elderly	Reduced number of falls Increased activities of daily living Muscle power
HIV/AIDS	Cognitive function
Liver disease	Lower incidence of severe infections Lower frequency of hospitalisation
Malignancy	Immunological benefits
Osteoarthritis	Increased activities of daily living[a] Improved osteoarthritis index[a]

[a]Nutritional supplement also containing immunoglobulin G (90 mg). Based on Stratton RJ, Green CJ, and Elia M (2003) *Disease-Related Malnutrition: An Evidence Based Approach to Treatment*. Oxford: CABI Publishing.

of malnutrition in the community setting. A systematic review of 78 randomized controlled trials (RCTs) (including 44 RCTs from the community setting) suggests oral nutritional supplements can improve energy and nutrient intakes, improve body weight (or attenuate weight loss), and improve a number of functional and clinical outcomes in various patient groups (**Table 2**). Meta-analysis of RCTs from both hospital and community settings suggests significantly lower mortality (odds ratio, 0.62; 95% confidence interval, 0.49–0.78) and complication rates (infections and postoperative complications) (odds ratio, 0.29; 95% confidence interval, 0.18–0.47) in patients given oral nutritional supplements (typically 1.05–2.5 MJ (250–600 kcal) daily).

For some patients, nutrition via the oral route is either unable to meet the nutritional requirements (e.g., patients with a poor appetite) or contraindicated (e.g., a cerebrovascular accident patient with aspiration and intestinal failure). For such patients, HETF and HPN may be required, although the treatment is usually initiated in hospital.

Artificial Nutrition Support: Home Parenteral Nutrition and Home Enteral Tube Feeding

Patients suffering from chronic conditions often prefer to be treated in the familiar surroundings of their home rather than in hospital. When the treatment involves sophisticated techniques, it is essential that either the patient or the caregiver is adequately trained to distinguish between problems that can be easily remedied at home and those that need expert advice and treatment in hospital. With the increasing pressure for hospital beds and the increasing cost of hospital care, many forms of treatment that were previously restricted to the hospital environment have extended to the community, including renal dialysis, cytotoxic drug therapy, HETF, and HPN. HETF has grown rapidly so that its prevalence in several developed countries is now several times greater than in hospital. In contrast, PN is still practiced less commonly outside hospital than in hospital and is likely to remain so in the foreseeable future. Both forms of treatment have led to the development of professional teams specialising in nutritional support in both the hospital and the community. These teams deal with problems ranging from simple day-to-day management issues to difficult ethical problems, such as concerning withholding or withdrawing nutritional support.

Origins and Development

The first report of HPN appeared in 1970 in North America, and in Europe the first reports appeared in the late 1970s. The number of people receiving HPN has increased considerably since then but remains substantially lower than for HETF (**Figure 2**).

HETF is a much older technique than HPN, with the first reports appearing centuries ago. Accurate information on the numbers of people receiving HETF is difficult to obtain because HETF tends to be initiated from many centres and centralized reporting and record keeping in most countries are not fully established. There has been rapid growth in HETF attributable to developments in tube technology (flexible fine bore tubes) and endoscopic procedures for placement of gastrostomy tubes (facilitating easier initiation and management of long-term feeding), as well as the development of home care services provided by commercial enteral

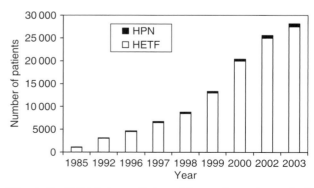

Figure 2 Estimated growth in point prevalence (amount of feeding taking place at a given point in time) in home enteral tube feeding (HETF) and home parenteral nutrition (HPN) in the United Kingdom.

feeding companies. In many developed countries there is considerably more ETF taking place in the community than in hospital. In Britain, there continues to be steady growth (10–20% per year) in the numbers of people receiving HETF, and in 2003, 21 527 people were registered with the British Artificial Nutrition Survey (BANS), with an estimated total number receiving HETF in excess of 25 000. As with HPN, HETF is less common in Europe than in North America and is practised much less in Eastern Europe, India, and China than in industrialized Western countries.

In addition to the differences in prevalence of HETF and HPN between countries, there may also be marked variations within countries. Even within one region of the United Kingdom (south and west regions) the number of individuals receiving HETF in 2002 within different primary care trusts varied from 82 to 632 per 1 million people. Similarly, considerable variation in the point prevalence of HPN was found to exist in different regions of the United Kingdom in 1999 (0 to 36 per 1 million). This large variation, which is unlikely to be due to chance, can be explained by variations in the availability of expertise and support staff, resources to fund such treatment, or local differences in attitudes/policies toward the use of artificial nutrition.

The wide variations in the prevalence of home artificial feeding throughout the world are related to health care economies. There is a relationship between expenditure on health care, as a percentage of gross domestic product (GDP), and the incidence of HPN and HETF. In India, Pakistan, and Africa, where spending on health is low, home artificial nutrition is less common. In Western Europe, where health care accounts for a greater proportion of GDP, home artificial nutritional support is more common. In the United States, with an even greater expenditure on health care, the prevalence of HPN and HETF is higher than anywhere else in the world.

Indications

Home enteral tube feeding The indications for HETF are different for adults and children. In adults, the most common indications are neurological disorders of swallowing resulting from cerebrovascular accidents, Parkinson's disease, and obstructive lesions of the upper gastrointestinal tract. These mainly affect older individuals so that in various countries approximately half of HETF is administered to individuals aged 65 years or older. In children, HETF is usually used in conditions that lead to failure to thrive, such as cerebral palsy, cystic fibrosis, congenital malformation, and metabolic disorders.

As with HPN, one of the main differences between countries in the indications for HETF concerns malignant disease. In North America, ~40% of people receiving HETF have been reported to have malignant disease, and up to ~70% in Italy. In the United Kingdom, the number of patients receiving HETF because of malignancy has steadily increased in both adults and children so that by 2000, 1 in 4 adults and 1 in 12 children who started HETF had cancer, usually of the upper gastrointestinal tract (mainly oesophageal, head and neck, and oropharyngeal). The age distribution of people receiving HETF is influenced by the indications. Because disorders of swallowing (strokes, motor neurone disease, and other neurological conditions) and cancer of the upper gastrointestinal tract tend to occur in older age groups, adults receiving HETF tend to be elderly (with more than 60% of those in the UK being older than 60 years and 46% older than 70 years). In recent years, there has been a trend to provide HETF to an older and more disabled population. Recent surveys in the UK suggest that approximately 50% of patients are house or bed bound and require total help to manage their tube feeding. Because the majority of these patients with high levels of disability are at home (spending <1% of their time in hospital), there are resource implications associated with the provision of health care by the underrecognized and underappreciated voluntary caregivers. Approximately 20% of those receiving HETF are children, and many children who started HETF because of cerebral palsy or congenital handicap continue tube feeding into adulthood.

Home parenteral nutrition The main indications for HPN are Crohn's disease, ischaemic bowel disease, motility disorders, or bowel and malignant disease. Patients receiving HPN are usually younger than those who receive HETF, although there is an overlap. There are also differences between the practice of HPN in different countries. One of the main differences concerns malignant disease. In the United States, 40–50% of patients receiving HPN have been reported to have cancer, and similar if not higher percentages have been reported in some European countries, such as Italy. Early reports from the United Kingdom and Denmark suggested that only a small proportion of HPN (~5%) involved patients with cancer, although this has increased with time. For example, in the United Kingdom it has steadily increased so that by 2003, one in seven patients starting HPN had cancer.

Table 3 Standards of practice for home enteral tube feeding (HETF)

Structure	Process	Outcome
There will be a training program for the health care professionals involved in the care of patients receiving HETF.	Discharge planning will be performed only by professionals who have the necessary experience or who have undertaken a course of training in the topic.	The patient has confidence in the hospital team planning his/her discharge.
There will be a model of care for patients needing HETF.	The members of the multidisciplinary team will be involved in writing the 'mission statement' on which the model is based.	The patient will know the benefits, aims and objectives of the HETF team.
There will be a relaxed, quiet area suitable for private discussion.	There will be a caring and compassionate atmosphere with adequate time for discussion.	The patient will feel able to express his/her fears and expectations.
The discharge planning documentation will include sections on domestic, family and social circumstances.	The nutrition team will evaluate, with the patient and family, how HETF will alter his/her way of life.	The patient will believe that the feeding system can be integrated into an acceptable way of life.
There will be written patient/carer learning goals for HETF.	A designated nurse or dietitian will be responsible for teaching the patient according to his/her individual capacity for learning.	The patient will be able to demonstrate the necessary skills and achieve all the learning goals.
There will be an instruction manual for HETF.	Information and procedures will be regularly updated in order to reflect developments and innovations in tube feeding, access, nutrients and delivery systems.	The patient will perform therapy based on current practice.
A relative, friend or appropriately trained health care professional will be available to deliver therapy if the patient is unable to do so.	The nurse/dietitian will help the patient identify the most appropriate carer. A community nurse will be given the opportunity to visit the patient in hospital and observe therapy before the patient is discharged.	The patient has confidence that safe care will be available at home.
Access to the gastrointestinal tract will be achieved by a tube suitable for long-term use.	The patient, nurse and doctor will choose the most appropriate tube and access site.	The patient will use a feeding tube which is acceptable and accessible.
There will be a policy for sharing care with the patient's General Practitioner (GP).	The GP will be contacted and a shared care protocol agreed.	The patient will know the responsibility of each health care professional.
Written information describing HETF will be available for the GP.	The hospital team will provide the GP with the information before the patient is discharged, together with the discharge date and on-call telephone numbers.	The patient will have confidence in his/her GP's knowledge of HETF.
There will be written procedures for the management of feeding tubes.	The nurse/dietitian will adapt the procedures according to the patient's physical skills and domestic circumstances.	The patient's daily life will not be restricted by prolonged inappropriate procedures.
There will be a written prescription for the enteral feed (and other prescribable items).	The patient's GP will be contacted and advised on how to prescribe the feed.	The patient will have the enteral feed available at home on the day of discharge.
There will be a list of the required equipment, e.g., syringes, connectors, administration sets, pump, drip stand, telephone.	Before discharge the patient's home health authority will be provided with the list and asked to arrange supply by making local arrangements or establishing a contract with a commercial supplier.	The patient will have all the necessary supplies in his/her home on the day of discharge.
There will be an on-call system for providing expert advice to the patient by telephone day and night.	The nurse/dietitian/doctor will explain the system to the patient and identify the professions involved.	The patient will know the names and telephone numbers of health care professionals to contact in case of emergency day or night.
Information will be available describing how the nutrient solutions and supplies will be provided following discharge.	The nurse/dietitian will explain the ordering system and discuss storage, depending on the patient's home circumstances.	The patient will know how to obtain supplies and store and dispose of unwanted material.
There will be a post-discharge monitoring protocol, established by the nutrition team.	Monitoring will be performed by a designated health professional as defined by the protocol.	The patient will know what the follow-up arrangements are.

There has also been an increase in age (due at least partly to the increasing use of HPN in patients with cancer and ischemic bowel disease) so that by 2003 nearly one-fourth of all patients receiving HPN in the United Kingdom were older than 60 years of age.

Organization

The organization and management of HETF and HPN has evolved over time. For example, delivery of feeds and equipment to the first patients who received HPN or HETF was undertaken by the hospitals that initiated the treatment. As the number of patients receiving such treatment increased, commercial organizations have established an organizational infrastructure for delivering feed and ancillary equipment through a national and international network. Some companies employ doctors, nurses, and other staff so that they can provide most of the care, although this practice varies from country to country. In many countries, there is joint care between commercial companies and the national health care systems.

HETF is initiated by many centers or hospitals, and some patients are followed up as outpatients. However, it is impractical to follow up many severely disabled patients in hospital, because they are house bound. Patients receiving HPN are often managed by centres with expertise in nutritional problems (e.g., in France, Denmark, and the United Kingdom). It has been suggested that all patients on HPN should be managed at such centers, but travelling to distant centers may require considerable time, effort, and expense. It is possible for patients to be managed more locally, especially if they are uncomplicated. It remains to be demonstrated if locally managed patients have better satisfaction and similar outcomes as those managed by larger centers. Of course, it is possible to have a system that combines local care and more distant specialist care when required.

Funding arrangements also vary. In several countries, home nutritional support is either totally or partially funded by the national health service, but payment may also be provided by private insurance and individual patients. The overall pattern of funding differs considerably among countries. Sometimes, confusion exists about the funding arrangements even in the same country, and this may limit and delay the use of HETF or HPN.

Patient organizations have developed in some countries, such as Patients on Intravenous and Nasogastric Nutrition Therapy (PINNT) in the United Kingdom. This organization provides support and information to people on home feeding, and it contributes to all levels of the operation of the British Association for Parenteral and Enteral Nutrition (BAPEN), through which it influences policy and decision making. Furthermore, since the feeding equipment for use at home was found to be impractical because it was originally designed for hospital use, PINNT has redesigned the equipment specifically for home use.

Standards of Care

Several surveys have identified inadequacies in training, support, and follow-up of patients receiving HETF and HPN. Specific problems include lack of written instructions about how to manage simple problems that may arise during feeding, lack of telephone contacts for use in emergency, lack of confidence, and inadequacy of equipment for home use. Such surveys have also highlighted the importance of a multidisciplinary approach and the need to undertake home visits to assess the status of severely disabled patients who cannot easily attend a hospital. Pressure on hospital beds has meant that some patients are discharged home before they have been adequately trained, and the care of such patients is sometimes passed on to other health care workers who have little experience of home nutritional support. Since HPN is relatively uncommon in the population, general practitioners may have never encountered patients on this form of therapy and are therefore poorly equipted to manage them. Patients' needs may change during the course of their treatment; therefore, there is a need to establish an organisational infrastructure for continuity of care for HETF and HPN over time and from one health care setting to another. Many hospitals do not have a nutrition team or policies that embrace the needs of people receiving artificial nutrition at home.

A series of guidelines for the management of artificial nutrition in the community have been developed by BAPEN (**Tables 3** and **4**). The guidelines cover aspects of training prior to discharge from hospital (although training can take place at home) and the support required from trained specialist staff once the patient is at home. A national and local organizational structure for delivering the support would aid the process.

Monitoring

The basic elements of monitoring are similar for both HETF and HPN. They include an assessment

Table 4 Standards of practice for home parenteral nutrition (HPN)

Structure	Process	Outcome
There will be a training program for health care professionals involved in the care of patients receiving HPN.	Discharge planning will be performed only by professionals who have the necessary experience or who have undertaken a course of training in the topic.	The patient has confidence in the hospital team planning his/her discharge.
There will be a model of care for patients needing home intravenous nutrition.	All members of the multidisciplinary team will be involved in writing the 'mission statement' on which the model is based.	The patient will know the beliefs, aims and objectives of the HPN Care Team.
There will be a relaxed, quiet area suitable for private discussion.	There will be a caring and compassionate atmosphere with adequate time for discussion.	The patient will feel able to express his/her fears and expectations.
The discharge planning documentation will include sections on domestic, family and social circumstances.	The nutrition team will evaluate with the patient and family how the HPN will alter his/her way of life.	The patient will believe that the feeding system can be integrated into an acceptable way of life.
There will be written patient/carer learning goals for HPN.	A designated nurse will be responsible for teaching the patient according to his/her capacity for learning.	The patient/carer will be able to demonstrate the necessary skills and achieve all the individual learning goals.
There will be an instruction manual for HPN.	Information and procedures will be regularly updated in order to reflect developments and innovations in venous access, nutrient solutions and delivery systems.	The patient will perform therapy based on current practice.
A relative, friend or appropriate health care professional will be available to deliver therapy if the patient is unable to do so (e.g., parent or guardian of a child).	The health care professional will help the patient to identify the most appropriate carer. The district nurse will be given the opportunity to visit the patient in hospital and observe therapy before the patient is discharged.	The patient has confidence that safe care will be available at home.
Venous access will be achieved by a central venous catheter suitable for long-term use.	The patient, nurse and doctor will choose the most appropriate catheter and access site.	The patient will use a central venous catheter that is acceptable and accessible.
There will be written procedures for the management of central venous catheters.	The nurse will adapt the procedures according to the patient's physical skills and domestic circumstances.	The patient's daily life will not be restricted by prolonged inappropriate procedures.
There will be a policy for sharing care with the patient's general practitioner (GP).	The GP will be contacted and a shared care protocol agreed.	The patient will know the responsibility of each health care professional.
Written information describing HPN will be available for the GP.	The hospital teams will provide the GP with the information before the patient is discharged, together with the discharge date, and on-call telephone numbers.	The patient will have confidence in his/her GP's knowledge of HPN.
There will be a written prescription for the nutrition solutions (and other prescribable items).	The patient's GP will be contacted and advised on how to prescribe the feed.	The patient will have the feeding solution available at home on the day of discharge.
There will be a list of the required equipment, e.g., refrigerator, infusion pump, syringes, sterile gloves, telephone.	Before discharge, the patient's home health authority will be provided with the list and asked to arrange supply by making local arrangements or establishing a contract with a commercial supplier.	The patient will have all the necessary supplies at home on the day of discharge.
There will be an on-call system for providing expert advice to the patient by telephone day and night.	The nurse will explain the system to the patient and identify the professions involved.	The patient/carer will know the names and telephone numbers to contact in case of emergency by day or night.
Information will be available describing how the nutrient solutions and supplies will be provided following discharge.	The nurse will explain the chosen supply system and discuss storage depending on the patient's home circumstances.	The patient will know how to obtain supplies, store them and dispose of unwanted material.
There will be a post-discharge monitoring protocol, established by the nutrition team.	Monitoring will be supervised by the nutrition team.	The patient will know the date of the first outpatient visit and what monitoring will be performed.

of the activity of the underlying disease, the nutritional and metabolic state of the patient, and complications associated with nutritional support (**Table 5**). The clinical history alerts the attending health professional to the general well-being, as well as the likelihood of specific problems, such as dehydration, electrolyte imbalance (e.g., diarrhoea), local infection (e.g., local redness and swelling near the

Table 5 Some complications associated with parenteral nutrition and enteral tube feeding

	Parenteral	Enteral tube feeding
Mechanical	Catheter malposition.	Tube malposition (e.g., into lung)
	Insertion trauma (e.g., pneumothorax, brachial plexus injury, cardiac arrhythmia)	Insertion trauma: drainage to stomach and bowel: peritonitis and peristomal leakage and inflammation
	Catheter blockage, kinking or occlusion	Tube blockage, e.g., kinking or occlusion
	Catheter embolus	
	Air embolus	
	Clot embolus (from catheter tip)	
	Lack of access site	
Feed/flow	Nutrient overload (e.g., hyperglycemia, infusional hyperlipidemia)	Diarrhea or constipation
		Bloated adbomen/cramps
		Regurgitation/aspiration of feed
Infections	Catheter-related sepsis	Infected feed administration set
	Infected feed/administration set	Infection around gastrostomy
Metabolic	Fluid and electrolyte disturbances	Fluid and electrolyte disturbances
	Hyperglycemia	Deficiency syndromes (rate with standard feeds given to typical patients)
	Deficiency syndromes, e.g., trace elements and vitamins	Hyper/hypoglycemia
	Nutrient overload (see above) and toxicity (e.g., some trace elements)	
Organ tissue dysfunction	e.g., Abnormal liver function, intestinal atrophy, metabolic bone disease	Mainly disease related, abnormal liver function
		Aspiration pneumonia
Psychological	Anxiety, depression, disturbance in self-image, social isolation	Anxiety, depression, disturbance in self-image, social isolation
Financial	Economic issues vary from centre to centre and country to country	Economic issues vary from center to center and country to country

catheter exit site or peristomal area), blocked tubes and catheters, and so on. Catheter-related sepsis is an important complication of PN, and aspiration pneumonia is an important complication of ETF. The patient/caregiver should have written instructions about basic procedures, which aim to reduce complication rates, and how to deal with simple problems and to recognize those that they cannot readily deal with. Specialist advice should be available 24 h a day. The frequency of complications depends at least partly on the support provided by health professionals.

Dietary intake should be monitored, especially in patients whose clinical status is changing. Appropriate dietary advice may facilitate return to normal oral feeding in some patients. In those with a swallowing difficulty, it may be necessary to assess whether swallowing has improved, with input from speech and language therapists, so that unnecessary HETF is not continued when full oral feeding becomes possible. Studies in the United Kingdom suggest that 15% of patients receiving HETF can revert to full oral feeding after 1 year. Blood tests should be carried out at intervals to check for metabolic stability and specific nutrient deficiencies (e.g., vitamins, minerals, and trace elements) and toxicities. The frequency with which tests are carried out depends on the patient (e.g., whether the patient is

receiving HETF or HPN), the duration of feeding, the extent of oral intake, and disease activity.

Outcome

The most important predictor of outcome in patients receiving home artificial nutritional support (enteral or parenteral) is the underlying disease. Therefore, mortality statistics strongly depend on the initial indications. Nevertheless, a few conclusions can be made. First, the complications associated with artificial nutritional support vary but are reported to be responsible for less than 3–5% of deaths. Second, the outcome is dependent not only on the type of disease but also on the stage of the disease (e.g., patients with advanced HIV who start HPN are only expected to survive a few months, whereas patients with less advanced disease are expected to survive longer). Third, the outcome of patients receiving HPN and HETF for a variety of conditions is available from the British Artificial Nutrition Survey (**Table 6**). For patients on HPN, overall mortality at 1 year is 11%, with 16% returning to oral feeding and the majority continuing with HPN. Patients with Crohn's disease often have a good prognosis (with 4% mortality and 38% returning to oral feeding within 1 year). For patients on HETF, typically an older patient group, mortality

Table 6 Twelve-month outcomes for patients receiving home parenteral nutrition (HPN) and home enteral tube feeding (HETF)

	Continuing		Discontinuing		
	Continues (%)	In hospital (%)	Transferred to oral (%)	Withdrawn/refused (%)	Died (%)
HETF					
All adults (n = 26 501)	45.7	0.6	16.2	1.1	36.3
– CVA (n = 9326)	49.2	0.5	11.5	0.8	38.0
– Oesophageal cancer (n = 2050)	26	0.7	22.6	2.0	48.8
All children (n = 5419)	72.9	0.6	18.7	0.9	6.8
– Cerebral palsy (n = 903)	87.5	0.3	5.2	0.9	6.3
– Congenital handicap (n = 561)	86.8	1.2	6.4	0.4	5.2
HPN					
All adults (n = 765)	71.2	0.4	15.7	1.7	11
All children (n = 68)	77.9	1.5	10.3	0	10.3

Based on British Artificial Nutrition Survey (2004).

is higher overall (36% at 1 year) and outcome varies according to age and condition. The outcome data for two common conditions in adults and children receiving HETF are shown in **Table 6**.

Assessments of quality of life, using EuroQol, suggest that the majority of patients receiving HETF and HPN have some problems (moderate or extreme) with mobility, self care, usual activities, pain/discomfort, and anxiety/depression (five EuroQol dimensions). Mean quality-of-life scores (0, 'worst imaginable health state'; 100, 'best imaginable health state') in adults receiving HPN (53 ± 18) are higher than those for adults receiving HETF (42 ± 27), but both are considerably lower than the scores obtained from the general population, even when adjusting for age. For HETF patients, quality-of-life scores have been found to be similar for those living at home and those in nursing care.

Intestinal Transplantation

In some patients with irreversible intestinal failure, intestinal transplantation can be considered as an alternative to long-term PN. The first intestinal transplantation in humans was undertaken in the early 1960s. Limitations in technical expertise and immunosuppressive therapy meant that none of the original patients survived beyond 76 days. From 1985 to 1990, a series of 20 patients were given cyclosporine but only 2 patients were able to resume normal nutrition and most of the grafts failed. The development of new immunosuppressive agents, particularly tacrolimus, resulted in renewed interest in intestinal transplantation. Furthermore, since 1990, there has been greater standardization of patient selection, operative procedures, and postoperative care mainly in centers specializing in intestinal transplantation. The total international experience is still limited, involving

less than 1000 transplants by 2004 (some of the transplants were isolated intestinal grafts, others were intestinal–liver transplants, and the remaining few were multivisceral transplants that included the intestine). Better graft and patient survival rates have been reported in the more experienced centers. In a series of 165 intestinal transplants at the University of Pittsburgh, patient survival was reported to be more than 75% at 1 year, 54% at 5 years, and 42% at 10 years. More than 90% of patients resumed an unrestricted oral diet.

It appears that intestinal transplantation has become a realistic life-saving option for some people who cannot be maintained on HPN. However, it is not yet the treatment of choice in patients who can be successfully maintained on HPN without noteworthy complications. Nor is it the treatment of choice in patients who are likely to deteriorate rapidly from other causes, such as aggressive multisystem disease, or likely to improve so that they can resume oral nutrition (e.g., patients with healing intestinal fistula or those with short bowel syndrome, in which benefits from intestinal adaptation may continue for up to 1–3 years). A better understanding of the immune response to the transplanted intestine and better immunosuppressive therapy, surgical techniques, and postoperative management are required. Appropriate selection and referral of patients to specialist centers are also important criteria that affect clinical outcomes.

Ethical Issues

The provision of nutritional support to people who are chronically sick, who have rapidly progressive disabling diseases, or who are terminally ill raises many ethical questions. Opinions about withholding or withdrawing artificial nutritional support vary from country to country because of different clinical, religious, and social beliefs and differences in national economies, some of which cannot support large-scale expensive long-term treatments. Thus, there is little home artificial nutrition in countries with poor economies. In more developed economies, the types of patients being fed may also vary considerably. For example, parenteral and enteral nutrition in patients with cancer are used more frequently in Italy than in the United Kingdom, suggesting that clinical attitudes to this type of nutritional support vary. The sanctity of human life is a belief that is strongly held by many religions, but when these conflict with medical judgment, public policies normally override personal religious beliefs. A common ethical controversy concerns the need to provide food and fluid to prolong life in severely disabled patients, such as those with severe neurological problems (e.g., cerebrovascular accident) or those approaching the end of their lives. Although health professionals have a duty to prolong life, it seems inappropriate to prolong suffering. There has been controversy as to whether the provision of food and fluid by a feeding tube placed in the stomach or small intestine should be regarded as an essential part of care or medical treatment. The highest legal authorities in countries such as the United States and England have ruled that this is medical treatment. From an ethical perspective, there is no difference between withholding and withdrawing treatment, but in practice it is often more difficult to withdraw treatment once it has begun than to not initiate it. Joint discussions at the outset between mentally capable patients, family members, and health care workers can do much to prevent future ethical dilemmas.

Conclusions

Home nutritional support, including both oral and artificial (enteral and parenteral) methods of feeding, is an important modality of treatment that is being used for an increasing number of people with disease and disability who are managed in the community. The identification of individuals who are at increased risk of malnutrition and who may benefit from additional nutritional support is a vital first step, which can be undertaken using a validated screening tool (such as MUST; **Figure** 1). Oral nutritional support, including liquid multinutrient supplements, is of value in improving the nutritional intake and functional well-being of patients with malnutrition in the community. Without ETF, many patients with persistent swallowing difficulties would die; similarly, without PN, many patients with persistent intestinal failure would not

survive. Although these forms of home therapy can be life-saving, they may restrict normal lifestyle and lead to life-threatening complications. These complications can be prevented or treated by establishing an adequate organizational infrastructure. This should include education and training of both health workers and patients/caregivers as well as a management structure that allows all patients to be followed up and, when necessary, admitting patients to the hospital for more intensive investigations and therapy. Ethical difficulties about withholding or withdrawing artificial nutritional support are likely to continue and to vary with time and from country to country. Intestinal transplantation is becoming a potentially realistic option for a few patients with irreversible intestinal failure who cannot be adequately maintained on long-term PN, but it has not yet become part of routine clinical care in the same way as renal transplantation has become routine in patients with renal failure, who would otherwise receive a lifelong treatment with dialysis.

See also: **Food Fortification**: Developed Countries; Developing Countries. **Malnutrition**: Secondary, Diagnosis and Management. **Nutritional Support**: Adults, Enteral; Adults, Parenteral; Infants and Children, Parenteral. **Supplementation**: Dietary Supplements; Developing Countries; Developed Countries.

Further Reading

British Medical Association (1999) *Withholding and Withdrawing Life-Prolonging Medical Treatment. Guidance for Decision Making.* London: British Medical Association.

Elia M (2003) *Screening for Malnutrition: A Multidisciplinary Responsibility. Development and Use of the 'Malnutrition Universal Screening Tool' ('MUST') for Adults.* Redditch, UK: BAPEN.

Elia M (Chairman), Russell CA, Stratton RJ, and British Artificial Nutrition Survey (BANS) Committee (2001) *Trends in Artificial Nutrition Support in the UK during 1996–2000.* Maidenhead, UK: BAPEN.

Elia M, Stratton RJ, Holden C *et al.* (2001) Home enteral tube feeding following cerebrovascular accident. *Clinical Nutrition* 20: 27–30.

Glencorse C, Meadows N, Holden C, and British Artificial Nutrition Survey (BANS) Committee (2003) *Trends in Artificial Nutrition Support in the UK between 1996 and 2002.* Redditch, UK: BAPEN.

Langnas AN (2004) Advances in small-intestine transplantation. *Transplantation* 77: S75–S78.

Lennard-Jones JEB (1998) *Ethical and Legal Aspects of Clinical Hydration and Nutritional Support.* Maidenhead, UK: BAPEN.

Moreno JM, Shaffer J, Staun J *et al.* (2001) Survey on legislation and funding of home artificial nutrition in different European countries. *Clinical Nutrition* 20: 117–123.

Stratton RJ and Elia M (1999) A critical, systematic analysis of the use of oral nutritional supplements in the community. *Clinical Nutrition* 18(supplement 2): 29–84.

Stratton RJ, Green CJ, and Elia M (2003) *Disease-Related Malnutrition: An Evidence Based Approach to Treatment.* Oxford: CABI Publishing.

Adults, Enteral

K N Jeejeebhoy, University of Toronto, Toronto, ON, Canada

Nutrients are normally taken by eating a diet composed of a variety of natural foods. In instances in which a normal oral diet cannot be taken, it becomes necessary to nourish the individual by either the enteral or parenteral (intravenous) route. In this article, the use of the enteral route is considered.

Definition of Enteral Nutrition

Enteral nutrition (EN) is the process of nourishing an individual by the administration of a liquid diet of defined composition, usually through nasogastric (NG), nasointestinal (NI), gastrostomy, or jejunostomy tubes (tube feeding). However, palatable enteral products may be taken as supplemental or complete enteral feeding by mouth.

Indications for Enteral Nutrition

Enteral nutrition is the preferred way of feeding patients who cannot eat, absorb, or use a normal diet in the presence of a usable gastrointestinal tract. The following are indications for EN:

1. Critical care patients, including those with trauma and burns, and also after major surgery.
2. Anorexia in patients with malignant disease, sepsis, liver and renal failure, and inflammatory bowel disease (IBD).
3. Upper gastrointestinal obstruction or ulceration of the pharynx, esophagus, stomach, and duodenum may prevent the ingestion of normal food. Examples of these conditions are cancer, central nervous system disorders, and stenosis following ulceration.
4. Pancreatic disease: In patients with pancreatitis it may be possible to feed a low-fat enteral formula through a NI route beyond the duodenum without causing increased disease activity or pain.

5. Short bowel and severe malabsorption: In controlled trials enteral diets are not better absorbed than normal food. Therefore, the presence of a short bowel per se is not an indication for enteral feeding. On the other hand, some patients with severe malabsorption may benefit from the use of elemental diets.
6. Inflammatory bowel disease: In IBD, enteral feeding is useful under the following situations:
   i. Profound anorexia preventing the ingestion of a normal diet.
   ii. Abdominal discomfort due to partial bowel obstruction or intestinal inflammation.
   iii. Growth retardation resulting from insufficient nutrient intake.
   iv. In Crohn's disease some controlled trials have suggested that enteral feeding induces a remission comparable to that seen with steroids.
7. Dementia: Patients unable to feed themselves because of profound mental changes.

Selection of Patients and Timing of Nutritional Support

The process of nutritional support should be an integrated continuum from normal diet to EN based on a plan. This plan should be developed at the moment of each patient's entry and implemented with modifications until discharge. It is undesirable to have to make an urgent decision on a weekend after realizing that the patient has been starving for the previous 2 weeks. I favor an approach in which the nutritionist examines the needs of each patient at entry and follows the algorithm given in **Figure 1**.

Target Nutrient Intake Possibly Achievable

The nutritionist discusses with the patient alternatives to dietary intake and the use of oral nutritional supplements that may include enteral diets taken by mouth. These supplements include liquid formula diets as well as specific supplements (e.g., potassium, magnesium, calcium, zinc, and vitamins). If during a trial period there is progressive improvement in intake or the patient meets the target, this process is continued. If the patient cannot meet the target or is clearly unable to progress toward it, then formal EN is started.

Target Nutrient Intake Achievement Failed or Impossible

These patients are prime candidates for NG or NI feeding if the gastrointestinal tract is normal, as in the case of critical care, anorexia (usually secondary

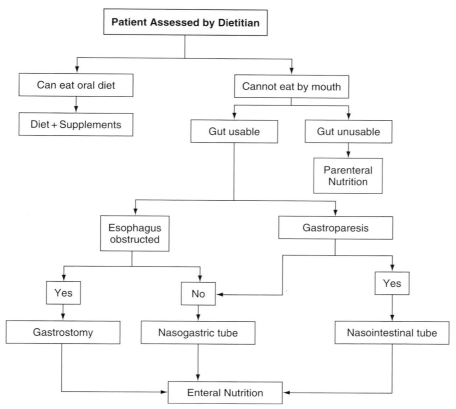

Figure 1 Algorithm for nutritional support.

to disease and malnutrition), neurological impairment preventing oral feeding, substantially increased requirements with relative anorexia (e.g., in burn cases), or chronic obstructive lung disease with severe dyspnea. However, for diseases of the pharynx, esophagus, or stomach or in cases of surgery of the esophagus, stomach, or pancreas, patients usually require intubation of the stomach or intestine by percutaneous gastrostomy or operative jejunostomy to allow feeding beyond the site of obstruction. If there is an abnormality of the intestinal tract, such as short bowel with more than 60 cm of available small intestine, IBD, or chronic partial bowel obstruction, diets must be delivered carefully with the aid of a pump to avoid surges of delivered fluid diets and consequent distension of the bowel. Despite careful selection, a proportion of patients expectantly fed via the nasogastric or nasoenteral route will show intolerance, complications, or inability to meet target nutrient intake without clinically unacceptable side effects. For example, in trials of patients with Crohn's disease, approximately 20% of patients could not tolerate nasogastric feeding. When EN fails or cannot be used for reasons given previously, then parenteral nutrition (PN) must be used.

Home Enteral Nutrition

In some patients, the oral route may be unusable for long periods of time or even permanently. This includes patients with indications given by Nos. 2, 3, and 5 in the list near the beginning of the article. In these patients, a percutaneous endoscopic gastrostomy is placed, and the patients are trained to feed themselves during the night and disconnect themselves during the day to go to school or work. This technique is invaluable to get patients with "gut failure" out of the hospital and rehabilitated.

Enteral Diets

The enteral diets are all complete and will meet the RNIs when fed to meet total energy requirements but may be deficient in meeting micronutrient requirements if given as supplements or in hypocaloric (not meeting total requirements) amounts. The types of diets are as follows:

1. Polymeric: Composed of whole proteins and oligosaccharides with fat partly as long-chain triglycerides and partly as medium-chain triglycerides. They are low in osmolality and palatable and can be taken by mouth.

Table 1 Specialized formulations

Formulation	Use
Branched-chain amino acids	Treat hepatic encephalopathy.
Glutamine	Reduce intestinal permeability, improve immunity, and promote mucosal regeneration.
ω-3 fatty acids	Reduce inflammatory response.
Arginine	Improve immunity.
High-fat diets	Reduce insulin requirements in diabetics. Reduce CO_2 output in patients with respiratory disease.

2. Peptide-based diets: The same as above but the protein is given in the form of peptides, which in theory are absorbed better than amino acids or proteins.
3. Elemental diets: They contain amino acids, are very low in fat, and the carbohydrate may be in the form of glucose. These diets are hyperosmolar and unpalatable. They are best given through a tube as a continuous infusion.
4. Special diets: They may be enriched in branched-chain amino acids, glutamine, ω-3 fatty acids, and arginine. Others have a high-fat content (**Table 1**).

Techniques of Administration

To ensure full calorie intake and to avoid gastrointestinal discomfort, enteral diets are best infused through a tube at a constant rate using a pump. The objective is to infuse at a rate that is equal to the rate of absorption so that intestinal distension does not occur. The diet should be stored in a sterile container so as to prevent bacterial growth while it is being infused. The routes of administration are as follows:

1. Nasogastric tube made of silicone rubber or polyurethane, 9–12 Fr in size: It is passed into the stomach and positioned in the antrum.
2. Nasointestinal tube: These tubes are similar to nasogastric tubes but longer. They are advanced under fluoroscopy into the duodenum. They may also be advanced by endoscopic guidance into the duodenum.
3. Percutaneous gastrostomy and buttons: Under sedation and local anesthesia, a gastrostomy can be placed using an endoscope. It can also be advanced into the duodenum. In long-term feeding the gastrostomy is replaced with a 'button' that is flush with the skin and can be intubated for feeding.
4. Percutaneous jejunostomy: This is placed at operation and can be used to feed into the intestine.

Evidence of the Benefits of Enteral Nutrition

EN has not been compared to standard care (SC) in the same systematic way as PN. Systematic reviews of EN compared to PN have consistently shown increased infectious complications with PN. However, all showed significantly elevated blood glucose in the PN group. It is likely that hyperglycemia was more frequent with PN because patients randomized to PN received more energy than those on EN, despite the intent to make both groups isocaloric. Data from a large controlled trial in intensive care unit (ICU) patients showed that keeping blood glucose below 7 mmol/l irrespective of the route of feeding significantly reduced mortality and multisystem organ failure arising from sepsis. This study indicated that hyperglycemia in the PN arm of the study would have significantly increased the risk of sepsis. None of these studies prove that EN is better than standard therapy; they show that it is less likely to cause infection than PN given without regard to the rigid control of blood glucose. This conclusion is supported by a large study (562 patients) comparing EN and PN that mirrors the conventional practice of NS. Using modest energy intake and avoiding hyperglycemia, the study showed that nutritional intake below 80% of the target was observed in 75% of randomized EN patients and 25% of randomized PN patients ($p < 0.001$). There was no significant differences in the incidence of septic morbidity between patients receiving PN and those given EN. The inability of EN to deliver target energy intake was also seen in several other trials, in which outcome was also no different between PN and EN.

Early Enteral Nutrition, Parenteral Nutrition, and Bacterial Translocation

In animal models, burns and trauma have been associated with the appearance of organisms in the mesenteric lymph nodes (MLNs). This process has been called bacterial translocation. Enteral feeding has been associated with reduced translocation in guinea pigs. In other animal studies, early enteral feeding reduced nitrogen loss and the level of catabolic hormones. However, human studies in patients who have been traumatized have not show any benefit of early (<24 h) enteral feeding. In addition, a prospective sampling of portal blood in trauma patients failed to confirm that translocation occurs in traumatized humans. A meta-analysis of early vs late enteral feeding showed no difference in outcome. In obese patients, a quasi-randomized trial showed that early feeding with a higher energy intake increased sepsis.

Special Formulations

Immunonutrition

Enteral formulations enriched in arginine, omega-3 fatty acids, and glutamine nucleotides are considered to enhance the immune response, and treatments with these formulations are collectively referred to as immunonutrition. The formulations under consideration vary in composition. They are distinguished by high (12–15 g/l) or low (4–6 g/l) arginine, the presence or absence of glutamine and nucleotides, and the concentration of omega-3 fatty acids. The proceedings of the summit on immune-enhancing enteral therapy concluded that immunonutrition should be given to malnourished patients undergoing elective gastrointestinal surgery and trauma patients with an injury severity score of ≥18 or those with an abdominal trauma index of ≥20. Despite lack of evidence, it was recommended for patients undergoing head and neck surgery and aortic reconstruction, those with severe head injury and burns, and for ventilator-dependent nonseptic patients. The summit did not recommend it for patients with splanchnic hypoperfusion, bowel obstruction distal to the access site, and after major upper gastrointestinal hemorrhage.

In contrast to the conclusions of the summit, systematic reviews of the evidence have given mixed results. The reviews suggested that although immunonutrition did reduce septic complications, the reduction did not result in reduced mortality. In a meta-analysis of 22 randomized controlled trials performed in 2419 critically ill or surgical patients, it was concluded that the amount of arginine in the formulations influenced the results. Taken as a whole, in critically ill patients there were no treatment effects on mortality or rates of infectious complications. In fact, there was a suggestion that in critical illness these formulations may increase mortality. To support this possibility, a trial suspended the use of immunonutrition in seriously ill patients after an interim analysis showed increased mortality with immunonutrition in these patients. However, in elective surgical patients immunonutrition reduced complications and length of stay. Since many trauma and septic patients may be critically ill, the recommendations made in the two publications referred to previously are at variance. Other meta-analyses have not separated critically ill and nonseptic patients and have concluded that immunonutrition reduced septic complications

and length of stay but criticized the component studies as being variable and overall not altering mortality.

Enteral Glutamine Supplementation

Glutamine is released into the circulation from muscle continuously in healthy people and especially in those with catabolic illness. The glutamine in the circulation is an important nutrient for immunocytes such as lymphocytes and for the mucosa of the intestine. In septic and malnourished patients, muscle glutamine is depleted, and it is hypothesized that in these patients the availability of glutamine for lymphocytes and the gut is reduced, resulting in increased risk of sepsis. Although enteral mixtures designed to improve immunity have given variable results, glutamine supplementation has not been shown to be harmful and has reduced complications in patients with bone marrow transplantation, after surgery, and in those with critical illness and burns.

Enteral Branched-Chain Amino Acid Formulations

Patients with hepatic encephalopathy have low levels of enteral branched-chain amino acids (BCAAs) and increased levels of phenylalanine and tryptophane. It has been postulated that since BCAAs compete with phenylalanine and tryptophane for transport through the blood–brain barrier, reduced levels of BCAAs promote the accumulation of these amino acids in the brain, where they are metabolized to false neurotransmitters that then cause encephalopathy. To reverse this state, BCAA-enriched formulas were developed, and in a meta-analysis of randomized controlled trials of these formulations in hepatic encephalopathy, they were shown to reduce the duration of encephalopathy in comatose patients.

Enteral Formulation Enriched in Protein

High-protein formulations are available to feed patients with adequate amounts of protein at a lower energy intake. These formulations are especially useful in patients who are critically ill and become hyperglycemic on standard formulations. Using high-protein formulations has allowed the administration of up to 2 g/kg protein in patients with protein losses, such as those with fistulas, burns, and abscesses, and in calorie-intolerant patients. One controlled trial has shown that a high protein intake reduces mortality in burn patients, whereas high energy intake in sepsis appears to increase mortality.

High-Fat Formulations

The average fat content of enteral formulations is approximately 30% of total energy. The main source of energy in these formulations is carbohydrate. The high carbohydrate has two relevant metabolic effects. First, it increases the need for insulin secretion. Second, when fed in amounts that exceed energy requirements, it increases CO_2 production. Diabetics potentially would therefore have reduced insulin requirements and a lower risk of hyperglycemia if fed high-fat formulations. Similarly, malnourished patients with chronic obstructive pulmonary disease (COPD) would have a lower risk of CO_2 retention if given a high-fat diet with a high calorie intake to promote weight gain. Therefore, high-fat formulations have been developed to feed patients with diabetes and COPD. However, there is little evidence that they are significantly better than standard formulations.

Enteral Omega-3 Fat Supplementation

Omega-3 fats are composed of polyunsaturated fatty acids, in which the first double bond 3 carbon atoms are located away from the methyl end of the fatty acid chain. The fatty acids found in fish oil, called eicosapentanoic and docosahexaenoic, are precursors of prostaglandins and thromboxanes that antagonize the prothrombotic effects of similar compounds derived from linoleic acid. In humans, when infused, they reduce the production of proinflammatory cytokines from stimulated mononuclear cells. They potentially have anti-inflammatory effects and have been shown in controlled trials to benefit patients with ARDS.

Enteral Nutrition with Probiotics

The administration of a probiotic, *Lacobacillus plantarum*, indicates that probiotics with EN may have a role in reducing septic complications in patients with pancreatitis and those after liver transplantation.

Optimizing Enteral Nutrition and Reducing Risk of Aspiration Pneumonia

Enteral feeding is associated with several factors that may result in reflux of gastric contents and aspiration: the supine position of the patient, the presence of a nasogastric tube, gastric contents, and delayed emptying of the stomach. Intuitively, placing the tip of the feeding tube into the intestine rather than the stomach should reduce aspiration, and the Canadian clinical practice guidelines recommend postpyloric feeding. On the other hand, a meta-analysis comparing gastric and postpyloric feeding did not show any significant difference in the incidence of pneumonia between patients fed into the stomach and those fed beyond the pylorus. Although enteral feeding is widely practiced as the route of choice, in a study of 103 patients admitted to an ICU who were observed prospectively for the development of nosocomial pneumonia, there was evidence that feeding contributed to pneumonia. In that study, a multivariate analysis concluded that continuous enteral feeding, but not the nasogastric tube, was an independent risk factor for nosocomial pneumonia and patients who developed pneumonia had a significantly higher mortality of 43.5% compared to 18.8% for those who did not develop pneumonia. Clearly, more studies need to be done to determine the best approach to prevent pneumonia.

The use of prokinetics is another way of promoting gastric emptying. In a placebo controlled randomized trial of 305 patients receiving enteral feeding, giving metoclopramide did not reduce the incidence of pneumonia. Erythromycin, a motilin receptor agonist, is another powerful prokinetic agent. In a randomized controlled trial the benefit of erythromycin was questionable. There was no difference in the rate of pneumonia between the placebo and erythromycin-treated patients. The previous studies unfortunately involved small numbers of patients, and there is a need for larger trials of small bowel feeding and prokinetics to establish their role in promoting enteral feeding and reducing the risk of aspiration.

Perioperative Enteral Nutrition

Infusing a diet enriched with arginine, omega-3 fatty acid, and RNA preoperatively and postoperatively has resulted in a significant reduction in total but not major complications. In patients undergoing abdominal surgery, progressive postoperative oral supplementation without formal EN reduces complications and raises the question as to whether EN, total parenteral nutrition (TPN), or immunonutrition are even necessary for the majority of patients. Complications can be reduced by introducing early sip feeding of liquid diets without formal EN.

A small but provocative study from India raises the same questions about the routine use of EN. Sixty postoperative patients were randomized to either a standard ward diet or a diet with a home-made liquid supplement (10 patients per group). They were also stratified to mild, moderate, and severe malnutrition groups of 20 patients each. There was no mortality in the study and patients were discharged after approximately 10 days. The supplemented groups received significantly more energy and protein. However, only in the severely malnourished patients was there a difference in the incidence of complications—7/10 in the control and 4/10 in the supplemented group. In the mild malnutrition group, there were 1/10 complications in each arm and 2/10 in the moderate malnutrition group. This study suggests that a very modest oral intake of supplements reduced complications but did so only in the severely malnourished group. It is likely that the aggressive nutritional support, as is practiced currently, may not be necessary and may even be detrimental in some situations. Larger randomized trials of oral supplements should be considered.

Enteral Nutrition and Head Injury

A systematic review of controlled trials of nutritional support in cases of head injury showed that the relative risk (RR) for death with early nutritional support was 0.67 (95% confidence interval (CI), 0.41–1.07), and the RR for death or complications at the end of follow-up was 0.75 (95% CI, 0.50–1.11). The findings suggested that early nutrition showed a trend toward reduced mortality and complications.

Nutritional Support of Bone Marrow Transplant Patients

A review found that although EN is the current standard for nutritional support, it has not found favor for patients undergoing bone marrow transplant because these patients have severe mucositis, often vomit the tube, and do not tolerate nasogastric tubes because of discomfort and ulceration. Veno-occlusive disease with encephalopathy may occur in bone marrow patients, which is another indication for TPN with branched-chain amino acids rather than EN. A controlled trial of EN versus TPN in bone marrow transplant patients showed that outcome was no different but body composition and magnesium levels were better maintained on TPN. In contrast, TPN patients had more fluid overload and hyperglycemia. It should be noted that 'enteral nutrition' in this trial was not tube feeding but a combination of snacks, diet counseling, and tube feeding. The authors concluded that TPN should be reserved for patients with severe mucositis. Review of the Cochrane

database concluded that the relative effectiveness of EN versus TPN could not be evaluated. In addition, patients with gastrointestinal failure should consider TPN with the addition of glutamine if EN is not possible.

Alcoholic Hepatitis and Enteral Nutrition

Seventy-one patients with severe alcoholic hepatitis were randomized to prednisone 40 mg/day or EN giving 2000 kcal/day for 28 days and then followed for 1 year or until death. The EN was a branched-chain-enriched diet and patients on steroid therapy were encouraged by dietitians to eat 2000 kcal/day with 1 g/kg/day of protein. No patients from the steroid arm dropped out, whereas 8/35 patients from the EN arm did not receive EN for the entire period but were included in the analysis (intent to treat analysis). It is of interest that all patients in the steroid arm ate 80% of the prescribed diet. Using intent to treat analysis, there were no differences in mortality or complications in the hospital between groups. After discharge, even when confounding variables were adjusted, the EN group had a significantly better survival. Since both groups seemed to receive the same energy intake, the reason for better long-term survival with EN needs further study. Was it because of the use of branched-chain amino acids or because steroid therapy had an undesirable catabolic effect?

Pancreatitis and Enteral Nutrition

Oral feeding is known to increase abdominal pain in patients with pancreatitis. Therefore, TPN has been used in these patients to 'rest' the pancreas. One study aimed to define the indications and evaluate the cost-effectiveness of nutritional support in a series of patients with pancreatitis. The patients were given nothing orally and only intravenous fluids for 48 h. Those who improved were fed orally (O group). The remainder were randomized to receive nutrients either infused into the jejunum (EN group) or by vein (TPN group). A total of 156 patients were included, of whom 75% improved (O) and were discharged within 4 days. In the randomized patients, 56% of the EN group received inadequate energy intake but were fed for a significantly shorter period (mean, 6.7 versus 10.8 days) and had less metabolic ($p < 0.003$) and septic complications ($p < 0.01$). More than 50% of TPN patients were hyperglycemic, in contrast to only approximately 15% of the EN group. Despite fewer complications in the EN group, the mortality was similar in the two groups. The authors concluded that hypocaloric enteral feeding is better than TPN. This study is similar to many others, showing that EN providing less than estimated energy intake is associated with reduced hyperglycemia and sepsis. The conventional interpretation is that the EN route reduces sepsis. The trial by van den Berghe et al. showed that irrespective of the route of nutritional support, control of hyperglycemia reduced mortality in the ICU. Their findings support the alternative explanation that the EN route protects the patient because it results in hypocaloric feeding, which prevents hyperglycemia. The study shows that EN can be given as a cheaper source of nutrition, but since EN was needed only for 6.7 days with less than adequate energy intake, it raises the question as to whether any nutritional support was required. Another important question is whether TPN should be hypocaloric rather than meet target energy intake in patients who are unable to take oral nutrition or EN for periods exceeding 7–10 days. In order to settle these issues, larger multicenter randomized trials are required.

See also: **Burns Patients**. **Colon**: Disorders; Nutritional Management of Disorders. **Diabetes Mellitus**: Dietary Management. **Eating Disorders**: Anorexia Nervosa; Bulimia Nervosa. **Microbiota of the Intestine**: Probiotics. **Nutritional Support**: Adults, Parenteral; Infants and Children, Parenteral. **Supplementation**: Dietary Supplements.

Further Reading

Alexander JW, MacMillan BG, Stinnett JD et al. (1980) Beneficial effects of aggressive protein feeding in severely burned children. *Annals of Surgery* **192**: 505–517.

Artigas AT, Dronda SB, Valles EC et al. (2001) Risk factors for nosocomial pneumonia in critically ill trauma patients. *Critical Care Medicine* **29**: 304–309.

Bertolini G, Iapichino G, Radrizzani D et al. (2003) Early enteral immunonutrition in patients with severe sepsis. Results of an interim analysis of a randomized multicentre clinical trial. *Intensive Care Medicine* **29**: 834–840.

De Jonghe B, Appere-de-Vechi C, Fournier M et al. (2001) A prospective survey of nutritional support practice in intensive care unit patients: What is prescribe? What is delivered? *Critical Care Medicine* **29**: 8–12.

Eyer SD, Micon LT, Konstantinides FN et al. (1993) Early enteral feeding does not attenuate metabolic response after blunt trauma. *Journal of Trauma* **34**: 639–643.

Gadek JE, DeMichele SJ, Karlstad MD et al. (1999) Effect of enteral feeding with eicosapentaenoic acid, gamma-linolenic acid, and antioxidants in patients with acute respiratory distress syndrome. Enteral Nutrition in ARDS Study Group. *Critical Care Medicine* **27**: 1409–1420.

Han-Geurts IJM, Jeekel J, Tilanus HW, and Brouwer KJ (2001) Randomized clinical trial of patient-controlled versus fixed regimen feeding after elective surgery. *British Journal of Surgery* **88**: 1578–1582.

Heyland DK, Dhaliwal R, Drover JW, Gramlich L, and Dodek P (2003) Canadian clinical practice guidelines for nutrition support in mechanically ventilated, critically ill adult patients. *Journal of Parenteral and Enteral Nutrition* **27**: 355–373.

Heyland DK, Novak F, Drover JW et al. (2001) Should immuno-nutrition become routine in critically ill patients? *Journal of the American Medical Association* **286**: 944–953.

Ibrahim EH, Mehringer L, Prentice D et al. (2002) Early versus late enteral feeding of mechanically ventilated patients: Results of a clinical trial. *Journal of Parenteral and Enteral Nutrition* **26**: 174–181.

Jeejeebhoy KN (2001) TPN potion or poison. *American Journal of Clinical Nutrition* **74**: 160.

Kudsk KA and Moore FA (chairpersons) (2001) Proceedings from the summit on immune-enhancing enteral therapy. *Journal of Parenteral and Enteral Nutrition* **25**: S1–S63.

Marik PE and Zaloga GP (2003) Gastric versus post-pyloric feeding: A systematic review. *Critical Care* **7**: R46–R61.

Montejo JC, Zarazaga A, Lopez-Martinez J and the Spanish Society of Intensive Care Medicine and Coronary Units (2003) Immunonutrition in the intensive care unit. A systematic review and consensus statement. *Clinical Nutrition* **22**: 221–233.

Moore FA, Moore EE, Poggetti R et al. (1991) Gut bacterial translocation via the portal vein: A clinical perspective with major torso trauma. *Journal of Trauma* **31**: 629–636.

Murray SM and Pindoria S (2002) Nutrition support for bone marrow transplant patients. *Cochrane Database of Systems Review* **2**: CD002920.

Naylor CD, O'Rourke K, Detsky AS, and Baker JP (1989) Parenteral nutrition with branched-chain amino acids in hepatic encephalopathy. A meta-analysis. *Gastroenterology* **97**: 1033–1042.

Nelson JK and Fleming CR (1990) Home enteral nutrition for adults. In: Rombeau JL and Caldwell MD (eds.) *Clinical Nutrition Enteral and Tube Feeding*, 2nd edn, pp. 450–462. Toronto: WB Saunders.

Saluja SS, Kaur N, and Shrivastava UK (2002) Enteral nutrition in surgical patients. *Surgery Today* **32**: 672–678.

Sanders DS, Carter MJ, D'Silva J et al. (2000) Survival analysis in percutaneous endoscopic gastrostomy feeding: A worse outcome in patients with dementia. *American Journal of Gastroenterology* **95**: 1472–1475.

Souheil A-Ai, Kimberly C, and O'Keefe SJD (2002) Hypocaloric jejunal feeding is better than total parenteral nutrition in acute pancreatitis: Results of a randomized comparative study. *American Journal of Gastroenterology* **97**: 2255–2262.

van den Berghe G, Wouters P, Weekers F et al. (2001) Intensive insulin therapy in the critically ill patients. *New England Journal of Medicine* **345**: 1359.

Woodcock NP, Zeigler D, Palmer MD et al. (2001) Enteral versus parenteral nutrition: A pragmatic study. *Nutrition* **17**: 1–12.

Yanagawa T, Bunn F, Roberts I, Wentz R, and Pierro A (2002) Nutritional support for head-injured patients. *Cochrane Database of Systems Review* **3**: CD001530.

Zaloga GP and Roberts P (1994) Permissive underfeeding. *New Horizons* **2**: 257–263.

Adults, Parenteral

J Binkley, S Daniell and G L Jensen, Vanderbilt
Center for Human Nutrition, Nashville, TN, USA

Parenteral nutrition (PN) is a compounded formulation of amino acids, dextrose, and lipid emulsions, along with electrolytes, multivitamins, and trace elements. The development of this form of nutrition intervention gave new hope to patients who suffered from intestinal compromise or failure.

PN had its modern beginnings in the mid-1960s as Dr. Stanley Dudrick and colleagues researched infusion of hypertonic glucose and protein solutions into the superior vena cava of beagle puppies. Normal growth and development of the beagles were maintained for 36 months using this approach. The first research that established the use of intravenous feedings in humans was reported by Dudrick and colleagues in 1969. From its early beginnings, PN was known as 'hyperalimentation,' with the belief that it was desirable to feed in excess of standard requirements. Years of clinical practice has shown that PN should be provided in more limited amounts in order to prevent some of the complications associated with its overzealous use.

This article focuses on components of PN for adult nutrition support, indications and contraindications for its use, implementation and monitoring for safety and efficacy, complications associated with use of PN, and consideration of its use for home patients. Prudent patient selection and careful monitoring will help to ensure the safe and effective administration of PN. A multidisciplinary approach to PN management is suggested to help optimize the use of this therapy.

Indications for PN

PN should be considered for patients when oral intake or enteral feedings are not possible or are contraindicated for a prolonged period of time. Enteral feedings are the preferred route of administration for specialized nutrition support for many reasons. Enteral feedings are more physiologic and facilitate maintenance of gastrointestinal integrity and function. In comparison with PN, enteral feedings are considerably less expensive and are associated with fewer serious adverse effects. Enterohepatic circulation and barrier function of the gastrointestinal mucosa can be preserved with even small quantities of enteral stimulation. Enteral

feedings are associated with a decreased incidence of bacterial translocation and associated sepsis in animal models. PN is indicated when the gastrointestinal tract is not functional, when the safe placement of an enteral feeding access device is not possible, or when the enteral route cannot adequately meet the nutritional needs of a patient. Table 1 lists common indications for PN. When enteral feedings cannot be established within 7–10 days, PN should be considered. Table 2 lists contraindications to the use of enteral feedings.

Bowel Rest

PN is often used when continued use of the gastrointestinal tract may not be advisable. PN may be selected for inflammatory bowel disease patients with severe acute exacerbations or for perioperative care. For patients with Crohn's disease, PN may aid the management of complications such as intestinal obstruction, fistula formation, short bowel syndrome, and severe diarrhea. Otherwise, enteral nutrition support is frequently used for nutrition support in inflammatory bowel disease with comparable efficacy.

PN can be used for bowel rest in severe acute pancreatitis, when its duration is anticipated to be more than 7–10 days. Various scoring systems are used to classify the severity of pancreatitis and together with sound clinical judgment can help to

Table 1 Common diagnoses with indications for PN

Perioperative support in severe malnutrition
Inflammatory bowel disease and related complications
Short bowel syndrome
Severe acute pancreatitis
Mechanical intestinal obstruction or pseudo-obstruction
High-output entercutaneous fistula
Prolonged postoperative ileus
Severe malabsorption
Bone marrow transplant/peripheral stem cell transplant
Severe hyperemesis gravidarum

Table 2 Contraindications to enteral nutrition

Diffuse peritonitis
Intestinal obstruction that prohibits use of the bowel
Intractable vomiting
Paralytic ileus
Intractable diarrhea
Gastrointestinal ischemia

Adapted from ASPEN Board of Directors and the Clinical Guidelines Task Force (2002) Guidelines for the use of parenteral and enteral nutrition in adult and pediatric patients. *Journal of Parenteral and Enteral Nutrition* **26**(1 supplement): 18SA.

assess the need for bowel rest with PN. Studies using nasojejunal or jejunostomy feeding tubes with elemental low-fat enteral formulas in patients with mild to moderate pancreatitis have demonstrated effectiveness. Patients who exhibit feeding intolerance with enteral nutrition should be considered for PN therapy.

Bowel rest may also be indicated for selected enterocutaneous fistulas, which can occur as a result of complicated Crohn's disease, gastrointestinal or abdominal abscesses, abdominal surgery or trauma, ischemia, or tumors or their accompanying treatment regimens such as chemoradiation. Bowel rest can help to promote potential closure of fistulas and can improve nutritional status of these patients. Depending on the output of the fistulas, many of these patients are at risk for malnutrition as well as dehydration and electrolyte abnormalities.

Perioperative Support in Severe Malnutrition

Increased morbidity and mortality risks are associated with malnourished surgical patients. The Veteran's Affairs Parenteral Nutrition Cooperative Trial evaluated the benefits of preoperative PN in patients with varying degrees of malnutrition. Significant benefit was demonstrated only among those patients who were severely malnourished (albumin <3.0 g/dl). Interestingly, an increased rate of infectious complications was observed in mildly and moderately malnourished patients receiving PN compared to the control group. If enteral access is available and feeds are tolerated, preoperative enteral nutrition support has been found to be equally effective when utilized for 7–14 days or longer in malnourished surgical patients. Early studies that suggested increased adverse outcomes with parenteral compared to enteral support were often based on management techniques that are no longer consistent with standard of practice, which included the overfeeding of macronutrients, rapid infusion rates, and a much less aggressive approach to the prevention of hyperglycemia. Therefore, many of the studies demonstrating more favorable outcomes with enteral support need to be repeated using current standards of care.

Postoperatively, in patients who have undergone intraabdominal procedures with extensive bowel manipulations, paralytic ileus is commonly observed. Use of narcotics or other pain medications, paralytic agents, and electrolyte abnormalities may also contribute to slow gastrointestinal motility and ileus. If a patient's gastrointestinal tract is not functional for more than 7–10 days, PN should be considered.

Gastrointestinal Inability to Absorb Adequate Nutrients

PN is indicated if the patient is unable to absorb adequate nutrients via the gastrointestinal tract. Short bowel syndrome can result from extensive bowel resection or dysfunction. Initially, fluid and electrolyte management is often the most critical aspect of nutrition care. Losses can be extensive. The resulting degree of malabsorption, and therefore the specific nutrition management requirements, depends on the remaining intestinal length or function, the presence or absence of large bowel continuity, and the presence or absence of the ileum. Enteral nutrition support is preferred over parenteral support; however, the adaptive phase for the remaining gastrointestinal tract often necessitates a period of PN requirement, often months to a few years. Sometimes patients with extensive bowel resection (less than 100 cm of remaining bowel) may require lifelong PN or small bowel transplantation.

Other Possible Indications for Use

The importance of adequate nutrition in pregnancy is widely recognized. Hyperemesis gravidarum (HG) is severe nausea and emesis that can persist throughout the gestation period, preventing the patient from receiving adequate calories and protein for fetal growth. HG usually occurs before the 20th week of gestation and is characterized by weight loss, changes in fluid and electrolyte status, and disturbances in acid–base balance. After attempting to achieve weight gain and resolution of symptoms with antiemetics, intravenous hydration, and diet modifications without success, specialized nutrition support with enteral feedings or PN may be appropriate for refractory cases. Enteral feedings are preferred, but PN is indicated if enteral feedings are not tolerated.

Another potential need for PN occurs in patients treated with high-dose chemotherapy with or without radiation, followed by hematopoetic stem cell transplantation. This treatment regimen may be associated with significant gastrointestinal side effects, including nausea, emesis, diarrhea, mucositis, esophagitis, xerostomia, and odynophagia. Nutritional compromise is possible due to the persistence of these symptoms for protracted time periods. Specialized nutrition support with enteral nutrition or PN may be indicated if patients are unable to maintain adequate oral intake or if they demonstrate persistent gastrointestinal side effects. PN has been suggested to improve posttransplantation survival, reduce disease relapse, and shorten hospital stay, although enteral feedings have also been successfully administered to such patients.

Nutrition Components of PN

Amino Acids

Amino acids yield 4 kcal/g when oxidized for energy. Nitrogen content varies somewhat, depending on the individual amino acid formulation and mixture of amino acids. Mixtures of buffered essential and nonessential amino acids are available as stock concentrations ranging from 3 to 20%. Specialty amino acid products are also available for specific disease states or pediatric populations. For example, formulations containing a higher concentration of branched-chain amino acids may be considered for patients with hepatic insufficiency with accompanying encephalopathy.

Dextrose

The carbohydrate energy source for PN is hydrated dextrose, which yields 3.4 kcal/g. Dextrose is available commercially in concentrations ranging from 2.5 to 70%. Dextrose solutions are acidic, and their osmolarity depends on concentration. Higher concentrations of dextrose must be administered directly into central veins instead of peripheral veins in order to prevent thrombophlebitis.

Lipid Emulsions

PN regimens include lipid emulsions as the source for fat calories and essential fatty acids. In the United States, commercially available intravenous lipid products contain largely n-6 long-chain fatty acids derived from vegetable oils. Long-chain lipid emulsions provide the most concentrated source of calories in PN (9 kcal/g). Other lipid-containing products are currently available in Europe, including lipid emulsions containing medium-chain fatty acids and structured triglycerides. The latter are custom synthesized triglycerides that contain both long-chain and medium-chain fatty acids on the same glycerol moiety. These lipid substrates may offer certain metabolic and immune tolerance advantages.

Controversy surrounds the use of intravenous lipid emulsions (IVLEs) due to early reports of adverse immune function and pulmonary effects in critically ill patients. These early reports of alterations in immune function were associated with excessive infusion rates or doses of IVLEs in comparison with today's standard dosing regimens. Concerns have also been raised that n-6 fatty acids may fuel inflammatory eicosanoid pathways. Lipids are contraindicated in patients with significant hypertriglyceridemia. When lipids are restricted, modest doses of lipids (30–40 g twice weekly) should be provided to prevent essential fatty acid deficiency (EFAD). Linoleic acid (18:3n6) and α-linolenic acid (18:3n3) are required to prevent EFAD. To prevent EFAD, 2–4% of calories should be provided as linoleic acid and 0.5% as α-linolenic acid.

Electrolytes

Specific patient electrolyte requirements can be determined and added, as feasible, to PN solutions. Usually, maintenance doses of electrolytes are determined and provided in daily amounts of electrolytes added to the PN solution. Additional repletion and replacement of losses can occur in electrolyte doses given outside the PN admixture. Sodium and potassium can be added as chloride or acetate, depending on acid–base needs. Physicochemical incompatibilities exist for large quantities of electrolytes added to the same PN formulation. In particular, calcium and phosphorus concentrations must be carefully scrutinized to prevent precipitation. Many factors may influence the solubility of these electrolytes in the PN solution, including the concentration of electrolytes, the pH of the final formula, temperature, and the presence of other components. A nutrition support pharmacist can be a resource to address compatibility concerns.

Multivitamins

Multivitamin preparations, including both water-soluble and fat-soluble vitamins, are available for inclusion in the PN admixture. These products have been formulated to meet the guidelines established by the American Medical Association Nutrition Advisory Group and the Food and Drug Administration. **Table 3** lists the composition of

Table 3 Contents of parenteral multivitamin preparations

Vitamin component	Current FDA requirements
Vitamin A	3300 IU
Vitamin D (ergocalciferol or cholecalciferol)	200 IU
Vitamin E (α-tocopherol)	10 IU
Vitamin K (phylloquinone)	150 µg
Vitamin C	200 mg
Folic acid	600 µg
Niacin	40 mg
Vitamin B_2	3.6 mg
Vitamin B_1	6 mg
Vitamin B_6	6 mg
Vitamin B_{12}	5 µg
Pantothenic acid	15 mg
Biotin	60 µg

standard adult multivitamin products. Some individual vitamin preparations, such as vitamin K, are available for injection as well.

Trace Elements

Intravenous trace element preparations are commercially available as single-entity products as well as a variety of combination products. Commonly used trace elements include zinc, copper, manganese, chromium, and selenium (**Table 4**). Other elements may be included as single additives.

Titration of Volume

Final fluid volumes of PN can be titrated to a desired amount using sterile water for injection. Concentrated substrates may be used to minimize volume of PN to provide the desired components. Typical PN volumes range from 800 to 2500 ml daily.

Compounding and Technical Requirements for PN

Access Devices and PN Concentrations

PN is administered into the venous system either through peripheral venous lines or through centrally placed access devices. Lower concentrations of dextrose and amino acids may be administered through peripheral veins for a short duration of therapy. Such formulas usually do not provide the patient's full nutrition needs, may require large volumes of fluid, and can only be used for short durations due to the difficulty of maintaining peripheral intravenous access. Osmolarity of peripheral formulas is best maintained at approximately 600 mOsm/l or less. This requirement means that peripheral PN formulas should contain no more than 5–10% dextrose and 3.5–5% amino acids. Potential complications of peripheral PN include phlebitis, infiltration, or fluid-overload issues. When higher concentrations of dextrose and amino acids are used, such as those generally needed to provide adequate daily nutrient requirements via PN, the hyperosmolar formula must be administered

Table 4 Contents of a common parenteral trace element preparation

Component	Dose
Zinc	5 mg
Copper	1 mg
Manganese	0.5 mg
Chromium	10 μg
Selenium	60 μg

directly into the superior or inferior vena cava to facilitate rapid dilution. Commonly used central venous catheters that may be used to administer PN include subclavian vein catheters, peripherally inserted central catheters, subcutaneously tunneled percutaneous catheters, or implanted subcutaneous infusion ports. Catheter type will be determined by expected duration of need, specific patient condition, patient care setting, as well as physician or patient preference.

Standard versus Individualized Preparations

Institutions or patient care providers may choose to provide PN solutions as standardized formulas or as customized admixtures, specially tailored to the individual's needs. Commercially available premixed PN solutions typically contain 5–25% dextrose and 2.75–5% amino acids, and they may vary by electrolyte content. Individualized formulations are selected to ensure the highest quality in patient safety and product efficacy; however, premixed solutions are often used in settings in which the demand for PN is low.

Two-in-One versus Total Nutrient Admixture

PN admixtures can be compounded by one of two methods: as a dextrose–amino acid solution with lipids infused separately or as a three-in-one formulation, also known as total nutrient admixture, in which all three macronutrients are combined in the same infusion bag. There are benefits and limitations with both methods, and the choice of administration depends on the care setting and institution or practitioner preference.

Cyclic PN

PN therapy may be infused continuously 24-h daily, or the same volume may be infused over a shorter period of time, such as a cycle of 12-h PN infusion and 12-h free of infusion. Infusion pumps can be programmed to adjust infusion rates according to the desired volumes and administration times. Continuous infusion is generally selected when PN is first initiated for an acutely ill patient. Benefits for a cyclic total PN regimen are particularly notable for long-term patients. A cycled PN regimen allows more mobility for the patient, thus enabling the patient to achieve a more active lifestyle. Limitations to a cycled PN regimen include fluid intolerance or glucose intolerance. When initiating a PN cycle, blood glucose concentrations should be checked to ensure that hyperglycemia or hypoglycemia is not an issue for the patient. Because of the potential for 'rebound hypoglycemia' upon abrupt cessation of infusion, the rate of administration is often tapered down at the end of the cycle to allow for downregulation of pancreatic release of insulin. Many infusion pumps have programmable taper functions.

Quality Control

Safety of PN solutions is a paramount objective and includes ensuring accuracy in compounding and avoiding both particulate matter and microbial contamination. PN solutions must be prepared using a strict aseptic technique in a class 100 environment using a laminar flow hood. All PN additives should always be added in the sterile environment to prevent risk of contamination. Many incompatibility issues exist when considering mixtures of PN solutions with other medications. Practitioners should assume that medications are incompatible unless data otherwise prove compatibility exists. Some medications have been demonstrated to be compatible as a component of PN solutions, such as heparin, regular insulin, H_2-receptor antagonists, and corticosteroids.

Calculating Nutritional Needs

Accurate height and weight measurements are important to make appropriate estimations of energy and protein needs. Several formulas exist to calculate ideal body weight (IBW). The following are commonly used:

$$Men = 50\,kg + 2.3\,kg \times each\,inch\,over\,5\,feet$$

$$Women = 45.5\,kg + 2.3\,kg \times each\,inch\,over\,5\,feet$$

Adjusted body weight can be calculated utilizing the following formula:

$$Adjusted\,body\,weight = IBW + 25\%\,of\,(actual$$
$$body\,weight - IBW)$$

Calculating Energy Needs

Calorie requirements are estimated to meet a patient's energy requirements, which are dependent on the patient's size, clinical condition, concurrent organ failure, and activity level. Determination of the appropriate energy prescription for a patient is crucial for meeting metabolic demands and helping to prevent erosion of lean body mass. Overzealous feeding is associated with significant risks, including difficulties with glucose control and other metabolic complications such as excessive carbon dioxide production. Common methods to estimate calorie requirements include simple weight-based

Table 5 Determination of energy needs

Condition	Need (kcal/kg)
Overnourished/obese	20 (upper end IBW)
Maintenance	25
Undernourished	30
Stressed/critically ill	25

IBW, ideal body weight.
Adapted from the National Advisory Group on Standards and Practice Guidelines for Parenteral Nutrition (1998) Safe practices for parenteral nutrition formulations. *Journal of Parenteral and Enteral Nutrition* **22**: 49–66.

algorithms (e.g., 25–30 kcal/kg body weight/day) (**Table 5**). The Harris–Benedict equations are also frequently used to estimate basal energy expenditure (BEE) using the following formulas:

$$Males: BEE\,(kcal) = 66.5 + [13.8 \times weight\,(kg)]$$
$$+[5 \times height\,(cm)]$$
$$-6.8 \times age\,(years)]$$
$$Females: BEE\,(kcal) = 655.1[9.6 \times weight\,(kg)]$$
$$+[1.8 \times height\,(cm)]$$
$$-[4.7 \times age\,(years)]$$

The BEE is then adjusted for the perceived degree of stress. Recent trends of providing fewer calories to seriously ill patients in order to prevent complications such as hyperglycemia, hypercapnia, and hepatic steatosis have been described as 'permissive underfeeding.' Trials have been conducted in obese hospitalized patients using hypocaloric regimens. These studies demonstrated that most patients achieved positive nitrogen balance and improved clinically with high-protein, hypocaloric PN formulations without experiencing significant adverse effects.

When an accurate assessment of energy needs is desired, indirect calorimetry may be considered. Such patients may include those who are otherwise difficult to assess or those who will require protracted nutrition support. A metabolic cart is used to measure oxygen consumption (VO_2) and carbon dioxide production (VCO_2). The modified Weir equation is used to estimate resting energy expenditure. The respiratory quotient (RQ) is determined as $RQ = VCO_2/VO_2$. The RQ gives an indication of net substrate oxidation, with $RQ > 1.0$ consistent with carbohydrate oxidation associated with overfeeding, and $RQ < 0.68$ consistent with lipid oxidation or starvation ketosis. Gas leaks or elevated FiO_2 requirements ($>0.60\%$) are common limitations to this approach.

Protein Requirements

Determining appropriate protein goals is important in order to help maintain lean body mass and to promote positive nitrogen balance. Initial requirements are adjusted by a subjective assessment of the patient's degree of catabolism and an evaluation of renal and hepatic function (Table 6). Subsequently, the protein prescription should be adjusted based on clinical response and continued reevaluation. The likelihood of achieving nitrogen balance or improvement in visceral protein status will depend on the degree of ongoing inflammatory response. Reductions in protein doses may be warranted in patients with significant hepatic failure with encephalopathy. Reductions may also be indicated for renal insufficiency, depending on the severity of renal failure and whether dialysis is initiated. For the morbidly obese patient, ideal body weight should be used to estimate protein needs.

Dextrose Prescription

Dextrose in PN solutions generally provides 40–60% of total energy requirements. Hyperglycemia is a common complication of PN due to diabetes, medications, or stress response, so the dextrose load is often initiated below goal until tolerance is demonstrated. The maximum glucose utilization rate is 5–7 mg/kg/minute. Doses that exceed this may result in glucose intolerance or hepatic steatosis. Studies have demonstrated that aggressive blood glucose management is associated with fewer septic complications in critically ill patients.

Fat Requirements

Fat calories usually comprise 20–30% of total PN energy. Doses may represent 0.5–1.0 g/kg body weight/day in the PN regimen. Patients with

Table 6 Estimation of protein needs

Condition	Need (g/kg/day)
Mild stress	1.0
Moderate stress	1.2–1.5
Severe stress	1.5–2
Acute renal failure, no dialysis	0.6
Hemodialysis/CVVHD	1.1–1.5
Peritoneal dialysis	1.2–1.5
Liver failure without encephalopathy	1.2–1.5
Liver failure with encephalopathy	0.4–0.6

Adapted from the National Advisory Group on Standards and Practice Guidelines for Parenteral Nutrition (1998) Safe practices for parenteral nutrition formulations. *Journal of Parenteral and Enteral Nutrition* **22**: 49–66.

preexisting lipid disorders should be evaluated for potential hypertriglyceridemia. Baseline triglyceride levels will aid the practitioner in safe determination of lipid dosing. Rapid piggyback lipid infusion with PN should be avoided in critically ill subjects.

Fluid Requirements

A patient's fluid intake and output should be considered when determining fluid requirements. Urinary losses, along with other losses such as diarrhea, nasogastric suction, emesis, fistula, or other drainage losses, can significantly increase the patient's need for additional fluid. In general, adult patients will need approximately 30 ml/kg body weight daily to meet volume requirements. Monitoring should include adequate urine output, skin turgor, and adequate mucous membrane hydration. Fluid overload in conditions such as compromised cardiac, hepatic, or renal function may dictate use of volume-concentrated formulations.

PN Implementation

Monitoring and Management

Appropriate monitoring of PN therapy is critical to ensure optimal nutrition therapy is achieved and to prevent complications of PN. Evolution of clinical course and patient condition may warrant changes in the frequency of tests and reevaluation of therapy. Additionally, as PN is transitioned to enteral feedings, tolerance should be monitored and PN should be weaned and discontinued.

PN tolerance should be carefully evaluated upon initiation of therapy. The managing practitioner should consider the patient's clinical condition and concurrent organ function, laboratory measurements, nutrition, and fluid status parameters. Laboratory measurements should include a complete metabolic profile and liver function tests at baseline and subsequent measurements after initiation of PN (Table 7). Electrolytes should be monitored daily until the patient is stable. Monitoring for acute care patients usually requires more frequent laboratory evaluations and more frequent changes to the PN formula than in long-term patients.

Evaluation of visceral proteins, such as albumin or prealbumin, has historically been an important part of nutrition assessment. These markers, however, may not adequately reflect an accurate picture of nutritional status or response to therapy because of other conditions, such as nephropathy, enteropathy, liver disease, or volume overload. Additionally, these visceral protein levels are often

Table 7 Suggested laboratory monitoring

Parameter	Baseline	Initiation	Critically ill patients	Stable patients
CBC with differential	Yes		Weekly	Weekly
PT, PTT	Yes		Weekly	Weekly
Electrolytes (Na, K, Cl, CO$_2$, Mg, Ca, PO$_4$, BUN, Cr)	Yes	Daily ×3	Daily	1 or 2 times per week
Serum triglycerides	Yes	Day 1	Weekly	Weekly
Transferrin or prealbumin	Yes		Weekly	Weekly
Serum glucose	Yes	Daily ×3	Daily	1 or 2 times per week
Capillary glucose		As needed	TID until consistently <200 mg/dl	As needed
Weight	Yes	Daily	Daily	2 or 3 times per week
Intake and output	Yes	Daily	Daily	Daily unless fluid status assessed by physical exam
ALT, AST, ALP, total bilirubin	Yes	Day 1	Weekly	Monthly
Nitrogen balance	As needed		As needed	As needed

Reprinted from Mirtallo JM. Introduction to parenteral nutrition. In: Gottschlich MM, ed. *The Science and Practice of Nutrition Support: A Case-Based Core Curriculum.* Dubuque, IA: KendallHunt Publishing Company; 2001: 221, with permission from the American Society for Parenteral and Enteral Nutrition (A.S.P.E.N.). A.S.P.E.N. does not endorse the use of this material in any form other than its entirety.

reduced by stress or injury due to a cytokine-mediated inflammatory response.

Because of significant protein binding, serum calcium levels should be evaluated in light of the patient's visceral protein status. The unbound calcium or 'ionized' calcium is physiologically active. Both bound and unbound calcium are included by standard serum calcium measurements. Laboratory testing for ionized calcium provides a more accurate depiction of calcium status in comparison to standard calcium samples.

Blood glucose levels should be carefully monitored throughout the course of PN infusion in order to detect and prevent hyperglycemia or hypoglycemia. Capillary blood glucose monitoring devices provide a convenient means of determining blood sugars. Blood capillary glucose levels should be obtained more frequently during the initial days of PN therapy and subsequently as needed for 'spot checks' or to verify glucose levels obtained by serum blood sampling. Insulin management may warrant a separate intravenous insulin infusion, subcutaneous coverage with sliding-scale insulin, or the addition of insulin as a component of PN. Because insulin needs are often acutely elevated in infection or stress, sliding-scale subcutaneous insulin or a separate insulin infusion may be used in combination with the addition of insulin to the PN.

Baseline triglyceride levels may be obtained prior to PN administration and periodically during the duration of therapy. Lipid doses should be reduced or held temporarily in adult patients with triglyceride levels >400 mg/dl. EFAD may develop after prolonged administration of PN without lipids;

therefore, at least weekly or biweekly doses should be considered for all patients.

Complications of PN

Short-term complications of PN therapy may be divided into three classes: mechanical, infectious, and metabolic. Longer term complications can include overfeeding, hepatobiliary complications, and metabolic bone disease.

Central catheter placement can be associated with serious mechanical complications, including pneumothorax, arrhythmias, catheter-related thrombosis, and catheter occlusion. Radiologic confirmation of line placement is necessary before initiating PN therapy. Catheter occlusion is the most common mechanical complication and may require thrombolytic treatment or line replacement. Catheter flushing protocols should be carefully followed to reduce risk of occlusion.

Infection due to catheter-related sepsis is another serious complication of PN that is associated with appreciable morbidity and cost. Prudent and meticulous catheter care and sterile technique should be emphasized. Catheter infections comprise a significant percentage of all nosocomial infections. Fever and unexplained hyperglycemia may be potential warning signs of catheter-related sepsis. It is important to note that there are frequently no external signs of catheter infection visible at the insertion site. Aseptic technique in manipulating the central line and related administration lines can help prevent introduction of infectious sources such as endogenous skin flora or contamination of the catheter hub. Appropriate methods and a sterile environment in compounding PN will reduce chances of contamination of the PN admixture during preparation. Treatment of catheter-related sepsis often includes access device removal and administration of appropriate antibiotic or antifungal therapy. With selected pathogens in patients with limited access options, salvage antimicrobial therapy may be considered to prevent the necessity of line removal.

The incidence of metabolic complications in PN patients is estimated to be 5–10%. Metabolic complications may include intolerance to fluid or macronutrients, or imbalances in electrolyte or vitamin and trace element homeostasis or function. Hyperglycemia is the most common complication associated with PN therapy.

Refeeding syndrome is a potential phenomenon of metabolic complications that may be observed when severely malnourished patients are re-fed in an overzealous manner. The rapid provision of macronutrients is associated with serum depletion and intracellular shifts of phosphorus, potassium, and magnesium as well as fluid retention and vitamin derangements. These abnormalities may result in the development of clinical sequellae such as arrhythmias, heart failure, respiratory failure, and death. Prevention of this phenomenon is achieved by identifying the patient at risk, repletion of electrolytes prior to initiation of nutrition support, and the slow advancement of PN with careful daily monitoring of electrolytes, including phosphorus and magnesium levels, as well as weights and fluid intake and output.

Electrolyte adjustments warrant close clinical evaluation. For example, hyponatremia can represent sodium deficiency or water excess. Electrolyte loss or shifts may occur from renal or gastrointestinal losses, hormonal imbalances, medication use, or acid–base disturbances. Accumulation of electrolytes may occur with fluid or acid–base shifts, renal insufficiency, or overzealous exogenous replacement. Generally, a consistent PN formula is recommended, with additional acute electrolyte replacements provided separately from the PN. Lower concentrations or even elimination of selected electrolytes from PN are often indicated in patients with renal failure.

Hepatobiliary complications, including steatosis and cholestasis, are associated with PN patients due to the lack of enteral stimulation and limited gastrointestinal motility. Cholestasis is universal in patients receiving PN for more than 6 weeks without enteral feedings. Transition to enteral or oral feedings will help prevent the potential development of gallstones associated with cholestasis. In adults, hepatic steatosis, or fatty liver, is generally associated with normal or mildly increased bilirubin levels and mild elevations in alkaline phosphatase and hepatic transaminases. In rare cases, hepatic steatosis may progress to steatohepatitis. In order to reduce the potential for hepatobiliary complications, the practitioner should attempt enteral feedings as soon as possible. Overfeeding with excessive lipid and dextrose loads should be avoided. The PN infusion can also be cycled to provide a rest period for the liver's macronutrient processing. Administration of a cholecystokinin–octapeptide may also help to reduce cholestasis.

Osteoporosis or osteomalacia may develop in long-term PN patients. Metabolic bone disease may develop due to underlying disease, inadequate intakes or malabsorption of calcium and vitamin D, corticosteroid therapy or other medications, and hypercalciuria. For selected long-term PN patients, treatment with bisphosphonates, calcium, and vitamin D should be considered to prevent the development of complications.

Home Parenteral Nutrition

Many patients are able to receive PN in the home setting. If the patient's medical condition is stable and careful patient selection has been employed, home parenteral nutrition (HPN) can be considered. The patient and caregiver must be able to be taught to use an infusion device, administer PN safely, and search for signs of infection, fluid issues, or other complications. Appropriate education should begin in the hospital and continue in the home setting. Psychosocial and socioeconomic issues, such as family support, private or government payer status, and patient emotional status, are important to consider when assessing the appropriateness of HPN.

Nocturnal administration of PN over 12 h can aid with patient mobility and quality of life and may also help to minimize hepatobiliary complications. Cycled PN infusion should generally begin in the inpatient hospital environment so tolerance of cycling can be safely evaluated. Since greater infusion rates are required for cycling, close monitoring during the transition phase is of particular importance for those with glucose or volume tolerance concerns.

Conclusions

PN offers a viable way to provide essential nutrients to individuals who are unable to use their gastrointestinal tracts effectively for a prolonged time period. Although this medical intervention is associated with significant risks, for many patients it can be a life-saving or life-prolonging therapy. Practitioners who manage patients who receive PN warrant specialized nutrition support training. PN management is most effective through a multidisciplinary approach, utilizing the expertise of physicians, pharmacists, dietitians, nurses, case managers, and social workers.

See also: **Energy**: Requirements. **Fatty Acids**: Metabolism. **Malnutrition**: Primary, Causes Epidemiology and Prevention; Secondary, Diagnosis and Management. **Nutritional Support**: In the Home Setting; Infants and Children, Parenteral. **Protein**: Requirements and Role in Diet. **Supplementation**: Dietary Supplements.

Further Reading

American Gastroenterological Association (2001) AGA technical review on parenteral nutrition. *Gastroenterology* **121**: 970–1001.

American Society for Parenteral and Enteral Nutrition Board of Directors and the Clinical Guidelines Task Force (2002) Guidelines for the use of parenteral and enteral nutrition in adult and pediatric patients. *Journal of Parenteral and Enteral Nutrition* **26**(1 supplement): 1SA–138SA.

Flancbaum L, Choban PS, Sambucco S *et al.* (1999) Comparison of indirect calorimetry, the Fick method, and prediction equations in estimating the energy requirements of critically ill patients. *American Journal of Clinical Nutrition* **69**: 461–466.

Heyland DK, MacDonald S, Keefe L *et al.* (1998) Total parenteral nutrition in the critically ill patient: A meta-analysis. *Journal of the American Medical Association* **280**: 2013–2019.

Horattas MC, Trupiano J, Hopkins S *et al.* (2001) Changing concepts in long-term central venous access: Catheter selection and cost savings. *American Journal of Infection Control* **29**(1): 32–40.

Klein CJ, Stanek GS, and Wiles CE (1998) Overfeeding macronutrients to critically ill adults: Metabolic complications. *Journal of the American Dietetic Association*, vol. 98: 795–805.

Klein S, Kinney J, Jeejeebhoy K *et al.* (1997) Nutrition support in clinical practice: Review of the published data and recommendations for future research directions. *Journal of Parenteral and Enteral Nutrition* **21**: 133–157.

McCowen K, Friel C, Sternberg J *et al.* (2000) Hypocaloric total parenteral nutrition: Effectiveness in prevention of hyperglycemia and infectious complications—A randomized clinical trial. *Critical Care Medicine* **28**: 3606–3611.

Mirtallo JM (2001) Introduction to parenteral nutrition. In: Gottschlich MM (ed.) *The Science and Practice of Nutrition Support: A Case-Based Core Curriculum.* Dubuque, IA: Kendall-Hunt.

Quigley EM, Marsch MN, Shaffer JL, and Markin RS (1993) Hepatobiliary complications of total parenteral nutrition. *Gastroenterology* **104**: 286–301.

Ranson JHC, Rifkin KM, Roses DF *et al.* (1974) Prognostic signs and the role of operative management in acute pancreatitis. *Surgical Gynecology & Obstetrics* **139**: 69–81.

Rombeau JL and Caldwell MD (eds.) (2001) *Parenteral Nutrition*, 3rd edn. Philadelphia: WB Saunders.

Shikora SA, Martindale RG, and Schwitzberg SD (eds.) (2002) *Nutritional Considerations in the Intensive Care Unit: Science, Rationale and Practice.* Dubuque, IA: Kendall-Hunt.

Solomon SM and Kirby DF (1990) The refeeding syndrome: A review. *Journal of Parenteral and Enteral Nutrition* **14**: 90–97.

Souba W (1997) Nutritional support. *New England Journal of Medicine* **336**: 41–48.

Task Force for the Revision of Safe Practices for Parenteral Nutrition (2004) Special report: Safe Practices for Parenteral Nutrition. *Journal of Parenteral and Enteral Nutrition* **28**: S39–S70.

Veterans Affairs Total Parenteral Nutrition Cooperative Study Group (1991) Perioperative total parenteral nutrition in surgical patients. *New England Journal of Medicine* **325**: 525–532.

Infants and Children, Parenteral

S Collier and C Lo, Children's Hospital, Boston, Harvard Medical School, and Harvard School of Public Health, Boston, MA, USA

Parenteral nutrition (PN) is a technique that allows provision of complete nutrient requirements intravenously, containing adequate amounts of energy, carbohydrate, protein, fat, minerals, and vitamins, while bypassing the gastrointestinal tract. It has allowed survival of many thousands of patients who cannot or will not eat or absorb enough to maintain their weight or nutritional balance because of disease or surgery. From its beginnings only approximately 30–40 years ago, it has expanded rapidly to become available for many patients, especially in the United States and then in Europe, but its expense and complications preclude wide availability in many countries. Before the availability of PN, as many as 30–50% of hospitalized patients had unrecognized malnutrition from chronic diseases and would remain for weeks without adequate nutrition to maintain weight or lean body mass, making them susceptible to infections and poor wound healing. Surprisingly, it has been difficult to demonstrate substantial reductions in morbidity or mortality with PN except in moderately or severely malnourished patients or those with long-term intestinal failure. It is difficult to estimate the exact impact, but a US registry, the Oley Foundation, enumerated 10 035 Medicare beneficiaries on home PN in 1992, giving a rough estimate of 40 000 patients on home PN in the United States. Approximately 15–20% of these patients were children.

One of the first attempts at PN was carried out by Sir Christopher Wren in 1656. He infused ale, opium, and beer intravenously into animals. Complete intravenous nutrition that we are most familiar with for patient support has been available for approximately 40 years. The research carried out by Dr. Stanley Dudrick and others allowed the support of the first pediatric patient on intravenous nutrition. The provision of intravenous nutrition was challenged by the development of several factors prior to its completed use in patient support, including catheter access, sterility of solutions, and the optimal form of each macro- and micronutrient.

Indications for Parenteral Nutrition

The often repeated adage continues to be true, "If the gut works, use it." However, there are many circumstances in which PN is necessary and life sustaining. The indications for use have not changed dramatically throughout the years since the development of PN. Congenital malformation of the intestine, specifically small bowel atresia, was the diagnosis the first time PN was used in the infant and young child. Congenital malformations of the gastrointestinal tract continue to be one of the leading reasons for its use. Other indications include severe malabsorption, intestinal dysmotility, other congenital defects, and patients with hematology–oncology diseases (**Table 1**).

Table 1 Conditions commonly requiring parenteral nutrition

Condition	Examples/comments
Surgical gastrointestinal disorders	Gastroschisis, omphalocele, tracheoesophageal fistula, intestinal atresias, meconium ileus, peritonitis, malrotation and volvulus, diaphragmatic hernia, prolonged postoperative ileus, Hirschsprung's disease, intestinal dysmotility
Short bowel syndrome	
Prematurity	
Congential heart disease	
Pancreatitis	
Gastrointestinal fistulas	
Bone marrow transplantation	
Acute intestinal disease	Antibiotic colitis, necrotizing enterocolitis, inflammatory bowel disease, chronic or secretory diarrhea
Hypermetabolic states	Burns, multiple trauma
Chronic idiopathic intestinal pseudo-obstruction	

Adapted from Hendricks KM, Duggan C, and Walker WA (eds.) (2000) *Manual of Pediatric Nutrition*, 3rd edn., London: BC Decker.

Dextrose

The primary source of energy during intravenous therapy is usually provided by dextrose (D-glucose). This is especially true in infants and children when higher energy requirements often necessitate glucose infusion rates of up to 15 mg/kg/min or more. Not until 1945 did Zimmerman report the first attempt at infusing intravenous solutions through a catheter placed in the superior vena cava. Experiments performed by Dudrick in beagle puppies advanced the glucose infusion solutions closer to what is utilized currently with hypertonic dextrose solutions. In current practice, hypertonic solutions are infused through a catheter with its tip centrally located in the superior vena cava or inferior vena cava. It continues to be the major energy component of intravenous support.

Initial doses of glucose should be approximately 5–7 mg carbohydrate/kg/min with incremental increases by 2–5 mg/kg/min. Frequent monitoring of blood glucose and urine for glucosuria is important to assess tolerance to increasing glucose infusion rates. It is important to avoid excessive carbohydrate intake to minimize complications from potential hyperglycemia with subsequent osmotic diuresis and over the long-term hepatic steatosis from increased fat synthesis that can occur with overfeeding. Hyperglycemia may ensue even without excess carbohydrate infusion in certain clinical situations, such as sepsis and renal failure, and also with the use of medications such as steroids. Glucose infusion rates should be decreased if hyperglycemia ensues; however, it may still be necessary to add insulin to control blood glucose to provide adequate support.

Protein

Another vital macronutrient that needed to be provided was protein. Initial experiments in the 1930s were done with plasma as the protein source, and investigators achieved positive nitrogen balance. In the early 1900s, research began on the development of protein hydrolysates and crystalline amino acids. Vitrum, a Swedish company, produced the first commercially available casein hydrolysate solution. It was developed by Arvid Wretlind, who hydrolyzed casein enzymatically and then dialyzed the mixture to remove large polypeptides. The crystalline amino acid solutions that we are more familiar with were first developed by Bansi in 1964. Wretlind went on to modify it further and eventually replaced the hydrolysates in the 1970s.

The development of amino acid solutions specifically for infants occurred in the early 1980s. These solutions provided conditionally required amino acids for the immature organ systems of premature infants and newborns. They were formulated based on the postprandial plasma amino acid levels of breast-fed infants. Special amino acid solutions for renal or liver failure are also available that have increased amounts of branched-chain amino acids. Studies on the solutions for liver failure have shown that they are probably beneficial in adult patients with encephalopathy. Glutamine is a much researched amino acid that could not initially be added to PN solutions due to shelf instability in liquid form. When added as a dipeptide, it has been found to be more stable. Not all studies have shown clear benefit to its addition in patients for gut adaptation or prevention of bacterial translocation.

The recommendation for initiation of protein is 1 g/kg/day and that for advancement is 1 g/kg/day to goal (**Table 2**). Blood urea nitrogen is monitored for tolerance to amino acid infusion.

Lipid Emulsions

Glucose was the only nonprotein source of energy until intravenous lipids were developed during the 1920s to the 1960s. The first emulsion available for clinical use was Lipomul, a cottonseed oil-based formulation. Because there were many adverse effects from its use, it was withdrawn from clinical use in the mid-1960s. After extensive testing, Wretlind developed Intralipid, a soybean-based emulsion, in 1961. It was well tolerated and is the most familiar intravenous fat emulsion currently available. It is available in 10, 20, and 30%

solutions. The advantage of the 20 and 30% solutions over the 10% solution is the lower ratio of phospholipids to triglyceride, which minimizes the increase in plasma lipoprotein X levels. Lipid emulsions provide essential fatty acids in addition to a concentrated energy source, which is particularly advantageous for patients requiring fluid restriction. Trials are under way on the use of emulsions that contain a blend of long-chain fat with medium-chain fats and those with fish oil blends. Also, structured fat emulsions are being studied for clinical use. These specialized emulsions may have advantages in patients with liver disease and those with sepsis.

Lipid emulsions are usually initiated at 1 g/kg/day and advanced to 2 or 3 g/kg/day or 30–50% of total energy. Serum triglyceride levels are monitored for tolerance. Hypertriglyceridemia may occur in situations of stress, sepsis, and renal and liver insufficiency/failure. In addition, a number of medications can cause hypertriglyceridemia. In these situations, a reduction in fat infusion is warranted, usually by infusing over 18–20 h instead of 24 h.

A minimum of 3–5% of total energy requirement is necessary to meet essential fatty acid requirements. In infants with indirect hyperbilirubinemia, it may be prudent to lower intravenous fat infusion to avoid potential risk of kernicterus since free fatty acids may displace bilirubin from albumin binding sites.

Micronutrients

To provide complete nutritional support, micronutrients, electrolytes, and minerals also need to be in the parenteral solution. The addition of adequate amounts of calcium and phosphate in one solution may be particularly problematic since precipitation may occur. Solubility guidelines are available that account for the brand and percentage of amino acids, which impact the pH of the solution. Compounding guidelines for the order of addition of calcium and phosphorus, amounts of other additives, and the temperature of the solution are other factors to optimize the solubility. Filters in the delivery system also help to minimize the risk of occlusion of the catheter if a solution should precipitate, especially with trimix solutions, in which lipids are mixed with the glucose/amino acid solution. Studies have evaluated the stability of the variety of nutrient components in trimix solutions.

Before the availability of vitamins and minerals, plasma levels of micronutrients decreased rapidly

Table 2 Pediatric parenteral nutritional requirements

	<2000 g	0–4 years	5–18 years
Energy (kcal/kg/day)	120	90–108	40–70
Protein (g/kg/day)	3–3.5	2.0–3.0	1–1.5
Fat (g/kg/day)	<3	<3	<2
Sodium (mEq/kg/day)	2–3	2–4	2–4
Potassium (mEq/kg/day)	2–3	2–4	2–4
Chloride (mEq/kg/day)	2–3	2–4	2–4
Calcium			
mEq/kg/day	3–4.5	2–3	0.5–2.5
mg/kg/day	60–90	40–60	10–50
Magnesium (mEq/kg/day)	0.35–0.6	0.25–0.5	0.25–0.5
Phosphate (mM/kg/day)	1.5–2.5	1–2	1–2
Zinc (μg/kg/day)	400	300	100
Selenium (μg/kg/day)	1–3	1–3	1–2
Trace elements (ml/l)	2	2	2
Multi vitamins (ml/day)	5	5	5–10

while infusing only macronutrients. The only commercial preparation initially available was a trace element solution that had iron and iodide. The first commercial preparation of multivitamins for intravenous use, introduced in the 1960s, lacked folic acid, vitamins B_{12} and K, and biotin. It also had very high concentrations of vitamins A and D and thiamin. Because of the variability in practice, there was increased risk of toxicity to vitamins A and D and deficiencies of other vitamins. Recommendations were made for intravenous pediatric and adult intravenous preparations in 1975. By 1978, there was a commercial multivitamin preparation that met these recommendations. Current preparations contain all vitamins for which there are Dietary Reference Intake values, with the exception of choline. A recent Food and Drug Administration mandate requires the addition of vitamin K to all preparations. Differences between the pediatric and adult forms of MVI include amounts of B vitamins and vitamin D (**Table 3**). There is currently no multivitamin preparation specifically for the premature infant. Dosing recommendations of Pediatric MVI for this group are based on weight (one-third vial for <500 g, two-thirds vial for 500–1000 g, and full vial for more than 1000 g).

A few trace element deficiencies have been noted in patients receiving long-term PN support. The first case of chromium depletion was reported in 1977, that of selenium deficiency in 1979, and that of molybdenum in 1981. There are now many trace element solutions available with a variety of combinations of minerals and that are appropriate to meet the needs of premature infants through the adult population. They are also available as single elements to tailor a solution as necessary. Contamination of trace elements can occur in parenteral solutions. Aluminum is one element that has been under scrutiny by the Food and Drug Administration mandate to minimize the amount patients receive for safety issues. It was initially found in high concentrations in the casein hydrolysates and continues to be found in high concentrations in a variety of intravenous preparations. Over time, aluminum can deposit in the bone, interfering with bone calcium uptake, and deposition in the brain may impair neurological development.

Metabolic Complications

Liver Disease

Although PN may be life sustaining, long-term use may be detrimental to the liver. The severity of injury ranges from reversible transaminase elevations to severe cholestasis and cirrhosis, especially in infants with short bowel syndrome. It is not clear whether this is due mainly to a nutrient deficiency, toxicity, or some physiological process missing because of the lack of enteral feeding. Prevention and treatment strategies continue to include minimizing or preventing episodes of sepsis, providing enteral feedings, moderating energy intake to provide for adequate growth but not to overfeed, cycling parenteral nutrition infusion, reduction of copper and manganese, use of an amino acid solution developed for infants, treatment/prophylaxis for bacterial overgrowth, and the use of ursodeoxycholic acid. Another drug that has been studied but is not available for clinical use is cholecystokinin, which promotes gallbladder contraction. A recent and controversial recommendation is the adjustment of the dose of intravenous lipid emulsion to ≤1 g/kg/day. Intravenous lipid emulsions are a rich source of linoleic acid, an omega-6 polyunsaturated fatty acid, and may enhance production of the proinflammatory cytokines. Increased leukotriene B4 synthesis by the hepatic macrophages will draw additional polymorphonuclear leukocytes that intensify the inflammatory response to endotoxin by release of reactive oxygen species.

Bone Disease

The development of osteopenia is another complication that is common with long-term PN support. The reasons are multifactorial and include relative immobility, inability to provide adequate calcium and phosphorus with solubility limitations, and hypercalciuria. It has also been suggested that the dose of vitamin D in the multivitamin preparation

Table 3 Comparison of parenteral multivitamin preparations for pediatric and adult populations

Vitamin	MVI Pediatric (Mayne)	Infuvite (Baxter) and MVI Adult with vitamin K (Mayne)
A (IU)	2300	3300
D (IU)	400	200
E (IU)	7	10
K (μg)	200	150
Ascorbic acid (mg)	80	200
Thiamine (mg)	1.2	6
Riboflavin (mg)	1.4	3.6
Niacin (mg)	17	40
Pantothenate (mg)	5	15
Pyridoxine (mg)	1	6
B_{12} (μg)	1	5
Biotin (μg)	20	60
Folate (μg)	140	600

may contribute to bone disease. Excessive vitamin D may suppress parathyroid hormone secretion and directly cause bone resorption. Although aluminum is still present in some intravenous solutions, including calcium gluconate, vitamins, and trace elements, the amounts are much less than those seen with the casein hydrolysates and are not believed to be a significant contributor to the development of metabolic bone disease. Prevention and treatment strategies include maximizing calcium and phosphorus in PN solutions, especially for growing children; providing enteral supplementation of these minerals as feasible; and providing weight-bearing physical therapy if possible.

Micronutrient Deficiency and Excess

If a patient is entirely PN dependent, certain micronutrients need to be provided. Some PN solutions require the addition of carnitine and selenium (if not provided in multi-trace element solutions) and iron dextran (if the patient is not receiving transfusions). All serum levels should be monitored on a monthly basis or every 6–12 months if in the long-term phase of support. There may be other micronutrients not yet identified that may be deficient in the purified PN solution, which is another reason to begin enteral feedings as soon as feasible. Monitoring for excess losses is also important. For example, with increased stool/ostomy losses, the patient may require increased zinc in the PN solution (Table 4).

Excess micronutrients can be caused by contamination, such as the case with aluminum, or clearance. Copper and manganese can accumulate and become directly hepatotoxic since both elements depend on the biliary pathway for excretion. Therefore, in the presence of cholestasis, there will be increased intrahepatic accumulation. Manganese has also been reported to deposit in brain tissue, so copper and manganese levels should be monitored routinely.

Catheter Complications

Complications with central venous catheters most frequently include obstructions, infections, and occasional leakage and perforation. Although PN can be temporarily provided through peripheral intravenous catheters, the high osmolarity of intravenous glucose–electrolyte solutions often causes phlebitis and loss of access. Therefore, long-term access requires placement of a central venous catheter placed via the internal or external jugular vein or a subclavian vein. There is also increased

Table 4 Suggested monitoring schedule for inpatients receiving parenteral nutrition

Parameter	Daily	Weekly[a]	Periodically[a]
Weight	x		
Fluid balance	x		
Vital signs	x		
Urine sugar	x		
Catheter site/function	x		
Laboratory (serum)			
Sodium		x	
Potassium		x	
Chloride		x	
Bicarbonate		x	
Glucose		x	
Urea nitrogen		x	
Creatinine		x	
Triglycerides		x	
Calcium		x	
Magnesium		x	
Phosphorus		x	
Albumin and/or prealbumin		x	
Transaminases		x	
Bilirubin		x	
Selenium			x
Copper			x
Zinc			x
Iron			x

[a]Or more often as necessitated by clinical course.
Adapted from Hendricks KM, Duggan C, and Walker WA (eds.) (2000) *Manual of Pediatric Nutrition*, 3rd edn., London: BC Decker.

placement of peripherally inserted catheters by a team of specially trained staff and/or an interventional radiologist. Tip position in the superior vena cava or right atrial junction should be verified radiographically to reduce complications from venous thrombosis or rare perforations. Central placement allows rapid dilution of hypertonic solutions in a large-diameter vein to minimize obstruction or thrombosis. Catheters for central venous access have been made of polyvinyl chloride, polyurethane, and silastic, often with a Teflon cuff to anchor the catheter subcutaneously. However, formation of a fibrin sheath is still common, often with a biofilm that may harbor infectious organisms and prevent penetration of antibiotics. Central catheter obstructions can often be visualized by ultrasound or inserting radio-opaque dye in the catheter. A thrombus can often be lysed with installation of a small bolus of tissue plasminogen activator. Long-term anticoagulation with coumadin, low-dose coumadin, or low-molecular-weight heparin has been advocated by some to avoid repeated catheter obstruction, venous thrombosis, superior vena cava obstruction, and potential pulmonary emboli.

Obstructions caused by precipitation of calcium phosphate salts or medications may be susceptible to installation of a small amount of dilute acid, and those due to fatty material may be dissolved with dilute ethanol. For long-term home parenteral use, some patients prefer the use of implantable ports, which can be accessed through the skin daily with a special needle. Recently, peripherally inserted central catheters have been used for periods up to 1 month or longer without requiring a surgical procedure.

Infections

Patients who require PN are often predisposed to infectious complications. The catheter hub is often the entry site, with skin flora such as *Staphylococcus epidermidis*, *Staphylococcus aureus*, or *Candida* being the most common organisms, along with gram-negative enteric bacteria possibly from bacterial translocation. Antibiotic treatment through the central line is often successful without replacement of the catheter using antibiotic combinations such as vancomycin and gentamicin or with an antibiotic lock.

Summary

Advancements in the technology, production, and manufacturing of intravenous solutions have progressed during the past 40 years. In addition to improvement in the solutions available for dextrose, amino acids, and lipid emulsions, there has been progress with the delivery systems, catheters, and sterile techniques for line and skin care to reduce overall complications.

Ongoing research and product development in areas associated with long-term PN support are vital for future patient management to be able to continue to provide optimal support with minimal risk for those patients for whom PN is life sustaining.

See also: **Aluminum. Amino Acids**: Chemistry and Classification. **Bone. Children**: Nutritional Requirements; Nutritional Problems. **Chromium. Copper. Infants**: Nutritional Requirements. **Lipids**: Chemistry and Classification. **Liver Disorders. Manganese. Protein**: Quality and Sources. **Selenium. Supplementation**: Developing Countries.

Further Reading

American Gastroenterological Association Clinical Practice Committee (2001) AGA technical review on parenteral nutrition. *Gastroenterology* 121: 970–1001.

American Society of Parenteral and Enteral Nutrition (ASPEN) (1993) Guidelines for the use of parenteral and enteral nutrition in adult and pediatric patients. *Journal of Parenteral and Enteral Nutrition* 17: 1–52.

Buchman A (2002) Total parenteral nutrition associated liver disease. *Journal of Parenteral and Enteral Nutrition* 26: S43–S48.

Dudrick SJ (2003) Early developments and clinical applications of total parenteral nutrition. *Journal of Parenteral and Enteral Nutrition* 27: 291–299.

Forchielli ML, Gura K, Anessi-Pessina E *et al.* (2000) Success rates and cost-effectiveness of antibiotic combinations for initial treatment of central venous line infections during total parenteral nutrition. *Journal of Parenteral and Enteral Nutrition* 24: 119–125.

Kaufman SS (2002) Prevention of parenteral associated liver disease in children. *Pediatric Transplantation* 6: 37–42.

Kinney JM (2000) *Clinical Nutrition Parenteral Nutrition*, 3rd edn., pp. 1–20. Philadelphia: WB Saunders.

Klein S, Kinney S, Jeejeebhoy K *et al.* (1997) Nutrition support in clinical practice: Review of published data and recommendations for future research directions. *Journal of Parenteral and Enteral Nutrition* 21: 133–156.

Kleinman RD, Barness LA, and Finberg L (2003) History of parenteral nutrition and fluid therapy. *Pediatric Research* 54: 762–772.

Oley Foundation (1994) *North American Home Parenteral and Enteral Nutrition Patient Registry, Annual Report with Outcomes Profiles 1985–1992*. Albany, NY: Oley Foundation.

Rombeau JL and Caldwell MD (1993) *Parenteral Nutrition*, 2nd edn. Philadelphia: WB Saunders.

Seidner DL (2002) Parenteral nutrition associated metabolic bone disease. *Journal of Parenteral and Enteral Nutrition* 26: S37–S42.

Shils ME (2000) Recalling a 63 year nutrition odyssey. *Nutrition* 16: 582–628.

Veterans Affairs Total Parenteral Nutrition Cooperative Study Group (1991) Perioperative total parenteral nutrition in surgical patients. New England Journal of Medicine 325: 525–532.

Vinnars E and Wilmore D (2003) History of parenteral nutrition. *Journal of Parenteral and Enteral Nutrition* 27: 225–232.

NUTRITIONAL SURVEILLANCE

Contents
Developed Countries
Developing Countries

Developed Countries

N R Sahyoun, University of Maryland, College Park, MD, USA

There has been increasing recognition in the past three decades that dietary intake patterns are associated with the development of chronic diseases and that improving nutritional intake may be a means of improving the well-being of the population and of reducing the cost of health care. Hence, nutritional surveillance has become an important topic on the health political agenda in many areas of the world and may become an integral part of surveillance systems. In addition, as new technology has enabled faster data collection and analysis, surveillance systems have evolved and become more sophisticated in the past decade.

This article defines nutrition surveillance and its usefulness. It also describes the types of surveillance activities and systems in place in the industrialized countries of Europe, the United States, Australia, New Zealand, and Canada. Emerging issues in nutrition and health are also discussed. Note that although the structures of surveillance systems in industrialized and developing countries have many similarities, the type of activities, target populations, and outcomes may be different. Thus, there is a need to describe the nutritional surveillance systems in place in industrialized countries separately.

Nutrition Surveillance and Its Usefulness

Nutrition surveillance is a system established to continuously monitor the dietary intake and nutritional status of a population or selected population groups using a variety of data collection methods whose ultimate goal is to lead to policy formulation and action planning. The term 'nutrition monitoring' is often used in addition to or interchangeably with 'nutrition surveillance' and is defined as surveillance that is carried out on selected individuals. In this article, the term nutrition surveillance is used to include all data collection methods that are described.

The information obtained through nutrition surveillance is used for three broad purposes: policy development, nutrition research, and monitoring. As **Figure 1** illustrates, there are strong interrelationships between these three purposes. Specifically, the information generated by nutrition surveillance activities is used to describe the nutritional status of the population and identify population groups at high nutrition risk. Programs are then targeted to those in need. The efficacy of the programs is assessed and nutrition policy developed. Trends in health status and food intake are monitored and food supply needs are estimated. Also, linkages between food consumption, nutritional status, and health status are examined. For example, normative data collected from surveys in the United States have been used to develop new growth charts, released in 2000, to monitor nutritional status and health of children. Similarly, the World Health Organization, using international data, is also in the process of developing new international growth charts. Monitoring trends in child

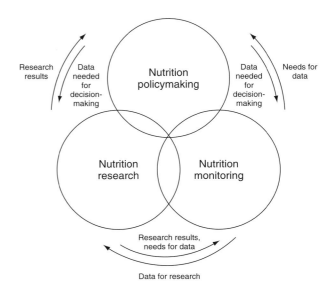

Figure 1 Relationships among nutrition policymaking, nutrition research, and nutrition monitoring. (From the US Department of Health and Human Services/US Department of Agriculture (1993) Ten-year comprehensive plan for the National Nutrition Monitoring and Related Research Program. *Federal Register* **58**: 32752–32806.)

growth helps to identify populations in need, evaluate nutritional and health interventions, and raise political awareness of nutritional problems.

Food fortification is another example of an interaction between monitoring, research, and policy, and it highlights the importance of nutrition surveillance systems. Folic acid supplementation, in addition to normal dietary folate intake, was recognized to significantly reduce the incidence of neural tube defects, one of the most common birth defects. This led to the mandatory fortification in 1998 of enriched grain products with folic acid in Canada and the United States. Survey data were used to determine the amount of folic acid that needed to be added to the food supply to provide beneficial effects without the harmful effect of potentially excessive intake. Surveys that examined the impact of folic acid supplementation showed a 19% reduction in neural tube defects. Continuous monitoring is essential to ensure that the added intake of folic acid does not have longer term negative impacts on the different population groups.

Nutrition Surveillance Systems

A nutrition surveillance system ideally collects information on all components in the relationship between food and health. This includes collecting data on food production, food supply and availability for consumption (national and household), food consumption patterns, dietary composition of foods, nutrient intake, nutrient utilization, and nutritional status. It also includes variables that may influence these processes, such as food culture, food security, lifestyle, knowledge, attitude and behavior toward food, and sociodemographic factors. **Figure 2** depicts the relationship of food to health outcome and illustrates the various levels of influence. A nutrition surveillance system would ideally obtain nutrition information along that continuum from food supply to health. At the core of a nutrition surveillance system is the collection of dietary intake patterns because they provide a basis for nutritional risk assessment. These dietary data include information obtained from the national food supply and from food consumption by households and by individuals. Each type of data collected corresponds to a different stage in the food distribution chain and is obtained by different methods. Some of these methods are described next.

Dietary Data Collection Methods

Food supply data Food supply data provide information on the type and amount of food available for human consumption to the country as a whole. The most common method of measuring this available food is through the use of food balance sheets. It is a method of indirectly estimating the amounts of food consumed by a country's population at a certain time. It provides data on food disappearance rather than on actual food consumption. It is calculated by using beginning and ending inventories, and the

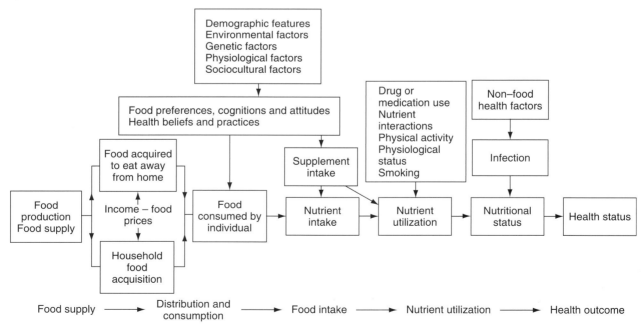

Figure 2 A conceptual model of the relationships of food to health. (Life Sciences Research Office, Federation of American Societies for Experimental Biology. Nutrition Monitoring in the United States – An Updated Report on Nutrition Monitoring. Washington, D.C.: U.S. Government Printing Office, 1989.)

difference is the amount of food consumed. The beginning inventory includes data on food production, imports and exports, and adjustments for non-human food consumption and an estimate of waste. Results are then converted to per capita basis food availability. To obtain the mean per capita annual consumption of food, total disappearance of food is divided by the country's population. Quantities of each food commodity are then multiplied by the appropriate nutrient values, and the results are expressed either in kilograms per year or in grams per day of individual food commodities and nutrient availability per person. No deduction is made for household food waste or the loss of nutrients in food preparation. Food is not distributed equally among a country's population, so this method only indicates the amount of food that leaves the food distribution system and is available for human consumption to the country as a whole. The best and most useful use of this data is to compare available food supply within and between countries and to monitor trends and forecast food consumption patterns over time. For example, **Table 1** illustrates the use of food balance sheets data and shows the worldwide and regional increase in the average supply of dietary fat from 1967–1969 to 1997–1999. Caution is needed, however, in comparing data between countries because food balance sheets, although compiled in a similar manner, may differ in food groupings, level of processing of commodities, and nutrient conversion of factors.

The Food Agriculture Organization (FAO) has published international food balance sheets yearly since 1949 and also covering the period 1934–1948. FAO food balance sheets are compiled from data supplied by approximately 200 countries. FAO uses the United Nations Population Division mid-year estimates of population size for its food balance sheet data and to calculate per capita values. International food balance sheets have also been compiled and published by the Organization for Economic Cooperation and Development on 23 countries (18 European countries, Australia,

Canada, Japan, New Zealand, and the United States), whereas the Commission of the European Communities (EURO-Stat) publishes data for its 12 member countries. In addition, individual countries publish their own data. For example, Canadian data on per capita food availability have been prepared annually by Statistics Canada since 1979. In the United States, annual estimates of commodity foods consumed by the civilian population are calculated and have been reported since 1909.

Food consumption by households Methods have been devised to obtain information on the availability of food and beverages for consumption by a household, family group, or institution. The basic concept is to collect the types and amounts of food that enter a household and that are available for consumption. These methods vary by the level of respondent burden and extent of recall expected, and there are four main ones: the food account, list-recall, inventory, and food record methods. Generally, the information is collected for a period of 7 days. In the food account method, the head of household records daily all types and quantities of food that enter the household within a 7-day period. In the list-recall method, the head of household is interviewed and must recall the foods used by the household on an 'as purchased' basis. The inventory and food record methods require daily recording of food acquired and of changes in the food inventory and also detailed weighing and measuring of food, placing a heavy burden on the respondent.

These household food consumption methods do not provide actual food intake by individuals within the household. Instead, individual food consumption and nutrient intake are calculated by dividing household food consumption by the number of members in the household regardless of age or sex. This information is then reported in terms of household income level, family size, and other general characteristics of interest. Several countries have used household methods for their national

Table 1 Supply of dietary fat by region

Region	Supply of dietary fat (g per capita per day)			
	1967–1969	*1977–1979*	*1987–1989*	*1997–1999*
World	53	57	67	73
North America	117	125	138	143
European Community	117	128	143	148
Oceania	102	102	113	113

Adapted from Food and Agriculture Organization of the United Nations (2003) *Diet, Nutrition and the Prevention of Chronic Diseases. Report of a Joint WHO/FAO Expert Consultation,* WHO Technical Report Series No. 916. Geneva: World Health Organization.

food consumption surveys. In Canada, household food consumption surveys were conducted at approximately 4-year intervals and then yearly since 1997. The United Kingdom originally used the household inventory method but in 1950 changed methods because it had too high of a respondent burden. In the United States, nationwide household food surveys started in the 1930s and used the household food record method, but in the 1980s household food consumption surveys collected food intake of individual household members in addition to household food expenditure. In Europe, an ongoing project of the European Union is to harmonize dietary exposure from household surveys to improve comparisons of these data between countries.

Food consumption by individuals Collecting information on dietary intake of individuals provides a level of detail that allows the exploration of relationships between dietary intake, nutritional status, and health outcomes. It also provides information on intake distribution and patterns by age, gender, and other well-defined criteria, thereby identifying population groups at risk. Individual dietary intake data is collected in a variety of ways. The three most common methods are food record, 24-h recall, and food frequency questionnaires (FFQs). Food records are used to measure dietary intake over a single time period, usually 3–7 days. Respondents are asked to measure and weigh their food intake. Although this method provides details on the amount and kind of food consumed, it places a heavy burden on respondents, requiring motivated, trained, and literate individuals. The 24-h dietary recall also requires a trained interviewer who asks and probes respondents on the kind and amount of all food and drink consumed during the previous day. This method is used to monitor group mean intakes in the population. It is currently recommended that a second recall be collected to better estimate the population distribution of usual intake of nutrients and to correct for reporting error. Methods of collecting this data have become progressively more sophisticated as computerized systems have been developed to include standardized probes and multiple passes of intake over the day to prompt recall. These innovations have led to improved estimates of nutrient intake. FFQs are most often self-administered instruments in which respondents are presented with a list of food items and asked to report usual frequency of consumption over a specific time period (usually 1 year). FFQs are designed to obtain data regarding usual intake, are less costly to administer and code than recalls or records, and vary in

the number of foods included in the food list. FFQs are semiquantitative and lack the detail of records or recalls.

Several variations of these methods of individual data collection have been devised. However, each of these dietary assessments provides advantages and limitations, and their applicability depends on the setting and the purpose of the data collected. Collecting individual dietary intake patterns is more time-consuming than collecting information on the food supply or household intake; however, most industrialized countries now collect these data or are making plans to do so. **Table 2** presents some of the surveys conducted by various industrialized countries and the method of dietary data collection selected by each country. The methods are quite varied, which limits comparability across surveys.

Examples of Nutrition Surveillance Activities

The 1990s saw a proliferation of nutrition surveys as local governments and international bodies such as the European Commission, the World Health Organization (WHO) and the International Union of Nutritional Scientists called for the establishment of a nutrition surveillance system. Most countries in Europe have a health interview survey, and some countries have a health examination survey as well. The dietary information gathered from these surveys varied considerably, from including one question on diet to including a FFQ. A few countries even measured nutritional biomarkers, whereas others did not collect any dietary intake data at all. Again, these methodological differences limit comparability of the results.

Most of the European Union member states have or are establishing a nutritional policy as an independent field of multidisciplinary research. The European Food Consumption Survey Method (EFCOSUM) was created as a project of the European Union Programme on Health Monitoring. One of its functions is to define a method for monitoring food consumption in nationally representative samples of all age–sex categories in Europe in a comparable way. It made recommendations about the best and most cost-effective data collection methods to use and the minimum variables needed to assess the nutritional status of populations. In addition, another objective of EFCOSUM is to indicate how to make existing food consumption data comparable and available to the health monitoring system. Also, WHO is stimulating regional and international networking and is strengthening community-based activities to prevent major

Table 2 Nationwide food consumption surveys with individual-based dietary intake data

Country	Year	Survey	Population (ages in years)	Sample size	Dietary method	Other information[a]
Australia	1983	National Dietary Survey of Adults	25–64	6295	24 h Rcl	A, BC, CE, MH
	1985	National Dietary Survey of Schoolchildren	10–15	5224	1d FR	A, BC, BP
	1995	National Nutrition Survey	2+	13 858	24 h Rcl (2nd 24 h Rcl from subsample) FFQ	A, BP
Canada	1970–1972	Nutrition Canada	0–65+	12 795	24 h Rcl, FFQ	A, BC, MH
	2004	National Population Health Survey	12+			
Europe						
Austria	1991–1994	Austrian Study on Nutritional Status (ASNS)	6–18	2173	7d FR	
	1993–1997	ASNS	19–65	2065	24 h Rcl, DH	A
	1998–2002	ASNS	19–60 55+	2580 645	24 h Rcl	A
Belgium	1980–1985	Belgium Interuniversity Research on Nutrition and Health	25–74	10 971	1d FR (DH in subsample)	A, BC, MH
	2003–2005	National Food Consumption Survey	All	3200 planned	24 h Rcl, FFQ	Fieldwork in 2004
Denmark	1985	Dietary Habits in Denmark	15–80	2442	DH	A
	1995	Danskernes Kostvaner	1–80	3098	7d FR	
	2000–2002	National Continuous Dietary Survey	4–75	1500 (2000) 1500 (2001) 1000 (2002)	7d FR	
Finland	1992	Dietary survey of Finnish adults (FINDIET 1992)	25–64	1861	3d FR	
	1997	Dietary survey of Finnish adults (FINDIET 1997)	25–64 65–74	2862 290	24 h Rcl	
France	1993–1994	Etudes Nationale des Consommations Alimentaires	2–85	1500	7d FR	A
	1998–1999	Individual National Food Consumption Survey	3–14 15+	1018 1985	7d FR	
Germany	1985–1989	National Nutrition Survey in Former West Germany	4–65+	24 632	7d FR KN, ATT, BH	A, BC
	1991–1992	National Nutrition Survey in East Germany	18–79	1897	DH	
	1998	German Nutrition Survey	18–79	4030	DH (4-week recall and FFQ)	
Ireland	1990	Irish National Nutrition Survey	10–65+	1214	DH	
	1997–1999	North–South Food Consumption Survey	18–64	1379	7d FR, ATT	A (self-reported)
	2003–2005	National Children's Food Survey	5–12	600		
Italy	1994–1996	INN-CA 1994–96	0–94	2734	7d FR	

Continued

Table 2 Continued

Country	Year	Survey	Population (ages in years)	Sample size	Dietary method	Other information[a]
The Netherlands	1987–1988	The Dutch National Food Consumption Survey (DNFCS-1)	1–85	5898	2d FR	A (self-reported)
	1992	The Dutch National Food Consumption Survey (DNFCS-2)	1–92	6218	2d FR	A (self-reported)
	1997–1998	The Dutch National Food Consumption Survey (DNFCS-3)	1–97	6250	2d FR	A (self-reported)
Norway	1993	National Dietary Survey	13	1705	FFQ	A (self-reported)
			18	1564	ATT, BH	
	1993–1994	National Dietary Survey among Adults NORKOST	16–79	3144	FFQ, ATT, BH	A (self-reported)
	1997	National Dietary Survey among Adults NORKOST	16–79	2672	FFQ, ATT	A (self-reported)
	1999	National Dietary Survey	6 and 12 months, 2 years	2400 2010	FFQ	
Portugal	1980	Portuguese Food Consumption Survey	1–65+	13 080	1d FR, 24 h Rcl, FFQ	A, BC,CE, MH
Sweden	1989	Household Food Survey, HULK	1–74	2036	7d FR	A (self-reported)
	1997–1998	Riksmaten	18–74	1215	7d FR	A (self-reported)
United Kingdom	1986–1987	The Dietary and Nutritional Survey of British Adults	16–64	2197	7d FR	A, BC, CE, BP
	1992–1993	National Diet and Nutritional Survey (NDNS)	1.5–4.5	1675	4d FR	
	1994–1995	NDNS	65+	1687	4d FR	A, BC, CE, BP
	1997	NDNS	4–18	1701	7d FR	
	2000–2001	NDNS	19–64	2000	7d FR, BH	A, BC, CE, BP
	2003–2005	Low Income Diet and Nutrition Survey		2000	7d FR	Fieldwork in 2003
New Zealand	1977	National Diet Survey	20–74	1938	24 h Rcl	A
	1989	Life in New Zealand Survey	15+	1702	24 h Rcl, FFQ, ATT, BH	A, BC, CE
	1997	National Nutrition Survey	15+	4636	24 h Rcl, FFQ, KN, ATT, BH	A, BC, CE
	2002	Children's Nutrition Survey	5–14	3200	24 h Rcl, FFQ, BH	A, BC
United States	1970–1974	National Health and Nutrition Examination Survey (NHANES I)	1–74	20 749	24 h Rcl, FFQ	A, BC, CE, MH
	1976–1980	NHANES II	1–74	20 322	24 h Rcl, FFQ	A, BC, CE, MH
	1988–1994	NHANES III	2 month+	33 994	24 h Rcl, FFQ	A, BC, CE, MH
	1999+	National Health and Nutrition Survey	2 month+	9965 (1999–2000) 5500 (2001) 5000 (planned/ year)	24 h Rcl, FFQ	A, BC, CE, MH Continuous data collection
	1992	NHANES I Epidemiologic Follow-Up Study	25–74	9281		Follow-up interviews of NHANES I participants in 1982, 1986, 1987

Continued

Table 2 Continued

Country	Year	Survey	Population (ages in years)	Sample size	Dietary method	Other information[a]
	1992	NHANES II Mortality Follow-Up Study				Mortality Follow-up of NHANES II participants
	1977–1978	Nationwide Food Consumption Survey		30 467	24 h Rcl, 2d FR	
	1987–1988	(NFSC)		25 100		
	1985–1986 (annual)	Continuing Survey of Food Intakes by Individuals (CSFII)	19–50 F 1–5 years 19–50 M	6400 3200 1100	24 h Rcl, 2d FR	
	1989–1991 (annual)	CSFII	All	15 192	24 h Rcl, 2d FR (subsample) KN, ATT, BH (subsample)	
	1994–1996 (annual)	CSFII	All	16 103	24 h Rcl, 2d FR (subsample) KN, ATT, BH (subsample)	
	1998		0–9	5559		

[a]Information other than sociodemographic. 24 h Rcl, 24-h dietary recall; 1d FR, 1-day food record; FFQ, food frequency questionnaire; DH, dietary history; KN, dietary knowledge; ATT, dietary attitude; BH, dietary behavior; A, anthropometry; BC, biochemical tests; BP, blood pressure; CE, clinical exam; MH, medical history; F, Female; M, Male.

noncommunicable diseases (NCDs) or chronic conditions. An international assessment of national capacity for the prevention and control of these diseases conducted in 2001 indicated that many countries lack policies to deal with the prevention of chronic diseases and lack legislation for food and nutrition.

The United States has the most extensive and comprehensive nutrition surveillance system in the world. Food consumption surveys were initiated in the 1930s and the surveillance system has expanded since then to include many cross-sectional and longitudinal surveys and surveillance systems. Due to the large number of surveys conducted in the United States, only a partial list is presented in **Table 2**. In 1990, the National Nutrition Monitoring and Related Research Program was established by the US Congress to strengthen food and nutrition data collection efforts via a 10-year plan. One of the outcomes of this effort was the establishment in 1999 of a continuous nutrition survey, the number one source of nutrition status information on the US population, which aims to collect a representative sample of 5000 individuals yearly. Similarly, in 1992, Australia launched a national food and nutrition policy for ongoing monitoring and surveillance of the food and nutrition system, which was established in 1998 and aimed to consolidate and strengthen data collection efforts. In Canada, the Canadian Community Health Survey began in

2000 to provide timely cross-sectional estimates of health determinants, health status, and the health system in a 2-year collection cycle. A nutrition component of the survey was implemented in 2004. The National Nutrition Survey of Japan has been conducted annually since 1946. Recently, Japan modernized the handling and processing of the data, which will allow for more rapid and greater data gathering capabilities and more accurate and timely reporting.

The assessment of nutritional status not only includes collecting dietary intake but also anthropometric measures, biochemical tests, and clinical examination. The measures of nutritional status collected in the different surveys vary considerably, as shown in **Table 2**. The simplest and most common anthropometric measures of nutrition status are height and weight, which are used to calculate body mass index, a widely accepted measure of overweight and obesity. Waist circumference and hip-to-waist ratio are also frequently measured to obtain an estimate of body fat distribution. Alternatively, a number of surveys have collected self-reported height and weight measures. Also, biological samples such as blood, urine, saliva, and hair have been collected, particularly in US surveys, as biomarkers of dietary intake to validate dietary data collection instruments, to relate to environmental exposure, and to study diet–health relationships. The selection of biomarkers for inclusion in a survey is subject to budgetary constraints and survey logistics as well as health and methodological priorities determined by each country. For example, Germany has analyzed blood for ferritin, minerals, and certain vitamins such as folate and vitamin B_{12}, whereas the United Kingdom has analyzed blood for folate and vitamins D and C. In an effort to prioritize and standardize data collection, EFCOSUM has recommended at a minimum the analysis of biomarkers for folate, vitamin D, iron, iodine, and sodium. Finally, the most common clinical measure incorporated in surveys is that for blood pressure. Additionally, self-reported or physician-reported medical conditions are frequently collected from survey participants. In the United States, a wide array of clinical exams are conducted as part of the National Health and Nutrition Examination Survey, including dental health and vision.

Emerging Nutrition and Health Issues

Several emerging health issues that are related to dietary intake and lifestyle choices have made it essential to track eating habits and nutritional status over time. For example, obesity is an escalating epidemic through the world among both children and adults and a major concern because of its health consequences. Obesity has been linked to an array of health disorders, such as type 2 diabetes, cardiovascular disease, and disability. In 1995, WHO estimated that there were approximately 200 million obese adults worldwide and 18 million children younger than 5 years old classified as overweight. As of 2000, the number of obese adults had increased to more than 300 million. In the United States, 64.5% of adults were classified as overweight in 1999–2000, up from 46.0% in 1976–1980. Also, the percentage of overweight children in the United States (aged 5–14 years) has doubled in the same period from 15 to 32%. In England, the prevalence of obesity has doubled since 1980. Australia, New Zealand, Canada, and European countries have all reported an increase in the proportion of obese adults and children. WHO has begun to formulate a Global Strategy on Diet, Physical Activity, and Health under a 2002 mandate from the World Health Assembly. The overall goal of the strategy is to improve public health through healthy eating and physical activity.

Another issue of emerging international importance is that both the number and the proportion of people 60 years of age or older are increasing in almost all areas of the world, and these worldwide trends are expected to continue. In 2002, there were an estimated 605 million older people in the world. **Table 3** shows the countries with the highest

Table 3 Countries with more than 10 million inhabitants in 2002 with the highest percentage of people older than age 60 years and projections for 2025

2002		2025	
Country	%	Country	%
Italy	24.5	Japan	35.1
Japan	24.3	Italy	34.0
Germany	24.0	Germany	33.2
Greece	23.9	Greece	31.6
Belgium	22.3	Spain	31.4
Spain	22.1	Belgium	31.2
Portugal	21.1	United Kingdom	29.4
United Kingdom	20.8	Netherlands	29.4
Ukraine	20.7	France	28.7
France	20.5	Canada	27.9

Data from the United Nations (www.who.int/hpr/ageing/ActiveAgeingPolicyFrame.pdf).

percentage of the population older than 60 years of age. As a consequence of this demographic change, NCDs have been estimated to account for approximately 60% of global deaths and 45% of the global burden of disease. Attention to this demographic change has resulted in changes in health policies in order to help the population achieve healthy and active aging. WHO has developed a policy framework that focuses on preventing and reducing the burden of disabilities and reducing the risk factors associated with NCDs. These policies include healthy eating and physical activity.

Research has consistently demonstrated that sufficient daily intake of fruit and vegetables could help prevent major NCDs, such as cardiovascular diseases, type 2 diabetes, obesity, and certain cancers. According to the 2002 World Health Report, up to 2.7 million lives could potentially be saved each year if fruit and vegetable consumption were increased. However, surveys conducted in Europe and the United States have indicated that the consumption of fruit and vegetables is lower than recommended for health. According to Kraisid Tontisirin, the director of FAO's Food and Nutrition Division, "FAO faces the challenge to increase worldwide awareness of the health benefits of increased fruits and vegetable consumption. To effectively promote more consumption of fruit and vegetables, prevailing diets need to be more systematically assessed for their nutrition and health implications."

These emerging issues linking nutrition and health outcomes reinforce the importance of developing and maintaining a nutrition surveillance system. However, direct and indirect methods of dietary data collection that can easily be applied in the field need to be developed further.

See also: **Dietary Intake Measurement**: Methodology; Validation. **Dietary Surveys**. **Folic Acid**. **Food Fortification**: Developed Countries; Developing Countries. **Nutritional Surveillance**: Developing Countries. **Pregnancy**: Prevention of Neural Tube Defects. **World Health Organization**.

Further Reading

Australian Centre for International and Tropical Health and Nutrition (2000) *Plan for the Development and Management of a National Food and Nutrition Monitoring and Surveillance System*, Australian Centre for International and Tropical Health and Nutrition, The University of Queensland, Herston, Australia. Available at ftp://www.sph.uq.edu.au/pdf.ftp/P1_0802_Long.pdf.

Briefel RR (2001) Nutrition monitoring in the United States. In: Bowman BA and Russell RM (eds.) *Present Knowledge in Nutrition*, pp. 617–635. Washington, DC: ILSI Press.

Canadian Community Health Survey (accessed 2004) www.statcan.ca/english/sdds/3226.htm.

EFCOSUM Group (2002) European Food Consumption Survey Method. *European Journal of Clinical Nutrition* **56**(supplement 2): S1–S94.

Food and Agriculture Organization of the United Nations (2003) *Diet, Nutrition and the Prevention of Chronic Diseases. Report of a Joint WHO/FAO Expert Consultation*, WHO Technical Report Series 916. Geneva: World Health Organization.

Margetts BM and Nelson M (1998) *Design Concepts in Nutritional Epidemiology*. New York: Oxford University Press.

New Zealand Ministry of Health (2003) *Food and Nutrition Monitoring in New Zealand*. Wellington, New Zealand: Ministry of Health.

U.S. Department of Health and Human Services/U.S. Department of Agriculture (1993) Relationship among nutrition policymaking, nutrition research, and nutrition monitoring. Tenyear comprehensive plan for the National Nutrition Monitoring and Related Research Program. *Federal Register* **58**: 32752–32806.

Woteki CE, Briefel RR, Klein CJ *et al.* (2004) Nutrition monitoring: Summary of a statement from an American Society for Nutritional Sciences Working Group. *Journal of Nutrition* **132**: 3782–3783. Data supplement available at www.nutrition. org/cgi/data/132/12/3782/DC1/1.

Developing Countries

L M Neufeld and L Tolentino, National Institute of Public Health, Cuernavaca, Mexico

Nutritional surveillance was defined in the previous article as a system established to continuously monitor the dietary intake and nutritional status of a population or selected population groups using a variety of data collection methods, with the ultimate goal of having a direct impact on actions to improve the situation. The challenges to meet this goal in developing countries are many, and they differ from those of more industrialized countries for a number of reasons. First, in most developing countries the prevalence of problems related to nutritional deficiency is higher than in industrialized countries and the prevalence varies greatly within and between regions and countries. Second, continuous national monitoring (e.g., through the health care system) is not well established in many countries and resources in many countries are scarce. Finally, during the past decade there has been a dramatic increase in the prevalence of overweight and obesity and their related morbidities. Together, the problems related to under- and overnutrition present unique challenges to national and international policymakers and heighten the need for nutritional surveillance systems that are able to provide useful information to policymakers.

To date, the major shortfall of nutritional surveillance has been the link between the data collected and its use in policy and programs, particularly in developing countries, where the need for nutrition interventions is great. Health and nutrition policies and programs should use information from nutritional surveillance systems to identify needs of specific populations within regions and countries and to help design appropriate interventions that address the relevant causes of these problems. This implies an open communication between those involved in data collection and those who would ultimately use the information. Unfortunately, the number of concrete examples in which this link has resulted in nutritional surveillance information being directly used to influence policy is still limited.

The responsibility for making nutritional surveillance action-oriented lies with all parties involved—donors, agencies or researchers involved in data collection and analysis, and policymakers. In many developing countries, the lack of existing information systems and limited local resources implies that external funds, often from donor agencies, will be required for surveillance activities. At all stages of planning, those responsible for data collection should interact directly with policymakers to ensure that the information is collected, analyzed, and presented in a way that is meaningful to them. Once data on the nutrition situation become available, policymakers should seek technical assistance from experts in the field to assist with the design of interventions with high potential for impact. Evaluation of policy and programs is essential to complete the cycle and permit new assessments and analyses based on these outcomes. This again implies the need for external funds in many cases. Researchers or national or international agencies may need to become advocates to promote dialogue with policymakers and to convince donors of the importance of this process.

The Nature of Nutritional Surveillance Data in Developing Countries

Information collected as part of a nutritional surveillance system should include not only documentation of the nutritional problems but also an analysis of their direct and indirect causes. A conceptual framework, such as that of UNICEF, for understanding the causes of malnutrition should be used to determine the types of information that are needed. The exact information needed therefore may be context specific, depending on what preexisting information is available. The following are examples: (1) If recent national data show an adequate national food supply, but a high prevalence of malnutrition in children younger than 5 years of age still exists in the country, information related to household food security, individual food consumption, as well as other causes of childhood malnutrition such as infections may be needed; and (2) if the prevalence of obesity has increased recently in a country, information on dietary intake and physical activity patterns will be needed to understand the causes of this increase and to design appropriate interventions.

Details of different methods to collect data at the national, household, and individual level are described in the previous article and will not be reviewed here. Rather, this article focuses on some of the specific strengths, limitations, and applications of each type of data as they apply to nutritional surveillance in developing countries and describes some additional methods that have been adapted for use in developing countries.

National Food Supply Data

The Food and Agriculture Organization (FAO) compiles and monitors food supply data for many developing countries. The estimates are typically based on food balance sheets supplied from each country's national records. The information is usually converted to per capita food availability and is presented for developing countries as a whole, by region, subregion, and for more than 100 individual countries. Information is also available for many countries (e.g., in Latin America—Mexico, Brazil, Argentina, and Chile) from national statistical institutes as well as regional statistical organizations (e.g., the Council for Statistics in Latin America). Much of this information can be accessed free of charge through local Internet sites.

Food supply data are essential to make comparisons between and across regions and to monitor trends. For example, according to the FAO food supply data, approximately 10% of the worlds' population now lives in countries where the food supply is low (<2200 kcal/person/day). This is down from 57% in the mid-1960s. Nonetheless, according to 2001 FAO data, there are still 30 countries with low food supply. Ideally, this type of information should be used to promote agricultural policies that will enhance food supply.

Despite these important uses, these data should be interpreted with caution, particularly in the developing country context. Although many countries show national increases in food supply, this does not address the issue as to how food is distributed within the country. Increases in access among the most vulnerable groups may not parallel increases in national production. Thus, although food supply data are useful for trend analysis, they should not be used to assess changes in food consumption or food security.

Trends toward a decline in the food supply can also be identified using food balance information. This may be a reflection of an unstable political environment or some severe natural disease that influenced food production. Ideally, this information should be used to influence agricultural policy to stimulate higher levels of production. However, war or other political strife may impede this process. The data should not be used to predict food shortages or famine because it is not useful to identify vulnerable groups within a population and because vulnerable groups may already be experiencing shortages by the time that this information is available and processed.

The quality of data used to generate food balance sheets can vary greatly between countries. In general, the methods are thought to underestimate total per capita energy availability in developing countries. In some countries, particularly those where small-holder agriculture is still common, this may be related to underestimates of true production due to a less centralized economy.

Household Food Consumption Data

The documentation of household food security in developing countries continues to be of great interest because of its relationship to specific health and nutrition indicators and as a means of monitoring the impact of political and environmental change on these outcomes. There have also been a number of efforts to document the impact of poverty alleviation programs on food security. Food security is often measured by quantifying household food consumption, which provides an estimate of the food available to be consumed on a per capita basis.

Traditional methods to assess household food consumption include those that collect data over a period of time, often 7 days, by asking the respondent to keep a record of food entering the home (food account method) or by quantifying the food consumed at each meal (household food record method). Other methods may include an inventory of food available in the home over a period of time or the list-recall method, whereby the respondent is asked to recall all food purchased, quantity, and purchase price over a given time. These methods have many limitations in a developing country. For example, respondents may have limited literacy and numeracy skills. In this case, field-workers would be responsible for data collection, resulting in increased survey time and costs. Many poor households have little or no food stores in the home and inventory methods may not provide an adequate estimate of household consumption. Furthermore, these methods often rely on telephone or costly house-to-house surveys, the resources for which may not be available. Thus, these types of household consumption methods have been excluded from many large-scale surveillance systems in developing countries and efforts have been made to develop more appropriate methods.

In the past decade or so, there has been considerable interest in dietary diversity as an indicator of household consumption. (The dietary diversity score is also used to assess intake of individuals. The principle is the same, but the respondent is asked to list all foods or food groups consumed by the individual.) This method provides qualitative information on all foods or food groups, including meals and snacks, that were consumed over a given period of time (often 1, 3, or 7 days) by all members of the household. Each food or food group is assigned a value based on its nutrient density, bioavailability, and typical portion size. Portion size is included because although some foods (e.g., nuts) may have high nutrient density, they are typically consumed in small quantities. Points are then summed and the adequacy of dietary diversity is assessed based on this score. Reasonable correlations have been found between dietary diversity, household socioeconomic status, and household consumption as assessed by more traditional methods. The major advantage of this type of instrument is that it is simple and less time-consuming than other household consumption methods, with important implications for its use in large surveys. Although the use of this type of instrument in nutritional surveillance systems is still limited, its potential as a simple method to assess and monitor household food security appears promising.

Individual Nutritional Status and Dietary Intake Data

Information on the dietary intake and nutritional status of individuals in a population is essential for monitoring trends in these indicators over time and in response to political and environmental changes, as a means of identifying groups for intervention, and to assess the impact of interventions on nutritional status of the population. Although dietary intake and simple anthropometric measurements, such as weight and height, have often been the focus of health and nutrition surveys, it is essential that other indicators of nutritional status such as micronutrient deficiencies also be documented because they continue to be important public health problems in most developing countries. Furthermore, as discussed previously, information on factors that are direct (e.g., the prevalence of infections) and indirect (e.g., maternal education and family socioeconomic status) causes of nutritional problems increases the usefulness of nutritional surveillance information for policymakers.

Many nutritional surveillance systems have dealt with this daunting list of indicators by focusing efforts on specific high-risk groups—a logical decision in light of limited resources. Thus, more information is available for children younger than 5 years of age and women of reproductive age than for olden children, adolescents, adult men, and older adults. With the increasing prevalence of overweight and obesity, particularly in school-age children and adults, this strategy may need to be modified. Although not evident in all developing countries, this paradox is particularly striking in some middle-income Latin American countries, such as Mexico and Chile, but is also documented in India and many other countries.

The coexistence of malnutrition and "over-" nutrition represents an important challenge to all those involved in nutritional surveillance. For funders, the population groups being monitored may need to be expanded, with important cost implications; malnutrition in children and pregnant and lactating women has not disappeared in developing countries with the increase in overweight and obesity. For those involved in data collection, these additional nutritional problems imply the development and validation of new instruments to measure causes of overweight and obesity (e.g., physical activity). For policymakers, the burden lies in the need for policies and programs that respond to two extremes of nutrition problems, often occurring in the same communities and even households. For example, programs designed to improve dietary intake in household members at risk for nutritional deficiencies (e.g., children younger than 2 years of age) should not cause an increase in energy intake among those members of the household at risk for overweight and obesity (e.g., school-aged children). Thus, program evaluations must be designed to detect both desirable and unexpected or undesirable outcomes.

The choice of which indicators are most appropriate for monitoring the nutritional status and dietary intake of the population depends on the country context and the specific objective of the surveillance system. For example, in countries where food shortages are common, indicators that are particularly sensitive to change, such as the prevalence and severity of malnutrition in children younger than 5 years of age, should be used. If the objective is to determine the impact of improving the nutritional status of a population in which stunting and anemia are the principal problems, then the prevalence of these should obviously be monitored.

Information on the intake and nutritional status of individuals is available from a variety of sources in developing countries. We present a description of the types of information available for children younger than 5 years of age (**Table 1**) and adults (**Table 2**) from a variety of information sources. Much of this information is obtained from large-scale multination health and nutrition surveys and from databases maintained by international organization, such as FAO and the World Health Organization (WHO). A number of countries conduct periodic nationally representative health and nutrition surveys, and information may also be available from smaller scale health and nutrition surveys and from routine growth monitoring and promotion programs. The following sections provide a brief discussion of each of these types of information in the developing country context.

Multination Health and Nutrition Surveys

During the past few decades, the Demographic and Health Surveys (DHS) have been conducted in many countries in all regions of the world. The DHS surveys are nationally representative surveys that include household and individual health and nutrition indicators. The surveys are large, typically 5000 to 30 000 households, and are conducted periodically, often at 5-year intervals. The data included in the survey vary slightly by country (**Tables 1** and **2**) but typically include as a minimum anthropometric measurements and hemoglobin concentration (prevalence of anemia) of children and women of reproductive age and breast-feeding and complementary feeding practices. One of the major strengths of the DHS surveys is that they use standard questionnaires that allow for

comparisons across survey years and between countries. Information from DHS surveys is readily available on the Internet.

The WHO Global Database on Child Growth and Malnutrition provides a compilation of information from nationally representative and smaller scale surveys conducted in a number of countries. In order to be included in the database, a number of criteria must be met for data collection, analysis, and presentation. This facilitates the comparison of information that has been collected in different countries and regions. Nutrition Country Profiles are also compiled by FAO and include national-, household-, and individual-level data. The national-level data are obtained from the United Nations global data banks and are supplemented for many countries by data from local institutions and independent experts. Considering this broad range of sources, many differences in methodology of data collection, analysis, and presentation may exist and should be taken into consideration when comparing data from different countries.

National Health and Nutrition Surveys and Small-Scale Surveys

Both the WHO and FAO databases may include information obtained from nationally representative health and nutrition surveys conducted by individual countries and from small-scale health and nutrition surveys. The former has the major advantage that data may be representative of the population in the country. The latter does not usually provide representative data but has the strength that the survey may be targeted to specific high-risk groups, thus providing data for those to whom policymakers may need to target interventions.

Information on nutritional status of individuals, particularly children, may also be collected at the local community level through national growth monitoring and promotion activities conducted as part of government or nongovernmental agency development activities. Many such activities stress a high level of local involvement in data collection and can be very useful to provide feedback for decisions on resource allocation that need to be made at a local level. Data can then be aggregated to higher administrative levels and can be used for regional and national resource allocation. Although this type of surveillance may not have the same level of data quality control as the larger, more heavily supervised surveys, they have the advantage of being readily available and may promote a higher level of community involvement.

Table 1 Surveys in developing countries with individual nutritional status data for children younger than 5 years of age

Region/country	Survey year	Age (years)	Sample size[a]	Data included	Source
Africa					
Benin	2001	0–4.99	5305	Anthropometry, dietary intake, use of nutritional supplements, micronutrient deficiencies (Fe, I, vitamin A), complementary feeding practices, fertility and birth interval, vaccine coverage, morbidity, mortality	DHS, FAO
Burkina Faso	1998–99	0–4.99	3792	Anthropometry, use of nutritional supplements, micronutrient deficiencies (Fe, I, vitamin A), complementary feeding practices, morbidity, mortality, sanitation	DHS
Congo	1997	0–4.99	NA	Anthropometry	FAO
Eritrea	2002	0–4.99	5241	Anthropometry, use of nutritional supplements, use of iodized salt, complementary feeding practices, parental education, vaccine coverage, morbidity, mortality, sanitation	DHS
Ethiopia	2000	0–4.99	9814	Anthropometry, use of nutritional supplements, micronutrient deficiencies (Fe, I, vitamin A), use of iodized salt, complementary feeding practices, fertility and birth interval, parental education, vaccine coverage, morbidity, mortality	DHS
Guinea	1999	0–4.99	2939	Anthropometry, complementary feeding practices, morbidity, mortality	DHS
Malawi	2000	0–4.99	9318	Anthropometry, use of nutritional supplements, use of iodized salt, complementary feeding practices, fertility and birth interval, parental education, vaccine coverage, morbidity, mortality, sanitation	DHS
Mali	2001	0–4.99	9408	Anthropometry, use of nutritional supplements, micronutrient deficiencies (Fe, I, vitamin A), use of iodized salt, complementary feeding practices, fertility and birth interval, parental education, vaccine coverage, morbidity, mortality, sanitation	DHS
Mauritania	2000–01	0–4.99	3554	Anthropometry, use and nutritional supplements, use of iodized salt, complementary feeding practices, morbidity	DHS
Mozambique	1997	0–2.99	4206	Anthropometry, complementary feeding practices	DHS
Namibia	2000	0–4.99	4123	Anthropometry, use and nutritional supplements, complementary feeding practices	DHS
Niger	2000	0–4.99	4616	Anthropometry	WHO

Continued

Table 1 Continued

Region/country	Survey year	Age (years)	Sample size[a]	Data included	Source
Rwanda	2000	0–4.99	6490	Anthropometry, use of nutritional supplements, micronutrient deficiencies (Fe, I, vitamin A), use of iodized salt, complementary feeding practices, fertility and birth interval, parental education, vaccine coverage, sanitation	DHS
Tanzania	1999	0–4.99	2582	Anthropometry, use of nutritional supplements, micronutrient deficiencies (Fe, I, vitamin A), use of iodized salt, complementary feeding practices, fertility and birth interval, parental education, vaccine coverage, morbidity, mortality, sanitation	DHS
Togo	1998	0–2.99	3260	Anthropometry	WHO
Uganda	2000–01	0–4.99	5604	Anthropometry, use of nutritional supplements, micronutrient deficiencies (Fe, I, vitamin A), use of iodized salt, complementary feeding practices, fertility and birth interval, parental education, vaccine coverage, morbidity, mortality, sanitation	DHS
Zambia	2001–02	0–4.99	5216	Anthropometry, use of nutritional supplements, micronutrient deficiencies (Fe, I, vitamin A), use of iodized salt, complementary feeding practices, fertility and birth interval, parental education, vaccine coverage, morbidity, mortality, sanitation	DHS
Zimbawe	1999	0–4.99	3559	Anthropometry	WHO
Asia and Southwest Pacific					
Bangladesh	2001	0–4.99	71 931	Anthropometry	WHO
Bangladesh	1999–2000	0–4.99	5421	Anthropometry, micronutrient deficiencies (Fe, I, vitamin A)	DHS
Bhutan	1999	0.5–4.99	2981	Anthropometry, micronutrient deficiencies (Fe, I, vitamin A)	FAO, WHO, NS
Cambodia	2000	0–4.99	3372	Anthropometry, use of nutritional supplements, micronutrient deficiencies (Fe, I, vitamin A), complementary feeding practices	DHS
China	2000	0–4.99	16 491	Anthropometry, use of nutritional supplements, micronutrient deficiencies (Fe)	FAO, WHO
Fiji	1993	0–4.99	618	Anthropometry, micronutrient deficiencies (Fe, I, vitamin A), complementary feeding practices	FAO, WHO, NS
India	1998–99	0–2.99	24 396	Anthropometry, micronutrient deficiencies (Fe, I, vitamin A)	FAO, WHO, NS
Lao People's Democratic Republic	2000	0–4.99	1347	Anthropometry, use of nutritional supplements, micronutrient deficiencies (I, vitamin A), complementary feeding practices	WHO, NS
Nepal	2001	0–4.99	6409	Anthropometry, dietary intake, use of nutritional supplements, complementary feeding practices	WHO, DHS, NS

Continued

Table 1 Continued

Region/country	Survey year	Age (years)	Sample size[a]	Data included	Source
Pakistan	1995	0–4.99	7368	Anthropometry, micronutrient deficiencies (I, vitamin A)	FAO, WHO
Papua New Guinea	1982–83	0–4.99	27 464	Anthropometry, complementary feeding practices, micronutrient deficiencies (I, vitamin A)	WHO, NS (rural)
Philippines	1998	0–4.99	24 308	Anthropometry	FAO, NS
Sri Lanka	1995	0.25–4.99	2782	Anthropometry, micronutrient deficiencies (Fe, I, vitamin A)	FAO, NS
Vanuatu	1996	0–4.99	1194	Anthropometry, dietary intake, micronutrient deficiencies (Fe, I, vitamin A)	FAO, NS
Vietnam	2000	0–4.99	94 469	Anthropometry	WHO
Vietnam	2001	0–2.99	1321	Complementary feeding practices	DHS
Near East					
Egypt	2003	0–4.99	5761	Anthropometry, use of nutritional supplements, dietary intake, micronutrient deficiencies (Fe, I, vitamin A), use of iodized salt, complementary feeding practices, vaccine coverage, morbidity	DHS
Iran	1998	0–4.99	2536	Anthropometry	FAO, WHO, NS
Jordan	2002	0–4.99	5484	Anthropometry, use of nutritional supplements, dietary intake, micronutrient deficiencies (Fe, I, vitamin A), complementary feeding practices	DHS
Morocco	1997	0–4.99	3555	Anthropometry	WHO
Turkey	1998	0–4.99	2677	Anthropometry, dietary intake, complementary feeding practices	DHS
Latin America and the Caribbean					
Antigua y Barbuda	1981	0–5.99	463	Anthropometry	WHO
Argentina	1995–96	0–5.99	16 981	Anthropometry, complementary feeding practices	WHO
Barbados	1981	0–4.99	597	Anthropometry, complementary feeding practices	NS
Bolivia	1998	0–4.99	5773	Anthropometry, use of nutritional supplements, micronutrient deficiencies (Fe, I, vitamin A), complementary feeding practices, fertility and birth interval, parental education, vaccine coverage, morbidity, mortality, sanitation	DHS
Brazil	1996	0–4.99	3815	Anthropometry, use of nutritional supplements, micronutrient deficiencies (Fe, I, vitamin A), complementary feeding practices, fertility and birth interval, parental education, vaccine coverage, morbidity, mortality, sanitation	DHS
Chile	2002	0–4.99	51 572	Anthropometry, complementary feeding practices	WHO
Colombia	2000	0–4.99	4060	Anthropometry, use of nutritional supplements, micronutrient deficiencies (Fe, I, vitamin A), use of iodized salt, complementary feeding practices, fertility and birth interval, parental education	DHS
Costa Rica	1996	1–6.99	1008	Anthropometry, use of nutritional supplements, micronutrient deficiencies (Fe, I, vitamin A)	NS

Continued

Table 1 Continued

Region/country	Survey year	Age (years)	Sample size[a]	Data included	Source
Dominica	1984	0–4.99	245	Anthropometry, complementary feeding practices	WHO
Dominican Republic	2002	0–4.99	2086	Anthropometry, use of nutritional supplements, micronutrient deficiencies (Fe, I, vitamin A), complementary feeding practices, fertility and birth interval, parental education	DHS
Ecuador	1998	0–4.99	2998	Anthropometry, complementary feeding practices	PAHO
El Salvador	2002–03	0.25–4.99	—	Anthropometry, complementary feeding practices	WHO
Guatemala	2002	0.25–4.99	6308	Anthropometry, use of nutritional supplements, micronutrient deficiencies (Fe, I, vitamin A), complementary feeding practices, fertility and birth interval, parental education	DHS
Guyana	1997	0–4.99	289	Anthropometry, complementary feeding practices	PAHO
Haiti	2000	0–4.99	6176	Anthropometry, use of nutritional supplements, micronutrient deficiencies (Fe, I, vitamin A), complementary feeding practices, fertility and birth interval, parental education	DHS
Honduras	2001	0.25–4.99	5613	Anthropometry	WHO
Jamaica	1999	0–4.99	574	Anthropometry, complementary feeding practices	PAHO
Mexico	1999	0–4.99	8011	Anthropometry, micronutrient deficiencies (Fe, Zn, I, vitamin A, vitamin C, folic acid), complementary feeding practices	NS
Nicaragua	2001	0–4.99	171	Anthropometry	World Bank
Panama	1997	0–4.99	2049	Anthropometry, complementary feeding practices	PAHO
Paraguay	1990	0–4.99	3389	Anthropometry, use of nutritional supplements, micronutrient deficiencies (Fe, I, vitamin A), complementary feeding practices, fertility and birth interval, parental education	DHS
Peru	2000	0–4.99	10 477	Anthropometry, use of nutritional supplements, micronutrient deficiencies (Fe, I, vitamin A), complementary feeding practices, fertility and birth interval	DHS
Trinidad & Tobago	2000	0–4.99	781	Anthropometry, complementary feeding practices	WHO
Uruguay	1992–93	0–4.99	11 521	Anthropometry, complementary feeding practices	SISVEN
Venezuela	2000	0–4.99	321 257	Anthropometry, complementary feeding practices	SISVAN

[a]Total sample size reported. Actual sample sizes differ by variable. All samples include both sexes.
Fe, anemia and/or iron deficiency; I, iodine deficiency; DHS, Demographic and Health Surveys; FAO, Food and Agriculture Organization of the United Nations; WHO, World Health Organization; NS, nationally representative health and/or nutrition survey not included in FAO or WHO database; PAHO, Pan American Health Organization; SISVEN, Sistema de Vigilancia Epidemiológica Nutricional [Nutritional Epidemiology Monitoring System]; SISVAN, Sistema de Vigilancia Alimentaria y Nutricional [Food and Nutrition Monitoring System].

Table 2 Surveys in developing countries with *per capita* consumption data and individual nutritional status data for adults

Region/country	Survey year	Age (years)	Sample size[a]	Data included	Source
Africa					
Benin	2001	15–49	2579	Anthropometry, dietary intake, micronutrient deficiencies (Fe), per capita consumption	FAO
Burkina Faso	1999	15–49	3416	Anthropometry, dietary intake, micronutrient deficiencies (Fe, I), per capita consumption	FAO, NS
Ethiopia	2000	15–49	13 447	Anthropometry	DHS
Guinea	1990	—	779	Anthropometry, dietary intake, micronutrient deficiencies (I), per capita consumption	FAO
Mali	2001	—	10 049	Anthropometry, micronutrient deficiencies (Fe, I)	DHS
Mauritania	1990	>18	2112	Anthropometry, dietary intake, micronutrient deficiencies (I), per capita consumption	FAO, NS
Namibia	1992	15–49	2249	Anthropometry, dietary intake, micronutrient deficiencies (Fe, I, vitamin A), per capita consumption	FAO
Niger	1995	18–60	NA	Anthropometry, dietary intake, micronutrient deficiencies (I), per capita consumption	FAO
Togo	1997	>19	375	Anthropometry, dietary intake, micronutrient deficiencies (I), per capita consumption	FAO
Zimbawe	1999–2000	15–49	5590	Anthropometry	DHS
Asia and Southwest Pacific					
Bangladesh	1996–97	15–49	3921	Anthropometry	FAO, DHS
Cambodia	1998	15–49	1109	Anthropometry	FAO
China	1996	>20	28 706	Anthropometry, dietary intake, micronutrient deficiencies (Fe, I) per capita consumption	FAO, NS
Fiji	1993	18–65	2573	Anthropometry, dietary intake, micronutrient deficiencies (Fe, I), per capita consumption	FAO, NS
India	1996	All	NA	Anthropometry, dietary intake, micronutrient deficiencies (Fe, vitamin A), per capita consumption	FAO
Lao People's Democratic Republic	2001	>15	5942	Anthropometry, dietary intake, use of nutritional supplements, micronutrient deficiencies (Fe), complementary feeding practices	FAO
Nepal	2001	15–49	7774	Anthropometry, dietary intake, use of nutritional supplements, micronutrient deficiencies (vitamin A), complementary feeding practices	DHS
Papua New Guinea	1997	21–50	1041	Anthropometry, dietary intake, per capita consumption	FAO
Philippines	1998	20–39	3123	Anthropometry	FAO, NS
Sri Lanka	1997	—	2624	Anthropometry, dietary intake, per capita consumption, micronutrient deficiencies (Fe)	FAO
Vanuatu	2000	20–60	800	Anthropometry	FAO
Viet Nam	1997	15–49	4212	Anthropometry, micronutrient deficiencies (vitamin A)	FAO, NS

Continued

Table 2 Continued

Region/country	Survey year	Age (years)	Sample size[a]	Data included	Source
Near East					
Egypt	2003	15–49	8078	Anthropometry, use of nutritional supplements, use of iodized salt	DHS
Iran	1995	20–74	NA	Anthropometry, dietary intake, per capita consumption, micronutrient deficiencies (Fe)	FAO
Jordan	2002	15–49	7682	Anthropometry, dietary intake, use of nutritional supplements, micronutrient deficiencies (Fe, I, vitamin A)	DHS
Morocco	1992	20–35	2751	Anthropometry, dietary intake, micronutrient deficiencies (I), per capita consumption	FAO
Turkey	1998	15–49	2183	Anthropometry, micronutrient deficiencies (I)	FAO
Latin America and the Caribbean					
Argentina	1990	19–64	504	Anthropometry, dietary intake, micronutrient deficiencies, per capita consumption	FAO
Bahamas	1988–89	15–64	1771	Anthropometry, dietary intake, micronutrient deficiencies, per capita consumption	FAO
Brazil	1996	15–49	2951	Anthropometry, dietary intake, micronutrient deficiencies, per capita consumption	FAO
Chile	1996	25–64	2127	Anthropometry, dietary intake, micronutrient deficiencies, per capita consumption	FAO
Colombia	2000	15–49	3070	Anthropometry, dietary intake, micronutrient deficiencies, per capita consumption	FAO
Costa Rica	1996	20–59	NA	Anthropometry, dietary intake, micronutrient deficiencies, per capita consumption	FAO
Cuba	1995	20–59	9815	Anthropometry, dietary intake, micronutrient deficiencies, per capita consumption	FAO
Dominican Republic	1997	15–49	2492	Anthropometry, dietary intake, micronutrient deficiencies, per capita consumption	FAO
Guatemala	1999	15–49	2585	Anthropometry, dietary intake, micronutrient deficiencies, per capita consumption	FAO
Jamaica	1999	25–74	2075	Anthropometry, dietary intake, micronutrient deficiencies, per capita consumption	FAO
Mexico	2000	20–99	45 200	Anthropometry, dietary intake, micronutrient deficiencies, per capita consumption	FAO, NS
Nicaragua	1999	15–49	4793	Anthropometry, dietary intake, micronutrient deficiencies, per capita consumption	FAO
Panama	1995	21–60	2448	Anthropometry, dietary intake, micronutrient deficiencies, per capita consumption	FAO
Peru	1997	15–49	9600	Anthropometry, dietary intake, micronutrient deficiencies, per capita consumption	FAO

Continued

Table 2 Continued

Region/country	Survey year	Age (years)	Sample size[a]	Data included	Source
Trinidad & Tobago	1999	>20	803	Anthropometry, dietary intake, micronutrient deficiencies, per capita consumption	FAO
Uruguay	1991	20–50	1079	Anthropometry, dietary intake, micronutrient deficiencies, per capita consumption	FAO
Venezuela	1997	20–50	14 084	Anthropometry, dietary intake, micronutrient deficiencies, per capita consumption	FAO

[a]Total sample size reported. Actual sample sizes differ by variable. All samples include both sexes with the exception of Costa Rica and Peru, for which data were found for women only.
Fe, anemia and/or iron deficiency; I, iodine deficiency; NA, not available; DHS, Demographic and Health Surveys; FAO, Food and Agriculture Organization of the United Nations; NS, nationally representative health and/or nutrition survey not included in FAO database.

See also: **Dietary Intake Measurement**: Methodology; Validation. **Dietary Surveys**. **Malnutrition**: Primary, Causes Epidemiology and Prevention; Secondary, Diagnosis and Management. **Nutritional Assessment**: Anthropometry; Biochemical Indices; Clinical Examination. **Nutritional Surveillance**: Developed Countries. **Obesity**: Definition, Etiology and Assessment. **United Nations Children's Fund**. **World Health Organization**.

Further Reading

Comisión Económica para América Latina y el Caribe [Council for Statistics in Latin America] (CEPAL) (2004) www.cepal.org. Accessed 23 September 2004.

Demographic and Health Surveys (2004) http://measuredhs.com. Accessed 27 September 2004.

Food and Agriculture Organization (FAO) (2004) *World Agriculture: Towards 2015/2030—An FAO Perspective.* http://www.fao.org/docrep/005/y4252e/y4252e04.htm. Accessed 21 September 2004.

Gibson RS (1990) *Principals of Nutritional Assessment.* New York: Oxford University Press.

Jonsson U (1995) *Towards an improved strategy for nutritional surveillance. Food and Nutrition Bulletin* **16**(2). [www.unu.edu/unupress. Accessed 20 September 2004].

Latham M (2004) *Human Nutrition in the Developing World.* http://www.fao.org/DOCREP/W0073e07.htm. Accessed 20 September 2004.

Rose D, Meershoek S, Ismael C *et al.* (2002) Evaluation of a rapid field tool for assessing household diet quality in Mozambique. *Food and Nutrition Bulletin* **23**: 181–191.

Ruel MT (2003) Operationalizing dietary diversity: A review of measurement issues and research priorities. *Journal of Nutrition* **133**: 3911S–3926S.

Sistema de Vigilancia Alimentaria y Nutricional [Food and Nutrition Monitoring System] (SISVAN) (2004) http://www.sisov.mpd.gov.ve/articulos/23/. Accessed 25 September 2004.

Sistema de Vigilancia Epidemiológica Nutricional [Nutritional Epidemiology Monitoring System] (SISVEN) (2004) http://165.158.1.110/english/sha/ururstp.htm. Accessed 25 September 2004.

WHO/FAO (2003) *Joint WHO/FAO Expert Consultation on Diet, Nutrition and the Prevention of Chronic Diseases.* Geneva: World Health Organization.

World Health Organization, Department of Nutrition for Health and Development (2004) *WHO Global Database on Child Growth and Malnutrition.* http://www.who.int/nutgrowthdb/. Accessed 22 September 2004.

NUTS AND SEEDS

J Gray, Guildford, UK

In botanical terms, the word 'nut' is used to describe a wide range of seeds, mostly from trees, with a tough, often lignified, seed coat or shell. True nuts include the chestnut, brazil nut, and hazelnut. In practice, these are usually classified together with certain other so-called nuts, for example the almond, cashew, and peanut, and other seeds which are all used in similar ways in the diet. Nuts and seeds come from a diverse range of different plants, so their nutritional composition is quite varied, but like most plant seeds they contain a food reserve designed to meet the needs of the developing plant embryo. In many nuts and seeds this is fat, but in others it is starch or other polysaccharides.

Therefore, these foods are concentrated sources of dietary energy, as well as sources of protein, unsaturated fatty acids, various micronutrients, and fiber (nonstarch polysaccharides, NSP).

Nuts and seeds have a wide range of uses. In the typical Western omniverous diet they tend to be used either as snack items or added as minor ingredient to savory and sweet dishes, but they have wider applications in vegetarian diets as important sources of protein and other nutrients. Certain nuts and seeds are also made into spreads, for example peanut butter and tahini (sesame seed spread).

Types

The major types of nuts and seeds grown for human consumption are shown in **Table 1**.

Nuts

Almond   The almond (*Prunus amygdalis* var. *dulcis*), sometimes called the sweet almond, is one of the oldest nut crops. It is believed to have originated in Southeast Asia but is now grown more widely, including in southern Europe, Africa, southern Australia, and California. It is closely related to peaches and plums, but in the almond, in contrast to these other fruits, the 'flesh' or mesocarp becomes hard and dry as it matures, and splits open to leave the thin shell or endocarp which contains the edible almond seed or 'nut.' The nuts are eaten fresh, often in the ground form in prepared dishes, as well as roasted and salted.

Another species, *Prunus amara* or the bitter almond, is inedible but is cultivated for its oil, which is also present in the sweet almond and in the kernels of apricots and peaches. This oil contains benzaldehyde, the essential oil, and hydrocyanic acid, from which the benzaldehyde is separated to be used in flavorings and perfumes.

Brazil nut   The triangular-shaped Brazil nut (*Bertholletia excelsa*) grows in large forests in the Amazon river basin in South America. The nuts are actually hard-shelled seeds which are produced in groups of between 12 and 30 within a large, hard, thick-walled woody fruit or pod. The sweet-tasting nut meat is consumed in the fresh state and Brazil nut oil may be extracted for use as a lubricant.

Cashew nut   The cashew (*Anacardium occidentale*) originated in Brazil but is now cultivated extensively in all tropical areas, notably in India and East Africa. The cashew fruit, which contains the seed or 'nut,' hangs at the end of what is referred to as the cashew 'apple'—the edible swollen fruit stem or pedicel. The fruit itself is kidney-shaped, about the size of a large bean, and has a two-layered shell. The outer layer of this shell contains a caustic oil that must be burned off before the nut is touched. The nuts are then roasted again or boiled to remove other toxic substances and the second shell is removed. The nuts may also be used as a source of oil.

Chestnut   The sweet or Spanish chestnut (*Castanea sativa*) is a native tree of southern Europe, believed to have been introduced into Britain by the Romans. The fruit consists of two to four compartmentalized seeds or burrs, covered with numerous needle-sharp branched spines and containing the seeds or 'nuts,' which are covered with a tough outer coat. The flesh of the nut is hard and inedible and is cooked, often by roasting or boiling, before being eaten. The cooking process changes the texture so that the chestnut becomes much softer than other nuts and more like a vegetable, largely as a result of its high carbohydrate content (see below).

Coconut   The coconut (*Cocos nucifera*) grows on the coconut palm, which is common in tropical areas throughout the world. The native origin of the palm is uncertain, as the nuts were easily dispersed between both islands and continents by ocean currents and by early explorers. The fruits are borne on the tree in clusters of about 15 to 20 and are enclosed in a thick outer husk and covered in a mass of fibers (the mesocarp and exocarp), which is normally removed when the coconut is harvested. The familiar hard shell of the coconut is the endocarp, or inner layer, of the mature ovary of the fruit, and within the shell is the actual seed, covered with a thin brown seed coat. The white coconut 'meat,' which can be eaten either fresh or desiccated, is actually part of the endosperm (storage tissue) of the seed. Coconut 'milk,' which is found in the unripe nut and is drunk or used in cooking, is the liquid form of the endosperm, which solidifies as the fruit ripens. The coconut meat may be dried

Table 1   Major types of nuts and seeds grown for human consumption

Almond	Pecan
Brazil	Pine nuts
Cashew	Pistachio
Chestnut	Walnut
Coconut	Pumpkin seeds
Hazelnut	Sesame seeds
Macadamia	Sunflower seeds
Peanut	

to produce copra, which is pressed to remove the coconut oil used widely as a food oil and in soap and cosmetic manufacture.

Hazelnut (cobnut; filbert) The most widely grown hazelnut (*Corylus avellana*) is a native of Europe, although about 10 different species of *Corylus* grow throughout Europe, North America, and Asia. There is evidence that these nuts were cultivated in Ancient Greece and collected by Mesolithic peoples. The shell of the hazelnut is the matured ovary wall of the flower and the edible nut meat within this is the matured embryo.

Macadamia nut The macadamia nut (*Macadamia integrifolia*, smooth-shelled; *M. tetraphylla*, rough-shelled) is native to eastern tropical Australia but was subsequently introduced to Hawaii, which is now the leading producer of these nuts, and also to parts of Africa and South America. It is the smooth-shelled variety that has been developed commercially. The edible kernel of the nut is the seed, consisting mostly of the cotyledons of the embryo. It is enclosed in a hard, thick, brown shell, which is itself encased in a fibrous husk that splits open when the husk dries. This occurs after the fruit falls, or when it is removed from the tree at maturity. After harvesting, the nuts are dried (to a moisture level of 1.5%), roasted (traditionally in coconut oil, or dry-roasted), and salted.

Peanut The peanut (*Arachis hypogaea*), sometimes referred to as the ground nut or monkey nut, originated in South America. Although referred to as a nut, it is in fact part of the legume family. The plant was introduced to Africa by early European explorers and to North America by the slave trade; it was also introduced to India and China. The name 'ground nut' derives from the fact that the flower withers after pollination to leave a stalk-like part of the plant, which pushes under the soil and carries the fertilized ovules in its tip. Underground, the tip continues to develop into the characteristic pod of the peanut, containing the seeds, or 'nuts.' The shape and size of the pod, and the number and color of the seeds, are variable, depending on the peanut cultivar. On a worldwide basis, two-thirds of the peanut crop is crushed for oil (arachis oil) and peanut products are used widely in both food processing, with peanut butter as an important product, and for animal feed. The peanut itself may be eaten fresh or roasted and salted.

Pecan The pecan (*Carya illinoinensis*) is a member of the walnut family, and the tree is classified botanically as a hickory. The tree is a native of North America, grown in the southern central states. After harvesting, the nuts are air-dried to remove 10–20% of their moisture. The nut is similar to the walnut, but with a more mild and sweet flavor. The pecan nut kernel is eaten fresh and in the US it is used widely in confectionery and baked goods.

Pine nuts Pine nuts or kernels are small edible seeds which are extracted from the cones of various species of pine. The most commonly eaten variety is that from the European stone pine (*Pinus pinea*), which is native to northern Mediterranean regions. The small, oil-rich seeds are encased in a hard shell. The seeds are sometimes referred to as pignolia nuts, whereas the seeds of the pinyon pines (*Pinus edulis* and *Pinus monophylla*), which grow in the southwestern US and in northern Mexico, are known as pinon nuts.

Pistachio nut The pistachio nut is the seed of the pistachio tree (*Pistacia vera*). It is a native of central Asia, Pakistan, and India, where it was cultivated 3000 years ago, and it has also been cultivated for many years in Mediterranean regions and more recently in California. The pistachio fruit is similar to a peach; the outer 'husk' (the exocarp and mesocarp of the fruit) encloses a hard but thin off-white shell (the endocarp). This splits open just before the nut matures to reveal the edible embryo, which consists mainly of two green cotyledons covered in a thin seed coat. The green nut kernels are highly prized and are eaten roasted and salted as well as in various Middle Eastern dishes.

Walnut The walnut (*Juglans* spp.) is the common name given to about 20 species of trees in this family. The most important species is *Juglans regia*—the English or Persian walnut—which is believed to have originated in Ancient Persia, later taken to Greece, and eventually distributed throughout the Roman empire. There are records of its growth in England in the sixteenth century. It was taken to America and called the English walnut to distinguish it from the native American black walnut (*Juglans nigrans*) and the butternut (*Juglans cinerea*), both of which have much thicker, less brittle shells. The walnut fruit has an outer leathery husk and an inner furrowed stone, which is the shell of the nut, within which is the edible seed.

Seeds

Pumpkin seeds The large flat seeds of the members of the pumpkin family (*Cucurbita maxima*; *C. moschata* and related species) can be dried and eaten raw, used in both sweet and savory cooked dishes, or roasted.

Sesame seeds   The sesame plant (*Sesamum indicum*), which is a native of Africa, grows in tropical and subtropical regions and is now common in Asia. The seeds are small and off-white in color. They may be eaten whole or used in confectionery and baked goods and as a source of oil used in cooking. The seeds are also ground to a paste called tahini.

Sunflower seeds   The sunflower (*Helianthus annus*) is a member of the Compositae or daisy family. It is believed to have originated in North America, where it was cultivated by the native Indians, and was introduced to Europe in the sixteenth century. The flat seeds may be dehusked and eaten raw or cooked, but the plant is generally cultivated for the oil they contain, which is a rich source of polyunsaturated fatty acids (see below), and is widely used for cooking and in margarine manufacture. The residual oil-cake is used for animal feed.

Macronutrient Content

Green nuts, as harvested, may contain 50% or more water, but these nuts must be cured or semidried for storage, so the moisture content of most nuts, as eaten, is low (1–6%). The exceptions are fresh coconut and chestnuts, with a moisture content of 45 and 52%, respectively. The water, macronutrient, and energy content of the nuts and seeds discussed in this article are shown in **Table 2**.

Fat

The total fat content of most nuts and seeds is high because, as the seed ripens, the fat store increases and its starch content declines. However, the amount of fat is quite variable, ranging from about 78% in the macadamia nut and 70% in the pecan to around 50–55% in nuts such as the almond, cashew, hazelnut, and pistachio, and as low as 3% in chestnuts. The fat content of the edible seeds is between 45 and 60%.

The different fatty acid fractions contained in these nuts and seeds are also quite variable, as shown in **Table 3**. The vast majority of nuts and seeds are rich in monounsaturated and polyunsaturated fatty acids. However, in some nuts, such as the peanut, hazelnut, and macadamia nut, monounsaturated fatty acids predominate, whereas in the walnut and in sunflower seeds polyunsaturated fatty acids predominate. The exception is the coconut, in which saturated fatty acids constitute the major fat fraction.

Carbohydrate

With the exception of the starch-rich chestnut (almost 37% carbohydrate), the carbohydrate content of most nuts is relatively low at around 3–7%. However, peanuts, cashews, pumpkin, and sunflower seeds contain more carbohydrate (13–19%). In most nuts and seeds this carbohydrate is a variable mixture of starch and sucrose, although in some there are small quantities of glucose and fructose as well, and in sunflower seeds there are some oligosaccharides.

Table 2   Water, macronutrient, and energy content of selected nuts and seeds (per 100 g, kernel only)

	Water (g)	Protein (g)	Fat (g)	Carbohydrate (g)	Energy	
					(kJ)	(kcal)
Almond	4.2	21.1	55.8	6.9	2534	612
Brazil	2.8	14.1	68.2	3.1	2813	682
Cashew	4.4	17.7	48.2	18.1	2374	573
Chestnut	51.7	2.0	2.7	36.6	719	170
Coconut	45.0	3.2	36.0	3.7	1446	351
Hazelnut	4.6	14.1	63.5	6.0	2685	650
Macadamia (salted)	1.3	7.9	77.6	4.8	3082	748
Peanut	6.3	25.6	46.1	12.5	2341	564
Pecan	3.7	9.2	70.1	5.8	2843	689
Pine nuts	2.7	14.0	68.6	4.0	2840	688
Pistachio (roasted, salted)	2.1	17.9	55.4	8.2	2485	601
Walnut	2.8	14.7	68.5	3.3	2837	688
Pumpkin seeds	5.6	24.4	45.6	15.2	2360	569
Sesame seeds	4.6	18.2	58.0	0.9	2470	598
Sunflower seeds	4.4	19.8	47.5	18.6	2410	581

Data from Holland *et al.* (1992).

Table 3 Total fat and fatty acid composition of selected nuts and seeds (g per 100 g, kernel only)

	Total fat	Saturated fatty acids	Monounsaturated fatty acids	Polyunsaturated fatty acids (total)	cis n-6 Polyunsaturated fatty acids	cis n-3 Polyunsaturated fatty acids
Almond	55.8	4.7	34.4	14.2	13.3	0.1
Brazil	68.2	16.4	25.8	23.0	22.9	0.1
Cashew	48.2	9.5	27.8	8.8	—[a]	—[a]
Chestnut	2.7	0.5	1.0	1.1	1.0	0.1
Coconut	36.0	31.0	2.0	0.8	0.5	0
Hazelnut	63.5	4.7	50.0	5.9	5.4	0.1
Macadamia (salted)	77.6	11.2	60.8	1.6	—[a]	—[a]
Peanut	46.1	8.2	21.1	14.3	—[a]	—[a]
Pecan	70.1	5.7	42.5	18.7	16.0	0.7
Pine nuts	68.6	4.6	19.9	41.1	—[a]	—[a]
Pistachio (roasted, salted)	55.4	7.4	27.6	17.9	—[a]	—[a]
Walnut	68.5	5.6	12.4	47.5	—[a]	—[a]
Pumpkin seeds	45.6	7.0	11.2	18.3	—[a]	—[a]
Sesame seeds	58.0	8.3	21.7	25.5	23.6	0.4
Sunflower seeds	47.5	4.5	9.8	31.0	—[a]	—[a]

[a]No data available.
Data from Holland *et al.* (1992) and The Ministry of Agriculture, Fisheries and Food.

Protein

The protein content of nuts is quite variable, but most nuts are considered to be a good source of protein. It is low (2–3%) in the chestnut and coconut, between 8 and 15% for most other nuts, but high (18–26%) in the cashew, pistachio, almond, and peanut, so that the amount of protein in many nuts is about the same as in meat, fish, or cheese. Pumpkin, sesame, and sunflower seeds are also rich in protein.

However, the proportions of indispensable amino acids in any one particular type of nut or seed, and in fact all plant foods, differ from those needed in the human diet, with one or sometimes more 'limiting amino acids.' In most nuts and seeds, with the exception of pistachio nuts and pumpkin seeds, it is lysine that is the limiting amino acid. Thus, although the total amount of protein in nuts and seeds may be high, these foods must be complemented by other sources of plant protein, such as legumes and/or animal sources of protein (meat, fish, eggs, milk, cheese), to ensure that the overall protein quality of the diet is adequate.

Micronutrient Content

The vitamin and mineral contents of the nuts and seeds discussed in this article are shown in **Tables 4** and **5**, respectively.

In general, nuts and seeds are a good source of the B vitamins, including folic acid, and of the tocopherols (vitamin E), although some, such as almonds, hazelnuts, and sunflower seeds, contain much more vitamin E than others. Nuts and seeds do not contain vitamin C, and many nuts have little or no vitamin A activity.

Nuts and seeds contain quite large amounts of many minerals. In particular, many nuts and seeds, especially sesame seeds, are good sources of calcium. They are also generally rich in potassium, magnesium and phosphorus, iron, and in trace elements such as copper, zinc, manganese, and others such as chromium. Brazil nuts are particularly rich in selenium.

Fiber Content

Compositional values for the total amount of fiber (nonstarch polysaccharides, NSP), and the different fiber fractions where available, are shown in **Table 6** for the nuts and seeds discussed in this article. It can be seen that nuts and seeds contain significant amounts of fiber, similar to the amounts found in vegetables and fruit. Although nuts and seeds do contain some soluble fiber, most of the fiber in these foods is of the insoluble type, much of which is cellulose. Of the insoluble noncellulosic polysaccharides, arabinose predominates in most nuts, although the coconut contains large quantities of mannose. Most nuts and seeds are likely to contain quite large amounts of lignin, particularly those with a tough seed coat such as sesame seeds, although actual values are not available.

Table 4 Vitamin content of selected nuts and seeds (per 100 g, kernel only)

	Carotene (μg)	Vitamin E (mg)	Thiamin (mg)	Riboflavin (mg)	Niacin (mg)	Vitamin B6 (mg)	Folate (μg)
Almond	0	23.96	0.21	0.75	3.1	0.15	48
Brazil	0	7.18	0.67	0.03	0.3	0.31	21
Cashew	6	0.85	0.69	0.14	1.2	0.49	67
Chestnut	0	1.20	0.14	0.02	0.5	0.34	N[a]
Coconut	0	0.73	0.04	0.01	0.5	0.05	26
Hazelnut	0	24.98	0.43	0.16	1.1	0.59	72
Macadamia (salted)	0	1.49	0.28	0.06	1.6	0.28	N
Peanut	0	10.09	1.14	0.10	13.8	0.59	110
Pecan	50	4.34	0.71	0.15	1.4	0.19	39
Pine nuts	10	13.65	0.73	0.19	3.8	N	N
Pistachio (roasted, salted)	130	4.16	0.70	0.23	1.7	N	58
Walnut	0	3.85	0.40	0.14	1.2	0.67	66
Pumpkin seeds	230[b]	N	0.23	0.32	1.7	N	N
Sesame seeds	6	2.53	0.93	0.17	5.0	0.75	97
Sunflower seeds	15	37.77	1.60	0.19	4.1	N	N

[a]Nutrient present in significant quantities but no reliable information available on the amount.
[b]Estimated value.
Data from Holland *et al.* (1992).

Table 5 Mineral and trace element content of selected nuts and seeds (per 100 g, kernel only)

	Sodium (mg)	Potassium (mg)	Calcium (mg)	Magnesium (mg)	Phosphorus (mg)	Iron (mg)	Copper (mg)	Zinc (mg)	Manganese (mg)	Selenium (μg)
Almond	14	780	240	270	550	3.0	1.00	3.2	1.7	4
Brazil	3	660	170	410	590	2.5	1.76	4.2	1.2	1530[a]
Cashew	15	710	32	270	560	6.2	2.11	5.9	1.7	29
Chestnut	11	500	46	33	74	0.9	0.23	0.5	0.5	Tr
Coconut	17	370	13	41	94	2.1	0.32	0.5	1.0	1[b]
Hazelnut	6	730	140	160	300	3.2	1.23	2.1	4.9	Tr
Macadamia (salted)	280	300	47	100	200	1.6	0.43	1.1	5.5	7
Peanut	2	670	60	210	430	2.5	1.02	3.5	2.1	3
Pecan	1	520	61	130	310	2.2	1.07	5.3	4.6	12
Pine nuts	1	780	11	270	650	5.6	1.32	6.5	7.9	N[c]
Pistachio (roasted, salted)	530	1040	110	130	420	3.0	0.83	2.2	0.9	6[b]
Walnut	7	450	94	160	380	2.9	1.34	2.7	3.4	19
Pumpkin seeds	18	820	39	270	850	10.0	1.57	6.6	N	6[b]
Sesame seed	20	570	670	370	720	10.4	1.46	5.3	1.5	N
Sunflower seeds	3	710	110	390	640	6.4	2.27	5.1	2.2	49[b]

[a]Range, 230–5300 μg per 100 g.
[b]Estimated value.
[c]Nutrient present in significant quantities but no reliable information available on the amount.
Data from Holland *et al.* (1992).

Toxins and Contaminants

Phytic Acid

Phytic acid (*myo*-inositol hexaphosphoric acid) is present in all seeds, where it is believed to act as a store of phosphate and trace elements for the developing plant embryo. The phytate content of the commonly eaten nuts and seeds is variable. In general, the oil seeds, such as sesame and sunflower, and a number of the tree nuts, have higher phytate levels than the leguminous peanut, although the oils expressed from the seeds do not contain phytate. The phytate content of the coconut and chestnut is particularly low.

Because of its molecular structure, phytic acid is a highly effective chelator, which forms insoluble complexes with mineral cations. Its presence in plant foods has led to concerns that it may reduce the bioavailability of various dietary minerals and trace elements, including calcium, magnesium, iron,

Table 6 Total dietary fiber, as measured by the Englyst method, and fiber fractions in selected nuts and seeds (g per 100 g, kernels only)

| | | | Fiber fractions | | |
| | | | Noncellulosic polysaccharide | | |
	Total fiber	Cellulose	Soluble	Insoluble	Lignin
Almond	7.4[a]	1.9[a]	1.1[a]	4.4[a]	N[b]
Brazil	4.3	1.6	1.3	1.4	N
Cashew	3.2	0.6	1.6	1.0	N
Chestnut	4.1	1.1	1.3	1.7	N
Coconut	7.3	0.8	1.0	5.5	N
Hazelnut	6.5	2.2	2.5	1.8	N
Macadamia (salted)	5.3	1.4	1.9	2.0	N
Peanut	6.2	2.0	1.9	2.3	N
Pecan	4.7	1.2	1.5	2.0	N
Pine nuts	1.9	N	N	N	N
Pistachio (roasted, salted)	6.1	1.3	2.7	2.1	N
Walnut	3.5	1.1	1.5	0.9	N
Pumpkin seeds	5.3	1.1	1.7	2.5	N
Sesame seeds	7.9	N	N	N	N
Sunflower seeds	6.0	1.4	1.8	2.8	N

[a]Estimated value.
[b]Nutrient present in significant quantities but no reliable information available on the amount.
Data from Holland *et al.* (1992).

zinc, and copper. Although nuts are rich in iron, there is evidence that the addition of nuts to a meal can have a substantial inhibitory effect on iron absorption, presumably because of their phytate and polyphenol content. However, it appears that this can be overcome by the addition of a source of vitamin C to the meal, thereby underlining the need to mix different groups of foods within a meal, particularly when plant foods are the main source of nutrition.

The significance of dietary phytate intake to overall mineral nutriture is still uncertain. It is likely that in a mixed diet of animal and plant foods, dietary phytate may be of less significance than among people consuming diets where plant foods are the sole source of nutrition (vegans). Available data suggest that the trace element status of most adult vegetarians is adequate, but because of increased requirements for growth, vegetarian children may be more vulnerable to the reduced bioavailability of minerals and trace elements, notably zinc, which could be a consequence of the ingestion of large amounts of phytate-containing plant foods.

Intolerances/Allergies to Nuts

Intolerances to nuts, or more specifically, allergies to nut proteins, occur in a relatively small minority of people. However, there is evidence that such adverse reactions have become more common, and the severity of the reaction that occurs in these sensitive individuals means that they must be taken very seriously. Peanuts are the most commonly cited cause of these severe reactions, estimated to affect between 0.1 and 0.2% of the population, but allergic reactions to tree nuts, incuding Brazil nuts, almonds, hazelnuts, and cashews, and also to sesame seeds, have been reported.

Contaminants

Nuts and seeds may be subject to mould growth during storage if the conditions are inappropriate. Certain moulds produce secondary metabolites which are toxic to humans and animals, known as the mycotoxins. Of these mycotoxins, the aflatoxins, notably aflatoxin B1, are produced by three closely related species of mould: *Aspergillus flavus*, *A. parasiticus*, and *A. nomius*. These moulds may contaminate various food commodities in tropical and subtropical regions, including tree nuts, but one of the most important crops to be affected is the peanut. Aflatoxins are acutely toxic to the liver and may also be involved in the etiology of human liver cancer in certain parts of the world. Ochratoxins, which are produced by other *Aspergillus* species, have also been found to contaminate nuts.

Some species of mould are able to proliferate within growing crops even before they are harvested, forming an endophytic relationship with the plant. This relationship has been found to exist between *Aspergillus parasiticus* and peanuts. It appears that when the plant is growing normally, no aflatoxin is produced by the mould, but when the plant is stressed, as occurs in drought conditions, then the mycotoxin may be produced. The concentrations of aflatoxins produced in this way are lower than would ensue from poor postharvest storage, but the economic consequences still may be considerable.

There are regulatory limits for the aflatoxin levels in foods. In the UK, the sale of nuts for direct consumption is prohibited if the aflatoxin content exceeds $4\,\mu g\,kg^{-1}$ or $10\,\mu g\,kg^{-1}$ for nuts which are to be subjected to further processing before being sold. A proportion of nuts imported into the UK, especially peanuts, are contaminated with aflatoxin. In 1994, 3% of samples examined under a European surveillance program were found to exceed the UK limit. Nonetheless, such findings should be kept in perspective: The numbers are low and their significance in public health terms, relative to other diet-related risks, is small.

Role in the Diet

Nuts and seeds can make a useful contribution to the dietary intake of macronutrients, notably protein and unsaturated fatty acids, micronutrients, dietary fiber, and energy. Although these commodities play a relatively minor role in the average Western diet, they are more important in the diets of Western vegetarians, especially vegans. Even on a worldwide basis, the nutritional contribution of nuts and seeds is relatively small: Plant foods are estimated to supply around 65% of edible protein, but only 8% of protein and 4% of total dietary energy is estimated to derive from pulses, oil crops, and nuts (Young and Pellett, 1994).

In the UK, average weekly household consumption of nuts and their products, as recorded by the National Food Survey, is about 14 g per capita, with only 11% of households purchasing these commodities; there are no separate data for nuts eaten as out of home snacks. Data from the Dietary and Nutritional Survey of British Adults indicate that average weekly intake of people consuming unsalted nuts and nut mixes is 63 g per week, but again only 12% of the adults surveyed were consuming these

commodities. Therefore, even for nutrients which are present in relatively large amounts in nuts, such as vitamin E, magnesium, and copper, these foods only provide about 1% of the average daily intake in the UK.

See also: **Dietary Fiber**: Physiological Effects and Effects on Absorption. **Fatty Acids**: Metabolism; Monounsaturated; Omega-3 Polyunsaturated; Omega-6 Polyunsaturated; Saturated; *Trans* Fatty Acids. **Folic Acid**. **Food Allergies**: Etiology. **Food Safety**: Mycotoxins. **Protein**: Quality and Sources. **Vegetarian Diets**.

Further Reading

Englyst HN, Bingham SA, Runswick SA, Collinson E, and Cummings JH (1988) Dietary fibre (non-starch polysaccharides) in fruit, vegetables and nuts. *Journal of Human Nutrition and Dietetics* 1: 247–286.

Gibson RS (1994) Content and bioavailability of trace elements in vegetarian diets. *American Journal of Clinical Nutrition* 59(supplement): 1223S–1232S.

Gregory J, Foster K, Tyler H, and Wiseman M (1990) *The Dietary and Nutritional Survey of British Adults*. London: HMSO.

Harland BF and Oberleas D (1987) Phytate in foods. *World Review of Nutrition and Dietetics* 52: 235–259.

Hartmann HT, Flocker WJ, and Kofranek AM (1981) *Plant Science. Growth, Development, and Utilization of Cultivated Plants*. Englewood Cliffs, NJ: Prentice Hall.

Holland B, Unwin ID, and Buss DH (eds.) (1992) *Fruit and Nuts. The First Supplement to McCance & Widdowson's The Composition of Foods*, 5th edn. London: The Royal Society of Chemistry.

Macfarlane BJ, Bezwoda WR, Bothwell TH *et al.* (1988) Inhibitory effect of nuts on iron absorption. *American Journal of Clinical Nutrition* 47: 270–274.

Ministry of Agriculture, Fisheries and Food (1994) *The Dietary and Nutritional Survey of British Adults—Further Analysis*. London: HMSO.

Morris ER (1993) Phytic acid. In: Macrae R, Robinson RK, and Sadler MJ (eds.) *Encyclopaedia of Food Science, Food Technology and Nutrition*, pp. 3587–3591. London: Academic Press.

Moss MO (1996) Mycotoxins. *Mycological Research* 100: 524–526.

Ryden P and Selvendran RR (1993) Phytic acid. In: Macrae R, Robinson RK, and Sadler MJ (eds.) *Encyclopaedia of Food Science, Food Technology and Nutrition*, pp. 3582–3587. London: Academic Press.

Young VR and Pellett PL (1994) Plant proteins in relation to human protein and amino acid nutrition. *American Journal of Clinical Nutrition* 59(supplement): 1203S–1212S.

OBESITY

Contents

Definition, Etiology and Assessment

A Pietrobelli, Verona University Medical School, Verona, Italy

Obesity is a situation of excess body fat accumulation, and a clinical diagnosis of obesity should be based on an accurate direct or indirect measure of total body fat. The most widely used measurement to define obesity in adults is body mass index (BMI; weight in kg/height in m^2). It is a predictor of body fat from a population perspective, but it has limitations on an individual level and is only a proxy measurement of body fat. BMI shows significant variations during childhood; thus, age- and gender-specific reference standards must be used, and in adolescents the pubertal status should also be evaluated. An expert committee convened by the International Obesity Task Force (IOTF) in 1999 determined that although BMI is not an ideal measure of adiposity, it has been validated against other measures of body fat and may therefore be used to define overweight and obesity in children and adolescents. Because it is not clear at which BMI level adverse health risk factors increase in children, the group recommended cutoffs based on age-specific values that project to the adult cutoffs of 25 kg/m^2 for overweight and 30 kg/m^2 for obesity. Using data from six different reference population (Great Britain, Brazil, The Netherlands, Hong Kong, Singapore, and the United States), Cole and colleagues derived centile curves that passed through the points of 25 and 30 kg/m^2 at age 18 years. **Table 1** is useful for epidemiological research because children and adolescents can be categorized as non-overweight, overweight, and obese using a single standard tool.

There are differences in body composition across adult ethic groups, with one study of whites and Asians showing a difference of 2 or 3 BMI units in adults with the same body composition. It has been found that African American, Mexican American, and Mohawk Indian children carry more central fat than white children. Several studies have compared the US NHANES criteria for defining overweight or obesity using age- and gender-specific 85th and 95th percentile cutoffs with those of the Centers for Disease Control and Prevention (CDC) using similar percentile cutoffs and the IOTF alternative set of cutoffs based on centiles passing through BMI 25 and 30 at age 18 years. Using the NHANES III data, the different methods (i.e., NHANES/WHO, CDC, and IOTF) give approximately similar results but with some discrepancies, especially among younger children.

Definition

Obesity is an increase in body fat. This increase in fat can be evenly distributed over the body, or it can be concentrated in specific regions. Differences in body fat distribution are gender specific. Women tend to deposit fat more on their buttocks (gynoid distribution), and men tend to deposit fat on their waist (android distribution).

Table 1 International cutoff points for body mass index (BMI) for overweight and obesity by sex between 2 and 18 years

Age (years)	BMI 25 kg/m²		BMI 30 kg/m²	
	Males	Females	Males	Females
2	18.41	18.02	20.09	19.81
2.5	18.13	17.76	19.80	19.55
3	17.89	17.56	19.57	19.36
3.5	17.69	17.40	19.39	19.23
4	17.55	17.28	19.29	19.15
4.5	17.47	17.19	19.26	19.12
5	17.42	17.15	19.30	19.17
5.5	17.45	17.20	19.47	19.34
6	17.55	17.34	19.79	19.65
6.5	17.71	17.53	20.23	20.08
7	17.92	17.75	20.63	20.51
7.5	18.16	18.03	21.09	21.01
8	18.44	18.35	21.60	21.57
8.5	18.76	18.69	22.17	22.18
9	19.10	19.07	22.77	22.81
9.5	19.46	19.45	23.39	23.46
10	19.84	19.86	24.00	24.11
10.5	20.20	20.29	24.57	24.77
11	20.55	20.74	25.10	25.42
11.5	20.89	21.20	25.58	26.05
12	21.22	21.68	26.02	26.67
12.5	21.56	22.14	26.43	27.24
13	21.91	22.58	26.84	27.76
13.5	22.27	22.98	27.25	28.20
14	22.62	23.34	27.63	28.57
14.5	22.96	23.66	27.98	28.87
15	23.29	23.94	28.30	29.11
15.5	23.60	24.17	28.60	29.29
16	23.90	24.37	28.88	29.43
16.5	24.19	24.54	29.14	29.56
17	24.46	24.70	29.41	29.69
17.5	24.73	24.85	29.70	29.84
18	25	25	30	30

Modified from Cole TJ, Bellizzi MC, Flegal KM and Dietz WH (2000) Establishing a standard definition for child overweight and obesity worldwide: International survey. *British Medical Journal* **320**(7244): 1240–1243.

Measures of Body Fatness

Studies of adipose tissue distribution, its causes, and its effects on morbidity and mortality are fundamental in the field of obesity. An ideal measure of body fat should be "precise with small measurement error; accessible, in terms of simplicity, cost, and easy to perform; acceptable to the subject; well documented with published reference values." There is no consensus as to which methods best define and describe adipose tissue and its distribution. Several studies have noted that the increased risk of obesity is related to mesenteric and portal depots of adipose tissue. However, subcutaneous adipose tissue, particularly around the hips and buttocks, appears not to increase health risk.

The different methods used to estimate total fat and adipose tissue are discussed next and presented in order of decreasing accuracy.

Cadaver analysis The main use of cadaver studies is to validate other methods that can be used to study patients *in vivo*.

Imaging techniques Total adipose tissue and its distribution can be quantified using imaging techniques such as computed tomography (CT) and magnetic resonance imaging (MRI). Both methods produce high-resolution cross-sectional images from signals resulting from exposure of the subject to an X-ray source (CT) or electromagnetic field (MRI). Total body fat volume, total fat mass, and percentage fat mass can be estimated. In addition to providing total adipose tissue, imaging techniques are able to separate adipose tissue into subcutaneous, visceral, and intraorgan components. An accuracy of better than 1% error for body fat measurement is possible with these techniques.

Dual-energy X-ray absorptiometry This method is based on the principle that transmitted X-rays at two energy levels are differentially attenuated by bone mass and soft tissue mass, and the soft tissue mass is subdivided into fat mass and lean mass. Reproducibility of dual-energy X-ray absorptiometry (DXA) is approximately 0.8% for bone, 1.7% for fat, and 2.0% for body weight. One concern regarding DXA is whether changes in soft tissue hydration influence body fat estimates. A few studies have shown small but systematic and predictable errors in DXA soft tissue composition analysis with body fluid balance changes. Using DXA, it is possible to obtain abdominal fat estimates. Unfortunately, these cannot be separated into subcutaneous and visceral components.

Bioimpedance analysis This method measures the resistance in the body to an imperceptible electrical current. The measurement is based on the relationship among the volume of the conductor (body), the conductor's length (height), and its electrical impedance. Bioimpedance analysis assumes fat mass is anhydrous and that conductivity reflects fat-free mass. Conceptually, a human devoid of adipose tissue could have minimum impedance, and impedance would increase to a maximum when all lean tissue is replaced by fat/adipose tissue. This approach estimates total body water, which can be transformed using appropriate formulas and in turn can estimate fat-free mass and hence fat mass.

Anthropometric measurements Anthropometric measurement can be used to estimate total body fat, regional fat, and fat distribution. Anthropometric measures of relative adiposity or fatness are BMI, skinfold thickness, waist, hip, and other girth measurements. BMI is widely used as an index of relative adiposity among children, adolescents, and adults. The World Health Organization classifies a person with a BMI of 25 kg/m^2 or higher as overweight, whereas a person with a BMI of 30 kg/m^2 or higher is classified as obese. This measurement has low observer error, low measurement error, and good reliability and validity. However, BMI may not be a sensitive measure of fatness in subjects who are short, tall, or who have highly developed muscle. There may also be racial differences in the relationship between proportion of body fat and BMI.

The amount of subcutaneous fat can be estimated by measuring thickness directly using a skinfold caliper at different sites on the body. The sites most often used are the upper arm (biceps and triceps), under the scapula (subscapular), and above the iliac crest (suprailiac). Increasing the number of measurement sites reduces errors and corrects for possible differences in fat distribution among individuals within the same age and gender group.

Anthropometric methods are also applicable as 'surrogate' measurements of visceral adipose tissue. Circumferences are more reliable than skinfolds, and in recent years the most widely used anthropometric technique has been the waist circumference. Waist circumference is measured at the minimum circumference between the iliac crest and the rib cage using an anthropometric tape. It is an indirect measure of visceral adiposity, which is strongly correlated with risk for cardiovascular disease in adults and an adverse lipid profile and hyperinsulinemia in children.

Etiology

Obesity is a multifactorial disease. The relative contributions of genetics and the environment to the etiology of obesity have been evaluated in several studies. Approximately 30–40% of the variance in BMI can be attributed to genetics and 60–70% to the environment. Clearly, the interaction between genes and the environment is fundamental. In a given population, some subjects are genetically predisposed to become obese, but the genotype may be expressed only with adverse environmental situations (i.e., high-fat, energy-dense diets and sedentary lifestyle).

Development of obesity occurs when caloric intake is higher than energy expended. Three metabolic factors have been reported to be predictive of weight gain: a low sedentary energy expenditure, a high respiratory quotient, and a low level of physical activity. Resting metabolic rate is highly correlated with fat-free mass. Sedentary lifestyle has an impact on weight gain. Several other factors are also associated with overweight. Gender, age, race, and socioeconomic status could influence weight gain, with overweight and obesity being more likely among women, older subjects, minority races, those with a low socio-economic status, and those with low levels of education.

It is well-known that obesity runs in families. In fact, high birth weight, maternal diabetes, and obesity in family members are factors that may influence the degree of adiposity. For a subject, if one parent is obese, the odds ratio is approximately 3 for obesity in adulthood, and if both parents are obese, the odds ratio increases to 10. There are critical periods of development for excessive weight gain. The duration of breast-feeding was found to be inversely associated with risk of being obese later in life, possibly mediated by physiologic factors present in human milk. Adolescence is another critical period for development of obesity. The risk of obesity persisting into adulthood is higher among obese adolescents than among younger children.

Lifestyle changes during the past several decades have affected childhood patterns of physical activity as well as diet. Leisure activity (e.g., television and computer games) is increasingly sedentary, and there is generally a decreased amount of routine physical activity. Taken together, these factors play a potential role in the development of the overweight epidemic.

Assessment for Therapy

One of the goals of assessment of overweight/obesity is to decide whom to treat. Three main issues must be evaluated: whether treatment is indicated, whether treatment is safe for the patient, and whether the patient is ready and motivated to lose weight. In addition, routine assessment of eating and activity patterns in adults as well as in children must be considered. Recognition of excessive weight gain relative to linear growth is essential throughout childhood.

Proper identification and classification of obesity through body composition assessment are important steps to initiate before beginning weight-loss treatment. Dietary management, physical activity, surgery, pharmacotherapy, and psychological and familial support must be considered together as part of obesity assessment. Before beginning a weight-loss program, patients should be evaluated for number and severity of cardiovascular risk factors. These conditions may require that treatment be initiated along with weight-loss strategies.

See also: **Adolescents**: Nutritional Requirements. **Body Composition**. **Children**: Nutritional Requirements. **Dietary Intake Measurement**: Methodology; Validation. **Obesity**: Fat Distribution; Childhood Obesity; Complications; Prevention; Treatment.

Further Reading

American Academy of Pediatrics (2003) Policy statement. Prevention of pediatric overweight and obesity. *Pediatrics* **112**: 424–430.

Anonymous (2004) Who pays in the obesity war. *Lancet* **363**: 339.

Aronne LJ (2002) Obesity as a disease: Etiology, treatment, and management consideration for the obese patient. *Obesity Research* **10**(S2): 95–130.

Dietz WH (2004) Overweight in childhood and adolescence. *New England Journal of Medicine* **350**: 855–857.

Eckel RH (2003) Obesity: A disease or a physiologic adaptation for survival. In: Eckel RH (ed.) *Obesity Mechanisms and Clinical Management*, pp. 3–30. Philadelphia: Lippincott Williams & Wilkins.

Friedrich MJ (2002) Epidemic of obesity expands its spread to developing countries. *Journal of American Medical Association* **287**: 1382–1386.

Hedley AA, Ogden CL, Johnson CL et al. (2004) Prevalence of overweight and obesity among U.S. children, adolescents, and adults, 1999–2002. *Journal of the American Medical Association* **291**: 2847–2850.

Heshka S and Allison DB (2001) Is obesity a disease? *International Journal of Obesity* **25**: 1401–1404.

Lobstein T, Baur L, and Uauy R (2004) Obesity in children and young people. A crisis in public health. *Obesity Reviews* **5**(S1): 1–104.

Ogden CL, Flegal KM, Carroll MD, and Johnson CL (2002) Prevalence and trends in overweight among U.S. children and adolescents, 1999–2000. *Journal of the American Medical Association* **288**: 1728–1732.

Peskin GW (2003) Obesity in America. *Archives of Surgery* **138**(4): 354–355.

Pietrobelli A and Heymsfield SB (2002) Establishing body composition in obesity. *Journal of Endocrinological Investigation* **25**: 884–892.

Pietrobelli A, Heymsfield SB, Wang ZM, and Gallagher D (2001) Multi-component body composition models: Recent advances and future directions. *European Journal of Clinical Nutrition* **55**(2): 69–75.

Pietrobelli A and Steinbeck KS (2004) Paediatric obesity. What do we know and are we doing the right thing? *International Journal of Obesity* **28**: 2–3.

Roux L and Donaldson C (2004) Economics and obesity: Causing the problem or evaluating solutions? *Obesity Research* **12**: 173–179.

Fat Distribution

J Stevens and K P Truesdale, University of North Carolina at Chapel Hill, Chapel Hill, NC, USA

In 1956, the French physician, Jean Vague, noted that an upper body, or masculine, fat distribution was associated with adverse health consequences. It has now been clearly demonstrated that obesity-related chronic diseases are associated with the location, as well as the amount, of adipose tissue on the body. Although the relative importance of total adiposity versus type of adiposity continues to be debated, the notion that an 'apple-shaped' (or android) body is associated with greater obesity-related health risks than a 'pear-shaped' (or gynoid) body is well accepted (**Figure 1**). Imaging techniques such as computed tomography (CT) allow measurement of visceral adipose tissue and layers of subcutaneous fat. Anthropometric studies do not provide precise measures of fat depots but nevertheless have provided clues to the causes and consequences of differences in fat distribution. Guidelines are being developed for the use of anthropometric assessments of fat distribution in clinical and public health settings.

Measurement of Fat Distribution

Fat patterning, the distribution of fat, is measured using either imaging or anthropometric

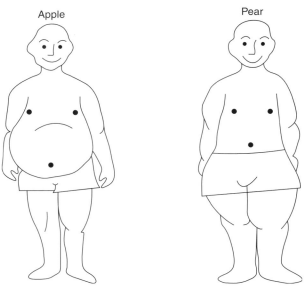

Figure 1 The apple (android) and pear (gynoid) body shapes.

techniques. Measurement has focused on assessment and differentiation of subcutaneous and intraabdominal (visceral) depots; however, recently measurement of fat residing in muscle has become of interest. Imaging techniques have the advantage of providing separate measurements of fat in these three different depots, but they remain too expensive for use in most clinical and community settings. Anthropometric measurements cannot provide a direct assessment of the amount of fat in different depots, but they can provide variables that correlate with assessments from imagining techniques and are quick, inexpensive, and noninvasive.

Imaging Techniques

Computed tomography and magnetic resonance imaging (MRI) are considered the most precise methods for measuring body fat distribution. MRI has the advantage of not exposing subjects to radiation. Dual energy X-ray is primarily used to measure bone mineral content and total body fat. This technique can measure total abdominal fat, but it cannot differentiate between visceral and subcutaneous fat.

Figure 2 shows two different cross-sectional images of the abdomen obtained by MRI. These images are constructed from 256×256 pixels, which vary from white to black with different shades of gray. Each pixel represents $2.4\,mm^2$. The fat regions are depicted as the lighter portions of the images. The subcutaneous fat area delineates the perimeter of the abdomen, whereas the visceral area is contained within the subcutaneous area. Figure 2A represents a cross section of an abdomen with a relatively small subcutaneous fat area in comparison with an enlarged visceral fat area. Figure 2B shows a subject with a small visceral fat-to-subcutaneous fat depot ratio.

CT scans have shown that approximately 12% of fat in normal weight subjects is among and inside muscles. Some researchers advocate considering this fat in a separate compartment, which, from a metabolic standpoint, is more closely related to visceral fat. Some researchers have suggested that subcutaneous fat be separated into deep and superficial layers separated by the 'fascia superficialis.'

Anthropometric Techniques

Anthropometric indices used to measure fat patterning include skinfold thicknesses, circumferences, sagittal diameter, and ratios such as

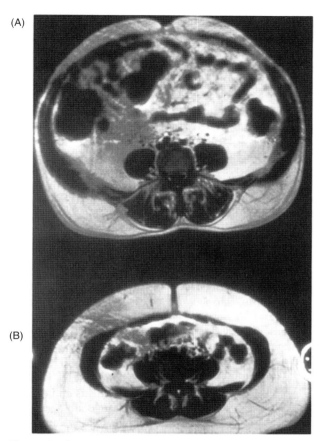

Figure 2 Cross-sectional images of the abdomen obtained by MRI. (A) Small subcutaneous fat area and enlarged visceral fat area. (B) Small visceral fat area in comparison with subcutaneous fat depot.

waist-to-hip, waist-to-thigh, waist-to-height, and subscapular-to-triceps skinfolds. Skinfold thicknesses and skinfold ratios have not been found to be very well correlated with metabolic measurements or with visceral fat and are not recommended for use as indicators of fat patterning. Numerous equations using combinations of anthropometric measurements to predict the amount of visceral fat have not offered substantial improvement over the simpler measurements, and an accurate equation has yet to be developed.

Waist circumference (WC) alone and waist-to-hip ratio (WHR) are the most popular anthropometric methods used to measure fat distribution in both clinical and community settings. Both measures are correlated with visceral fat, with a correlation coefficient (r) generally ranging from 0.5 to 0.8. It is problematic that there is no uniform method of defining the location at which the waist and hip measurement should be assessed (Table 1). Waist

Table 1 Anatomical locations used to measure waist and hip circumferences

Waist circumference
One-third between the xyphoid process and umbilicus
Narrowest part of torso
Midway between xyphoid process and umbilicus
Midway between lower rib and iliac crest
One inch (~2.5 cm) above umbilicus
Level of umbilicus
Level of iliac crest
Immediately below the lowest rib
Immediately above the iliac crest

Hip circumference
Largest horizontal circumference around the buttocks
Level of iliac crest
Maximal circumference between superior border of iliac crest
    and thigh region 4 cm below superior iliac crest

circumferences measured at four sites (immediately below the lowest rib, at the narrowest point, midpoint between the lowest rib and the iliac crest, and immediately above the iliac crest) have been compared and found to differ from each other. Other work has shown that the highest correlations with risk factors were obtained when WHR was calculated as the waist measured at the point midway between the lower rib margin and iliac crest (approximately 1 inch (~2.5 cm) above the umbilicus) or when the waist was measured at the umbilicus and hips measured at the widest point of the buttocks. Although two different waist measurements have been demonstrated to perform equally well, the bony landmark measurement (the point midway between the lower rib margin and iliac crest) may be preferred since the umbilicus may shift position when an individual gains or loses weight. The World Health Organization (WHO) has recommended measuring the waist at the midpoint between the lowest rib and the iliac crest, whereas immediately above the iliac crest is the site recommended by the National Institutes of Health (NIH).

Sagittal diameter, the height of the abdomen measured with the subject in the supine position, can be measured anthropometrically or by imaging. **Figure 3** shows a technique for the anthropometric measurement of sagittal diameter using a caliper. Measurement is usually taken at the largest supine anteroposterior diameter between the xyphoid process and umbilicus. Some studies have found sagittal diameter to be a better indicator of visceral fat than WHR. Correlations between sagittal diameter and amount of visceral fat range from $r = 0.51$ to $r = 0.87$, with higher correlations occurring when sagittal diameter is measured using imaging

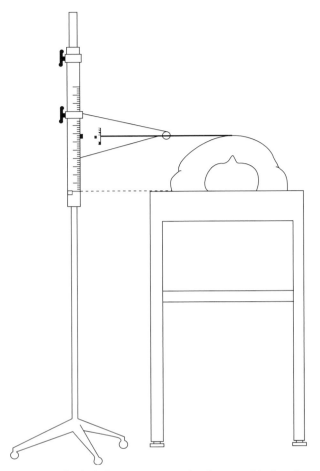

Figure 3 Sagittal diameter measured anthropometrically using calipers.

techniques. In general, correlations tend to be higher in men than women.

Metabolic Characteristics of Visceral and Subcutaneous Fat

The main function of adipose tissue is to store and break down fat based on energy excess or need, respectively. The uptake of fat is regulated by the enzyme lipoprotein lipase (LPL). This enzyme hydrolyzes triacylglycerols into free fatty acids, which can then be transported into the adipocyte and reesterified for storage. Greater LPL activity is associated with greater accumulation of fat. In premenopausal women, its activity is higher in the gluteal–femoral adipose areas than in the abdominal areas. The opposite is true in men, in whom LPL activity is the same or higher in the abdominal adipose areas than in the gluteal–femoral regions.

The breakdown of fat (lipolysis) is regulated by the enzyme hormone-sensitive lipase (HSL). This enzyme releases free fatty acids, which are then released into the bloodstream and taken up by tissues, with the exception of the brain and red blood cells, for energy use or storage. The rate of basal lipolysis is higher in gluteal–femoral fat tissue than in abdominal tissue in both men and women. This may be due to greater cell size in that region. In the abdominal area, basal lipolysis is higher in subcutaneous fat than in visceral fat. However, when stimulated hormonally, rates of lipolysis may differ between men and women. Lipolytic rates have been shown to be higher in the visceral compared to the subcutaneous region in men, whereas the opposite trend is seen in women.

Regulators of Lipolysis and Fat Storage

The processes of lipolysis and fat storage are regulated by hormonal factors, which either enhance or suppress the activities of HSL and LPL. Through the action of glucocorticoid receptors, glucocorticoids enhance LPL activity and promote abdominal deposition of fat. The density of glucocorticoid receptors is greater in the visceral abdominal depot than in the subcutaneous abdominal depot. Therefore, an increase in glucocorticoid secretion is associated with increases in abdominal fat deposition compared to other fat depots.

Insulin favors fat storage by increasing LPL and decreasing HSL activity. Insulin has stronger antilypolytic effects in adipose located in the abdominal region compared to the femoral regions in both men and women. Paradoxically, insulin binding is stronger in the gluteal–femoral region than the abdominal region. Therefore, it has been hypothesized that insulin regulates lipolysis at the postreceptor level.

Catecholamines regulate lipolysis through α_2- and β-adrenoreceptors. The β-adrenoreceptors increase lipolysis, whereas the α_2-adrenoreceptor inhibits it. Although both the α_2- and the β-adrenoreceptors coexist in adipose tissue, they are regionally specific such that there may be an excess of one type of receptor relative to the other in various adipose regions. The lipolytic effect of catecholamines is 10–20 times greater in the abdominal region than in the gluteal–femoral region, as marked by a two-fold increase in the number of β-adrenoreceptors in both sexes. The lipolytic action of catecholamines is more pronounced intraabdominally than in the abdominal subcutaneous tissue. Sex differences are displayed with the α-adrenoreceptor. Although the number of receptors is similar in both sexes, the sensitivity of the receptors is reduced by a factor of 10–15 in the abdominal compared with the gluteal–femoral region.

Sex hormones, such as estrogen, testosterone, and progesterone, also affect the balance of fat accumulation/mobilization, although their effects vary in men and women and the mechanisms are not clearly understood. Studies show that estrogen decreases LPL expression and activity in adipose tissue. It has been shown that testosterone stimulates lipolysis by increasing the number of β-adrenoreceptors. Estrogen and progesterone, on the other hand, stimulate fat storage and inhibit lipolysis, preferentially in the gluteal–femoral area compared to the abdominal area.

An increased androgenic profile is associated with upper body fat accumulation in women, but studies on men are conflicting. Significant inverse associations between fat distribution and testosterone have been found in population studies on men. Reduced visceral fat has also been observed when testosterone treatment was administered to men. These findings challenge the hypothesis that an androgenic hormone profile contributes to a more 'male type' of fat pattern and the associated metabolic sequelae.

The controversy over the effect of sex hormones on fat distribution is complicated by the metabolism of sex hormones. Sex hormone-binding globulin (SHBG) binds circulating testosterone and estrogen. Decreased SHBG concentration may be associated with an android shape. Therefore, studies need to distinguish between total circulating and unbound sex hormones and SHBG.

Sequelae of Altered Metabolism in Visceral Fat

Intraabdominal adipose tissue has metabolic characteristics that are different from those of adipose tissue from other sites. These differences seem to be most pronounced in the regions that are drained by the portal circulation. These 'portal adipose tissues' have a sensitive system for the mobilization of free fatty acids due to a preponderance of β-adrenergic receptors and little α-adrenergic inhibition.

The hypothesis has been advanced that the heightened responsiveness of intraabdominal fat to lipolytic agents results in increased lipolysis with venous drainage of the released free fatty acids directly to the liver. These fatty acids may contribute to increases in triacylglycerol synthesis and hyperinsulinemia secondary to decrements in insulin degradation. Hyperinsulinemia could produce insulin resistance and eventually type 2 diabetes in susceptible individuals. However, the hypothesis that increased release of free fatty acids from intraabdominal adipose tissue leads to insulin resistance through effects on the liver lacks supporting evidence *in vivo*.

The proposed mechanism of action of fat patterning on metabolic syndrome is linked to hyperinsulinemia. Hyperinsulinemia may lead to increased blood pressure through increased sympathetic stimulation of the vessels, heart, and kidneys. In addition, insulin resistance combined with a relative increase in androgenic activity may lead to an unfavorable lipid profile. In addition to the effects of free fatty acids on insulin and glucose, an increased visceral depot decreases the activity of LPL. This causes an increase in very low-density lipoprotein (VLDL) secretion and a decrease in its catabolism. The production of high-density lipoprotein (HDL) therefore decreases, the transfer of lipids (i.e., VLDL to LDL and HDL) increases, and an enrichment of triacylglycerols results.

In obesity and type 2 diabetes, there is an increased content of lipids within and around muscle fibers. Researchers have suggested that the accumulation of triacylglycerols within the skeletal muscle may play an important role in insulin resistance. In obese individuals with elevated amounts of visceral adipose tissue, there is a strong correlation between visceral adipose tissue and insulin resistance independent of subcutaneous (abdominal and nonabdominal) adipose tissue and cardiovascular fitness. It has been suggested that the discrepancies in the literature regarding the independent effect of visceral or subcutaneous adipose tissue on insulin resistance are due to the large variations of abdominal obesity within the study populations.

Leptin is a hormone that is produced in the adipose cells and can act on the hunger center in the hypothalamus to reduce hunger and appetite and thereby lower food intake. Plasma leptin levels are correlated with body fat. Researchers have discovered a leptin receptor gene that is responsible for obesity due to the mutation or absence of the gene. This condition is extremely rare in humans. In general, in obese humans the leptin levels are elevated (hyperleptinemia).

There is a progressive increase in plasma levels during puberty in girls due to the increase in body fat during this period and in response to the effect of estrogens. Circulating leptin levels tend to decrease in response to testosterone in boys, thus resulting in higher plasma leptin levels in women compared to men. Leptin levels are also affected by insulin and glucocorticoids.

Correlates and Possible Determinants of Fat Distribution

A large number of studies have examined correlations between fat distribution and genetic, behavioral, and physiological variables. Many factors, including heredity, overall fatness, gender, age, smoking, alcohol consumption, physical activity, and ethnicity, are associated with either an android or a gynoid shape. The underlying reasons for the observed associations between these variables and fat patterning remain to be elucidated. Correlates of fat distribution are important to understand since they may confound relationships between fat patterning and physiological outcomes or morbidity or mortality outcomes. There is evidence that body shape and amount of visceral fat are partially determined by genetics. After eliminating effects of age and overall fatness, studies have shown that heritable factors can account for as much as 20–50% of the variability in waist-to-hip ratio.

Fat distribution becomes more central or android as overall fatness increases. The correlation between overall fatness and fat patterning indices ranges from $r = 0.5$ to 0.9, depending on which measure of fat patterning is used. The more obese an individual, the more difficult it is to measure the waist and hip circumferences and the higher the measurement error.

Fat distribution has long been known to vary by gender, with men more android (apple shaped) than women, who are more gynoid (pear shaped). Men have a higher WHR and significantly more intra-abdominal adipose tissue than women. During weight gain in normal weight men, fat is preferentially deposited abdominally in the subcutaneous and visceral regions—proportionately more in the upper compared to the lower abdomen. In men, little fat is deposited in the gluteal–femoral regions until they become obese. Women have a higher percentage of body fat and higher proportion of fat in the gluteal–femoral regions than men. The gender differences are sufficiently large that recommended cutpoints for indices of fat distribution must be gender specific.

Aging is accompanied by changes in both weight and fat distribution. The largest increase in body weight occurs between young adulthood and middle adulthood. Independent of weight gain, abdominal fat increases with aging. This increase tends to be most pronounced between young adulthood and middle age in men and between middle age and old age in women (related to menopausal status).

Although cigarette smokers tend to be leaner than nonsmokers, they have more central adiposity (as indicated by larger waist circumference and WHRs) compared to nonsmokers, after the effects of age and body mass index (BMI) are eliminated. Furthermore, WHR increases progressively with an increase in the number of cigarettes smoked daily. The WHR increases with increasing 24-h cotinine excretion, indicating that central fat accumulation is dependent on the dose of smoke inhaled. Some studies have found a more androgenic hormone profile in cigarette smokers, although this finding has been inconsistent. Increased cortisol secretion, an endocrine response to stressors associated with upper body fat deposition, may explain some of the association between smoking, alcohol consumption, and fat distribution.

Although alcohol consumption has been postulated to be correlated with fat distribution, studies have been inconclusive. There is evidence that beer and spirits are associated with higher levels of WHR, whereas wine is not. Not only frequency but also intensity of alcohol consumption may be important. One study showed that frequency of alcohol consumption was inversely associated, but intensity was positively associated, with abdominal adiposity (measured by sagittal diameter), even after the effects of age, education, physical activity, smoking, and grams of alcohol had been controlled. After combining the effects of frequency and intensity, the high frequency (daily) but low intensity (<1 drink/day) group had the lowest sagittal diameter, whereas the low frequency (<weekly) but high intensity (>3 drinks/day) group had the largest sagittal diameter.

Physical activity is inversely correlated with fat distribution in both men and women. Negative associations exist between WHR and various sports and exercise indices after controlling for the effects of BMI, smoking, and education. There is evidence that activity may be associated with a preferential mobilization of abdominal fat. Endurance training has been shown to increase aerobic fitness and decrease body mass and fat mass. Resistance training results in an increase in fat-free mass and muscle strength.

Fat distribution varies by ethnicity. African Americans have less visceral fat than whites at the same BMI, whereas Asians have a larger percentage of visceral fat. At the same BMI, African Americans have greater bone density and muscle mass than whites. Asians have smaller body frames, less muscle mass, and a larger percentage of fat mass at the same BMI as African Americans and whites. A study comparing migrant and British-born South Asian women to a general population of women in Scotland found that after controlling for the effect of age, migrant South Asians had larger waist circumference and WHR. However, after also controlling for physical activity, cigarette smoking, alcohol consumption, and parity, only WHR remained different between the two groups.

Fat Distribution and Disease Risk

Numerous studies have examined associations between fat patterning and mortality and morbidity.

Since fat distribution is correlated with age as well other risk factors for disease, such as smoking, alcohol consumption, physical activity, and menopause in women, it is important to control for the effects of these variables in order to obtain an estimate of the independent effect of central obesity on morbidity. The impact of some of these correlates of fat distribution may be subtle and unlikely to seriously distort relationships between fat patterning and disease. However, age, the ultimate risk factor for disease and death, is sufficiently highly correlated with fat distribution to result in substantial distortion. Similarly, cigarette smoking is related adequately strongly to fat patterning and to various diseases and outcomes to make analyses that do not adjust for smoking difficult to interpret.

The large correlation between fat patterning and overall adiposity also influences the interpretation of results, making it difficult to differentiate between the two effects. Some researchers compare the size of the correlation between fat distribution (usually measured as WHR) and total adiposity (usually measured as BMI) in an attempt to show the relative importance of each. Others examine effects within tertiles (or other categories) of BMI and WHR simultaneously or test for an independent effect of WHR or BMI in multiple regression models that include both variables. In the latter type of analysis, the associations of both WHR and BMI with an outcome can be greatly reduced or even disappear because of collinearity between the two measures.

Researchers have found positive correlations between fasting glucose, insulin, blood pressure, total cholesterol, LDL cholesterol, and triacylglycerols using imaging techniques, sagittal diameter, waist circumference, and WHR in most, but not all, studies. Visceral fat and HDL cholesterol are inversely associated. The strength of the associations varies but tends to be largest for triacylglycerols. Associations are reduced after controlling for BMI and age.

There is strong evidence to link waist circumference and WHR with the risk of developing type 2 diabetes, even after eliminating the effects of age, smoking, BMI, and other important correlates. An individual who is obese (>150% ideal body weight) and has an elevated WHR (>0.8) may have as much as a 10-fold increased risk for developing type 2 diabetes compared with an individual who is of normal weight (<120% ideal body weight) and has a low WHR (<0.72).

Elevated WHR has been positively associated with cardiovascular disease in some population studies, although not as consistently as diabetes. Scientists have recognized that several of the cardiovascular disease risk factors, including abdominal obesity, cluster in individuals. This cluster of risk factors is referred to as metabolic syndrome. The other risk factors in metabolic syndrome are insulin resistance/glucose intolerance, dyslipidemia (high triaclyglycerols and low HDL cholesterol), and high blood pressure.

Applications

Waist circumference can be used to assess obesity-related health risks in public health and clinical settings. Because it consists of only one measurement instead of two, it introduces less measurement error than WHR. A large waist has been shown to reflect both generalized obesity and centralized body fat distribution, which suggests that waist circumference could replace both BMI and WHR as a simple indicator of the need for weight management. Also, waist circumference tends to be more highly correlated with visceral fat than WHR.

It has been shown that hip circumference alone is inversely associated with cardiovascular disease risk after controlling for age, BMI, smoking, and waist circumference. Therefore, some predictive information may be lost if hip circumference is not assessed. If an index of body shape, independent of total body fatness, is desired the WHR may be preferred over waist alone because it is less highly correlated with total adiposity. Waist-to-hip ratio is a widely accepted form of fat patterning assessment. It is a good predictor of disease and metabolic disorders, with an increasing WHR indicating increased risk. Cutpoints used to define elevated WHR range from 0.90–1.00 in men to 0.80–0.90 in women.

Guidelines for the use of waist circumference in combination with BMI have been issued by NIH and WHO. NIH guidelines use BMI cutoffs for an initial assessment of overweight and obesity and recommend waist circumference cutoffs as a supplementary indicator of health risk. Increased relative risk for the development of obesity-associated risk factors in most adults is predicted for adults within the BMI range of 25–35 when the waist is ≥ 102 cm (40 in.) in men and ≥ 88 cm (35 in.) in women.

Conclusions

The relationship of body fat distribution to metabolic abnormalities and disease has now been well recognized. Individuals with a more android than gynoid body shape tend to have a more adverse metabolic profile and an increased risk for type 2 diabetes and cardiovascular disease.

Although much has been learned about fat distribution, there are several issues that need further exploration. The question of whether body type can be changed through behavior needs to be more fully addressed. Standardized anthropometric measurements need to be established, and the implications of differences in fat distribution among ethnic groups need to be elucidated. A better understanding of the risks associated with fat residing in muscle is needed, and this information must be integrated with what is known about visceral and subcutaneous fat. Finally, more research is needed to identify mechanisms of action. An increased abdominal depot may not necessarily be the cause of metabolic disturbances but an effect of underlying genetic and endocrine abnormalities.

See also: **Adipose Tissue. Body Composition. Diabetes Mellitus**: Etiology and Epidemiology; Classification and Chemical Pathology. **Exercise**: Beneficial Effects. **Hyperlipidemia**: Overview; Nutritional Management. **Lipids**: Chemistry and Classification. **Obesity**: Definition, Etiology and Assessment.

Further Reading

Aronne LJ and Segal KR (2002) Adiposity and fat distribution outcome measures: Assessment and clinical implications. *Obesity Research* **10**(supplement 1): 14S–21S.

Bosello O and Zamboni M (2000) Visceral obesity and metabolic syndrome. *Obesity Review* **1**: 47–56.

Deurenberg P, Deurenberg-Yap M, and Guricci S (2002) Asians are different from Caucasians and from each other in their body mass index/body fat per cent relationship. *Obesity Review* **3**: 141–146.

Jakicic JM, Donnelly JE, Jawad AP *et al.* (1993) Association between blood lipids and different measures of body fat distribution: Effects of BMI and age. *International Journal of Obesity* **17**: 131–137.

Kelley DE, Goodpaster BH, and Storlien L (2002) Muscle triglyceride and insulin resistance. *Annual Review of Nutrition* **22**: 325–346.

Lean MEJ, Han TS, Bush H *et al.* (2001) Ethnic differences in anthropometric and lifestyle measures related to coronary heart disease risk between South Asian, Italian and general-population British women living in the west of Scotland. *Internation Journal of Obesity* **2001**: 1800–1805.

Lissner L, Björkelund C, Heitmann BL, Seidell JC, and Bengtsson C (2001) Larger hip circumference independently predicts health and longevity in a Swedish female cohort. *Obesity Research* **9**: 644–646.

Molarius A and Seidell JC (1998) Selection of anthropometric indicators for classification of abdominal fatness—A critical review. *International Journal of Obesity* **22**: 719–727.

National Institutes of Health, National Heart Lung and Blood Institute (1998) Clinical guidelines on the identification, evaluation, and treatment of overweight and obesity in adults. The Evidence Reports. *Obesity Research* 6(supplement 2): 53S. [Available at www.nhlbi.nih.gov/guidelines]

Seidell JC, Kahn HS, Williamson DF, Lissner L, and Valdez R (2001) Report from a Centers for Disease Control and Prevention workshop on use of adult anthropometry for public health and primary health care. *American Journal of Clinical Nutrition* 73: 123–126.

Smith SR, Lovejoy JC, Greenway F *et al.* (2001) Contribution of total body fat, abdominal subcutaneous adipose tissue compartments, and visceral adipose tissue to the metabolic complications of obesity. *Metabolism* 50: 426–435.

Stevens J, Couper D, Pankow J *et al.* (2001) Sensitivity and specificity of anthropometrics for the prediction of diabetes in a biracial cohort. *Obesity Research* 9: 696–705.

Turcato E, Bosello O, Francesco V Di *et al.* (2000) Waist circumference and abdominal sagittal diameter as surrogates of body fat distribution in the elderly: Their relation with cardiovascular risk factors. *International Journal of Obesity* 24: 1005–1010.

Wang J, Thornton JC, Bari S *et al.* (2003) Comparisons of waist circumferences measured at 4 sites. *American Journal of Clinical Nutrition* 77: 379–384.

Childhood Obesity

E M E Poskitt, London School of Hygiene and Tropical Medicine, London, UK

This article discusses obesity in children and adolescents with regard to prevalence, epidemiology, clinical features, and management/prevention. Obesity not associated with a recognized underlying clinical condition is the focus of this article since this represents far the majority of children with obesity. However, obesity associated with congenital or acquired medical conditions is discussed briefly. Management and prevention are also discussed.

Obesity is increasing in prevalence among children in virtually all developed countries. In the United Kingdom, 8.5% (twice the rate of 10 years ago) of 6-year-old and 15% (three times the rate of 10 years ago) of 15-year-old children are obese. Childhood obesity is also increasing in prevalence among the affluent in less well-developed countries. Since it has been estimated that in Western countries one-third of obese adults were obese in childhood, and since both adult and adolescent obesity carry significant risk of health complications, obesity in childhood is currently seen as a concern for families, communities, and nations.

Body Composition in Childhood and Definition of Childhood Obesity

Obesity is an excess of body fat. However, the percentage of body weight that is fat varies normally throughout childhood (**Table 1**). The infant is born with modest amounts of fat. More than 50% of the energy in breast milk comes from fat, and young infants lay down fat very rapidly so that in the 4 or 5 months that it takes a normal infant to double birth weight, the weight of fat in the body has tripled. By 6 months of age, infants are increasing weight-bearing activity and fat deposition slows relative to lean tissue growth. From 1 year onward, there is a natural process of slimming with less fat than lean tissue deposited so that the child of 5 years often has a lower percentage body weight as fat than at any other time in life. This is followed by the 'adiposity rebound,' when fat deposition accelerates only to slow again with the onset of the pubertal growth spurt in males. In pubertal girls, very brief slimming early in the female growth spurt is followed by vigorous fat deposition particularly around the breasts and hips.

Assessment of Overweight and Obesity in Childhood

Precise methods of estimating body fat are complicated and expensive. There are no accepted age-related 'norms' for percentage body weight as fat in childhood. For these reasons, anthropometric indices involving weight and height are widely used to estimate relative fatness. Such methods are relatively simple, noninvasive, well tolerated, and can be used in clinical practice and large population studies. However, they provide only indirect measures of fatness.

Weight can be related to height and age in various ways. Until recently, there was no consensus

Table 1 Percentage of body weight as fat at different ages in childhood

Age (years)	% body weight as fat	
Birth	11[a]	
0.3	25[a]	
1.0	24[a]	
	Males	*Females*
5	12.5[b]	15.3[b]
10	17.6[b]	16.0[b]
15	11.4[b]	23.3[b]

[a]Fomon SJ (1974) *Infant Nutrition. 2nd edition*, Philadelphia: WB Saunders, p. 69.
[b]Widdowson EM (1974) *Changes in body proportions and compositions during growth*.
In Davis JA, Dobbing J. *Scientific Foundations of Paediatrics*. London: Wm Heinemann. pp. 152–63.

definition of overweight/obesity from weights in relation to height and age. In adults, body mass index (BMI; weight in kg/(height in m)^2) is used as a proxy for fatness. A BMI >25 kg/m^2 (overweight) is associated with a significant increase in the risk of mortality and with an increased prevalence of complications of obesity. In childhood, BMI varies with age in a nonlinear fashion. Since at different ages children tend to retain their growth positions in relation to those of their peers, the International Obesity Task Force has defined childhood overweight and obesity as those points on the BMI centile, or standard deviation, for age distribution charts that, if followed to the age 18, would meet the adult cutoff points for overweight and obesity (BMI, 25 and 30 kg/m^2). This definition involves no direct assessment of body fat or lean body mass for age. It needs evaluating against other evidence of excessive body fat and the prevalence of complications of obesity, particularly since it presumes a constant prevalence of obesity in childhood at every age, which clinically seems unlikely. Nevertheless, the method does allow the opportunity to compare relative fatness between different studies and to demonstrate changes in population distribution of BMI for age over time.

Waist circumference is widely used in adult assessment of obesity because high waist circumference is associated with increased abdominal fat and increased risk for the morbid complications of obesity in adult life. Consensus regarding cutoff points for normal waist circumference measurements in childhood has not been reached, but high (compared with age-related populations) waist circumferences do seem to predispose to developing obesity comorbidities.

Risk Factors for Childhood Obesity

There is no clear evidence that obese individuals eat more or exercise less than their nonobese peers. Methods of measuring energy intakes and outputs are not precise when used over time and in community settings. The range of normal requirements and normal basal metabolic rates is large and obscures the energy imbalances of individuals. However, for the individual, obesity occurs when energy intake (food) exceeds the energy expenditure (basal metabolism, physical activity, growth, counteracting infection, maintaining body temperature, and thermodynamic action of food).

Familial Obesity

Most studies from developed countries show that approximately 80% of obese children have at least one parent, and 40% have both parents, overweight or obese. Twin and adoption studies indicate that genetic factors play a role in this family predisposition to obesity, although lifestyles almost certainly also influence familial similarities in habitus. In most cases of familial obesity, there is no recognised genetic explanation or apparent Mendelian inheritance, suggesting a genetic susceptibility expressed in an obesogenic environment.

Socioeconomic and Environmental Deprivation

Although it is the affluent who tend to become obese in countries undergoing industrialization, it is children from socioeconomically deprived environments in Europe and from families in which child care and nurture are poor irrespective of income who show the greatest predisposition to obesity.

Early Feeding

There is no consistent evidence that breast feeding protects children from later obesity. Any associations between breast feeding and a low prevalence of obesity may simply indicate that both obesity and a low prevalence of breast feeding are common in socioeconomically deprived communities. Furthermore, breast feeding is not a passive process but one that involves maternal emotions and close mother–child contact. The process of feeding and recognizing readiness to feed may teach a mother subtle subconscious understanding of her child's needs. Thus, the process of breast feeding may have positive influences on mothers' attitudes to child nurture—attitudes that are less readily acquired through formula feeding. Likewise, studies of early weaning, although occasionally showing evidence of an association with later obesity, are certainly not consistent in finding relationships between weaning practices and later overweight. Early feeding studies can never be double-blind controlled, and differences may only reflect common aspects of nurture rather than specific effects of a particular infant feeding procedure.

Diet and Dietary Change

Studies from several countries suggest that the childhood obesity epidemic has developed despite secular trends toward lower energy intakes by children. These estimates may have failed to account for recent increases in food eaten outside the home in the United Kingdom and other countries. The eating habits of most families in industrialized countries have changed during the past 30 years in ways that seem likely to make it easy for individuals to overeat. Foods are readily available and children have money to buy them. Much advertizing of snack foods is aimed at children. Manufactured foods have varied forms and packaging. Small differences in flavor or appearance may reduce the satiety effect usually associated with eating large amounts of the same food. Most snacks aimed at children and the well-advertised prepared-before-sale meals are energy dense and high in saturated fats, refined carbohydrates, and sugar. In addition, the portion sizes in restaurants and of confectionery items have increased. It is too easy to eat without being aware of energy intake.

Physical Activity

Trends to lower energy expenditure, as well as dietary change, must have significance for the development of obesity. Opportunities for vigorous physical activity in sport have declined in many schools and communities, but the increase in long periods of almost complete inactivity (such as when watching television) may be having greater effects on children's nutritional status than the loss of relatively brief periods of intense activity. Studies in the United States and Mexico indicate that in adolescent boys obesity increases in proportion to the hours spent watching television.

Characteristics of Obese Children

Children without Recognizable Pathology

Obese prepubertal children are relatively tall for age (many in the upper quartile and most in the upper half of the population distribution for height). Advanced growth may be associated with advanced maturity of bones (advanced bone age), early onset of puberty, and cessation of growth with only average stature in adult life. However, some children remain tall and obese into adult life, and others slim dramatically with the adolescent growth spurt. It is not clear whether obesity drives accelerated maturation or whether obesity is one manifestation of a predisposition to exuberant growth of both lean and fat tissue also expressed by early puberty.

Obesity Associated with Recognized Medical Condition

There are conditions in which obesity is part of a recognized genetic defect, clinical syndrome, or acquired pathological condition (**Table 2**). Together, these conditions account for only a very small

Table 2 Specific conditions associated with obesity in childhood

Conditions	Inheritance	Clinical example
Congenital conditions		
Congenital obesity	Single gene defect affecting leptin metabolism	Congenital leptin deficiency
		Leptin receptor defect
		Prohormone convertase-1 defect
		Melanocortin-4 receptor defect
		Peroxisome proliferators activated receptor
		POMC deficiency
Inherited syndromes associated with childhood obesity	Autosomal dominant	Biemond's syndrome
	Autosomal recessive	Alstrom's syndrome
		Bardet–Biedl syndrome
		Biemond's syndrome (some)
		Carpenter's syndrome
		Cohen's syndrome
	X-linked recessive	Borjeson–Forssman–Lehmann syndrome
Inherited syndromes affecting mobility	X-linked recessive	Duchenne muscular dystrophy
	Polygenic inheritance	Spina bifida
Inherited disorders of growth	Autosomal dominant	Achondroplasia
Chromosomal abnormalities	Deletion or uniparental disomy for q11–q13 fragment of chromosome 15	Prader–Willi–Labhart syndrome
	Trisomy 21	Down's syndrome
	Abnormalities of sex chromosomes	Klinefelter's syndrome
		Turner's syndrome
Acquired conditions		
	Hormonal abnormalities	Hypothyroidism
		Growth, hormone deficiency
		Cushing's syndrome
		Polycystic ovarian syndrome
	Hypothalamic damage	Hydrocephalus
		Meningoencephalitis
	Drug treatment	Steroid treatment
		Sodium valproate

proportion of obese children. With the exception of very rare single gene defects in leptin metabolism, obesity is a secondary feature in these conditions and presentation is usually for some other aspect of the condition. Single gene defects affecting leptin are associated with progressive gross obesity from early life and may respond with dramatic fat loss with leptin treatment. Where obesity is only a part of a spectrum of abnormalities, common associated features are short stature, developmental delay, and craniofacial and other bony abnormalities.

Chromosomal abnormalities are more frequent causes of a predisposition to obesity. Prader–Willi syndrome, due to deletion or uniparental disomy of part of the long arm of chromosome 15, is associated with characteristic facies, small hands and feet with tapering fingers, hypogonadism, early hypotonia, difficulty feeding, and initially failure to thrive. From the second year of life many of these children show voracious appetite, progressive obesity, and negative behavior (stealing food and refusing to follow a diet). Many also commonly have psychodevelopmental problems with moderate mental retardation that exacerbates the difficulties maintaining normal weight for height and age. Gross obesity commonly leads to early death associated with hypoventilation (Pickwickian syndrome) and/or complications of type 2 diabetes mellitus.

Down's syndrome children are also prone to develop obesity in late childhood and adolescence. This is generally unrelated to recognized pathophysiological explanations for the obesity, although the syndrome is associated with an increased incidence of autoimmune thyroiditis and hypothyroidism (which exacerbates obesity).

Obesity may be an associated feature of other pathology in childhood. Endocrine problems, such as hypothyroidism and Cushing's syndrome, lead to obesity, but linear growth retardation does also, which often draws attention to the problem before obesity is severe. Hypothalamic damage (e.g., hydrocephalus and meningoencephalitis) and problems leading to immobility (e.g., spina bifida and Duchenne's muscular dystrophy) may also predispose to obesity. Nonpathological childhood obesity is usually associated with normal intelligence, relatively tall stature before puberty, and no overt abnormalities, so brief assessment of growth, general health, and intelligence usually distinguishes obese children for whom investigation for possible underlying pathology is required.

Complications of Childhood Obesity

Childhood obesity used to be considered relatively free of serious medical complications compared to adult obesity, although psychological consequences were recognised as common. Today, many obese children and adolescents show evidence of significant pathophysiological changes. Thus, the increasingly gross obesity of children and adolescents in North America, western Europe, and some other affluent societies has become a matter of major public health concern.

Cosmetic Problems

Orthopedic problems Flat feet and knock knee, perhaps related to the excess weight and need to internally rotate the knees to accommodate fat thighs when bringing the legs together, are common and can lead to ungainly gait. Slipped upper femoral epiphysis is a more serious problem, which is particularly common in overweight young adolescents and may also be associated with hormonal abnormalities such as hypothyroidism.

Skin problems Intertrigo, seborrheic eczema, and thrush are common in the thick heavy skinfolds of severely obese children. Pink or pale cutaneous striae, distinct from the purplish striae resulting from thinning of subcutaneous tissues in Cushing's syndrome, are common on the abdomen and upper limbs and may be a source of embarrassment. Hirsutes (abnormal facial and body hair) occurs particularly in adolescent girls with polycystic ovarian syndrome, which is associated with obesity and insulin resistance. Acanthosis nigricans, a velvety, pigmented, thickening of the skin usually at the back of the neck, is another important marker for insulin resistance, affecting up to 90% of children with type 2 diabetes mellitus.

Psychological problems Some overweight/obese children maintain high self-esteem and have little concern about their body image. These children may excel in sports in which their excess weight and tall stature are advantageous. However, many obese and overweight children have low self-esteem, dissatisfaction with their body image, and difficulty with peer relationships. Often, they underachieve at school. For some obese children, psychological problems antedate the obesity. Low self-esteem and difficulty with peer relationships have led to withdrawal, inactivity, and seeking solace in food. For other obese children, however, obesity is the prime cause of their psychological problems. Studies using silhouettes of figures with different body builds show that most children perceive obese silhouettes very negatively, preferring those portrayed by slimmer figures as friends.

Severe Complications

Adult obesity The extent to which childhood obesity progresses to adult obesity depends on the ages of children and adults at the time of study, the severity of obesity, the duration of obesity, and the family history of obesity. In one study fewer than 20% of males younger than 17 years of age remained obese as 35-year-old adults, whereas 20–39.9% of females younger than 17 years of age were still obese at 35 years of age. The probability of being obese at age 35 increased with increasing age and increasing BMI in childhood at the time of study. Where there is a strong family history of obesity in adult life, it seems likely that the obese child will follow the family pattern. Progression from child to adult obesity still only accounts for a minority of obese adults, although with the increasing prevalence of childhood obesity, this may change since it is highly unlikely that equal proportions of fat and thin children become obese adults.

Type 2 diabetes mellitus and the metabolic syndrome Although hyperinsulinemia has long been recognized from research studies in obese children, overt type 2 diabetes mellitus has been considered a rarity in childhood until recently. Studies in the United States show that among grossly obese children, type 2 diabetes mellitus is now disturbingly common, not only in adolescence but also in children younger than 10 years old. The problem is less common, but certainly present, in Europe also. Although hyperinsulinemia seems most prevalent in obese children from the Indian subcontinent, hyperinsulinemia and overt type 2 diabetes mellitus are also described in obese Caucasian children. Seventy-five percent of UK children with type 2 diabetes mellitus are overweight and 50% have a family history of type 2 diabetes mellitus. Girls are proportionally more likely (3:2) to develop type 2 diabetes than boys.

The metabolic syndrome (insulin resistance syndrome; syndrome X) is a clustering of problems associated with resistance to insulin and/or hyperinsulinemia that includes obesity, high central (i.e., intra- and peri-abdominal) distribution of fat, hypertension, and dyslipidemia. Females with polycystic ovarian syndrome also show clustering of these features. The criteria for diagnosis of the insulin resistance syndrome in childhood have not been defined, but some obese children show clustering of extreme values for the parameters of the metabolic syndrome. Hypertension, hyperinsulinemia, and dyslipidemia in obese children are indications for vigorous intervention to prevent morbidity and early mortality.

Pickwickian syndrome Very severe obesity may be associated with hypoventilation and/or upper respiratory obstruction with sleep apnoea. (The sleepy fat boy in Charles Dicken's *Pickwick Papers* is the origin of the syndrome's name.) Underventilation leads to increased circulating carbon dioxide levels, which may precipitate pulmonary hypertension and right-sided heart failure. Rising circulating carbon dioxide levels may result in the respiratory centre of the brain ceasing to respond to carbon dioxide buildup and instead responding to falling oxygen levels as stimulus to breathe. Thus, if affected individuals are given oxygen because of increasing cyanosis, the stimulus to breathe may be removed with potentially disastrous consequences.

Management

Goals

Ideally, the goal of fat reduction in obesity should be to restore normal body composition and retain it for the rest of life. However, evidence suggests that morbidity and mortality are reduced with even small reductions in excess fat. Thus, loss of some excess fat and the pursuit of healthy eating and activity may be beneficial even if normal fatness is not restored. Parents and children need realistic guidance on achievable goals and on the time required to achieve them. Fat reduction programs should be sustainable, able to maintain normal linear growth, and follow overall healthy lifestyle practices.

For young children, it may not be necessary to lose weight since the normal rates of weight and height gain mean that keeping weight stationary while linear growth occurs allows children to grow 'into their weight.' However, most children presenting for help with obesity are so overweight that it would require years of static weights for current weights to decrease to normal for their heights. Gradual weight reduction should aim for weight losses of approximately 500–1000 g/month. Dramatic weight losses suggest excessive energy deficit with perhaps reduced lean tissue deposition, shorter adult height, and potentially reduced peak bone mass. The fattest children are unlikely to ever achieve normal BMI for age and normal fatness, but they need to be encouraged that significant fat reduction will improve their self-image, ability to exercise, and reduce late complications of obesity.

Dietary Management

Treatment must alter energy balance so that energy intakes are less than energy expenditures in metabolism and activity. Diets should be adequate for protein and micronutrients. They should aim to *change the quality and energy density* of the food eaten more than *reduce the quantity* of food eaten, although reducing the amount of snacking will probably be appropriate (**Table 3**). There is no consistent evidence that reduction of any particular energy source is more effective than any other in promoting fat loss, so 'balanced diets' conforming to the 'healthy diet' principles of WHO and many governments should be followed.

Physical Activity

More time is spent in relatively minor activity than in strenuous physical activity, so policies that increase energy expenditure in activity must include reductions in sedentary 'activities.' People, not only children, tend to eat more when they are inactive

Table 3 Management of childhood obesity: dietary measures

Purpose of action	Policy	Action
Organize eating	Control number of eating events	Restrict eating to recognized meal and snack periods with perhaps two snacks only for children and three snacks for adolescents
	Eat meals, as a family whenever possible, at table rather than in front of the television	Where possible, eat meals prepared at home and served on a plate rather than ready-to-eat, microwaved individual meals
Be aware of the nutrient content of meals	Meals prepared at home	Where possible, prepare meals at home so that the cook at least is aware of the nutritional makeup of the meal
	Precooked/ready to eat meals	Read the nutritional information given on the packet and observe not only the content/100 g but also the weight (and thus nutrient content) of the food bought and fed to each member of the family
Reduce the energy content of the food intake	Portion sizes	Portion sizes can be reduced—using smaller plates may make this less obvious; avoid second helpings
	Change the form of food used to low-energy density versions	Use 'low-calorie' margarines, spreads, mayonnaise, yoghurts, soups, baked beans, etc.
		Use semi-skimmed milk, sugar-free fruit squashes, etc.
		Grill and bake and boil without added fat rather than frying foods
	Avoid added fats and sugars	Do not add fats to vegetables when preparing them for table
		Avoid (or reduce) added sugar to stewed fruit dishes; sweeteners dissolved in boiled water can be used instead if necessary
Reduce energy content of drinks	Fruit juices, etc.	Eat whole fruit rather than fruit juices (which are usually many fruits compressed and often with added sugar)
		Use 'low-calorie' fruit squashes
		Preferably drink water
		Avoid added sugar
	Tea, coffee, etc.	Try to avoid sweeteners so as to accustom child to less sweet tastes
Increase satiety	Increase intake of foods that require chewing, that take time to eat, or that increase satiety	Increase vegetable, salad, and fruit intake
		Increase whole-meal cereal intake
		Encourage 'jacket' potatoes, boiled potatoes rather than chips, crisps, and mashed potatoes
	Take more time over meals	Eat as a family when possible to allow social interaction during eating, slower eating, and thus greater sense of satiety after the meal

Table 4 Management of childhood obesity: increasing energy expenditure

Purpose	Type of action
Reduce sedentariness	Reduce time spent watching television
	Develop interests/hobbies that give children things to occupy them at home and that may give them activities outside the home
	Encourage children to participate in family life by helping parents around homes, doing simple domestic tasks, running up- and downstairs to fetch for other members of family, etc.
Increase activity in everyday life	Walk or cycle rather than go by car whenever possible
	Use public transport rather than car so at least have to walk to bus stop
	Use stairs rather than elevators and escalators when practical
	Walk up escalators
	Do short walking errands for family as much as possible
	Send child out into garden for activity when he or she comes home from school before doing homework, etc.
Increase family activity	Make a habit of going for walks, taking part in physical activity in garden or parks, etc. in leisure time
	Plan activities during holidays and weekends
Encourage and support child to participate in physical activity at school	Obese children may be very successful at swimming (but may be too self-conscious to wear bathing suit)
	Dancing and aerobics may be more acceptable than contact sports, especially for girls
Increase energy expenditure as heat	Reduce home heating a few degrees to increase need for energy to keep warm in cold weather
	Encourage family to become accustomed to relatively cool environments

and relaxing rather than when they are occupied and active. Keeping children from being bored or from spending their leisure time watching television, when food can be consumed almost unnoticed, should reduce eating opportunities. Overweight children should be encouraged to take up hobbies in order to keep their minds off eating. **Table 4** outlines how their physical activity can be increased without necessarily subjecting them to the often perceived misery of sports and gym (although these should also be encouraged). Embarrassment and fear of ridicule as well as the high energy expenditure required for activity on the sports field are exacerbated by mechanical difficulties associated with gross weight.

Television

It is important to reduce time spent watching television for most of these children. Energy utilization is very low when viewing, and much advertising is aimed at encouraging children to eat foods that are energy dense, high in fat, and of low satiety. Viewing as a family should be encouraged, with the television in the living room rather than in children's bedrooms, so parents are involved in their children's viewing and can advise on the significance and nature of advertizements. Viewing time should be limited, but wise negotiation rather than didactic action will probably be necessary to avoid intrafamily conflict. Indeed, parents should be involved in children's slimming regimens, particularly because so many parents

are overweight. Many children who watch television express preference for other activities but indicate that they are not given the opportunities to participate in other activities. Children cannot be expected to implement slimming behavior if an obesogenic family lifestyle continues unchanged around them.

Very severe childhood obesity (particularly if accompanied by a life-threatening complication such as Pickwickian syndrome) may require more dramatic interference than described previously. Very low-energy diets have been used quite successfully for short-term weight reduction. However, such diets are intrusive, carry some risk for nutrition and growth, and unacceptable to many obese. No drugs are currently approved for treatment of obesity in childhood. Drug treatment has not been associated with notable successes in the past.

Prevention of Obesity in Childhood

The prevention of obesity involves creating lifestyle changes at the family, school, community, and national level. Initiatives need to be affordable and sustainable so that those most at risk of obesity are reached and feel ownership of community programmes. **Table 5** suggests changes needed to reduce the obesogenic factors in the current Westernized environment. If the obesity epidemic is to be halted, governments and international industries have to work with communities to bring about effective change.

Table 5 Possible national and community measures to reduce epidemic of childhood obesity in Western societies

Purpose	Action
Reduce snacking on energy-dense foods	Act to reduce all advertising of energy-dense foods to children
	Possibly ban advertising to children on television
	Remove sweetened drinks and confectionery dispensing machines in schools
	Review foods on sale at school
Increase children's and parents' knowledge of nutrient content of foods	Programmes to educate parents and children on interpreting nutrition labels on foods
	Consider indicating energy content of foods in terms of minutes/hours of activity necessary to balance energy intake from food
	Practical nutrition teaching in schools
Encourage intake of whole foods, fruits and vegetables, and home-prepared foods so there is more awareness of content of foods eaten	Consider subsidising fresh fruits/vegetables and whole-meal cereals and making them more accessible in deprived communities
	Teach families how to cook rather than purchase ready-to-eat meals
Reduce energy intakes generally	Review nutritional content of school dinners
	Develop policies to encourage and make consumption of whole foods, fruits, and cereals attractive and fashionable to children
Increase energy expenditure in activity	Increase play areas, safe parks, and playing fields in communities
	Consider opening school playing fields off hours and on holidays
	Develop safe integrated community transport systems so children can use public transport
	Develop bike paths
Increase energy expenditure in heat	Reduce environmental temperature of public places by a few degrees; encourage people to wear more clothes if they find this uncomfortable

See also: **Adolescents**: Nutritional Problems. **Appetite**: Psychobiological and Behavioral Aspects. **Breast Feeding**. **Children**: Nutritional Requirements; Nutritional Problems. **Diabetes Mellitus**: Etiology and Epidemiology. **Exercise**: Beneficial Effects. **Food Choice, Influencing Factors**. **Nutritional Assessment**: Anthropometry; Clinical Examination. **Obesity**: Definition, Etiology and Assessment; Fat Distribution; Complications; Prevention; Treatment. **Socio-economic Status**. **Weight Management**: Approaches.

Further Reading

Burniat W, Cole TJ, Lissau I, and Poskitt EME (2002) In *Child and adolescent obesity: causes and consequences; prevention and management*. Cambridge: Cambridge University Press.

Cole TJ, Bellizzi MC, Flegal KM, and Dietz WH (2000) Establishing a standard definition for child overweight and obesity worldwide: international survey. *British Medical Journal* **320**: 1–6.

Dietz WH and Gortmaker SL (1985) Do we fatten our children at the television set: Obesity and television viewing in young children and adolescents. *Pediatrics* **75**: 807–812.

Farooqi IS and O'Rahilly S (2000) Recent advances in the genetics of severe childhood obesity. *Archives of Disease in Childhood* **83**: 31–34.

Lissau I and Sorensen TIA (1994) Parental neglect during childhood and increased risk of obesity in young adulthood. *Lancet* **343**: 324–327.

Lobstein T, Baur L, and Uauy R (eds.) (2003) *Childhood obesity. The new crisis in public health*. Report to WHO. London: IASO International Obesity Task Force.

Power C, Lake JK, and Cole TJ (1997) Measurement and long term health risks of child and adolescent fatness. *International Journal of Obesity* **21**: 507–526.

Reilly C, Methven E, McDowell ZC, Hacking B, Alexander D, Stewart L, and Kelnar CJH (2003) Health consequences of obesity. *Archives of Disease in Childhood* **88**: 748–752.

Complications

A Ahmed and R L Atkinson, Obetech Obesity Research Center, Richmond, VA, USA

Obesity is a serious chronic disease associated with complications and comorbidities that involve most systems of the body (**Table 1**). The common factor in all obese people is the presence of excess adipose tissue stores and an increased percentage of body fat. Even in the absence of complications and comorbidities, obesity increases the risk of early mortality. It has been estimated that there are 300 000 obesity-related deaths in the United States each year. In addition to medical complications, obesity is associated with psychological and social problems that may overshadow the medical problems in the quality of life for many obese people.

Table 1 Complications of obesity

Metabolic complications
Metabolic syndrome
Type 2 diabetes
Insulin resistance, hyperinsulinemia
Dyslipidemia
Gout
Abnormalities of hormones and other circulating factors
– Growth hormone
– Hypothalamic–pituitary–adrenal axis
– Cytokines
– Renin–angiotensin system
– Leptin
– Ghrelin
Diseases of organ systems
Cardiac and vascular diseases
– Coronary heart disease
– Hypertension
– Congestive heart failure
– Cerebrovascular disease
– Thromboembolic disease
Respiratory system abnormalities
– Obesity–hypoventilation syndrome
– Sleep apnea
Digestive system abnormalities
– Gall bladder disease
– Hepatic disease
Reproductive system abnormalities
– Hormonal complications: males
– Hormonal complications: females
– Obstetric complications
Nervous system
– Pseudotumor cerebri
– Adiposis dolorosa
– Alzheimer's disease
Immune system dysfunction
Skin disease
Eye disease
Cancer
Breast
Uterus
Gallbladder
Colon
Prostate
Others
Mechanical complications of obesity
Arthritis
Increased intraabdominal pressure
Surgical complications:
Perioperative risks: anesthesia, wound complications, infections
Incisional hernias
Psychosocial complications
Psychological complications
Social complications
Economic impact

Role of Distribution of Body Fat in the Complications of Obesity

The distribution of excess adipose tissue contributes to the complications of obesity. Obese individuals may be classified as those whose excess fat is deposited in the upper body versus those with increased lower body obesity. Upper body obesity may be localized to the subcutaneous space versus the intraabdominal space (visceral fat). Waist circumference and the ratio of waist to hip circumferences correlate with the morbidity and mortality of obesity. Individuals with increased visceral fat, as measured by the cross-sectional area on computed tomography or magnetic resonance imaging, are at greater risk for systemic complications of obesity compared to people with fat localized to abdominal subcutaneous depots or to the lower body. The mechanisms of these differences are not clear, but research has shown that visceral fat has a higher triglyceride turnover rate and releases greater amounts of fatty acids into the circulation than do other adipose tissue depots. Since blood vessels from the visceral fat drain into the portal vein, some investigators postulate that exposure of the liver to high levels of free fatty acids produces insulin resistance, which is known to be correlated with many of the complications of obesity described here. There are significant racial differences in deposition of visceral fat. Asians and Hispanics tend to selectively deposit fat in the abdominal cavity with excess energy intake, whereas blacks have less visceral fat than other groups.

Metabolic and Organ System Complications of Obesity

Obesity is a syndrome that resembles premature aging. Multiple metabolic, hormonal, and organ system dysfunctions occur in aging. Similar changes occur in obesity, but at an earlier age. This section reviews generalized metabolic changes that occur with obesity and discusses individual organ systems.

Metabolic Syndrome

The term 'metabolic syndrome' has been given to a cluster of abnormalities that classically include insulin resistance, glucose intolerance, hypertension, and dyslipidemia. Several other abnormalities, such as sleep apnea, gout, and pseudotumor cerebri, have been associated with insulin resistance and the metabolic syndrome.

Type 2 Diabetes

A strong association of obesity with the prevalence of type 2 diabetes mellitus (DM) is well documented. The risk of developing type 2 DM increases with the degree and duration of obesity—as much as 50-fold with severe obesity. The US National Diabetes Commission reported that the risk of diabetes doubles for every 20% of excess body weight. The risk of type 2 DM is greater with visceral obesity. Type 2 DM is frequently associated with other complications, such as hypertension and dyslipidemia, resulting in additive risks for atherosclerosis and cardiovascular disease. Poor glycemic control in type 2 DM may lead to severe microvascular complications, including nephropathy, retinopathy, and neuropathy. Weight loss is a very effective treatment for type 2 DM and can prevent the onset of type 2 DM in susceptible individuals. Type 2 DM, once very rare in children, has increased greatly in prevalence with the obesity epidemic.

Insulin Resistance and Hyperinsulinemia

'Insulin resistance' refers to the phenomenon of insensitivity of the cells of the body to insulin's actions. Different tissues may have different insulin sensitivities. For example, adipose tissue may be more sensitive to insulin than muscle tissue, thus favoring the deposition of fatty acids in adipose tissue and diminished fatty acid oxidation in muscle. Insulin resistance is usually associated with hyperinsulinemia. Hyperinsulinemia is an independent marker that predicts the development of atherosclerosis. A causal relationship between hypertension and hyperinsulinemia has not been well established. Hypertension associated with hyperinsulinemia could be due to increased renal sodium retention, increased intracellular free calcium, increased sympathetic nervous system activity, or increased intraabdominal pressure due to increased visceral fat deposition.

The mechanisms of insulin resistance with increasing obesity are not clear, but increased production of cytokines such as tumor necrosis factor-α (TNF-α) and interleukin-6 (IL-6) is thought to play a role. Basal insulin levels increase with the degree of overweight, perhaps due to increased insulin secretion and/or reduced clearance by the liver. A reduced receptor number and/or post–insulin receptor defects may play a role in insulin resistance. Both basal hyperinsulinemia and insulin resistance decrease with weight reduction.

Dyslipidemia

Obesity, particularly visceral obesity, is associated with increased serum levels of cholesterol, triglycerides, low-density lipoproteins (LDL), very low-density lipoproteins (VLDL), apolipoprotein B, and reduced levels of high-density lipoprotein (HDL) cholesterol.

Every 10% increase in relative body weight is associated with a 12 mg/dl increase in serum cholesterol concentration. The correlation of serum cholesterol with body mass index (BMI = kg/m^2) is greater for men than women. Increased serum triglycerides with weight gain may be due to increased intake of fats, hyperinsulinemia, and impaired removal of triglycerides into tissues because of low levels of lipoprotein lipase activity. Insulin resistance promotes lipolysis and increased circulating free fatty acids, which enhance the formation of VLDL in the liver. Dyslipidemia contributes to increased atherosclerosis in obesity. Weight reduction usually reduces serum cholesterol and triglycerides, increases HDL cholesterol, and may reduce atherosclerosis.

Gout

Serum uric acid and the prevalence of gout correlate positively with BMI. High serum uric acid levels correlate with insulin resistance and an increased risk of atherosclerotic cardiovascular disease in obesity. Serum uric acid levels may temporarily increase with acute weight loss, but they usually decrease with large amounts of weight loss. The lower uric acid levels are maintained with continued weight loss.

Abnormalities of Hormones and Other Circulating Factors

Growth hormone Obesity is typically accompanied by a decrease in growth hormone (GH) levels and an increase in growth hormone binding protein levels. An inverse relation exists between GH levels and percentage fat mass. GH levels fall with increasing age. GH is released by the anterior pituitary and affects lipid, carbohydrate, and protein metabolism. GH also controls the rate of skeletal and visceral growth. GH is lipolytic in adipose tissue. Animal studies show enhanced catecholamine-induced lipolysis and increased β-adrenoreceptors in adipocytes of GH treated animals. The rises in GH after meals, with sleep, and in response to secretogogues such as arginine or levodopa are blunted in obese people. GH stimulates secretion of insulin-like growth factor-1 (IGF-1). However, IGF-1 is increased in obesity, suggesting a difference in sensitivity to GH. The defects in GH and IGF-1 are reversed by weight reduction.

The hypothalamic–pituitary–adrenal axis The hypothalamic–pituitary–adrenal (HPA) axis may be abnormal in obesity. Patients with Cushing's syndrome display a number of clinical features that resemble those seen in patients with the metabolic syndrome, including abdominal obesity, insulin resistance, impaired glucose homeostasis, hypertension, and lipid abnormalities. These similarities led to the hypothesis that a dysregulation of the HPA axis in the form of functional hypercortisolism could potentially be a cause for abdominal obesity and its different metabolic consequences. High levels of emotional or physical stress are thought to increase cortisol secretion or turnover and thereby increase visceral obesity.

Another potential mechanism involves the peripheral metabolism of cortisol. The enzyme 11-β-hydroxysteroid dehydrogenase, which converts steroid precursors to cortisol, is expressed in adipose tissue. With increasing obesity, more cortisol is derived from cortisone in adipose tissue due to the increased activity of this hormone. Urine studies in obesity also show an increase in the ratio of tetrahydrocortisol to tetrahydrocortisone, indicating a relative increase in the pathways leading to cortisol formation.

Cytokines Adipose tissue secretes a number of cytokines, such as TNF-α and interleukins, which may play a role in fat metabolism and insulin resistance. TNF-α has been shown to alter basal and glucose-stimulated insulin secretion and to produce insulin resistance in isolated cell lines. Adipocytes also produce IL-6, −10, and −11, which stimulate C-reactive protein, a systemic marker of inflammation. All of these ILs are increased in obesity. IL-6 and its subsequent inflammation have been postulated to play an etiologic role in the increased risk of thromboembolism observed in obese patients. Adipose tissue is also capable of producing plasminogen activator inhibitor-1, which may play a role in the increased risk of thromboembolism. Plasma IL-8 is increased in normoglycemic obese subjects and is related to fat mass and to TNF-a levels. Circulating IL-8 is also acutely upregulated by hyperinsulinemia. An increase in circulating IL-8 may be one of the factors linking obesity with greater cardiovascular risk.

Renin–angiotensin system Several components of the renin–angiotensin system are expressed by the adipose tissue. Angiotensinogen levels are increased and have been linked to hypertension and increased cardiovascular risk in obesity.

Leptin Leptin, the product of the *ob* gene, is made predominantly in adipose tissue. Leptin receptors are present in the hypothalamus. Leptin was postulated to act as a signal from adipose tissue to the brain to regulate fat stores. However, serum leptin levels correlate positively with body fat stores and

are higher in obese people. Females have higher serum leptin levels than males, but this association does not appear to be due to estrogen levels. Leptin is found in greater concentrations in abdominal subcutaneous fat compared to visceral fat. The mechanisms for these differences are not known, but it is possible that this may play some role in the differential metabolic responses of subcutaneous and visceral fat.

Ghrelin Ghrelin is a potent growth hormone secretagogue that is produced mainly by the stomach. Administration of ghrelin increases food intake, and ghrelin levels increase with dieting and weight loss. However, serum ghrelin has a negative correlation with percentage body fat, so levels in obese people are lower than in nonobese people.

Diseases of Organ Systems

Atherosclerotic and Arteriosclerotic Vascular Diseases

Diseases of the vascular system provide the greatest contribution to the increased mortality associated with obesity. In both sexes, the excess mortality due to vascular disease increases linearly with BMI greater than 25 kg/m^2. The vascular complications of obesity can be categorized into five major groups: coronary heart disease, hypertension, congestive heart failure, cerebrovascular disease, and thromboembolic disease.

Coronary heart disease Longitudinal studies show a positive correlation of BMI with coronary heart disease (CHD), and obesity is an independent predictor of CHD. However, in the presence of other risk factors, such as hypertension, high serum cholesterol and triglycerides levels, low serum HDL cholesterol levels, and insulin resistance, all of which are increased by obesity, the risk of atherosclerotic CHD increases dramatically. Weight loss reduces all of these risk factors associated with cardiovascular disease, but because long-term reductions in body weight have been difficult to achieve, there are few long-term studies of changes in cardiovascular mortality due to weight loss. A very low-fat diet (10% of total calories as fat) has been shown to reduce the size of atherosclerotic plaques in coronary arteries. Such low-fat diets almost invariably produce weight loss.

Hypertension The prevalence of hypertension among overweight adults in the United States is 2.9 times higher than that of nonoverweight individuals.

Every 10-kg increase in body weight is associated with an increase of 3 and 2 mm Hg in systolic and diastolic blood pressures, respectively. Persistent hypertension can contribute to the development of left ventricular hypertrophy, coronary ischemia, and stroke.

The etiology of the association between hypertension and obesity is unclear. The following are some of the mechanisms offered to explain the association between obesity and hypertension:

Hyperinsulinemia due to insulin resistance leading to increased renal reabsorption of sodium
Sodium retention due to a decreased renal filtration rate, increased intraabdominal pressure, and/or increased plasma renin activity
Increased sympathetic nervous system activity

Except in long-standing cases, weight reduction is usually accompanied by a decrease in blood pressure. The reductions in blood pressure with weight loss are not dependent on decreases in salt intake. Many studies have shown that even modest weight losses, in the range of 5–10% of initial body weight, may produce reductions or even normalization of blood pressure in obese individuals.

Congestive heart failure Total blood volume increases with excess body weight. Higher oxygen consumption in obesity and increased blood flow to the splanchnic bed and adipose tissue increase cardiac output. Also, the transverse diameter of heart, thickness of the posterior wall, and thickness of the interventricular septum increase with body weight. Left ventricular mass is a stronger predictor of morbidity and mortality than blood pressure. A combination of these factors may result in the congestive heart failure seen in severely obese people. The heart rate, stroke volume, blood volume, cardiac output, and left ventricular work return to normal with weight reduction. One study that compared weight loss by dieting to treatment with antihypertensive drugs demonstrated a greater improvement in cardiac hypertrophy with weight loss, despite similar reductions in blood pressure.

Cerebrovascular disease Obesity-related atherosclerosis and arteriosclerosis increase the risk of cerebrovascular disease and strokes. Obesity is an independent risk factor for strokes, even in the absence of other comorbidities.

Thromboembolic disease The risks of venous stasis, deep vein thrombosis, and pulmonary embolism are increased in obesity, particularly in people with abdominal obesity. Lower extremity venous disease may result from increased intraabdominal pressure, impaired fibrinolysis, and the increase in inflammatory mediators described previously.

Respiratory System

Obesity is associated with reduced lung volume, altered respiratory patterns, and an overall reduction in the compliance of the respiratory system, including a diminished vital capacity and total lung capacity. More severe obesity is associated with the 'obesity–hypoventilation syndrome,' which is characterized by excessive daytime sleepiness and hypoventilation. The increased work required to move the chest wall, a decrease in arterial oxygenation in the lungs, and a diminished sensitivity of the respiratory center to the stimulatory effect of carbon dioxide are postulated to contribute to the obesity–hypoventilation syndrome.

The obesity–hypoventilation syndrome may be associated with, or exacerbated by, obstructive sleep apnea, a syndrome characterized by repeated collapse of the upper airway and cessation of breathing with sleep. Obstructive sleep apnea occurs when the tongue obstructs the glottis and prevents entry of air into the trachea. Up to 50% of massively obese people have sleep apnea. The risk of arrhythmias and sudden death increases during apneic episodes. Weight reduction usually reduces the severity of sleep apnea, and massive weight reduction, such as that after gastric bypass surgery, eliminates the disease in most patients.

Digestive System

Gallbladder disease The risk of gallbladder disease, particularly gallstone formation, is increased in obesity and occurs with greater frequency in women. The prevalence of gallbladder disease in obese individuals increases with age, body weight, and parity. The etiology of increased gallstones is unclear, but genetic factors play a role. Increased cholesterol production, which leads to increased excretion of cholesterol in bile, is known to occur in obesity and correlates with increases in body weight. Many obese people skip meals and the reduced number of meals may result in less frequent emptying of the gallbladder. The resulting bile stasis may contribute to gallstone formation. Although long-term weight loss and maintenance may reduce the occurrence of gallbladder disease, the risk of gallstone formation actually increases during the active weight loss phase. The etiology of this increase is thought to be the mobilization of cholesterol from adipose tissue during rapid weight loss. This increased load of cholesterol in the circulation produces supersaturation of the bile, leading to gallbladder sludge in approximately 25% of patients and to symptomatic disease in approximately 1–3%. Treatment with ursodeoxycholic acid reduces or eliminates the risk of gallstone formation during weight loss.

Hepatic disease

Abnormalities in hepatic function are commonly reported in obese people. Fatty liver, due to increased concentrations of fatty acids, diglycerides, and triglycerides in hepatocytes, is reported in obese people. The frequency of fatty liver has been reported to be as high as 94% in very obese subjects. A small number of very obese subjects will develop micronodular cirrhosis. Abnormal liver enzymes on laboratory screening are very common in obese people and do not require further evaluation unless they are markedly elevated. Weight loss results in disappearance of the excess fat and normalization of the liver function tests.

Reproductive System

Hormonal Complications: Males Obese men have elevated levels of plasma estrone and estradiol that correlate with the degree of obesity. Plasma total testosterone and free testosterone (the biologically active moiety) are reduced in obese men, and the reductions correlate negatively with the degree of obesity. The reduced levels of free and total testosterone are not generally accompanied by hypogonadism or a decrease in libido, potency, or sperm count in obese men. Free and total plasma testosterone levels normalize upon significant weight reduction. Also, estrogen levels are normalized if individuals attain normal weight but not if the weight loss is modest and significant obesity persists.

Hormonal Complications: Females Obese women have normal levels of total plasma estradiol but reduced levels of sex hormone binding globulins (SHBG). Thus, free estradiol (the biological active moiety) is significantly elevated. The high levels of free estradiol are postulated to increase the risks of endometrial and breast cancer and to reduce fertility. Estrone, derived in adipose tissue from androgen precursors, is also increased in obesity. Obesity in women is associated with the polycystic ovary syndrome (PCOS), characterized by hyperestrogenism, hyperandrogenism, polycystic ovaries, oligomenorrhea or amenorrhea, hirsutism, and infertility. Women with PCOS also have insulin resistance and are at high risk for developing impaired glucose tolerance and diabetes mellitus. Weight loss usually normalizes SHBG and estradiol levels for individuals with simple obesity, but weight loss may not restore fertility to patients with severe PCOS.

Obstetric complications Obesity increases the risk of complications during pregnancy and child birth. Increased body weight, hypertension, and fluid retention during pregnancy can lead to toxemia of pregnancy. Heavier women have a longer duration of labor and a greater frequency of abnormal labor and caesarian sections.

Nervous system

Pseudotumor cerebri This syndrome is characterized by increased intracranial pressure, headaches, blurred vision or loss of vision, and papilledema. It is most common in massively obese individuals and may be seen in association with sleep apnea or with the obesity–hypoventilation syndrome. It may be associated with retinal hemorrhage or loss of vision from severe papilledema. Some investigators believe that increased intraabdominal pressure with massive obesity is an etiologic factor for pseudotumor cerebri. Major weight loss, particularly after obesity surgery, results in dramatic improvement.

Adiposis dolorosa This is a syndrome of unknown etiology characterized by pain in subcutaneous adipose tissue. Adiposis dolorosa occurs predominantly in postmenopausal women (female: male ratio of about 30:1) and has been described over all areas of the body. The painful areas of fat may occur as subcutaneous lumps on physical examination, but more commonly there are no differences from normal adipose tissue. The disease usually begins gradually with mild pain and tenderness of the area involved, but it may progress to severe pain, particularly with movement or exercise. Intravenous infusions of lidocaine are reported to relieve pain short term or even permanently. The mechanism involved in the relief of pain from lidocaine is unknown.

Alzheimer's disease Obesity has been linked to an increased prevalence of Alzheimer's disease. The etiology of this increase is unknown.

Immune System

Animal studies have shown an increased rate of infection and mortality in obese dogs compared to lean animals experimentally infected with canine distemper virus. Cell-mediated immune response is impaired in obese individuals. Maturation of monocytes into macrophages after *in vitro* incubation is significantly less for obese compared to lean subjects. Impaired cell-mediated immune response in children was demonstrated to be due to subclinical deficiencies of zinc and copper. The impairment in the immune response was reversed after 4 weeks of zinc and copper supplements. As described previously, there are changes in numerous cytokines with obesity. The role of these changes in immune function is not clear.

Skin

Obese people may have several disorders of the skin. The most common is stasis changes of the skin of the lower legs in massively obese people. The etiology of this finding is venous stasis, edema, and breakdown of the skin. Fragilitas cutis inguinalis is a condition of fragile skin in the inguinal area of obese people. This condition is diagnosed by stretching the skin of the inguinal area. A linear tear appears at right angles to an applied force that is insufficient to tear the skin of a normal person. This condition is unrelated to the sex and age of the person.

Acanthosis nigricans, seen occasionally in obesity, is characterized by darkening of the skin in the creases of the neck, axillary regions, and over the knuckles. An association between acanthosis nigricans and insulin resistance is reported in people who have circulating antibodies to the insulin receptors. Since acanthosis nigricans also may be associated with highly malignant cancers such as intraabdominal adenocarcinomas, physicians should be alert to this possibility and not attribute the condition simply to the presence of obesity.

Eye Disease

Obesity is associated with an increased prevalence of cataracts. People with abdominal obesity are at greater risk than those with lower body obesity, insulin resistance may be involved in the pathogenesis of cataract formation, and diabetes is a well-known risk factor.

Cancer

Obesity increases the risk of cancers of the breast, colon, prostate, endometrium, cervix, ovary, kidney, and gallbladder. Studies have also found a somewhat increased risk for cancers of the liver, pancreas, rectum, brain, esophagus, and non-Hodgkin's lymphoma.

Although there are many theories about how obesity increases cancer risk, the exact mechanisms are not known. The mechanisms may be different for different types of cancer. Also, because obesity develops through a complex interaction of heredity and lifestyle factors, researchers may not be able to determine whether the obesity or other factors led to the development of cancer.

Mechanical Complications of Obesity

Arthritis

Obesity is frequently complicated by degenerative arthritis (DJD). Increased body weight leads to trauma of the weight-bearing joints and speeds the development of osteoarthritis in obesity. Knee and hip joints are particularly affected. However, obese patients have increased DJD of the hands, perhaps due to cytokines produced by adipose tissue, which may damage the cartilage in joints. Flattening of the arc of the planter surface of the feet (flat feet) occurs more frequently in obese people, presumably due to the stress of carrying excess body weight. Flat feet may lead to unsteady gait and aches and pains after walking. Increased fat deposition, particularly in the abdominal region, can change the natural curvature of the spine, causing lordosis and resulting in backache in obese people.

Intraabdominal Pressure

In severely obese people, the excess visceral fat is thought to increase intraabdominal pressure. Animal research shows that experimentally induced acute increases in intraabdominal pressure to the levels seen in the abdomens of very obese people cause increases in pleural pressure, intracranial pressure, and central venous pressure. The investigators postulated that in humans, increased intraabdominal pressure may contribute to hypertension, insulin resistance and type 2 DM, obesity–hypoventilation syndrome, pseudotumor cerebri, incisional hernia, and urinary incontinence. Massive weight loss following obesity surgery normalizes the increased intraabdominal pressure and reduces or eliminates all the symptoms listed previously.

Surgical Complications

Obese patients are at an increased risk of surgical and perisurgical complications, including an increased risk of complications and death from anesthesia, longer operating times, delayed wound healing, increased postoperative wound infections and pneumonia, and a higher frequency of incisional hernias after surgeries involving the abdominal wall. Many surgeons recommend weight reduction before elective surgery, but there are few data to document that acute weight reduction improves the outcome of surgery.

Psychosocial Complications

Psychological Complications

Obesity is associated with negative emotions, low self-esteem, decreased marital satisfaction, and body image disparagement. All of these conditions and beliefs show improvement with weight reduction.

Dieting efforts correlate positively with the prevalence of eating disorders, particularly binge eating. A correlation of eating disorders with abuse of drugs and alcohol has been shown. In strictly dieting female college freshmen who were not alcohol abusers at baseline, the frequency of alcohol abuse was reported to increase after 1 year compared to nondieters.

Social Complications

Obesity carries a social stigma that dramatically affects the quality of life for obese individuals, particularly for women. Factors contributing to the social bias against obese people are beliefs that obesity is due merely to overeating and therefore obese people must lack will power. Many members of the general public, and even health professionals, ignore the evidence for the genetic contribution to obesity, believe that obese people are responsible for their own plight, and believe that they do not deserve sympathy for their disability. Despite similar intelligence (as judged by IQ values and the Scholastic Aptitude Test scores), a significantly lower number of obese females were admitted to certain colleges compared to nonobese females. The choice of mates is adversely affected by obesity. Obese individuals tend to marry mates with less education and from a lower socioeconomic class. It is more difficult for an obese person to find a job or to be promoted once hired, so lower earnings and a lower socioeconomic status are correlated with obesity. Obese employees are viewed as less competent, less productive, inactive, disorganized, and less successful by employers.

The bias against obesity has been shown to begin in early childhood. Obese children are considered lazy, stupid, slow, and self-indulgent by both children and adults. Because of these societal attitudes, many obese children and adolescents have lower self-esteem than do their nonobese counterparts.

Economic Impact

In the United States, the direct cost of obesity has been estimated at more than $100 billion per year. The indirect costs of early retirement and increased risk for disability requiring financial support are also considerable. Because obese people have more health problems, health care costs for the obese are higher than for nonobese individuals.

See also: **Arthritis**. **Cholesterol**: Sources, Absorption, Function and Metabolism; Factors Determining Blood Levels. **Coronary Heart Disease**: Lipid Theory; Prevention. **Cytokines**. **Diabetes Mellitus**: Etiology and Epidemiology; Classification and Chemical Pathology; Dietary Management. **Gout**. **Hypertension**: Dietary Factors. **Lipoproteins**. **Obesity**: Definition, Etiology and Assessment; Fat Distribution; Childhood Obesity; Prevention; Treatment.

Further Reading

Atkinson RL (1982) Intravenous lidocaine for the treatment of intractable pain of adiposis dolorosa. *International Journal of Obesity* 6: 351–357.

Bjorntorp P (1993) Visceral obesity: A 'civilization syndrome.' *Obesity Research* 1: 206–222.

Flegal KM, Carroll MD, Ogden CL, and Johnson CL (2002) Prevalence and trends in obesity among U.S. adults, 1999–2000. *Journal of the American Medical Association* 288(14): 1723–1727.

Grundy SM and Barnett JP (1990) Metabolic and health complications of obesity. *Disease of Month* 36: 641–731.

Klein S and Romijn JA (2003) Obesity. In: Larsen PR, Kronenberg HM, Melmed S, and Polonsky KS (eds.) *Williams Textbook of Endocrinology*, 10th edn, pp. 1619–1641. New York: Saunders.

Kottke TE, Lambert A, and Hoffman RS (2003) Economic and psychological implications of obesity epidemic. *Mayo Clinic Proceedings* 78: 92–94.

Ousman Y and Burman KD (2002) *Endocrine Function in Obesity*. Available at http://endotext.com/obesity/obesity12/obesityframe12.htm.

Sugerman HJ, Felton WL 3rd, Salvant JB Jr, Sismanis A, and Kellum JM (1995) Effects of surgically induced weight loss on idiopathic intracranial hypertension in morbid obesity. *Neurology* 45: 1655–1659.

Tataranni PA and Bogardus C (2003) Obesity and diabetes mellitus. In: Porte D Jr, Sherwin RS, and Baron A (eds.) *Handbook of Diabetes Mellitus*, 6th edn, pp. 401–413. New York: McGraw-Hill.

Zumoff B and Strain GW (1994) A perspective on the hormonal abnormalities of obesity: Are they cause or effect? *Obesity Research* 2: 56–67.

Prevention

T P Gill, University of Sydney, Sydney, NSW, Australia

There can be little doubt that obesity has become a major public health and economic problem of global significance. According to World Health Organization (WHO) estimates, approximately 1 billion people throughout the world were overweight in 2002 and more than 300 million of these were obese. Prevalence rates continue to rise rapidly in all areas of the world, including low-income countries, and obesity-associated illness are now so common that they are replacing the more traditional public health concerns, such as undernutrition and infectious disease, as the most significant contributors to global ill health.

The health impact of obesity is considerable, and obesity impacts on both quality and length of life. Overweight and obesity are associated with a wide range of chronic conditions, such as diabetes, hypertension, cardiovascular disease (CVD), and certain cancers, as well as non-life-threatening but painful conditions, such as arthritis, back pain, and breathlessness. Obesity also places enormous financial burdens on governments and individuals and accounts for a significant proportion of total health care expenditure in developed countries. Analyses suggest that obesity is fast approaching cigarette smoking as the major preventable cause of mortality.

In recent years, our understanding of the epidemiology and causation of obesity has improved dramatically and there is an acceptance that urgent action is required to address the problem. However, there are very few examples of successful, large-scale obesity prevention initiatives from any area of the world. Despite these limitations, sufficient understanding has been gained from smaller scale obesity prevention initiatives together with experiences from the management of other epidemics of noncommunicable diseases to allow effective planning and implementation of obesity prevention programs to proceed.

Principles of Obesity Prevention

Rational for Obesity Prevention

There are a number of reasons why prevention is likely to be the only effective way of tackling the problem of overweight and obesity. First, obesity develops over time, and once it has done so, it is very difficult to treat. A number of analyses have identified the limited success of obesity treatments (with the possible exception of surgical interventions) to achieve long-term weight loss. Second, the health consequences associated with obesity result from the cumulative metabolic and physical stress of excess weight over a long period of time and may not be fully reversible by weight loss. Third, the proportion of the population that is either overweight or obese in many countries is now so large that there are no longer sufficient health care resources to offer treatment to all. It can be argued, therefore, that the prevention of weight gain (or the

reversal of small gains) and the maintenance of a healthy weight would be easier, less expensive, and potentially more effective than to treat obesity after it has fully developed.

Objectives of Obesity Prevention

There remains a great deal of confusion regarding the appropriate objectives of an obesity prevention program. It is often assumed that to be effective, any intervention to address the problem of excess weight in the community should result in a reduction in the prevalence of overweight and obesity. However, such an objective is unrealistic and may be counterproductive. Most communities are experiencing significant increases in the average weight of the population as a result of a sizeable energy surplus resulting from reduced energy expenditure combined with an increased energy intake. This is leading to rapidly escalating rates of overweight and obesity. To reverse this trend will require not only the removal of this energy surplus but also the creation of a negative energy balance that will need to be maintained by the whole population for a significant period of time. Few (if any) interventions are capable of reducing energy intake, or increasing energy expenditure sufficiently, or are sustained long enough and with sufficient reach to achieve this effect. More appropriate objectives would relate to a reduction in the level of weight gain or the maintenance of weight stability in adults and the achievement of appropriate growth and development in children. The achievement of these objectives would result in a slowing in the rate of increase, followed by stabilization and then an eventual decline in the level of overweight and obesity in the community.

However, even the goal of weight stability within a population may be difficult to achieve in the short term because it would require the maintenance or reestablishment of energy balance in time of significant energy surplus. Therefore, it may be necessary to identify more sensitive short- and medium-term outcomes to evaluate obesity prevention programs. Such process outcomes may relate to the achievement of appropriate changes in energy intakes or outputs, food or physical activity behaviors, or changes to the environment that are significant enough to positively impact upon the achievement of energy balance.

Importance of Weight Gain Prevention in Adults

There are a number of important reasons why it is preferable to focus on weight gain prevention as the key individual and population objective of obesity prevention initiatives in adults (**Box 1**). The association between elevated body mass index (BMI) and increased risk of ill health is clear and consistent.

Box 1 Why focus on weight gain prevention?

- Weight gain in adulthood carries an independent risk of ill health.
- Risk for chronic disease begins to increase from low BMI levels and significant weight gain can occur within normal limits.
- Extended periods of weight gain are difficult to reverse.
- Weight gain in adulthood is mostly fat gain.
- The relationship between absolute BMI and health risk varies with age and ethnicity but no such variations occur in the relationship between weight gain and ill health.
- A focus on weight gain prevention avoids exacerbation of inappropriate dieting behaviors.
- Weight maintenance can serve as a first stage goal for weight treatment programs.
- The message is equally relevant to all sections of the adult population.
- It avoids further stigmatization of people with an existing weight problem.
- It avoids reference to poorly understood terms such as 'healthy weight.'

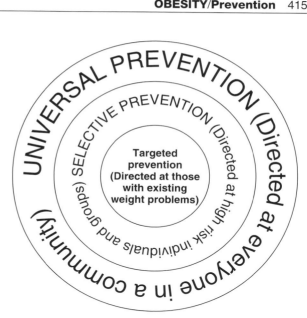

Figure 1 Levels of obesity prevention intervention. (Adapted from Gill TP (1997) Key issues in the prevention of obesity. *British Medical Bulletin* **53**(2): 359–388.)

However, research has demonstrated that weight gain per se is also associated with increased health risk, and that this risk is independent of absolute BMI (provided a person is not underweight). A number of studies have shown strong relationships between weight gain and increasing levels of diabetes, hypertension, gall bladder disease, and coronary heart disease. Therefore, a large weight gain in a lean individual may carry equivalent risk to maintaining a stable but slightly elevated BMI in an overweight individual. The combination of an elevated BMI and ongoing weight gain, however, leads to greatly magnified levels of risk.

Who Should Obesity Prevention Strategies Target?

Deciding where to invest limited time and resources in obesity prevention is a difficult task but finite health resources make this a necessity. WHO has identified three distinct but equally valid and complementary levels of obesity prevention (**Figure 1**). The specific 'targeted' approach directed at very high-risk individuals with existing weight problems is represented by the core of the figure, the 'selective' approach directed at individuals and groups with above average risk is represented by the middle layer, and the broader universal or populationwide prevention approach is represented by the outer layer. This replaces the more traditional classification of disease prevention (primary, secondary, and tertiary), which can be confusing when applied to a complex multifactorial condition such as obesity.

Universal prevention is the domain of public health, whereas selective and targeted prevention

are predominantly dealt with in community and health care service settings. Community settings include schools, colleges, worksites, community centers, and shopping outlets.

Whole Community

Overweight and obesity are public health problems of relevance to the whole community and require strategies that focus on populationwide change rather than attempting to address individuals or small groups in isolation of the community in which they live. An effective population strategy needs to both improve population knowledge about obesity and its management and reduce the exposure of the community to obesity-promoting factors in the environment. Action at a population level requires coordination at a central level and the investment of resources to be maintained over a long period of time to achieve population change.

Family Focus

There are numerous reasons why children should be a major focus of any obesity prevention strategy. There is strong evidence that a high proportion of overweight or obese children will become obese adults. Childhood obesity also has immediate effects on health, and weight-related conditions are becoming more prevalent and their effect more pronounced as the rates of childhood obesity increase. However, children grow rapidly and increase the level of lean body mass as they age, and so reducing or keeping fat mass constant allows the normalization of weight over time. Thus, childhood (particularly younger children) is a period during which prevention efforts have a higher chance of success.

However, children also have little direct control over the environment in which they live. Parents and other caregivers mostly control decisions regarding the food available and the opportunities for activity. In addition, the behaviors of parents and other siblings have a profound effect on the diet and physical activity behaviors of children. For this reason, it is preferable to focus childhood obesity prevention efforts on the family environment rather than directly on children.

High-Risk Groups

There are a number of groups that appear to be at higher risk of developing overweight and obesity (**Table 1**). These groups warrant special attention and include the following:

- Those with a family history of weight problems
- Socially disadvantaged and isolated communities
- Certain ethnic groups
- Smokers who have recently quit smoking
- Those who have recently lost weight

In addition, there are certain times in a person's life when the person is more prone to weight gain (**Table 1**). These age groups could be considered for selective prevention interventions. These times include the following:

Prenatal
Adiposity rebound (5–7 years)
Adolescence
Early adulthood
Pregnancy
Menopause

Table 1 Identifying at-risk groups for obesity

Critical ages and life stages	Reason for increased risk
Prenatal	There is evidence that in utero development has permanent effects on later growth and energy regulation.
Adiposity rebound (5–7 years)	Body mass index begins to increase rapidly after a period of reduced adiposity during preschool years. Food and activity patterns change as a result of exposure to other children and school. Early and rapid weight rebound often precedes the development of obesity.
Adolescence	Period of increased autonomy that is often associated with irregular meals, changed food habits, and periods of inactivity during leisure combined with physiological changes that promote increased fat deposition, particularly in females.
Early adulthood	Early adulthood usually correlates with a period of marked reduction in physical activity. In women this usually occurs between the ages of 15 and 19 years but in men it may be as late as the early 30s.
Pregnancy	Excessive weight gain during pregnancy often results in retention of weight after delivery, particularly with early cessation of breast feeding. This pattern is often repeated after each pregnancy.
Menopause	In Western societies weight generally increases with age but it is not certain why menopausal women are particularly prone to rapid weight gain. The loss of the menstrual cycle does affect food intake and reduce metabolic rate slightly.
High-risk groups	
Family history of weight problems	There is no longer any doubt that given the same environment some individuals are more prone to depositing fat. The basis of these differences in individual susceptibility to obesity is yet to be fully elucidated but is believed to involve a number of physiological processes associated with fat deposition and oxidation and involuntary energy expander.
Certain ethnic groups	In NSW, recent migrants from southern Mediterranean countries and the Middle East are more likely to be obese and their children are more likely to develop a more severe form of obesity that to immediate health consequences.
Socially or economically disadvantaged	In NSW, there is an inverse association between income and education level and obesity which is most pronounced among women and children. It is argued that cheaper foodstuffs are usually high in fat and energy dense and those with less financial resources spend more time in sedentary activities such as watching TV.
Recent successful weight reducers	Successful weight reduction is usually followed by the regain of one-half to one-third of the weight loss over the following year. It is believed that biological and behavioral processes act to drive body weight back to baseline levels.
Recent past smokers	Smokers are usually thinner than nonsmokers because smoking tends to depress appetite, increase the basal metabolic rate, and, after each cigarette, induce a surge in heart and metabolic rate. The effect on metabolism of smoking 24 cigarettes per day has been estimated at approximately 200 kcal per day.

Adapted from Gill TP (1997) Key issues in the prevention of obesity. *British Medical Bulletin* **53**(2): 359–388.

Those with an Existing Weight Problem

In developing weight gain prevention strategies, it is important not to neglect those with an existing weight problem who could benefit from more intensive efforts to help prevent further weight gain.

Key Elements of a Weight Gain Prevention Plan

Weight gain and obesity develop when the energy intake from food and drink exceeds energy expenditure from physical activity and other metabolic processes. It is often assumed that the prevention of weight gain should focus solely on attempting to alter these behaviors within individuals and communities. However, research has consistently shown that numerous and diverse factors, including environmental and social factors, influence the behaviors that lead to excessive weight gain. Addressing aspects of the obesogenic (obesity-promoting) environment, as well as individuals' eating and physical activity patterns, is considered to be critical to the success of any obesity prevention program.

The 2003 WHO report on diet, nutrition, and the prevention of chronic disease undertook a detailed review of the literature and identified a range of key factors that either increase or decrease the risk of weight gain and the development of obesity (Table 2). These factors were rated on the quality of evidence available to support their contributory role. This analysis serves as a very useful guide as to the focus of weight gain prevention initiatives.

Diet and Physical Activity Behaviors

The WHO analysis identified a number of key dietary and physical activity behaviors, amenable to change, that could conceivably influence energy balance sufficiently to contribute to the prevention of weight gain and obesity. Behaviors that reduced the risk of obesity included regular physical activity, high dietary fiber intake, and possibly breast-feeding and low glycemic index diets. Behaviors that increased the risk of obesity included a high intake of energy-dense foods, a high intake of sugar-sweetened drinks and juices, time spent in sedentary behaviors, and possibly large portion sizes, a high intake of fast foods, and a restrained eating pattern.

The area of dietary and physical activity antecedents to weight gain and obesity is still poorly understood and new research findings, which help clarify our understanding, are being presented on a regular basis. In addition, different behaviors are more prevalent or pronounced in different regions of the world. It is therefore difficult to give definitive recommendations on the most important and useful behaviors to target in obesity prevention strategies. However, strong evidence exists to support the inclusion of some key behaviors.

Reducing Energy Intake

Reducing the intake of high energy-dense foods (i.e., foods high in fat/sugar)   There is a high level of agreement that the overconsumption of energy-dense foods is a major contributor to excess energy intake and weight gain and that restriction of energy-dense food items is a useful strategy for the prevention of weight gain. However, discussion continues as to whether fat or refined carbohydrate is the major contributor to energy density in the modern diet and thus should be the target of programs to control weight. The debate is being fuelled by dietary data from many developed countries that show that dietary fat intakes have leveled out or declined

Table 2 Summary of the strengths of evidence of factors that may promote or protect against weight gain and obesity

Evidence	Decreases risk	Increases risk
Convincing	Regular physical activity	High intake of energy-dense foods[a]
	High dietary fiber intake	Sedentary lifestyle
Probable	Home and school environments that support healthy food choices for children	Heavy marketing of energy-dense foods and fast-food outlets
	Promoting linear growth	Adverse social and economic conditions in developed countries (especially for women)
		Sugar-sweetened soft drinks and juices
Possible	Low glycemic index foods	Large portion sizes
	Breast-feeding	High proportion of food prepared outside of home
		Rigid restraint/periodic disinhibition eating patterns
Insufficient	Increased eating frequency	Alcohol

[a]Energy-dense foods are high in fat/sugar and energy-dilute foods are high in fiber and water, such as vegetables, fruits, legumes, and whole grain cereals.
Adapted from WHO (2003) *Joint WHO/FAO Expert Report on Diet, Nutrition and the prevention of Chronic Disease*, WHO Technical Report Series 916. Geneva: WHO.

slightly and intakes of carbohydrates have increased dramatically. However, research has shown that dietary fat (along with water and fiber) is a major contributor to the energy density of foods and that ad libitum low-fat diet plans are an effective dietary approach to weight gain prevention or moderate weight loss. There is also strong evidence that excess carbohydrate, particularly high glycemic index carbohydrate, contributes to weight gain and its restriction aids weight loss and improves cardiovascular risk factor profiles.

Increasing the intake of high-fiber, energy-dilute foods (especially vegetables and fruits)   There is less evidence on the effectiveness of increasing the intake of energy-dilute foods such as vegetables and some fruits in the diet. Such a strategy would assist weight gain prevention only if the inclusion of such foods leads to a reduction in the intake of more energy-dense alternatives and thus creates a reduction in energy intake. Few studies have addressed this issue in a comprehensive manner, but the additional health benefits of these foods makes such a strategy low risk in nutritional terms.

Reducing the consumption of sugar-sweetened soft drinks and juices   Evidence is accumulating from a variety of studies that energy consumed as sweetened drinks is less well compensated for than energy consumed as solid food. Longitudinal studies have also indicated that sweetened drinks (soft drinks or sodas) are associated with weight gain in both children and adults. Recent work has also demonstrated that the simple strategy of reducing the intake of sweetened drinks can be effective in preventing or limiting inappropriate weight gain.

Reducing the level of food prepared outside of the home   The proportion of food purchased and consumed at food outlets outside of the home has increased dramatically in recent decades in both developed and developing nations. In the United States, approximately 40% of the household food budget is spent on food eaten away from home, and much of this is spent at fast-food outlets. A number of analyses have linked increased consumption of fast food with increased risk of obesity. Although few studies have evaluated the effect of reducing the consumption of fast food, it would seem to be a valuable strategy with few nutritional negatives.

Reducing portion sizes   The portion size of packaged foods and snacks, as well as restaurant serving sizes, has increased rapidly in recent times and has been identified as an important factor in the consumption of excess energy. Evidence suggests that people will consume the portion of food they are provided rather than respond to satiety signals to stop eating and leave food. Also, as the serving size increases, the ability of consumers to estimate accurately how much they have consumed decreases. Reducing portion sizes is a simple but immediately effective mechanism for reducing energy intake.

Increasing Energy Expenditure

Regular physical activity   Although it is difficult to obtain accurate assessments of physical activity, there is little doubt that energy expenditure from activity has decreased in the past 50 years in most countries throughout the world. In contrast to popular belief, participation rates in organized leisure-time physical activity have increased in recent times in many countries. This supports the contention that the greatest contributor to this reduction in energy expenditure is associated with substantial changes in occupational and incidental physical activity. Changes in employment patterns and work practices together with a reliance on motorized transport and the removal of almost all manual labor from our daily lives have led to a dramatic reduction in daily physical exertion.

Studies that have examined the association between physical activity and weight gain and the impact of increasing physical activity on weight gain prevention have been limited by the ability to accurately measure physical activity and to engage people in sufficient levels of physical activity to prevent weight gain. However, there is sufficient evidence to support an important role for increasing physical activity in any weight gain prevention strategy, although questions remain about how much exercise is necessary and what type of exercise is appropriate to promote. The issue of the amount of extra time that people should spend in moderate physical activity to prevent weight gain remains hotly debated, but it is clearly substantially more than the 30 minutes on 5 or more days each week recommended by experts to reduce cardiovascular disease risk. The type of exercise that should be the focus of weight gain prevention strategies is also under review. It has been suggested that the most effective ways to include regular physical activity in daily living are through increased incidental activity, increased participation in active recreation, and increased use of active transport.

Reduced time spent in sedentary behaviors (especially TV watching) Changes in societal structures and improvements in technology have allowed a reduction in time spent at work or on domestic chores, leaving a greater proportion of the day for leisure. At the same time, most of the entertainment options developed to fill this time, such as watching television, playing video games, and using computers, are sedentary activities that require very little energy expenditure. These forms of entertainment, which initially complemented other forms of leisure activity, are occupying more hours of the day and are displacing more active pursuits and games. As a consequence, a number of studies have identified clear links between time spent in this sedentary behavior and weight gain. However, it is important to make a distinction between a lack of physical activity and sedentary behavior because their mechanisms for impacting on body weight may be different and a person with a high level of physical activity can also have a high level of sedentary behavior. Although the precise pathway by which sedentariness influences weight gain is not known, it is believed to involved both a reduction in physical activity and an increase in dietary energy intake through inappropriate food intake that is often stimulated by and accompanies sedentary activities.

Some studies in children have shown that programs that seek to reduce time spent in sedentary behaviors are more effective in controlling weight than programs that aim to increase physical activity alone. In some cases, a simple program to reduce the amount of time spent watching television was sufficient to significantly limit inappropriate weight gain in children.

Creating Supportive Environments

The external physical, social, political, and economic environments in which people exist have a profound effect on their attitudes and behaviors. Each day, people interact with a wide range of services, systems, and pressures in settings such as schools, the workplace, home, restaurants, and fast-food outlets. In addition, laws, policies, economic imperatives, and the views of governments, industry, and society as a whole influence these settings. Each of the features of this complex system, which shapes the environment in which we live, has the capacity to inhibit or encourage appropriate dietary and physical activity patterns. The availability of open space, access to public transport, the design of suburbs, access to buildings, the perceived level of safety, provision of lighting, and many other

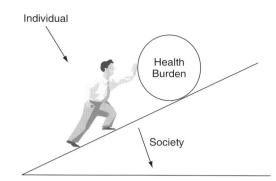

Figure 2 Influence of societal and environmental factors on development of obesity. (From House of Commons Health Committee (2004) *Obesity: Third Report of Sessions 2003–04. Volume 1. Report Together with Formal Minutes.* London: The Stationery Office Ltd.)

factors influence our capacity and desire to be more physically active in our daily lives. Similarly, advertising pressures, access to appropriate food choices, school food policies, and nutrition information and labeling all potentially influence food selection. Today, there is also a large commercial drive to promote obesogenic behaviors (cars and food are the two most advertised products on television).

Trying to motivate people to make healthy choices when the external environment works against such behaviors is a recipe for failure. **Figure 2** illustrates the role that the social environment plays in assisting or inhibiting personal behavior choices made by individuals, which ultimately impact upon their health. Great success is likely to be achieved by creating a supportive environment and then promoting the healthy dietary and physical activity choices within such an environment.

Lessons from Past Prevention Efforts

Obesity Prevention Programs

A number of systematic reviews have assessed the current scientific literature on programs addressing the prevention of obesity in both children and adults and have identified only a limited number of evaluated programs. The reviews concluded that there was simply too small a body of research conducted in a limited number of settings to provide firm guidance on consistently effective interventions. However, reviews of childhood obesity prevention initiatives indicated that certain approaches appear to be associated with greater success. Intensive intervention in small groups was a successful management strategy in children, as was involving the entire the family. Reducing levels of inactivity was successful at both treating and preventing weight gain. Some interventions that increased time spent in formal physical activity were successful in controlling weight gain, but generally multicomponent programs that addressed a range of strategies were deemed to hold the most promise.

There was general agreement that efforts should be heavily oriented toward preventing obesity in children because of the greater likelihood of success at a younger age. More effort needs to be directed at creating environmental and policy changes that will support the adoption of behaviors conducive to weight control rather than simply relying on education approaches.

Large-Scale Community Coronary Heart Disease and Diabetes Prevention Trials

Conducting large-scale, communitywide trials to address the prevention of obesity is a very expensive and difficult process; consequently, evidence of this nature is very limited. However, a number of large CVD and diabetes prevention trials have included weight as an intermediary outcome, which can also provide useful information about effective strategies to address obesity, and have demonstrated that it may be possible to prevent weight gain if not reduce weight at a population level.

The results of early large-scale community CVD prevention trials, such as the Stanford Three Community and Five Community studies as well as the Minnesota Heart Health Program, had limited impact on weight status and reinforced the difficulty of preventing weight gain in the community. However, later programs, such as the Pawtucket Heart Health Program, were able to make a modest impact on weight gain in the intervention community after 10 years. These programs demonstrate the time lag that can be expected between the implementation of a truly communitywide program and the extent of behavior change likely to be required to impact upon the weight status of the community. It has been suggested that unless weight is the primary outcome of the intervention, it is unlikely that sufficient focus will be placed on achieving the level of change required to impact on energy balance and community weight status.

Strong and consistent evidence of the success of large-scale weight gain prevention initiatives has been obtained from diabetes prevention trials that have addressed the progression to diabetes in people identified as glucose intolerant. Four large-scale trials have produced significant reductions in the rate of

diabetes by focusing on exercise and diet, which resulted in small weight losses of approximately 3 or 4 kg on average. The largest trial conducted in the United States found that advice to reduce the energy and fat in the diet together with modest increases in physical activity, which was reinforced with regular follow-up from a 'coach,' led to an average weight loss of 5.6 kg and 58% reduction in the number of people progressing from impaired glucose tolerance to diabetes.

Lessons from Other Prevention Efforts

Although the number of successful large-scale obesity prevention programs is limited, there is a wealth of information from past public health programs that can be used to address other chronic diseases and risk factors. The International Obesity Task Force identified 10 key principles on which efforts to prevent obesity at a population level should be based. These are presented in **Box 2** and are drawn from experiences addressing cardiovascular disease, smoking, alcohol and drug problems, dental disease, road accidents, and other public health issues.

Although much has yet to be elucidated about the development of obesity and its effective management and prevention, there is a consensus that action to address the problem must not be delayed. Efforts to prevent weight gain need to be well

---

Box 2   IOTF principles for the development of population obesity prevention initiatives

1. Education alone is not sufficient to change weight-related behaviors. Environmental and societal intervention is also required to promote and support behavior change.
2. Action must be taken to integrate physical activity into daily life, not just to increase leisure time exercise.
3. Sustainability of programs is crucial to enable positive change in diet, activity, and obesity levels over time.
4. Political support, intersectoral collaboration, and community participation are essential for success.
5. Acting locally, even in national initiatives, allows programs to be tailored to meet real needs, expectations, and opportunities.
6. All parts of the community must be reached, not just the motivated healthy.
7. Programs must be adequately resourced.
8. Where appropriate, programs should be integrated into existing initiatives.
9. Programs should build on existing theory and evidence.
10. Programs should be properly monitored, evaluated, and documented. This is important for dissemination and transfer of experiences.

Source: Kumanyika S, Jeffery RW, Morabia A *et al.* (2002) Obesity prevention: The case for action. *International Journal of Obesity* **26**(3): 425–436.

designed, comprehensive, and appropriately evaluated so that the knowledge base improves with each new program.

See also: **Coronary Heart Disease**: Prevention. **Diabetes Mellitus**: Etiology and Epidemiology. **Energy**: Requirements. **Exercise**: Beneficial Effects. **Obesity**: Definition, Etiology and Assessment; Childhood Obesity. **Weight Management**: Approaches; Weight Maintenance. **World Health Organization**.

Further Reading

Campbell K, Waters E, O'Meara S *et al.* (2002) Interventions for preventing obesity in children. *Cochrane Database Systematic Review* 2: CD001871.

Dietz W and Gortmaker S (2001) Preventing obesity in children and adolescents. *Annual Review of Public Health* 22: 337–353.

Douketis J, Feightner J, Attia J *et al.* (1999) Periodic health examination, 1999 update: 1. Detection, prevention and treatment of obesity. *Canadian Medical Association Journal* 160(4): 513–525.

Egger G and Swinburn B (1997) An 'ecological' approach to the obesity pandemic. *British Medical Journal* 315(7106): 477–480.

French S, Story M, and Jeffery RW (2001) Environmental influences on eating and physical activity. *Annual Review of Public Health* 22: 309–335.

Gill TP (1997) Key issues in the prevention of obesity. *British Medical Bulletin* 53(2): 359–388.

House of Commons Health Committee (2004) *Obesity: Third Report of Sessions 2003–04. Volume 1. Report Together with Formal Minutes.* London: The Stationery Office Ltd.

James WPT and Gill TP (2004) Prevention of obesity. In: Bray G, Bouchard C, and James WPT (eds.) *Handbook of Obesity: Clinical Applications*, 2nd edn. New York: Marcel Dekker.

Kumanyika S, Jeffery RW, Morabia A *et al.* (2002) Obesity prevention: The case for action. *International Journal of Obesity* 26(3): 425–436.

NHS Centre for Reviews and Dissemination (2002) The prevention and treatment of childhood obesity. *Effective Health Care Bulletin* 7(6).

Saris W, Blair S, van Baak MA *et al.* (2003) How much physical activity is enough to prevent unhealthy weight gain? Outcome of the IASO 1st Stock Conference and consensus statement. *Obesity Reviews* 4: 101–114.

Story M (1999) School-based approaches for preventing and treating obesity. *International Journal of Obesity and Related Metabolic Disorders* 23(supplement2): S43–S51.

US Surgeon General (2001) *The Surgeon General's Call to Action to Prevent and Decrease Overweight and Obesity.* Washington, DC: Office of the Surgeon General.

World Health Organization (2000) *Obesity: Preventing and Managing the Global Epidemic. Report of a WHO Consultation*, WHO Technical Report Series 894. Geneva: WHO.

World Health Organization (2003) *Joint WHO/FAO Expert Report on Diet, Nutrition and the Prevention of Chronic Disease*, WHO Technical Report Series 916. Geneva: WHO.

Treatment

E C Uchegbu, Royal Hallamshire Hospital, Sheffield, UK
P G Kopelman, Queen Mary's, University of London, London, UK

Introduction

Increasing body weight is associated with increasing health risks (**Table 1**). Randomized controlled trials demonstrate that weight reduction reduces these health risks and confirm the value in treating overweight and obesity.

Obesity is a chronic disease of multiple etiologies characterized by an excess of adipose tissue. Recent research has begun to unravel the biochemical and genetic factors implicated in its etiologies. As a result of the factors that determine its severity, health risks, and response to therapy, treatment must be tailored to specific needs. The ability of a treatment to maintain long-term weight reduction is as important as its ability to cause the initial weight loss. In several studies inability in maintaining the lowered weight is the cause of the treatment failure.

Nevertheless, a successful program should also lead to an improvement in the quality of life, self-esteem, social functioning, anxiety, and depression.

Several professional, governmental, and other organizations have drawn up guidelines for obesity management. These strategies for providing care to the obese patient provide useful evidence-based guidance for clinical management.

Health Risks due to Overweight/Obesity

Increasing body fatness is accompanied by profound changes in physiological function. These changes are, to a certain extent, dependent on the regional distribution of adipose tissue. Generalized obesity results in alterations in total blood volume and cardiac function while the distribution of fat around the thoracic cage and abdomen restricts respiratory excursion and alters respiratory function. The intra-abdominal visceral deposition of adipose tissue, which characterizes upper body obesity, is a major contributor to the development of hypertension, elevated plasma insulin concentrations and insulin resistance, hyperglycemia, and hyperlipidemia. The alterations in metabolic and physiological function that follow an increase in adipose tissue mass are predictable when considered in the context of normal homeostasis.

Table 1 Obesity-associated diseases and conditions

Disorder	Associated diseases and conditions
Cardiovascular disorders	Coronary heart disease
	Hypertension
	Cerebrovascular disease
	Deep vein thrombosis
	Pulmonary embolism
Respiratory disorders	Obstructive sleep apneas
	Obesity hypoventilation syndrome
	Breathlessness
Gastrointestinal disorders	NASH (nonalcoholic steatohepatitis)
	Cirrhosis
	Gallstones
	Colorectal cancer
	Hiatus hernia/gastroesophageal reflux
Renal disorders	Proteinuria
Reproductive disorders	Primary ovulatory infertility
	Development of gestational diabetes
	Increased risk of neural tube defects
Musculoskeletal disorders	Osteoarthritis
	Gout
	Nerve entrapment
Genitourinary	Endometrial cancer
	Prostate cancer
	Stress incontinence
Metabolic and endocrine disorders	Artherogenic lipid profile
	Insulin resistance
	Type 2 diabetes mellitus
	Polycystic ovary syndrome
	Postmenopausal breast cancer
	Hirsuitism
Skin disorders	Acanthosis nigricans
	Lymphoedema
	Sweat rashes

Ethnicity has an impact on body fat distribution and adipose tissue metabolism. Overweight currently is defined as a body mass index (BMI) $>25\,\mathrm{kg\,m^{-2}}$ and obesity as a BMI $>30\,\mathrm{kg\,m^{-2}}$. The evidence for this is drawn from large population studies that suggest people with a BMI of $19{-}25\,\mathrm{kg\,m^{-2}}$ have the lowest mortality. However, there have been proposals to define race-specific standards according to ethnic background. Specifically, Asians have greater visceral fat and associated morbidity than do Caucasians. A BMI as low as $23\,\mathrm{kg\,m^{-2}}$ may be associated with weight-related diabetes or insulin resistance in these groups. For any given weight category, the presence of certain complications moves the individual into a higher health risk category. Evaluation of such risks should be part of the intervention program.

Patient Selection

Obesity and overweight are chronic conditions. Short-term programs are likely to be ineffective, with rapid weight regain once treatment is stopped. Treatment programs must be for the longer term and include measures to prevent relapse. Preventing further weight gain in those at risk should also form part of obesity management and help ensure an appropriate use of resources. Those at risk will include moderately overweight subjects and those who have upper body obesity. Weight loss is indicated in adults with a BMI of more than $25\,\mathrm{kg\,m^{-2}}$ and/or abdominal girth of more than or equal to $102\,\mathrm{cm}$ in males and more than or equal to $88\,\mathrm{cm}$ in females. Additional important treatment areas include weight gain in infancy, adolescence, and pregnancy. A family history of obesity or associated diseases, fat distribution, and risks for coronary heart disease are individually important factors that may influence treatment mode.

Treatment Aims and Realistic Weight Loss Goals

Treatment aims to improve health and well being and decrease the risks of ill health later in life, through reducing the amount and possibly distribution of body fat. The success or failure of any treatment program may be judged by an arbitrarily chosen weight or percentage weight loss. Hence, the evidence that modest degrees of weight loss produce significant health gain influences the success or failure of any treatment. With this background it is logical to redefine successful treatment in terms of a decrease in the severity of obesity rather than a return to normal weight. Even weight stabilization without weight loss represents a modestly successful outcome compared to the natural history of obesity, which is progressive weight gain. A weight loss of between 5 and 10% of the initial body weight is associated with clinically useful improvements in terms of blood pressure, plasma cholesterol, and a significant improvement in diabetic control (see **Table 2**). Weight loss should be approached incrementally with new weight goals negotiated with the patient if the original target is achieved. Goals for older patients (>65 years) will be different from those who are young; data suggest that a population becomes heavier with age whereas the risk from obesity does not increase proportionately.

Dietary Treatment of Obesity

The primary determinant of weight loss is energy deficit. Short-term weight loss has been achieved by

Table 2 Benefits of 10 kg weight loss

Condition	Health benefit
Mortality	Fall of more than 20% in total mortality
	Fall of more than 30% in diabetes-related death
	Fall of more than 40% in obesity-related cancer death
Blood pressure	Fall of 10 mm Hg systolic blood pressure
	Fall of 20 mm Hg diastolic blood pressure
Diabetes	Fall of 50% in fasting glucose
	Reduces risk of developing diabetes by 50%
Lipids	Fall of 10% in total cholesterol
	Fall of 15% in LDL cholesterol
	Fall of 30% in triglycerides
	Rise of 8% in HDL cholesterol

Adapted with acknowledgment from the Scottish Intercollegiate Guidelines Network (SIGN) Obesity in Scotland: integrating prevention with weight management. A national clinical guideline recommended for use in Scotland. Edinburgh (1996).

energy reduction in diets of varied macronutrient composition. Obesity is a chronic and relapsing disease; hence, it is the long-term efficacy of these dietary strategies in maintaining lowered weight (and minimizing the risk of diet-related chronic diseases) that is of fundamental importance.

Types of Dietary Treatment

There are several dietary strategies available both in a clinical and commercial setting. These diets vary greatly in the degree of caloric restriction, relative amounts of macronutrients (protein, carbohydrate, fat), medical supervision, scientific basis, and cost. These diets can be broadly divided into:

- low-calorie diets ($\geq$3400 kJ (800 kcal) day^{-1}, typically 3400–6300 kJ (800–1500 kcal) day^{-1})
- very low-calorie diets (<3400 kJ (800 kcal) day^{-1})

Traditionally, low-calorie diets that incorporate various methods for restricting food intake have been recommended for weight management.

Such treatment requires a period of supervision for at least 6 months. A review of 48 randomized control trials (RCTs) shows strong and consistent evidence that an average weight loss of 8% of the initial body weight can be obtained over 3–12 months with a low-calorie diet (LCD) and this weight loss causes a decrease in abdominal fat, the adipose tissue deposition that is associated with the highest disease risk. Very low-calorie diets (VLCD) have been shown to reduce weight at a greater rate in the first 2–3 months compared to low-calorie diets but have not been associated with superior maintenance of lost weight after a year. A review of weight loss trials of LCD and VLCD with available follow-up during 2–7 years showed that long-term weight loss in most trials is in the range of 2–6 kg.

Low-fat, high-carbohydrate diets Low-fat, high-carbohydrate diets have played a central role in the dietary management of overweight and obesity. Generally, these strategies aim to provide a macronutrient composition of 25–35% energy from fat, 45–60% from total carbohydrate, and 15–20% from protein, thereby moving individuals towards national dietary guidelines (COMA reports). A review of controlled clinical trials demonstrated that a 10% reduction of dietary fat leads to a ~3–4-kg weight loss in normal overweight subjects and ~5–6-kg weight loss in the obese. Evidence from a recent systematic review suggests that a low-fat diet is equally as effective in achieving long-term weight loss in overweight and obese subjects as alternative dietary strategies. Low-fat high-carbohydrate diets may have a role in weight maintenance. Combined with physical activity and behavioral strategies, the American Diabetes Prevention Program and the Finnish Diabetes Prevention Trial demonstrated maintenance of modest weight loss (3–4 kg) with a marked reduction in the risk of developing type 2 diabetes mellitus over a 4-year study period.

Low glycemic index diets The glycemic index (GI) is a dietary concept originally developed for the therapy of diabetes, which has recently become popular despite scant evidence of its effectiveness in weight management. The GI is a property that describes the effect of carbohydrate from a given food on postprandial blood glucose. It is measured by comparing the blood glucose response of the test food with that of a reference food (usually white bread). Low-GI foods are more slowly absorbed leading to an attenuated and prolonged insulin and metabolic response to foods; it is suggested that more moderate blood glucose and metabolic response may sustain satiety and energy balance to a greater extent than larger metabolic shifts would.

Epidemiological analyses link low-GI load diets to a more favorable lipids profile and reduced incidence of type 2 diabetes mellitus and cardiovascular disease. Evidence from interventional studies supports the benefits of low-GI diets in reducing the risks of coronary heart disease and diabetes but there are no long-term studies that have evaluated its weight-loss efficacy. Therefore, it is appropriate to promote the constituents of a low-GI diet (increased legumes, wholegrain cereals, and fruit consumption) as part of a well-balanced hypo-caloric diet for the long-term management of obesity and its metabolic complications.

High-protein, low-carbohydrate diets High-protein diets have recently been popularized as a means of rapid weight loss despite the lack of objective evidence in long-term efficacy and safety. Typically, these diets offer wide latitude in protein food choices, and are restrictive in other food choices (mainly carbohydrate). Animal protein rather than plant protein is advocated leading to a higher intake of total fat – mainly saturated fat and cholesterol. Many of the popular high-protein diets promote protein intake of 28–64% of dietary energy, which exceeds established requirement of 10–15%, and severely limit carbohydrate dietary energy to 3–10%. A recent popular high-protein, low-carbohydrate diet, the Atkins diet, provides on average 27% energy from protein, 5% energy from carbohydrates, and 68% energy from fat. The diet results in the avoidance of important staple foods, such as bread, pasta, rice, potatoes, and cereals, as well as foods high in sugars. Consumption of fruits, vegetables, whole grains, and low-fat dairy products, foods associated with lowering blood pressure and protecting against cancer and heart disease, are all limited.

The initial weight loss in high-protein diets is high due to fluid and glycogen loss related to low carbohydrate intake, overall caloric restriction that is encouraged by structured eating plans, restricted range of foods allowed, and limited tolerance of high-protein foods. This often promotes a misconception about weight loss by suggesting that it is not related to total energy intake but is due to exclusion of certain foods.

A recent systematic review of the efficacy of low-carbohydrate, high-protein diets demonstrates that the amount of weight loss is principally associated with decreased caloric intake rather than reduced carbohydrate content. Researchers have yet to establish whether individuals can maintain long-term weight loss with a high-protein, low-carbohydrate diet because of the short duration of these studies, and long-term adverse effects are also unknown. Possible negative effects include increased risks of cardiovascular disease, renal disease, cancer, osteoporosis, and compromised vitamin and mineral status.

Energy prescribed diet This dietary strategy determines the daily energy requirement for weight loss by calculating energy expenditure, adjusting for physical activity, and subtracting an energy deficit to induce weight loss –usually 2100–2520 kJ (500–600 kcal) for 0.05 kg weight loss. As a result the prescribed diet will often be in excess of 3400–6300 kJ (800–1500 kcal). The popularity of this approach relates to the findings of improved compliance in those advised on a 2520 kJ (600 kcal) deficit diet compared to a traditional fixed energy intake of 5040 kJ (1200 kcal) day^{-1}.

Formulas and meal replacements Meal replacements are another category of calorie-controlled diets. These include nutritional fortified shakes, snack bars, and low-calorie frozen meals. An entire meal or snack is replaced with a portion controlled prepackaged meal or drink that provides approximately 840–1260 kJ (200–300 kcal), although formulations and nutrient content vary. Meal replacements are designed to be eaten with additions of conventional foods that supply dietary fiber, other nutrients, additional calories, and water. Most weight loss programs that use meal replacements recommend replacing two meals and one snack a day to lose weight and then replacing one meal per day to maintain weight loss. This strategy generally provides 5040–6729 kJ (1200–1600 kcal) day^{-1} and the regular meal should meet the recommendations of a healthy diet.

A recent meta-analysis that summarized the efficacy of this approach compared to conventional energy-restricted diets suggests that it is an effective weight-loss strategy both in the short and long term in a clinical trial setting. There is no information about the efficacy outside a clinical trial where meal replacement products need to be purchased, and are frequently discontinued at an early stage.

Very low-calorie diets Very low-calorie diets are formula foods; they are designed to provide larger and more rapid weight loss than the standard low-calorie diets. They are commonly given in liquid form to completely replace usual food and snack intake providing in the region of 1890–3400 kJ (450–800 kcal) day^{-1}. To reduce the potential risks from loss of lean body tissue, VLCDs are enriched in protein of high biologic value and also includes the full complement of recommended daily allowance for vitamins, minerals, electrolytes, and fatty acids. However, diets providing such low-energy intakes are often associated with a feeling of fatigue, constipation, nausea, and diarrhea. A most serious complication associated with VLCD is the development of symptomatic cholelithiasis associated with the rapid weight loss (1–2 kg week^{-1}).

Owing to the potential adverse effects of these diets, they are generally reserved for short-term treatment in individuals who are moderately to severely obese (BMI >35 kg m^{-2}) and who have failed at more conservative approach to weight loss, in particular in those with medical conditions that may respond to weight loss such as obstructive sleep apnea, type 2 diabetes mellitus, or prior to surgical procedure.

Weight regain is common with the reintroduction of food. Studies show that in the long term, VLCDs are no more effective than more modest dietary restriction.

Commercial Slimming Organizations and Products Such organizations are profit-making ventures. However, they have been shown to be economical, practical, and an effective way of providing care for a large number of moderately obese people in the community. Weekly meetings serve to encourage and reinforce active participation by members, who learn through the exchange of ideas within the group. Weight losses achieved by commercial groups are comparable to those seen in general practice or hospital outpatient clinics. When behavioral techniques are added to the basic program of balanced diet, the results are further improved.

Over recent years there has been increasing use of weight loss-related web sites on the Internet, which are directed mainly at females. The content and structure of these web sites vary widely. They often lack professional contact and the expertise to deal with medical complications.

Behavior Treatment

Behavior therapy provides an important approach to losing and maintaining weight. The focus is on behaviors related to body weight, namely food intake and physical activity. It serves to identify the abnormal eating behaviors and life style developed over the years and helps to unlearn them and allow body weight to return to normal. The behavior techniques used include self-monitoring, stimulus control, and, recently, cognitive therapy, which involves identifying and changing negative thoughts.

The key difference between behavioral methods and other forms of treatment is that the individual must take responsibility for initiating and maintaining treatment rather than relying on external forces.

There are several elements of behavioral treatment (see **Table 3**). Evidence from RCTs confirms that behavioral strategies reinforce changes in diet and physical activity in obese subjects to produce weight loss of 10% over 4 months to 1 year. Longer term followup shows a return to baseline in the absence of continuing behavioral intervention.

Eating patterns and behaviors are, to a greater extent, acquired by learning, and for this reason there has been much interest in modifying the behavior within the family setting. Obese children are more likely than nonobese children to become obese adults. Behavior therapy seems to be effective in arresting this process in some children.

Exercise and Physical Activity

Exercise produces fat loss in obese and normal weight subjects, although losses rarely exceed 5% of body

Table 3 Elements of behavioral treatment

Element	Intervention strategy
Self-monitoring	Observe, record, and provide feedback on: • food consumption (food diary) • physical activity (activity diary, pedometer) • weight record
Goal setting	Realistic weight-loss goals Separate short-term from long-term goals Focus on health benefits
Stimulus control	Identify and modify environmental barriers: • healthy eating, normalize eating pattern • increasing daily energy using activities
Problem solving	Handling emotional issues and social events: • examine situation • choose a solution and implement it • evaluate the outcome
Cognitive change	Changing inaccurate belief about weight loss • examine thought and feelings • challenge inaccurate ones • use positive self-affirmations

weight. For any given weight loss, fat-free mass (FFM) is better preserved in exercising than non-exercising subjects: this is likely to be important in the long term because FFM is the best predictor of resting metabolic rate, which is the largest contributor to daily energy expenditure for all but active athletes.

There are other beneficial effects of exercise that are independent of its effects on weight loss. Regular exercise reduces blood pressure, improves insulin sensitivity, both in association with or independent of weight loss. Favorable effects on the atherogenic lipid profiles have also been reported with exercise and physical training in obese subjects. Such benefits are substantial and should be emphasized to all patients; however, persuading an obese person to participate in regular physical activity and to maintain exercise as a part of daily routine is not easy.

One of the most consistent findings in studies of physical activity is enhanced weight maintenance for at least 2 years from the start of the intervention. It is not necessary to increase maximal oxygen uptake in the obese to derive benefit from exercise: metabolic evidence of fitness is achieved with less vigorous exercise.

Physical activity recommendations suggest 30 min of moderate activity on at least 5 days of the week. This level of activity is associated with improved fitness and protection from cardiovascular diseases. When using exercise solely as a strategy for weight reduction, longer duration of daily activity of a moderate intensity lasting 45–60 min is required.

Reduction in the time spent in sedentary behaviors (such as television watching) is an important strategy for increasing physical activity and energy expenditure. Similarly, encouraging findings have been observed in children and adolescents advised to include more lifestyle activity (e.g., walking versus car use) compared to those with traditional programs of activity.

Drug Treatment of Obesity

Rationale

Diet restriction even when combined with behavioral therapy and increased exercise is often unsuccessful in achieving weight loss and maintenance in obese subjects. Obesity is not a single disorder but a heterogeneous group of conditions with multiple causes. Although genetic differences are of undoubted importance, the marked rise in the prevalence of obesity is best explained by behavioral and environmental changes that have resulted from technological advances. In such circumstances, it is appropriate to consider pharmacological treatment as an adjunct to the other treatment modalities.

In broad terms a pharmacological agent can cause weight loss by reducing energy intake or absorption/ and by increasing energy expenditure. Current drug treatment of obesity is directed at reducing energy/ food intake either by an action on the gastrointestinal system or via an action through the central nervous system control of appetite and feeding.

Selection of Patients

Pharmacological treatments of obesity have had a controversial history and are still regarded with skepticism and suspicion by some medical practitioners. This results from experiences with older agents that turned out to have serious side effects and were withdrawn as a result. Current agents approved for use have been shown to be safe and effective both in weight reduction and in the improvement of comorbidities of obesity. Nevertheless, it is important that doctors who prescribe such drugs are fully familiar with the mode of action and potential risks.

Several sets of guidelines have been developed for the use of drugs in the treatment of obesity. In the UK, The Royal College of Physicians' guidance on the use of anti-obesity drugs suggests that it may be appropriate to consider use of drugs after at least 3 months of supervised diet, exercise, and behavioral management. Exceptionally, this period may be shortened when the clinician judges that drug treatment is justified at an earlier stage due to over-riding medical circumstances. **Table 4** lists the criteria that should be applied to judge the suitability of a patient for drug treatment.

Table 4 Criteria for selecting obese patients suitable for obesity drug treatment

- Drug treatment may be appropriate where diet and exercise have not achieved acceptable weight loss relative to medical risk
- In such patients drug treatment may be appropriate for:
  - those whose BMI is more than 30
  - those with established comorbidities whose BMI is more than 27, if the drug license permits
- Weight-lowering drugs should be targeted at those at high risk from obesity, not obesity alone

The following groups will have priority for drug treatment
- Patients with established comorbidities such as type 2 diabetes, hypertension, and dyslipidemia
- Patients who are physically restricted by their weight either because of breathlessness or arthritis
- Patients considered to be at high risk – for example, those with a family history of overweight or obese parents who died prematurely from CHD or developed type 2 diabetes with complications

The criteria applied to the use of an anti-obesity drug are similar to those applied to the treatment of other relapsing disorders. It is important to avoid offering anti-obesity drug therapy to patients who are seeking a 'quick fix' for their weight problem. The initiation of drug treatment will depend on the clinician's judgement about the risks to an individual from continuing obesity. It may be appropriate after at least 3 months of supervised diet, exercise, and behavioral management, or at a subsequent review, if a patient's BMI is equal to or greater than $30\,kg\,m^{-2}$ and weight loss is less than 10% of the presenting weight. In certain clinical circumstances it may also be appropriate to consider anti-obesity drug treatment for those patients with established comorbidities whose BMI is $27\,kg\,m^{-2}$ or greater if this is permitted by the drug's licence (see **Figure 1**). An anti-obesity drug should not be prescribed for a patient whose BMI is less than that specified in the product licence for the drug – the licence indication does not presently take account of the morbidity from obesity seen in certain populations at a lower BMI.

The experience from the use of anti-obesity drugs during 12–24 month randomized controlled trials indicate that approximately 50% of the actively treated patients respond as judged by 5–10% reduction in body weight maintained over 12 months. The weight loss occurs in the 'responder' group within 12 weeks. This indicates a suitable time period when a response to drug treatment can be identified and a decision taken to continue the medication. Continuing assessment of drug therapy for efficacy and safety is essential. If the drug is efficacious in helping a patient to lose and/or maintain weight loss, and there are no serious side effects, it may be continued.

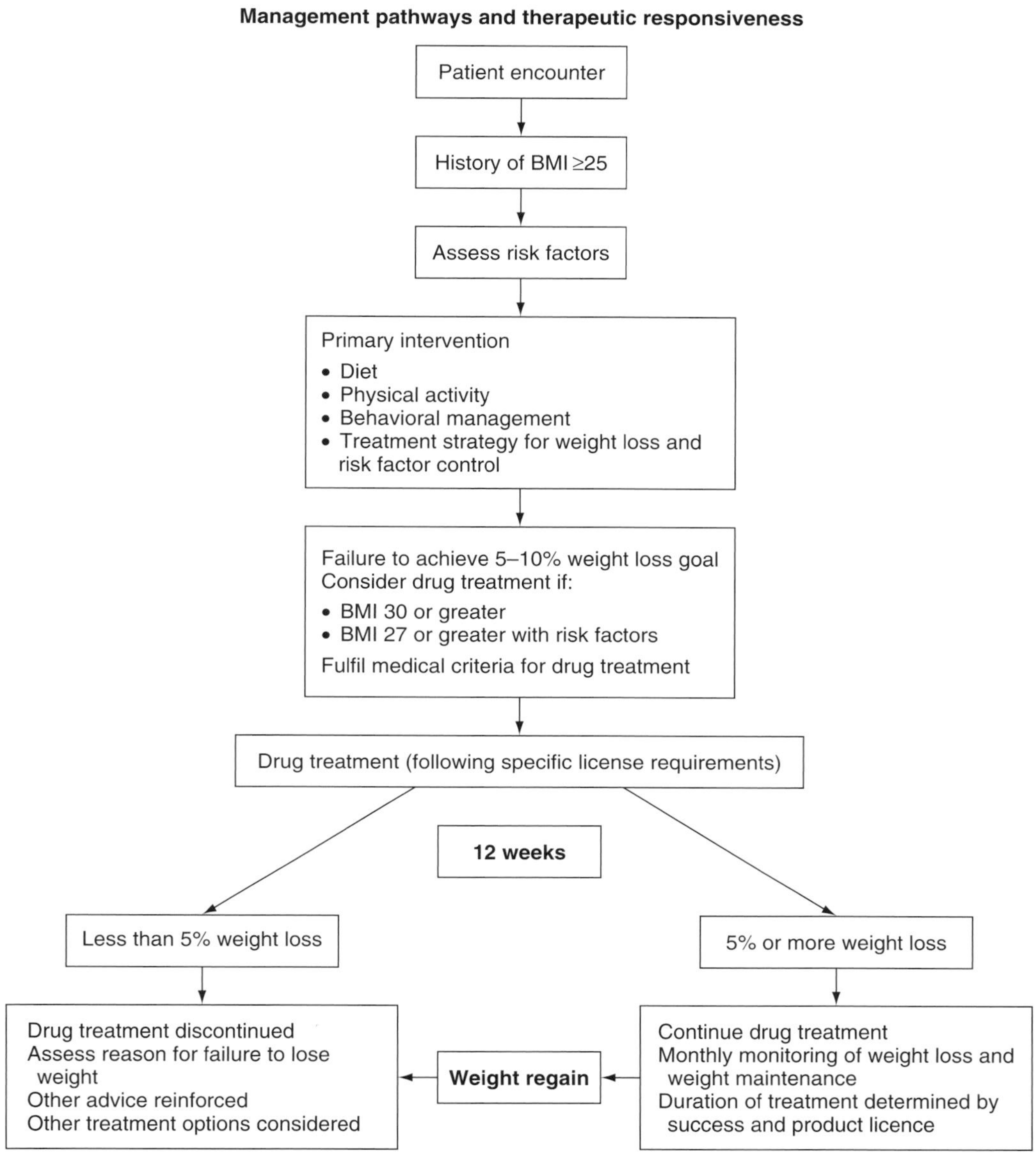

Management pathways and therapeutic responsiveness

Figure 1 A management pathway for the appropriate prescription of an anti-obesity drug. (Adapted with permission from RCP Guidelines 2003.)

If not, it should be discontinued. Once a weight loss target has been achieved, there should be an opportunity for re-negotiation of a new target, if indicated, and/or long term monitoring with reinforcement.

Types of Drugs

The two categories of anti-obesity medication currently licensed for use in obese subjects are:

1. Those that act on the gastrointestinal system (pancreatic lipase inhibitors) as malabsorption agents to inhibit nutrient absorption.

2. Those that act on the central nervous system primarily to reduce hunger perception.

Drugs acting on the gastrointestinal system

Orlistat Orlistat is a gastric and pancreatic lipase inhibitor that reduces the absorption of dietary fat in a dose-dependent manner. At the therapeutic dose of 120 mg three times a day, it blocks the absorption of about 30% of dietary triacylglycerol resulting in an energy deficit of 850 kJ (200 kcal) day^{-1} for an individual on an average diet of 9240 kJ (2200 kcal) day^{-1} with 40% of calories from fat.

Adverse effects of orlistat are predominantly related to its gastrointestinal action of fat malabsorption and can be associated with a modest reduction in fat-soluble vitamins (A, D, E, and K). However, clinical deficiency has not been reported in clinical trials. Nevertheless, it is recommended that patients taking orlistat receive vitamin supplements. Patients may complain of loose or liquid stool, fecal urgency, anal leakage, and infrequently fecal incontinence due to undigested fat. These adverse effects become less common with longer duration of treatment suggesting that patients learn to avoid high-fat meals to avoid these side effects hence enforcing behavioral change. This may well contribute to the therapeutic effects of orlistat treatment. Orlistat is minimally absorbed (less than 1%) and systemic events are negligible.

Drugs acting on the central nervous system These drugs are commonly referred to as appetite suppressants, which is only one of their actions. Some of these agents have been proven to enhance satiety and slow gastric emptying; and an increase in energy expenditure has also been suggested. They act by increasing the neurotransmitter activity in the brain centers that regulate food intake.

Sibutramine Sibutramine enhances the sensation of satiety after a meal by its central action as a serotonin and/or epinephrine re-uptake inhibitor. Sibutramine is a beta-phenethylamine and is well absorbed following oral administration. It undergoes extensive first pass metabolism in the liver to produce two pharmacologically active metabolites that have long elimination half-lives of 14–16 h.

Side effects commonly reported in clinical trials include dry mouth, constipation, anxiety, rhinitis, and insomnia but these rarely led to withdrawal from the study. The noradrenergic actions of the drug may cause an increase in blood pressure and heart rate in some patients or prevent the expected fall in these parameters with weight loss. It should not be given in patients with uncontrolled hypertension. It should not be given concomitantly with monoamine oxidase inhibitors, nor other centrally acting anorexic drugs, or sympathomimetic agents including cold remedies such as pseudoephedrine.

Phentermine and diethylpropion Published evidence of the use of phentermine and diethylpropion indicates short-term induction of weight loss that is frequently followed by weight regain on cessation of the drug. There are no recently published randomized controlled trials of the drugs demonstrating efficacy beyond 26 weeks. Both drugs remain restricted to 3 month's use in the terms of their product license.

Rimonabant (SR 141716) Rimonabant is a selective central cannaboid (CB1) receptor antagonist. It is an appetite suppressant in advanced development for obesity treatment. The rationale behind this drug is to reduce appetite by blocking cannaboid receptors in the hypothalamus. The central cannaboid (CB1) receptors are believed to play a role in controlling food consumption and the phenomena of dependence/habituation.

Preliminary results from a 2-year international multicenter study confirm its effectiveness in weight reduction, reduction in waist circumference (a marker of the dangerous abdominal obesity), and improvements in lipids and glycemic profiles. The study also confirmed its good safety profile. The side effects reported were mainly mild and transient and most frequently involved nausea, diarrhea, and dizziness.

Rimonabant has potential as a treatment for smoking cessation because the central cannaboid system is also involved in the body's response to tobacco dependence.

Prescribing guidelines for anti-obesity drugs

Anti-obesity drugs should be prescribed in an appropriate clinical setting that includes systems for monitoring and follow-up of progress. The choice of anti-obesity drug is largely dependent on the experience of the prescriber in using one or another agent (see **Table 5**). For the two agents currently recommended for use there are no good clinical studies that have directly compared them or have explored which particular patient will benefit more from one than the other. A drug should not be considered ineffective because weight loss has stopped, provided the lowered weight is maintained.

The Elderly and Children

There is limited information about the use of anti-obesity drugs in patients over the age of 75 years. In such circumstances, the accepted practice is to aim for weight maintenance rather than weight loss. Neither drug is licensed for use in children.

Surgical Treatment for Obesity

Surgical treatment is an appropriate intervention for the management of morbid obesity. Criteria for selection of patients suitable for surgery are listed in **Table 6**.

Table 5 Comparison of actions and indications for use of sibutramine and orlistat

	Sibutramine	Orlistat
Mode of action	Promotes satiety Enhancing effect on thermogenesis	Dietary fat malabsorption
Indication	Adjunct to diet in obese patients with BMI $\geq 30\,kg\,m^{-2}$ without comorbidities or BMI $\geq 27\,kg\,m^{-2}$ with comorbidities	Adjunct to diet in obese patients with BMI $\geq 30\,kg\,m^{-2}$ without comorbidities or BMI $\geq 28\,kg\,m^{-2}$ with comorbidities
Suitable for	Those with uncontrollable appetite Frequent snackers Nocturnal eaters Those with need for immediate weight loss for medical reasons Those without contraindication to its use (specifically cardiac abnormalities or elevated blood pressure, i.e., >145/95 mm Hg) Patients with low HDL cholesterol	Those who have lost at least 2.5 kg through diet and lifestyle modification Patients requiring longer term behavioral changes whose dietary assessment suggests high-fat intake Patients with impaired glucose tolerance Those with elevated LDL cholesterol Chronic malabsorption Cholestasis
Specific contraindication	Tourette syndrome Cardiovascular disease Congestive cardiac failure Hypertension Hyperthyroidism, phaechromocytoma Pregnancy, breastfeeding	Pregnancy, breast feeding
Duration of treatment	Not more than 1 year	Maximum of 2 years

Types of Obesity Surgery

At least 30 surgical techniques have been developed for the treatment of obesity. Superficial cosmetic removal of adipose tissue (liposuction) will not be considered because it has no lasting benefit and it is not regarded as a treatment for obesity. Jaw wiring (intermandibular fixation) can restrict intake of food but it is no longer recommended for surgical treatment of obesity due to a lack of long-term efficacy.

The operative procedures currently used for the surgical treatment of obesity are outlined below.

Gastric restriction Gastric restriction can by achieved by gastroplasty or gastric banding. Gastroplasty techniques involve the fashioning of a proximal pouch of the stomach by vertical stapling and a constrictive band opening, thereby restricting the gastric volume to approximately 15–20 ml that empties into the remainder of the stomach.

Gastric banding involves the external 'pinching off' of the upper part of the stomach with a band usually made of Dacron. A modification of the gastric banding is an inflatable circumgastric band attached to a subcutaneous reservoir that allows access by a hypodermic syringe to inject or withdraw fluid thereby tightening or enlarging the bandwidth. This operation can be performed laparoscopically, significantly improving the perioperative safety of operating for the severely obese patients.

Gastric restriction operations require strict dietary compliance because an intake of high caloric liquids or soft foods are not inhibited by the narrow outlet and may explain a failure to lose weight. The advantage of these techniques is very low operative mortality (<1%) and relative lack of long-term nutritional deficiencies. The reported excess weight loss after 3–5 years is between 40 and 60% but there is a slow regain thereafter.

Gastric by-pass A 20–30-ml pouch is created by staples and connected to the jejunum transected 50 cm from the ligament of Treitz (Roux-en-Y gastric bypass). It results in weight loss by both restrictive and malabsorptive mechanisms. Published evidence confirms this procedure produces greater weight loss compared to gastric restrictive techniques but more frequent adverse effects including 'dumping' and nutritional deficiency may accompany it. Its operative mortality is approximately 1%.

Table 6 Criteria for patient selection

- BMI $\geq 40\,kg\,m^{-2}$
- BMI $\geq 35\,kg\,m^{-2}$ with serious comorbidity demonstrated to be responsive to weight loss
- Failure to achieve weight loss with conventional means
- Able to lose weight prior to surgery
- Have no evidence of psychiatric disease or maladaptive eating behaviors
- Absence of endocrine disorders that can cause morbid obesity
- Psychological stability:
  - Absence of alcohol and drug abuse
  - Understanding of how surgery achieves weight loss
  - preoperative psychological evaluation for selected patients

Biliopancreatic diversion Biliopancreatic diversion includes a gastric resection and diversion of the biliopancreatic juice to the terminal ileum to reduce the absorption of nutrients. In this operation, an entero-entero anastomosis is performed between the proximal limb of the transected jejunum and ileum, 50–100 cm proximal to the ileocecal valve.

Biliopancreatic diversion achieves up to 78% excess weight loss at 5 years. Nutritional deficiencies are relatively common (between 5 and 40% of patients for the longer term). In addition, alterations in bowel movements are frequent with 3–5 motions, commonly offensive, occurring each day.

Efficacy of Surgical Treatment for Obesity

Surgery is usually successful in inducing substantial weight loss in the majority of obese patients. This is achieved primarily by a necessary reduction in calorie intake.

In a review of RCT comparing different treatment strategies of obesity, surgery resulted in greater weight loss (23–28 kg more weight loss at 2 years) with improvement in quality of life and comorbidities.

The Swedish Obese Subjects (SOS) study demonstrated long-term beneficial effects on cardiovascular risk factors. The development of type 2 diabetes mellitus is most favorably influenced with a 14-fold risk reduction in those obese patients undergoing surgical treatment.

A Multidisciplinary Approach to the Management of Overweight and Obesity

Published evidence confirms that patients do better whatever the treatment when seen more frequently and for a greater length of time. Moreover, strategies that involve expertise incorporating dietetic, behavioral, and exercise experts as well as physicians and surgeons are also more successful in sustaining weight loss. This underlines the importance of a multidisciplinary approach. Treatment programs should include a system for regular audit and the provision for change as a result of the findings. Any center that claims to specifically provide expertise in weight management should incorporate the essential elements outlined in Table 7.

Strategies for Weight Loss Maintenance

Preventing regain of fat losses is the major challenge of weight maintenance. A program to enable the individual to maintain their lowered weight

Table 7 Essential elements of an appropriate setting for obesity management

- Trained staff directly involved in the running of the weight loss program. These staff (medical, nursing, and other healthcare professionals) should have attended courses on the management of obesity and must be given the opportunity to continue their education
- Printed program for weight management that includes clear advice on diet, behavioral modification technique, physical exercise, and strategies for long-term lifestyle changes. Such a program may include a family and/or group approach
- Suitable equipment, in particular accurate and regularly calibrated weighing scale and stadiometer
- Specific weight-loss goals for patients with energy deficit being achieved by moderating food intake and increasing physical expenditure
- Documentation of individual patients' health risks. This will include BMI, waist circumference, blood pressure, blood lipids, and cigarette smoking and comorbid conditions
- A clearly defined follow-up procedure that involves collaboration between the different settings of care, and provides regular monitoring and documentation of progress, along with details of criteria for judging the success of weight loss. This will allow a weight loss program to be properly supported, medical conditions to be monitored, and problems or issues to be addressed at the earliest opportunity. It is also advisable to have a checklist of possible adverse drug effects, e.g., anxiety, disturbances of sleep, breathlessness, depression, and diarrhea.

must follow any successful weight loss. Published evidence suggests that a combination of dietary and physical activity modifications and reinforcement of behavioral methods are the most effective in the long term. These modifications needs to be integrated and accepted as a way of life and the responsibility for following this must lie with the patient.

See also: **Coronary Heart Disease**: Prevention. **Diabetes Mellitus**: Dietary Management. **Energy**: Balance. **Exercise**: Beneficial Effects; Diet and Exercise. **Hunger. Hyperlipidemia**: Overview. **Obesity**: Definition, Etiology and Assessment; Fat Distribution; Prevention.

Further Reading

Astrup A, Ryan L, Grunwald GK *et al.* (2000) The role of dietary fat in body fatness: evidence from a preliminary meta-analysis of ad libitum low fat dietary intervention studies. *British Journal of Nutrition* 83(supplement 1): S25–S32.

Bravata DM, Sanders I, Huang J *et al.* (2003) Efficacy and safety of low carbohydrate diets. A systematic review. *JAMA* 289(14): 1837–1850.

Bray GA, Bouchard C, and James WPT (eds.) (1998) *Handbook of Obesity*. New York: Marcel Dekker.

British Nutrition Foundation (1999) *Obesity*. London: Blackwell Science.

Colquitt J, Clegg A, Sidhu M *et al.* (2003) Surgery for morbid obesity (Cochrane Review). In: *The Cochrane Library*, issue 3. Oxford: Update Software.

National Institutes of Health (NIH), National Heart, Lung, and Blood Institute (NLLBI) (1998). *Clinical Guidelines on the Identification, Evaluation, and Treatment of Overweight and Obesity: the Evidence Report.* Washington: US Government Press.

Department of Health (1991) *Dietary Reference Values for Food Energy and Nutrients for the United Kingdom: Report on Health and Social Subjects*, vol. 41. London: HMSO.

Frost G, Masters K, King C *et al.* (1991) A new method of energy prescription to improve weight loss. *Journal of Human Nutrition and Dietetics* 4: 369–373.

Haddock CK, Poston WSC, Dill PL *et al.* (2002) Pharmacotherapy for obesity: a quantitative analysis of four decades of published randomised clinical trials. *International Journal of Obesity* 26: 262–273.

Harvey EL, Glenny AM, Kirk SF, and Summerbell CD (1999). A systematic review of interventions to improve health professionals' management of obesity. *International Journal of Obesity* 23: 1212–1222.

James WPT, Astrup A, Finer N *et al.* for the STORM Study Group (2000). Effect of Sibutramine on weight management after weight loss: a randomised trial. *Lancet* 356: 2119–2125.

Klem M, Wing R, McGuire H *et al.* (1997). A descriptive study of individuals successful at long-term maintenance of substantial weight loss. *American Journal of Clinical Nutrition* 66(2): 239–246.

Kopelman PG (2000) Obesity as a medical problem. *Nature* 404: 635–643.

Kopelman PG and Stock M (eds.) (1999) *Clinical Obesity.* London: Blackwell Science.

National Task Force on the Prevention and Treatment of Obesity (2002). Medical care for obese patients: advice for health care professionals. *American Family Physician* 65: 81–88.

Robert SB (2000) High glycaemic index foods, hunger and obesity: Is there a connection. *Nutrition Review* 58: 163–169.

Royal College of Physicians of London (2003) *Anti-Obesity Drugs. Guidance on Appropriate Prescribing and Management.* London: RCP.

Sjostrom CD, Peltonem M, Wedel IT *et al.* (2000) Differentiated long-term effects of intentional weight loss on diabetes and hypertension. *Hypertension* 36(1): 20–25.

Sjostrom L, Rissanen A, Andersen T *et al.* (1998) Weight loss and prevention of weight regain in obese patients: a 2-year, European, randomised trial of Orlistat. *Lancet* 352: 167–172.

Oils *see* **Fats and Oils**

OLDER PEOPLE

Contents

Physiological Changes

N Solomons, Center for Studies of Sensory Impairment, Aging and Metabolism (CeSSIAM), Guatemala City, Guatemala

The Aging of the Population and its People

The maximal human life span is about 120 years. Approaching this degree of longevity, however, was not a prominent feature in the evolutionary phases of our species, *Homo sapiens*. The imperative was to survive the various mortal hazards long enough to reproduce and provide initial care for the offspring. The twenty-first century has ushered in an unprecedented longevity. The life expectancy of infants born today in Western Europe or Japan is over 75 years. The most rapidly increasing population segment in the world today is the centenarian. By the year 2020, there will be over 1 billion people over 60 years of age, constituting 13.3% of the global population, and three-quarters of them will be living in developing countries.

Many people are living a long time, but not all of them are healthy and functional throughout their lifespan. Chronic disability and the cost of health services and custodial care are a growing burden on the economies of developed and developing countries alike. In order to understand the pathological aspects of advancing age, the normative pattern of changes in physiological function in older persons is an essential benchmark.

The Nature of Senescence

Aging has been described as "a series of time-related processes that ultimately bring life to a close," that is, a process of physiological 'wearing out.' Physiology is the basis of human functionality, as well as of our susceptibility to disease. The late gerontologist, Nathan Shock, established the principle of a progressive decline in physiological reserves as a consequence of 'normal' aging, recognizing that the rate of decline differed markedly among the body's organ systems. In fact, one cannot really separate the concept of the physiology of older persons from the physiology of the aging process itself. Similarly, the high prevalence of chronic diseases in older persons challenges our ability to discriminate 'normative' senescence from pathophysiological changes.

The origin of physiological changes in older persons begins within the domain of cellular senescence. The extension to tissue and organ levels originates in what we interpret to be the physiological changes of human aging. Major advances in our cellular and molecular understanding of basic aging processes have been made in recent years.

Cellular Senescence

In most tissues, with the notable exception of neural tissue, healthy cells are replicating cells, which are capable of mobilizing at least 20 enzymes and proteins that must be preassembled to initiate DNA synthesis for cell division. An irreversible state of growth arrest known as replicative senescence is the fundamental basis of cellular aging. Such senescent cells remain viable and metabolically active, but their genomic function and protein expression are distinct from that of normal, proliferating cells. Iron accumulates in senescent cells, possibly contributing to the greater oxidative stress and cellular dysfunction seen in senescent cells. Senescent cells also express proinflammatory enzymes, an internal process that could possibly contribute to the aging process; intercellular adhesion molecules, which are part of the inflammatory response, are overexpressed in association with senescent cells and aging tissue.

Telomeres and Telomerase

Telomeres are small units composed of the tandem DNA repeats and associated proteins, which cap the end of linear chromosomes and are responsible for maintaining chromosome length. They provide stability to the chromosome and protect against DNA loss associated with cellular replication. The mechanism of replicative arrest of senescent cells has been related to changes in the function of telomerase, a nuclear enzyme that synthesizes and maintains the telomeres. Shortening and uncapping of these structures, related to the number of past cell divisions, renders the DNA strand incapable of replication.

Apoptosis

Another factor involved in aging at the cellular level is the orderly 'retirement' of cells. For every cell that divides in, another would somehow have to make space for the extra cell in order to maintain numerical stability in the organ. This is achieved by a process of programed cell death, known as 'apoptosis.' Cell senescence disrupts these apoptotic processes. Necrosis, by contrast, is cell death due to injury or noxious stimuli. Diseases of aging may favor the necrotic process.

Mitochondrial Senescence and Oxidative Stress

The intracellular mitochondria, organelles involved in energy metabolism, are central to the process of cell senescence. They are also involved in regulating thermogenesis, calcium buffering, and integrating apoptosis. With aging, mitochondria become less efficient, in part due to mutations in the cell nucleus, derepressing the expression of proteins that compete with mitochondrial function. This disrupts energy metabolism for the cell and makes the mitochondria more porous, releasing reactive oxygen species into the rest of the cell. The mitochondrial production of reactive oxygen species is inversely proportional to longevity in animals. The oxidative activity also damages the mitochondria themselves. Mitochondria have their own DNA strands, and these accumulate mutations with age. In tissues dependent on progenitor (stem) cells, mitochondrial DNA mutations can disrupt replication.

Free radicals and reactive oxidative species can produce mutations in nuclear material and oxidize proteins and lipids throughout the cells. Aging involves an accumulation of oxidative damage at the cellular level, if not an increase in its intensity as well. The thiol-containing antioxidant mechanisms, typified by glutathione but represented by a number of sulfur-containing species, represent an important buffer against intracellular free radicals, but decline with age due to downregulation of their synthetic enzymes. Confirming the cellular trend to oxidative stress in aging cells, clinical biomarkers of oxidation and antioxidant mechanisms reveal that systemic oxidative stress increases with aging characterized by lower concentrations of vitamins E and C and carotenes as well as lower activities of Cu-Zn-superoxide dismutase, catalase, and glutathione peroxidase.

Physiological Changes Occurring in Tissues and Organ Systems with Human Aging

Physiology has classically been organized around organ systems. According to this convention, the important features of the age-associated changes are enumerated and synthesized, with implications for human nutrition.

Integumentary Tissues

The integumentary tissues (skin, hair, nails) cover and protect the body. Two of the more classical and reproducible manifestations of aging can be seen in this system. The depigmentation of hair to gray or white is an almost universal aging effect given sufficient survival. Wrinkling of the skin, due to alteration in connective tissue composition, is another consequence of aging; it should be assessed by the changes in skin texture only in the non-sun-exposed regions of the body. Beyond the cosmetic consequences of the aging integumentary tissues, wound healing is a health-relevant consideration. Healing of wounds is slower with increasing age, but the resulting scars have the same tensile strength. Reduced recruitment of vessels of the microvascular is a function of aging.

The skin is an endocrine organ. Vitamin D is produced from the conversion of 7-hydroxy-cholesterol to cholecalciferol in the dermis of the skin. The efficiency of vitamin D decreases with age, such that older persons need a longer exposure to solar radiation to produce a given quantity of the vitamin.

Pulmonary and Respiratory System

Compliance of the chest wall changes with age, which gets stiffer and less compliant. The muscular force of the diaphragm is reduced with advancing years. The combination of these two factors reduces the maximal amount of air that can be moved into and out of the lungs. This diminution in the so-called forced vital capacity (FVC) of the lungs occurs as one gets older. There is less compliance, less recoil, and greater dead space. The original lung capacity, however, is sufficient to allow for sufficient gas exchange throughout life in the absence

of underlying pulmonary disease. Nonetheless, the longitudinal Framingham Heart Study found an association between decrease in lung capacity and all-cause mortality.

The hygiene of the respiratory airways is somewhat compromised by a decreasing function of the microcilia of the bronchial epithelial cells. Since this mechanism is used to clear microbial pathogens, it has a direct influence on host defenses. Finally, since the basis of the respiratory system is an exchange of gases (oxygen, carbon dioxide, trace gases) with the bloodstream, any cardiovascular changes involving the right-side chambers of the heart will influence the overall gas-exchange efficiency for the body.

Cardiovascular and Circulatory System

For this system, it is necessary to separate the aging effects on the cardiac muscle and its apparatus from the aging of the vessels of the circulatory system, which transports blood to and from the heart. A characteristic of aging is a diminished resting cardiac output, which can have the combined bases of lower force of the cardiac muscle and a lesser oxygen demand for metabolism with diminished active-cell mass. Aging of the myocardium reduces its capacity for cellular repair and replacement. With aging, elevations of noradrenaline (norepinephrine) associated with downregulation of beta-1 receptors mimics the process of the failing heart. The compliance of the arteries emanating from the heart decreases with age. Stiffening of these vessels produces a progressive rise in the systolic blood pressure.

It is the circulation through smaller blood vessels and the generation of new vessels (neovascularization) that is a major concern with advancing years. The process of angiogenesis, through which new blood vessels are formed, is impaired during aging. The integrity of endothelial cells lining the vessels, the cascade of coagulation factors, and growth factors and neurochemical mediators and their respective receptors are all altered by aging in the neovascularization processes.

Oral Cavity and Alimentary Tract

The digestive tract is subject to functional changes with aging. Beginning in the oral cavity, loosening and loss of teeth is a frequent companion of aging. Saliva secretion decreases leading to relative degrees of xerostomia or dry mouth.

Reduced parietal cell function develops in older persons, but prior *Helicobacter pylori* infections are now thought to be a major cause of hypochlorhydria in later life. An important nutritional consequence of reduced gastric acid secretion is a lesser biological availability of iron. Since iron stores are generally replete in both men and women in later life, this has little practical nutritional impact. The reduced secretion of gastric intrinsic factor, however, contributes to vitamin B_{12} deficiency, which is an important nutritional problem of older persons.

The capacity of the liver for biliary secretion and the pancreas for digestive enzyme and bicarbonate secretion begins adult life with a >90% excess of the necessary minimum. Secretory function declines with increasing age, but rarely falls below the minimal reserve capacity. The metabolic and detoxifying capacity of the human liver also has a reserve capacity and is not usually compromised by normal aging.

Intestinal motility is reduced with aging as a result of functional changes in the visceral nerves. With decreased transit the residence time of the chyme on the absorptive surfaces is longer, compensating for any senescence in the mucosal uptake itself. The reduction in motility produces the most noticeable and notorious of the manifestations of intestinal health in older persons, namely reduced frequency of defecations.

Musculoskeletal System

Bone mineral content declines with age; this aging process is known as 'osteopenia.' (It should be distinguished from the related pathological process in which bone architecture is altered, producing 'osteoporosis.') From the peak in the third and fourth decades, a 30% average decline in bone mineral density occurs through the ninth decade. In women, there is well-characterized acceleration of the rate of bone mineral loss immediately following the menopause. Decreasing levels of anabolic hormones may be associated with musculoskeletal atrophy and decrease in function that is observed in older women. This change in skeletal mineralization with aging is not associated with any apparent change in vitamin D nutriture as reflected in circulating levels of the vitamin.

The joints of the body undergo changes with the senescence of replacement of the cartilaginous substance, complicated by the pathological effects of cumulative use over the life span.

Recently, increasing attention has been given to the loss of muscle strength and substance with increasing age. Sarcopenia loss of lean body mass skeletal muscle mass replacement by fat mass Decreased creatinine-to-height ratio in normative aging in healthy subjects diminished grip strength is a function of age. [Reduction in muscle mass (sarcopenia obesity) is an important determinant of physical function and metabolic rate.]

Renal and Urogenital System

That renal creatinine and inulin clearance decreases with aging has been demonstrated for decades. These functional changes in filtration are associated with changes in the glomerular structure in the kidney. Circulatory senescence decreases blood flow to the kidneys, which further reduces the efficiency of renal clearance. The reserve capacity of these organs is such, however, that age-associated glomerular decline *per se* does not compromise the net excretion of nitrogenous waste.

Urine flow at the outlet is another aging consideration. The male urogenital system undergoes a characteristic aging change in the hypertrophy of the prostate gland, associated with decreased secretion of prostatic fluid. The anatomical consequence is a constriction in the passage through which urine flows from the bladder.

Gonads and Reproductive System

It has been aptly stated by Harman that: "It is clear that aging results in alterations of endocrine physiology, which in turn appear to contribute to development of the senescent phenotype." Aging is associated with a decrease in pituitary hormone secretions. This decline explains, in part, the reduction in gonadal hormone production with aging. Primary aging of the testes and ovaries themselves accounts for the remainder of the changes. As the ovaries have a finite number of eggs, ovulation can only continue through the number of cycles that correspond to the original store of ova. Menopause ensues with the characteristic cessation of estrogenic hormone secretion. In both sexes, gonadal androgenic hormone production declines with consequent effects on libido.

Endocrine Systems and Metabolism

As stated above, the pituitary gland is the hub of endocrine regulation. Important among the decline stimulation within the axis is that growth hormone (GH) secretion declines with increasing age, a condition termed 'somatopause.' The changes in the growth hormone/insulin-like growth factor axis with aging produce changes in function, metabolism, and body composition analogous to the pathological growth hormone deficiency seen in younger adults. Another change with age is the efficiency with which physical activity stimulates the secretion of GH.

The availability of hormones is not the only variable in endocrine signaling. Cellular and intracellular receptor function is complementary. An attractive explanation for the disordering of hormonal axes is oxidative damage to cell membranes, compromising the function of receptors.

Basal and resting metabolism and diet-induced thermogenesis are all reduced with increasing age. Changes in body composition, and the replacement of lean tissue with fat and the increasing visceral distribution of fat, as well as decreasing physical activity, influence these metabolic changes of aging. Basal metabolic rate (BMR) declines in aging more than can be attributed to body composition changes and intracellular mitochondrial senescence may explain part of this discrepancy. For practical purposes, the standard oxygen consumption value equivalent to one metabolic equivalent (MET), that is, $3.5\,ml\,min^{-1}\,kg^{-1}$, is not appropriate for elderly people.

Hematopoietic and Immune System

The formation of new red and white blood cells and platelets is one of the most proliferation-dependent physiological processes of the body. The various classes of circulating white cells are the underpinning of the host defense system, together with tissue macrophages, hepatic proteins, and the alimentary tract's mucosa.

Hematological aging The blood-forming organ is the bone marrow. Aging is associated with fatty infiltration of the marrow spaces in the long bones, but enough marrow remains to support the turnover of erythrocytes and red blood cell lines. The circulating red blood cell mass does not normally change with advancing age, nor does the normative peripheral white cell count or platelet number. As noted, iron stores tend to be abundant in later life; nutritional problems influencing red blood cell production are based on alterations in gastric function (vitamin B_{12} malabsorption), which result in a macrocytic (megaloblastic) anemia.

Immunological aging Circulating phagocytic white blood cells counts do not reduce with aging but aging does influence the innate host defense system. Mucosal barrier functions are influenced by aging of the gut in its interaction with microflora. Although not reduced in number, aged macrophages and neutrophils have blunted intracellular signaling by specific receptors, decreased metabolic functions, and impaired bacterial killing. Production of superoxide anion, chemotaxis, and orderly apoptosis of neutrophils is also disrupted by the disordered signaling. The tumor cell-destroying capacity of natural killer (NK) cells in the elderly is diminished.

More profound changes occur in the adaptive immune functions, which rely on the memory (T cell) lymphocytic cell line. Life-long antigen exposure induces increases in the number of memory T cells, but with enhanced reactivity against self-antigens, priming the individual for autoimmune disease. In healthy adults, IgA concentration increases by $0.2\,g\,l^{-1}$ per decade throughout life. The T lymphocytes, however, respond more poorly to ongoing antigen assault in later life. Thymic involution associated with neural and hormonal changes of aging is an impediment to T-cell maturation in older persons. The basis of intrinsic function deficits of memory cells, on the other hand, has been ascribed to defective signaling and includes hyporesponsiveness to mitogen-stimulated proliferation and decrease in genetic suppression, allowing increased stimulation of inflammatory cytokines; the balance between pro- and anti-inflammatory cytokines shifts with aging, favoring the inflammatory pole, especially with the greater expression of interleukin 6. This has a negative systemic effect on bone metabolism, as well as dysregulating overall immune function.

Aging of mitochondria in the immune cell lines produces increased intracellular reactive oxygen species burdens. Finally, there is diminished programed death (apoptosis) of immune cells and dysregulation of apoptosis-dependent functions.

Central and Peripheral Nervous System

The integration of all senses and origins of all systemic coordination is a function of the brain and central nervous system. This is the one system in which proliferation of the primary cells (neurons) is not an issue after early childhood, although the supportive, nerve-tending (glial) cells continue to depend on replication and apoptosis for normal function.

Central nervous system The neurons of the brain continue to divide only through to the second year of life. Thereafter, the goal is to preserve the number and health of the cerebral nerve cell mass. Myelination of axons of nerve cells must be maintained throughout life. This is the function of the supporting cells (oligodendrocytes), which over 40 years continue to differentiate into myelin-producing cells. Free radicals pose a threat to these axon-tending cells, whose metabolic demands for producing the brain's cholesterol and maintaining its array of myelin sheaths render them particularly vulnerable to stress.

Positron emission tomography (PET) imaging of the aging brain has revealed and mapped the plethora of changes in blood flow and neurotransmitter metabolism that occurs with advancing years.

Special senses The special senses related directly to the cranial nerves (vision, hearing, taste, and smell) experience age-related change. With respect to vision, the most typical of all biological aging changes is presbyopia, or the loss of accommodation function for the ocular lens with loss of capacity of the associated musculature. The consequence is loss of near-vision, which leads to the need for reading glasses or bifocal spectacles. A more important aging change related to the lens is the opacification that leads to cataract formation. The eye is designed to translate light energy into visual images, but the energy of light, particularly the ultraviolet β rays of solar energy, damages ocular tissue. Thus, there is as a strong environmental component to the disarranging of the laminar stacking of the fibrillar proteins of the lens, which imparts its clear, transparent basis; consumption of diets high in antioxidant vitamins has been associated with the delay in cataract formation.

Age-related hearing loss is a feature of biological aging. It affects the cochlear neural structures and leads to loss of acuity, especially for higher pitched tones. It is speculated that apoptosis of the most vital neural cells drives this hearing loss, based on mutations in the mitochondria due to life-long free-radical stress.

Taste and smell acuity decline with aging, both in sensitivity and in accuracy of recognition. Since these combined senses account for the recognition of flavors, their diminution with age could affect appetite and reduce the enjoyment of meals.

Cognitive function The intellectual, reasoning, and memory functions of the cerebral cortex decline with increasing age. This has been a universal observation in general elderly populations. The debate is whether this is a consequence of neurodegenerative diseases (pathological change) or a biological correlate of aging (senescence). Continued intellectual stimulation has been posited as an approach to retard cognitive decline, and a role for B-complex vitamins and antioxidants has been advanced.

Peripheral nervous system Vibratory perception in the peripheral extremities is the classical index of peripheral nervous decline with aging. Less well appreciated is the effect of aging on pain perception, in which there can be a numbing of sensation or, less commonly, an accentuation of perception. Pain perception from the visceral organs is often dulled, which can have adverse implications for the early detection of organic diseases. All of the peripheral nerve dysfunction can result from the compensatory sprouting of axonal limbs to compensate for the loss of motor neurons. This is well directed at first, but with further aging the synaptic connections are poorly directed and motor function suffers as a consequence.

Drug Metabolism

The metabolism of drugs and pharmacological agents is not the purview of any single organ system. Older persons tend to be prescribed increasing numbers of medications with advancing age. Important changes in drug metabolism occur with aging. Metabolism and disposition of drugs changes with age. This involves age-associated decrease in function of some, but not all, cytochrome P450 enzymes. Among the pharmacokinetic and pharmacodynamic changes that occur with advancing age are reductions in renal and hepatic clearance and an increased effective half-life of lipid-soluble drugs. The older population shows increased sensitivity to some psychotropic drugs and anticoagulants, with the frail elderly being more susceptible than healthy elders.

Synthesis and Conclusion

The number of older people is increasing in all regions and all societies of the world. Advancing age produces senescent changes in cellular function that are reflected in a declining capacity of all physiological systems. The increased prevalence of disease in older populations Aging is a major risk factor for disease but does not necessarily lead to age-related diseases.

All physiological systems are intrinsically interrelated in maintaining the health and function of the organism. Aging is associated with a loss of complexity in the dynamics of many physiological systems. It has been speculated that the basis for the syndrome of frailty in older persons may result from a reduced ability to adapt to internal and external stresses of daily life due to the loss of dynamic coordination among the interrelated physiological systems.

The alterations in physiological functions with aging have important implications for absorbing, retaining, and utilizing nutrients. The extent to which dietary patterns and nutrient intakes are accelerating or retarding the rates of functional decline is a matter of ongoing investigation in gerontological nutrition and physiology.

See also: **Aging. Brain and Nervous System. Cytokines. Older People**: Nutritional Requirements; Nutrition-Related Problems; Nutritional Management of Geriatric Patients. **Osteoporosis. Vitamin K**.

Further Reading

Ahluwalia N (2004) Aging, nutrition and immune function. *Journal of Nutrition, Health and Aging* 8: 2–6.

Balin AK (ed.) (1994) *Practical Handbook of Human Biologic Age Determination*. Boca Raton: CRC Press.

Harman SM (2004) What do hormones have to do with aging? What does aging have to do with hormones? *Annals of the New York Academy of Science* 1019: 299–308.

Hayflick L (2003) Living forever and dying in the attempt. Experimental Gerontology 38: 1231–1241.

Hutchinson ML and Munro HN (1986) *Nutrition and Aging: Bristol-Meyer Nutrition Symposia*, vol. 5. Academic Press.

Leveille SG (2004) Musculoskeletal aging. *Current Opinion in Rheumatology* 16: 114–118.

Lipsitz LA (2004) Physiological complexity, aging, and the path to frailty. *Science of Aging Knowledge Environment* 16: 16.

Mishra SK and Misra V (2003) Muscle sarcopenia: an overview. Acta Myol 22: 43–47.

Park HL, O'Connell JE, and Thomson RG (2003) A systematic review of cognitive decline in the general elderly population. *Internation Journal of Geriatric Psychiatry* 18: 1121–1134.

Timiras PS (1994) *Physiological Basis of Aging and Geriatrics*, 2nd edn. Baton Raton: CRC Press.

Nutritional Requirements

N Solomons, Center for Studies of Sensory Impairment, Aging and Metabolism (CeSSIAM), Guatemala City, Guatemala

Human Aging and Nutrition

The World Health Organization defines the 'elderly' as persons of 60 years of age and older. The elderly constitute a rapidly expanding segment of populations in both developed and developing countries. This is the combined result of ever-longer survival and dramatic reductions in fertility rates. Regardless of age, people must respond to their feelings of hunger and thirst by consuming foods and beverages. This eating and drinking behavior also serves to provide the nutrients to nourish the body. The amount of a nutrient that must be ingested and absorbed to maintain an adequate and appropriate body composition varies with age across the life span, depending on basic underlying physiological and metabolic processes specific to the chronological stage of life. The degree to which we retain and conserve, or excrete or degrade, absorbed nutrients is influenced by chronological age and biological aging.

As a consequence of this new demographic reality, attention is being focused belatedly on gerontology and its nutritional biology; this, in turn, is reflected in very recent efforts to refine our knowledge of the amounts of various macro- and micronutrients that the aging body requires (nutrient requirements) and of the amounts that must be consumed in the diet to provide for sufficient uptake of these nutrients (nutrient recommendations).

Successful Aging, Normative Aging, and Frailty

From an epidemiologic and demographic, as well as an economic and humanitarian standpoint, the ideal contribution of life-long nutrition would be to a situation of 'compression of morbidity,' first enunciated by J. Fries. It strives to keep individuals free of chronic illness, functional, and independent until the final moments of their lives, and thus reduces the burden of disability and dependency suffered by individuals, their families, and the society that contributes to their maintenance to a minimum.

A disclaimer has traditionally been appended to the official pronouncements of recommended nutrient intakes; whether they are from national or international expert panels, the prescriptions are meant to apply to 'healthy' individuals. Nutrient needs in disease conditions are considered to be a clinical matter, and are related to the pathologies in question.

When it comes to older persons, the exigency of being 'healthy' becomes immediately problematic. Advanced age is associated with increased susceptibility to chronic and degenerative illnesses. Most persons over 60 years of age have two or three chronic illnesses diagnosed, and are receiving multiple medications. Maintaining a rigid definition of healthy for application of nutrient recommendations in later life would exclude almost everyone from coverage by nutrient-intake standards.

In fact, the older the cohort of individuals examined, the more heterogeneous are individuals of the same chronological age in their physical and cognitive functioning. Over the last two decades, general domains of classifications have come into usage to embrace the heterogeneity of aging populations: successful aging; usual aging; and frailty. Successful aging has been defined as multidimensional, "encompassing the avoidance of disease and disability, the maintenance of high physical and cognitive function, and sustained engagement in social and productive activities." It may involve aspects of resilience and wisdom, as well. Usual aging involves an accumulation of ailments and loss of function that is typical of older persons surviving to later life. Frailty is the far extreme of disability and dependency associated with major physical and cognitive decline in which disease and senescent processes become irreversibly established.

A prominent and optimistic school of thought suggests that exposures to behavioral and environmental factors that modify risk of disease and dysfunction determine one's position in these alternative outcomes in the aging process. In this view, more optimal nutrient intake, food selection, and life-style choices could reduce the heterogeneity, retaining more individuals in the successfully aged category for most of their life span. Others consider that genetic constitution may be as important in determining the course of aging as any positive or negative influences during our lifetime.

Overview of Specific Factors of Aging Influencing Nutritional Requirements

The discussion of nutrient requirements and recommended dietary intakes of nutrients in older persons has proceeded on both the theoretical and empirical level. Since the peak years for human reproduction occur before advanced middle age, and well before older age begins, the forces of selective reproduction cannot exert themselves for Darwinian selection of traits favoring longevity in the evolution for any traits related to longevity *per se* or physiological sustained function. Hence, there is little evolutionary selection for nutrient requirements to achieve advanced age or for long-term survival. It is more for the preservation of comfort and function for those surviving to advanced age that optimization of nutritional intakes for the elderly would apply, that is for humanitarian and public health importance in the face of the physiological and anatomic changes of senescence.

As early as the 1970s, nutritional scientists advanced the proposition that requirements for different macro- and micronutrients changed with age. A large number of conjectures based on an emerging scientific understanding of senescent physiology have been advanced. It has been suggested that the decreased physical activity and physical conditioning associated with the body composition changes attendant to aging, sets the stage for alterations in requirements in both amounts and relative proportions of protein and the energy-yielding macronutrients. Decreased gastric secretory capacity has a negative influence on the absorption of calcium, iron, and vitamin B_{12}. Changing intestinal motility and digestive function evoked considerations of distinct increases and decreases of nutrients to compensate for the senescence of the intestinal tract, with particular interest in dietary fiber. Attention to compensatory intake for all of the nutrients involved in skeletal mineralization has come to the fore in relation to the recognized tendency to bone mineral loss with advancing age.

The immune and host defense system has been the focus of gerontological nutrition. Increased intakes of both vitamin E and zinc, well above the normally recommended level, have stimulated certain immune functions in studies involving older volunteers. Cognitive function declines with advancing age, and it has even been suggested that adjustment of nutrient intake can favorably affect the retention of memory and cognitive function in older persons. The adequate intake of B-complex vitamins, particularly those related to homocysteine metabolism (vitamin B_{12}, folic acid, vitamin B_6, riboflavin), are associated with mental function in older age. It has also been suggested that older individuals need more *n*-3 fatty acids for preserving cerebral cellular anatomy related to cognition.

Nutrient Intake Recommendations in Later Life

Comprehensive recommendations for macro- and micronutrients with differential attention to older persons have arisen from a collaboration between the US and Canada, and from expert panels serving the United Nations System. Each panel has set out its methodology and definitions and then presented tables of quantitative estimates. The recommendations for persons considered elderly in the respective systems are outlined below.

Definitions Surrounding Recommended Intakes of Nutrients

An important advance in establishing nutrient intake recommendations relates to the semantics. There has been a refining of the operational definitions of terms related to nutrient intakes. Recommended nutrient intakes (RNIs) are set by the agencies of the United Nations (UN) System and are considered to be the intakes of nutrients required to satisfy the requirements of nearly all healthy persons of a given age, sex, and physiological condition, and should be universal for all regions of the globe.

The Food and Nutrition Board of the Institute of Medicine in the US took a new approach in 1997 in which they applied the new dietary reference intakes (DRI) to micro- and macronutrient intakes. This work was undertaken jointly with Canada. It began with an assessment, where possible, of the estimated average requirement (EAR). This is defined as "the average daily nutrient intake level estimated to meet the requirement of half the healthy individuals in a particular life stage and gender group." The EAR is critical for an assessment of the risk of a nutrient deficiency problem at the population level. The traditional criterion used for decades, the recommended dietary allowance (RDA), is preserved. It is defined in the DRI process as "the average daily nutrient intake level sufficient to meet the nutrient requirement of nearly all (97 to 98 percent) healthy individuals in a particular life stage and gender group." When an EAR cannot be established from which to derive a formal RDA, the DRI process has a 'fall-back' category known as adequate intake (AI); this is defined as "a recommended average daily nutrient intake level based on observed or experimentally determined approximations or estimates of nutrient intake by a group (or groups) of apparently healthy people that are assumed to be adequate." A new classification scheme involving a range of intakes was created specifically for energy, electrolytes, and liquids: the acceptable macronutrient distribution ranges (AMDRs).

For the first time, a specific and well-defined process to delimit levels of excess intake of nutrients and dietary substances was defined by the DRI process as the upper tolerable intake levels (UL). The UL is "the highest average daily nutrient intake level likely to pose no risk of adverse health effects to almost all individuals in the general population." It is considered that as intake increases above the UL, the potential risk of adverse effects increases. To date, the UN System's process has dealt much less explicitly with issues of excessive intake of nutrients and dietary substances.

Established Recommended Intakes for Older Persons

In earlier versions of the RDAs for the US population (up to the 10th edition in 1989), the nutrient recommendations for all healthy adults over 51 years of age were combined as a single value. For the UN System, the age threshold in the early editions was 50 years or older. Concerted efforts to refine our understanding of nutrient requirements for older adults have been made over the past two decades. This allowed the US-Canada DRI process to establish categories for men and women aged 70 years and older. For the WHO/FAO process, a specific estimation for individuals over 65 years has been provided in the 2002 micronutrient recommendations.

Given the magnitude of the theoretical considerations regarding senescence and aging physiology that have been raised by various authors, what is really surprising is the paucity of specific instances in which the recommended intakes of nutrients for men or women in the 'elderly category' are considered to be different from persons in the next youngest age category. Composite tables for men (**Table 1**) and women (**Table 2**) are given for all of the nutrients and dietary substances expressed in the US-Canada DRIs and in the UN system for RNIs.

Macronutrients In the DRI system, a universal, individual protein requirement was established as 0.80 g of good-quality protein per kilogram of body weight per day independent of age. No evidence for altered protein requirements with older age has been found. Moreover, it is recommended that the contribution of protein to total energy intake should not exceed 30%. The US Food and Nutrition Board also established an amino acid pattern in 2002. It specifies the density (mg per g protein) of seven indispensable (essential) amino acids (histidine, isoleucine, leucine, lysine, threonine, tryptophan, and valine) and for two amino acid combinations (methionine + cysteine, phenylalanine + tyrosine). This pattern is universal from age 1 year to the extremes of older age without modification.

It has long been recognized that energy recommendations cannot be made on a group basis, as each individual has his or her own daily energy requirement dependent on the amount of energy one is forced to expend with metabolic reactions, food processing, and physical exertion. In the DRI process, this is recognized in an effort to individualize the estimation of energy intake. Estimated energy requirement (EER) is based on the amount of energy needed to maintain energy balance in relation to one's total energy expenditure. The DRI process for the US and Canada has published general EER equations (multidimensional nomograms) by which a reasonable estimate of an individual energy requirement can be calculated. There are general equations for adult men and women (over 19 years of age), based on consideration of physical activity level, weight, and height. In addition, there is an age term in the general EER, which is attached to a negative (minus sign) term in the equation. This signifies that energy requirements decline as a function of advancing years.

Although dietary fiber is not considered to be an 'essential' nutrient, the DRIs give a recommended level for intake. Curiously, in light of the active discussion of the role of fiber for the elderly in colonic function, the recommendations for intake by men decline from 38 to 30 g per day and in women from 25 to 21 g per day after 50 years. These are continued throughout the 70 year period, as well. This is a consequence of the fiber recommendations being pegged to total average energy intake.

Table 1 Nutrient intake recommendations for older males

	UL^a	ERA^a	RDA/AI^aAMDR^a	RNI^b
Macronutrients				
Water (l)	–	–	**2.1**^{c}	–
Carbohydrate (g)	–	100	120	–
Protein (g)	–	46	56	–
Total fat (g)	–	–	20–35	–
n-6 PUFA (g)	–	–	14^c	–
n-3 PUFA (g)	–	–	1.6^c	–
Dietary fiber (g)	–	–	**30**	–
Vitamins				
Vitamin A (RAE)	3000	625	900	600 (μg RE)
Vitamin D (mg)	50	–	**15**^{c}	**15**
Vitamin E (mg α-tocopherol)	1000	12	15	10 (mg α-TE)
Vitamin K (μg)	–	–	120^c	65
Vitamin C (mg)	2000	75	90	45
Thiamin (mg)	–	1.0	1.2	1.2
Riboflavin (mg)	–	1.1	1.3	1.3
Niacin (mg)	35	12	16	16
Vitamin B_6 (mg)	100	1.4	1.7	1.7
Biotin (mg)	–	–	30^c	–
Pantothenic acid (mg)	–	–	5^c	5
Folic acid (μg)	1000	320	400	400
Vitamin B_{12} (μg)	–	2.0	2.4	2.4
Choline (mg)	3500	–	550^c	–
Elements				
Sodium (g)	2.3	–	1.2^c	–
Potassium (mg)	–	–	4.7^c	–
Chloride (g)	3.6	–	1.8^c	–
Calcium (mg)	2500	–	**1200**^{c}	**1300**
Phosphorus (mg)	**3000**	580	700	–
Magnesium (mg)	(350)	350	420	**230**
Iron (mg)	45	6	8	14^d
Zinc (mg)	40	9.4	11	7.0^e
Iodine (μg)	1100	95	150	130
Copper (mg)	10	0.7	0.9	–
Fluoride (mg)	10	–	4^c	–
Manganese (mg)	11	–	2.3^c	–
Chromium (μg)	–	–	**30**^{c}	–
Selenium (μg)	400	45	55	34
Molybdenum (μg)	2000	34	45	–

^{a}In DRIs 70 years plus is considered as 'older'.
^{b}In UN System (WHO/FAO/IAEA) 65 years plus is considered as 'older'.
^{c}Recommendation in the form of adequate intake.
^{d}Assumes a 10% bioavailability of iron from the diet.
^{e}Based on the assumption of a moderate bioavailability of zinc.
The figures in **bold** denote recommendations specifically modified for ageing (see text).
UL, upper tolerable upper intake level; EAR, estimated average requirements; RDA, recommended dietary allowance; AI, adequate intake; AMDR, acceptable macronutrient distribution range; RNI, recommended nutrient intake; PUFA, polyunsaturated fatty acids; RAE, retinol activity equivalents; RE, retinol equivalents; α-TE, alpha-tocopherol.

Water It is recommended in the DRI as an adequate intake (AI) that males over the age of 70 require 2.6 l and females 2.1 l of water per day; this is a decline from the 51–70-year age group, where the daily water intake recommendations were 3.7 l and 2.6 l, respectively. It is further suggested that males and females over 70 years of age derive 81% of their daily water allowance from beverages and 19% as the metabolic water from foods. This is consistent throughout adulthood from age 19 years. Hence, there is no consideration of a higher requirement for water intake with older age. With respect to the electrolytes, no differences in AIs exist across the ages in adulthood.

Micronutrients A number of recommendations (RDAs or AIs) change with advancing age in the DRI system; this is indicated by the bold type in

Table 2 Nutrient intake recommendations for older females

	UL	ERA[a]	RDA/AI[a]AMDR[a]	RNI[b]
Macronutrients				
Water (l)	–	–	**2.6[c]**	–
Carbohydrate (g)	–	100	120	–
Protein (g)	–	38	46	–
Total fat (g)	–	–	20–35	–
n-6 PUFA (g)	–	–	11[c]	–
n-3 PUFA (g)	–	–	1.3[c]	–
Dietary fiber (g)	–	–	**21**	–
Vitamins				
Vitamin A (RAE)	3000	500	700	600 (μg RE)
Vitamin D (mg)	50	–	**15[c]**	**15**
Vitamin E (mg α-tocopherol)	1000	12	15	7.5 (mg α-TE)
Vitamin K (μg)	–	–	90[c]	55
Vitamin C (mg)	2000	60	75	45
Thiamin (mg)	–	0.9	1.1	1.1
Riboflavin (mg)	–	0.9	1.1	1.1
Niacin (mg)	35	11	14	14
Vitamin B$_6$ (mg)	100	1.3	1.5	1.5
Biotin (mg)	–	–	30[c]	–
Pantothenic acid (mg)	–	–	5[c]	5
Folic acid (μg)	1000	320	400	400
Vitamin B$_{12}$ (μg)	–	2.0	2.4	2.4
Choline (mg)	3500	–	425[c]	–
Elements				
Sodium (g)	2.3	–	1.2[c]	–
Potassium (mg)	–	–	4.7[c]	–
Chloride (g)	3.6	–	1.8[c]	–
Calcium (mg)	2500	–	**1200[c]**	**1300**
Phosphorus (mg)	**3000**	580	700	–
Magnesium (mg)	(350)	265	320	**190**
Iron (mg)	45	5	**8**	11[d]
Zinc (mg)	40	6.8	8	4.9[e]
Iodine (μg)	1100	95	150	110
Copper (mg)	10	0.7	0.9	–
Fluoride (mg)	10	–	3[c]	–
Manganese (mg)	11	–	1.8[c]	–
Chromium (μg)	–	–	**20[c]**	–
Selenium (μg)	400	45	55	26
Molybdenum (μg)	2000	34	45	–

[a]In DRIs 70 years plus is considered as 'older'.
[b]In UN System (WHO/FAO/IAEA) 65 years plus is considered as 'older'.
[c]Recommendation in the form of adequate intake.
[d]Assumes a 10% bioavailability of iron from the diet.
[e]Based on the assumption of a moderate bioavailability of zinc.
The figures in **bold** denote recommendations specifically modified for ageing (see text).
UL, upper tolerable upper intake level; EAR, estimated average requirements; RDA, recommended dietary allowance; AI, adequate intake; AMDR, acceptable macronutrient distribution range; RNI, recommended nutrient intake; PUFA, polyunsaturated fatty acids; RAE, retinol activity equivalents; RE, retinol equivalents; α-TE, alpha-tocopherol.

Tables 1 and 2. The change in recommendations occurs at either age 50 or 70 years. In women over 50 years, the RDA for dietary iron decreases from 18 mg to 8 mg day^{-1}; there is no change in requirement for the 70 year plus age group. This lower value is the recommendation for adult men of all ages. The fact that the menopause allows women to replete iron stores depleted by an adulthood of monthly menstrual blood loss accounts for this lower RDA in older women.

The senescence of the skeletal system and the reduction of bone mineral content with age is a major nutritional concern in gerontological nutrition. In recent revisions of the recommendations, evidence for the need for increases in both vitamin D and calcium for older persons has led to changes in the estimates of requirements for these nutrients in later life. Within the DRI system the RDA for vitamin D for males and females over 70 years is 15 mg. The

RDA for adults over 50 years is 10 mg and for young adults is 5 mg. Similar increases in vitamin D intake with age are recommended by the FAO/WHO. With respect to calcium, the recommended levels increase from 1000 mg for younger adults to 1200 mg at age 50 and beyond in the DRI system, and from 1000 to 1300 mg in the FAO/WHO standards. These are justified based on the higher propensity for skeletal fractures after 70 years of age associated with epidemiological evidence of widespread vitamin D deficiency in this age group, and evidence showing a reduction in bone loss with daily calcium intakes exceeding 1000 mg after mid-life.

With respect to chromium it is interesting that the estimation for AI declines with advancing age. The AI for persons over 70 in the DRI is the same as that for individuals between 51 and 70, but it is $5 \mu g \, day^{-1}$ higher for the 19–50 age range. This reduction is tied to the lower energy demands for individuals over 50 years of age.

The upper tolerable upper intake level (UL) for phosphorus in the DRI system is $3000 \, mg \, day^{-1}$ for both men and women over 70 years as compared to $4000 \, mg \, day^{-1}$ for adults in the 19–70 age group. This lower tolerance is explained by the greater prevalence of impaired renal function in advanced old age.

Magnesium intake recommendations in the FAO/WHO guidelines decline for individuals over 65 years by $30 \, mg \, day^{-1}$ compared to those in the 51–65 years age group. An anomalous finding for the magnesium RDA in the DRI system, which applies to all adult age groups, is that the UL for magnesium has been set at 350 mg. This is only 30 mg higher than the 320 mg daily recommended for older women, and is 70 mg lower than the 420 mg daily intake recommended for older men.

Dietary Guidelines for Health, Function, and Disease Prevention

Concomitant to recommendations for daily nutrient intake based on requirements, guidance and orientation for the pattern of selection of nutrient sources among the food groups have emerged as so-called 'dietary guidelines.' They are often accompanied by an icon or emblem, such as a pyramid in the US, a rainbow in Canada, and a Hindu temple in India, each of which expresses the general tenets of the dietary guidelines in a visual manner. A quantitative prescription, or some notion of balance among foods and food groups, is the basis of dietary guidelines; there is also often a proscription for foods considered to be harmful or noxious.

The additional susceptibility of older persons to chronic degenerative diseases makes adherence to these healthful dietary patterns, throughout the periods in the life span preceding the older years, more relevant. Recent epidemiological research has shown that compliance or behavior concordant with healthy eating guidelines are associated with lower later life incidences of certain cancers, cataracts, diabetes, hypertension, stroke, and cardiovascular diseases, as well as overall survival. There is intense interest in whether and how diet and nutrition influence the maintenance of cognitive function with aging.

Robert Russell and colleagues constructed a food guidelines pyramid, which specifically focused on the health of the elderly. Among the elements and tenets that differed from the standard US pyramid are the following recommendations: to drink additional water and liquid; to increase consumption of dietary fiber; and to consider dietary supplements such as calcium and vitamin E. Otherwise, selecting the same requisite serving portions of the specific food groups, and avoiding excess sugar, salt, and separated fats as indicated by the conventional guidelines emblem is recommended for the older population as well.

It is generally conceded that the major benefits for prevention of nontransmissible disease to be derived from adopting a healthful life style and dietary habits will accumulate over a lifetime; hence, beginning such practices at as early an age as possible will yield the greatest benefits. In this context, the application and emphasis of dietary guidelines specifically for the elderly is controversial and as yet unresolved. One school of opinion, one shared by Russell and coworkers, holds the view that the benefits of adhering to dietary guidelines are continuous, and actively protect from metabolic and neoplastic diseases even in the latter stages of the life span. The alternative proposition suggests that long-term survivorship is a manifestation of a superior genetic constitution resistant to chronic diseases. The very fact of survival to advanced age is a suggestion that the survivor's dietary practice will neither prejudice nor further protect health.

Barriers to Meeting Recommended Nutrient Intakes and Healthful Dietary Intake Patterns by Older Persons

The late Professor Doris Calloway, in the early 1970s, commented: "People eat food, not nutrients." This highlights the paradoxes in considering and enumerating the objectives of dietary intake at the level of the chemical composition, while most members of the general public are uninformed as to the nutrient composition of the foods and beverages in their diets.

Elderly persons face a number of challenges in meeting their recommended nutrient intakes. In the first instance, they are likely to be those with the least sophisticated or available knowledge of the nutrients required and the food sources to provide them. The social, economic, and physiological changes imposing on the lives of persons surviving to advanced age pose logistical problems for their selecting and purchasing a diet. Economic dependency and the limited incomes of older persons may restrict their access to high-quality foods. Social isolation, depression, and impaired mobility, as well as chewing difficulties may limit the variety of items included in the diet with advancing age. In some circumstances, it may be that free-living and independent elders are relatively less able to optimize their nutrient intake and dietary pattern compared to more dependent individuals served or fed in institutional settings.

The exigencies of consuming a healthful diet for the prevention of chronic diseases, emphasizing a plant-based diet rich in whole grains, fruits and vegetables, limits the nutrient selection that would be obtained from an even wider variety of foods and food-groups. Specific essential fatty acids, and certain minerals (calcium, zinc, selenium) and some vitamins are far less nutrient dense in foods of vegetal origin, setting a dilemma between consuming for nutrient adequacy and prevention of degenerative disease.

The widespread fortification of processed foods with micronutrients by the food industry in industrialized nations could mitigate much of the risk of insufficient nutrient intakes. Fortification of foods with iron may be more disadvantageous than beneficial to older persons whose iron reserves for nutritional purposes should normally be amply filled. A higher intake of iron puts a strain on the intestinal regulatory capacity and would tend toward excessive iron storage with any oxidative consequences for health that may result. National programs of fortification of grain flours and cereal products with folic acid for the prevention of neural tube defects in pregnancies are proliferating; mathematical models of how this policy may in fact increase the masking of macrocytic anemias due to vitamin B_{12} deficiency associated with senile gastric atrophy have been generated for European elderly populations.

Future Considerations

The DRI recommendations are specifically derived for the populations of the US and Canada in North America. The RNIs of the UN System are meant to be universal across the entire world. The slight majority of the living elderly are currently to be found in the low-income, largely tropical regions of the world in which 80% of the global population reside; this shift is due to rise rapidly over the next two decades. A number of caveats apply to the estimation of nutrient intake recommendations for the elderly across the world. If the "applies only to healthy individuals" disclaimer were applied to the developing world, then virtually no older people would qualify as eligible for coverage by any nutrient recommendations system. However, rather than abandon the effort for nutrient intake guidance, an attempt should be made to take into account the influences of life-long climatic issues (heat, humidity) and ecological factors (parasites, recurrent infections) on nutrient needs in later life.

Nature versus nurture issues will also continue to be debated with regard to nutrient requirements, especially in later life. Of course, with the recent assembling of the genetic code, the issues of 'nutrigenomics' and 'nutrigenetics' theoretically could soon be brought to bear on understanding individual variation in needs for and tolerances of essential and nonessential nutrients and dietary bioactive substances. The significance of this potential for the already aged person is likely to be limited for two reasons. First, the accumulative effects of nutrient imbalance will already have been established. Second, the economic and intellectual wherewithal to access and execute such individualized prescriptions for nutrient intakes and dietary patterns will likely escape the majority of older persons with limited financial means. Hence, further refinements in recommended intakes for older persons are likely to remain at the level of this segment of the population as a group and will involve establishing evidence that increased intakes of specific nutrients will have health-protective effects or function-enhancing properties, and that the effective upper tolerable levels/limits for certain nutrients in later life are lower than those for younger members of the adult population.

See also: **Ascorbic Acid**: Physiology, Dietary Sources and Requirements. **Bone. Calcium. Chromium. Cobalamins. Fatty Acids**: Omega-3 Polyunsaturated. **Folic Acid. Food Fortification**: Developed Countries. **Older People**: Nutrition-Related Problems; Nutritional Management of Geriatric Patients. **Riboflavin. Supplementation**: Role of Micronutrient Supplementation. **Vitamin B$_6$. Vitamin E**: Physiology and Health Effects. **Zinc**: Physiology.

Further Reading

Blumberg J (1997) Nutritional needs of seniors. *Journal of American College of Nutrition* **16**: 517–523.

Drewnowski A and Warren-Mears VA (2001) Does aging change nutrition requirements? *Journal of Nutrition in Health and Aging* **5**: 70–74.

Food and Nutrition Board/World Health Organization (2002) *Recommended Nutrient Intakes*. Geneva: WHO.

Fries JF (2002) Successful aging–an emerging paradigm of gerontology. *Clinics Geriatric Medicine* **18**: 371–382.

Hartz SC, Russell RM, and Rosenberg IH (1992) *Nutrition in the Elderly. The Boston Nutritional Status Survey*. London: Smith-Gordon.

Institute of Medicine, Food and Nutrition Board (2000) *Dietary Reference Intakes. Applications in Dietary Assessment*. Washington, DC: National Academy Press.

Rowe JW and Kahn RL (2000) Successful aging and disease prevention. *Advances in Renal Replacement Therapy* **7**: 70–77.

Russell RM, Rasmussen H, and Lichtenstein AH (1999) Modified Food Guide Pyramid for people over seventy years of age. *Journal of Nutrition* **129**: 751–753.

Russell RM (2000) The aging process as a modifier of metabolism. *American Journal of Clinical Nutrition* **72**(supplement 2): 529S–532S.

Solomons NW (2002) Nutrition and the extremes of life: dilemmas and enigmas of advanced old age. *Asia Pacific Journal of Clinical Nutrition* **11**: 247–250.

World Health Organization/Tufts University School of Nutrition and Policy (2002) *Keep Fit for Life: Meeting Nutritional Needs of Older Persons*. Geneva: WHO.

Nutrition-Related Problems

C P G M de Groot and W A van Staveren, Wageningen University, Wageningen, The Netherlands

The population older than 55 years of age is increasing rapidly throughout the world. In industrialized countries, the proportion of elderly people will increase by approximately 1% per year; in developing countries an increment of approximately 3% per year is expected. The nutritional needs of this population will require increasingly more attention from professionals working in the food industry as well as in health care.

Aging is defined as all physiological changes that occur from conception until old age and ultimately death. In this article, the term is restricted to changes that occur in adulthood, when growth has stopped.

On the one hand, nutrition is considered one of the key determinants in the process of aging. On the other hand, age-related changes take place in body appearance, in functional capacity and in the body's capacity to adapt to physical stress that affects nutritional needs.

It is difficult to distinguish between changes due to old age *per se* and changes that are the consequences of disease. In this article, the effects of aging on body composition, including energy needs and problems of over- and underweight, bone mass, and water balance are discussed. Physiological functions of the digestive system, malabsorption, nutrient drug interactions, and consequences for nutritional requirements are described, together with the high-risk micronutrients and early warning signs for malnutrition.

Changes in Body Composition and Energy Needs

Fat-Free Mass and Energy Needs

One of the truly age-driven phenomena is the loss of muscle mass and strength, called sarcopenia. It is distinct from muscle loss (cachexia) caused by inflammatory disease or from weight loss and attendant muscle wasting caused by starvation or advanced disease. Regardless of major differences between individuals, aging-related changes in body composition with time are universal. In addition to changes in lean tissue, this also holds for changes in fat mass, body water, and bone mass.

Throughout middle age, body mass tends to increase due to an accumulation of fat, preferentially intra-abdominally. Thereafter, usually after 60 years of age, it declines in association with loss of lean tissue. Diminution of physical activity enhances the changes in body composition occurring with aging, which in turn affect physical function. Ultimately, these processes result in a lower requirement for energy.

The total demand for energy is dominated by the energy needed per day to maintain vital functions, the basal metabolic rate (BMR), representing 60–70% of total energy expenditure. Most of the remainder (approximately 25%) is needed to cover the costs of physical activities. The BMR declines with age by up to 5% per decade. It is the decrease in lean tissue with age that determines this decline. One of the most important preventive measures in this process is the maintenance of physical activity. This helps to maintain lean body mass, physical fitness, and the requirement for energy.

Partly as a response to reduced energy needs, the energy intakes of affluent populations decline with age. This decline in food intake involves a decrease in meal size and a reduction in between-meal snacks. Morley called this physiologic decline in food intake "anorexia of aging." This type of anorexia may be considered partially as a response to reduced energy needs but also partially as a dysregulation of food intake. Roberts *et al.* studied energy regulation in young and older adults by deliberately overfeeding and underfeeding their subjects. After a period of underfeeding, young people compensated by overeating when fed ad libitum. However, the older adults did not compensate. The same holds following a period of overfeeding; the older adults did not compensate with a reduction in food intake when fed ad libitum.

Anorexia of aging places an increasing number of elderly people at risk for malnutrition because the opportunities for providing an adequate dietary nutrient intake are very limited when total food consumption becomes low (e.g., <6.3 MJ (1500 kcal) (**Figure 1**). Current recommendations for daily energy intake are approximately 9 MJ for elderly men and approximately 8 MJ for elderly women. Institutionalized elderly people or the elderly who are sick are especially likely to fail to achieve such intakes.

For health reasons, it is important that elderly people avoid becoming underweight. Although losing weight may be favorable at younger ages and being overweight is a known health risk in adults, there is evidence that low body weight and loss of body weight in the elderly are more strongly associated with risk of mortality (**Figure 2**). This is clearly shown by data from the Survey in Europe

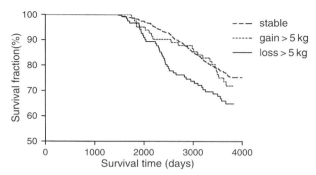

Figure 2 Probability of survival for participants from the SENECA study with and without weight change in the first 4 years. (Reproduced from Thomas D (ed.) (2002) Undernutrition in older adults. *Clinics in Geriatrics* **18**(4), with permission of WB Saunders.)

on Nutrition and the Elderly, a Concerted Action (SENECA). Weight loss (>5 kg over 4 years) seemed to be predictive for survival. It is even more important to be slightly overweight than underweight for people older than age 70 years. Therefore, except for those who are obese, elderly people should be encouraged to maintain an adequate energy intake. According to the SENECA study, 20–25% of the relatively healthy participants failed to do so: Approximately 8% lost and 16% gained at least 5 kg of body weight over a period of 4 years. When appetite is reduced, an increase in meal frequency may not only help to promote energy intakes but also prevent blood glucose levels from declining steeply.

Body Water, Dehydration, and Medication

Because lean tissue has a high water content, there is a decrease in total body water—especially extracellular water—with advancing age from 80% at birth to 60–70% after age 70 years. In addition, older people experience diminished sensation of thirst, and urinary concentrating ability declines as a function of age. Thus, older people have an increased risk of dehydration, particularly when diuretic or laxative medicines are used or in the presence of some diseases common in old age, such as diarrhea, renal disease, and infection with fever. Because water is essential to all biological functions, fluid intakes during old age should be at least 1700 ml per day. In the body, water acts as a diluent for water-soluble drugs. Given the decrease in body water with age, older people may need lower dosages of water-soluble drugs than younger adults to achieve the desired therapeutic effect and to avoid drug toxicity.

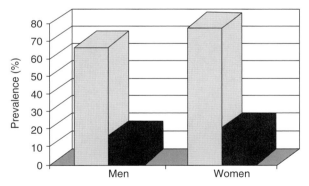

Figure 1 Prevalence of inadequate intake of at least one nutrient among elderly people whose daily energy intake is less than 6.3 MJ (gray bars) and for those whose energy intake exceeds 7 MJ (black bars). (From De Groot CPGM, van Staveren WA, Dirren H *et al.* (eds.) (1996). SENECA, nutrition and the elderly in Europe. Follow-up study and longitudinal analysis. *European Journal of Clinical Nutrition* **50**(supplement 2):127, with permission from Macmillan Press Limited.)

Bone Mass and Nutritional Factors

Throughout life, bone mass changes, with a maximum (peak bone mass) achieved by age 25–30 years and bone loss occurring after the fourth decade. Higher calcium intakes in childhood and early adulthood result in a 3–8% greater bone mass later in life, thereby improving the key factor in the osteoporotic process and the age-associated risk of fractures. In women, there is a perimenopausal increase in the rate of bone loss that persists after menopause following a decline in oestrogen production (**Figure 3**).

Factors other than age and sex that are associated with low bone mass include low body weight, smoking, alcohol consumption, reduced physical activity, low calcium absorption, and secondary risk factors such as the use of steroids. Although there is still uncertainty about the quantitative role of nutritional factors in the pathogenesis of osteoporosis, preventive measures include adequate calcium intakes (probably even in old age) and exposure to sunlight to ensure vitamin D adequacy and/or dietary supplementation with vitamin D. Restricted sunlight exposure, reduced capacity of the skin to produce vitamin D, and low vitamin D intake make elderly people prone to vitamin D deficiency.

Nutritionally Related Problems and the Digestive System

Taste

The number of taste buds varies widely from person to person but does not decline with age. Taste perception and the perceived flavor of foods decrease, but this is affected by many factors, including diminishing smell, age-related changes in the olfactory system, the integration of the central nervous system, medication, oral hygiene, and nutrition (**Figure 4**). Inadequate intakes of zinc, copper, nickel, and some vitamins have been associated with decreased perception of flavor of food.

Stomach

Atrophic gastritis is common in elderly people, resulting in hypochlorhydria and reduced gastric secretion. There is no consensus whether atrophic gastritis and the decrease in gastric acid secretion are normal processes of aging or a result of *Helicobacter pylori* infection. Independent of the cause, lack of gastric acid may interfere with the optimal absorption of nutrients. In the case of vitamin B_{12}, this may have clinical consequences. The mechanism for the reduced absorption of vitamin B_{12} is not clear, but protein-bound colabamin absorption is reduced in the elderly with atrophic gastritis or hypochlorhydria and this situation can be reversed with free vitamin B_{12} (the crystalline form) administration. Again, the prevalence of vitamin B_{12} deficiency is higher in *H. pylori* infection and eradication of this bacteria may correct vitamin B_{12} levels.

Small Intestine

Transit time is not changed in the elderly; however, their slower gut motility may cause stasis, with

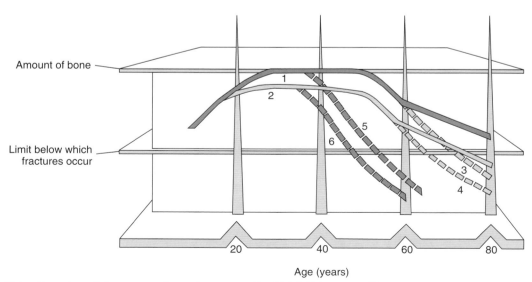

Figure 3 Rate of bone loss: 1, bone mass change in women with a high initial amount of bone and an average loss after menopause; 2, bone mass change in women with a low initial amount of bone and an average loss after menopause; 3 and 4, bone mass change in women with high losses after menopause; 5 and 6, bone mass change in women with an early menopause or after surgical removal of ovaries. First fractures occur approximately 10 years after menopause.

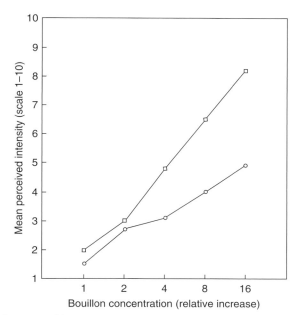

Figure 4 Mean responses of perceived intensity of bouillon flavor judged by a group of 23 elderly subjects (circles) and 32 young subjects (squares). (From Graaf C, Polet P and van Staveren WA (1994) Sensory and pleasantness of food flavors in elderly subjects. *Journal of Gerontology: Psychological Sciences* **94**: 93–99.)

bacterial overgrowth and malabsorption. The latter also may be caused by a reduced mucosal surface due to poor oxygenation of the tips of the villi as a result of a decreased blood supply from a low cardiac output. Decreased absorption is most frequently observed for electrolytes, lactose, vitamin D, and calcium. Absorption of digested food takes place by diffusion and by active transport across membranes. Adequate fluid must be available for absorption to proceed. The dehydrated state of the aged can reduce the capacity of the gut to absorb digested food.

Colon

The mucosal and muscle layers of the colon may atrophy, resulting in weakening of the muscle wall. Reduced motility of the colon allows prolonged exposure of feces to water absorption and drying. Reduced bulk results in further reduction of the stimulus to muscle contraction and will lead to constipation. This may be enhanced by a diet lacking dietary fiber, little physical activity, and poor tone of abdominal muscles.

Liver

Liver reserves of vitamins A, D, and B_{12} are unlikely to be diminished. Protein synthesis and especially the synthesis of vitamin K-dependent factors are reduced. However, it is not clear if this affects vitamin K requirements.

Gastrointestinal System

Elderly people are more prone to nutritional deficiencies that cause significant functionally deleterious consequences. The gastrointestinal system has been identified as an important cause of these problems. However, the mild functional and anatomic age-related changes do not seem to explain the incidence of malnutrition in the elderly. Rather, the lower functional reserve may accelerate nutritional problems under pathological challenge.

Nutrient and Drug Interactions

Many elderly people use drugs. In Europe, 83% of 'apparently healthy' people in the previously mentioned SENECA study use an average of two types of drugs, with antihypertensives (33%), analgesics (31%), diuretics (24%), sleeping pills (18%), and psychotropic drugs (17%) taken most often. Many drugs taken by the elderly can interfere with nutritional status. The possible effects include suppression or stimulation of appetite and impaired nutrient absorption and metabolism. For example, lisdiuretics can have adverse effects on calcium metabolism, salicylates can increase the need for vitamin C, and some types of antihypertensives act as antagonists of vitamin B_6. Negative consequences of laxatives, often taken by the elderly, include interference with nutrient absorption. Dietary interventions may help to reduce the intake of drugs. There is evidence that moderate sodium restriction prevents or delays the development of hypertension. Also, limiting alcohol intake provides protection because approximately 10% of cases of hypertension in men have been attributed to alcohol. Culinary skills become important to ensure that elderly people continue to find eating enjoyable, especially because increases in olfactory and taste thresholds occur with aging (**Figure 4**).

Risks for Malnutrition

Elderly people most at risk of developing malnutrition are those who eat little because of poverty, disability resulting from chronic geriatric disease, or a combination of these factors. Malnutrition is found in elderly people living in their homes if they are indigent, isolated, or homebound because of their own disability or the serious illness of their partner. Ten main risk factors for noninstitutionalized elderly can easily be identified and acted on by nonmedical personnel (**Table 1**). It must be understood that each risk in **Table 1** is only a potential

Table 1 Early warning signs for malnourishment

Medical and physiological factors

Recent unintended weight change of approximately
  >5% in the preceding month
Disease, polypharmacy or long-term medication
Immobility
High alcohol consumption

Psychological factors

Bereavement and/or depression or loneliness
Mental confusion
Poor nutrional knowledge

Socioenvironmental factors

Lack of sunlight
Low budget for food
Missed meals or snacks

danger sign; each has to be considered in relation to others. It should be stressed, however, that malnutrition is much more common in the elderly in long-term care, especially those who are unable to feed themselves.

Recommended Nutrient Intakes and High-Risk Nutrients in the Elderly

Recommended nutrient intakes for the elderly and very old may be set with different objectives. The values may serve either diagnostic or prescriptive purposes. Today, gerontologists and nutritionists are interested in the amount of nutrient that it takes to prevent a chronic disease from occurring rather than the amount of nutrient it takes to prevent a deficiency state. Most countries have their own set of requirements and age specificity may differ. In **Table 2** values are given as published by the Institute of Medicine (USA and Canada) for the oldest age group, mostly 70 years and older. The values should be accepted cautiously, with the proviso that change may be desirable when new information on nutritional needs of the elderly becomes available; for elderly patients who belong to particular disease groups, including mental diseases; for elderly people using specific drugs; and for elderly

Table 2 Recommended daily allowances (RDA) and observed problems for selected food components

Component	RDA[a]	Problems
Energy (MJ)		
Men	9–11	Low energy intake (<6.3 MJ) is highly correlated with insufficient micronutrient supply.
Women	8–10	
Protein (g/kg body weight)	0.8	Protein turnover may be lower than in young adults, which indicates lower requirement. However, the efficiency of protein synthesis is decreased.
Vitamin A (μg)		
Men	900	Risk of toxicity from megadoses in supplements.
Women	700	
Vitamin D (μg)	15	Requirement is increased in old age owing to insufficient synthesis with little or no exposure to UV light.
Thiamin (mg)		
Men	1.2	Special attention in those who eat little and elderly with alcoholic problems.
Women	1.1	
Riboflavin mg		
Men	1.3	Those consuming few animal products, especially milk, may be at risk.
Women	1.1	
Vitamin B_6 (mg)		
Men	1.7	Requirement may be higher when using antihypertensive drug hydralazine.
Women	1.5	
Folate (μg)	400	Extra attention for patients with atrophic gastritis and patients using a number of medicines.
Vitamin B_{12} (μg)	2.4	Vegans and patients with hypochlorhydria and atrophic gastritis have high risk; some drugs may interact.
Vitamin C (mg)		
Men	90	Increased requirements for patients using salicytes. Be alert for low vitamin C supply when using cooked meals from catering services and insufficient supply of fresh fruits.
Women	75	
Calcium (mg)	1.2	High-risk groups include elderly people using little or no milk and milk products and patients using lisdiuretica and some other drugs.
Iron (mg)	8	With reduction in lean body mass, iron requirement may be decreased. However, occult blood loss may increase requirement.
Iodine (μg)	150	Supply often inadequate; in some places enriched products (salt) should be used.
Water (ml)	1500–2000	Attention to fluid intake is necessary.

[a]Values derived from recent reports of the Institute of Medicine's Food and Nutrition Board (1999–2002), except RDAs for energy and water. The latter data are derived from the Expert Group Nutrition and the Elderly, The Netherlands (1995).

people using specific diets that may reduce the absorption of some nutrients.

Dietary Guidelines

Dietary surveys do not indicate that dietary guidelines for the elderly should be totally different from those for younger adults. Emphases in the program, however, should be different. Nutrition education programs for the elderly should give priority to drinking habits and to promoting the consumption of foods that are good sources of calcium, zinc, magnesium, potassium, folate, and vitamin B_6. Thus, recommendations should focus on the importance of daily consumption of (green) vegetables, fruit, wholegrain products and fortified cereals, and (low-fat) milk and milk products, and they should emphasize the nutritional value of fish and legumes. Because greater variety is associated with higher nutrient intakes in the elderly, the recommendation to eat a wide variety of foods is also important. Studies have emphasized that a healthy diet as well as other lifestyles, such as being moderately physically active and not smoking, are still important at an older age.

The Use of Dietary Supplements

The few studies on dietary supplementation among elderly people suggest that, as for younger adults, those elderly who need supplements do not use them, whereas the elderly consuming a diet with a high nutrient density use supplements. Food supplements include specially formulated preparations containing vitamins, minerals, and protein or a combination of these and other ingredients. Unnecessary use of supplements should be discouraged because consumption of megadose levels (amounts exceeding 10 times the recommended daily allowance) of various nutrients may cause adverse health effects. However, there are situations in which supplements have a role to play. For example, vitamin D would be indicated for the housebound elderly, and vitamin B_{12}, folate, potassium, or other nutrients may be a necessary supplement in disease conditions or when certain drugs are used that influence nutrient absorption, utilization, or excretion. In addition, suitable supplementation provides a means for improving the nutritional status of malnourished elderly or preventing nutritional deficiencies in people who are at risk.

See also: **Body Composition**. **Bone**. **Colon**: Nutritional Management of Disorders. **Dental Disease**. **Dietary Guidelines, International Perspectives**. **Drug–Nutrient Interactions**. **Energy**: Balance. **Liver Disorders**. **Malabsorption Syndromes**. **Older People**: Physiological Changes; Nutritional Requirements; Nutritional Management of Geriatric Patients.

Further Reading

De Groot CPGM, van Staveren WA, Dirren H *et al.* (eds.) (1996) SENECA, nutrition and the elderly in Europe. Follow-up study and longitudinal analysis. *European Journal of Clinical Nutrition* 50(supplement 2): 127.

Department of Health (1992) *The Nutrition of Elderly People*, Report on Health and Social Subjects No. 43. London: HMSO.

Expert Group Nutrition and the Elderly (1995) *Nutrition of the Elderly*. The Hague: Netherlands Food and Nutrition Council.

Haveman-Nies A, de Groot CPGM, and van Staveren WA (2003) Relation of dietary quality, physical activity and smoking habits to 10 year changes in health status in older Europeans in the SENECA study. *American Journal of Public Health* 3: 318–322.

Hazzard WR, Bierman EL, Blass JP *et al.* (1994) *Principles of Geriatric Medicine and Gerontology*, 2nd edn. New York: McGraw-Hill.

Rosenberg IH and Sastre A (2002) *Nutrition and Aging*, Nestle Nutrition Workshop Series, Clinical & Performance Program, vol. 6. Basel: Karger.

Schürch B and Scrimshaw NS (eds.) (2000) Impact of human aging on energy and protein metabolism and requirements. *European Journal of Clinical Nutrition* 54(supplement 3): S1–S165.

Thomas D (ed.) (2002) Undernutrition in older adults. *Clinics in Geriatrics* 18(4).

Nutritional Management of Geriatric Patients

M-M G Wilson and J E Morley, St Louis University, St Louis, MO, USA

Undernutrition

Overwhelming evidence implicates undernutrition as a major index of increased mortality in older adults. Undernourished elders admitted to acute facilities are more likely to develop complications, resulting in increased length of stay and healthcare costs. Rehabilitative efforts are less rewarding as patients often fail to return to baseline functional status and are more likely to require long-term placement or emergency readmission.

Free-living older persons with suboptimal nutritional status are at increased risk of dependence on care givers as a result of compromised activities of daily living. Additionally, convincing evidence exists linking undernutrition with an increased incidence of frailty, gait instability, falls, hip factures, immune dysfunction, delayed wound healing, and decreased cognitive function. Nevertheless, nutritional assessment and dietary management are often overlooked when health professionals evaluate geriatric patients.

As many as one-third of older adults in the US may be undernourished However, early clinical detection and appropriate intervention occur in less than one-tenth of cases. Health-care providers must remain astutely aware that geriatric health maintenance mandates efficient nutritional evaluation, surveillance, and prompt intervention.

Diagnosis and Evaluation of Undernutrition

Anthropometry

Several anthropometric indices have been proffered for the evaluation of undernutrition in older adults. These include:

- body weight less than 80% of the ideal body weight for height and age;
- weight loss exceeding 10% of baseline weight in the preceding 6 months; or
- body mass index less than 17.

Erroneously, the normative references for most of these criteria are younger subjects.

Within the older population the usefulness of this index is hampered by the lack of age-adjusted reference values. Reference values applicable in younger adults are not suitable for use in older persons as sarcopenia, age-related skin changes, and vertebral osteoporosis with height loss confound such norms. Within the older population, intentional weight loss resulting from dietary restriction should not discourage comprehensive nutritional assessment, as recent evidence indicates that both voluntary and involuntary weight loss in older persons portend similar adverse health outcomes.

Calculation of the body mass index (BMI) is considered to be one of the most objective anthropometric indices, as it permits correction of body weight for height. The BMI, calculated by dividing the weight in kilograms by the height in meters squared, is based on the proven premise that weight in the younger adult increases proportionately with height. However, this concept is false in older persons as height is significantly affected by age-related changes. Loss of height with aging occurs secondary to shortening of the axial skeleton due to age-related osteoporosis, degenerative disc changes, vertebral thinning, and kyphoscoliosis. Furthermore, using height as an anthropometric index is impractical in nonambulant and bed-bound persons. Nevertheless, clinical use of the BMI in the older population has been preserved by the development of adapted nomograms. Such nomograms are based on the determination of BMI using surrogate parameters of height adapted from the appendicular skeleton, which is relatively unaffected by age-related osseous changes. These parameters include total arm length, arm span, erect forearm length, and knee to floor height.

Skin fold thickness measurements are also used as anthropometric indices of total body fat in younger adults. However, the precise relationship between skin fold thickness and total body fat is unpredictable, as is the response of subcutaneous fat to undernutrition. Furthermore, in the older adult, the accuracy of this technique is confounded by age-related qualitative and quantitative changes in body fat. Altered compressibility of body fat has also been shown to occur with aging, rendering skin fold thickness measurements unreliable for use in older adults. Measurement of mid-arm circumference is another frequently used anthropometric index. However, several factors influence muscle bulk including exercise, disease, and genetic factors. In the older person this index is of doubtful clinical utility.

Several factors confound the use of anthropometric indices, underscoring the importance of serial measurements. These allow for quantification of response to intervention and also enhance accuracy of data interpretation by utilizing intrasubject comparison. More accurate methods of body composition analysis are available but are unlikely to be suitable for routine clinical use. These include computerized tomography, bioelectrical impedance, nuclear magnetic resonance imaging, *in vivo* neutron activation analysis, dual energy X-ray absorptiometry (DEXA) and direct photon absorptiometry (DPA). Because of alterations in body water with aging, the value of bioelectrical impedance is questionable. The DEXA technique is excellent but the migration of body fat to the abdomen with aging may result in an underestimation of body fat in older persons. DPA is based on analysis of tissue attenuation of photons transmitted at two different energy levels. This technique permits measurement of different tissue compartments. Both fat mass and fat-free mass can be measured using this technique. Currently, these methods are used almost exclusively for research purposes. Most of these emerging techniques are very expensive and have not been validated for use in clinical settings. Therefore, for practical clinical purposes, the most cost-effective nutritional parameter of proven clinical utility in older adults remains serial body weight measurements.

Biochemistry

Hypoalbuminemia is often erroneously used as an index of undernutrition. However, the diagnostic specificity of this index is poor. Serum albumin levels are determined by a complex interplay between nutritional intake, total body albumin distribution, and several pathological changes that alter the biosynthetic and catabolic rates of albumin. In the acutely ill or stressed older person, cytokine release suppresses albumin and prealbumin synthesis. Additionally, the release of catabolic counter-regulatory hormones in stressful situations reduces albumin synthesis even further. Direct downregulation of albumin gene expression also occurs in situations of acute stress. Paradoxically, undernutrition itself may result in a compensatory reduction in albumin catabolism, yielding inappropriately high albumin levels. Although serum albumin is a poor index of undernutrition, hypoalbuminemia is linked with frailty, excess comorbidity and increased mortality in older adults. Thus, the clinical relevance of hypoalbuminemia lies in the identification of a high-risk subset of older persons in whom early and aggressive nutritional intervention is crucial.

Several other biochemical indices are used as nutritional markers. However, like albumin, they lack diagnostic specificity and have relatively long half-lives, which limit their value in the serial evaluation of undernutrition. Insulin-like growth factor 1 is considered to have the greatest positive predictive value as it has been shown to correlate well with nutritional status even during periods of acute stress. Added advantages of this index are a relatively short half-life of 2–6 h and a rapid response to fasting and refeeding. Nonetheless, routine use of this assay in the evaluation of undernutrition is precluded by cost. Overall, for practical clinical purposes, the use of biochemical markers in routine nutritional geriatric management is cost-ineffective and unreliable.

Hematology

Anemia of chronic disease resulting directly from undernutrition is a recognized clinical entity. Studies have identified reduced erythropoiesis and alterations of erythrocyte function in undernourished persons that respond to nutritional repletion. Iron and folate deficiency anemias may also result from inadequate micronutrient intake in undernourished persons.

Measurement of the total lymphocyte count (TLC) is helpful mainly in the stratification of the severity of undernutrition. A TLC of less than $1200 \times 10^6 1^{-1}$ indicates mild undernutrition while counts less than $800 \times 10^6 1^{-1}$ are usually found in severely undernourished persons.

Recognizing Causative Factors of Undernutrition

Age-related physiological reduction in appetite, 'anorexia of aging,' is well documented. Several factors have been implicated in the genesis of this phenomenon. Evidence suggests that the decrease in lean body mass, energy expenditure, and metabolic rate that occurs with advancing age may partially account for the reduction of food intake in healthy older persons. Age-related reduction in olfactory and gustatory receptor sensitivity may compromise the hedonic qualities of meals, further reducing the desire to eat. Similarly, age-related alterations in hormonal and neurotransmitter-mediated function may also play a role in suppressing food intake. Animal studies suggest that aging results in a reduction in the opioid feeding drive and an increase in the satiating effect of cholecystokinin. This may lead to the ingestion of smaller meals and prolonged periods of satiety between meals. More recently ghrelin, a hunger-inducing peptide hormone, has been shown to decrease with age. Similarly, older hypogonadal men have inappropriately high levels of leptin, a satiation-inducing peptide hormone.

The occurrence of a variety of pathological factors superimposed on the background of age-related physiological changes may further compromise nutritional status in the older adult (**Table 1**). Existing data suggest that as many as one-third of undernourished older persons suffer from untreated depression. Neuro-vegetative symptoms in depressed older persons often result in anorexia, social withdrawal, reduced motivation, and decreased activity, all of which can compromise nutritional intake. The use of appropriate antidepressants very often reverses these symptoms, resulting in an increase in food intake and restoration of adequate nutritional status. Choice of antidepressants is crucial in the management of depressed, older undernourished persons. The popularity of selective serotonin reuptake inhibitors in younger persons has led to their increasing use in the older population. However, in older persons the efficacy of such agents in improving mood may be marred by adverse gastrointestinal effects, such as nausea, vomiting, and diarrhea, which may further compromise nutritional status. Thus, where such agents are used, careful monitoring of nutritional status is mandatory. Mirtazapine is a useful antidepressant that is unrelated to selective serotonin

Table 1 Common and uncommon causes of undernutrition in older persons

Reduced food intake
Anorexia
Ill-fitting dentures
Periodontal disease
Oropharyngeal disease
Orofacial dyskinesias

Psychosocial factors
Depression
Eating disorders
Bereavement
Social isolation
Low financial income

Physical/mental disability
Persistent tremors
Dyskinesia/dyspraxia
Arthritides
Parkinsonism
Cerebrovascular disease
Dementia
Behavioral disorders

Increased nutrient metabolism
Hyperthyroidism
Phaeochromocytoma
Wandering, agitation
Movement disorders
Hemiballismus

Reduced nutrient utilization
Malabsorption syndrome
Chronic inflammatory bowel disease
Gluten enteropathy

Gastroesophageal disease
Inflammatory
Neoplastic
Dysmotility

Multifactorial
Chronic bronchitis, emphysema
Cardiac failure
Malignant disease
Substance abuse

reuptake inhibitors, tricyclics, or monoamine oxidase inhibitors (MAOI). Mirtazapine belongs to the piperazino-azepine group of compounds. Available evidence suggests that Mirtazapine has an additional orexigenic and anti-emetic effect, which may increase energy consumption. Electroconvulsive therapy is a viable option in depressed persons with severe anorexia. Evidence exists in support of the efficacy of this treatment modality in restoring appetite following failure of pharmacological agents.

Minor dysphoric changes may adversely affect nutritional status and warrant intervention. Over 30% of older community-dwelling persons live alone, usually as a result of bereavement or migration of younger family members. Meals are often eaten alone and the lack of social interaction during meal preparation and consumption can compromise the recreational and hedonic aspects of dining. Consequently, such elders are poorly motivated to prepare and eat meals. Particular attention should be paid to the recreational aspects of mealtimes, and older persons should be encouraged to socialize during meals. This can be accomplished in a variety of ways. Participation in dining clubs, where available, should be encouraged. Arrangements can also be made for older persons to dine at senior citizens' centers. Ambulant senior citizens should be encouraged to eat out, if this is preferred.

Effective nutritional intervention mandates due consideration of financial and socioeconomic factors. Approximately one-third of the older population live below the poverty line and many experience difficulty with the purchase of food items necessary to ensure a balanced diet. Inadequate transportation, limited mobility, and poorly accessible shopping facilities may be added limiting factors. Social and community agency services should be considered where relevant, and an attempt should be made to provide appropriate assistance.

A wide variety of prescribed drugs can cause anorexia, nausea, and other symptoms of gastrointestinal distress in older persons, rendering medication review an important component of nutritional management. Digoxin, theophylline, and nonsteroidal anti-inflammatory agents are frequent culprits in this regard. Enquiry must also be made into the use and tolerance of self-prescribed medication. Offending drugs, once identified, must be discontinued. Iatrogenesis also contributes to undernutrition by way of therapeutic diets. Low-cholesterol and low-salt diets are often prescribed to older persons on the basis of data extrapolated from younger persons. There is currently little evidence to suggest that these diets are of any benefit to older persons when used as primary prevention strategies. Available data actually indicate increased mortality in older adults with low-cholesterol levels. Evidence suggests that hypocholesterolemia may reflect increased cytokine expression in acutely ill and frail older adults. Thus, restrictive diets in older persons should be discouraged, as they often reduce palatability and consequently discourage food intake. Health professionals should also make enquiries regarding self-prescribed diets. Studies indicate that the older population is more susceptible to food fads and advertised commercial diets, which are often unbalanced and of dubious benefit. Prolonged ingestion of such diets can result in marked undernutrition.

A wide variety of medical illnesses require focused therapeutic intervention in order to maintain or restore adequate nutritional status. Degenerative and neurological diseases can significantly impair mobility and physical function. The use of adapted appliances and cutlery in such cases may improve manual dexterity and preserve the ability to self-feed. In older persons with severely impaired function, who are unable to cook, meal delivery services ('meals on wheels') may be an acceptable alternative to home-cooked meals. Tooth loss is another important risk factor for undernutrition. Periodontal disease and edentulism are highly prevalent among the geriatric population and can impair masticatory ability. Older persons who have lost teeth, experience pain on mastication, or receive inadequate dental care should be carefully screened and offered appropriate therapy. The use of dentures may improve food intake. However, where dentures are poorly tolerated, alteration in the consistency of meals is helpful. Dysphagia occurs commonly in older persons with degenerative and vascular neurological conditions such as dementia, Parkinsonism, and cerebrovascular disease. A bedside swallowing evaluation should be an integral component of nutritional evaluation, followed by a modified barium swallow with fluoroscopy in cases where significant dysphagia is identified. In most cases oral food intake will remain possible, with appropriate modifications regarding swallowing technique, feeding precautions, and food consistency.

Health professionals often wrongly assume that older adults possess adequate knowledge of basic dietetic practice and nutritional studies. There is evidence to suggest that the nutritional attitudes and knowledge of undernourished older persons may be inadequate, particularly with regard to food preparation. Dietary education and counseling are crucial components of nutritional intervention in undernourished older persons who retain the responsibility for preparing their own meals. Such counseling should be targeted towards identifying deficits in basic dietary knowledge and the correction of poor nutritional practices.

Nutritional Assessment Tools

Arrays of nutritional screening tools have been developed to facilitate the identification of older persons at risk for undernutrition. The Nutrition Screening Initiative (NSI) in the US stemmed from a collaborative effort between family physicians, dietitians, and the National Council of Aging. This is a three-tiered tool formulated to assist in the detection of older persons at risk for nutritional compromise and subsequent direction of such persons toward the appropriate level of care. The first level of screening is designed to be initiated by the patient or primary care giver. Persons identified to have an increased risk of undernutrition

are then referred for evaluation by healthcare or social services personnel. This constitutes the second level of screening. The identification of factors that may warrant medical intervention will prompt referral to a physician for further evaluation. The NSI is of proven value as an epidemiological tool and serves to increase the awareness of patients and care givers to undernutrition. However, its usefulness within orthodox settings may be hampered by the number of personnel and services required, which may constitute a significant drain on available resources. Added drawbacks to the use of this tool for the individual patient are the lack of professional supervision at initiation and reliance on patient compliance in adhering to the specified clinical pathway protocol.

The Mini Nutritional Assessment (MNA) is a comprehensive and simple tool designed to evaluate the nutritional status of older persons. This is the first well-validated nutritional screening instrument and is recommended for use in people aged over 75 years. Cross-validation indicates that nutritional assessment using this tool will accurately evaluate and categorize nutritional status in about 75% of older persons without the need for further biochemical tests or clinical assessment. The MNA scoring system permits the stratification of older adults into three categories: well-nourished, at risk of undernutrition, and undernourished. An advantage of the MNA is that it can easily be used by a wide range of health professionals in a variety of clinical settings that cater for both free-living and institutionalized older persons. Several other tools are of practical value in the clinical setting. Morley has developed a useful screening tool known by the acronym SCALES (Table 2). This uses basic biochemical and anthropometric indices to identify older adults at risk of undernutrition, and can be readily incorporated into serial evaluation of the older person in

Table 2 SCALES: screening tool for the early detection of patients at risk of protein-energy undernutrition

Parameter	Score 1 point	Score 2 points
Sadness	GDS 10–15	GDS >15
Cholesterol	<4.65 mmol l^{-1} (180 mg dl^{-1})	<4.14 mmol l^{-1} (1660 mg dl^{-1})
Albumin	<40 g l^{-1} (4 g dl^{-1})	<35 g l^{-1} (3.5 g dl^{-1})
Loss of weight	<1 kg (2 lb) in 1 month	<2.7 kg (6 lb) in 6 months
Eating problems	Cognitive impairment or physical limitations	Cognitive impairment and physical limitations
Shopping problems	Inability to shop or prepare a meal	

Patients scoring over 3 are at risk. GDS, geriatric depression score.

Table 3 MEALS ON WHEELS: common causes of undernutrition in older persons

Medication (e.g., digoxin, theophylline, psychotropic drugs)
Emotional (depression)
Anorexia, alcoholism
Late-life paranoia
Swallowing disorders
Oral and dental disease
No money (absolute or relative poverty)
Wandering (dementia, behavioral disorders)
Hyperthyroidism, hyperparathyroidism
Entry problems (malabsorption)
Eating problems
Low-salt or low-cholesterol diets
Shopping and food preparation problems

different clinical settings. The simple mnemonic MEALS ON WHEELS, also devised by Morley, may prove useful in prompting consideration of the risk factors and common causes of nutritional compromise (**Table 3**).

More recently, the Council of Nutrition Appetite Questionnaire has been validated for the evaluation of appetite in older adults. A unique feature of this appetite assessment tool is the ability to predict significant weight loss (**Table 4**).

Oral Nutritional Repletion

Appropriate treatment of the underlying causes of undernutrition should be accompanied by oral nutritional supplementation in persons who are able to eat. Objective quantitative baseline assessment of food intake is mandatory. This is best achieved by the maintenance of a food diary, in which the patient records all food items consumed over a 72-h period. Review of the food diary also permits evaluation of food preferences and eating patterns. The goal of nutritional supplementation should be the consumption of the recommended daily allowance of macronutrients and micronutrients. Several predictive equations have been derived for the purpose of determining the optimal energy intake for each individual. However, it remains unclear as to what extent corrections have been made for age-related physiological changes in nutritional requirements and energy expenditure. The Benedict-Harris equation is perhaps the best known and most frequently applied. Using this equation, the required daily energy intake in kilocalories is derived as follows:

- Men: $66 + 13.7W + 5H - 6.8A$
- Women: $665 + 9.6W + 1.8H - 4.7A$

where W is the weight in kilograms, H is the height in centimeters, and A is the age in years. Upward adjustment is required by factors ranging from 1 to

Table 4 The Council of Nutrition Appetite Questionnaire

1. My appetite is:
1. very poor
2. poor
3. average
4. good
5. very good

2. When I eat:
1. I feel full after eating only a few mouthfuls
2. I feel full after eating about a third of a meal
3. I feel full after eating over half a meal
4. I feel full after eating most of the meal
5. I hardly ever feel full

3. I feel hungry:
1. rarely
2. occasionally
3. some of the time
4. most of the time
5. all of the time

4. Food tastes:
1. very bad
2. bad
3. average
4. good
5. very good

5. Compared to when I was younger, food tastes:
1. much worse
2. worse
3. just as good
4. better
5. much better

6. Normally I eat:
1. less than one meal a day
2. one meal a day
3. two meals a day
4. three meals a day
5. more than three meals a day

7. I feel sick or nauseated when I eat:
1. most times
2. often
3. sometimes
4. rarely
5. never

8. Most of the time my mood is:
1. very sad
2. sad
3. neither sad nor happy
4. happy
5. very happy

Instructions: Complete the questionnaire by circling the correct answers and then tally the results based upon the following numerical scale: A = 1, B = 2, C = 3, D = 4, E = 5. The sum of the scores for the individual items constitutes the CNAQ score. Scoring: If the CNAQ score is less than 28, there is an increased risk of significant weight loss over the next 6 months.

1.5, to compensate for increased activity or pathologically stressful conditions.

For practical clinical purposes, a total daily energy intake of $147 \, \text{kJ kg}^{-1}$ ($35 \, \text{kcal kg}^{-1}$) achieves efficient nutritional repletion. Recent dietary guidelines emphasize an overall healthy and balanced dietary pattern that includes a wide variety of fruits, vegetables, and grain products. Specifically, at least 5 daily servings of fruits and vegetables and 6 daily servings of grain products, including whole grains. Low-fat dairy products, fish, legumes, poultry, and lean meats are encouraged. Guidelines also suggest at least two servings of fish per week.

The current recommended daily allowance for protein is at least $1 \, g \, kg^{-1}$ body weight. However, acutely stressful or hypercatabolic conditions mandate an increase in protein intake to about $1.5 \, g \, kg^{-1}$. Generally, compliance with these dietary guidelines achieves the dual purpose of ensuring optimal macronutrient and micronutrient intake. This obviates the need for the routine prescription of pharmacological multivitamin preparations in undernourished persons, unless specific signs of micronutrient deficiency are evident.

Nutritional supplementation with regular or fortified natural food items is the ideal mode of nutritional repletion. This possesses the advantages of familiarity, palatability, and cost-effectiveness. Where the patient is reluctant or unable to consume the required total energy intake in natural food items, commercially formulated nutritional supplements are a reasonable alternative. The choice of preparation should be based on palatability and patient preference unless underlying medical conditions such as lactose or gluten intolerance have to be considered. Patients with malabsorption syndromes should be given hydrolyzed preparations to enhance nutrient absorption. Regardless of the preparation used, an attempt should be made to vary flavors, as age-related sensory-specific satiety may limit intake if only one flavor is used. Erroneously, nutritional supplements are often administered with meals. Recent evidence indicates that liquid supplements are more effective in increasing daily energy intake when administered at least 1 h before meals. Data shows that when supplements are administered with meals, a suppressant effect on food consumption is evident. Thus, older adults on nutritional supplements should receive these between meals to maximize net energy intake. Ultimately, in persons with severe undernutrition, the focus should be on energy intake and patient food preference, not on optimal proportions of macronutrient and micronutrient intake. Frequently, efforts to ensure a balanced diet necessitate the use of food items that may compromise palatability and result in a counterproductive reduction in food intake.

Enteral Tube Feeding

Enteral or parenteral modes of nutrient delivery are often used in people who are unable to eat or swallow. In the presence of a functioning gastrointestinal tract, enteral feeding is more appropriate due to the lower incidence of complications, more efficient nutrient utilization, increased cost-effectiveness, and greater ease of administration. Additionally, small bowel hypoplasia and alterations in gastrointestinal secretions may result from prolonged parenteral nutrition. Nasogastric and nasoenteric tubes should be reserved for short-term nutritional support in persons who may be able to resume oral feeding within 14 days, in order to avoid the significant morbidity associated with the use of nasal tubes. In persons in whom prolonged enteral intake is anticipated, gastrostomy or jejunostomy tubes may be considered.

In patients who retain normal gastrointestinal absorptive function, regular meals may be puréed and delivered through large-bore feeding tubes. A variety of polymeric enteral feeding formulas are also available; these are of relatively low viscosity, rendering them particularly suitable for delivery through small-bore tubes, which are usually more comfortable and aesthetically pleasing. In persons with malabsorption, hydrolyzed predigested formulae are available. Specific formulations also exist for people with special nutritional requirements due to diseases such as diabetes mellitus or renal or respiratory failure.

In older people, large volume bolus tube feedings may be associated with a greater risk of aspiration. Thus, where possible, continuous infusions of feeds are preferred. In order to further reduce the risk of aspiration pneumonia, it is recommended that the patient is positioned in a 30° head-up incline during feedings. Feeds may be infused over a 24-h period or over 14–18 h with a nocturnal break. The latter infusion schedule is often advocated on the grounds that it mimics normal eating patterns more closely. In addition, the absence of a nocturnal feed-free period has been shown to obliterate the physiological diurnal variation in insulin, cortisol, and glucagons secretion. Maximal nutrient utilization is also encouraged by daytime feed infusions as gastric emptying occurs more rapidly during the day. Continuous infusion of enteral tube feeds should be initiated at a rate of $30 \, ml \, h^{-1}$ using half-strength feeds. If tolerated, full-strength feeds may then be introduced at the same rate and increased by $25 \, ml \, h^{-1}$ every 8–12 h until the recommended daily energy intake is achieved. Despite the popularity of enteral tube feeding, emerging evidence indicates that the medical risks of percutaneous endoscopic gastrostomy (PEG) tube feeding may outweigh the risks. Studies in older adults with dementia fail to demonstrate any reduction in comorbidity or mortality with PEG feeding. Similarly, available data fails to demonstrate any significant improvement in functional status, nutritional status, or quality of life with this method of feeding. Thus, health providers should set realistic goals for patients and family members who opt for PEG feeding. Ultimately, the indications and benefits of PEG tube placement are more likely to be based on personal psychosocial, cultural, or ethical preferences.

Parenteral Nutritional Repletion

In the older person with a nonfunctioning gastrointestinal tract, parenteral nutrition may be unavoidable. All patients receiving parenteral nutrition must be monitored closely for adverse effects. For short-term intravenous nutritional repletion, peripheral parenteral nutrition may be used. Low osmolality nutritional preparations, with a low risk of toxicity to soft tissue, are best suited for this purpose. There is a paucity of data regarding the safety and efficacy of most peripheral parenteral nutritional products for periods exceeding 14 days. Thus, where longer periods of intravenous feeding are required, total parenteral nutrition through a large central vein is indicated. Standard total parenteral formulations comprising 25% dextrose, 5% amino acids, electrolytes, and trace elements in optimal amounts are suitable for use in most patients. During prolonged parenteral nutrition, lipid emulsion supplements should be added to prevent deficiency of essential fatty acids.

Pharmacological Management of Undernutrition

Older patients with a poor response to treatment of underlying causes and nutritional supplementation may benefit from orexigenic agents (**Table** 5).

Table 5 Orexigenic agents

Megesterol acetate
Mirtazapine
Dronabinol (delta-9-tetrahydrocannabinol)
Corticosteroids
Loxiglumide (Cholecystokinin antagonist)
Oxoglutarate
Anabolic agents (testosterone, anadrol)
Oxandrin
Growth hormone
Cyproheptadine

Megestrol acetate is a synthetic progestogen approved for use by the Food and Drug Administration (FDA) as an orexigenic agent in patients with Acquired Immune Deficiency Syndrome (AIDS) and cancer-related anorexia and cachexia. Recent evidence indicates that megesterol acetate is also an effective orexigenic agent in geriatric patients. Thromboembolic disease and adrenal suppression are rare complications, but patients should be monitored closely for these events.

Dronabinol (delta-9-tetrahydrocannabinol), the active ingredient of *Cannabis sativa*, is another FDA-approved orexigenic agent for use in patients with Acquired Immune Deficiency Syndrome (AIDS). Dronabinol is also an effective orexigenic and antiemetic in patients receiving cancer chemotherapy. Additional evidence indicates that dronabinol induces weight gain in persons with dementia, although research has yet to determine whether weight gain in such patients is due to increased energy intake or reduced agitation with improved behavior and consequently decreased energy expenditure. Side effects of dronabinol in older adults include delirium, euphoria, and increased somnolence. The latter two qualities may favor the use of dronabinol as an orexigenic agent in palliative care.

One third of depressed older adults manifest with weight loss. Effective antidepressant therapy should result in weight gain in this subset of patients. Notably, the choice of antidepressant therapy may influence body weight reuptake. Selective serotonin (5-hydroxytryptamine, 5-HT) inhibitors, such as fluoxetine, can cause significant weight loss at the onset of therapy. Evidence in younger adults suggests that this is a transient phenomenon with baseline body weight being restored as treatment progresses. However, age-related changes in energy regulation and adaptation to chronic disease may delay or prevent return to baseline body weight in older patients. Mirtazapine has proved useful in the management of depressed patients with weight loss. Mirtazapine is a well-tolerated and effective antidepressant that inhibits presynaptic alpha$_2$ adrenergic receptors and postsynaptic 5-HT2 and 5-HT3 receptors. Mirtazapine has been shown to induce an earlier increase in appetite and subsequent weight gain in older depressed persons with weight loss.

Several agents previously touted as effective orexigenic agents, such as human growth hormone, have fallen out of favor. The administration of human growth hormone to healthy older adults has been shown to increase muscle bulk. However, significant side effects such as carpal tunnel syndrome, gynecomastia and hypoglycemia were noted; furthermore, the increase in muscle bulk failed to produce a parallel increase in muscle strength. Inadequate data regarding the safety and efficacy of growth hormone administration precludes routine clinical use. Similarly, the role of insulin-like growth factor (IGF-I) in the management of undernutrition is questionable. Although the data suggest that exogenously administered IGF-I may enhance nitrogen retention, gluconeogenesis, and maintenance of normal gastrointestinal function, evidence-based outcome studies are lacking.

Abundant data exist regarding the role of anabolic steroids in the management of undernutrition. However, current evidence supports the restriction of testosterone therapy as an orexigenic agent to hypogonadal undernourished men. As a general rule, pharmacological treatment should be considered second-line therapy and reserved for patients who have failed to respond to nonpharmacological measures.

Managing Undernutrition in the Community Setting

With increasing emphasis on home healthcare, the number of community-dwelling persons requiring alternative modes of feeding has increased. Special consideration and appropriate modification of therapeutic regimens may be required in such cases to ease the care giver or personal burden.

If enteral tube feeding is provided at home, continuous infusion may limit the patient's mobility and functional independence. This method also has the disadvantage of requiring immediate access to technical support, in the event of mechanical failure of the infusion pump. Thus, care givers and patients may find intermittent bolus feeding a more convenient and less daunting task. To minimize the aspiration risk, intermittent bolus feeds should be administered, where possible, with the patient in a seated position. Patients should also be encouraged to remain seated for at least 1 h after feeds. Some active older people resent the social inconvenience and embarrassment of tube feeding during daytime hours, and may prefer overnight enteral infusions of hypercaloric feeds. Hypercaloric feeds contain twice the amount of equal volumes of regular enteral feeds, thereby permitting the provision of adequate nutritional support over shorter periods.

Parenteral nutrition within the home is fraught with all the hazards of intravenous therapy. Thus, availability of skilled services to monitor such therapy is critical. Additionally, adequate care giver and social support is mandatory for patients receiving this mode of nutritional repletion at home.

Health providers involved in home delivery of enteral and parenteral nutritional therapy will need to develop and implement comprehensive therapeutic programs incorporating skilled nursing and dietary services to ensure safe and effective treatment.

Managing Undernutrition in Long-Term Care Institutions

Therapeutic strategies for managing undernourished institutionalized older adults are similar to those used within the community, though perhaps due to readily available medical supervision, enteral and parenteral modes of feeding are used more often. The comparatively formal structure of the nursing home environment has the added advantage of encouraging closer supervision of therapy and stricter nutritional surveillance.

A major drawback to oral nutritional repletion in institutionalized older persons is the restricted variety of meals. This can usually be circumvented by involving the residents in menu development and, where feasible, granting permission for meals of the residents' choice to be supplied by family or friends. Residents of nursing homes are often less functional than their peers and thus may be more dependent on assistance for their basic activities of daily living. When the ability to self-feed is compromised, it is imperative that all meals are supervised and assistance with feeding rendered where necessary. Many residents are persistent wanderers, and may expend a considerable amount of energy in this exercise. In such patients an appropriate increase in their daily energy intake is required to prevent weight loss. Similar adjustments may be required for residents with persistent involuntary movements or severe agitation.

Long-term care institutions must preserve the social and recreational aspects of meals; all too often, mealtimes are reduced to clinical, sanitized, and isolated events. Within the nursing home environment mealtimes are best managed as a component of recreational therapy. Socialization and the preservation of each resident's dignity should be encouraged during meals. Nursing facilities should also attempt to mimic community resources by making food items available outside scheduled mealtimes, from vending machines and snack carts.

Nutritional surveillance programs are crucial to the success of established intervention strategies within nursing homes. Quality indicators, preferably employing anthropometric indices, should be defined to monitor the success of intervention strategies. Continuous quality improvement and total quality management programs must also be implemented as critical components of effective nutritional intervention strategies. Finally, the development of nutrition focus groups and the use of interdisciplinary intervention strategies directed at increasing nutritional intake and preventing undernutrition should be encouraged.

Micronutrient Deficiency

In older people at risk of nutritional compromise, micronutrient supplementation deserves special attention, in order to forestall the development of micronutrient deficiency (**Table 6**). The clinical features of established vitamin deficiency are well recognized. The first recourse in the management of micronutrient deficiencies should be the provision of a well-balanced diet. In the presence of a functioning gastrointestinal tract, an adequate diet containing the recommended daily allowance of each micronutrient effectively prevents and corrects deficiency states. However, the failure to consume the required amount of food may warrant the use of oral pharmacological micronutrient supplements. Vitamin B_{12} deficiency may be considered unique in this regard as, traditionally, replacement therapy has been administered parenterally. However, available evidence suggests that food-cobalamin deficiency may be the most common cause of vitamin B_{12} deficiency in older adults. In this condition cobalamin cannot be extracted from ingested food, although free cobalamin is readily absorbed as absorptive function is normal and intrinsic factor is present in adequate quantities. Thus, in persons with vitamin B_{12} deficiency resulting from food-cobalamin deficiency,

repletion may be adequately achieved by oral replacement therapy.

There is a rising trend toward dietary supplementation with pharmaceutical preparations containing large doses of vitamins and minerals, based on conclusions drawn from the results of several studies. Available evidence derived from human and animal studies indicates that antioxidant micronutrients, mainly vitamins A, C and E, may play a role in boosting immunity, preventing neoplastic disease, and preventing or retarding the progression of several degenerative diseases, such as atherosclerosis. Vitamins E and C have also been shown to reduce low-density lipoprotein (LDL) cholesterol levels and increase high-density lipoprotein (HDL) levels, in addition to lowering fasting plasma insulin levels and improving insulin efficiency. Epidemiological studies have suggested a protective role for antioxidants such as vitamin C, vitamin E, β-carotene, and glutathione in macular degeneration and cataracts. Nevertheless, evidence derived from other epidemiological studies suggests that antioxidants may lack significant benefit. Studies are ongoing in an attempt to resolve this controversy.

In older adults reduced cutaneous synthesis and enteric absorption of vitamin D increases the risk of vitamin D deficiency. Reduced renal responsiveness to parathormone is an added risk factor. At least $500 \, \text{IU} \, \text{day}^{-1}$ of vitamin D are required to prevent significant osteoporosis in postmenopausal women. Institutionalized patients with reduced exposure to sunlight are at higher risk of vitamin D deficiency due to reduced cutaneous synthesis. The role of calcium supplementation in the prevention of osteoporosis is also well accepted. Additional evidence suggests that inadequate dietary calcium consumption may play a role in the genesis of colorectal cancer and hypertension.

Table 6 Vitamins: recommended daily allowances (RDAs) and clinical features of deficiency states

	RDA	Deficiency states
Vitamin A	600–700 μg	Decreased immunity to infections, xerophthalmia, night blindness
Niacin	12–16 mg	Pellagra (dermatitis, dementia, diarrhea), glossitis, cheilosis
Pyridoxine	1.6–2 mg	Dermatitis, delirium, peripheral neuropathy, glossitis
Riboflavin	1.1–1.3 mg	Glossitis, cheilosis, normochromic anemia
Thiamin	0.8–0.9 mg	Beriberi, Wernicke's encephalopathy, Korsakoff's psychosis
Cyanocobalamin	5 μg	Megaloblastic anemia, optic atrophy, peripheral neuropathy, subacute combined degeneration of the cord, dementia
Ascorbic acid	40 mg	Hyperkeratosis, petechial hemorrhages, mucosal bleeding, lethargy
Vitamin D	10 μg	Osteomalacia, osteoporosis
Vitamin E	8–10 mg	Peripheral neuropathy, ataxia, hemolytic anemia
Folate	200 μg	Megaloblastic anemia, cognitive dysfunction
Vitamin K	65–80 mg	Spontaneous hemorrhage, hypothrombinemia

NE, niacin equivalent; RE, retinal equivalent.

Currently, the safety of large pharmacological doses of micronutrient supplements in humans remains to be established. In spite of this, a considerable proportion of the older population consumes large doses of these supplements as a primary preventive health measure. The risk of long-term supplementation with high doses of micronutrients, particularly in the presence of age-related changes, cannot be ignored, and few studies have addressed this issue specifically. Due caution must be exercised, even with the use of micronutrients such as vitamin D and calcium where clinical benefits have been clearly established. The complications of over-enthusiastic calcium and vitamin D supplementation include hypercalcemia, nephrocalcinosis, milk-alkali syndrome, ectopic calcification, and rebound gastric acidity. Calcium supplementation may also chelate iron compounds and precipitate iron deficiency. With regard to vitamin A, available data have identified an increase in absorption and reduced peripheral clearance of this vitamin in older adults, therapy increasing the risk of vitamin A toxicity. Similarly, older persons on long-term iron therapy, particularly in the absence of proven iron deficiency, are at increased risk for the development of secondary hemochromatosis.

On the basis of existing evidence, the use of pharmacological doses of vitamin and mineral supplements is probably best restricted to low-potency supplements and reserved for persons with established micronutrient deficiency who are unable to eat an adequate diet. Close monitoring of such patients for adverse effects is mandatory.

Obesity

Men aged 55–64 years have the highest prevalence of overweight for males in the US (71.7%). Although the prevalence drops with age, the prevalence of overweight among men and women over 75 years is still considerable (52% and 44%, respectively). At all ages, African Americans have a higher prevalence of overweight and obesity.

With aging there is increasing upper and central body fat distribution. This trend is accelerated in women following menopause. In women aged 55–69 years, central obesity has been demonstrated to be correlated with greater coronary artery disease mortality as well as total mortality. Even with weight loss, the waist to hip ratio remained an important predictor of mortality in elderly women. Leptin is a hormone produced by fat cells. In women, leptin levels rise in middle age in concert with the increase in fat mass and then fall in late old age as fat mass declines. In men, leptin levels

increase progressively from 65 years onwards. This may be due to age-related hypogonadism. In older men, testosterone replacement therapy decreased leptin levels.

As food intake declines with aging, obesity in old age is probably due to other factors. All three components of energy output – resting metabolic rate, thermic energy of feeding, and physical activity – decline with aging; thus the pathogenesis of obesity in old age appears to be predominantly due to altered energy output rather than to increased food intake.

While moderate degrees of overweight appear to confer minimal increased mortality in the older population, those above 130% of average body weight have an increased risk of death even at extreme ages. Most of the complications of obesity in older persons are similar to those seen in younger persons. Certain effects of obesity appear more commonly in older persons; for instance, functional decline is more common compared with younger persons. This is often associated with a 'fear of falling.' This syndrome is particularly common in older urban-dwelling adults and may lead to voluntary restriction of physical activity and consequent frailty. The prevalence of diabetes mellitus increases with age, due in part to the increased fat mass in middle age onwards. Obesity markedly increases the prevalence of sleep apnea in older persons. Overweight increases the rate of progression of osteoarthritis and its effects on function. In nursing homes, obesity has been associated with an increase in pressure ulcers. Increasing weight increases claudication in older persons with peripheral vascular disease.

Management of obesity in older persons usually should focus on enhancing functional status and increasing physical activity as opposed to aggressive caloric restriction. Available evidence linking aggressive weight loss in older adults with increased mortality mandates close monitoring during treatment. Surgery for obesity is not appropriate in older adults as the risks of bariatric surgery outweigh the benefits. For similar reasons, the use of thermogenic and anorexic agents should be avoided. Thus, a combination of exercise, healthy eating, and behavior modification is the cornerstone of therapy in older persons. Older obese adults need to be carefully monitored for the development of sarcopenia, visceral protein depletion, and increasing frailty. Due attention should also be given to micronutrient supplementation.

See also: **Antioxidants**: Diet and Antioxidant Defense. **Body Composition**. **Nutritional Assessment**: Anthropometry. **Nutritional Support**: Infants and

Children, Parenteral. **Obesity**: Definition, Etiology and Assessment.

Further Reading

de Groot CP, Enzi G, Matthys C, Moreiras O, Roszkowski W, and Schroll M (2002) Ten-year changes in anthropometric characteristics of elderly Europeans. *Journal of Nutrition, Health and Aging* 6(1): 4–8.

Glick MR (2000) Rethinking the role of tube feeding in patients with advanced dementia. *New England Journal of Medicine* 342: 206–210.

Guigoz Y and Vellas B (1997) The Mini-nutritional assessment for grading the nutritional state of elderly patients, presentation of the MNA, history and validation. *Facts, Research and Intervention Geriatric Newsletter: Nutrition* 6: 2.

Krumholz HM, Seeman T, and Merrill SS (1994) Lack of association between cholesterol and coronary heart disease mortality, morbidity and all-cause mortality in persons older than 70 years. *JAMA* 272: 1335–1340.

Mitchell S, Kiely DK, and Lipsitz LA (1998) Does artificial enteral nutrition prolong the survival of institutionalized elders with chewing and swallowing problems. *Journal of Gerontology* 53A(3): M207–M213.

Morley JE and Thomas DR (1999) Anorexia and aging: pathophysiology. *Nutrition* 15(6): 499–503.

Morley JE, Thomas DR, and Wilson MG (2001) Appetite and orexigenic drugs. Position Paper Council of Nutrition in Long Term Care. *Annals of Long-Term Care* Supplement: 2–12.

Position of the American Dietetic Association (2000) Nutrition, aging and continuum of care. Journal of the American Dietitic Association 100(5): 580–595.

Reynolds MW, Fredman L, Langenberg P, and Magaziner J (1999) Weight, weight change, mortality in a random sample of older community-dwelling women. Journal of the American Geriatric Society 47(12): 1409–1414.

Thomas DR, Ashmen W, Morley JE, and Evans WJ (2000) Nutritional management in long-term care: development of a clinical guideline. Council for Nutritional Strategies in Long-Term Care. *Journal of Gerontology and Medical Science* 55(12): M725–M734.

Wilson MG and Morley JE (2004) Nutritional assessment and support in chronic disease. In: Bales CW and Ritchie CS (eds.) *Handbook of Clinical Nutrition in Aging*, pp. 77–103. Humana Press Inc.

Osteomalacia *see* **Vitamin D**: Rickets and Osteomalacia

OSTEOPOROSIS

K O O'Brien, Johns Hopkins University, Baltimore, MD, USA

Optimal dietary intake is essential for bone health. During childhood and the pubertal growth spurt, nutrients are needed to fully consolidate skeletal mass and to ensure the attainment of a peak bone mass consistent with one's genetic potential. After peak bone mass is obtained, nutrition continues to play an essential role in skeletal health. If intakes of key nutrients are not consumed at required levels, mineral may be lost from bone or essential bone proteins may not be fully functional.

Osteoporosis and osteopenia are substantial public health problems. Low bone mass (osteopenia and osteoporosis) and vitamin D deficiency are currently substantial public health problems. Osteopenia is defined when adult bone mineral density values are 1–2.5 SD below the mean peak value observed in a young adult. If the deficit in bone is more pronounced, and bone mineral density falls 2.5 SD or more below that observed in a young adult, this is defined as osteoporosis. Approximately 200 million people worldwide have osteoporosis. Many more have suboptimal bone mass and are at increased risk of developing this disease. Vitamin D deficiency in adults can also impair bone mineralization and lead to osteomalacia (in adults) or rickets (if evident in pediatric age groups prior to the completion of longitudinal bone growth). Insufficient bone mass and impaired bone mineralization increases the risk of fractures at considerable cost and loss of quality of life. Because bone loss is not fully reversible, the most effective strategies for reducing osteoporosis should focus on prevention, with nutrition playing a key role.

Dietary Intake and Body Mass

A balanced diet is important to promote health and to maintain an appropriate body weight. An

Table 1 Nutritional and lifestyle parameters that may influence bone health

Minerals	Vitamins/ hormones	Lifestyle and environmental factors	Dietary components
Calcium	Vitamin D	Body mass index	Protein
Phosphorus	Vitamin K	Exercise	Soy/ phytoestrogens
Magnesium	Vitamin A	Cigarette smoking	Fatty acids
Sodium	Vitamin C	Alcohol intake	Homocysteine
Zinc	Vitamin B_{12}		
Copper	Vitamin B_6		
Iron	Folate		
Boron			
Manganese			
Fluorine			
Potassium			
Silicon			

individual's body weight is one of the strongest determinants of bone mass because of the skeleton's responsiveness to the load that is placed on it. Individuals with small body frames or those who are excessively thin have an increased risk of osteoporosis due to a lower overall skeletal reserve to draw on for calcium needed to offset the annual loss of bone that occurs later in life. At the extreme end of this spectrum, individuals with anorexia nervosa are at risk of osteoporosis because of alterations in hormonal status and amenorrhea in addition to insufficient dietary intake of nutrients required for bone health.

Although higher body weight is typically associated with a greater skeletal mass, obese individuals may sequester nutrients needed for skeletal health, such as vitamin D, in adipose tissue. Bariatric surgery as a treatment for morbidly obese individuals is becoming more common and leads to a loss of both body weight and bone mass. The long-term impact of this surgery on skeletal health is not yet fully elucidated, and it remains unclear if the amount of bone lost following surgery is solely a response to the decrease in body weight or if it is also associated with other adverse consequences of this surgery on bone health.

Although overall caloric intake impacts body weight, many nutrients and dietary components have been studied in relation to their impact on bone health (**Table 1**). Several of these key nutrients and components of the diet and their roles in bone health and skeletal homeostasis are detailed next.

Calcium

Calcium is the most abundant mineral found in bone and comprises approximately 33% of bone mineral.

Optimal calcium intakes are essential across the life cycle to meet the daily intrinsic requirements of calcium required for skeletal growth and to offset urinary, dermal, and endogenous fecal calcium losses. When dietary intakes of calcium are not sufficient to maintain circulating calcium concentrations and/or when the losses of calcium from the body are excessive, bone calcium will be resorbed to maintain calcium homeostasis. Because calcium is essential for the structural integrity of bone, deficiencies or inadequate intakes of this mineral will have a detrimental impact on bone mass and quality.

Skeletal mass peaks at approximately age 20–30 years, with much of this gain occurring during the pubertal growth spurt. Nearly 50% of adult bone mass is accumulated during the pubertal growth spurt. Thus, this period of skeletal accretion can be viewed as a window of opportunity to maximize skeletal mass. Calcium supplementation studies in children have found increased bone mass with supplementation, an effect that is most pronounced when implemented during the prepubertal period. It is not clear to what degree calcium supplementation during the pubertal growth spurt results in a net gain in peak bone mass or if it solely influences the tempo at which peak bone mass is achieved. To account for the importance of this nutrient in bone mineralization, the recommended adequate intake of calcium is highest (1300 mg or 2.5 mmol.day) between the ages of 9 and 18 years.

Calcium supplementation has also been found to have beneficial effects on bone health in adults and may have the greatest impact in individuals whose habitual dietary calcium intakes are less than 400 mg (10 mmol)/day. To account for a decreased efficiency of intestinal absorption coupled with increased losses of calcium in older individuals, recommended calcium intakes increase to 1200 mg (30 mmol)/day in those age 50 or older. As discussed in more detail later, due to the prevalence of vitamin D deficiency in the elderly, oral vitamin D supplements up to 800 IU/day may also be required in order for the impact of calcium supplementation to be evident.

Several epidemiological studies have found significant relationships between an individual's lifelong intake of milk and subsequent risk of fracture. The degree to which this effect is a consequence of increased calcium intake or due to other nutritional components of milk and dairy products requires further study.

Despite the importance of calcium in bone mineral acquisition and maintenance, calcium intakes fall below the recommended level for the majority of age groups, with intake being particularly low for adolescent girls and adult and elderly women. It is often difficult to increase consumption of calcium in certain age groups due to low intakes of dairy products or to other factors, such as lactose intolerance, dieting, or altered appetite and food consumption patterns in groups such as the elderly. To increase the calcium content of the diet, nonfat milk powder yogurt or cheese, can be added to a number of recipes to increase the calcium content of the food without adversely affecting taste. An increasing variety of calcium-fortified food products are now also available. Individuals with lactose intolerance may improve intake of calcium by use of lactose-free dairy products or lactase pills. Increasing calcium intake from dietary versus supplemental sources also increases the intake of many other nutrients needed for bone health, including protein, magnesium, zinc, phosphorus, and vitamin D. For this reason, dietary approaches to increase calcium intake should be promoted over the use of calcium supplements alone. Despite these benefits, in some instances it may be necessary to utilize calcium supplements to achieve recommended intake levels.

Several forms of calcium supplements are commercially available. Existing supplemental forms differ slightly with respect to their relative calcium content per tablet and their absorbability; however, the magnitude of these differences is minor and may not be biologically significant. Caution should be used when relying on natural sources of calcium (such as those prepared from bone meal, limestone, or oyster shells) because these preparations may also contain heavy metals such as lead. Several calcium supplements also contain additional nutrients required for bone health, including vitamins D and K. Because the fraction of calcium absorbed falls as calcium intake increases, little additional benefit per dose is achieved when taking supplemental calcium sources containing more than 500 mg (12.5 mmol) per dose.

Magnesium

More than half of the magnesium found in the body is located in bone. In addition to its presence in bone, magnesium is important in calcium metabolism and bone health because it is required for parathyroid hormone secretion. Parathyroid hormone (PTH) is integral to bone health because it increases the production of the active form of vitamin D (1,25-dihydroxyvitamin D) and plays a role in the tubular reabsorption of calcium and phosphorus.

Although magnesium deficiency is associated with abnormalities in vitamin D metabolism, hypocalcemia, and impaired PTH secretion, epidemiological studies linking magnesium intakes to measures of skeletal health have produced conflicting results. Some studies report significant associations between dietary magnesium intake and bone mineral density, but others have not supported this finding. Relationships between magnesium status and bone mass may be more challenging to elucidate due to the lack of a highly sensitive indicator of magnesium status.

Studies have indicated that typical magnesium intakes in healthy adolescents may not be sufficient to maintain magnesium balance. Data on the impact of magnesium supplementation on bone mass remain controversial. While some studies have found magnesium supplementation to result in positive effects on bone mass, others have reported no significant benefit. Additional studies are needed to clarify these discrepancies and to assess the net effect of magnesium status and supplementation on bone metabolism. Because dietary intakes fall below recommended levels in several age groups and because of the known relationships between magnesium and hormones integral to bone health, increased attention should be focused on optimal magnesium intakes in relation to bone homeostasis.

Zinc and Copper

Zinc and copper play important roles in bone metabolism and bone health in part due to the roles they play as cofactors for various enzymes required for the synthesis or modification of bone matrix constituents. Zinc is a cofactor for a myriad of enzymes in the body, including alkaline phosphatase. Alkaline phosphatase is synthesized by osteoblasts and is essential for bone mineralization. Zinc also plays a role in the osteoblast via its involvement in aminoacyl-tRNA synthetase. Copper is a necessary cofactor for lysyl oxidase, an enzyme involved in collagen cross-linking. Both copper and zinc are found as components of superoxide dismutase, and they may protect bone from oxidative damage. Genetic defects that cause zinc deficiency (acrodermatitis enteropathica) or copper deficiency (Menkes' disease) result in growth retardation, stunting, and impaired bone growth.

Although more research on the roles of zinc and copper in bone health and fracture risk is clearly needed, the importance of these nutrients in skeletal health should be recognized and optimal intakes should be promoted in relation to skeletal homeostasis.

Vitamin D

Vitamin D is particularly important for bone health because of the role it plays in calcium homeostasis.

The active form of vitamin D stimulates the synthesis of calcium binding protein in the intestine to facilitate calcium transport across the intestine. Vitamin D also plays a regulatory role in renal calcium reabsorption and in calcium release from bone.

Vitamin D can be obtained from the diet (although only vitamin D-fortified milk and fatty fish provide substantial amounts) or is made in the skin following exposure to sunlight. Deficiency of this vitamin is increasingly recognized as an issue of concern across all age groups of the US population from neonates to the elderly. This deficiency is due to a combination of inadequate dietary intake (dairy products provide the largest dietary contribution to vitamin D intake) and to inadequate sunlight exposure. Rickets is increasing among exclusively breast-fed minority infants in the United States. This is thought to be due to the low vitamin D content of human milk combined with insufficient endogenous dermal synthesis. Vitamin D deficiency in adults results in osteomalacia and secondary hyperparathyroidism, increasing bone resorption and the risk of osteoporosis.

Lack of sufficient endogenous production of vitamin D in the skin is influenced by geographical location (more northern latitudes have a shorter season during which the wavelength needed for vitamin D synthesis is available), increased use of sunscreen and cosmetics and skin care products containing sunscreen (sunscreens with SPF values of 8 or greater block the dermal production of vitamin D), and lifestyle factors that decrease exposure to sunlight.

Studies suggest that the optimal serum concentration of vitamin D may be markedly higher (>30 ng/ml) than that traditionally used to define vitamin D deficiency (<10–15 ng/ml). If these increased levels are eventually accepted as optimal target concentrations, an even greater fraction of the population will have suboptimal status of this vitamin.

Supplementation with vitamin D and calcium has been found to be effective in decreasing fracture incidence. Several studies in older adults have found significant relationships between vitamin D status (as determined by 25-hydroxyvitamin D concentrations) and both musculoskeletal function and risk of sarcopenia. Combined vitamin D and calcium supplementation in the elderly may also decrease the risk of falling. Individuals with low dairy product intake, those living in northern latitudes, or those with inadequate sunlight exposure may need to rely on supplemental sources of vitamin D to maintain circulating concentrations at optimal levels required to promote bone health.

Vitamin K

Many proteins are dependent on vitamin K for the carboxylation of γ-carboxyglutamyl (Gla) residues. Several of these vitamin K-dependent proteins play integral roles in the bone matrix. Osteocalcin, one of the vitamin K-dependent proteins, is the most abundant noncollagenous protein in bone. Osteocalcin contains three Gla residues that require vitamin K for carboxylation. The ability of osteocalcin to bind to the hydroxyapatite fraction of bone is dependent on its degree of carboxylation. Deficiency of vitamin K increases the fraction of undercarboxylated osteocalcin in the circulation. In addition to osteocalcin, other vitamin K-dependent proteins (including matrix Gla protein and protein S) are found in bone and cartilage. Research is needed to elucidate the impact of vitamin K deficiency on risk of osteoporosis and fracture. Because of the known relationship between vitamin K and several crucial bone proteins, optimal status of this vitamin should be achieved to promote skeletal health.

Phosphorus

Phosphorus is another mineral that functions as an integral component of bone. Bone contains 85% of the phosphorus found in the body, and together calcium and phosphorus comprise the major fraction of bone mineral. Although sufficient phosphorus intakes are necessary to support bone mineralization, phosphorus homeostasis can be maintained across a range of intakes and ratios of calcium to phosphorus in the diet.

There is considerable controversy regarding the potential impact of elevated phosphorus intake from soda on bone health. Although concern has focused on the phosphoric acid and phosphorus content of soda in relation to calcium retention, the major impact of these products on bone health may be their displacement of other more nutritive beverages (such as milk) from the diet. Because increased soda consumption may increase the risk of excess weight gain and displace other more nutritive beverages from the diet, excessive soda intakes should be a cause for concern, especially in children and adolescents during the peak period of bone acquisition.

Sodium

Although many components of the diet play direct roles in bone mineralization, nutrients such as sodium are known to influence the retention of other nutrients required for optimal bone health. Sodium is one of the strongest determinants of urinary calcium excretion. Increased dietary sodium intake elevates urinary calcium losses, with every 2300 mg (100 mmol) increase in dietary sodium increasing the urinary excretion of calcium by approximately 40 mg (1 mmol). Thus, excessive intakes of sodium (such as those that may occur in individuals who consume large amounts of processed food, salt food heavily, or consume foods high in sodium) increase the obligatory losses of calcium from the body. During the growth phase this could potentially limit the amount of calcium that can be utilized for bone mineralization. The long-term impact of variation in sodium intake on bone mass and fracture risk has been difficult to quantify because of a lack of sufficient information on how dietary effects on urinary sodium loss are counterbalanced and because other dietary components may modify this response.

Protein

Protein is essential for the formation of the organic matrix of bone and optimal intakes are required for normal skeletal development and growth. The importance of protein in bone health is well-known; however, there are conflicting reports on the relative impact of extremes of protein intake on bone health. Many proteins are rich in sulfur amino acids. The resulting protein-induced acid load must be buffered before excretion from the body. Calcium is a positive cation and can be utilized to buffer increased dietary acid loads from high protein intakes. On average, for every 1-g increase in dietary protein intake, urinary calcium excretion increases by approximately 1 mg.

Differences in habitual protein intakes have been related to bone mass and risk of fracture. Many studies have reported positive relationships between increased animal protein intake and bone health. Higher animal protein intakes in the elderly have been associated with reduced bone loss. Other research has supported a positive association between higher animal protein intake and both greater bone mineral density and decreased risk of hip fractures. Studies have found that although urinary calcium excretion increases in response to acute increases in protein intake, intestinal calcium absorption also increases by an amount nearly comparable to that lost in urine. Insufficient intakes of protein can adversely impact muscle mass and function. In addition, low dietary protein intake has been associated with reductions in serum insulin-like growth factor-1 (IGF-1) concentrations. IGF-1 plays an essential role in skeletal health via its impact on osteoblast formation and bone growth.

In contrast to the many studies that have found positive relationships between protein intake and bone health, other data suggest that high protein intakes may have a detrimental impact on bone mass and fracture risk and it is likely that extremes of protein intake, both high and low, may have adverse consequences on bone homeostasis. To clarify these conflicting findings, more research is required to address the relative impact of the quantity and type of protein on skeletal health.

Phytoestrogens

Phytoestrogens are dietary components that have a chemical structure similar to that of endogenous estrogens. The primary phytoestrogens in the diet are obtained from soybean isoflavones (including genistein and daizein). These compounds appear to be able to weakly mediate some the genomic and nongenomic effects of estrogen and may function as agonists or antagonists, depending on the tissue and type of estrogen receptor involved. To date, supplemental sources of these compounds have not been found to decrease fracture risk. Additional clinical trials will assist in determining the long-term impact of phytoestrogens on bone health and fracture risk.

Homocysteine

For some time, it has been known that individuals with a genetic defect in homocysteine metabolism (homocystinuria) have an increased risk of early onset osteoporosis. However, only recently has attention focused on the potential impact of circulating homocysteine concentrations on bone health among the general population. This interest is based on studies that have reported significant relationships between serum homocysteine concentrations and increased risk of fracture in adults. The strength of the relationship observed is substantial and is similar to the relationship found between serum homocysteine concentrations and cardiovascular disease. The mechanisms responsible for the impact of homocysteine concentrations on fracture risk are not known. Increased homocysteine concentrations could possibly interfere with normal collagen production, but studies have not found a significant relationship between serum homocysteine concentrations and bone mineral density, and the impact of elevated homocysteine concentrations on bone health may be indirect. Further research will assist in identifying the mechanisms and relationships between homocysteine and bone health and the degree to which this relationship is influenced by folate, vitamin B_{12}, and vitamin B_6 status. Because of the other known adverse consequences of elevated serum homocysteine concentrations, additional incentive to monitor and promote reductions in this amino acid in relation to bone health is warranted.

Other Lifestyle Factors

Other lifestyle choices, such as smoking, alcohol abuse, and physical activity, also impact overall bone health. Excessive alcohol intake is a risk factor for low bone mass. This finding may be a consequence of poor dietary quality in chronic alcoholics and may also be related to adverse effects of excessive alcohol intake on osteoblast function. Cigarette smoking also adversely impacts bone health. Smokers may be leaner, and female smokers may experience an earlier menopause and have lower postmenopausal estrogen levels. Smoking may also have adverse effects on bone cells either directly or indirectly through an increase in oxidative stress.

Exercise is known to positively influence bone mass. During exercise, the strain placed on bone stimulates local bone responses to positively influence the balance in bone remodeling. Many studies have found positive associations between exercise and bone mass at a number of sites, especially the hip and the spine. The impact of exercise on bone mass is related to the intensity of the exercise and is associated with the degree to which it increases the habitual physical activity level of the individual. The impact of exercise on bone mass is also influenced by diet and may be most efficacious when calcium intake is optimal. Exercise not only impacts bone mass but also influences muscle strength, muscle mass, balance, and coordination. These improvements in muscle strength may also lead to improvements in posture, balance, flexibility, coordination, and gait stability that decrease the risk of falls.

Nutrient–Gene Interactions

Optimal nutrition is needed to supply the necessary substrates for bone; however, other parameters also influence the impact of a given nutrient on bone health. A substantial amount of bone mineral acquisition (up to 80%) is genetically determined. An individual's ability to utilize a given nutrient intake is influenced by his or her genetic makeup.

Many candidate genes have been associated or linked with the risk of osteoporosis or fracture, including genes coding for hormones (PTH), receptors (including PTH, vitamin D, estrogen, glucocorticoid, and calcitonin receptors), cytokines and growth factors (including IGF-1, transforming growth factor-β, epidermal growth factor, interleukin-4, and interleukin-6), and bone matrix proteins (such as osteocalcin, collagen type 1 ($\alpha 1$ and $\alpha 2$), and collagen type 11 ($\alpha 1$)). Although many of these genes have obvious roles in bone metabolism, other candidate genes (such as those coding for apolipoprotein E and methylenetetrahydrofolate reductase) have less obvious relationships to bone mass.

Several studies have found interactions between genotype, nutrient level, and environmental factors. For instance, the impact of exercise on bone can be influenced by the habitual dietary calcium intake and the individual's genotype (such as the vitamin D receptor genotype). Further research on the genetic control of bone mineral acquisition and loss will be invaluable in targeting groups at risk for low bone mass and may eventually be useful in setting genotype-specific intakes of bone-related nutrients to maximize skeletal health throughout the life cycle.

Best Practices to Prevent Osteoporosis

In summary, several practices can be adopted to assist in the prevention of osteoporosis. From a nutritional standpoint an emphasis should be made on adequate intakes of calcium, vitamin D and a balanced diet that meets the requirements of other essential bone-related minerals and nutrients (detailed in **Table 1**). A healthy body weight should be achieved and maintained throughout the life cycle. Age-appropriate physical activity and exercise programs should be promoted to maintain fitness, muscle strength and weight bearing activities. Lifestyle habits that adversely impact bone health, including smoking and excessive alcohol intake, should be avoided. Individuals with risk factors known to increase the risk of low bone mass should discuss these concerns with their physician to identify the need for bone density screening. Appropriate screening will allow for the initiation of medical interventions to maintain or build existing bone mass and reduce the subsequent risk of fragility related fractures. Attention to bone health and adoption of bone healthy habits should be initiated during childhood and maintained throughout the lifecycle to promote lifelong attainment of skeletal health.

See also: **Bone**. **Calcium**. **Copper**. **Magnesium**. **Phosphorus**. **Protein**: Requirements and Role in Diet. **Sodium**: Physiology. **Vitamin D**: Rickets and Osteomalacia. **Vitamin K**. **Zinc**: Physiology.

Further Reading

Branca F (2003) Dietary phyto-oestrogens and bone health. *Proceedings of the Nutrition Society* **62**: 877–887.

Bugel S (2003) Vitamin K and bone health. *Proceedings of the Nutrition Society* **62**: 839–843.

Heaney RP and Weaver CM (2003) Calcium and vitamin D. *Endocrinology and Metabolism Clinics of North America* **32**(1): 181–194.

Holick MF (2003) Vitamin D: A millennium perspective. *Journal of Cellular Biochemistry* **88**: 296–307.

Holick MF and Dawson-Hughes B (eds.) (2004) *Nutrition and Bone Health*. Totowa, NJ: Humana Press.

Institute of Medicine (1998) *Calcium, Phosphorus, Magnesium, Vitamin D, and Fluoride. Dietary Reference Intakes.* Washington, DC: National Academy Press.

Lowe NM, Fraser WD, and Jackson MJ (2002) Is there a potential therapeutic advantage to copper and zinc for osteoporosis? *Proceedings of the Nutrition Society* **61**: 181–185.

Prentice A (2004) Diet, nutrition and the prevention of osteoporosis. *Public Health Nutrition* **7**(1A): 227–243.

Tucker KL (2003) Dietary intake and bone status with aging. *Current Pharmaceutical Design* **9**: 2687–2704.

Wolf RL, Zmuda JM, Stone KL *et al.* (2000) Update on the epidemiology of osteoporosis. *Curr Rheumatol Rep* **2**: 74–86.

Oxidant Damage *see* **Antioxidants**: Observational Studies; Intervention Studies

PANTOTHENIC ACID

C J Bates, MRC Human Nutrition Research, Cambridge, UK

Absorption, Transport and Storage, Status Measurement

A considerable proportion of the pantothenic acid (vitamin B_5, see **Figure 1**) that is present in food eaten by animals or humans exists as derivatives such as coenzyme A (CoA) and acyl carrier protein (ACP). Compared with the crystalline vitamin, only about half of the vitamin in food is thought to be absorbed. The pantothenic acid in its derivatives in food is largely released as free pantothenic acid or pantetheine by pancreatic enzymes, and is then absorbed along the entire length of the small intestine by a combination of active transport and passive diffusion, of which the active transport process seems to predominate at physiological intakes. This active transport process is dependent on sodium, energy and pH and is saturable: the K_m is $c.$ 17 μM and V_{max} is $c.$ 1000 pmol cm^{-2} h^{-1}, with minor variations among species. The transport pathway is shared by biotin in colonic epithelial cells, and it appears to be regulated by an intracellular protein kinase C-mediated pathway. Calmodulin is also implicated in cellular pantothenic acid transport pathways.

In mice, it was found that usual dietary pantothenate levels did not affect the rate of absorption of a standard pantothenate dose, i.e., there was no evidence for feedback adaptation of the absorption pathway to low or high intakes, and it is assumed that the same is true in other species, including humans. However, there is some evidence from rat studies that the extent of secretion of enzymes degrading CoA into the gut lumen may partially limit the availability of pantothenic acid from CoA.

In humans, studies of urinary excretion of pantothenic acid after oral intakes of either free pantothenic acid or of the pantothenic acid present in food have indicated a relative availability of $c.$ 50% from the food-borne vitamin. Urinary excretion of pantothenate was $c.$ 0.8 mg day^{-1} when a pantothenate-deficient diet was eaten, rising to 40–60 mg day^{-1} at a high daily intake of l00 mg day^{-1}. At intermediate intakes, in the range 2.8–12.8 mg day^{-1}, the urinary excretion rate varied between 4 and 6 mg day^{-1}. Excretion of less than 1 mg day^{-1} is considered low. Urinary excretion rates reflect recent intakes perhaps more closely than most other biochemical indices.

The contribution of the gut flora to the available pantothenate for humans is unknown, but there is some evidence that bacterial synthesis of the vitamin may be important in animals, especially ruminants, since severe deficiency can only be achieved by using antibiotics or antagonists. Clinical conditions such as ulcers or colitis can adversely affect pantothenate status and excretion rates, and dietary fiber may affect its absorption.

After a dose of ^{14}C-labeled pantothenate, about 40% of the dose appears in muscle tissue and about 10% in the liver, with smaller amounts occurring elsewhere. The differential affinities of the various different tissues determines their individual contents of the coenzyme derivatives, CoA and ACP, since there is no other major store of the vitamin anywhere in the body. Most organs, including placenta, exhibit evidence of a unidirectional active transport process for the intracellular accumulation of pantothenate, which is dependent on sodium, energy, and pH. In placenta (and probably elsewhere) this transport process is also shared by biotin and by some of its analogs, which can exhibit competitive inhibition. The only tissues that have been shown to differ with respect to transport mechanisms are red cells and the central nervous system.

The uptake and efflux of pantothenate into and out of red blood cells is unaffected by sodium, energy, or pH. Red cells contain pantothenate, 4-phosphopantothenate, and pantetheine, but they do not contain mitochondria, or carry out CoA-dependent processes. The function of the pantothenate derivatives found in red cells is unknown, but their formation clearly results in higher concentrations of total pantothenate in red cells than in plasma, and red cell (or whole blood) total pantothenate is considered a better status index, and is more predictably related to

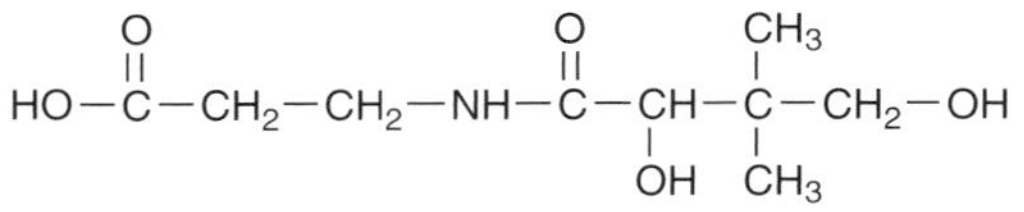

Figure 1 Structure of pantothenic acid.

intake, than is serum or plasma pantothenate. A concentration less than $1\,\mu mol\,l^{-1}$ of pantothenate in whole blood is considered low; the normal range is $1.6–2.7\,\mu mol\,l^{-1}$. Pantothenate in serum appears to be a very short-term marker and it is not well correlated with changes in intake or status.

Concentrations in body fluids are traditionally measured by microbiological assay using *Lactobacillus plantarum*. If CoA is present, enzymatic hydrolysis is needed to liberate free pantothenic acid for the microbiological assay. Other assay methods reported include gas chromatography (after conversion to a volatile derivative), radioimmunoassay (RIA), or enzyme-linked immunoabsorbent assay (ELISA).

Unlike several other B vitamin precursors of cofactors, pantothenate is not entirely converted to coenzyme forms inside the cell, and metabolic 'trapping' is therefore less dominant than it is for some other B vitamins. There is some evidence that the free pantothenate in tissues is more closely related to dietary pantothenate than the coenzyme forms are; the latter are relatively protected during periods of dietary deficiency or of low intakes. Uptake of pantothenate from plasma into most tissues is proportional to the plasma concentration because the active transport process is nowhere near saturated at typical plasma concentrations of $c.\ 10^{-6}\,M$.

Pantothenate is required for the hepatic acetylation of drugs by its presence in acetyl CoA, and it has been shown that pantothenate deficiency can impair this process; moreover, 20–60% of human populations are slow acetylators, varying with their ethnic grouping. Whether this function can be used to develop a functional test for pantothenate status is an intriguing but unresolved question.

Metabolism and Turnover

The primary role of pantothenic acid is in acyl group activation for lipid metabolism, involving thiol acylation of CoA or of ACP, both of which contain 4-phosphopantotheine, the active group of which is β-mercaptoethylamine. CoA is essential for oxidation of fatty acids, pyruvate and α-oxogutarate, for metabolism of sterols, and for acetylation of other molecules, so as to modulate their transport characteristics or functions. Acyl carrier protein, which is synthesized from apo-ACP and coenzyme A, is involved specifically in fatty acid synthesis. Its role is to activate acetyl,

malonyl, and intermediate chain fatty acyl groups during their anabolism by the biotin-dependent fatty acid synthase complex (i.e., acyl-CoA: malonyl-CoA-acyl transferase (decarboxylating, oxoacyl and enoyl-reducing, and thioester-hydrolyzing), EC 2.3.1.85).

The organ with the highest concentration of pantothenate is liver, followed by adrenal cortex, because of the requirement for steroid hormone metabolism in these tissues. Ninety-five per cent of the CoA within each tissue is found in the mitochondria. However, the initial stages of activation of pantothenate and conversion to CoA occur in the cytosol. It was originally believed that the final stages of CoA synthesis must occur within the mitochondria, but later evidence indicated that transport across the mitochondrial membrane is, after all, possible. β-oxidation within the peroxisomes is also CoA-dependent, and is downregulated by pantothenate deficiency.

The pathways of conversion of pantothenic acid to CoA and to ACP are summarized in **Figure 2**. There are three ATP-requiring reactions and one CTP-requiring reaction in the synthesis of CoA. The rate of CoA synthesis is under close metabolic control by energy-yielding substrates, such as glucose and free fatty acids (via CoA and acyl CoA) at the initial activation step, which is catalyzed by pantothenate kinase (ATP: pantothenate 4-phosphotransferase, EC 2.7.1.33). This feedback control is thought to be a mechanism for conservation of cofactor requirements. There are also direct and indirect effects of insulin, corticosteroids, and glucagon, which result in important changes in tissue distribution, uptake, etc. in persons with diabetes. The mechanisms involved here are complex and not yet fully understood; however insulin represses and glucagon induces the enzyme.

A rare genetic disease, Hallervorden-Spatz syndrome, has recently been shown to result from deficiency of pantothenate kinase, and is now alternatively known as pantothenate kinase-associated neurodegeneration (PKAN). Dystonia, involuntary movements, and spasticity occur, and although there is no cure, some palliative treatment is possible.

In genetically normal people, fasting results in a reduction of fatty acid synthase activity with loss of the coenzyme of ACP, which thus achieves the desired objective of a shift away from fatty acid synthesis, towards breakdown. This interconversion of apo-ACP and holo-ACP is thus a very important process for the short-term regulation of fatty acid synthesis.

Deficiency of sulfur amino acids can result in reduced CoA synthesis; likewise copper overload can (by interfering with sulfur amino acid function) also reduce CoA synthesis.

Excretion of free pantothenate in the urine is the primary excretion route in humans; in other mammals

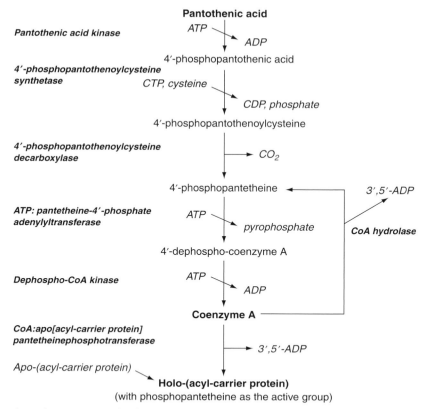

Figure 2 Synthetic pathway between pantothenic acid, coenzyme A, and acyl carrier protein.

the glucuronide or glucoside may be excreted. There is little evidence of degradation to simpler products, and pantothenic acid appears to be very efficiently conserved in animals. Some bacteria can cleave it to yield pantoic acid and β-alanine. A potentially useful breakdown product of CoA is taurine, formed via cysteamine. This amino acid is an essential nutrient for some carnivorous animals such as cats.

When dietary intakes are low, the majority of the circulating vitamin, which is filtered in the kidney tubules, is absorbed by the same type of sodium-dependent active transport process that also occurs at most other sites in the body. Retention of a test dose of pantothenate is, as expected, greater in partially depleted subjects, than in saturated ones. Secretion into breast milk is proportional to intake and to blood levels of the vitamin; therefore, dietary supplements taken by the lactating mother generally increase the breast milk content of the vitamin.

Metabolic Function and Essentiality

As noted above, the biochemical functions, and hence the basis for the dietary requirement of pantothenic acid, arise entirely from its occurrence as an essential component of CoA and of ACP, which cannot be synthesized *de novo* in mammals from simpler precursors.

In addition to the now well-established roles of CoA in the degradation and synthesis of fatty acids, sterols, and other compounds synthesized from isoprenoid precursors, there are also a number of acetylation and long-chain fatty acylation processes which seem to require CoA as part of their essential biological catalytic sites, and which are still being explored today. The acetylation of amino sugars, and some other basic reactions of acetyl-CoA and succinyl-CoA in intermediary metabolism, have been known since the 1980s. However, the addition of acetyl or fatty acyl groups to certain proteins in order to modify and control their specific and essential properties is a more recent discovery. The first category of these modifications comprises the acetylation of the N-terminal amino acid in certain proteins, which occurs in at least half of all the known proteins that are found in higher organisms. The specific amino acids that are recipients of these acetyl groups are most commonly methionine, alanine, or serine. The purposes of this terminal acetylation process are not entirely clear and may be multiple, including modifications of function (e.g., of hormone function), of binding and site recognition, of tertiary peptide structure, and of eventual susceptibility to degradation. Another possible site of protein acetylation is the side chain of certain internal lysine residues, whose side chain ε-amino group may become acetylated in some proteins, notably the basic histone proteins of the cell nucleus, and the α-tubulin proteins of the cytoplasmic microtubules, which help to determine cell shape and motility. Its essential role in the synthesis of α-tubulin appears to be a particularly important one.

Proteins can also be modified by acylation with certain long-chain fatty acids, notably the 16-carbon saturated fatty acid, palmitic acid, and the 14-carbon saturated fatty acid, myristic acid. Although structurally very similar to each other, these two fatty acids seek entirely different protein locations for acylation and also have quite different functions. They have recently been explored with particular emphasis on viral and yeast proteins, although proteins in higher animals, in organs such as lung and brain, can also become acylated with palmityl moieties. Palmitoyl CoA is also required for the transport of residues through the Golgi apparatus during protein secretion. It is believed that these protein acylations may enable and control specific protein interactions, especially in relation to cell membranes, and proteins that are palmitoylated are generally also found to be associated with the plasma membrane. Signal transduction (e.g., of the human β_2-adrenergic receptor) is one process that appears to be controlled by palmitoylation, and other palmitoylated proteins possess some structural importance, for example in the case of the protein–lipid complex of brain myelin. Clearly, these subtle protein modifications, all of which depend on CoA and hence on pantothenic acid, have a wide-ranging significance for many biological processes, which is still being actively explored.

Pantothenic acid is essential for all mammalian species so far studied, namely humans, bovines, pigs, dogs, cats, and rodents, as well as for poultry and fish. Pantothenate deficiency signs in animals are relatively nonspecific and vary among species. Deficiency in young animals results in impaired growth, and requirement estimates based on maximum growth rates are between 8 and 15 mg per kg diet. Rats that are maintained on a diet low in pantothenate exhibit reduced growth, scaly dermatitis, alopecia, hair discoloration and loss, porphyrin-caked whiskers, sex organ disruption, congenital malformations, and adrenal necrosis. Deficient chicks are affected by abnormal feather development, locomotor and thymus involution, neurological symptoms including convulsions, and hypoglycemia. Pigs exhibit intestinal problems and abnormalities of dorsal root

ganglion cells, and several species suffer nerve demyelination. Fish exhibit fused gill lamellae, clumping of mitochondria, and kidney lesions. Signs specific for pantothenate depletion are not well characterized for humans. A syndrome that included 'burning feet' has been described in tropical prisoner-of-war camps during World War II, and it was said to respond to pantothenic acid supplements; however this was likely to have been a more complex deficiency. A competitive analog of pantothenate, ω-methyl pantothenate, interferes with the activation of pantothenic acid; it also produces burning feet symptoms, Reye-like syndrome, cardiac instability, gastrointestinal disturbance, dizziness, paraesthesia, depression, fatigue, insomnia, muscular weakness, loss of immune (antibody) function, insensitivity to adrenocorticotrophic hormone, and increased sensitivity to insulin. Large doses of pantothenate can reverse these changes. One of the earliest functional changes observed in mildly deficient rats was an increase in serum triacylglycerols and free fatty acids, presumably resulting from the impairment in β-oxidation. Paradoxically, CoA levels are relatively resistant to dietary pantothenate deficiency; however there are some inter-organ shifts in pantothenate in certain metabolic states.

As noted above, CoA is required for Golgi function, involved in protein transport. Pantothenate deficiency can therefore cause reductions in the amounts of some secreted proteins. Other metabolic responses to deficiency include a reduction in urinary 17-ketosteroids, a reduction in serum cholesterol, a reduction in drug acetylation, a general reduction in immune response, and an increase in upper respiratory tract infection.

Recently, some studies of wound healing and fibroblast growth have indicated that both pantothenic acid and ascorbic acid are involved in trace element distribution in the skin and scars of experimental animals, and that pantothenic acid can improve skin and colon wound healing in rabbits. It is not yet known whether these observations are relevant to wound healing in humans.

Requirements

In the UK, National Food Survey records suggest that during recent decades mean adult daily pantothenate intakes have been consistently in the range of 4–6 mg. Since there is little evidence for the magnitude of minimum requirements in humans, the UK committee responsible for the revision of dietary reference values in 1991 suggested that intakes in the range 3–7 mg day^{-1} can be considered as adequate (although no specific values for the reference nutrient intake, estimated average requirement or lower reference nutrient intake for pantothenate were set). The US adequate intake (AI) for pantothenic acid is currently set at $5\,mg\,day^{-1}$ for adults; $4\,mg\,day^{-1}$ for children aged 9–13 years; $3\,mg\,day^{-1}$ for 4–8 years, and $2\,mg\,day^{-1}$ for 1–3 years. There was insufficient evidence to set an estimated average requirement (EAR), a recommended daily allowance (RDA), or a tolerable upper intake level (UL).

There are few studies in communities where intakes are likely to be low; indeed, pantothenic acid is so widely distributed in human foods that it is unlikely that any natural diets with a very low content will be encountered. Some variations in status among communities have been described, but these do not define requirements. In a group of adolescents in the USA, daily pantothenate intakes were around $4\,mg$; total blood pantothenate was in the 'normal' range of c. 350–$400\,ng\,ml^{-1}$, and intakes were correlated with red cell pantothenate ($r = 0.38$) and with urinary pantothenate ($r = 0.60$), both $P < 0.001$. In adults, these correlations were less strong.

During pregnancy and lactation there is some evidence that requirements may increase. As for most water-soluble vitamins, maternal blood levels do decrease significantly on normal diets during pregnancy, and the mean daily output of the vitamin in breast milk in the US is of the order of 2–$6\,mg$. The adequate intake (AI) in the USA is $6\,mg\,day^{-1}$ during pregnancy and $7\,mg\,day^{-1}$ during lactation. It has been suggested that infant formulas should contain at least $2\,mg$ pantothenate per liter and the AI for infants is $1.7\,mg\,day^{-1}$ from birth to 6 months and $1.8\,mg\,day^{-1}$ from 7 to 12 months of age.

Dietary Sources and High Intakes

Pantothenate is widely distributed in food; rich sources include animal tissues, especially liver, and yeast, with moderate amounts occurring in whole grain cereals and legumes (see **Table 1**). It is fairly stable during cooking and storage, although some destruction occurs at high temperatures and at pH values below 5 or above 7. Highly processed foods have lower contents than fresh foods. Commercial vitamin supplements containing pantothenate usually contain the calcium salt, which is crystalline and more stable than the acid.

Synthesis by gut flora in humans is suspected but not yet proven; the rarity of diet-induced deficiency has been attributed to contributions from gut flora sources.

There is some evidence that pantothenic acid supplements may be beneficial for treatment of rheumatoid arthritis and for enhancement of athletic performance, specifically in running. Pantethine, the disulfide dimer of pantetheine, may have cholesterol-

Table 1 Pantothenate content of selected foods

Food	mg per 100 g wet wt	mg per MJ
Meat, offal, and fish		
Stewed minced beef	0.36	0.41
Grilled pork chop	1.22	1.58
Calf liver, fried	4.1	5.59
Lamb's kidney, fried	4.6	5.87
Cod, grilled	0.34	0.85
Dairy products		
Cow's milk, full cream	0.58	2.12
Cheese, cheddar	0.50	0.29
Yogurt (whole milk, plain)	0.50	1.50
Boiled chicken's egg	1.3	2.12
Human milk	0.25	0.87
Fruits		
Apples, eating, flesh and skin	trace	trace
Oranges, flesh	0.37	2.34
Pears, flesh and skin	0.07	0.41
Strawberries, raw	0.34	3.01
Dried mixed fruit	0.09	0.08
Vegetables		
Potatoes, boiled, new	0.38	1.18
Carrots, boiled, young	0.18	1.94
Brussel sprouts, boiled	0.28	1.83
Cauliflower, boiled	0.42	3.59
Onions, fried	0.12	0.18
Grains, grain products, nuts		
White bread	0.40	0.43
Wholemeal bread	0.60	0.65
Rice, boiled, white	0.10	0.17
Cornflakes	0.30	0.19
Baked beans in tomato sauce	0.18	0.51
Peanuts, plain	2.66	1.14

Compiled from Food Standard Agency (2002) McCance and Widdowson's *The Composition of Foods*, 6th Sixth Summary edn. Cambridge: Royal Society of Chemistry, © Crown copyright material is reproduced with the permission of the Controller of HMSO and Queen's Printer for Scotland.

lowering properties. The mechanisms of these reported effects are unclear and they require further investigation and verification. A homolog of pantothenate, pantoyl γ-aminobutyrate (hopanthenate), which can act as a pantothenate antagonist, has been used to enhance cognitive function, especially in Alzheimer's disease. It acts on GABA receptors to enhance acetylcholine release and cholinergic function at key sites in the brain.

There is little or no evidence for any toxicity at high intakes: at daily intakes around $10\,g$ there may be mild diarrhea and gastrointestinal disturbance, but no other symptoms have been described. Pantothenate has been prescribed for various chronic disorders, but is not known to be useful in high doses.

See also: **Cofactors**: Organic. **Energy**: Metabolism. **Fatty Acids**: Metabolism. **Lactation**: Dietary

Requirements. **Lipids**: Chemistry and Classification. **Nutritional Assessment**: Biochemical Indices.

Further Reading

Bender DA (1992) Pantothenic acid. *Nutritional Biochemistry of the Vitamins*, ch. 12, pp. 341–359. Cambridge: Cambridge University Press.

Bender DA (1999) Optimum nutrition: thiamin, biotin and pantothenate. *Proceedings of the Nutrition Society* **58**: 427–433.

Institute of Medicine (2000) *Dietary Reference Intakes for Thiamin, Riboflavin, Niacin, Vitamin B₆, Folate, Vitamin B₁₂, Pantothenic Acid, Biotin and Choline*, pp. 357–373. Washington, DC: National Academy Press.

Miller JW, Rogers LM, and Rucker RB (2001) Pantothenic acid. In: Bowman BA and Russell RM (eds.) *Present Knowledge in Nutrition*, 8th edn., ch. 24. pp. 253–260. Washington, DC: ILSI Press.

Plesofsky NS (2001) Pantothenic acid. In: Rucker RB, Suttie JW, McCormick DB, and Machlin LJ (eds.) *Handbook of Vitamins*, 3rd edn., ch. 9. pp. 317–337. New York: Marcel Dekker Inc.

Plesofsky-Vig N and Brambl R (1988) Pantothenic acid and coenzyme A in cellular modification of proteins. *Annual Review of Nutrition* **8**: 461–482.

Plesovsky-Vig (2000) Pantothenic acid. In: Shils ME, Olson JA, Shike M, and Ross AC (eds.) *Modern Nutrition in Health and Disease*, 9th edn., ch. 25. pp. 423–432. Baltimore: Williams & Wilkins.

Smith CM and Song WO (1996) Comparative nutrition of pantothenic acid. *Journal of Nutritional Biochemistry* **7**: 312–321.

Swaiman KF (2001) Hallervorden-Spatz syndrome. *Pediatric Neurology* **25**: 102–108.

Tahiliani AG and Beinlich CJ (1991) Pantothenic acid in health and disease. *Vitamins and Hormones* **46**: 165–227.

van den Berg H (1997) Bioavailability of pantothenic acid. *European Journal of Clinical Nutrition* **51**: S62–63.

PARASITISM

P G Lunn, University of Cambridge, Cambridge, UK

Introduction

In common with all other animals, human beings are susceptible to a range of parasitic organisms. The most important and commonest of these have been with man for countless years and have become so well adapted that in most cases man is their major if not only host. Although parasitic infections occur throughout the world, it is in the wet tropics and subtropics where they are found at their greatest prevalence and intensity. Most developing countries are also located in these areas and the consequent poverty, poor hygiene, and inadequate sanitation augment the favorable environmental conditions to enhance proliferation of these organisms. Only those that are known to interfere with host nutritional status will be discussed in this article.

Parasitic infections of the gastrointestinal tract are among the commonest diseases in the world (**Table 1**) and in most developing countries there has been little improvement in prevalence rates for many years. Indeed in some cases, e.g., schistosomiasis, local prevalence has been increasing with expanding irrigation schemes. Their association with poverty ensures that these diseases occur in areas where poor child growth and malnutrition are common and where there are persistent health problems. While there is no doubt that severe infections of any parasite can result in severe illness or even death of the host, such cases are rare even in areas of high prevalence and the norm is for low to moderate parasite numbers, which result in few, if any overt clinical symptoms. Nevertheless, by causing subtle reductions in appetite, digestion and absorption; by increasing chronic inflammation, and by inducing

Table 1 Estimated world prevalence of parasites important to human nutrition

	Approx. prevalence (millions)
Helminth parasites	
Ascaris lumbricoides (roundworm)	1500
Necator americanus and *Ancyclostoma duodenale* (hookworms)	1300
Trichuris trichiura (whipworm)	1100
Schistosoma haematobium, S. japonicum, and *S. mansoni*	200
Strongyloides stercoralis and *S. fülleborni*	200
Protozoal parasites	
Giardia intestinalis	200 symptomatic cases, total much higher
Entamoeba histolytica	400 but may be much higher
Cryptosporidium spp.	?

Data from Crompton, DWT (1999) How much human helminthiasis is there in the world? *Journal of Parasitology* **85**: 397–403; Olsen BE, Olson ME, and Wallis PM (2002) *Giardia: The Cosmopolitan Parasite*. Wallingford, UK: CABI; Haque R et al. (2003) Current concepts: amebiasis. *New England Journal of Medicine* **348**: 1565–1573.

nutrient loss, particularly of iron and protein, it is believed that such low-level but long-term infections contribute to the persistently poor nutritional state of many, especially children, in the developing world.

The most important parasites of man are from two main groups: the helminth worms and protozoans. Although several hundred different species have been described, the vast majority of infections are caused by relatively few.

Mechanisms of Parasite–Host Nutrition Interactions

Gastrointestinal parasites interfere with the nutrition of their host by one or more of the following mechanisms (**Figure 1**).

Loss of Appetite, Anorexia

Loss of appetite is a common feature in many illnesses and not only those involving the gastrointestinal tract. It is now thought that much of the appetite loss in disease is mediated by one or more cytokines released by lymphocytes as part of the body's response to tissue damage or invasion. Additionally, however, parasitized individuals often complain of symptoms such as nausea, abdominal pain, flatulence, and distension and discomfort, while the protozoal infections are associated with vomiting, diarrhea, or dysentery, all of which can be expected to reduce appetite.

Maldigestion and Malabsorption

Several GI parasites are well placed to interfere with these processes so it is not surprising that maldigestion and/or malabsorption of fat, protein, and carbohydrate as well as many of the micronutrients has been reported during infection. Structural damage to the mucosa of the intestine, such as the flattening or thickening of villi, or villus atrophy, will reduce the absorptive surface area. Damage to the cells diminishes their absorptive properties and limits active transport processes, while accelerated

replacement of damaged cells may result in immature mucosal cells with reduced enzymatic and transport capacity. Food that is not fully digested and absorbed in the small intestine will enter the large bowel where excessive colonic fermentation may result in diarrhea.

Nutrient Losses

Accelerated loss of nutrients from the body is probably the most important mechanism by which parasitic infections compromise the nutritional status of their host. Nutrient losses arise both directly and indirectly.

Direct losses occur during the feeding of the blood-sucking and tissue-invading parasites. Blood and tissue ingested by the worms forms part of the loss but the lesions caused by feeding and burrowing activity continue to ooze blood and tissue fluids after the parasites have moved on. Similarly, the passage of schistosome eggs through the tissues of the bladder or intestine is often accompanied by tissue damage and blood loss. Increased turnover and accelerated shedding of parasite-damaged enterocytes into the lumen of the GI tract is another mechanism of increased nutrient loss. Even though some of the nutrients lost into the lumen may be reabsorbed, the process is far from complete. Vomiting or diarrhea causes loss of electrolytes and important trace elements such as zinc.

Indirect losses arise from stimulation of the host's immunological and inflammatory mechanisms that are mobilized to combat the infection and repair tissue damage. Localized inflammation at the site of the parasite activity, often accompanied by lymphocytic infiltration of tissues cause further damage to the mucosa, augmenting maldigestion, malabsorption, and nutrient losses as more damaged cells are shed. Activation of the systemic inflammatory system, i.e., the acute phase response, is a general reaction of the body to pathogen invasion or tissue damage. It results in a widespread cytokine-mediated catabolic response. Growth slows or ceases, muscle tissue is broken down to provide substrates for gluconeogenesis and the repair of damaged cells, and a negative nitrogen balance ensues. Anorexia occurs and there are increased losses of amino acids, minerals, and vitamins in the urine and feces.

Competition for Nutrients

Competition for nutrients is generally unlikely owing to the considerable difference in biomass of the host and parasite. However, the tapeworm, *Diphyllobothrium latum*, does compete for vitamin B_{12} taken in the diet. The worm concentrates large amounts of this vitamin in its own tissues, depriving the host and in some cases leading to megaloblastic anemia.

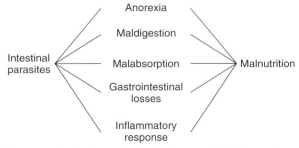

Figure 1 Mechanisms of parasite–host nutrition interactions.

Parasite Epidemiology and Impact on Host Nutrition

Clinical Studies

Much of our knowledge of the impact of parasitism on host nutrition (**Table 2**) comes from hospital studies of heavily parasitized patients. Irrespective of the organism involved, nutritional status and anthropometric indices of such severely ill patients are invariably poor on admission but quickly improve following treatment. Such data must however be interpreted with caution. In developing countries, malnourished individuals admitted to hospital rarely suffer from a single parasitic infection; viral and bacterial pathogens and other parasitoses are frequently present as are frank dietary deficiencies. Patients are routinely dosed with wide-range antibiotics and anthelmintics and given high-quality rehabilitation diets, so, in general, neither the cause of their symptoms nor the basis for recovery can be established with certainty.

Helminth Parasites

Ascaris lumbricoides (**roundworm**) About 73% of all infections by this worm are estimated to occur in Asia with many countries having prevalence rates greater than 50%. In some rural areas over 90%

Table 2 Parasite interference with host nutrition

Parasite	Symptom	Nutritional effect
Ascaris lumbricoides	Anorexia and abdominal pain	Growth retardation, weight loss
	Malabsorption syndrome	Reduced fat and nitrogen uptake
		Reduced vitamin A status
	Lactose intolerance	Growth retardation, weight loss
	Acute-phase response	Growth retardation, weight loss
Hookworm	Anorexia and abdominal pain	Growth retardation, weight loss
	Diarrhea	Growth retardation, weight loss
	Blood loss	Iron deficiency, anemia
	Protein-losing enteropathy	Hypoalbuminemia, edema
Schistosoma spp.	Anorexia	Growth retardation, weight loss
	Diarrhea	Growth retardation, weight loss
	Blood loss	Iron deficiency, anemia
	Plasma protein loss	Hypoalbuminemia
	Acute-phase response	Growth retardation, weight loss
Trichuris trichiura	Anorexia	Growth retardation, weight loss
	Abdominal pain and vomiting	Growth retardation, weight loss
	Diarrhea and dysentery	Loss of trace elements, e.g., zinc
		Growth retardation, weight loss
	Blood loss	Iron deficiency, anemia
	Plasma protein loss	Hypoalbuminemia, edema
	Acute phase response	Growth retardation, weight loss
Strongyloides spp.	Anorexia	Growth retardation, weight loss
	Abdominal pain and vomiting	Growth retardation, weight loss
	Malabsorption syndrome	Reduced fat absorption
	Protein-losing enteropathy	Hypoalbuminemia, edema
	Acute-phase response	Growth retardation, weight loss
Giardia intestinalis	Anorexia	Growth retardation, weight loss
	Diarrhea and vomiting	Loss of trace elements
	Malabsorption syndrome	Reduced fat absorption
		Reduced vitamin A status
	Mucosal disruption	Lowered disaccharidase activity
		General maldigestion
	Acute-phase response	Growth retardation, weight loss
Cryptosporidium spp.	Anorexia	Growth retardation, weight loss
	Abdominal pain	Growth retardation, weight loss
	Diarrhea and vomiting	Loss of trace elements
	Mucosal disruption	Lowered disaccharidase activity
		General malabsorption
	Acute-phase response	Growth retardation, weight loss
Entamoeba histolytica	Diarrhea and dysentery	Fluid and electrolyte loss
		Electrolyte imbalance
		Loss of trace elements
	Acute-phase response	Growth retardation, weight loss

of children harbor the infection. It is less prevalent in Africa (about 12% of all cases) and in central and southern America (about 8% of all cases). It is uncommon but still present in some rural areas of Europe and southeastern parts of the US. Adult *A. lumbricoides* live in the lumen of the upper part, i.e., the jejunum, of the small intestine. The worms live for some 12–20 months and females grow to 20–35 cm in length and 3–6 mm in diameter. An adult female discharges 200 000–240 000 eggs per day into the lumen and these pass out of the body in the feces. Infection occurs by oral ingestion of eggs from fecally contaminated food, water, hands, kitchen utensils, or play things. Both the prevalence and intensity of infection with *A. lumbricoides* increase rapidly during early childhood and although prevalence often remains high throughout life, intensity of infection tends to peak in the 5–15 years age range.

Despite the large size of these worms, mild to moderate infections are generally well tolerated with few, if any, overt symptoms. Clinical studies give inconsistent results. Although anorexia, abnormal mucosal histology, decreased absorption of fat and carbohydrate, reduced lactase activity, decreased transit time, reduced nitrogen retention, reduced vitamin A absorption, and lower vitamin A status have all been reported, they are by no means present in all cases. These abnormalities are in keeping with a stimulation of the host's immune and inflammatory mechanisms and it seems likely that occurrence of these symptoms depends on whether such mechanisms have been initiated. Why the immune and inflammatory response should be initiated in some cases of *A. lumbricoides* infection but not others is not known, but it may be at least partly due to genetics.

Hookworms Although 13 different human hookworm parasites have been listed, only two species, *Necator americanus* and *Ancyclostoma duodenale*, are responsible for virtually all cases of hookworm disease in humans. The two worms are similar in appearance, feeding pattern, and life history. Man is their only known host. *Necator americanus* is the only species seen in North America and it predominates in central and southern America, central Africa, southern India, Indonesia, and the South Pacific. *Ancyclostoma duodenale* is found in Mediterranean Europe, the Middle East, North Africa, Pakistan, Iran, and northern India. Both species occur in parts of Brazil, India and Africa, throughout Southeast Asia, Indonesia and the Pacific islands.

Adult worms live in the upper part of the small intestine and eggs are discharged into the lumen. Up to 10 000 (*N. americanus*) or 25 000 (*A. duodenale*) eggs per day can be produced and are passed out in the feces. Eggs hatch within 48 h and the larvae are free living for 2–3 weeks but then must reach a host or die. Adult female *A. duodenale* are 10–13 mm in length, *N. americanus* 9–11 mm, and the males about 2 mm shorter. *Necator americanus* can live for up to 5 years.

Both prevalence and intensity of infection increase with age in childhood up to about 10–15 years, and then remain constant during adulthood. High prevalence is associated with inadequate or unhygienic disposal of feces, which contaminates the soil. Lack of footwear, a common state in developing countries, allows feet to come in contact with infective larvae.

Loss of blood, particularly of its iron content, is the most important pathological feature of hookworm infection. Iron deficiency anemia is one of the commonest deficiency diseases in the world and there is no doubt that hookworms contribute significantly to the estimated two billion individuals who suffer from this problem. Through its feeding activity, each *N. americanus* worm causes the loss of about 0.03 ml of blood per day, while the larger *A. duodenale* accounts for approximately 0.15 ml per day. Part of this loss is blood ingested by the worm, but each time the worm moves to a new site, perhaps up to six times per day, the lesions continue to ooze blood into the lumen.

Daily blood loss from an individual passing 2000 eggs per gram of feces has been estimated at 4.3 ml (containing 2.0 mg of iron) and 8.9 ml (4.2 mg of iron) for *N. americanus* and *A. duodenale*, respectively. Although the intestine will reabsorb approximately 35% of this iron, daily losses will be 1.3 and 2.7 mg of iron, respectively. Assuming that only 10% of dietary iron is absorbed, an increased dietary intake of 13 mg and 27 mg, respectively, is required to make good these losses. As most diets contain only 15–20 mg of iron per day and some 10–15 mg of this is needed to cover daily metabolic requirements, intake would need to at least double to replace the loss from even this moderate hookworm load. In developing countries this is rarely possible, so without iron supplements, iron stores are soon depleted and iron deficiency anemia ensues. In lighter infections, subclinical iron deficiency is shown by low plasma ferritin and iron concentration, low transferrin saturation, and elevated erythrocyte protoporhyrin content.

Protein is also lost into the lumen of the small intestine during hookworm disease. Estimates of plasma loss vary considerably and values over 100 ml (containing 6–7 g of protein) per day have been recorded, although much of this may be reabsorbed. Nevertheless, moderate to heavy hookworm infections are associated with hypoalbuminemia, hypoproteinemia, edema, and kwashiorkor, especially in areas where the protein content of the diet is low.

Schistosomes The three commonest species responsible for disease are *Schistosoma haematobium*, *S. mansoni*, and *S. japonica*, with some individuals in Africa harboring two species. Urinary schistosomiasis, found mainly in Africa and some eastern Mediterranean countries, is caused by *S. haematobium*. Infection with either *S. mansoni* (found in Africa, the Middle East, parts of South America, and the Caribbean) or *S. japonica* (occurs in China, the Philippines, and Indonesia) results in intestinal schistosomiasis. These worms live in blood vessels: *S. haematobium* in the vesicle venules of the urinary bladder with the other two species infecting the mesenteric veins adjacent to the intestines. Adults live in male/female pairs and damage is caused by passage of eggs through the tissues into either the bladder (*S. haematobium*) or the gut lumen. Eggs leave the body in the urine or feces. If they reach fresh water, they hatch to produce miracidia, which must find a suitable snail host. After entering the snail, the parasites multiply by asexual reproduction, eventually producing free-swimming cercaria that are infective to man. Infection is by skin penetration during contact with fresh water containing cercaria. Egg production starts some 2–3 weeks after infection. The parasite lives for 3–8 years. The prevalence of this parasite in many developing countries is increasing as irrigation schemes allow the intermediary snail hosts to extend their range.

Iron deficiency anemia associated with blood loss occurs in both urinary and intestinal schistosomiasis. Although blood loss can be severe in heavy *S. haematobium* infection, in a study of nonhospitalized children with low to moderate infection, iron losses ranged from 120 to 500 μg day^{-1}, increasing with rising egg count. This is less than losses due to hookworm, but dietary iron consumption would need to increase by about a third to compensate. In areas where iron status is poor, the extra burden due to *S. haematobium* will undoubtedly contribute to the onset of anemia. Intestinal schistosomiasis caused by *S. mansoni* can also result in iron deficiency but it is generally less severe than that seen in hookworm disease. Little data is available for *S. japonicum* infection, but its effect appears to be similar to *S. mansoni*.

The poor nutritional status of infected individuals may be related to anorexia, diarrhea, and activation of the inflammatory mechanisms of the host. Blood cytokine concentrations are raised in schistosomiasis causing growth faltering and weight loss.

Trichuris *trichiuris* (whipworm) This helminth is widespread throughout the tropics and subtropics. Most cases of infection (63% of the worldwide total) occur in Asia, with 11% in Africa and 14% in the Americas; however, a few cases are still seen in the US, Western Europe, and Japan.

Man is the principal host of the parasite, which lives in the large intestine. Adults are 3–5 cm in length and are whip shaped; the long thin anterior end is embedded in the mucosa, with the thicker posterior end in the lumen. Worms feed on mucosal cells but may also ingest red and white blood cells. Eggs leave the host in feces and embryonate in the soil. Infection occurs by oral ingestion of embryonated eggs on fecally contaminated food, hands, or utensils. They hatch in the small intestine and larvae develop in the villi before moving down to the large intestine. Egg production starts 30–90 days after ingestion.

In some rural areas the prevalence can exceed 90% and although prevalence remains high throughout life, peak intensity usually occurs between the ages of 5 and 15 years.

This helminth causes loss of blood and iron from the large intestine of its host by its burrowing and feeding activities. More than 3000 worms have been found in heavy *T. trichiuris* infection and such individuals do have marked iron deficiency anemia. However, in the majority, where worm counts rarely exceed 100, the infection is usually asymptomatic. Plasma protein loss can also be substantial in heavy infections but although plasma albumin values are frequently reduced, hypoproteinemic edema is rare.

Heavy infections are characterized by persistent dysentery, abdominal pain, nausea, vomiting, and tenesmus leading to rectal prolapse. Appetite is reduced and raised plasma cytokines and acute-phase proteins indicate activation of host immune and inflammatory mechanisms. Loss of nutrients including zinc and other trace elements in the persistent dysentery and vomiting may further lower nutritional status.

Strongyloides stercoralis This worm has a worldwide distribution but is found predominantly in the tropics. Prevalence rates are uncertain as detection of the larvae by direct fecal examination (the method usually employed) gives a considerable underestimate. Prevalence rates of up to 85% have been reported but are uncommon. In parts of Africa, a closely related worm, *Strongyloides fülleborni* is often more common than *S. stercoralis*.

Adult worms are about 2.7 mm in length and are usually found in the duodenum and upper jejunum. Eggs are passed into the lumen but most hatch while still in the GI tract. Although the majority of larvae pass out in the feces, some penetrate the wall of the intestine and reinfect the host, a situation known as autoinfection. Larvae passed with the feces live in the soil and grow into adults of both sexes. Eggs are laid and larvae hatch within 1–2 weeks. They metamorphose to an infective stage when they must either locate a host or die. Infection is usually by skin penetration. Because of the autoinfection process, infection with this parasite can last indefinitely and severe disease can suddenly appear many years after an individual has left an endemic area.

The impact of this worm on nutritional status has not been clearly defined. Heavily infected subjects have a severe small intestinal illness with anorexia, abdominal pain, nausea, diarrhea, and vomiting. There is some evidence for a malabsorption syndrome, steatorrhea is often present, but it is not seen in all cases. A substantial protein-losing enteropathy can occur, resulting in severe hypoalbuminemia and kwashiorkor-like oedema. Protein loss arises from a combination of the burrowing activity of the worms and a local inflammatory reaction from the host. The little information on *S. fülleborni* infection suggests it has a similar impact on host nutrition.

Special features of helminth parasites Helminth infections all exhibit certain characteristic features by which they differ from most other infective organisms:

1. In contrast to most infective organisms, most helminths cannot reproduce within the host; each worm has to gain individual access to the host, usually by ingestion or skin penetration.
2. Intensity of infection shows an overdisperse distribution; it is usual for 20% of an infected population to harbor 80% of the parasites. Thus, a large majority of individuals will have only light infections and show few if any symptoms.
3. Some individuals appear to be predisposed to have heavy worm burdens; they quickly reacquire a heavy load after eradication of their original infection. Household and family clustering of high parasite loads is also seen. Clearly such differences might be explained on the basis of increased exposure of individuals and family groups due to particularly unhygienic living conditions or greater occupational risk. However,

increased host genetic susceptibility has recently been demonstrated to account for between 21 and 44% of the observed variance in infection intensity.
4. Infection by several different parasites at the same time (polyparasitism) is extremely common in many areas.
5. Re-infection following deworming occurs very quickly because of considerable contamination of the environment by the large numbers of eggs produced by the parasites. In a study in Myanmar, preinfection prevalence of *A. lumbricoides* was reached only 6–8 months after deworming.

Protozoal Parasites

Giardia intestinalis (= lamblia) This organism is a common parasite of the human gastrointestinal tract and is found in all parts of the world. Although its prevalence is greatest in developing countries where hygiene facilities are poor, outbreaks of giardiasis continue to occur in many developed countries. It has a simple life history. The trophozoite (the active form in the intestine) lives in the duodenum and jejunum of the host where it attaches to the enterocytes by means of a ventral disk. It reproduces rapidly by mitotic division and in heavy infections can cover large areas of the mucosa. Some trophozoites encyst; a protective wall forms around the organism, and the cysts pass out in the feces. Cysts are directly infective and after ingestion by a new host, the organisms emerge to establish a new infection. Disease can follow the ingestion of as few as 10 cysts which, given moist conditions, are viable for several months.

In developed countries, most infections can be traced to contaminated water, but direct person-to-person transmission has been documented. In developing countries, poverty-related unsanitary conditions and inadequate disposal of feces promote oro-fecal spread of the parasite, but contaminated water is also likely to be important. The large number of cyst-producing individuals with asymptomatic infection constitutes a reservoir of *G. intestinalis*. In addition, some animals are known to harbor *Giardia* and may be a source of human giardiasis.

Infection with *G. intestinalis* can be associated with a wide range of symptoms: from mild, self-limiting watery diarrhea to persistent foul-smelling diarrhea with vomiting, abdominal pain and distension, and a severe malabsorption syndrome. However, many infected individuals (from 20 to 84% of infected cases) remain asymptomatic. It is not clear why the parasite can cause such a range of degrees of illness.

The nutritional impact varies with both the severity and duration of the symptoms. In the early stages, anorexia is of major importance, but if the disease persists, intestinal aspects compound the situation. In at least 50% of symptomatic patients there is malabsorption of fat, carbohydrates, protein, and micronutrients (particularly vitamin A) associated with structural and functional abnormalities in the small intestine. Damage to the mucosa can range from little to subtotal villus atrophy, but most subjects have mild villus shortening and increased crypt depth. The abnormalities are associated with a reduction in disaccharidases, notably lactase activity and in lowered intraluminal concentrations of the hydrolytic enzymes trypsin, chymotrypsin, and lipase. The small intestinal barrier function is compromised, allowing translocation of potentially antigenic macromolecules into the body with consequent stimulation of the immune and inflammatory mechanisms resulting in growth retardation. Little is known about the nutritional effects of nonsymptomatic giardiasis.

Cryptosporidium parvum and other *Cryptosporidium* species

These organisms have only been recognized as human parasites since 1976. They have a worldwide distribution but in developed countries they generally causes a self-limiting disease, which occurs most commonly in child institutions and in people working with animals. However, water-borne outbreaks have occurred in which large numbers of people have become infected. Cryptosporidiosis is much more prevalent in developing countries where it is mainly a disease of children. The parasites live in the upper part of the small intestine, attached to the mucosal cells from which they feed.

Both sexual and asexual reproduction occurs in the host and cysts are produced, most of which pass out in the feces. However, some excyst while passing through the gastrointestinal (GI) tract resulting in autoinfection that can prolong the disease long after the original source of infection has been eliminated. Infection is by ingestion of cysts in fecally contaminated food, water, or utensils, or from unhygienic contact with infected persons. Continued exposure is facilitated by the many infected individuals who remain asymptomatic while passing cysts. *Cryptosporidium* spp., including *parvum*, also occur in many animals and can be transmitted to humans.

Most infected individuals remain asymptomatic, but in others, acute or chronic diarrhea associated with vomiting, abdominal pain, dehydration, and fever can occur. Immunocompromised and previously malnourished cases tend to have more severe and prolonged disease.

The nutritional impact of the infection depends on the severity and duration of the infection but growth retardation and lowered nutritional indices occur in asymptomatic cases as well as those with symptoms. Structural damage to the mucosa of the small intestine is seen, with shortened and fused villi and lengthening of the crypts due to accelerated cell division to replace damaged cells. Surface area is greatly reduced and the immature enterocytes have lower enzymatic and transport activity than mature cells. The resulting maldigestion, malabsorption, and stimulation of the host immune and inflammatory mechanisms are likely to account for the adverse nutritional effects. In children, growth remains poor for many months after infection has resolved. The nutritional status of asymptomatic individuals appears to be compromised by less extreme expression of these same mechanisms.

Entamoeba histolytica

This ameba has a very wide distribution but is most commonly found in developing countries where lack of hygienic facilities exacerbate fecal contamination of water, food, and hands. The organism is exclusive to humans; there are no animal hosts. These parasites generally infect the large intestine where they can cause severe disease by invading mucosal tissues.

The life cycle is simple: adult amebae reproduce asexually forming substantial colonies and in some cases cause ulcerative lesions in the mucosa. Some organisms encyst and pass out with the feces. Following ingestion of the cysts by another host, the amebae emerge when the cyst reaches the large bowel. The organism can also invade other organs, notably the liver, resulting in a life-threatening illness.

Although this parasite can cause life-threatening diarrhea and dysentery in some, most infected individuals remain free of symptoms. In others, persistent diarrhea can continue for months, interspersed with periods of apparently normal bowel function. As the parasite is most commonly found in the large intestine, there is little interference with food digestion and absorption and its main effect on nutrition seems to be due to loss of trace elements and electrolytes in watery stools. In more severe cases, blood is also lost in this way but amounts are small. Infection is associated with inflammation of the large bowel (colitis) indicating that host immune and inflammatory mechanisms have been stimulated and this may account for reports of hypoalbuminemia.

Community and Intervention Studies

Iron Deficiency and Iron Deficiency Anemia

A close relationship between the level of hookworm infection and severity of anemia has been observed in many cross-sectional field studies. Similar, though generally less severe, levels of anemia have been associated with intensity of schistosome species and *T. trichiura* disease. The cause and effect relationship suggested by this data has been confirmed by longitudinal investigations of iron status following anthelmintic administration. Community studies in Kenya, India, and Papua New Guinea have recorded substantial increases (up to $6 \, gl^{-1}$) in hemoglobin concentration between 4 and 8 weeks after treatment for hookworm. These marked improvements were seen even when parasite loads were not completely eliminated. Effective treatment of severe *Schistosoma and T. trichiura* infections also results in much improved iron status.

Growth and Protein-Energy Malnutrition

Although clinical studies confirm that these parasites have the potential to interfere with growth and nutritional status, evidence that they are a major cause of the widespread stunting and protein-energy malnutrition seen in developing countries is not as conclusive as may be expected. This may be because most infected individuals in a community will have only low to moderate parasite loads and whether a particular disease is important in precipitating malnutrition on a community or public health scale will depend on whether or not such low level infections impact on nutritional status. Information has come from two types of study: (1) cross-sectional surveys; and (2) longitudinal, placebo controlled intervention studies in which nutritional improvements are sought following the use of antiparasite drugs.

A large number of cross-sectional community studies have associated parasitic infection with growth deficits and poor anthropometric indices. Schistosomiasis has long been associated with poor growth, and an extreme condition, schistosomiasis dwarfism, in which physical and sexual development were severely retarded was reported to be quite common in China until the 1950s. Most recent studies of mild to moderate infection with all three schistosome species confirm an association with poor nutritional status that is more marked in girls, but the degree of impairment is variable between different regions and at best can only explain a small part of the total nutritional deficit of the subjects. Hookworm infection is similarly associated with poor appetite, slower growth, and lowered nutritional indices, all of which become more marked with increasing severity of iron deficiency anemia. Iron supplementation of hookworm-infected children has been reported to improve appetite and growth performance as well as iron status, suggesting that the lowered nutritional status may be secondary to iron deficiency rather than a direct effect of the parasite. Growth retardation seen in moderate to heavy *T. trichiura* infection may be similarly explained, although heavier burdens of this worm frequently cause dysentery, which can result in loss of essential trace elements such as zinc.

The impact of the protozoal parasites *Giardia* and *Crytosporidium* on nutritional status has been less well studied, but infection appears to be associated with persistent diarrheal disease and prolonged growth faltering even after apparent elimination of the parasites. Moreover, these parasites, unlike the helminths, are very common in children during the first 2 years of life when growth is at its greatest. Growth-retarding infections at this time of life, particularly in developing countries, appear to compromise growth throughout the whole growth period, thus the impact of these parasites on nutritional status may be far greater than currently appreciated. This is certainly an area requiring more research.

The results of these cross-sectional studies have been reinforced by longitudinal community-wide studies of nutritional improvement following reduction or eradication of parasite burden with anthelmintic drugs. The results of such studies have, however, been less than convincing. Successful treatment of heavily poly-parasitized Kenyan children harboring hookworm, *A. lumbricoides* and *T. trichiura*, with albendazole resulted in improvements in weight, arm circumference, and skinfold thickness and was associated with increased appetite and fitness. Statistical analysis of this data implicated hookworm as being the most important in compromising nutritional status. Weight gain above placebo-treated counterparts averaged 1.3 kg per 6 months, and added about 3% points to a weight-for-age of approximately 80%. However, similar studies in many parts of the world in subjects with lower intestinal helminth burdens have reported only small improvements, whereas others found no change at all in nutritional status indices following successful deworming. Treatment of schistosomiasis in Kenyan, Brazilian, and Filipino children showed only small improvements in nutritional status, e.g., in Kenya, the per cent weight-for-age only increased from 72.9 to 74.9% following eradication with praziquantel. A recent meta-analysis of these studies concluded that deworming did improve nutritional status, but that the effect was small.

Overall, both community and intervention studies do suggest that elimination of GI parasites would improve growth and anthropometric status of children in developing countries but that such improvement would be limited. This contrasts with the very substantial improvement in iron status and iron deficiency anemia that follows effective treatment of organisms causing blood loss.

Treatment and Prognosis

Table 3 shows the drugs most commonly used in treatment of these parasitic infections. Anthelmintic drugs have improved dramatically during the last 20 years and are now highly effective; in most cases a single course of treatment will result in parasite eradication. However, immunocompromised hosts, including malnourished children, may require more extensive courses of therapy to completely eliminate the infection. This is particularly the case in the treatment of cryptosporidiosis. Iron supplements are usually provided where blood loss has resulted in iron deficiency anemia.

Recovery from infection is usually complete and rapid as most parasites do not cause lasting damage to their host. Schistosomiasis is the exception and can result in permanent granuloma formation in several tissues, particularly the liver and spleen, which may become life threatening.

Prevention

Although drugs are now available to eradicate infections, unless the home environment changes, most individuals will soon become reinfected. The transmission of all the parasites discussed occurs most commonly through close contact between the host and infected human feces, either orally or by skin penetration. The basic requirement for prevention is an efficient and hygienic mode of disposal of feces, improved facilities in the home, for example clean running water, concrete floor to the home, plus a knowledge of basic hygiene. Use of footwear and avoidance of contact with water likely to contain schistosome cercaria would help. For the foreseeable future, however, such control measures are quite unrealistic in most developing countries and the alternative may be the large-scale, nation-wide use of anthelmintics to regularly deworm all individuals in endemic areas. School-based regular treatment programmes can be effective. Safe, effective, and relatively cheap drugs are now available and their use in this way could substantially reduce the level of helminth disease throughout the developing world. Such programs can be expected to result in a marked reduction in the prevalence and severity of iron deficiency anemia but in most situations, to have a relatively small impact on child growth, stunting, and incidence of protein-energy malnutrition.

See also: **Anemia**: Iron-Deficiency Anemia. **Cytokines**. **Diarrheal Diseases**. **Infection**: Nutritional Interactions. **Iron**. **Zinc**: Physiology.

Further Reading

Cooper ES, Whyte-Alleng CAM, Finzi-Smith JS, and MacDonald TT (1992) Intestinal nematode infections in children: the physiological price paid. *Parasitology* **104**: S91–S103.

Crompton DWT (1999) How much human helminthiasis is there in the world? *Journal of Parasitology* **85**: 397–403.

Crompton DWT (2000) The public health importance of hookworm disease. *Parasitology* **121**: S39–S50.

Crompton DWT and Nesheim MC (2002) Nutritional impact of intestinal helminthiasis during the human life cycle. *Annual Review of Nutrition* **22**: 35–59.

Dickson R, Awasthi S, Williams P, Demellweek C, and Gamer P (2000) Effects of treatment for intestinal helminth infection on growth and cognitive performance in children: systematic review of randomised trials. *British Medical Journal* **320**: 1697–1701.

Grove DI (1996) Human strongylodiosis. *Advances in Parasitology* **38**: 251–309.

Haque R, Huston CD, Hughes M *et al.* (2003) Current concepts: amebiasis. *New England Journal of Medicine* **348**: 1565–1573.

Lunn PG and Northrop-Clewes CA (1993) The impact of gastrointestinal parasites on protein-energy malnutrition in man. *Proceedings of the Nutrition Society* **52**: 101–111.

O'Lorcain P and Holland CV (2000) The public health importance of *Ascaris lumbricoides*. *Parasitology* **121**: S51–S71.

Olson BE, Olson ME, and Wallis PM (2002) *Giardia: The Cosmopolitan Parasite* Wallingford, UK: CABI.

Solomons NW (1993) Pathways to the impairment of human nutritional status by gastrointestinal pathogens. *Parasitology* **107**: S19–S35.

Table 3 Drugs of choice for parasitic infections

Infection	Drug
Ascariasis	Mebendazole, albendazole, pyrantel pamoate
Hookworm infection	Mebendazole, albendazole
Schistosomiasis	Praziquantel, metrifonate, niridazole, oltipraz
Trichuriasis	Mebendazole, albendazole
Strongyloidiasis	Thiobendazole, ivermectin
Giardiasis	Metronidazole, tinidazole, secnidazole, furazolidone, albendazole
Cryptosporidiosis	Nitazoxanide, spiramycin, clindamycin,
Amebiasis	Metronidazole, secnidazole, paromomycin, nitazoxanide

Stephenson LS (1993) The impact of schistosomiasis on human nutrition. *Parasitology* **107**: S107–S123.

Stephensen LS, Holland CV, and Cooper ES (2000) The public health significance of *Trichuris trichiura*. *Parasitology* **121**: S73–S95.

Stephenson LS, Latham MC, and Ottesen EA (2000) Malnutrition and parasitic helminth infections. *Parasitology* **121**: S23–S38.

Tzipori S (2002) Cryptosporidiosis: current trends and challenges. *Microbes and Infection* **4**: 1045–1080.

Pathogens *see* **Infection**: Nutritional Interactions; Nutritional Management in Adults

PELLAGRA

C J Bates, MRC Human Nutrition Research, Cambridge, UK

History of Pellagra: Recognition, Causes, and Treatment

The following historical summary is based mainly on Carpenter's excellent compendium of key pellagra-related publications published in 1981. Pellagra (meaning 'rough' or 'raw' skin) was common in western Europe (e.g., France and Italy) and especially the southern United States until the early decades of the twentieth century. It has been estimated that it claimed approximately half a million lives between the early eighteenth century and 1930, with as many as 10 000 deaths in the United States in 1929 alone. The typical signs and symptoms of human pellagra are summarized in **Table 1**.

The characteristic signs and symptoms of pellagra were given the name 'mal de la rosa' in 1720 by doctors working in the Asturia region of Spain, and it was very common in Italy at the end of the eighteenth century. As early as 1810, one European description concluded that the disease was neither contagious nor hereditary but was probably caused by a poor diet, especially diets in which grain such as corn (i.e., sweet corn) was the principal staple. The concept of a 'protein' deficiency, as distinct from the characteristic body-wasting calorie deficiency of common famines, was proposed in approximately 1850, and a good hospital diet was shown to have positive curative effects. As early as 1860, however, one observer commented that poor Mexican peasants whose diet was mainly corn based did not exhibit pellagra, and he attributed this to

their practices of roasting the corn with lime and of preventing mould growth.

Table 1 Signs and symptoms of niacin deficiency in man and animals

Human deficiency[a]
Loss of appetite and weight
Dermatosis (hyperpigmentation, hyperkeratosis, desquamation of the epidermis, especially where frequently exposed to strong sunlight)
Anorexia
Achlorhydria
Angular stomatitis, cheilosis, magenta tongue
Diarrhea
Anemia
Neuropathy (headache, dizziness, tremor, neurosis, apathy)
Death in severe and prolonged cases

Blacktongue in dogs and cats
Pustules in mouth and excessive salivation, darkening and necrosis of tongue
Diarrhea

Pigs
Neurological lesions affecting ganglion cells; histopathology of nerves
Anemia
Degeneration of intestinal mucosa and diarrhea

Rats
Reduced growth rate
Alopecia
Damage to peripheral nerves (cells and axons)

Birds (e.g., chickens and ducks)[b]
Inflammation of the upper gastrointestinal tract
Dermatitis
Diarrhea
Poor growth of feathers; bowed and weakened legs

[a]All animal species lose appetite and weight when deficient, but the characteristic skin lesions that are observed in human pellagra are rarely seen in other species. Some deficiency symptoms have been produced in other primates (e.g., monkeys).
[b]Ruminants are usually resistant to pellagra, except when forced to produce high quantities of milk or lean tissue.

For the next approximately 50 years, the 'toxin' theory of pellagra causation held sway, and there were government-backed campaigns in Europe to prevent mould growth (in Italy) and to reduce the population's reliance on corn as a staple (in France). In Europe, the prevalence of pellagra was clearly declining sharply (by the beginning of the twentieth century) just as it was beginning to emerge as a major new scourge in the southern United States. A plethora of conflicting hypotheses in the United States included poor sanitation, infection, insect-borne disease, and toxins from bacteria or moulds, but the largely correct 'poor diet' hypothesis was completely ignored until Joseph Goldberger, during the period from 1914 until his death in 1929, carried out classical and definitive controlled feeding studies, both in human convicts and in an animal model, causing 'blacktongue,' a corn diet-induced condition that could be induced in dogs (**Table 2**). Although the exact relationship of the diseases that Goldberger described, and then produced in his animal model, to classical human pellagra remains controversial, the most important outcome of his studies was that pellagra was now seen not as an infectious disease but as primarily a diet-related one, and it was recognized that it and similar diseases could unequivocally be induced by monotonous, poor-quality diets. Families who kept a cow were relatively protected.

Funk's newly formulated hypothesis about essential 'vitamines' and Gowland Hopkins' concept of 'accessory food factors', both of which were emerging at about the same time as Goldberger's studies, set the scene for a focused hunt for a specific organic substance that would be present in the 'curative' diets and which might thereby be identified as the elusive 'pellagra-preventive' (PP) that was thought to be present in the preventative and curative foods. Goldberger classified a range of foods according to their PP properties and found that dried yeast and a water-soluble extract from yeast were both curative, even in small quantities. During the 1930s, following the elucidation of the role of the pyridine nucleotides in food energy metabolism and release, the central roles of nicotinic acid and nicotinamide were elucidated and were equated with the curative PP factor present in the curative food extracts. The term 'niacin' was then coined because 'nicotinic acid' appeared to be etymologically associated with tobacco and was therefore considered to be unsuitable as the name for an essential dietary factor.

Complex Causation

Although pellagra in dogs and humans usually responds well to supplements of pure niacin, there are several further strands to the story that complicate the idea that all the characteristics and manifestations of pellagra can be explained as the result of a simple dietary deficiency of a single water-soluble factor (i.e., vitamin) identified as the molecule niacin. First, it soon became clear that the total niacin content of different foods, as measured by chemical analysis, was not necessarily a good guide to their pellagra-producing or preventing properties. During the 1940s, it was shown that in rats (which respond to pellagragenic diets by a reduced growth rate but not by skin lesions) high dietary tryptophan levels could substantially reduce the requirement for dietary niacin. Tryptophan was then shown to be equally effective in humans in reducing the pellagragenic properties of poor diets.

Table 2 History of the recognition of pellagra, and its probable causes, in human populations

1. A poorly understood disease (dermatitis, gastrointestinal and mental signs/symptoms) appeared first in Europe in the eighteenth and nineteenth centuries and then in the southern United States in the 1910s and was named 'pellagra' (= raw/rough skin).
2. Favored causal hypotheses (USA) initially included infection, mouldy grain and insects.
3. In 1914–1916, Joseph Goldberger disproved the infection hypothesis by self-experimentation and then producing pellagra in prisoners fed mainly corn diets.
4. In the 1920s, he developed the "blacktongue" model of pellagra in dogs, with corn diets.
5. In the 1930s, nicotinic acid was isolated as a pure water-soluble compound ('vitamin') of known structure from yeast and liver extracts, able to cure pellagra and blacktongue.
6. In the mid-twentieth century, niacin was shown to be bound as an unavailable part of the large chemical complex 'niacytin' in corn. Heating in alkaline environment (e.g., Mexican tortillas) can liberate this bound niacin.
7. Intermediary metabolism studies revealed that niacin can be produced from tryptophan in the body. Pellagragenic diets are therefore low in tryptophan as well as niacin. The concept of 'niacin equivalents,' usually [mg niacin plus one-sixtieth of mg tryptophan] in food, developed. Human requirements are estimated.
8. The Indian cereal 'jowar' shown to be pellagragenic. Some, but not all, studies have implicated its high leucine content.
9. Niacin and riboflavin deficiencies often coexist; therefore, the signs and symptoms of 'pellagra-like' disease are often attributable to multiple vitamin deficiencies, of which niacin and riboflavin are usually the most important.
10. Certain inborn errors of metabolism (genetic defects) or iatrogenic effects of drugs can mimic pellagra signs, symptoms, and metabolic defects.

Soon after this, the complex metabolic pathway linking tryptophan to niacin and to the pyridine nucleotide coenzymes was elucidated. Between 34 and 86 mg tryptophan in human diets is now considered to be equivalent to 1 mg niacin, with a mean conversion ratio of 60 mg tryptophan per 1 mg niacin used universally to calculate the niacin equivalents (NE) value of any diet. This is recognised to be a much better index of the anti-pellagra potency of a diet than its niacin content *per se*.

However, this was only one part of the complex etiology of pellagra. The causes of the signs of pellagra in human populations, and indeed also in Goldberger's experimental studies, were and are likely to be a complex mixture of B vitamin deficiencies, of which niacin and tryptophan content are indeed the dominant effectors, but riboflavin is also an important component, followed sometimes by thiamin, vitamin B_6, and possibly vitamin B_{12} and some other nutrients including zinc and iron. The antivitamin effects of certain toxins, especially mould toxins, cannot be ruled out, and several bacterial, fungal, and other toxins have been shown to be capable of depleting cellular levels of NAD(P). In addition, and perhaps most important for corn and the other grain diets, the niacin present in corn and other grains is often chemically bound into a macromolecular complex that is sometimes called niacytin, from which the niacin cannot readily be released by digestive enzymes in the gastrointestinal tract but which requires heat and alkali treatment during food preparation (as in the preparation of Mexican tortillas, which involves lime and heat treatment) so as to make it adequately bioavailable.

In India, the millet-type cereal called 'jowar' is frequently associated with pellagra signs and symptoms, even though it is apparently a reasonably good source of available niacin and tryptophan. Studies have suggested an association with its high leucine content, which may impair the conversion of tryptophan to niacin coenzymes. However, the aetiology of this association remains controversial and unresolved. Balance studies in humans have failed to show a consistent effect of either leucine or vitamin B_6 supplementation on the excretion of the metabolites of tryptophan, which is a sensitive test for imbalanced tryptophan conversion pathways.

Oestrogenic hormones can affect the conversion of tryptophan to niacin coenzymes, and this is thought to be the causal basis for the observation that women (except during pregnancy) seem to be considerably more susceptible to pellagra than men.

Several commonly used drugs also have anti-niacin (iatrogenic) effects in man. Perhaps the most important is isoniazid, which is commonly used in the treatment of tuberculosis. It inhibits kynureninase activity (an enzyme in the tryptophan conversion pathway) by inactivating the enzyme's essential cofactor, pyridoxal phosphate, derived from vitamin B_6. There are several other metabolic interconnections between niacin and vitamin B_6, such that any interference with vitamin B_6 metabolism is likely to affect niacin economy as well. Since up to 60% of Asian Indians are genetically slow acetylators (i.e., deactivators) of isoniazid, the use of this drug in Indians is especially apt to cause pellagra symptoms. The anti-Parkinsonism drugs Carbidopa and Benseride can also cause pellagra symptoms, and in people taking these, there is a reduced rate of excretion of the niacin metabolite N-methylnicotinamide. Another niacin antagonist is N-acetyl pyridine, which can cause neurological symptoms and histological damage to the hippocampus in some animals.

There are also several inborn errors of metabolism that can result in pellagra-like symptoms in man. Although none of these are very common, the best known is Hartnup's disease, an autosomal recessive condition in which the cellular transport of tryptophan (and other neutral amino acids) is impaired so that tryptophan is rapidly lost in the urine through failure of renal tubular reabsorption. Patients respond well to supplementation with niacin or with tryptophan peptides but not to free tryptophan, which cannot be well absorbed and retained. Other inborn errors of tryptophan economy that can result in pellagra include the vitamin B_6-responsive condition xanthurenic aciduria, hydroxykynurenuria, tryptophanuria (i.e., tryptophan dioxygenase deficiency), and another linked to an increased activity of the enzyme picolinate carboxylase. All these conditions are rare but informative inborn errors of metabolism affecting the tryptophan–niacin metabolic pathway. Tumors of the enterochromaffin cells, which synthesise excessive amounts of 5-hydroxytryptophan and 5-hydroxytryptamine, can also result in pellagra since hyperactivity of this pathway can result in the diversion of tryptophan away from the alternative pathway that converts it to the niacin coenzymes.

High-Risk Groups in Present-Day Society

Today, the most high-risk group for development of pellagra signs and symptoms in Western society is chronic alcoholics, whose diets are often poor, and in addition are subject to liver damage from alcohol abuse and its cellular toxicity. Certain forms of psychosis, including depression and schizophrenia, are associated with abnormalities of the tryptophan metabolism pathways, including those involved in the formation of 5-hydroxytryptamine (serotonin) and 5-hydroxytryptophan in the central nervous system. Some of these may benefit from modulation of these pathways by drugs and/or supplements. People with AIDS may exhibit some impairment of NAD production, which may in turn respond to niacin supplements as a support treatment, and high-dose nicotinic has been used as one of many alternative treatments for people with cardiovascular disease. In the developing world, pellagra is most commonly encountered in certain African countries (e.g., refugees in Malawi) and areas of India and China.

Biochemical Status Assays: Recommended Intakes

The detection of subclinical niacin deficiency and the confirmation of a clinical deficiency require the objective measurement of biochemical status (and, if possible, of dietary intake, which is usually a more time-consuming task) in order to provide confirmatory evidence, especially because the typical clinical signs and symptoms of pellagra are not entirely specific and pathognomic. Biochemical status estimates can be used to characterize a population, particularly any high-risk subgroups, and to monitor the efficacy of any anti-pellagra interventions. For most micronutrients, robust, specific, and sensitive blood component status assays have been developed. However, for niacin the only promising blood-based assay, namely of intracellular pyridine nucleotide (NAD(P)) concentrations, has not been developed into a definitive and generally accepted biochemical status assay with well-defined normal ranges and a demonstrated association between low concentrations and clinical

deficiency signs and symptoms. It has been suggested that a ratio of NAD to NADP below 1.0 in erythrocytes may provide evidence of niacin deficiency, but this requires confirmation.

The practical measurement of niacin status has mainly depended on urinary assays of the excretory products of niacin metabolism, namely N^1-methyl nicotinamide (NMN), N^1-methyl-2-pyridone-5-carboxamide (2-pyridone), and N^1-methyl-4-pyridone-3-carboxamide (4-pyridone), which can be quantitatively estimated by high-performance liquid chromatography separation followed by UV absorption–detection. The Interdepartmental Committee on Nutrition for National Defense has selected as the preferred principal index of niacin status an NMN excretion rate of 5.8 μmol (0.8 mg) per day in 24 h urine samples as defining the junction between biochemical deficiency and sufficiency. If only casual (spot) urine samples are available, then the ratio of NMN to 2-pyridone may provide a useful alternative index, and one study suggested that <8.8 μmol of the combined excretion of NMN plus 2-pyridone can be considered as defining borderline adequacy, corresponding to a niacin intake in the region of 6 mg NE/day. The average adult NE requirement has been estimated from depletion–repletion studies to be approximately 5.5 mg NE/1000 kcal food energy/day, and thus with a 20% allowance for individual variation to cover the needs of the majority of healthy individuals, an RNI (UK) of approx. 6.6 mg NE/1000 kcal (4200 kjoule) food energy/day translates into the broad ranges of UK RNI values that are shown in **Table 3**. In the USA, the basis for the calculation is

Table 3 Reference and recommended intakes of niacin equivalents[a]

Age group	United Kingdom[b]		United States[c]
	LRNI (mg niacin equivalents/day)	RNI	RDA (mg niacin equivalents/day)
0–6 months	2	3	2
6–12 months	3–4	4–5	4
12 months–13 years	5–10	8–15	6–12
Adult	8–12	13–18	14–16
Lactation	10	15	17

[a]One niacin equivalent (mg NE) is equivalent to 1 mg niacin or one-sixtieth of the tryptophan consumed. Since the mean energy intake increases with age, and differs between the sexes after puberty, there is a corresponding difference in the absolute values for each population group. This table provides only a simplified summary of the published values.
[b]UK values are calculated on the basis of an LRNI (Lower Reference Nutrient Intake) of 4.4 mg NE/1000 kcal food energy and an RNI (Reference Nutrient Intake) of 6.6 mg NE/1000 kcal, both of which are constant for all population groups. The LRNI is intended to cover the needs of the lower 2.5% of a healthy population, whereas the RNI is intended to cover 97.5% of a healthy population.
Source: Department of Health (1991) *Report on Health and Social Subjects No. 41. Dietary Reference Values for Food Energy and Nutrients for the United Kingdom.* London: HMSO.
[c]The US RDA values are intended to cover the needs of 97.5% of a healthy population and are set 30% above the Estimated Average Requirements. Source: Food and Nutrition Board (1998) *Dietary Reference Intakes for Thiamin, Riboflavin, Niacin, Vitamin B₆, Folate, Vitamin B₁₂, Pantothenic Acid, Biotin and Choline.* Washington, DC: National Academy Press.

now somewhat different, but nevertheless, the US RDA ranges shown in **Table 3** are generally similar to the UK RNIs.

Glossary

Niacin Combination of nicotinamide and nicotinic acid.

Niacin equivalents (NE) mg niacin plus one-sixtieth of mg tryptophan in a defined quantity (e.g., mg/100 g or mg/d) of food or diet.

Niacytin A macromolecular complex of niacin found in some cereals, notably maize (sweet corn), which is poorly bioavailable but liberates niacin on heating with alkali. Mexican tortillas are cooked by heating maize flour with lime, which liberates the niacin in a bioavailable form.

Jowar An Indian cereal (staple) that is associated with high pellagra risk and is rich in the amino acid leucine, but which contains only a marginally adequate amount of niacin + tryptophan.

Isoniazid A drug used in the treatment of tuberculosis that antagonizes vitamin B_6 and is associated with pellagra symptoms, especially in Asian Indians.

Carbidopa, Benseride Anti-Parkinsonism drugs that can cause pellagra-like symptoms.

N-acetyl-pyridine A niacin antagonist, studied in animals.

NAD, NADH, NADP, NADPH The pyridine nucleotide coenzymes containing niacin that are involved in many essential hydrogen transfer reactions of intermediary metabolism, namely nicotinamide adenine dinucleotide (oxidized and reduced forms) and nicotinamide adenine dinucleotide phosphate (oxidized and reduced forms).

NMN N^1-methyl nicotinamide, a degradation product of niacin found in the urine.

2-pyridone, N^1-methyl-2-pyridone-4-carboxamide, another degradation product of niacin, is also found in the urine.

RDA Recommended Dietary Amount of a named nutrient, being the daily amount needed to cover the needs of the majority, usually 97.5% (i.e., mean plus 2 standard deviations) of the members of a healthy population of each defined age group and sex in the USA. RNI (Reference Nutrient Intake) is the UK equivalent of the RDA. (EAR: Estimated Average Requirement; LRNI: Lower Reference Nutrient Intake (UK only), which is the amount need to cover only that 2.5% of the population with the lowest requirements for the named nutrient).

Pellagra A human disease that is often equated with a clinical niacin deficiency but may have more complex causes.

Hartnup's disease A genetic disease of humans that exhibits some features similar to those of pellagra but that results from an impaired membrane transport of tryptophan.

Blacktongue Induced niacin deficiency disease in dogs, an animal model for human pellagra.

Units Niacin or niacin equivalents in food are usually expressed as milligrams per 100 g, usually of wet weight of food. Concentrations of analytes in tissues, blood, or urine are usually expressed in SI units (e.g., μmol/l or $\mu mol\,l^{-1}$).

See also: **Cereal Grains**. **Drug–Nutrient Interactions**. **Niacin**. **Riboflavin**. **Thiamin**: Physiology. **Vitamin B_6**.

Further Reading

Anonymous (1987) Pellagra treated with tryptophan. *Nutrition Reviews* **45**: 142–151.

Bender DA (1992) Niacin. In *Nutritional Biochemistry of the Vitamins*, pp. 184–222. Cambridge: CUP.

Carpenter KJ (ed.) (1981) *Pellagra: Benchmark papers in History of Biochemistry*, vol. 2. Stroudsberg, PA: Dowden, Hutchinson & Ross.

Carpenter KJ and Lewin WJ (1985) A reexamination of the composition of diets associated with pellagra. *American Journal of Clinical Nutrition* **115**: 543–552.

Combs GF Jr (1998) Niacin. In *The Vitamins. Fundamental Aspects in Nutrition and Health*, 2nd edn., pp. 312–331. New York: Academic Press.

Cook NE and Carpenter KJ (1987) Leucine excess and niacin status in rats. *Journal of Nutrition* **117**: 519–526.

Fu CS, Swendseid ME, Jacob RA, and McKee RW (1989) Biochemical markers for assessment of niacin status in young men: Levels of erythrocyte niacin coenzymes and plasma tryptophan. *Journal of Nutrition* **119**: 1949–1955.

Henderson LM (1983) Niacin. *Annual Review of Biochemistry* **3**: 289–307.

Horwitt MK, Harvey CC, Rothwell WS, Cutler JL, and Haffron D (1956) Tryptophan–niacin relationship in man. *Journal of Nutrition* **60**(supplement 1): 1–43.

Jacob RA (2001) Niacin. In *Present Knowledge in Nutrition*, 8th edn., pp. 199–206. Washington, DC: ILSI Press.

Multiauthor symposium (1981) Pellagra. *Federation Proceedings* **40**: 1519–1537.

Sauberlich HE (1999) Niacin (nicotinic acid, nicotinamide). In *Laboratory Tests for the Assessment of Nutritional Status*, 2nd edn., pp. 161–174. Boca Raton, FL: CRC Press.

Van Eys J (1991) Nicotinic acid. In: Machlin LJ (ed.) *Handbook of Vitamins*, vol. 2, pp. 311–340. New York: Marcel Dekker.

Pesticides *see* **Food Safety**: Pesticides

Phenylketonuria *see* **Inborn Errors of Metabolism**: Nutritional Management of Phenylketonuria

---

Phosphate *see* **Small Intestine**: Structure and Function

PHOSPHORUS

J J B Anderson, University of North Carolina, Chapel Hill, NC, USA

The consumption of a diet sufficient in phosphorus, in the form of phosphate salts or organophosphate molecules, is critical for the support of human metabolic functions. Too much phosphorus, in relation to too little dietary calcium, may contribute to bone loss, and too little phosphorus along with too little dietary calcium may not adequately maintain bone mass, especially in the elderly. Therefore, under normal dietary conditions, dietary phosphorus is used for numerous functions without any concern; it is only when too much or too little phosphorus is ingested that skeletal problems may arise. Certainly, elderly subjects need to consume sufficient amounts of phosphorus, like calcium, to maintain bone mass and density, but too much phosphorus may contribute to inappropriate elevations of parathyroid hormone (PTH) and bone loss. It is not clear where most elderly subjects fall along this continuum of intake patterns. This article discusses the mechanisms by which phosphate ions impact on calcium and also on bone tissue.

Calcium–Phosphate Interrelationships

Although phosphorus in the form of phosphate ions is essential for numerous body functions, its metabolism is intricately linked to that of calcium because of the actions of calcium-regulating hormones, such as PTH and 1,25-dihydroxyvitamin D, on bone, the gut, and the kidneys. Adequate phosphorus and calcium intakes are needed not only for skeletal growth and maintenance but also for many cellular roles, such as energy production (i.e., adenosine triphosphate (ATP)). Phosphate ions are incorporated in many organic molecules, including phospholipids, creatine phosphate, nucleotides, nucleic acids, and ATP.

Dietary Sources of Phosphorus

Animal products, including meats, fish, poultry, eggs, milk, cheese, and yogurt, are especially rich in phosphorus, as phosphates, but good amounts of phosphorus can be obtained from cereal grains and many vegetables, including legumes. Because of the abundance of phosphorus in the food supply, deficiency is highly unlikely except perhaps late in life when some elderly individuals consume little food. An extremely rare deficiency disease, phosphate rickets, in infants has been reported to result from inadequate phosphorus intake.

In the United States, mean phosphorus intakes approximate 1200–1500 mg per day in adult males and 900–1200 in adult females. In addition, phosphate additives used in food processing and cola beverages are also consumed, but the quantities are not required by food labeling laws to be given on the label so that the actual additional amounts consumed can only be estimated. Phosphate additives used by the food industry may be found in baked goods, meats, cheeses, and other dairy products.

Table 1 Calcium and phosphorus composition of common foods

Food category	Phosphorus mg/serving	Calcium mg/serving	Ca:P ratio (wt:wt)
Milk, eggs, and dairy			
Cheddar cheese, 1 oz.	145	204	1.4
Mozzarella cheese-part skim, 1 oz.	131	183	1.4
Vanilla ice milk, 1 cup	161	218	1.4
Lowfat yogurt, 1 cup	353	448	1.3
Skim milk, 8 oz.	247	301	1.2
Skim milk-Lactose reduced, 8 oz.	247	302	1.2
Vanilla ice cream, 1 cup	139	169	1.2
Vanilla soft-serve ice cream, 1 cup	199	225	1.1
Egg substitute, frozen, 1/4 cup	43	44	1.1
Chocolate pudding, 5 oz.	114	128	1.1
Processed American cheese, 1 oz.	211	175	0.8
Lowfat cottage cheese, 1 cup	300	200	0.7
Processed cheese spread, 1 oz.	257	129	0.5
Instant chocolate pudding, 5 oz.	340	147	0.4
Soy milk, 8 oz.	120	10	0.1

A conservative estimate is that most adults in the United States consume an extra 200–350 mg of phosphorus each day from these sources and cola beverages. Therefore, the total phosphorus intakes for men and women are increased accordingly. Because the typical daily calcium intake of males is 600–800 mg and that of females is 500–650 mg, the Ca:P ratios decrease from approximately 0.5–0.6 to less than 0.5 when the additive phosphates are included. As shown later, a chronically low Ca:P dietary ratio may contribute to a modest nutritional secondary hyperparathyroidism, which is considered less important in humans than in cats. **Table 1** provides representative values of calcium and phosphorus in selected foods and the calculated Ca:P ratios. Only dairy foods (except eggs), a few fruits, and a few vegetables have Ca:P ratios that exceed 1.0.

Recommended intakes of phosphorus have been set for adults in the United States at 900 mg per day for men and 700 mg per day for women.

Intestinal Absorption of Phosphates

Because phosphate ions are readily absorbed by the small intestine (i.e., at efficiencies of 65–75% in adults and even higher in children), a prompt increase in serum inorganic phosphate (Pi) concentration follows within an hour after ingestion of a meal begins. (Calcium ions or Ca^{2+} are much more slowly absorbed.) The increased serum Pi ($HPO_4^=$) concentration then depresses the serum calcium ion concentration, which in turn stimulates the parathyroid glands to synthesize and secrete PTH. PTH acts on bone and the kidneys to correct the modest decline in Ca^{2+} and homeostatically return it to the set level. Reports suggest that an elevation of serum Pi ionic concentration directly influences PTH secretion independently of hypocalcemia. These meal-associated fluctuations in Pi and Ca^{2+} are part of normal physiological adjustments that occur typically three or more times a day.

Pi ions are thought to be absorbed primarily by transcellular mechanisms that involve cotransport with cations, especially sodium (Na^+). These rapid mechanisms account for the uptake of Pi ions in blood within 1 h after ingestion of a meal. The blood concentration of Pi is less tightly regulated than the serum calcium concentration. Wider fluctuations in serum Pi concentrations reflect both dietary intakes and cellular releases of inorganic phosphates.

Most Pi absorption by the small intestine occurs independently of the hormonal form of vitamin D. The reported role of 1,25-dihydroxyvitamin D in intestinal Pi transcellular absorption is somewhat unclear because of the normally rapid influx of Pi ions after a meal, but this hormone may enhance the late or slower uptake of Pi ions. Paracellular passive absorption of Pi ions may also occur, but the evidence for this is limited.

Phosphate Homeostatic Mechanisms

The blood concentrations of Pi ions are higher early in life and then decline gradually until late life. The normal range for adults is 2.7–4.5 mg/dl (0.87–1.45 mmol/l). The percentage distributions of the blood fractions of phosphorus compared to those

Table 2 Approximate percentage (%) distributions of calcium and phosphate in blood

Serum fraction	Calcium	Phosphate
Ionic	50–55%	55–60%
Protein-Bound	45–50	10–13
Complexed	0.3–0.6	30–35

of calcium are given in **Table 2**. The homeostatic control of this narrow concentration range of Pi is maintained by several hormones, including PTH, $1,25(OH)_2$ vitamin D, calcitonin, insulin, glucagon, and others, but the control is never as rigorous as that of serum calcium. In contrast to calcium balance, which is primarily regulated in the small intestine by $1,25(OH)_2$ vitamin D, Pi balance is mainly regulated by the phosphaturic effect of PTH on the kidney, primarily the proximal convoluted tubule. In this sense, Pi regulation is less critical than that of calcium, which may result from the presence of multiple stores of this ion distributed throughout the body (i.e., bone, blood, and intracellular compartments).

A major regulator of Pi is PTH, whose role has been fairly well uncovered. PTH increases bone resorption of Pi (and calcium ions), it blocks renal tubular Pi reabsorption following glomerular filtration (whereas PTH favors calcium reabsorption), and it enhances intestinal Pi absorption (and calcium absorption) via the vitamin D hormone, $1,25(OH)_2$ vitamin D. Other hormones have more modest effects on serum Pi concentration.

Functional Roles of Phosphates

Several major roles of Pi ions have been briefly noted (i.e., intracellular phosphate groups for cellular energetics and biochemical molecules as well as for the skeleton and teeth (structures)). Other important functions also exist. For example, in bone tissue phosphates are critical components of hydroxyapatite crystals, and they are also considered triggers for mineralization after phosphorylation of type 1 collagen in forming bone. Serum phosphates, $HPO_4^=$ and $H_2PO_4^-$, also provide buffering capacity that helps regulate blood pH and also cellular pH.

Considerable cellular regulation occurs through the phosphorylation or dephosphorylation of Pi ions under the control of phosphatase enzymes, including protein kinases. These cell regulatory roles of Pi ions coexist with regulatory functions involving calcium ions, but Pi ions are much more widely distributed within cells and cell organelles than Ca ions.

Insulin affects Pi ions by increasing their intracellular uptake, although temporarily, for the prompt phosphorylation of glucose. Insulin may also influence the use of Pi ions when insulin-like growth factor-1 acts to increase tissue growth or other functions. Because of the broad uses of Pi ions in structural components, energetics, nucleic acids, cell regulation, and buffering, there is an overall generalization that these versatile yet critical ions support life.

Phosphate in Health and Disease

Phosphate balance in adults is almost always zero, in contrast to calcium balance, which is usually negative, because of the effective action of PTH on renal tubules to block Pi reabsorption. In late life, however, intestinal phosphate absorption decreases and the serum phosphate concentration declines. These physiological decrements may contribute to disease, especially to increased bone loss and osteopenia or more severe osteoporosis. Typically, these changes in Pi balance are also accompanied by similar changes in calcium balance. Too little dietary phosphorus and too little dietary calcium may be determinants of low bone mass and density and, hence, increased bone fragility. The usual scenario invoked to explain osteoporosis in old age, however, is that too little dietary calcium in the presence of adequate dietary phosphorus stimulates PTH release and bone loss (**Figure 1**).

Three human conditions that involve abnormal Pi homeostasis need explanation.

Aging and Renal Function

The serum concentration of Pi increases with a physiological decline in renal function associated with aging (but not renal disease per se). Healthy individuals excrete approximately 67% of their absorbed phosphate via the urine and the remainder via the gut as endogenous secretions. As the glomerular filtration capacity of the kidneys declines, the serum Pi concentration increases and more Pi is retained by the body. PTH secretions increase but the typical serum PTH concentrations, although elevated, remain within the upper limits of the normal range, at least for a decade or so. Thereafter, however, serum Pi and PTH both continue to climb as renal function declines and increased rates of bone turnover lead to measurable bone loss. This situation probably affects millions in the United States each year as they enter the 50s and proceed into the 60s; many of these individuals are overweight or obese and have the metabolic syndrome, which

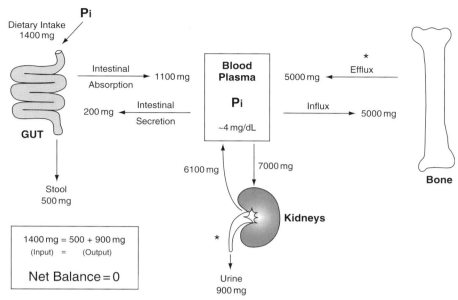

Figure 1 Phosphorus homeostasis and balance. The intestine, kidneys, and bone are organs involved in phosphate homeostasis. Fluxes of phosphate ions between blood and these organs are shown. Note the high fluxes in and out of bone each day. To convert phosphorus values from g to mmol, multiply by 32.29; from mg/dl to mmol/l, multiply by 0.3229. *Steps enhanced by parathyroid hormone. (Adapted with permission from Anderson JJB, Sell ML, Garner SC, and Calvo MS (2001) Phosphorus. In: Bowman BA and Russell R (eds.) *Present Knowledge in Nutrition*, 8th edn, p. 282. Washington, DC: International Life Sciences Institute Press.)

may negatively impact renal function. As the syndrome worsens, many of these individuals will progress to chronic renal failure and renal secondary hyperparathyroidism.

Nutritional Secondary Hyperparathyroidism

This mild condition has not been fully assessed in any longitudinal studies lasting as long as 1 year. The initiating event is a chronic low-calcium and high-phosphorus intake (low Ca:high P ratio) that leads to a chronic elevation of serum PTH. Elevations in PTH stimulate osteoclastic bone resorption and declines in bone mass and density. This condition has only been studied experimentally using human subjects for 28 days, but the chronic increases in PTH and vitamin D hormone suggest that even a lowering of the Ca:Pi ratio below 0.5—in this study to ~0.25—resulted in adverse effects. Longer term studies are needed to determine if bone losses occur under this chronic dietary regimen.

Renal Secondary Hyperparathyroidism

The true secondary hyperparathyroidism of chronic renal failure (CRF) has been extremely difficult to treat by clinicians because of high Pi and PTH concentrations in this condition. Traditional treatment includes the use of binders (chemical) to prevent Pi absorption from the small intestine. In recent years, a calcium-sensing receptor (CaR) in the parathyroid glands has been identified and drugs are being developed that will trick the CaR into thinking that serum calcium is normal rather than depressed, thereby reducing PTH secretion. A reduction in PTH then helps in the conservation of bone tissue since bone loss is such a severe problem in CRF patients.

Conclusions

The general view of dietary phosphorus, supplied in foods as phosphates, is that too much relative to calcium skews the Ca:P ratio to much less than 0.5. Another view, however, has been emerging that suggests that many elderly subjects, especially women, have very low phosphorus intakes in addition to low calcium intakes and that they may benefit from increased consumption of both calcium and phosphate from foods and supplements. In dietary trials designed to reduce fractures of elderly women and men, especially nonvertebral fractures, calcium plus vitamin D has been the treatment, but at least one trial that used calcium phosphate plus vitamin D has shown significant reduction in fractures over 18 and 36 months of follow-up. Further studies are needed to target the role of phosphate ions in reducing fractures among the elderly.

See also: **Aging**. **Bone**. **Calcium**.

Further Reading

Anderson JJB, Sell ML, Garner SC, and Calvo MS (2001) Phosphorus. In: Bowman BA and Russell R (eds.) *Present Knowledge in Nutrition*, 8th edn. Washington, DC: International Life Sciences Institute Press.

Baker SS, Cochran WJ, Flores CA *et al.* (1999) American Pediatrics Committee on Nutrition. Calcium requirements of infants, children, and adolescents. *Pediatrics* **104**: 1152–1157.

Brot C, Jorgensen N, Jensen LB, and Sorensen OH (1999) Relationships between bone mineral density, serum vitamin D metabolites and calcium:phosphorus intake in healthy perimenopausal women. *Journal of Internal Medicine* **245**: 509–516.

Calvo MS, Kumar R, and Heath HH III (1990) Persistently elevated parathyroid hormone secretion and action in young women after four weeks of ingesting high phosphorus, low calcium diets. *Journal of Clinical Endocrinology and Metabolism* **70**: 1340–1344.

Calvo MS and Park YM (1996) Changing phosphorus content of the US diet: Potential for adverse effects on bone. *Journal of Nutrition* **126**: 1168S–1180S.

Chapuy MC, Arlot ME, Duboeuf F *et al.* (1992) Vitamin D_3 and calcium to prevent hip fractures in elderly women. *New England Journal of Medicine* **327**: 1637–1642.

Garner SC (1996) Parathyroid hormone. In: Anderson JJB and Garner SC (eds.) *Calcium and Phosphorus in Health and Disease*, pp. 157–175. Boca Raton, FL: CRC Press.

Goulding A, Cannan R, Williams SM *et al.* (1998) Bone mineral density in girls with forearm fractures. *Journal of Bone and Mineral Research* **13**: 1143–1148.

Harnack L, Stang J, and Story M (1999) Soft drink consumption among US children and adolescents: Nutritional consequences. *Journal of the American Dietetic Association* **99**: 436–441.

Institute of Medicine, Food and Nutrition Board (1997) *Dietary Reference Intakes: Calcium, Phosphorus, Magnesium, Vitamin D and Fluoride*. Washington, DC: National Academy Press.

Khosla S, Melton LJ III, Dekutoski MB *et al.* (2003) Incidence of childhood distal forearm fractures over 30 years: A population-based study. *Journal of the American Medical Association* **290**: 1479–1485.

Ritter CS, Martin DR, Lu Y *et al.* (2002) Reversal of secondary hyperparathyroidism by phosphate restriction restores parathyroid calcium-sensing receptor expression and function. *Journal of Bone and Mineral Research* **17**: 2206–2213.

Shea B, Wells G, Cranney A *et al.* (2002) VII. Meta-analysis of calcium supplementation for the prevention of postmenopausal osteoporosis. *Endocrine Reviews* **23**: 552–559.

Slatopolsky E, Dusso A, and Brown A (1999) The role of phosphorus in the development of secondary hyperparathyroidism and parathyroid cell proliferation in chronic renal failure. *American Journal of Medical Sciences* **317**: 370–376.

Uribarri J and Calvo MS (2003) Hidden sources of phosphorus in the typical American diet: Does it matter in nephrology? *Seminars in Dialysis* **16**: 186–188.

Vinther-Paulsen N (1953) Calcium and phosphorus intake in senile osteoporosis. *Geriatrics* **9**: 76–79.

Wyshak G (2000) Teenaged girls, carbonated beverage consumption, and bone fractures. *Archives of Pediatric and Adolescent Medicine* **154**: 610–613.

Wyshak G and Frisch RE (1994) Carbonated beverages, dietary calcium, the dietary calcium/phosphate ratio, and bone fractures in girls and boys. *Journal of Adolescent Health* **15**: 210–215.

Physical Activity *see* **Exercise**: Beneficial Effects; Diet and Exercise

---

PHYTOCHEMICALS

Contents
Classification and Occurrence
Epidemiological Factors

Classification and Occurrence

A Cassidy, School of Medicine, University of East Anglia, Norwich, UK

There is a considerable body of evidence to suggest that populations that consume diets rich in fruits and vegetables, whole-grain cereals, and complex carbohydrates have a reduced risk of a range of chronic diseases. This has led to the suggestion that the diversity of substances found in food, particularly plant-derived or plant-based foods, may underlie the protective effects that are attributed to diets high in fruits and vegetables and other plant foods. Although fruits and vegetables are rich sources of micronutrients and dietary fiber, they also contain a wide variety of secondary metabolites, which provide the plant with color, flavor, and antimicrobial and insecticide properties. Many of these substances have been attributed a wide array of properties but have yet to be recognized as nutrients in the conventional sense. Many of these potentially protective plant compounds, termed phytochemicals, are receiving increasing attention. Phytochemicals, also known as phytonutrients, are plant-based compounds that exert numerous physiological functions in mammalian systems. Many of them are ubiquitous throughout the plant and as a result are present in our daily diet. Among the most important classes are the flavonoids, which are classified based on their chemical and structural characteristics. This article focuses on the different classes of phytochemicals and their relationships to human diseases.

Phytochemicals: General

Plants synthesize a wide array of compounds that play key roles in protecting plants against herbivores and microbial infection and as attractants for pollinators and seed-dispersing animals, allelopathic agents, UV protectants, and signal molecules in the formation of nitrogen-fixing root nodules in legumes. Although they have long been ignored from a nutritional perspective, the function of these compounds and their relative importance to human health are gaining significant interest.

Phytochemicals comprise a wide group of structurally diverse plant compounds, which are predominantly associated with the cell wall and widely dispersed throughout the plant kingdom. They are secondary plant metabolites, characterized by having at least one aromatic ring with one or more hydroxyl groups attached. The nature and distribution of these compounds can vary depending on the plant tissue, but they are mainly synthesized from carbohydrates via the shikimate and phenylpropanoid pathways. They range in chemical complexity from simple phenolic acids, such as caffeic acid, to complex high-molecular-weight compounds, such as the tannins, and they can be classified according to the number and arrangement of their carbon atoms. In plants, they are commonly found conjugated to sugars and organic acids and can be classified into two groups, flavonoids and nonflavonoids. The most researched group of compounds to date is the flavonoids, and this article focuses on this group.

Flavonoids

Flavonoids constitute a large class of phytochemicals that are widely distributed in the plant kingdom, are present in high concentrations in the epidermis of leaves and skin of fruits, and have important and varied roles as secondary metabolites. More than 8000 varieties of flavonoids have been identified, many of which are responsible for the colors of fruits and flower. They are found in fruits, vegetables, tea, wine, grains, roots, stems, and flowers and are thus regularly consumed by humans. Although it has been widely known for centuries that derivatives of plant origin possess a broad spectrum of biological activities, it was first suggested that flavonoids may be important for human health in the 1930s when it was observed that a fraction from lemon juice could decrease the permeability of arteries and partially prevent symptoms in scorbutic pigs. At the time, it was suggested that these compounds should be defined as a new class of vitamins, vitamin P, and the substance responsible for the effects was identified as the flavonoid rutin. However, the data were not generally accepted and the term vitamin P was abandoned in the 1950s. There was renewed interest in flavonoids when a potentially protective role for flavonoids in relation to heart disease in humans was reported. Since that time, there has been a surge of interest in the potential role of flavonoids in human health, with research suggesting antioxidant effects, hormonal actions, antiinfectious actions, cancer-preventative effects, the ability to induce chemical defense enzymes, and actions on blood clotting and the vascular system. However, concrete evidence that they positively influence human health is lacking, and adverse effects have also been reported for some polyphenols. The main subclasses of flavonoids are flavones, flavonols, flavan-3-ols, isoflavones, flavanones, and anthocyanidins (**Figure 1** and **Table 1**).

Other flavonoid groups that are thought to be less important from a dietary perspective are the dihydroflavones, flavan-3,4-diols, coumarins, chalcones, dihydrochalcones, and aurones. The basic flavonoid skeleton can have numerous constituents; hydroxyl groups are usually present at the 4-, 5-, and 7- positions. Sugars are very common, and the majority of flavonoids exist naturally as glycosides. The presence of both sugars and hydroxyl groups increases water solubility, but other constituents, such as methyl or isopentyl groups, render flavonoids lipophilic.

Although many thousands of different flavonoids exist, they can be classified into different subclasses. The main subclasses that are important from a human health perspective are the flavones,

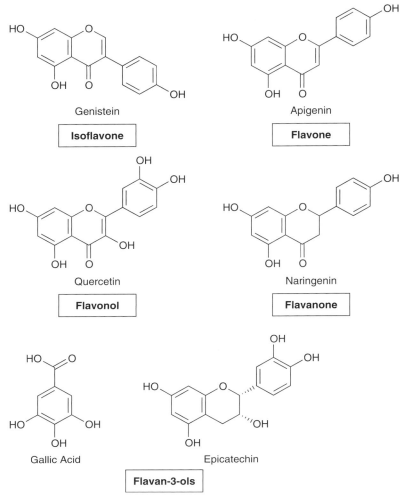

Figure 1 Structures of the major subclasses of flavonoids.

flavonols, flavan-3-ols, isoflavones, flavanones, and anthocyanidins (**Figure 1**).

Flavonols

These are arguably the most widespread of the flavonoids because they are dispersed throughout the plant kingdom. The distribution and structural variations of flavonols are extensive and have been well documented. Extensive information on the different flavonols present in commonly consumed fruits, vegetables, and drinks is available; however, there is wide variability in the levels present in specific foods, in part due to seasonal changes and varietal differences. The most common flavonols are kaempferol, quercetin, isorhamnetin, and myricetin.

Flavones

Flavones have a close structural relationship to the flavonols, but unlike flavonols they are not

widely distributed in plants. The only significant occurrences in plants are in celery, parsley, and a few other herbs, and they predominantly occur as 7-O-glycosides (e.g., luteolin and apigenin). In addition, polymethoxylated flavones have been found in citrus fruits (e.g., nobiletin and tangeretin).

Flavan-3-ols

Flavan-3-ols, often referred to as flavanols, are the most complex class of the flavonoids because they range from simple monomers (catechin and its isomer epicatechin) to the oligomeric and polymeric proanthocyanidins, which are also known as condensed tannins. Proanthocyanidins can occur as polymers of up to 50 units, and when hydroxylated they can form gallocatechins or undergo esterification to form gallic acid. Red wine contains oligometric proanthocyanidins derived mainly from the seeds of black grapes. Green tea is also a rich source of

Table 1 Principal dietary sources of flavonoids

Flavonoid	Compound	Food source
Flavonol	Quercetin, kempferol, myricetin	Onion, apple, broccoli, tea, olives, kale, cranberry, lettuce, beans (green, yellow)
Flavone	Luteolin, apigenin	Olives, celery
Flavan-3-ol	Catechin, epicatechin	Tea, red wine, apple
Flavanone	Naringenin, hesperidin	Citrus fruit
Anthocyanidins	Cyanidin, delphinidin, malvidin, petunidin	Grapes, cherries
Chalcones, dihydrochalcones		Heavily hopped beer, tomatoes (with skins), cider, apple juice
Isoflavone	Genistein, daidzein	Soy

Information from Hollman PC, Katan MB (1997) Absorption, metabolism and health effects of dietary flavonoids in man. Biomed Pharmacother **51**(8): 305–10.
Scalbert A, Williamson G (2000) Dietary intake and bioavailability of Polyphenols. J Nutr **130** (8S Suppl): 2073S–85S.

flavan-3-ols, principally epigallocatechin, epigallocatechin gallate, and epicatechin gallate. However, during fermentation of tea leaves the levels of catechins decline and thus the main components of black tea are high-molecular-weight thearubigins, whose structures are derived from flavonoids but are unknown. The catechins are widespread, but the main sources in the diet come from tea, wine, and chocolate.

Anthocyanins

Anthocyanins are widespread in nature, predominantly in fruits and flower tissues, in which they are responsible for the red, blue, and purple colors. They are also found in leaves, stems, seeds, and root tissue. In plants, they protect against excessive light by shading leaf mesophyll cells. Additionally, they play an important role in attracting pollinating insects. The most common anthocyanins are pelargonidin, cyanidin, delphinidin, peonidin, petunidin, and malvidin, which are predominantly present in plants as sugar conjugates.

Flavanones

The flavanones are the first flavonoid products of the flavonoid biosynthetic pathway. They are characterized by the presence of a chiral center at C2 and the absence of the C2–C3 bond. The flavanone structure is highly reactive, and they have been reported to undergo hydroxylation, glycosylation, and O-methylation reactions. Flavanones are present in high levels in citrus fruits, with the most common glycoside known as hesperidin (hesperetin-7-o-rutinoside), which is present in citrus peel. Interestingly, flavanone rutinosides are tasteless, whereas the flavanone neohesperidoside conjugates (e.g., neohesperidin) from bitter orange and naringenin (naringenin-7-o-neohesperidoside) from grapefruit peel have an intensely bitter taste.

Isoflavones

Isoflavones are flavonoids, but they are also called phytoestrogens because of their oestrogenic activity. Structurally, they exhibit a similarity to mammalian oestrogens and bind to oestrogen receptors α and β. Apart from basic structural similarities, the key to their estrogenic effect is the presence of the hydroxyl groups on the A and B rings. They are classified as oestrogen agonists but also as oestrogen antagonists since they compete with oestrogen for their receptor. They have also been demonstrated to exert effects that are independent of the oestrogen receptor.

Current Estimates of Intake

Diets rich in plant-derived foods can provide more than 1 g of phenolic compounds per day, although there are major international and interindividual differences in exposure. Flavonols, flavones, and flavan-3-ols constitute the three major subclasses of flavonoids, and a significant amount of information on the content of selected flavonoids from these subclasses in fruits and vegetables has been obtained using high-performance liquid chromatography techniques. The other subclasses are flavanones, anthocyanidins, and isoflavones.

Given the differences in dietary intake, particularly for fruits and vegetables, between populations, it is not surprising that the relationships between the predominant flavonoids and their sources will vary between populations, nor is it unexpected that there will be wide inter- and intraindividual variations in intake of the individual subclasses of the flavonoids. Flavonol intake was estimated to be highest in a Japanese population group (64 mg/day) and lowest in Finland (6 mg/day). International comparisons of dietary sources also reflect this variation, but only a few sources of flavonoids are responsible for most of the intake. Red wine was the main source of the flavonol quercetin in Italy, tea was the main source in Japan and The Netherlands, and onions were the most significant contributor to intake in Greece, the United States, and the former Yugoslavia (**Table 1**).

Table 2 Estimated dietary intake of flavonoid subclasses in different countries

Flavonoid subgroup	Estimated intake (mg/day)			
	Denmark	Holland	Finland	Japan
Flavonol	1.5–8.6	1–17	1.1–7	16.4
Flavone	1–2	2	No data	0.3
Flavan-3-ol	45	50	8.3	40
Flavanone	7.1–9.3	No data	8.3–28.3	No data
Isoflavone	<1	No data	No data	50
Anthocyanidins	6–60	No data	No data	No data

The estimated daily intake of flavonoids, including catechins and anthocyanins, is >50 mg for all the countries presented in **Table 2**, and realistically intake is probably higher than 100 mg/day if data on all flavonoid groups were available. If this intake is compare to daily intakes of other dietary antioxidants, such as vitamin C (80 mg/day), vitamin E (8.5 mg/day), and β-carotene (1.9 mg/day), it is clear that flavonoid intakes exceed or are at least comparable to those of other established antioxidants, indicating that these compounds constitute an important part of dietary intake of antioxidants.

Absorption and Metabolism of Flavonoids

The flavonols and flavones are generally present in plants in the form of glycosides and as such are water-soluble. Thus, some of the flavonol glycosides may be absorbed intact in the small intestine or hydrolyzed by mucosal enzymes and absorbed as aglycones. However, those that pass through the small intestine unabsorbed or reenter the gut from the bile become available for bacterial metabolism in the colon.

The colon contains numerous microorganisms and as a result it has significant capacity for catalytic and hydrolytic reactions. These colonic bacteria produce enzymes that are capable of stripping flavonoid conjugates of their sugar moieties, enabling free aglycones to be absorbed. The enzymes produced by colonic bacteria can also break down the flavonoids into simple compounds, resulting in the production of a range of derivatives, some of which may be more biologically active than the parent compound. This is an important area for future research because the metabolism of flavonoids is influenced by intestinal microflora and these metabolic reactions may result in deactivation of bioactive compounds or activation of previously inactive compounds. It is therefore critical to identify the bacteria involved in

these transformation reactions and define their relative importance and occurrence in the human gut to gain a better understanding of the transformation processes.

Other key body compartments that are important in defining the metabolism of flavonoids are the liver and, to a lesser extent, the small intestine and kidney, in which the biotransformation enzymes are located. Flavonols and flavan-3-ols are primarily metabolized in the colon and liver.

The evidence for absorption of intact flavonoid glycosides is weak. Recent data showing β-glucosidase activity in the small intestine, together with the absence of intact glycosides in plasma and urine, strongly suggest that only free flavonoid aglycones are being absorbed. In addition, data also indicate that there is a more rapid and efficient absorption of flavonoids originating from glucosides than from other glycosides or free aglycones. This suggests that dietary sources containing high levels of glucose-bound flavonoids are more likely to have potential health benefits than foods containing other flavonoid glycosides.

Bioavailability of Flavonoids

Critical to a food's 'nutritional' value is whether the 'nutrient' or compound is provided in a bioavailable form from the food. Flavonoids therefore may have to be absorbed from the large intestine if they are to exert a potential health effect. Early data from animal studies suggested that flavonoids were only absorbed to a limited degree because gut microflora preferentially destroyed the heterocyclic rings of the compounds before absorption occurred in the small intestine. However, an increasing number of studies suggest that the bioavailability of flavonoids is greater than was previously recognized, although increases in the concentrations of flavonoids and its associated metabolites in plasma and urine do not necessarily mean that they have significant effects *in vivo*. There are few data on their intracellular location and mechanism of action. Thus, a key area for future research will be to clarify the absorption, bioavailability, and metabolism of a range of flavonoid compounds.

Potential Mechanisms of Action

The effect of flavonoids on enzymatic, biological, and physiological processes has been extensively studied, but few studies have attempted to determine the actual compound or metabolite responsible for the observed effects. Much of the *in vitro* data assume that the biological activity originates from the flavonoid ingested, without taking into consideration the biotransformations that may occur following ingestion and metabolism, as it is well established that following ingestion they are transformed into a range of structurally distinct compounds.

In interpreting the mechanistic data, it is also important to remember that little attention has been paid to the physiological relevance of the concentration used in the *in vitro* model systems. Thus, in some instances biological effects have been shown at concentrations that are unachievable *in vivo*; therefore, the biological relevance of these mechanisms to humans is questionable.

Since flavonoids are complex groups of compounds with variable structures and activities, it is unlikely that they exert their biological effects by common mechanisms. However, since it is also now established that the pathophysiological processes leading to the development of cardiovascular disease and cancer are complex, this means that there are many potential sites and stages at which bioactive plant compounds present in food could act to potentially reduce the formation of cancerous cells or the atherosclerotic plaque in cardiovascular disease. Elucidating the underlying mechanisms of how flavonoids work is a key aim for nutrition research.

In vitro experimental systems suggest that flavonoids can scavenge oxygen-derived free radicals; exert antiinflammatory, antiallergic, and antiviral effects; and have anticarcinogenic properties.

Potential Health Effects

There is substantial epidemiological evidence that populations that consume diets rich in plant foods have a reduced risk of cardiovascular disease and various cancers, and the potential role of bioactive compounds in plants in this association is gaining significant attention within nutrition research. Identification of the role of flavonoids in the primary mechanisms that may protect against cellular damage may yield clues to slowing aspects of the aging process and postpone age-related diseases.

Most research on flavonoids and health has focused on quercetin due to its antioxidant potency and potential role in cardiovascular disease. However, the diverse and broad nature of flavonoids means that subclasses other than the flavonols may be more important to human health since they appear to be more bioavailable and thus have a greater potential to protect against the various

mechanisms involved in aging and disease development.

Cardiovascular Health

The stimulus for much of the research on the role of flavonoids in human health was derived from epidemiological studies, particularly a study suggesting that dietary flavonoids may protect against cardiovascular disease. During the past decade, a significant amount of research has examined the effect of flavonoids in foods and pure flavonoid compounds at various stages in the atherosclerosis process.

A significant proportion of the research on flavonoids has concentrated on their antioxidant actions, and their capacity to act as antioxidants remains their best described biological property to date. Their antioxidant ability is well established *in vitro*, and *in vivo* animal data also suggest that consumption of compounds such as rutin or red wine extracts, tea, or fruit juice lowers oxidative products such as protein carbonyls, DNA damage markers, and malonaldehyde levels in blood and a range of tissues.

The flavones and catechins appear to be the most powerful flavonoids at protecting the body against reactive oxygen species. Although the mechanisms and sequence of events by which free radicals interfere with cellular functions are not fully understood, one of the most important events may be lipid peroxidation, which results in cellular damage. Flavonoids may prevent such cellular damage by several different mechanisms, including direct scavenging of free radicals such as superoxides and peroxynitrite, inhibition of nitric oxide, or antiinflammatory effects.

Cancer

The specific mechanisms by which individual dietary components can alter the cancer process remain poorly understood. However, mechanisms underlying the carcinogenesis process are understood sufficiently so that model systems to evaluate the ability of a specific compound to inhibit or promote processes that may prevent or delay cancer development can be predicted. Phytochemcials can act at a variety of sites relevant to the development of the cancer cells. They may inhibit carcinogen activation, induce hepatic detoxification pathways, exert antioxidant effects/metal chelation properties, enhance immune response, induce apoptosis, and alter hormonal environment.

From a mechanistic perspective, evidence suggests that flavonoids have the potential to alter the cancer development process by several different mechanisms. These include inhibition of the metabolic activation of carcinogens by modifying the expression of specific phase I and II enzymes, acting as antioxidants, inhibiting protein kinase C, interfering with expression of the mutated *ras* oncogene, and influencing other redox-regulated aspects of cell proliferation.

In addition to *in vitro* data, it is also well established that certain flavonoids can protect against chemically induced and spontaneously formed tumors in animal models. However, despite the significant amount of experimental evidence indicating that specific flavonoids have potent anticarcinogenic effects, the available epidemiological data are contradictory. Some ecological, cohort, and case–control studies suggest that tea consumption lowers the risk of developing cancer, whereas other investigations have failed to find such an association. The inconclusive nature may relate to poor information on dietary intake of flavonoids.

Safety

Although flavonoids may have potential health effects, the function of many of these compounds in the plant is to discourage attack by fungal parasites, herbivores, and pathogens. As a result, it is not surprising than many are toxic and mutagenic in cell culture systems, and excessive consumption by animals or humans may cause adverse metabolic reactions. However, the concentrations used in cell culture experiments in general tend to exceed the levels that are achievable *in vivo* following dietary consumption. Results of recent studies using β-carotene supplements should reinforce the need to proceed with caution in using flavonoid supplements, where levels could easily exceed doses obtained from normal dietary intake. For the majority of the identified phytochemicals, there are limited data on the 'safe level' of intake or optimal level of intake for health benefits, and it is critical that these margins be more clearly defined in future research.

Conclusions

There is increasing evidence that flavonoids may be protective against a number of age-related disorders. Data suggest that diets high in flavonoids may not only reduce the risk of cardiovascular disease and cancer but also, by protecting against cellular damage, may slow aspects of the aging process and improve quality of life by postponing age-related diseases. There is still much to be uncovered about their bioavailability, metabolism, mode of action,

and optimal doses or, indeed, the actual compounds responsible for the health effect. Research has focused on foods as well as individual components of food to help us further our knowledge. Given the limited information to date, there are no recommended dietary intakes for phytochemicals, but people should consume a wide variety of foods that incorporate the various phytochemicals to maximize disease prevention. Further research is required to define optimal doses for potential health effects and to define safe levels of intakes for many of these phytochemicals. Many of these compounds should be viewed as pharmaceutical compounds because although they occur naturally, they still require the same levels of proof of efficacy and safety in use as synthetic pharmaceutical agents.

See also: **Antioxidants**: Diet and Antioxidant Defense; Observational Studies; Intervention Studies. **Cancer**: Epidemiology and Associations Between Diet and Cancer; Effects on Nutritional Status. **Coronary Heart Disease**: Prevention. **Fruits and Vegetables**. **Phytochemicals**: Epidemiological Factors. **Tea**. **Whole Grains**.

Further Reading

BNF (2003) Plants: Diet and health. In: Goldberg G (ed.) *The Report of the BNF Task Force*. Oxford: Blackwell. [ISBN 0-632-05962-1].

Bravo L (1998) Polyphenols: Chemistry, dietary sources, metabolism, and nutritional significance. *Nutrition Reviews* 56: 317–333.

Cassidy A, DePascual S, and Rimbach GH (2003) Molecular mechanisms by which isoflavones potentially prevent atherosclerosis. *Expert Reviews in Molecular Medicine* 5: 1–9.

Day AJ and Williamson G (2001) Biomarkers for exposure to dietary flavonoids: A review of the current evidence for identification of quercetin glycosides in plasma. *British Journal of Nutrition* 86(supplement 1): S105–S110.

Dragsted LO (2003) Antioxidant actions of polyphenols in humans. *International Journal for Vitamin and Nutrition Research* 73: 112–119.

Duthie G and Crozier A (2000) Plant-derived phenolic antioxidants. *Current Opinion in Clinical Nutrition and Metabolic Care* 3: 447–451.

Hasler CM and Blumberg JB (1999) Phytochemicals: Biochemistry and physiology. Introduction. *Journal of Nutrition* 129: 756S–757S.

Hertog MG, Kromhout D, Aravanis C *et al.* (1995) Flavonoid intake and long-term risk of coronary heart disease and cancer in the seven countries study. *Archives of Internal Medicine* 155: 381–386.

Hollman PC and Arts ICW (2000) Flavonols, flavones and flavonols—Nature, occurrence and dietary burden. *Journal of the Science of Food and Agriculture* 80: 1081–1093.

Hollman PC and Katan MB (1999) Health effects and bioavailability of dietary flavonols. *Free Radical Research* 31(supplement): S75–S80.

Nielsen SE, Freese R, Kleemola P *et al.* (2002) Flavonoids in human urine as biomarkers for intake of fruits and vegetables. *Cancer Epidemiology Biomarkers and Prevention* **11**: 459–466.

Nijveldt RJ, van Nood E, Van Hoorn DE *et al.* (2001) Flavonoids: A review of probable mechanisms of action and potential applications. *American Journal of Clinical Nutrition* **74**: 418–425.

Setchell KD and Cassidy A (1999) Dietary isoflavones: Biological effects and relevance to human health. *Journal of Nutrition* **129**: 758S–767S.

Epidemiological Factors

H Wiseman, King's College London, London, UK

There is considerable interest in the role that dietary phytochemicals may play in the protection of human health. This article considers the epidemiological evidence for the health protective effects of phytochemicals such as flavonoids, phytoestrogens, glucosinolates, and their derivatives and allium organosulfur compounds, particularly against cancer and heart disease. Possible health benefits of the soya isoflavone phytoestrogens to brain (especially cognitive function) and bone health are also considered together with the importance of their metabolism by the gut microflora (conversion of daidzein to equol) (**Table 1**). The possible mechanisms of action of these phytochemicals and others of related interest are also considered.

Epidemiological Sources of Evidence Indicating Potential Health Benefits of Phytochemicals

Flavonoids

Flavonoids are a group of more than 4000 polyphenolic compounds found in many plant foods.

This group includes the flavonols such as quercetin, flavanols (or catechins, including catechin, epicatechin, epigallocatechin, and epigallocatechin gallate), flavones such as apigenin, and flavanones and anthocyanadins.

Until recently, the extent of absorption and bioavailability of flavonoids was somewhat unclear. Studies with ileostomy patients have shown that humans can absorb significant amounts of quercetin and that glycosides can be absorbed from the small intestine. Absorption of quercetin glucosides was 52%, absorption of pure quercetin was 24%, and that of quercetin rutinoside was 17%. This shows that not only can the glycone form of quercetin be absorbed but also absorption of the glucoside was greater than that of both the aglycone and the rutinoside, showing absorption to be enhanced by conjugation with glucose.

Epidemiological evidence suggests that dietary flavonoids, such as the quercetin, kaempferol, myricetin, apigenin, and luteolin found in tea, apples, onions, and red wine (usually as glycoside derivatives of the parent aglycones), may help to protect against coronary heart disease (CHD). The main epidemiological evidence comes from the Zutphen Elderly study and the Seven Countries Study. In the Zutphen Elderly study (805 men aged 65–84 years), the mean baseline flavonoid intake was 25.9 mg daily and the major sources of intake were tea (61%), onions (13%), and apples (10%). Flavonoid intake, which was analyzed in tertiles, was significantly inversely associated with mortality from CHD, and the relative risk of CHD in the highest versus lowest tertile of flavonoid intake ($\geq$28.6 vs <18.3 mg/day) was 0.42 (95% confidence interval, 0.20–0.88).

The Zutphen Elderly study thus suggests that regular flavonoid consumption, as part of the food matrix, may reduce the risk of death from CHD in elderly men. This study also provides evidence for flavonoid-mediated protection against stroke.

Table 1 Overview of epidemiological data relating to the role of soybean products in breast cancer risk

Study	Soybean product	Findings	Estimate of relative risk
Case–control[a]	Soybean protein	↓ Risk	0.43
	Soybean:total protein	↓ Risk	0.29
Case–control	Soybean	Not significant	[b]
Prospective	Miso soup	↓ Risk	0.46
Prospective	Miso soup	↓ Risk[c]	[b]
	Tofu	↓ Risk[c]	[b]

[a]Premenopausal women only.
[b]Could not be calculated.
[c]Decreased risk was only found to be significant for the baseline period 1971–1975.
Adapted from Messina MJ, Persky V, Setchell KDR and Barnes S (1994) Soy intake and cancer risk: A review of the *in vitro* and *in vivo* data. *Nutrition and Cancer* **21**: 113–131.

Dietary flavonoids (particularly quercetin) were inversely associated with stroke incidence. The relative risk of the highest versus the lowest quartile of flavonoid was 0.27 (95% confidence interval, 0.11–0.70). Black tea contributed approximately 70% to flavonoid intake and the relative risk for a daily consumption of 4.7 cups or more of tea versus less than 2.6 cups of tea was 0.31 (95% confidence interval, 0.12–0.84). This study also found that intake of catechins, whether from tea or other sources (e.g., chocolate), may reduce the risk of ischemic heart disease but not stroke. In the Rotterdam study (a large population-based study of men and women aged 55 or older), an inverse association was found between tea and flavonoid (quercetin, kaempferol, and myricetin) intakes and the incidence of myocardial infarction.

In 16 cohorts of the Seven Countries Study, the average long-term intake of flavonoids was inversely associated with mortality from CHD (**Table 2**). Surprisingly, flavonoid intake, did not appear to be an important determinant of cancer mortality in this study. This is in contrast to the anticarcinogenic effects observed in animal models and in human cancer cells *in vitro*. An inverse association between tea consumption and the incidence of some cancers has been reported in a prospective cohort study of 35 369 postmenopausal women. Inverse associations with increasing frequency of tea drinking were seen for cancers of the digestive tract and the urinary tract. The relative risk for women who reported drinking ≥2 cups (474 ml) of tea per day compared to those who never or only occasionally drank tea was 0.68 (95% confidence interval, 0.47–0.98) for digestive tract cancers and 0.4 (95% confidence interval, 0.16–0.98) for urinary tract cancers. Another epidemiological study reported a reduced risk of gastric cancer from drinking 10 cups or more daily of green tea. Tea, especially green tea, is particularly rich in catechins, such as epicatechin, epigallocatechin, and epigallocatechin gallate, in addition to flavonols such as quercetin.

The association between flavonoid intake and chronic diseases has been studied in Finland in 10 054 men and women. The incidence of cerebrovascular disease was lower at higher kaempferol, naringinin, and hesperetin intakes. Asthma incidence was lower at higher quercetin, naringinin, and hesperetin intakes. Men with high quercetin intakes had a lower lung cancer incidence, and men with higher myricetin intakes had a lower prostate cancer risk.

Flavonol and flavone intakes have been studied in the United States in health professionals (37 886 men and 78 886 women) using a semiquantitiative food frequency questionnaire. Of the flavonols and flavones investigated, quercetin contributed 76% in men and 73% in women. The mean flavonol and flavone intake was 20–22 mg/day, and onions, tea, and apples contributed the greatest amounts of flavonols and flavones. This information should prove useful in the investigation of the role of flavonoids in disease prevention.

Phytoestrogens

Phytoestrogens are phytochemicals found in a number of edible plants. The highest levels of dietary intakes of phytoestrogens are found in countries with a low incidence of hormone-dependent cancers. The main phytoestrogens in the human diet are the isoflavonoids and the lignans. Isoflavonoids include the isoflavones genistein, daidzein, and glycitein and occur mainly (as glycosides of the parent aglycone) in soybeans (*Glycine max*), a wide range of soy products, and to a lesser extent in other legumes. The main source of plant lignans are various seeds, such as linseed (secoisolariciresinol), sesame seed

Table 2 Data from the Seven Countries Study: Flavonoid (flavonol and flavone) intakes of middle-aged men in various countries in approximately 1960 and contribution of different foods to total flavonoid intake

Country	Flavonol and flavone intake (mg/day)	Quercetin intake (mg/day)	Tea (%)	Fruit and vegetables (%)	Red wine (%)
The Netherlands	33	13	64	36	0
Japan	64	31	90	10	0
United States	13	11	20	80	0
Finland	6	6	0	100	0
Croatia	49	30	0	82	18
Serbia	12	10	0	98	2
Greece	16	15	0	97	3
Italy	27	21	0	54	46

Adapted from Hertog MGL and Hollman PCH (1996) Potential health effects of the dietary flavonol quercetin. *European Journal of Clinical Nutrition* **50**: 63–71.

(matairesinol), and various grains (matairesinol and secisolariciresinol).

The incidence of breast and prostate cancer is much higher in Western countries than in Far Eastern ones, where there is an abundance of dietary phytoestrogens. Populations in the Far East have been consuming soyabean for centuries. In contrast, Western cultures and diets have only started to adopt soy foods much more recently. Western-style soy foods are produced by modern processing techniques in large soybean-processing plants. Traditional soy foods, made from soybeans, include both nonfermented and fermented foods. The nonfermented soy foods include soy milk and the soy milk product tofu and also whole-fat soy flour, soy nuts, whole dry beans, and fresh green soybeans. Traditional fermented soy foods include soy sauce, tempeh, natto, miso, and fermented tofu and soy milk products. Soy milk is the name given to the aqueous extract derived from whole soybeans. A cup of soy milk is thought to contain approximately 40 mg of isoflavones. In soybeans, textured vegetable protein, and tofu (soybean curd), there are high levels of the conjugated isoflavones called daidzin and genistin. In contrast, in the fermented soybean products such as miso, nearly all the isoflavones are present in their unconjugated forms called genistein and daidzein.

After ingestion, the glycones daidzin and genistin are hydrolyzed by gut bacterial glucosidases and by mammalian intestinal lactase phlorizin hydrolase to release the aglycones genistein and daidzein. These may be absorbed or further metabolized. Although most studies suggest that the bioavailabilities of genistein and daidzein are similar, some indicate greater bioavailability for genistein. Daidzein can be metabolized by the gut microflora to form the isoflavan equol (oestrogenic and more potent antioxidant than daidzein) or O-desmethylangolensin (O-DMA; nonoestrogenic), whereas genistein is metabolized to the nonoestrogenic p-ethyl phenol. In studies, only approximately 35% of subjects are able to convert daidzein to equol. Interindividual variation in the ability to metabolize daidzein to equol could thus influence the potential health protective effects of soya isoflavones. Equol is produced in greater amounts by subjects who consume diets that are low in fat and high in carbohydrate and fiber. Developmental changes in isoflavone metabolism occur, and although isoflavone absorption and the ability to convert daidzein to O-DMA develop early in infancy, equol production appears much later.

The lignan phytoestrogen precursors matairesinol and secisolariciresinol are present in foods as glycosides and are converted by gut bacteria to the two main mammalian lignans enterolactone and enterodiol, respectively, which are weakly oestrogenic. Matairesinol undergoes dehydroxylation and demethylation directly to enterolactone, whereas secisolariciresinol is converted to enterodiol, which can then be oxidized to enterolactone. After absorption, enterolactone and enterodiol are converted to their β-glucuronides and eventually excreted in urine.

In humans, omniverous subjects usually have quite low levels of isoflavonoid excretion. The Japanese (males and females) have the highest levels of isoflavonoid excretion in subjects following macrobiotic, vegan, and lactovegetarian diets. Urinary lignan excretion is higher in Finland compared to the United States and Japan. In assessing exposure to the protective effects of phytoestrogens, urinary excretion rates should be considered in combination with actual plasma levels. In some Japanese men, the plasma biologically active sulfate + free lignan fraction was similar or even higher than in Finnish men.

Urinary excretion of phytoestrogens can be used as a measure of intake and thus possible exposure and possible protection against cancer. Low urinary excretion of enterolactone in breast cancer patients was found in an epidemiological case–control study in Australia. Prospective studies from Finland and Sweden have shown low plasma concentrations of enterolactone to be associated with a high risk of breast cancer. However, the Swedish study also found a greatly increased risk of breast cancer in the highest quintile of enterolactone concentrations. A plasma enterolactone concentration of 30–80 nmol/l is therefore probably protective against breast cancer. Production of equol is associated with a decreased risk of breast cancer, and production of large amounts of equol is associated with an increased ratio of 2-hydroxyestrone to 16α-hydroxestrone in urine and this has been suggested to decrease breast cancer risk.

Japanese women and women of Japanese origin living in Hawaii but who consume a diet similar to the traditional Japanese diet (rich in soy products) have a low breast cancer incidence and mortality. Women in the Far East who have low rates of breast cancer are thought to consume approximately 30–50 times more soy products than women in the United States. A case–control study in Singapore found that premenopausal women who consumed 55 g of soy per day had a 50% reduced risk of breast cancer compared to women who infrequently consumed soy foods. A high intake of miso soup has been associated with a reduced risk of breast cancer in Japanese women. In prospective trials, a trend toward an inverse association between intake of tofu and subsequent risk of breast cancer and an inverse association between intake of miso soup and development of breast cancer have been found. However, a large prospective study in Japan did not show any effect of soy consumption on breast cancer risk, although this may be because dietary intake was studied in adult women rather than in children or adolescents. A number of studies in rodents have indicated that a protective effect of a soy isoflavone-rich diet may occur only if soya is consumed before puberty or during adolescence. Soy, if consumed throughout life, appears to protect against breast cancer, particularly if consumed before and during adolescence. Soy isoflavones may decrease breast cancer risk by influencing the menstrual cycle and endogenous sex hormone concentrations. In some but not all studies, increased concentrations of sex hormone binding globulin leading to lower free sex hormone concentrations and a longer menstrual cycle were observed.

A trend toward protective effects against prostate cancer of tofu but not miso has been shown in a large group (approximately 8000) of men of Japanese ancestry in Hawaii followed for 20 years. The latency period for prostate cancer appears to be lengthened in these men, who have a low mortality from prostate cancer. However, the incidence of *in situ* prostate cancer in autopsy studies is similar to that of men in Western countries. The consumption of soy isoflavones by these men may be responsible for this long latency period. This probably means that they die of other causes, including old age, before the prostate cancer can develop to a life-threatening stage. The three most recent studies all suggest that soy intake does protect against prostate cancer. Two studies showed that reduced risk is related to consumption of soy foods and one was a prospective study that showed that consumption of soy milk more than once a day was protective against prostate cancer.

Although soy and isoflavonoids appear not to protect against colon cancer, lignans or lignan-rich foods can protect against colon cancer development in animal models. There is also increasing evidence for cardioprotective effects, bone protective effects, and possibly cognitive benefits of phytoestrogens, and these are under investigation. A lower incidence of heart disease has been reported in populations consuming large amounts of soy products, often in combination with oily fish consumption, which also has cardioprotective benefits. Increased bone mineral density has been found in epidemiological studies in women with high dietary intakes of soy isoflavones. The incidence of dementia has been reported to be lower in Asian countries, particularly Japan, where consumption of soy isoflavones is high. Although one epidemiological study found an association between high intakes of tofu and cognitive impairment, other factors, including age and education, may explain this possible increased risk among tofu consumers.

Brassica Glucosinolates and Their Derivatives

Glucosinolates (previously known as thioglucosides) are sulfur-containing phytochemicals found in cruciferous or brassica vegetables, such as broccoli, cabbage, kale, cauliflower, and Brussels sprouts. Although approximately 100 different glucosinolates are found in the plant kingdom, only approximately 10 are found in brassica vegetables. They are also found in other plant foods. Degradation products of glucosinolates include other organosulfur compounds, such as the isothiocyanates and dithiothiols. Glucosinolate degradation products also include indoles.

Epidemiological data suggest that the relatively high content of glucosinolates and related compounds may be responsible for the observed protective effects of brassica vegetables in the majority of the 87 case–control studies and 7 cohort studies that have been carried out on the association between brassica consumption and cancer risk (**Tables 3–5**). In the case–control studies, 67% of studies showed an inverse association between consumption of brassica vegetables and risk of cancer at various sites. If individual brassica vegetables are considered, then the values for the number of studies that showed an inverse association between consumption of brassica vegetables and risk of cancer at various sites are as follows: broccoli, 56%; Brussels sprouts, 29%; cabbage, 70%; and cauliflower, 67%. The cohort studies showed inverse associations between broccoli consumption and the risk of all types of cancer taken together; between the consumption of brassicas and risk of stomach cancer and the occurrence of second primary cancers; and between the consumption of cabbage, cauliflower, and broccoli and the risk of lung cancer. Overall, it appears that a high consumption of brassica vegetables is associated with a decreased risk of cancer. The associations were most consistent for stomach, lung, rectal, and colon cancer. The epidemiological literature also provides some support for the hypothesis that high intakes of brassica vegetables can reduce risk of prostate cancer. Further epidemiological research is required to separate the cancer protective effects of brassica vegetables from those of vegetables in general.

Allium Organosulfur Compounds

There is increasing epidemiological evidence that other organosulfur compounds in addition to those derived from glucosinolates can protect against

Table 3 Case–control studies of stomach, colon, and rectal cancer showing inverse, null, or positive associations for the consumption of different types of phytochemical-rich fruit and vegetables

Fruit or vegetable type	No. of studies								
	Stomach cancer[a]			Colon cancer[b]			Rectal cancer[c]		
	Inverse	Null	Positive	Inverse	Null	Positive	Inverse	Null	Positive
Fruit	14	3	0	5	2	1	3	0	1
Citrus fruit	11	1	0	2	1	3	4	1	0
Tomatoes	9	1	1	4	0	2	3	2	1
Vegetables	11	0	0	8	0	1	2	0	2
Raw vegetables	10	0	0	3	0	1	—	—	—
Allium vegetables	9	1	1	4	1	1	2	0	1
Cruciferous vegetables	—	—	—	8	3	1	5	0	0
Green vegetables	8	0	0	4	1	0	—	—	—
Legumes	7	0	2	1	2	2	—	—	—
Carrots	7	1	1	—	—	—	4	0	1

[a]Data summarize the results from 31 studies (both statistically significant and nonsignificant results included).
[b]Data summarize the results from 21 studies (both statistically significant and nonsignificant results included).
[c]Data summarize the results from 13 studies (both statistically significant and nonsignificant results included).
Adapted from Steinmetz KA and Potter JD (1996) Vegetables, fruit and cancer prevention: A review. *Journal of the American Dietetic Association* **96**:1027–1039.

Table 4 Case–control studies of lung, breast, and pancreatic cancer showing inverse, null, or positive associations for the consumption of different types of phytochemical-rich fruit and vegetables

Fruit or vegetable type	No. of studies								
	Lung cancer[a]			Breast cancer[b]			Pancreatic cancer[c]		
	Inverse	Null	Positive	Inverse	Null	Positive	Inverse	Null	Positive
Fruit	8	0	0	3	0	1	6	1	0
Citrus fruit	—	—	—	1	0	2	1	2	0
Tomatoes	4	0	0	—	—	—	—	—	—
Vegetables	7	0	0	—	—	—	5	1	0
Raw vegetables	—	—	—	—	—	—	2	1	0
Green vegetables	9	0	0	5	1	0	—	—	—

[a]Data summarize the results from 13 studies (both statistically significant and nonsignificant results included).
[b]Data summarize the results from 13 studies (both statistically significant and nonsignificant results included).
[c]Data summarize the results from nine studies (both statistically significant and nonsignificant results included).
Adapted from Steinmetz KA and Potter JD (1996) Vegetables, fruit and cancer prevention: A review. *Journal of the American Dietetic Association* **96**: 1027–1039.

cancer. Allium species such as garlic (*Allium sativum*) and onions (*Allium cepa*) are a rich source of organosulfur compounds, such as the diallyl sulfides. There is epidemiological evidence from the Netherlands Cohort Study (120 852 men and women 55–69 years of age) for a strong inverse association between onion consumption and incidence of stomach carcinoma. However, the consumption of leeks and the use of garlic supplements were not associated with stomach carcinoma risk. The relative risk for stomach carcinoma in the highest onion consumption category (≥0.5 onions/day) was 0.50 (95% confidence interval, 0.26–0.95) compared to the lowest consumption category (no onions/day). However, this study did not support an inverse association between the consumption of onions and leeks and the use of garlic supplements and the incidence of male and female colon and rectal carcinoma. There is only limited epidemiological evidence concerning the beneficial influence of garlic organosulfur compounds on cardiovascular disease.

Potential Importance of Flavonoids to Human Health: Molecular Mechanisms of Action

Flavonoids possess a broad spectrum of biological actions ranging from anticarcinogenic to antiinflammatory, cardioprotective, immune-modulatory, and

Table 5 Cohort and case–control studies of all types of cancer showing inverse, null, or positive associations for the consumption of different types of phytochemical-rich fruit and vegetables

Fruit or vegetable type	All types of cancer[a]		
	Inverse	Null	Positive
Fruit	29	12	5
Citrus fruit	26	8	6
Tomatoes	35	5	10
Vegetables	55	4	9
Raw vegetables	33	4	2
Allium vegetables	27	3	4
Cruciferous vegetables	38	8	8
Green vegetables	61	5	13
Legumes	14	6	16
Carrots	50	7	7

[a]Data summarize the results from 194 studies (both statistically significant and nonsignificant results included).
Adapted from Steinmetz KA and Potter JD (1996) Vegetables, fruit and cancer prevention: A review. *Journal of the American Dietetic Association* **96**: 1027–1039.

antiviral. The mechanisms by which flavonoids cause these effects may include induction of the activity of some important enzymes while inhibiting the activity of others. Modulation of membrane function, including the activity of membrane-bound enzymes, through a protective membrane antioxidant action is likely to be of prime importance.

Membrane function is understood to be of vital importance to many cellular processes, including the role of membrane enzymes and receptors in cell growth and signalling. Membrane function may be influenced by dietary components directly by altering membrane fluidity or indirectly by protection against the free radical-mediated process of membrane lipid peroxidation. This can arise from oxidative stress and result in oxidative membrane damage. Flavonoids such as quercetin and myrecetin have been widely found to inhibit membrane lipid peroxidation. Flavonoids inhibit lipid peroxidation *in vitro* by acting as chain-breaking antioxidants: They donate a hydrogen atom to lipid radicals, thus terminating the chain reaction of lipid peroxidation. Additionally, flavonoids can act as metal chelating agents. Furthermore, kaempferol-3-O-galactoside protected mice against bromobenzene-induced hepatic lipid peroxidation. The relative potencies of flavonoids as antioxidants is governed by a set of structure–function relationships: In general, optimum antioxidant activity is associated with multiple phenolic groups, a double bond in C2–C3 of the C ring, a carbonyl group at C4 of the C ring, and free C3 (C ring) and C5 (A ring) hydroxy groups. It is of related interest that consumption of 300 ml of either black or green tea greatly increased

plasma antioxidant capacity in 10 volunteers. This suggests that normal levels of tea consumption could provide sufficient flavonoids to achieve a potentially health protective effect.

There is increasing evidence for the role of free radicals in the oxidative DNA damage implicated in carcinogenesis. The ability of flavonoids to act as antioxidants may contribute to the anticancer effects observed in animal models and human cells in culture *in vitro*, which could potentially be important to human health despite the current lack of epidemiological evidence and the finding that consumption of flavonoids in onions and black tea (providing 91 mg/day of quercetin for 2 weeks) by young healthy male and female subjects had no effect on oxidative DNA base damage in leucocytes. Quercetin has been shown to have growth inhibitory effects *in vitro* on breast cancer cells, colon cancer cells, squamous cell carcinoma cell lines, acute lymphoid and myeloid leukemia cell lines, and a lymphoblastoid cell line. These effects appear to be mediated *via* binding to cellular type 2 oestrogen binding sites. Furthermore, when the ability of two citrus flavonoids, hesperetin and naringenin (found in grapefruit mainly as its glycosylated form naringin), and three noncitrus flavonoids to inhibit the proliferation and growth of a human breast cancer cell line was investigated, the concentrations required to achieve 50% inhibition ranged from 5.9 to 56 μg/ml. The effectiveness of the citrus flavonoids was enhanced by using them in combination with quercetin, which is widely distributed in other foods. Quercetin fed to rats in the diet at levels of 2% or 5% inhibited the incidence and multiplicity of chemical carcinogen-induced mammary tumors. Mammary tumorigenesis in rats was delayed in the groups given orange juice (rich in citrus flavonoids together with other phytochemicals and nutrients) or fed the naringin-supplemented diet compared with the other groups. A number of the phenolic compounds of green tea, including the catechins, have been shown to inhibit tumour formation in rats induced by N-methyl-N'-nitro-N-nitrosoguanidine and also mutation induced by aflatoxin and benz(a)pyrene.

Quercetin has been shown to inhibit the activity of two enzymes that play an important role in mammary cell growth and development, tyrosine protein kinase activity and phosphoinositide phosphorylation, and it also inhibits protein kinase C, which is vital in the regulation of cellular proliferation. Blockade of the tyrosine kinase activity of the EGR receptor leading to growth inhibition and apoptosis in pancreatic tumor cells have been reported for quercetin and luteolin. Furthermore, inhibition of tumor growth through cell cycle arrest and induction of apoptosis by quercetin are thought to be functionally related to activation of the tumor suppressor protein p53. In addition, quercetin has been shown to regulate the growth of endometrial cancer cells (Ishikawa cell line) via suppression of EGF and the cell cycle protein, cyclin D1. A further mechanism for the antiproliferative action of quercetin may be via perturbation of microtubule functions such as polymerization through the binding of quercetin to tubulin, which induces conformational changes.

A number of mechanisms have been proposed for the protection by flavonoids against CHD, including antioxidant activity. Oxidative damage to low-density lipoprotein (LDL) (particularly to the apoprotein B molecule) is considered to be an important stage in the development of atherosclerosis: It is a prerequisite for macrophage uptake and cellular accumulation of cholesterol leading to the formation of the atheromal fatty streak. Flavonoids such as quercetin are effective inhibitors of *in vitro* oxidative modification of LDL by macrophages or copper ions. Although consumption of flavonoids in onions and black tea (providing 91 mg/day of quercetin for 2 weeks) by young healthy male and female subjects had no effect on plasma F_2-isoprostane concentrations (a biomarker of *in vivo* lipid peroxidation) or on resistance of LDL to copper–ion-induced oxidation, flavonoids in red wine have been reported to protect LDL against oxidative damage. The antioxidant properties of flavonoids may contribute to the reduced risk of CHD in wine drinkers, the so-called French paradox. Resveratrol, another phenolic phytochemical found in wine, has been shown to protect LDL against oxidative damage and appears to protect against cancer in animal models. Further studies on this interesting compound are clearly warranted.

Quercetin displays potent antithrombotic effects: It inhibits thrombin and ADP-induced platelet aggregation *in vitro*, and this may be through inhibition of phospholipase C activity rather than through inhibition of thromboxane synthesis. Flavonoid binding to platelet membranes may inhibit the interaction of activated platelets with vascular endothelium. In addition, quercetin elicits coronary vasorelaxation that is endothelium independent. The antioxidant activity of flavonoids may also prevent the damaging action of lipid peroxides generated by activated platelets on endothelial nitric oxide and prostacyclin, which both inhibit platelet aggregation and have vasodilatory activity.

The activity of flavonoids as inhibitors of the viral enzyme reverse transcriptase also suggests that they may be beneficial in the control of retroviral infections such as AIDS.

Possible adverse effects on human health should also be considered. Quercetin was reported to induce bladder cancer in rats when administered in the diet at a level of 2%. These results were not confirmed in another study, however, which used quercetin at levels reaching 10%. It should be noted that under certain *in vitro* conditions flavonoids and other phenols can act as prooxidants and cause DNA damage. However, phenols have complex pro- and antioxidant effects *in vitro*, depending on the assay system used, and it is often difficult to predict their net effect *in vivo*. For example, many synthetic and dietary polyphenols (including quercetin, catechin, gallic acid ester, and caffeic acid ester) can protect mammalian cells from the cytotoxicity induced by peroxides such as hydrogen peroxide. Although tea is a good source of flavonoids, phenolic compounds including tannins and also polyphenols and phenol monomers are good inhibitors of iron absorption, which could contribute to the nutritional problem of iron deficiency. In general, it is unlikely that sufficiently toxic quantities of any particular flavonoid could be consumed from the diet, which contains many diverse varieties of flavonoids in varying quantities.

Potential Importance of Phytoestrogens to Human Health: Molecular Mechanisms of Action

The probable beneficial effects of phytoestrogens against breast cancer are likely to be mediated via numerous mechanisms. However, it has not been fully established whether the protective effects of soya and cereals result from their phytoestrogen content or from some other effect.

Many studies utilising breast cells in culture such as the oestrogen-sensitive MCF-7 cell line show that phytoestrogens (genistein was used in most of studies) stimulate tumor growth at low concentrations while inhibiting growth at higher concentrations. Genistein is a potent and specific *in vitro* inhibitor of tyrosine kinase action in the autophosphorylation of the epidermal growth factor (EGF) receptor and is thus frequently used as a pharmacological tool. The EGF receptor is overexpressed in many cancers, particularly those with the greatest ability for metastasis, and it has therefore often been assumed that some of the anticancer effects of genistein are mediated *via* inhibition of tyrosine kinase activity. However, this is likely to be an oversimplification of the true *in vivo* situation.

Although genistein is a much better ligand for oestrogen receptor β (ERβ) than for the ERα (20-fold higher binding affinity), it can also act as an oestrogen agonist via both ERα and ERβ in some test systems. Mechanisms other than those involving oestrogen receptors are likely to be involved in the inhibition of cell proliferation by genistein because genistein inhibits both the EGF-stimulated and the 17β-oestradiol-stimulated growth of MCF-7 cells. Although studies have shown that exposure to genistein can reduce the tyrosine phosphorylation of cell proteins in whole cell lysates, studies using cultured human breast and prostate cancer cells have not confirmed that genistein has a direct effect on the autophosphorylation of the EGF receptor. Many other mechanisms of anticancer action for isoflavones and genistein in particular have been suggested, including inhibition of DNA topoisomerases, cell cycle progression, angiogenesis, tumor invasiveness, and enzymes involved in oestrogen biosynthesis. They also include effects on the expression of DNA transcription factors c-*fos* and c-*jun*, on reactive oxygen species, on oxidative membrane damage and oxidative damage *in vivo*, and on the negative growth factor, transforming growth factor-β (TGF-β).

Although cholesterol lowering is probably the best documented cardioprotective effect of soya, vascular protection is also likely to contribute and may be mediated via a number of mechanisms. Soya isoflavones are likely to contribute to the cardioprotective benefits of soya.

ERβ is the predominant ER isoform expressed in the rat, mouse, and human vascular wall. In the rat carotid injury model, following endothelial denudation of rat carotid artery, ERα is expressed at a low level, whereas the expression of ERβ increases by greater that 40-fold and treatment of ovariectomized female rats with genistein provides a similar dose-dependent vasculoprotective effect in this model to that observed with 17β-oestradiol. However, studies in ERβ knockout mice have shown that ERβ is not required for oestrogen-mediated inhibition of the response to vascular injury and suggest that either of the two known oestrogen receptors (or another unidentified one) is sufficient to protect against vascular injury.

Vascular protection could also be conferred by the ability of genistein to inhibit proliferation of vascular endothelial cells and smooth muscle cells and to increase levels of TGF-β. TGF-β helps maintain normal vessel wall structure and promotes smooth muscle cell differentiation while preventing their migration and proliferation. Genistein has been shown to increase TGF-β secretion by cells in culture, and increased TGF-β production may be a

mediator of some of the cardioprotective effects of soya isoflavones.

Antioxidant action is one of the mechanisms that may contribute to the vascular protective effects of soya isoflavones. Antioxidant properties have been reported for isoflavones both *in vitro* and *in vivo*. In a randomized crossover study of young healthy male and female subjects consuming diets that were rich in soy that was high (56 mg total isoflavones/day: 35 mg genistein and 21 mg daidzein) or low in isoflavones (2 mg total isoflavones/day), each for 2 weeks, plasma F_2-isoprostane concentrations were significantly lower after the high-isoflavone dietary treatment than after the low-isoflavone dietary treatment. The lag time for copper–ion-induced LDL oxidation was significantly longer.

Increased resistance to LDL oxidation has also been reported in a 12-week single open-group dietary intervention with soy foods (60 mg total isoflavones/day) in normal postmenopausal women. A randomized crossover study in hyperlipidemic male and female subjects consuming soya-based breakfast cereals (168 mg total isoflavones/day) and control breakfast cereals, each for 3 weeks, reported decreased oxidized LDL (total conjugated diene content) following consumption of the soy-based breakfast cereal compared to the control.

Effects of soya isoflavones on arterial function, including flow-mediated endothelium-dependent vasodilation (reflecting endothelial function) and systemic arterial compliance (reflecting arterial elasticity), may contribute to vascular protection and these have been measured in a number of studies. A randomized double-blind study administering either soy protein isolate (118 mg total isoflavones/day) or cesin placebo for 3 months to healthy male and postmenopausal subjects (50–75 years of age) showed a significant improvement in peripheral pulse wave velocity (reflecting peripheral vascular resistance and one component, together with systemic arterial compliance, of vascular function) but worsened flow-mediated vasodilation in men and had no significant effect on the flow-mediated vasodilation in postmenopausal women.

Some beneficial effects following dietary intervention with soy isoflavones have been observed on bone health, and the mechanism is likely to be via an oestrogenic action, particularly because ERβ is highly expressed in bone, although this requires further investigation. Consumption by postmenopausal women (6-month parallel group design) of soy protein (40 g/day providing either 56 mg isoflavones/day or 90 mg isoflavones/day) compared to caesin and nonfat dry milk (40 g/day) produced significant increases in bone mineral content (BMC) and bone mineral density (BMD) in the lumbar spine (but not in any other parts of the body) only in the higher isoflavone (90 mg/day) group compared to the control group. In a long-term study, consumption by postmenopausal women (2-year parallel group design) of isoflavone-rich soy milk (500 ml/day providing 76 mg isoflavones/day) compared to isoflavone-poor soy milk control (providing 1 mg isoflavones/day) resulted in no decline in BMC and BMD in the treatment group compared to significant losses in the control group. The ability to produce equol was associated with a better response to the treatment.

Some beneficial effects following dietary intervention with soy isoflavones have been observed on the cognitive function aspect of brain health, and the mechanism is likely to be via an oestrogenic action, particularly because ERβ, in addition to ERα, is expressed in brain. Although other mechanisms may contribute, they remain to be elucidated. Consumption by young healthy male and female subjects (parallel group design) of a high-soy diet (100 mg isoflavones/day for 10 weeks) compared to a low-soy diet (0.5 mg isoflavones/day) resulted in improved cognitive function, including significantly improved short-term and long-term memory and mental flexibility. These improvements were found in males and females. Consumption by postmenopausal women (parallel group design, placebo controlled) of a dietary supplement (soy extract containing 60 mg isoflavones/day for 12 weeks) resulted in improved cognitive function, particularly improved long-term memory.

Phytoestrogens can cause infertility in some animals and thus concerns have been raised over their consumption by human infants. The isoflavones found in a subterranean clover species (in Western Australia) have been identified as the agents responsible for an infertility syndrome in sheep. No reproductive abnormalities have been found in peripubertal rhesus monkeys or in people living in countries where soy consumption is high. Indeed, the finding that dietary isoflavones are excreted into breast milk by soy-consuming mothers suggests that in cultures in which consumption of soy products is the norm, breast-fed infants are exposed to high levels without any adverse effects. Isoflavone exposure soon after birth at a critical developmental period through breast feeding may protect against cancer and may be more important to the observation of lower cancer rates in populations in the Far East than adult dietary exposure to isoflavones. Although some controversy exists as to whether soy-based infant formulas containing isoflavones pose a health risk, a review of studies on the use of soy milk in infants suggests that there is no real basis for concern. Toxicity from isoflavones may arise from their action as alternative substrates for the enzyme thyroid peroxidase, and people in Southeast Asia would be protected by the dietary inclusion of iodine-rich seaweed products.

Potential Importance of Glucosinolate Derivatives and Related Compounds to Human Health: Molecular Mechanisms of Action

There may be some important health protective effects of glucosinolate derivatives and related compounds. The hydrolytic products of some glucosinolates have been shown to display anticancer properties. Glucosinolates are hydrolyzed following exposure to the endogenous plant enzyme myrosinase (also found in the gut microflora) to form isothiocyanates. Isothiocyanates are biologically active compounds with anticancer properties and are more bioavailable than glucosinolates.

A metabolite of glucobrassicin (3-indoylmethylglucosinolate), indole-3-carbinol has been shown to inhibit the growth of human tumors of the breast and ovary. Furthermore, indole-3-carbinol may modulate the oestrogen hydroxylation pathway such that a less potent form of oestradiol is produced, thus conferring protection against oestrogen-related cancers.

Consumption of Brussels sprouts (300 g/day of cooked sprouts) for 1 week has been shown to increase rectal glutathione S-transferase -α and -π isoenzyme levels. Enhanced levels of these detoxification enzymes may partly explain the epidemiological association between a high intake of glucosinolates in cruciferous vegetables and a decreased risk of colorectal cancer. It is likely that genetic polymorphisms and associated functional variations in biotransformation enzymes, particularly in glutathione S-transferases, will alter the cancer preventative effects of cruciferous vegetables.

Compounds including the isolated glucosinolate sinigrin and aqueous extracts of cooked and autolyzed Brussels sprouts (rich in glucosinolate degradation products) decreased hydrogen peroxide-induced DNA stand breaks in human lymphocytes and thus exerted a DNA-protective effect. Oral adminiatration of sinigrin has been shown to induce apoptosis and suppress aberrant crypt foci in the colonic mucosa of rats treated with 1,2-dimethylhydrazine. Similar effects were observed with oral administration of freshly prepared Brussels sprout juice, rich in glucosinolate breakdown products including isothiocyanates.

Isothiocyanates can prevent the formation of chemical carcinogen-induced tumors of the liver, lung, mammary gland, stomach, and oesophagus in animal models. The anticarcinogenic effects of isothiocyanates may be mediated by a combination of mechanisms, including inhibition of carcinogen activation by cytochromes P450: This could be achieved by both direct inhibition of enzyme catalytic activity and downregulation of enzyme levels and induction of phase 2 enzymes such as glutathione transferases and NAD(P)H:quinone reductase (these detoxify any remaining DNA-attacking electrophilic metabolites generated by phase 1 enzymes). Dietary glucosinolates and their breakdown products have been tested as anticarcinogens in terms of their ability to induce the anticarcinogenic phase 2 enzyme marker quinone reductase in murine Hep a1c1c7 cells, and the relative activities observed were found to be dependent on the nature of the side chain of the parent glucosinolate.

Phenethyl isothiocyanate protects mice against nitrosoamine-induced lung tumorigenesis. It also modulates the activity of phase 1 and phase 2 xenobiotic-metabolizing enzymes, resulting in the inhibition of the oxidative activation of a number of chemical carcinogens.

The isothiocyanate sulforophane is a particularly potent inducer of detoxification enzymes. A novel isothiocyanate-enriched broccoli has been developed that has an enhanced ability to induce phase 2 detoxification enzymes in mammalian cells compared to standard commercial broccoli.

Undesirable goitrogenic effects have been identified for isothiocyanates and other hydrolytic products of glucosinolates. Furthermore, in contrast to the anticancer effects of brassica vegetables discussed previously, a number of genotoxic effects have also been demonstrated in bacterial and mammalian cells. In bacterial assays (induction of point mutations in *Salmonella* TA98 and TA100 and repairable DNA damage in *Escherichia coli* K-12), juices from eight brassica vegetables tested caused genotoxic effects in the absence of metabolic activation. The order of potency was Brussels sprouts > white cabbage > cauliflower > green cabbage > kohlrabi > broccoli > turnip > black raddish. In mammalian cells, structural chromosome aberrations were observed with some of the juices, with the most potent being Brussels sprouts and white cabbage, and genotoxic effects were accompanied by decreased cell viability. The isothiocyanate-containing fraction (and other breakdown products of glucosinolates) of these brassica juices was found to contain 70–80% of the total genotoxic activity of the juices. The flavonoid- and other phenolic-containing fraction had a much weaker effect. In related studies, the isothiocyanates, allyl isothiocyanate and phenethyl isothiocyanate, were found to be more than 1000-fold more cytotoxic in a Chinese hamster ovary cell line than their parent glucosinolates (sinigrin and gluconasturtiin, respectively). Phenethyl isothiocyanate also induced genotoxic effects (chromosome aberrations and sister chromatid exchanges).

More data are required before an overall recommendation can be made regarding the likely beneficial or otherwise influences of glucosinolates (and their derivatives) on human health.

S-Methyl Cysteine Sulfoxide

S-methyl cysteine sulfoxide is another sulfur-containing phytochemical found in all brassica vegetables, in addition to glucosinolates. Both S-methyl cysteine sulfoxide and methyl methane thiosulfinate (its main metabolite) can block genotoxicity, induced by chemicals, in mice. S-methyl cysteine sulfoxide is thus likely to contribute to the observed ability of brassica vegetables to protect against cancer in both human and animal studies. It is of interest that a hydrolytic product of S-methyl cysteine sulfoxide was linked in the 1960s to the severe hemolytic anemia or kale poisoning observed in cattle in Europe in the 1930s.

Potential Importance of Other Phytochemicals to Human Health: Molecular Mechanisms of Action

Allium Organosulfur Compounds

Allium organosulfur compounds may be phyotchemicals of importance to human health by acting as antioxidants, thus protecting against free radical-mediated damage to important cellular targets such as DNA and membranes implicated in cancer and neurodegenerative diseases and aging. Protection against oxidative damage to LDL and cellular membranes could also protect against cardiovascular disease. Aged garlic extract (AGE) inhibits lipid peroxidation and the oxidative modification of LDL, reduces ischemic/reperfusion injury, and enhances the activity of the cellular antioxidant enzymes superoxide dismutase, catalase, and glutathione peroxidase. AGE also inhibits the activation of the oxidant-induced transcription factor NF-κB. Investigation of the major organosulfur compounds in AGE identified highly bioavailable water-soluble organosulfur compounds with antioxidant activity, such as S-allylcysteine and S-allylmeracptocysteine.

Organosulfur compounds such as diallyl sulfide may also protect against cancer by modulation of carcinogen metabolism, and this may involve altered ratios of phase 1 and phase 2 drug-metabolizing enzymes. Various garlic preparations including aged garlic extract have been shown to inhibit the formation of nitrosamine-type carcinogens in the stomach, enhance the excretion of carcinogen metabolites, and inhibit the activation of polyarene carcinogens. Inhibitory effects of organosulfur compounds on the growth of cancer cells *in vitro*, including human breast cancer cells and melanoma cells, have been observed. Modulation of cancer cell surface antigens, associated with cancer cell invasiveness, has been observed, and in some cases cancer cell differentiation can be induced. AGE can reduce the appearance of mammary tumors in rats treated with the powerful carcinogen dimethyl benz(*a*)anthracene (DMBA), which is activated by oxidation by cytochromes P450 to form the DNA binding form of DMBA diol epoxide, resulting in DNA legions and cancer initiation. The antibacterial activity of these allium compounds may also prevent bacterial conversion of nitrate to nitrite in the stomach. This may reduce the amount of nitrite available for reacting with secondary amines to form the nitrosamines likely to be carcinogenic particularly in the stomach.

Allium organosulfur compounds appear to possess a range of potentially cardioprotective effects. In one study, 432 cardiac patients were divided into a control group (210) and a garlic-supplemented group (222), and garlic feeding was found to reduce mortality by 50% in the second year and by approximately 66% in the third year. Furthermore, the rate of reinfarction was reduced by 30 and 60% in the second and third year, respectively. It should be noted that only a small number of patients in both groups experienced the end event of death or myocardial infarction, and a much larger scale study is needed. AGE lowers cholesterol and triglycerides in laboratory animals and can reduce blood clotting tendencies. It has been suggested that garlic supplementation at a level of 10–15 g of cooked garlic daily could lower serum cholesterol by 5–8% in hypercholestrolemic individuals. However, there may be more important cardioprotective effects of garlic. In animal studies, AGE suppressed the levels of plasma thromboxane B_2 and platelet factor levels, which are important factors in platelet aggregation and thrombosis. In rats, frequent low doses (50 mg/kg) of aqueous extracts of garlic or onions (onion was less potent) produced significant antithromotic activity (lowering of thromboxane B_2) without toxic side effects.

Aqueous extracts of raw garlic also inhibited cyclooxygenase activity in rabbit platelets, again contributing to an antithrombotic effect. In addition, AGE and S-allyl cysteine and S-allyl mercaptocysteine have antiplatelet adhesion effects. Platelet adhesion to the endothelial surface is involved in atherosclerosis initiation. Furthermore, S-allyl mercaptocysteine inhibits the proliferation of rat aortal smooth muscle cells, another important atherosclerotic process. Indeed, this antiproliferative effect on smooth muscle cells may be indicative of a possible antiangiogenic ability in relation to prevention of tumor growth and metastasis.

Saponins

Saponins are another steroidal phytochemical of interest that may, in addition to isoflavone phytoestrogens, contribute to the health protective effects of soya products. Soyabeans have a high saponin content and soyabean saponins have been shown to have a growth inhibitory effect on human carcinoma cell *in vitro*, probably by interacting with the cell membrane and increasing membrane permeability. The proposed anticarcinogenic mechanisms of saponins include normalization of carcinogen-induced cell proliferation, direct cytotoxicity, bile acid binding, and immune-modulating effects. Of particular interest is the finding that saponins actively interact with cell membrane components: They possess surface active characteristics because of the amphiphillic nature of their chemical structure. Thus, they can act to alter cell membrane permeability and cellular function. Soybean saponins have been reported to inhibit hydrogen peroxide damage to mouse fibroblast cells and thus may protect human health through antioxidant-mediated mechanisms.

Saponins from ginseng root (*Panax ginseng C.A. Mey.*) may also be important. Antioxidant effects have been reported for total ginseng saponins and its individual saponins (ginsenosides Rb1, Rb2, Rc, and Rd; others include Re and Rg1). Furthermore, ginsenosides Rb1 and Rb2 protected cultured rat myocardiocytes against superoxide radicals, and the mechanism for this may involve induction of genes responsible for antioxidant defences rather than radical scavenging. Ginsenosides stimulate endogenous production of nitric oxide in rat kidney, and this may contribute to the observed antinephritic action of these compounds and suggest a protective role in the kidney. Furthermore, it has been suggested that the observed cardioprotective effects of ginsenosides in animal models may be mediated by nitric oxide release. In addition, ginsenoside enhanced release of nitric oxide from endothelial cells, particularly from perivascular nitric oxidergic nerves in the corpus cavernosum of animal models, may partly account for the reported aphrodisiac effects of ginseng. Also, ginsenosides have been shown to have beneficial effects on inferior human sperm motility and progression. It is of interest that regulation of lipid metabolism by ginseng has been reported, and although the mechanism of action remains unclear, it is likely that the peroxisome proliferator-activated receptor-α is involved.

Other Phytochemicals of Interest

A wide range of other phytochemicals may have important beneficial effects on human health if consumed in sufficient amount to be efficacious. In many cases, their full spectrum of molecular actions remains to be elucidated. Nevertheless, the following phytochemicals and their main botanical sources are deemed worthy of mention.

The phytochemicals dihydrophthalic acid, ligustilide, butylidene, phthalide, and n-valerophenone-O-carboxylic acid have been isolated from Angelica root (*Angelica sinensis*). They are likely to contribute to the observed circulatory modulating effects of Angelica root, including increasing coronary flow, modulation of myocardial muscular contraction, and antithrombotic effects.

Phytochemicals extracted from licorice (*Glycyrrhiza glabra L.*) include glycyrrhetic acid, glycyrrhizic acid (the sweet principle of licorice), and an active saponin glycyrrhizin (a 3-O-diglucuronide of glycyrrhetic acid). In rats, dietary supplementation with 3% licorice elevated liver glutathione transferase activity, suggesting a potential detoxification and anticancer effect of these phytochemicals because glutathione transferase catalyses the formation of glutathione conjugates of toxic substances for elimination from the body. Antibacterial, antiviral, antioxidant, and antiinflammatory effects have also been reported for these compounds. Indeed, glycyrrhizin has been reported to inhibit HIV replication in cultures of peripheral blood mononuclear cells taken from HIV-seropositive patients.

Phytochemicals found in ginkgo (*G. biloba*) leaves, including ginkgolic acid, hydroginkgolic acid, ginkgol, bilobol, ginon, ginkgotoxin, ginkgolides (A–C), and a number of flavonoids common to other plants, such as kaempferol, quercetin, and rutin, are currently attracting attention for their possible effects on circulation, particularly cerebral circulation, and this may improve brain function and cognition. Indeed, ginkgo, ginseng, and a combination of the two extracts have been found to improve different aspects of cognition in healthy young volunteers. A number of studies have reported that extracts of ginkgo leaves enhanced brain circulation, increased the tolerance of the brain to hypoxia, and improved cerebral hemodynamics. It has been suggested that these effects are mediated via calcium ion flux over smooth cell membranes and via stimulation of catecholamine release. In addition, protection against free radical-mediated retinal injury has been reported; thus, other antioxidant-mediated protective effects on human health are also possible. Damage to mitochondrial DNA could play a role in neurodegenerative diseases such as Alzheimer's disease and Parkinson's disease. There is limited evidence for significant improvements in CHD patients following treatment with a daily dose equivalent to 12 mg total ginkgetin. Ginkgolide B-activated inhibition of glucocorticoid production has been reported and is likely to result from specific transcriptional suppression of the adrenal peripheral-type benzodiazepine receptor gene in rats. This suggests that ginkgolide B may be useful pharmacologically to control excess glucocorticoid formation.

See also: **Cancer**: Epidemiology and Associations Between Diet and Cancer. **Cereal Grains. Coronary Heart Disease**: Prevention. **Fruits and Vegetables**. **Phytochemicals**: Epidemiological Factors. **Tea.**

Further Reading

Adlercreutz CHT (2002) Phyto-oestrogens and cancer. *Lancet Oncology* 3: 32–41.

Arts IC, Hollman PC, Feskens EJ, Bueno de Mesquita HB, and Kromhout D (2001) Catechin intake might explain the inverse relationship between tea consumption and ischemic heart disease: The Zutphen Elderly Study. *American Journal of Clinical Nutrition* 74: 227–232.

Beatty ER, O'Reilly JD, England TG et al. (2000) Effect of dietary quercetin on oxidative DNA damage in healthy human subjects. *British Journal of Nutrition* 84: 919–925.

File SE, Jarrett N, Fluck E et al. (2001) Eating soya improves human memory. *Psychopharmacology* 157: 430–436.

Gupta K and Panda D (2002) Perturbation of microtubule polymerization by quercetin through tubilin binding: A novel mechanism of its antiproliferative activity. *Biochemistry* 41: 13029–13038.

Kim H, Xu J, Su Y et al. (2001) Actions of the soy phytoestrogen genistein in models of human chronic: Potential involvement of transforming growth factor β. *Biochemical Society Transactions* 29: 216–222.

Knekt P, Kumpulainen J, Jarvinen R et al. (2002) Flavonoid intake and risk of chronic diseases. *American Journal of Clinical Nutrition* 76: 560–568.

Mithen R, Faulkner K, Magrath R et al. (2003) Development of isothiocyanate-enriched broccoli and its enhanced ability to induce phase 2 detoxification enzymes in mammalian cells. *Theoretical Applied Genetics* 106: 727–734.

O'Reilly JD, Mallet AI, McAnlis GT et al. (2001) Consumption of flavonoids in onions and black tea: Lack of effect on F_2-isoprostanes and autoantibodies to oxidized LDL in healthy humans. *American Journal of Clinical Nutrition* 73: 1040–1044.

Rowland IR, Wiseman H, Sanders TAB, Adlercreutz H, and Bowey EA (2000) Interindividual variation in metabolism of soy isoflavones and lignans: Influence of habitual diet on equol production by the gut microflora. *Nutrition and Cancer* 36: 27–32.

Shapiro TA, Fahey JW, Wade KL, Stephenson KK, and Talalay P (2001) Chemoprotective glucosinolates and isothiocyanates of broccoli sprouts: Metabolism and excretion in humans. *Cancer Epidemiology Biomarkers and Prevention* 10: 501–508.

Thomson M and Ali M (2003) Garlic [allium sativum]: A review of its potential use as an anticancer agent. *Current Cancer Drug Targets* 3: 67–81.

Wiseman H (2000) The therapeutic potential of phytoestrogens. *Expert Opinion in Investigational Drugs* 9: 1829–1840.

Wiseman H, Goldfarb P, Ridgway T, and Wiseman A (2000) *Biomolecular Free Radical Toxicity: Causes and Prevention.* Chichester, UK: John Wiley.

Wiseman H, O'Reilly JD, Adlercreutz H *et al.* (2000) Isoflavone phytoestrogens consumed in soy decrease F_2-isoprostane concentrations and increase resistance of low-density lipoprotein to oxidation in humans. *American Journal of Clinical Nutrition* 72: 395–400.

Phyto-estrogens *see* **Phytochemicals**: Classification and Occurrence; Epidemiological Factors

Polyunsaturated Fatty Acids *see* **Fatty Acids**: Omega-3 Polyunsaturated; Omega-6 Polyunsaturated

POTASSIUM

L J Appel, Johns Hopkins University, Baltimore, MD, USA

The major intracellular cation in the body is potassium, which is maintained at a concentration of approximately 145 mmol/l of intracellular fluid but at much lower concentrations in the plasma and interstitial fluid (3.8–5 mmol/l of extracellular fluid). The high intracellular concentration of potassium is maintained via the activity of the Na^+/K^+-ATPase pump. Because this enzyme is stimulated by insulin, alterations in the plasma concentration of insulin can affect cellular influx of potassium and thus plasma concentration of potassium. Relatively small changes in the concentration of extracellular potassium greatly affect the extracellular/intracellular potassium ratio and thereby affect nerve transmission, muscle contraction, and vascular tone.

In unprocessed foods, potassium occurs mainly in association with bicarbonate-generating precursors such as citrate and, to a lesser extent, with phosphate. In processed foods to which potassium is added and in supplements, the form of potassium is potassium chloride. In healthy people, approximately 85% of dietary potassium is absorbed. Most potassium (approximately 77–90%) is excreted in urine, whereas the remainder is excreted mainly in feces, with much smaller amounts excreted in sweat. Because most potassium that is filtered by the glomerulus of the kidney is reabsorbed (70–80%) in the proximal tubule, only a small amount of filtered potassium reaches the distal tubule. The majority of potassium in urine results from secretion of potassium into the cortical collecting duct, a secretion regulated by a number of factors including the hormone aldosterone. An elevated plasma concentration of potassium stimulates the adrenal cortex to release aldosterone, which in turn increases secretion of potassium in the cortical collecting duct.

Acid–Base Considerations

A diet rich in potassium from fruits and vegetables favorably affects acid–base metabolism because these foods are also rich in precursors of bicarbonate. Acting as a buffer, the bicarbonate-yielding organic anions found in fruits and vegetables neutralize noncarbonic acids generated from meats and other high-protein foods. In the setting of an inadequate intake of bicarbonate precursors, excess acid in the blood titrates bone buffer. As a result, bone becomes demineralized and calcium is released. Urinary calcium excretion increases. This state has been termed a 'low-grade metabolic acidosis.' Increased bone breakdown and calcium-containing kidney stones are adverse clinical consequences of excess diet-derived acids. Diets rich in potassium with its bicarbonate precursors might prevent kidney stones and bone loss. In processed foods to which potassium is added and in potassium supplements, the conjugate anion is typically chloride, which cannot act as a buffer.

Adverse Effects of Insufficient Potassium

Severe potassium deficiency, which most commonly results from diuretic-induced potassium losses, is characterized by a serum potassium concentration of less than 3.5 mmol/l. The adverse consequences of hypokalemia are cardiac arrhythmias, muscle weakness, and glucose intolerance. Moderate potassium deficiency, which commonly results from an inadequate dietary intake of potassium, occurs without hypokalemia and is characterized by increased blood pressure, increased salt sensitivity, an increased risk of kidney stones, and increased bone turnover. An inadequate intake of dietary potassium may also increase the risk of stroke and perhaps other cardiovascular diseases.

Kidney Stones and Bone Demineralization

Because of its effects on acid–base balance, an increased dietary potassium intake might have favorable effects on kidney stone formation. In one large observational study of women (**Figure 1**), there was a progressive inverse relationship between greater intake of potassium and incident kidney stones. At a median potassium intake of 4.7 g/day (119 mmol/day), the risk of developing a kidney stone was 35% less compared to that for women with an intake of <2.0 g/day (52 mmol/day). In the one available trial, an intake of approximately 3.6–4.7 g/day (92–120 mmol/day) of potassium in

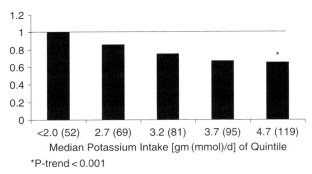

*P-trend < 0.001

Figure 1 Relative risk of kidney stones during 12 years of follow-up by quintile of potassium intake in 91 731 women. (Data from Curhan GC, Willett WC, Speizer FE, Spiegelman D, and Stampfer MJ (1997) Comparison of dietary calcium with supplemental calcium and other nutrients as factors affecting the risk of kidney stones in women. *Annals of Internal Medicine* **126**: 497–504.)

the form of potassium citrate reduced the risk of recurrent kidney stones.

Epidemiologic studies have consistently documented that increased potassium intake is associated with greater bone mineral density. In trials, supplemental potassium bicarbonate reduced bone turnover as manifest by less urinary calcium excretion and by biochemical evidence of greater bone formation and reduced bone resorption. However, no trial has tested the effect of increased potassium or diets rich in potassium on bone mineral density or clinical outcomes related to osteoporosis.

Elevated Blood Pressure

High levels of potassium intake are associated with reduced blood pressure. Observational data have been reasonably consistent in documenting this inverse relationship, whereas data from individual trials have been less consistent. However, three meta-analyses of these trials have each documented a significant inverse relationship between potassium intake and blood pressure in nonhypertensive and hypertensive individuals. In one meta-analysis, average net systolic/diastolic blood pressure reductions associated with a net increase in urinary potassium excretion of 2 g/day (50 mmol/day) were 4.4/2.4 mmHg. Typically, greater blood pressure reductions from potassium occur in African Americans compared to non-African Americans. Most of the trials that tested the effects of potassium on blood pressure used pill supplements, typically potassium chloride.

A high potassium intake has been shown to blunt the rise in blood pressure in response to increased salt intake. The term 'salt-sensitive blood pressure' applies to those individuals or subgroups who experience the greatest reduction in blood pressure when salt intake is reduced. One metabolic study of 38 healthy, nonhypertensive men (24 African Americans and 14 non-African Americans) investigated the effect of potassium supplementation on the pressor effect of salt loading (5.7 g/day of sodium (250 mmol)). Before potassium was supplemented, 79% of the African American men and 26% of the non-African American men were termed 'salt sensitive,' as defined by a salt-induced increase in mean arterial pressure of at least 3 mmHg. There was a progressive reduction in the frequency of salt sensitivity as the dose of potassium was increased. In the African Americans with severe salt sensitivity, increasing dietary potassium to 4.7 g/day (120 mmol/day) reduced the frequency of salt sensitivity to 20%, the same percentage as that observed in non-African American subjects when their potassium intake was increased to only 2.7 g/day (70 mmol/day).

Other studies indicate that potassium has greater blood pressure lowering in the context of a higher salt intake and lesser blood pressure reduction in the setting of a lower salt intake. Conversely, the blood pressure reduction from a reduced salt intake is greatest when potassium intake is low. These data are consistent with subadditive effects of reduced salt intake and increased potassium intake on blood pressure.

Cardiovascular Disease

The beneficial effects of potassium on blood pressure should reduce the occurrence of blood pressure-related cardiovascular disease. Potassium may also have protective effects that are independent of blood pressure reduction. This possibility has been tested in experimental studies conducted in rodents. In a series of animal models, the addition of either potassium chloride or potassium citrate markedly reduced mortality from stroke. Interestingly, these reductions occurred when blood pressure was held constant. Such data indicate that potassium has both blood pressure-dependent and blood pressure-independent properties that are cardioprotective.

In many, but not all, epidemiologic studies, an inverse relationship between dietary potassium intake and subsequent stroke-associated morbidity and mortality has been noted. A few observational studies have also shown an inverse association between potassium intake and coronary heart disease. In a 12-year follow-up of 859 men and women enrolled in the Rancho Bernardo Study, a significant inverse relationship between potassium intake and subsequent risk of stroke-related mortality was documented. Similarly, during the course of 8 years of follow-up in 43 738 US men in the Health Professionals Follow-Up Study, there was a significant inverse relationship between baseline potassium intake and stroke after adjustment for established cardiovascular disease risk factors, including blood pressure and caloric intake (**Figure 2**). In this study, a median potassium intake of 4.3 g/day (110 mmol/day) was associated with a 41% reduced risk of stroke in comparison to those with a median intake of 2.4 g/day (61 mmol/day). Consistent with these studies are other observational studies that have repeatedly documented a reduced risk of stroke from an increased intake of fruits and vegetables.

Adverse Effects of Excess Potassium Intake

In the generally healthy population with normal kidney function, a high potassium intake from foods poses no risk because excess potassium is

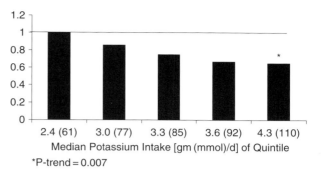

Figure 2 Relative risk of ischemic stroke by quintile of potassium intake in 43 738 men. (Data, from Ascherio A, Rimm EB, Hernan MA *et al.* (1998) Intake of potassium, magnesium, calcium, and fiber and risk of stroke among U.S. men. *Circulation* **98**: 1198–1204.)

readily excreted in the urine. In contrast, supplemental potassium can lead to acute toxicity in healthy individuals. Also, in individuals whose urinary potassium excretion is impaire a potassium intake less than 4.7 g/day (120 mmol/day) is appropriate because of adverse cardiac effects (arrhythmias) from hyperkalemia. Drugs that commonly impair potassium excretion are angiotensin converting enzyme inhibitors, angiotensin receptor blockers, and potassium-sparing diuretics. Common medical conditions associated with impaired potassium excretion are diabetes, chronic renal insufficiency, end stage renal disease, severe heart failure, and adrenal insufficiency. Elderly individuals are at increased risk of hyperkalemia because they often have one or more of these conditions or take one or more of the medications that impair potassium excretion.

Recommended Potassium Intake, Current Intake, and Dietary Sources

On the basis of available data, an Institute of Medicine committee set an Adequate Intake for potassium at 4.7 g/day (120 mmol/day) for adults. This level of dietary intake should maintain lower blood pressure levels, reduce the adverse effects of salt on blood pressure, reduce the risk of kidney stones, and possibly decrease bone loss. Current dietary intake of potassium is considerably lower than this level.

Humans evolved on a diet that was rich in potassium and bicarbonate precursors and low in salt. However, contemporary Western-style diets have the opposite pattern—that is, relatively low content of potassium and high content of salt. Based on intake data from the Third National Health and Nutrition Examination Survey (NHANES-III,1988–1994), the percentage of men and women who consumed equal to or more than 4.7 g/day (120 mmol/day) was less than 10 and 1%, respectively. Median intake of potassium in the United States ranged from 2.8 to 3.3 g/day (72 to 84 mmol/day) for adult men and 2.2 to 2.4 g/day (56 to 61 mmol/day) for adult women. The median potassium intake of non-African Americans exceeded that of African Americans. Because African Americans have a relatively low intake of potassium and a high prevalence of elevated blood pressure and salt sensitivity, this subgroup would especially benefit from an increased potassium intake.

Dietary intake surveys typically do not include estimates from salt substitutes and supplements. However, less than 10% of those surveyed in NHANES-III reported using salt substitutes or a reduced-sodium salt. Because a high dietary intake of potassium can be achieved through diet rather than pills and because potassium derived from foods also comes with bicarbonate precursors, as well as a variety of other nutrients, the preferred strategy to achieve the recommended potassium intake is to consume foods rather than supplements.

Dietary sources of potassium, as well as bicarbonate precursors, are fresh fruits, fruit juices, dried fruits, and vegetables. Although meat, milk, and cereal products contain potassium, their content of bicarbonate precursors does not sufficiently balance the amount of acid-forming precursors, such as sulfur amino acids, found in higher protein foods. The typical content of potassium-rich foods is displayed in **Table 1**. Salt substitutes currently available in the marketplace range from 0.4 to 2.8 g/teaspoon (11–72 mmol/teaspoon) of potassium, all as potassium chloride.

Conclusion

Potassium is an essential nutrient that is required for normal cellular function. Although humans evolved on diets rich in potassium, contemporary diets are quite low in potassium. An increased intake of potassium from foods should prevent many of the adverse effects of inadequate potassium intake, which are higher blood pressure levels, greater salt sensitivity, increased risk of kidney stones, and possibly increased bone loss. An inadequate potassium level may also increase the risk of stroke. In view of the high prevalence of elevated blood pressure, stroke, and conditions related to bone demineralization (i.e., osteoporosis and kidney stones) in the general population, individuals should strive to increase their consumption of potassium-rich foods, particularly fruits and vegetables.

Table 1 Foods rich in potassium

Food	Portion size	Potassium content, g (meq)
Beans		
Cooked dried beans	1/2 cup	0.4 (10.7)
Lima beans	5/8 cup	0.4 (10.8)
Fruit		
Apple	1 medium	0.1 (2.8)
Apricots	3 medium	0.3 (7.2)
Banana	6 in.	0.4 (9.5)
Cantaloupe	1/4 medium	0.3 (6.4)
Dates	10 pitted	0.6 (16.6)
Orange	1 small	0.3 (7.7)
Peach	1 medium	0.2 (5.2)
Prunes, dried	10 medium	0.7 (17.8)
Raisins	1 tablespoon	0.1 (2.0)
Watermelon	1 slice	0.6 (15.4)
Fruit juices		
Grapefruit	1 cup	0.4 (10.4)
Orange	1 cup	0.5 (12.4)
Pineapple	1 cup	0.4 (9.2)
Tomato	1 cup	0.5 (13.7)
Vegetables		
Corn	1 ear	0.2 (5.0)
Potato		
– White	1 boiled	0.3 (7.3)
– Sweet	1 boiled	0.3 (7.7)
Tomato	1 medium	0.4 (9.4)
Squash, winter	1/2 cup boiled	0.5 (11.9)
Meats		
Hamburger	1 patty	0.4 (9.8)
Rib roast	2 slices	0.4 (11.2)
Fish (e.g., haddock)	1 medium fillet	0.3 (8.0)
Milk		
Skim milk	8 oz.	0.3 (8.5)
Whole milk	8 oz.	0.4 (9.0)

See also: **Bone**. **Electrolytes**: Acid-Base Balance. **Hypertension**: Etiology; Dietary Factors; Nutritional Management. **Osteoporosis**.

Further Reading

Ascherio A, Rimm EB, Hernan MA *et al.* (1998) Intake of potassium, magnesium, calcium, and fiber and risk of stroke among U.S. men. *Circulation* 98: 1198–1204.

Bazzano LA, Serdula MK, and Liu S (2003) Dietary intake of fruits and vegetables and risk of cardiovascular disease. *Current Atherosclerosis Reports* 5: 492–499.

Curhan GC, Willett WC, Speizer FE, Spiegelman D, and Stampfer MJ (1997) Comparison of dietary calcium with supplemental calcium and other nutrients as factors affecting the risk of kidney stones in women. *Annals of Internal Medicine* 126: 497–504.

He FJ and MacGregor GA (2001) Beneficial effects of potassium. *British Medical Journal* 323: 497–501.

Institute of Medicine (2004) *Dietary Reference Intakes for Water, Potassium, Sodium, Chloride and Sulfate*. Washington, DC: National Academy of Sciences.

Lemann J, Bushinsky D, and Hamm LL (2003) Bone buffering of acid and base in humans. *American Journal of Physiology* 285: F811–F832.

Morris RC Jr, Sebastian A, Forman A, Tanaka M, and Schmidlin O (1999) Normotensive salt-sensitivity: Effects of race and dietary potassium. *Hypertension* 33: 18–23.

Whelton PK, He J, Cutler JA *et al.* (1997) Effects of oral potassium on blood pressure. Meta-analysis of randomized controlled clinical trials. *Journal of the American Medical Association* 277: 1624–1632.

Poultry *see* **Meat, Poultry and Meat Products**

PREGNANCY

Contents
Role of Placenta in Nutrient Transfer
Nutrient Requirements
Energy Requirements and Metabolic Adaptations
Weight Gain
Safe Diet for Pregnancy
Dietary Guidelines and Safe Supplement Use
Prevention of Neural Tube Defects
Pre-eclampsia and Diet

Role of Placenta in Nutrient Transfer

P Haggarty, Rowett Research Institute, Aberdeen, UK

Introduction

The main nutritional role of the placenta is to provide the correct mix of nutrients in sufficient quantities to support fetal growth and development throughout pregnancy. It has to do this whilst coping with wide variations in maternal nutrient intake between pregnancies and temporal variations within a pregnancy. The effective barrier to nutrients within the placenta is a single layer of cells called the syncytiotrophoblast, which close to term is around 4 μm thick with a total exchangeable surface area of around 10–15 m^2. This membrane represents a nutritional 'bottleneck' where competition for nutrient transporters and metabolic selectivity allows the placenta to regulate the nutrient mix within the fetal circulation to one best suited to fetal development. In addition to its role as a simple nutrient transporter the placenta also acts as an extra fetal organ for many metabolic transformations with the feto-placental unit working as a metabolic whole. Adaptive mechanisms within the placenta allow the mother to meet the nutrient demands of the growing fetus whist consuming apparently poor diets during pregnancy. The fetus itself plays an active role in regulating key aspects of placental metabolism and nutrient transfer function to meet its own nutrient requirements.

Under normal circumstances the nutrient transfer capacity of the human placenta exceeds the fetal requirement and a considerable proportion of transport function would have to be lost before it became limiting for fetal growth. Although relatively rare, intrauterine growth restriction resulting from uteroplacental insufficiency does occur. However, this is a complicated syndrome in which almost all aspects of placental and fetal metabolism are altered and it may not simply be due to a limitation of placental nutrient transfer capacity.

Fetal Nutrient Requirements

Prenatal development can usefully be divided into two periods: the embryonic period, which covers the first 8 weeks of life, and the fetal period, which lasts from the 9th week of gestation until term. During the latter period the fetus is entirely dependent on the placenta for its supply of nutrients. The fetus has an absolute requirement for the same essential nutrients as the adult but the adequacy of supply is particularly critical during *in utero* life when all the structures of the body are being established. In addition, because of the particularly high demand for some strictly nonessential nutrients these may be considered as 'conditionally essential' if the rate of utilization exceeds the fetal capacity for *de novo* synthesis.

The placenta has to maintain the supply of all nutrients at a rate adequate to allow unrestricted fetal growth. It also has to provide an appropriate mix of nutrients to meet the needs of the fetus at the different stages of pregnancy. For example, in the first two-thirds of pregnancy the fetus deposits mainly protein, while in late gestation fat takes over as the dominant form of deposition (**Figure 1**).

The availability of individual nutrients to the fetus depends not only on the maternal dietary intake but also on the function of the placenta and the many physiological and biochemical adaptations that occur during pregnancy (**Figure 2**). An understanding of placental function and its interaction with diet is essential to the setting of appropriate dietary guidelines for pregnancy.

The Human Placenta

The human placenta is a hemochorial, villous type where the maternal blood enters the intervillous space via the spiral arteries and flows directly around the terminal villi of the fetal circulation without any intervening maternal vessel wall. The surface area available for exchange gradually increases throughout pregnancy until it reaches around 10–15 m^2 in the last trimester (**Figure 1**). The nature of the exchangeable surface of the placenta also changes throughout gestation with the mature intermediate villi appearing towards the end of the second trimester and the terminal villi, which represent the main site of feto-maternal exchange, appearing a few weeks later. The rate of fetal blood delivery to the placenta (umbilical flow) also changes markedly during pregnancy and is approximately linearly related to fetal weight, and hence the fetal nutrient requirement, throughout gestation (**Figure 1**).

Anatomically, the human placenta is a large structure typically weighing around half a kilogram. However, its physical bulk belies the flimsy nature of the separation between the maternal and fetal

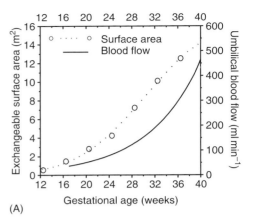

(A)

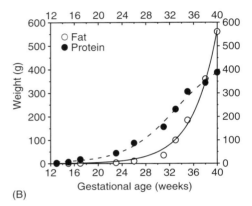

(B)

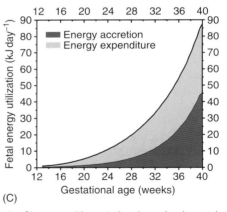

(C)

Figure 1 Changes with gestational age in placental exchangeable surface area and umbilical blood flow (A), accretion of fat and protein in the fetus (B), and the components of fetal energy requirements (C). (Reproduced with permission from: Sutton MS, Theard MA, Bhatia SJ, Plappert T, Saltzman DH, and Doubilet P (1990) Changes in placental blood flow in the normal human fetus with gestational age. *Pediatric Research* **28**: 383–387;Widdowson EM (1968) Growth and composition of the fetus and newborn. In: Assali NS (ed.) *The Biology of Gestation*, pp. 1–49 New York: Academic Press; Sparks JW (1984) Human intrauterine growth and nutrient accretion. *Seminars in Perinatology* **8**: 74–93.)

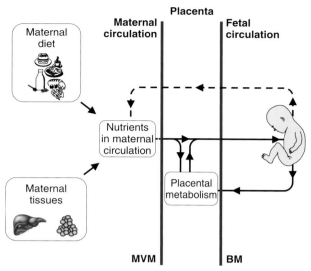

Figure 2 Nutrient exchanges between the maternal circulation, placenta, and fetus.

circulations, which consists of only two cell layers; the syncytiotrophoblast and the capillary endothelium. The endothelium allows the passage of nutrients through pores within the interendothelial cleft and therefore is not a significant barrier to nutrient passage. The effective barrier between the maternal and fetal circulation is provided by a thin trophoblastic cover in the form of a syncytium (a tissue in which the cytoplasm of constituent cells is continuous), known as the syncytiotrophoblast. Between 10 weeks and term the thickness of the villous trophoblast falls from around 10 µm to 4 µm and the overall maternofetal diffusion distance from 40 µm to 5 µm. Any substance crossing between the maternal and fetal circulation has to pass though this barrier, which consists of two membranes: the micovillous membrane (MVM) facing the maternal blood and the basal membrane (BM) facing the fetal blood. The surface area of the maternal-facing MVM is around 5–6 times that of the fetal-facing BM. There are other cell types and structures within the placenta, such as maternal myometrium and decidua, connective tissue, Hofbauer cells, and persisting cytotrophoblast cells, which contribute to the metabolic activity and nutrient requirements of the placenta but which are not thought to be significant barriers to transport.

Methods Used to Study Placental Function

Direct measurement of placental nutrient transport function in human pregnancy is practically and ethically extremely difficult to achieve. All of the

available techniques have drawbacks and involve a trade-off between physiological relevance and the quality of the information derived. There is a very small number of reports of studies where stable isotope-labeled amino acids and fatty acids have been administered to the mother and their appearance measured in the cord blood. These studies have the potential to provide information on dynamic placental nutrient transfer rates *in vivo* but their interpretation is severely constrained by the number of sequential cord blood samples that can be taken, and the conclusions have therefore been necessarily tentative. Placental function is often inferred by measurements of concentration differences in the maternal and fetal circulations. The most sophisticated of these involve measurements of arterio-venous differences across the umbilical cord at Caesarean section before the cord is cut but such studies are therefore only carried out in very late gestation. Cord blood levels may also be measured following delivery or, more informatively, at earlier stages of development using the invasive method of cordocentesis. However, an important disadvantage of any 'snapshot' of cord blood nutrient concentrations is that these are the net result of both placental delivery and fetal utilization.

Because of the problems with interpretation of results from *in vivo* studies a number of *in vitro* approaches have been developed. These include the dually perfused placenta, which retains the cellular structure and metabolic activity of the syncytiotrophoblast and the placental vascular structure but allows the nutrient composition of the maternal and fetal circulation to be controlled and transfer rates to be measured dynamically using isotopic tracers. The problems with this *ex vivo* technique are that the placenta tends to be very mature, the efficiency of perfusion cannot be assumed to exactly mimic the *in vivo* situation, and the composition of the maternal and fetal perfusates are not truly physiological. More detailed but less physiologically relevant to absolute rates of transfer are vesicles formed from the syncytiotrophoblast, which are particularly well suited to the study of nutrient transport mechanisms under highly controlled conditions. The most reductionist methodology involved the identification and characterization of individual transport proteins.

The Mechanisms of Placental Nutrient Transport

The transport of individual nutrients across the placenta generally depends on the same principles

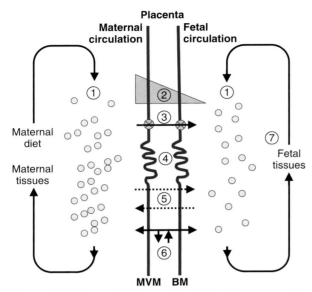

Figure 3 Factors affecting nutrient transfer across the syncytiotrophoblast. These include: (1) maternal and fetal blood flow; (2) the nutrient concentration gradient across the syncytiotrophoblast; (3) the concentration of transport proteins to facilitate or actively transport nutrients; (4) the exchangeable surface area; (5) the rate of diffusion of some nutrients across membranes without the intervention of transport proteins; (6) metabolism (utilization and *de novo* synthesis) within the placenta; and (7) the rate of nutrient utilization by the fetal tissues.

and the presence of the same or similar transport systems to those in the tissues and organs of the adult, although there are some additional factors specific to the placenta (**Figure 3**). In particular, unlike most tissues in the adult where either uptake or export dominate at any given time, the syncytiotrophoblast whose primary function is transport has to do both simultaneously.

The placental transport systems for the macronutrients (carbohydrate, fat, and protein) have been extensively studied. Glucose transport within the placenta appears to be mediated exclusively by the GLUT1 transporter, which has been located on both the MVM and BM. GLUT3 and GLUT4 are also present in the placenta but not in the syncytiotrophoblast itself. They are located on the vascular endothelium and the intravillous stromal cells, respectively. The syncytiotrophoblast also contains a wide range of amino acid transporters: system A, ASC, Asc, B^0, $b^{0,+}$, L, N, Gly, y^+, y^+L and X_{AG} and β. A number of fatty acid-binding proteins are also found in the placenta. Of these proteins FAT/CD36 and FATP have been located to both the MVM and BM but there is also a placenta-specific protein (p-FABPpm), which has been located exclusively on the MVM. This p-FABPpm is similar in size ($\sim$40 kDa) to the ubiquitous FABPpm found in

most mammalian cells but it has a different amino acid composition.

The driving force that results in the net transfer of nutrients to the fetus is different for different nutrients and this is reflected in their transplacental gradients (**Figure 4**). Where the nutrient concentrations are lower in the cord than maternal blood this has been cited as a reason to supplement the mother but in many cases it is precisely this gradient that drives placental nutrient transfer. Glucose is thought to flow down a concentration gradient from the mother to the fetus and this process of 'facilitated diffusion' is mediated by GLUT1. Unlike glucose the concentration of most amino acids in the fetal circulation is greater than that in the maternal circulation suggesting some form of active transport. For many amino acids the concentration is even higher within the placenta than the fetal circulation and the key gradient generating step for amino acids is the active transport across the MVM. The amino acids can then diffuse down a concentration gradient into the fetal circulation, and to some extent back to the mother. The concentration of water-soluble vitamins and lactate in the fetal circulation also exceeds that in the maternal circulation.

Like glucose, the fats and fat-soluble vitamins also flow down a concentration gradient from the mother to the fetus mediated by the various fatty acid transport proteins. However, unlike glucose or the amino acids, fat-soluble compounds can also cross the syncytiotrophoblast, and all other membranes for that matter, by simple diffusion and partition without the intervention of a carrier protein. The role of the fatty acid-binding proteins appears to be to improve the efficiency of this process. The key factor in understanding the driving force for the placental transfer of fat-soluble nutrients is that these compounds are only sparingly soluble in water (13 μM for C18:0 at 37 °C) and have to be transported in the plasma in hydrophobic binding sites on carrier proteins. The partition of fats between the maternal and fetal circulations is largely determined by the relative abundance of available hydrophobic binding sites within those compartments. Since only NEFA are thought to cross membranes it is the NEFA concentration gradient that is most relevant to the transplacental flow of fatty acids. The concentration of NEFA in the maternal plasma at term is around 3 times that in the fetal circulation but the concentration of its primary carrier protein, albumin, is actually 10–20% higher in the fetal circulation. This results in a ratio of NEFA to albumin on the fetal side of the placenta of around a quarter of that on the

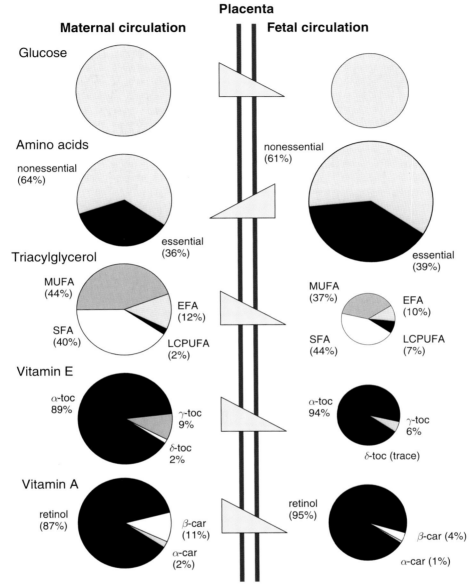

Figure 4 The relative concentration of nutrients in the maternal and fetal circulations. The concentration differences for each nutrient class are represented by the area of the circle in the fetal circulation relative to the maternal circulation. Apart from glucose the relative concentrations of individual nutrients within the nutrient groups are shown as segments of the circle. For triglyceride the fractions are saturated (SFA) monounsaturated (MUFA), essential (EFA), and long-chain polyunsaturated fatty acids (LCPUFA). For vitamin E the fractions are α-tocopherol (α-toc), γ-tocopherol (γ-toc), and δ-tocopherol (δ-toc). For vitamin A the abbreviated fractions are β-carotene (β-car) and α-carotene (α-car). (Reproduced with permission from: Berghaus TM, Demmelmair H, and Koletzko B (1998) Fatty acid composition of lipid classes in maternal and cord plasma at birth. *European Journal of Pediatrics* **157**: 763–768; Kiely M, Cogan PF, Kearney PJ and Morrissey PA (1999) Concentrations of tocopherols and carotenoids in maternal and cord blood plasma. *European Journal of Clinical Nutrition* **53**: 711–715; Cetin I., Marconi AM, Bozzetti P, Sereni LP, Corbetta C, Pardi G, and Battaglia FC (1988) Umbilical amino acid concentrations in appropriate and small for gestational age infants: a biochemical difference present *in utero*. *American Journal of Obstetrics and Gynecology* **158**: 120–126; Bozzetti P, Ferrari MM, Marconi AM, Ferrazzi E, Pardi G, Makowski EL, and Battaglia FC (1988) The relationship of maternal and fetal glucose concentrations in the human from midgestation until term. *Metabolism* **37**: 358–363.)

maternal side at term. The fat-soluble vitamins (A, E, and D) are also present in the fetal circulation in lower concentrations than in the maternal circulation. These materno-fetal concentration differences for the macronutrients develop gradually throughout gestation.

It is less easy to generalize about the transplacental gradient for minerals as some are at a

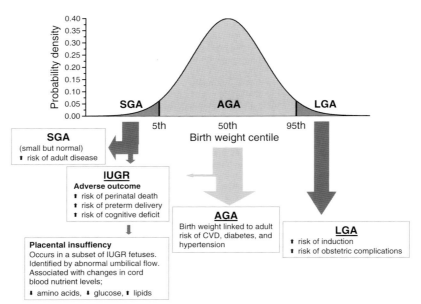

Figure 5   The normal distribution of birth weights and relative risks associated with babies that are small for gestational age (SGA), appropriate for gestational age (AGA), large for gestational age (LGA) and those subjected to intrauterine growth retardation (IUGR), and the relationship to placental insufficiency.

lower concentration in the fetal circulation (Se, Cu, Ba), some are higher (Ca, Zn, Be, Rb), and some are about the same (Co, Mg, Mo, Sn, Bi, Cd, Cs, La, Li, Pb). Iron is particularly important during pregnancy and its concentration in the fetal venous blood leaving the placenta is almost 3 times that of the maternal serum. Iron is transported in the serum on the transport protein transferrin and, like the fats and fat-soluble vitamins, its rate of transfer may be influenced by the availability of free binding sites.

Placental Selectivity

One of the key functions of placental nutrient transport is to maintain the most appropriate balance of nutrients in the fetal circulation and the balance of nutrients transferred by the placenta may be as important as the overall transfer capacity in influencing the pattern of fetal growth. Nutrients such as the fatty acids and amino acids occur in many forms yet they are translocated across membranes by a relatively small number of transporter molecules. This nutritional 'bottleneck' results in competition for transfer and the possibility of placental selectivity. An example of the resulting change in nutrient quality can be seen in the increase in the relative proportion of the essential to nonessential amino acids in the fetal circulation compared to the maternal circulation (**Figure 4**). The same is true of the fat-soluble vitamins where the relative concentration of the most biologically

active form is increased in the fetal circulation. In the case of the fatty acids it is the long-chain polyunsaturated fatty acids (LCPUFA) such as arachidonic acid (20:4 n-6; AA) and docosahexaenoic acid (22:6 n-3; DHA) that perform most of the essential functions in the fetus. Although the overall concentration of the lipid classes are greatly reduced in the fetal circulation the critical LCPUFA make up a greater proportion of total fatty acid in the fetal circulation. In the case of the fatty acids the placenta has multiple mechanisms including preferential binding of LCPUFA by p-FABPpm, selective uptake by the syncytiotrophoblast, intracellular metabolic channeling of individual fatty acids, and selective export to the fetal circulation, which allow it to preferentially deliver DHA and AA to the fetal circulation.

Placental Metabolic Activity

Although the barrier between the maternal and fetal circulation is effectively only one cell thick, the placenta is a substantial organ made up of many cell types. It is extremely active metabolically and has its own requirement for nutrients and this is consistent with the observations that the surface area of the maternal-facing membrane (MVM) is around 5 times greater than that of the fetal-facing membrane (BM), that the concentration of expression of GLUT1 is greater on the MVM, that the MVM contains additional fatty acid binding proteins that are not present on the BM, and that the amino acid transporters act to produce the maximum amino acid gradient across the MVM. The metabolic transformations within the placenta are intimately linked to fetal metabolism and represent another way in which the placenta can regulate nutrient transport availability within the fetal circulation.

In late pregnancy the overall contribution of fat to whole body oxidation is reduced and this is thought to result from the preferential utilization of carbohydrate and amino acids such as glutamate as an energy source in the feto-placental unit and the sparing of fatty acids to maximize fetal accretion of the critical LCPUFA in particular. The interrelationships between the placenta and fetus are particularly complex for the amino acids. The placenta is a net user of serine, glutamate, leucine, isoleucine, and valine and there is significant interconversion of alanine, pyruvate, and lactate between the placenta and fetal tissues. The concentration of lactate in the fetal circulation is considerably greater than that in the maternal circulation and a considerable proportion of the glucose taken up by the placenta is converted into lactate prior to export into the fetal circulation for use by the fetus. The placenta takes up serine from both the maternal and fetal circulation, converting this into glycine and exporting it into the fetal circulation for oxidation by the fetal liver and there is significant cycling of glutamate and glutamine between the placenta and fetal liver. This partition of the various segments of metabolic pathways between the placenta and fetal tissues is a general phenomenon and in many respects the feto-placental unit can be considered as a metabolic whole with the placenta acting as an extra fetal organ in addition to its role as a simple nutrient transporter. Metabolic activity in the feto-placental unit is also responsive to nutrient supply and fetal demand. For example, AA is an important precursor of the prostacyclins, prostaglandins, thromboxanes, and leukotrienes, which play key roles in pregnancy. When the maternal circulation of AA is low there is net uptake from the fetal circulation to maintain placental synthesis of these compounds.

Placental Buffering of Maternal Dietary Intake

In cases where the increased demand for nutrients during pregnancy is not met by the diet alone the shortfall may be made up from the maternal stores and the placenta may play a role in orchestrating some of the maternal nutritional adaptations in pregnancy. For example, placentally derived leptin is a potent stimulator of lipolysis and there is evidence that the rate of export into the maternal circulation is controlled to allow the placenta to modulate its own substrate supply in response to the fetal demand for fats. The various homeostatic mechanisms within the placenta and their interaction with maternal physiological adaptations during pregnancy act to ensure a constant supply of substrate to the fetus, free of large diurnal fluctuations corresponding to the timing of maternal meals, and to protect the fetus against a transiently poor intake during critical periods of fetal growth. These adaptations help the mother to meet the full fetal requirement for nutrients such as LCPUFA and iron whilst consuming apparently poor diets.

Placental Insufficiency and Fetal Growth

Potentially the most important public health issue relating to pregnancy is the epidemiological association between birth weight and adult disease susceptibility (cardiovascular disease, diabetes, and hypertension). The highest risk is associated with the lowest birth weight but, because of the nature of the normal distribution, in terms of the numbers potentially affected in adult life, it is the small variations in the normal birth weight range that have the largest public health implications. A causal connection between birth weight and adult disease has been proposed in the 'fetal origins' hypothesis, which is that fetal undernutrition in middle to late gestation leads to disproportionate fetal growth and programs later disease susceptibility. The close association between birth weight and placental weight has led to speculation that the placenta may limit fetal growth within the normal weight range. However, the available evidence suggests that the capacity of the human placenta to transport macronutrients exceeds the fetal requirement and that a considerable proportion of transport function would have to be lost before it became limiting for fetal growth.

True intrauterine growth restriction (IUGR) resulting from utero-placental insufficiency is a serious pathology that is associated with a greatly increased risk of adverse outcomes including perinatal mortality and morbidity, impaired mental, visual and aural development, autism, and cerebral palsy. IUGR is often detected indirectly by measuring abnormal umbilical artery flow velocity waveforms and/or abnormal fetal heart rate. The abnormal waveforms are thought to result from increased vascular resistance associated with abnormal arteriolar tree and villi branching and a reduction in the villous capillary tree. Pregnancies in which these abnormalities are observed are also associated with fetal hypoxia and reduced concentrations of glucose and amino acids in the fetal circulation and reduced activity of the system A amino acid transporter within the placenta. However, *in vitro* studies have shown that the hypoglycemia observed in some IUGR fetuses is not caused by a decreased glucose transport capacity within the placenta (expression and activity of GLUT1) and IUGR fetuses are actually hypertriglyceridemic compared to their appropriately grown counterparts. The fetal blood concentrations of the trace elements are also either normal or elevated in IUGR. Thus, while it is possible that the placenta from IUGR fetuses may limit the supply of amino acids there is no evidence that placental delivery is the first limiting factor in the supply of glucose, lipids, or trace elements. IUGR is a complicated syndrome in which almost all aspects of placental and fetal metabolism are altered and many researchers have emphasized the primary importance of the fetal hypoxia and its effects on fetal metabolism rather than a simple limitation of placental nutrient transfer capacity.

There is considerable uncertainty about the magnitude of the problem of IUGR. The lowest 5% of weight-for-gestational-age babies (defined according to well-nourished fetal growth centile charts) are referred to as small for gestational age (SGA) but babies in this range need not be growth retarded but may be naturally small and have no increased risk of adverse outcome. A further complication is that a baby born within the normal birth weight range could have suffered growth retardation *in utero* if its genetic potential was for a higher birth weight. The true incidence of IUGR resulting from uteroplacental insufficiency is therefore unknown but if it is defined in relation to umbilical flow or fetal heart rate abnormalities then it is only a fraction of even those in the lowest 5% of weight-for-gestational-age that are affected by uteroplacental insufficiency. At the other end of the spectrum babies that are large-for-gestational-age (LGA) are at higher risk of adverse obstetric outcomes and early developmental problems but there is no evidence that LGA or macrosomic babies are produced as a result of a primary alteration in the placenta.

The Role of the Fetus

The nutrient composition of the human diet varies enormously among populations yet the healthy human newborn is essentially the same the world over. The available evidence points to extensive homeostatic mechanisms at work within the placenta to ameliorate some of the variation in the quality of the maternal diet by regulating the mix of nutrients to the developing fetus. However, these mechanisms can only operate on the nutrients already available in the maternal circulation. The maternal diet and maternal circulating concentrations of many nutrients are major determinants of the concentrations in the fetal circulation and the fetus clearly has the ability to cope with relatively large variations in nutrient availability in the cord blood. The fetus also plays an active role in regulating placental nutrient transfer. The rate of placental nutrient transport is directly influenced by the transplacental concentration gradient, which is in turn largely determined by the rate of uptake by the fetal tissues. Another major determinant of placental nutrient transfer is the umbilical blood flow, which is approximately linearly related to the fetal weight, and hence the fetal nutrient requirement, throughout gestation. Finally, the most intimate connection between the fetus and the placenta is the way in which different parts of metabolic pathways and cycles are distributed between the placenta and fetal tissues, mainly the fetal liver. Thus, whilst the placenta has to provide the correct mix of nutrients in sufficient quantities to support fetal growth and development throughout pregnancy it is the fetus itself that ultimately regulates many key aspects of placental nutrient transfer function.

Acknowledgements

The author acknowledges the support of SEERAD.

See also: **Early Origins of Disease**: Fetal. **Low Birthweight and Preterm Infants**: Causes, Prevalence and Prevention. **Pregnancy**: Nutrient Requirements; Energy Requirements and Metabolic Adaptations; Safe Diet for Pregnancy.

Further Reading

Cetin I (2003) Placental transport of amino acids in normal and growth-restricted pregnancies. *European Journal of Obstetrics, Gynecology, and Reproductive Biology*, 110(supplement 1): S50–S54.

Dutta-Roy AK (2000) Transport mechanisms for long-chain polyunsaturated fatty acids in the human placenta. *American Journal of Clinical Nutrition* 71: 315S–322S.

Gagnon R (2003) Placental insufficiency and its consequences. *European Journal of Obstetrics, Gynecology, and Reproductive Biology* 110: S99–S107.

Haggarty P (2002) Placental regulation of fatty acid delivery and its effect on fetal growth – a review. *Placenta* 23(supplement A): S28–S38.

Hay WW Jr (1995) Metabolic interrelationships of placenta and fetus. *Placenta* **16**: 19–30.

Illsley NP (2000) Glucose transporters in the human placenta. *Placenta* **21**(1): 14–22.

Jansson T, Ylven K, Wennergren M, and Powell TL (2002) Glucose transport and system A activity in syncytiotrophoblast microvillous and basal plasma membranes in intrauterine growth restriction. *Placenta* **23**(5): 392–399.

Kaufmann P and Scheffen I (1998) Placental development. In: Polin RA and Fox WW (eds.) *Fetal and Neonatal Physiology*, pp. 59–70. W.B. Philadelphia: Saunders Company.

Marconi AM, Paolini C, Buscaglia M, Zerbe G, Battaglia FC, and Pardi G (1996) The impact of gestational age and fetal growth on the maternal-fetal glucose concentration difference. *Obstetrics and Gynecology* **87**: 937–942.

Pardi G, Marconi AM, and Cetin I (2002) Placental-fetal interrelationship in IUGR fetuses – a review. *Placenta* **23**(supplement A): S136–141.

Sparks JW (1984) Human intrauterine growth and nutrient accretion. *Seminars in Perinatology* **8**: 74–93.

Regnault TR, de Vrijer B, and Battaglia FC (2002) Transport and metabolism of amino acids in placenta. *Endocrine* **19**(1): 23–41.

Nutrient Requirements

L H Allen, University of California at Davis, Davis, CA, USA

Providing pregnant women with their nutrient needs is a public health priority in both wealthier and poorer countries, although the local resources to attain this objective may vary widely. The inability to meet nutrient requirements during pregnancy can have serious and often long-term adverse effects on development during the fetal and postpartum period and on maternal health. Most of the research that provides information on nutrient requirements during pregnancy has been conducted in industrialized countries, although trials in developing countries have been important in revealing the adverse effects of maternal nutrition and the benefits of nutrient interventions. In general, even in wealthier countries there is an unacceptably high rate of pregnancy complications that may be prevented by improved maternal nutrition, including anemia, low birth weight, birth defects, and preeclampsia. The situation is far worse in poorer regions of the world, however.

The most recent and best described recommended intakes of nutrients during pregnancy are those of the Institute of Medicine, developed for the United States and Canada, and these are the main set presented in this article (**Table 1**). The recommendations for the United Kingdom were published in 1992 and are discussed here when recommendations differ substantially from those of the Institute of Medicine. Many other countries have their own sets of recommendations, as do organizations such as the Food and Agriculture Organization/World Health Organization and the European Economic Community.

The set of Dietary Reference Intake (DRI) recommendations developed by the Institute of Medicine includes several values. The Estimated Average Requirement (EAR) is the intake required to meet the nutrient needs of 50% of a population group (e.g., pregnant women). It is an important value for two reasons. First, it is the value used to estimate the prevalence of inadequate intakes of a nutrient in a population group; the percentage of a group consuming less than the EAR of a nutrient is the percentage with an inadequate intake. For energy, the Estimated Energy Requirement is equivalent to the EAR. Second, the Recommended Dietary Allowance (RDA) is calculated by adding two standard deviations (usually unknown but assumed to be 20%) to the EAR. The RDA should meet the requirements of 97.5% of a population group. The Tolerable Upper Level (UL) for a nutrient is the intake above which there is a risk of adverse effects.

Table 1 shows the RDA for nonpregnant women and the EAR, RDA, and UL for pregnant women.

Energy

Maternal energy requirements increase during pregnancy due to higher basal energy expenditure as well as energy deposition in maternal and fetal tissues. Basal metabolism of the mother is higher due to the increased work by the lungs and heart and because of the metabolism of the fetus and uterus. A longitudinal study by Butte *et al.* found that basal metabolic rate increased by 10.7 ± 5.4 kcal per week of gestation, mostly in the second and third trimesters. On average, the fetus requires approximately 168 kcal/day. The substantial variability in basal energy expenditure among individual women is caused mainly by differences in fat-free mass (including maternal skeletal muscle mass and fetal tissue). The cumulative increase in basal energy expenditure during pregnancy is positively correlated with maternal fatness and weight gain. Energy requirements for the thermic effect of feeding are not different from those of nonpregnant women, nor is there much change in the total energy cost of activity. Although the increasing body weight of the mother means that the energy cost of each activity is higher, the net effect is cancelled out by the fact that after approximately 25 weeks of gestation

Table 1 Recommended Dietary Allowances (RDAs) for nonpregnant and pregnant women and Estimated Average Requirements (EARs) and Upper Limits of nutrients for pregnant women[a]

	AI/RDA,[b]adult woman	EAR, pregnancy	AI/RDA,[b]pregnancy	Upper Limit, pregnancy
Energy (kcal)	2200	2500	—	—
Energy (MJ)	9.2	10.5	—	—
Protein	50	+21	+25	None
Vitamins				
Vitamin A (μg retinol activity equivalents)	800	550	770	3000
Vitamin D (μg)	5	—	5	50
Vitamin E (mg α-tocopherol)	15	12	15	1000
Vitamin K (μg)	90	—	90	None
Vitamin C (mg)	75	70	85	2000
Folate (μg dietary folate equivalents)	400	520	600	1000 from fortified food + supplements
Thiamin (mg)	1.1	1.2	1.4	None
Riboflavin (mg)	1.1	1.2	1.4	None
Vitamin B_6 (mg)	1.3	1.6	1.9	100 as pyridoxine
Niacin (mg NE)	14	14	18	35
Vitamin B_{12} (μg)	2.4	2.2	2.6	None
Pantothenic acid (mg)	5	—	6	None
Biotin (μg)	30	—	30	None
Choline (mg)	425	—	450	3500
Minerals and trace elements				
Calcium (mg)	1000	—	1000	2500
Phosphorus (mg)	700	580	700	3500
Magnesium (mg)	320	300	360	+350 as supplement
Iron (mg)	18	22	27	45
Zinc (mg)	8	9.5	11	40
Iodine (μg)	150	160	220	1100
Copper (μg)	900	800	1000	10 000
Selenium (μg)	55	49	60	400
Chromium (μg)	25	—	30	None
Fluoride (mg)	3	—	3	10
Manganese (mg)	1.8	—	2	11
Molybdenum (μg)	34	40	50	2000

[a]Dietary Reference Intakes published by the Institute of Medicine, National Academy Press, for the United States and Canada (http://www.nap.edu).
[b]Values are RDAs except for vitamins D and K, pantothenic acid, biotin, choline, calcium, chromium, fluoride, and manganese, where value is an Adequate Intake (AI).

women tend to become less active. The longitudinal study by Butte *et al.* suggests that energy expenditure in physical activity decreases by approximately 100–200 kcal/day in women with a low or normal body mass index prior to pregnancy and by an average of more than 400 kcal/day in those with a high body mass index (>26 kg/m²).

In deriving the recommendations for the United States and Canada, the Estimated Energy Requirement (EER) during pregnancy is accepted to be the sum of the Total Energy Expenditure (TEE) of the nonpregnant woman, measured using a doubly labeled water technique, plus an estimated median change in TEE of 8 kcal/week, plus 180 kcal/day to cover energy deposited in maternal and fetal tissues. In the first trimester of pregnancy, TEE changes little and weight gain is small, so the energy requirement is increased only during the second and third trimesters. There is no RDA or UL because energy intakes greater than the EER would lead to undesirable weight gain.

The EER for pregnancy is as follows:

Trimester 1: nonpregnant EER + 0 kcal

Trimester 2: nonpregnant EER
+ 160 kcal (based on 8 kcal/week × 20 weeks) + 180 kcal

Trimester 3: nonpregnant EER
+ 272 kcal (based on 8 kcal/week × 34 weeks) + 180 kcal

Note that these formulae present average requirements in trimesters 1 and 2. If a more precise estimate of requirements is needed at a specific stage of gestation, instead of the mean increment of 160 kcal in trimester 1 and 272 kcal in trimester 2, the actual weeks of gestation can be multiplied by 8 kcal per week.

The UK recommendation is for an additional 200 kcal (0.8 MJ)/day above the prepregnant EAR but only in the last trimester. The recommendation is lower than that in the United States and Canada, in part because of the observation that the actual increase in energy intake during pregnancy is usually small.

Protein

The turnover of body protein is higher after approximately 13 weeks of pregnancy, and the mother adjusts by losing less nitrogen as urea even during the first trimester. A woman who gains 12.5 kg of body weight has deposited 925 g of protein, the fetus gains 440 g, the uterus 166 g, expanded maternal blood volume contains 81 g, the placenta 100 g, and the increment in extracellular fluid 135 g. The mother probably stores some additional protein in her body, presumably in muscle. The EAR for all age groups is 0.88 g/kg/day protein or 21 g of additional protein/day. The RDA is 1.1 g protein/kg/day or 25 g/day.

One-third of the 925 g total protein deposition during the 40 weeks of pregnancy occurs in the second trimester and two-thirds in the third trimester. By the end of the third trimester, the US–Canada recommendations assume that an additional consumption of 17 g protein/day is required to meet the needs for protein deposition, and since about half of this occurs during the second trimester this amounts to 8 g/day. It is also assumed that no additional protein is needed in trimester 1, but for the last two trimesters consumption of an additional 21 g/day (a total of 1.1 g/kg/day) is recommended. Recommended protein intakes for UK women are that an additional 6 g should be consumed during all three trimesters.

No UL has been set for protein, including for pregnancy, in the US–Canada recommendations due to lack of data on harmful effects. However, some earlier studies noted adverse pregnancy outcomes when high-protein supplements were given to relatively well-nourished pregnant women, so caution in this regard is certainly warranted.

Vitamins

Folic Acid

Maternal folate requirements increase markedly during pregnancy due to the utilization of the vitamin in cell division in the mother and fetus, single-carbon transfer reactions, and deposition in the fetus. Approximately a decade ago, research including randomized controlled trials finally proved that the risk of women giving birth to an infant with a neural tube defect (NTD) was significantly reduced if they consumed folic acid supplements prior to conception through approximately the first 4–6 weeks of pregnancy—during the time of neural tube closure. Some women are at greater risk of producing an infant with this birth defect, especially when their folate intake is rather low. Because such women are unaware of this risk unless they have had a previous NTD delivery, the recommendation is that all women who are capable of becoming pregnant consume at least 400 μg of folic acid daily from supplements, fortified food, or both in addition to consuming food folate from a varied diet.

In pregnancy, the recommendation is for all women to consume an additional 200 μg dietary folate equivalents daily (approximately 100 μg of folic acid as a supplement, which is more than twice as bioavailable as folate in food) in addition to the RDA for the nonpregnant woman of 400 μg/day. This amount was shown to prevent plasma homocysteine from becoming elevated during pregnancy and to maintain normal folate concentration in red blood cells. The UL of 1000 μg/day, the same as for nonpregnant women, is set to avoid potential exacerbation of vitamin B_{12} deficiency.

In the United Kingdom, the recommendation is substantially lower—an intake of 100 μg folate daily in addition to the recommendation of 200 μg/day for the nonpregnant, nonlactating woman. The UK committee's recommendation was based on the assumption that 100 μg/day will maintain plasma and erythrocyte folate concentrations at least at the level of those of nonpregnant women. Prevention of NTDs was not discussed, probably in part because the results of folic acid intervention trials were not clear at the time the recommendations were set.

In addition to its importance for lowering risk of NTDs in the periconceptional period, there is evidence that adequate folate status, which is important for maintaining normal plasma homocysteine concentrations, lowers the risk of other delivery problems and birth defects, including preeclampsia, preterm delivery, very low birth weight, club foot, and placental abruption. In the United States, Canada, and many other countries (more than 20 in Latin America alone), wheat flour is fortified with folic acid to ensure adequate folate status for pregnant women.

Other B Vitamins

Several B vitamin deficiencies cause homocysteinemia, notably folic acid, vitamin B_{12}, riboflavin, and vitamin B_6. Importantly, homocysteinemia is associated with adverse pregnancy outcomes. In a large retrospective study in Norway, for example, women in the highest 25% of plasma homocysteine concentrations had significantly more placental abruption, stillbirths, very low-birth-weight and preterm infants, preeclampsia, club foot, and NTDs in their offspring compared to women with values in the lowest 25%. Supplementation with folic acid up to 500–600 μg/day lowers plasma homocysteine, but few studies have been done on the other B vitamins. Of these, it is most difficult for poor women to obtain their dietary vitamin B_{12} requirement because this vitamin in found only in animal source foods, such as meat and dairy products.

The recommended intakes of most B vitamins and choline are increased above nonpregnant values as shown in **Table 1** The increases are based on evidence for higher maternal requirements (in the case of thiamin, riboflavin, niacin, and vitamin B_6) and for fetal and placental deposition of the vitamin (thiamin, riboflavin, niacin, vitamin B_6, vitamin B_{12}, and choline). UL values, the same as for nonpregnant women, have been set for niacin when consumed as nicotinic acid in supplements based on a 'flushing' reaction and for choline based on cholinergic reactions and a fishy body odor.

Vitamin A

The increment in vitamin A requirements during pregnancy is based on the amount of the vitamin that is found in fetal liver at birth. The liver content is assumed to be 36 μg, mostly accumulated during the last 3 months of gestation. Using an estimated 70% absorption of the vitamin from the maternal diet, the EAR is 50 μg above the requirement for the nonpregnant woman, whereas the RDA is 20% higher (60 μg).

In wealthier regions of the world, vitamin A deficiency during pregnancy is rare. Rather, there is more concern about the potentially adverse effects of consuming excessive amounts of the vitamin. Based on the potential for retinol excess to cause birth defects (malformations), especially if high doses are consumed early in pregnancy, a UL of 3000 μg/day is set for all women who may become pregnant as well as those who are pregnant. This intake is unlikely to be achieved with natural food, although it would be possible if large amounts of liver, foods fortified with the vitamin, or supplements were consumed. One situation in which this

restrictive UL becomes important is in the context of developing countries where high-dose vitamin A supplements are provided to postpartum women and their infants as part of the Expanded Program on Immunization, National Vitamin A Days, or similar programs. It is accepted that it is only safe to provide these high-dose supplements to the mother during the first 6 weeks postpartum, in case she becomes pregnant again.

Nevertheless, it is important to provide pregnant women with their recommended intake of the vitamin because one major study in Nepal showed a 40% reduction in infection-related maternal mortality by supplementing the women with approximately their RDA as retinol per week. Supplementation with β-carotene reduced mortality by 49%, and it is a nontoxic alternative. Additional trials to confirm the benefits of maternal supplementation with the vitamin in deficient populations are ongoing.

Vitamin D

In the form of 25(OH) cholecalciferol, vitamin D is transferred from the mother to the fetus in relatively small amounts that do not appear to cause maternal depletion. Those women who obtain adequate exposure to ultraviolet light do not need higher amounts during pregnancy. However, if usual intake declines below 150 IU (3.8 μg)/day at high latitudes (where there is little ultraviolet radiation in the winter, such as in France), evidence of low maternal 25(OH) cholecalciferol and infant depletion has been observed at delivery.

The recommendation for both adolescent and adult women is to continue to consume the amount recommended as adequate (the Adequate Intake (AI)) for nonpregnant women, 5 μg (200 IU/day). The UL of 50 μg (2000 IU/day) is the same as before pregnancy, based on prevention of high serum calcium concentrations. In the United Kingdom, the recommended intake is higher at 10 μg/day, which is probably appropriate based on its generally more northern latitude (thus less ultraviolet radiation) and lower synthesis of the vitamin in skin.

Vitamin C (Ascorbic Acid)

The EAR for nonpregnant women is based on the intake that attains the maximum neutrophil concentration of ascorbic acid. Maternal plasma vitamin C concentrations decline during pregnancy, probably as a result of normal hemodilution. Oxidized ascorbic acid is transferred from the maternal circulation to the fetus, where it is retained in the reduced form. Although vitamin C deficiency in pregnancy is rare in most situations, it has been associated with premature rupture of the membranes, increased risk of infections, preterm birth, and eclampsia. Smokers have lower levels of ascorbic acid in their serum and amniotic fluid. Based on the amount known to prevent infants from developing scurvy, the EAR is increased by 10 mg/day to 66 mg/day for those 14–18 years old and to 70 mg/day for adult women, and the RDA is 80 and 85 mg/day for these groups, respectively. The recommended intake is also increased by 10 mg/day in the United Kingdom. Women who smoke more than 20 cigarettes per day and regular aspirin users may require twice as much, as may heavy users of alcohol and street drugs. The UL of 2000 mg/day is based on prevention of diarrhea and gastrointestinal disturbances that occur with high intakes.

Vitamin E

There is no increase in the recommended intake of vitamin E during pregnancy, so the RDA remains at 15 mg of α-tocopherol/day for all ages. There have been no reports of deficiency of vitamin E during pregnancy nor any evidence of benefit from maternal supplementation. The UL is 1000 µg/day of any form of the vitamin taken as a supplement, extrapolated from data showing that high levels cause hemorrhaging in rats.

Minerals

Calcium

It has become recognized relatively recently that changes in maternal calciotropic hormones and calcium metabolism (i.e., increased intestinal absorption and reduced urinary excretion) enable the fetus to be supplied with adequate amounts of this mineral, and that little change in maternal intake is needed. There is no correlation between the number of pregnancies a woman has and her risk of bone fracture, so the maternal skeleton does not serve as the calcium reservoir for the fetus. Thus, for the United States and Canada there is no increase in recommended calcium intakes for pregnancy and the AI recommendation remains at 1300 mg/day for women aged 14–18 years and 1000 mg/day for the 18- to 51-year-old group. In the United Kingdom, the recommendation is also that no increase in intake is required during pregnancy, although the level of intake for nonpregnant, nonlactating women is considerably lower at 700 mg/day.

In a series of 14 randomized, controlled calcium intervention studies in different countries, increasing calcium intake in the range of 375–2000 mg/day reduced maternal blood pressure and the risk of pregnancy-induced hypertension and preeclampsia by 30–40%, with a greater effect in populations that consumed diets relatively low in calcium. The multicenter Calcium for Preeclampsia Prevention trial on 4589 pregnant women in the United States found no such benefits of a 2000 mg/day supplement, presumably because of reasonably high usual intakes of the mineral. It is possible that women at higher risk of pregnancy-induced hypertension, such as those with very low calcium intakes or adolescents, may benefit from calcium supplementation.

The UL for calcium in pregnancy is the same as that for the nonpregnant woman, 2500 mg/day. This safe level is set based on documented cases of 'milk-alkali syndrome,' in which there is high blood calcium, renal failure, and sometimes metabolic alkalosis as a result of chronic consumption of high calcium intakes.

Phosphorus

The efficiency of phosphorus absorption increases by 15% during pregnancy. The term infant contains approximately 17 g of phosphorus at birth, mostly in bone and water. The physiological adaptations of the mother that increase calcium retention also help to supply the fetus with more phosphorus. There is no evidence that the EAR needs to increase over that recommended for the nonpregnant women, so the RDA for women aged 14–18 years is 1250 mg/day and for those aged 19–50 years it is 700 mg/day. Based on the need to avoid high serum phosphorus concentrations, and the fact that phosphorus absorption is more efficient in pregnancy, the UL is set at 3500 mg/day, slightly lower than the 4000 mg/day for nonpregnant women.

Magnesium

It is assumed that the gain in fat-free mass in pregnancy (7.5 kg) is associated with a greater deposition of magnesium. If this tissue contains 470 mg/kg, after adjustment for a bioavailability of 40%, the EAR is an increase of 35 mg/day for pregnant women of all ages, and the RDA is 10% higher than this; for women aged 14–18 years, the EAR and RDA respectively are 335 and 400 mg; for those aged 19–30 years, these values are 290 and 350 mg; and for those 31–50 years, they are 300 and 360 mg. In the United Kingdom, there is no increment for magnesium in pregnancy based on the assumption that phosphorus metabolism becomes more efficient to meet fetal needs.

The UL for magnesium in pregnancy is set at 350 mg/day taken as a supplement, based on the potential for higher doses of magnesium salts to cause an osmotic diarrhea.

Iron

Incremental iron requirements for the mother and fetus are relatively well established, although how these requirements should be met is more controversial. It is generally accepted that the mother needs to absorb an additional 6 mg/day to supply the amount retained by the fetus (300 mg) and placenta (60 mg) and that used to synthesize additional maternal erythrocytes (450 mg) and replace blood loss during delivery (200 mg). Some iron is saved by the lack of menstruation in pregnancy. The fetus obtains iron from the placenta in a process that involves iron transfer from maternal transferrin to transferrin receptors on the placenta, endocytosis of holotransferrin, and release of iron into the fetal circulation. Maternal iron absorption and transfer to the fetus increases during the second and third trimesters. This process is upregulated if the mother is iron deficient, although in recent years it has become apparent that maternal iron deficiency does reduce the amount of fetal iron stored at birth and available to the fetus during the first months of life.

The EAR for pregnancy is set at 23 mg/day for adolescents and 22 mg/day for adult women, and the RDA is 27 mg/day for both groups. Although the requirement is mainly in the last trimester, it is important to build iron stores early and to avoid high doses later, so the higher intake recommendation is distributed throughout pregnancy. The UL is the same as that for the nonpregnant woman and is based on the need to avoid gastrointestinal distress.

It has been calculated that the maternal diet can supply enough iron to meet these increased needs during pregnancy, especially if maternal iron stores are adequate at conception. For this reason, the United Kingdom does not recommend that iron intake be increased during pregnancy, except when there is evidence of iron deficiency anemia. Iron deficiency anemia is a relatively common occurrence during pregnancy, especially in the following situations: Maternal iron status is poor at conception, and maternal diet is low in absorbable iron including heme iron from meat, fish, and poultry. The World Health Organization estimates that approximately 18% of women in industrialized countries and 35–75% of those in developing countries develop iron deficiency anemia during pregnancy. In the United States, the Centers for Disease Control

and Prevention reports that anemia affects 10% of low-income women in the first trimester, 14% in the second, and 33% in the last, with a much higher proportion of women becoming iron depleted by term. Accepted cut points for adequate hemoglobin concentration are 110 g/l in trimesters 1 and 3 and 105 g/l in trimester 2 due to midpregnancy hemodilution.

In most countries, iron supplements are recommended routinely for all pregnant women. Benefits clearly include reduction of anemia risk, improved maternal and iron status that can persist through the early postpartum period, and possibly some protection against low birth weight. The amount recommended has been reduced from former levels of 60–120 mg to 30 mg for nonanemic women and 60 mg for anemic women. The World Health Organization recommends 60 mg/day plus 400 µg folic acid, starting as soon as pregnancy is confirmed, but recognizes that 30 mg/day may be as effective as 60 mg/day. The folic acid recommendation was originally set based on older studies showing development of folate deficiency anemia in women. Although the risk of this anemia is probably low on a global scale, folic acid supplementation is recognized to have other potential benefits. Some countries still recommend iron supplementation only when pregnant women become anemic. There has also been considerable controversy concerning the best time to start supplementation.

Zinc

The estimated additional zinc required for pregnancy is approximately 100 mg, equivalent to 5–7% of the mother's body zinc, part of which is obtained through more efficient intestinal zinc absorption. Approximately half of this is deposited in the fetus. The EAR for pregnant women is based on an additional requirement of 2.7 mg/day during the last 10 weeks of gestation. The UL is based on evidence of impaired copper status at high intakes, as for nonpregnant women. No increment is recommended for pregnancy in the UK report, based on the assumption that needs can be met through adjustments in maternal zinc metabolism.

Zinc plays critical roles in cell division, hormone metabolism, protein and carbohydrate metabolism, and immunocompetence. Because zinc deficiency in pregnant animals causes birth defects and fetal growth retardation, there has been considerable effort to determine the effects of human zinc status on pregnancy outcome, especially in developing countries, where zinc intakes are often inadequate. In an analysis of 12 randomized, controlled intervention trials, only 2 (1 in India and 1 in the United States) found that zinc supplementation increased birth weight and reduced preterm delivery risk, whereas 6 found no effect. In the United States study, a positive effect was found in low-income, obese African American women with below average plasma zinc concentrations. Trials in Peru and Bangladesh showed no such benefits. In general, however, meeting recommended zinc intakes is more difficult but more critical for women whose diets are low in animal source foods and higher in fiber. High intakes (supplements) of iron and calcium may also impair zinc absorption and therefore increase requirements.

Iodine

In the many countries with endemic iodine deficiency, which include parts of the United States, Canada, and substantial areas of Europe and many other industrialized and developing countries, there is clear potential for the harmful effects of this deficiency to emerge during pregnancy. The most damaging effect of iodine deficiency is on the brain of the fetus since iodine is required for thyroid hormone, which in turn affects myelination and function of the developing central nervous system. The clinical expression of severe maternal iodine deficiency during pregnancy is cretinism, including severe mental retardation, deaf mutism, short stature, and spasticity. Injections of iodized oil before midpregnancy have markedly reduced cretinism and neonatal mortality in areas of severe iodine deficiency. In most countries, Universal Salt Iodization has reduced the prevalence of cretinism substantially, but milder indications of maternal deficiency persist even in Western Europe, including countries such as Belgium.

The EAR for pregnancy is set at 150 μg/day and the RDA at 160 μg/day for the United States and Canada based on the amount needed to prevent increased thyroid size in previously deficient women. The UL is 1100 μg/day, the same as for nonpregnant, nonlacting women, and it is based on the need to avoid elevated thyroid-stimulating hormone concentrations.

Trace Elements: Copper, Selenium, Chromium, Fluoride, Manganese, and Molybdenum

Copper is required for the function of many enzymes, primarily oxidases. In pregnancy, an increased intake of this mineral is recommended to cover deposition of approximately 18 mg/day, most of which is in fetal liver. The UL (10 000 μg/day) is the same as for nonpregnant women, based on the need to prevent the liver damage that occurs with high intakes.

Recommended intakes of selenium for adults are based on the criterion of maximizing plasma glutathione peroxidase activity. Based on an estimated selenium content of the fetus of 1000 μg, across pregnancy this would require that an additional 4 μg/day be consumed. The EAR is therefore increased from 45 to 49 μg/day and the RDA from 55 to 60 μg/day. The UL is determined on the basis of hair loss and brittle nails, which occur at higher levels of intake, and is the same as that set for nonpregnant women. An intake of 60 mg/day is also recommended throughout pregnancy in the United Kingdom, which is the same as the prepregnancy value for that population.

Chromium is required for normal insulin metabolism. There are no data from which to derive a recommendation for pregnancy, so an increase of 5 μg/day is recommended (as an AI) based on the additional weight and tissue chromium gained in pregnancy. No UL was set due to lack of documented adverse effects in humans.

For fluoride, there is no evidence that increasing the AI in pregnancy above that for the nonpregnant woman would benefit fetal tooth or bone content or afford protection against later tooth decay in the child. The UL is set at 10 mg/day to avoid fluorosis (discoloration of tooth enamel, joint pain, and skeletal abnormalities).

Manganese is required for bone formation and the normal metabolism of amino acids, lipids, and carbohydrates. The AI for pregnancy, estimated from the manganese content of maternal weight gain, is 2 mg/day. The UL is based on avoidance of elevated blood manganese and neurotoxicity, and it is not increased for pregnancy.

Recommended molybdenum intakes, based on the mineral's role as a cofactor for several enzymes, increase by 16 mg/day in pregnancy to cover the increment in fetal and maternal weight. The UL is derived from adverse reproductive effects seen in animals.

Water and Electrolytes

The US–Canada recommended intake of water for pregnant women is based on median intake from a large national survey in the United States. The AI of 3 l/day is anticipated to come from foods (0.7 l) and beverages (2.3 l). No UL was set because individuals stop drinking once their intake is adequate.

The AI for sodium in pregnancy is 1500 mg/day based on an intake level to cover daily losses, provide adequate intakes of other nutrients, and maintain normal function. The UL of 2300 mg/day is based on the adverse effects of higher intakes on blood pressure in susceptible members of the population.

The AI for potassium in pregnancy (4.7 g/day) is set at a level that will lower blood pressure, reduce the extent of salt sensitivity, and minimize the risk of kidney stones. There is no evidence that adverse effects of potassium are seen with high intakes from food and no UL was set, but potassium supplements can cause high blood potassium in some chronic diseases, such as renal disease and type 1 diabetes.

Summary

In the US–Canada recommendations, the recommended intakes are increased for most, but not all, nutrients during pregnancy. However, the recommendations are often based on less than ideal experimental data, in part due to the difficulty of conducting experiments on pregnant women.

For most nutrients, it is likely that some population groups may have higher requirements than those recommended in **Table 1**, notably women bearing more than one fetus or adolescents (see the Institute of Medicine volumes for specific recommendations for this age group). In order to meet the recommended nutrient increases, dietary quality often needs to be improved during pregnancy. It is often advised that pregnant women should also take iron supplements and/or a multiple vitamin–mineral supplement. The specific benefits of supplementation in pregnancy, optimal timing, and optimal doses are still somewhat controversial and the subject of ongoing research. Currently, some countries recommend routine supplementation for all pregnant women, whereas others recommend supplementation only when there is evidence of anemia, other nutritional deficiencies, a poor diet, or other problems such as drug or alcohol abuse.

See also: **Anemia**: Iron-Deficiency Anemia. **Ascorbic Acid**: Physiology, Dietary Sources and Requirements. **Calcium. Choline and Phosphatidylcholine. Chromium. Cobalamins. Copper. Folic Acid. Iodine**: Physiology, Dietary Sources and Requirements. **Iron. Magnesium. Manganese. Phosphorus. Potassium. Pregnancy**: Energy Requirements and Metabolic Adaptations; Safe Diet for Pregnancy. **Protein**: Requirements and Role in Diet. **Sodium**: Physiology.

Vitamin A: Physiology; Biochemistry and Physiological Role. **Vitamin B$_6$. Vitamin E**: Metabolism and Requirements. **Zinc**: Physiology.

Further Reading

Allen LH (2000) Anemia and iron deficiency: Effects on pregnancy outcome. *American Journal of Clinical Nutrition* **71**(supplement): 1280S–1284S.

Allen LH (2001) Pregnancy and lactation. In: Bowman BA and Russell RM (eds.) *Present Knowledge in Nutrition*, 8th edn, pp. 403–415. Washington, DC: ILSI Press.

Berry RJ, Li Z, Erickson JD *et al.* (1999) Prevention of neural-tube defects with folic acid in China. China–U.S. Collaborative Project for Neural Tube Defect Prevention. *New England Journal of Medicine* **341**: 1485–1490.

Butte NF, Wong WW, Treuth MS, Ellis KJ, and O'Brian Smith E (2004) Energy requirements during pregnancy based on total energy expenditure and energy deposition. *American Journal of Clinical Nutrition* **79**: 1078–1087.

Institute of Medicine, six volumes on Dietary Reference Intakes. http://nap.edu

Kaiser LL and Allen LH (2002) Position of the American Dietetic Association: Nutrition and lifestyle for a healthy pregnancy outcome. *Journal of the American Dietetic Association* **102**: 1479–1490.

Murphy MM, Scott JM, Arija V, Molloy AM, and Fernandez-Ballart JD (2004) Maternal homocysteine before conception and throughout pregnancy predicts fetal homocysteine and birth weight. *Clinical Chemistry* **50**: 1406–1412.

Prentice A (2000) Maternal calcium metabolism and bone mineral status. *American Journal of Clinical Nutrition* **71**: 1312S–1316S.

Scholl TO, Hediger ML, Bendich A *et al.* (1997) Use of multivitamin/mineral prenatal supplements: Influence on the outcome of pregnancy. *American Journal of Epidemiology* **146**: 134–141.

Energy Requirements and Metabolic Adaptations

G R Goldberg, MRC Human Nutrition Research, Cambridge, UK

The subject of energy metabolism in human pregnancy has received extensive consideration for more than 60 years, dating back to early work that assessed the contribution of fetal metabolism to the overall energy costs of pregnancy. Since then, the emphasis of much work has been on separating and quantifying the different components of gestational energy needs and on establishing appropriate recommendations for the energy requirements of pregnant women, with the intention to quantify average amounts. Deviations from average values were mostly regarded as undesirable biological or measurement noise that needed to be

Table 1 Protein and fat deposition during pregnancy for a reference woman[a]

Site	Protein		Fat		Water (kg)	Total	
	kg	MJ (kcals)	kg	MJ (kcals)		kg	MJ (kcals)
Fetus	0.44	12.76 (3050)	0.44	20.24 (4840)	2.41	3.29	33.00 (7890)
Placenta	0.10	2.90 (690)	0.04	0.18 (43)	0.54	0.64	3.08 (740)
Amniotic fluid	0.003	0.09 (21)	0.00	0.00	0.79	0.79	0.09 (21)
Uterus	0.17	4.81 (1150)	0.04	0.18 (43)	0.80	0.97	5.00 (1200)
Breasts	0.08	2.35 (560)	0.12	0.55 (130)	0.30	0.40	2.90 (690)
Blood	0.14	3.92 (940)	0.02	0.92 (220)	1.29	1.44	4.84 (1157)
Water	0.00	0.00	0.00	0.00	1.50	1.50	0.00
Subtotal	**0.93**	**26.83 (6400)**	**0.48**	**22.08 (5280)**	**7.63**	**9.04**	**48.9 (11 700)**
Fat stores	0.07	1.94 (460)	2.68	123.10 (29 400)	0.60	3.35	125.04 (29 900)
Total	**0.99**	**28.77 (6900)**	**3.16**	**145.18 (34 700)**	**8.24**	**12.38**	**173.94 (41 600)**

[a]Adapted from Prentice AM, Spaaij CJK, Goldberg GR *et al.* (1996) Energy requirements of pregnant and lactating women. *European Journal of Clinical Nutrition* **50**(supplement 1): S82–S111.

overcome by studying large samples of women to get a more precise estimate of the mean values. These inter-individual variations in the metabolic responses to pregnancy are increasingly recognized as biologically significant 'plasticity' that has true adaptive value in enabling women to carry a pregnancy to term under a wide range of nutritional conditions. The shorter and longer term consequences of such adaptations are being explored as part of fetal and infant origins of adult disease hypotheses.

Extra Energy Costs of Pregnancy

The question of how much extra dietary energy a pregnant woman needs is closely linked to the question of the amount of weight she should gain during pregnancy. This in turn is linked to her age and to her prepregnant body mass index as a proxy for energy status.

Hytten and Leitch's theoretical estimations of the overall energy costs of human pregnancy published more than 30 years ago have subsequently been experimentally validated as reasonable average values, and they have been adopted by many national and international bodies as a partial basis for developing recommended energy intakes in pregnancy. The costs can be divided into three main components: the energy deposited as new tissue in the conceptus, the energy deposited as fat, and the energy required to maintain this new tissue.

Tissue Deposition

Weight gain during pregnancy consists of the fetus, placenta, and amniotic fluid (the products of conception) and the extra growth of several maternal tissues. The deposition of fat in pregnancy is

presumed to help meet the extra energy demands of lactation. The total energy deposited as new tissue, excluding maternal fat, averages approximately 49 MJ (11 700 kcal). If an average maternal fat gain of 2.6 kg is assumed, then the estimate of the total energy deposited as new tissue during an average pregnancy is approximately 174 MJ (41 600 kcal) (**Table 1**).

Maintenance Energy Costs of Pregnancy

Because of the increase in tissue mass, the body's oxygen consumption also increases during pregnancy. Estimates suggest that the increase in oxygen consumption is equivalent to an extra 187 (45), 414 (100), 620 (148), and 951 (230) kJ/day (kcal) at 0–10, 10–20, 20–30, and 30–40 weeks of gestation, respectively. The total maintenance cost for an average human pregnancy is approximately 150 MJ (35 800 kcal) (**Table 2**).

Table 2 Increases in oxygen consumption during pregnancy[a]

	ml/min			
	10 weeks	20 weeks	30 weeks	40 weeks
Cardiac output	4.5	6.8	6.8	6.8
Respiration	0.8	1.5	2.3	3.0
Kidneys	7.0	7.0	7.0	7.0
Breasts	0.1	0.6	1.2	1.4
Uterus	0.5	1.2	2.2	3.6
Placenta	0	0.5	2.2	3.7
Fetus	0	1.1	5.5	12.4

[a]Adapted from Hytten FE (1991) Nutrition; Weight gain in pregnancy. In: Hytten F and Chamberlain G (eds.) *Clinical Physiology in Obstetrics*, 2nd edn. Oxford: Blackwell Scientific.

Theoretical Total Metabolic Costs of Pregnancy

Compared to many other mammals, humans have a relatively small and usually single infant, which develops during a long gestation period. The energy stress to the mother is therefore low per unit time. The 49 MJ of energy deposited as the products of conception represents only 4 or 5 days of food intake for the mother. Humans also differ from most other mammals because their large fat stores can help meet some of these costs. The theoretical total metabolic costs (i.e., due to extra tissue and increased metabolism) of pregnancy are approximately 335 MJ (80 000 kcal), or 1.25 MJ/day (300 kcal). This value does not make any allowance for changes (increases or decreases) in energy expended on physical activity. It is assumed that the majority of the energy costs of human pregnancy are met by behavioral adjustments in energy metabolism rather than increased energy intake. This assumption has formed the basis for energy intake recommendations, some of which are summarized in **Table 3**. It should be noted that the 1985 estimates used by WHO/FAO/UNU are under revision. Future recommendations may separate the obligatory costs (e.g., by fixed increments for basal metabolic rate (BMR) and tissue deposition) and differences in physical activity (based on PAL values).

Longitudinal Studies of the Energy Costs of Pregnancy

Fat Deposition

The increase in maternal fat stores is by far the largest contributor to the energy cost of tissue deposition. It is also the most variable. Although the average increase for a well-nourished woman who has an uncomplicated pregnancy and healthy infant is approximately 3 kg, a large number of studies have reported ranges of −2 to 8 kg and standard deviations of 2–4 kg. There is also a wide range in fat deposition between different populations, particularly when those from developed and developing countries are compared. Fat is very energy dense and therefore changes in body fat stores have a large impact on the energy costs of pregnancy. A loss of 2 kg saves approximately 78 MJ (18 600 kcal), whilst a gain of 8 kg costs approximately 312 MJ (74 600 kcal). Women most likely to need an energy reserve to help meet the costs of lactation are often those who are least able to deposit spare energy as fat in pregnancy. Conversely, women who store large amounts of fat during pregnancy are least likely to need to use it during lactation. They are often able to increase food intake and/or decrease physical activity instead.

Table 3 Examples of current recommendations for energy intakes during pregnancy

	Trimester(s)	Increment, MJ/day (kcal/day)	Total for pregnancy, MJ (kcal)	Qualifying comments
FAO/WHO/UNU (1985)	All	1.20 (300)	336 (80 300)	
	All	0.84 (200)	235 (56 150)	For healthy women who reduce activity Energy and protein requirements are undergoing revision (interim report published 2004)
United Kingdom (1991)	3rd	0.80 (190)	74 (17 000)	Underweight women and those not reducing activity may need more
United States and Canada (2002)	1st	Adult EER + 0		For women aged 19–50 years
	2nd	Adult EER + 160 kcal (8 kcal/ week × 20 weeks) + 180 kcal		EERs for pregnant adolescents are based on EER for 14- to 18-year-olds
	3rd	Adult EER + 272 kcal (8 kcal/ week × 34 weeks) + 180 kcal		EER is based on total energy expenditure in the nonpregnant state; increments for pregnancy are 8 kcal/week for total energy expenditure and 180 kcal/day for tissue deposition

EER, estimated energy requirement.

Studies have shown that excess energy intake during pregnancy results in excess maternal weight (and fat) gain. Postpartum retention of excess fat has implications for the development of obesity and its comorbidities such as type 2 diabetes.

Basal Metabolic Rate

The cumulative increase in BMR can comprise a large part of the total energy costs of pregnancy. Although 150 MJ is a good estimate of the average energy cost of maintenance for a well-nourished woman, there is a very wide range. This has an important influence on the extra daily requirements for individual women. Studies in which BMR has been measured every 6 weeks from prepregnancy to 36 weeks of pregnancy have shown very marked differences. In some women, there is the expected response to pregnancy—an immediate and progressive increase in BMR. In other women, BMR actually decreases or increases only slightly in the early stages of pregnancy and does not increase substantially until late gestation. This offsets the later increase in BMR such that there is actually a slight net saving of energy over the entire gestation period in some of these 'energy-sparing' women. The total net cost of maintenance, estimated as the cumulative area under the curve represented by the rise in a mother's BMR above the prepregnancy baseline metabolic rate, is negative or only very small. Data indicate that this between-subject variability is found in women from both well-nourished and marginally-nourished populations. However, 'energy-sparing' and 'energy-profligate' responses dominate in marginally and well-nourished women, respectively. There is a more than 5-fold range between the most energy-profligate and the most energy-sparing women.

In addition to the wide variability in changes in BMR between individual women, there are also wide variations between different populations. Well-nourished affluent women from developed countries tend to show an energy-profligate increase in BMR. In marginally nourished thinner women from developing countries the increase in BMR is delayed and/or preceded by a decline in early pregnancy. The total maintenance costs of pregnancy in these studies range from +210 MJ (+50 000 kcal) to −45 MJ (−11 000 kcal).

Diet-Induced Thermogenesis

A reduction in diet-induced thermogenesis (DIT) may be a mechanism by which energy is saved during pregnancy. However, when expressed as a proportion of energy intake, DIT remains essentially unaltered during pregnancy and any changes are small and unlikely to be biologically significant.

Energy Cost of Activities

Results from a number of longitudinal studies have shown that the cost of non-weight-bearing activity changes little until very late pregnancy. From approximately 35 weeks, the gross costs (which include changes in BMR) increase by approximately 11% and net costs by approximately 6%. The gross and net costs of weight-bearing exercise (treadmill walking and standardized step testing) remain fairly constant during the first half of pregnancy and then increase progressively by approximately 15–20% at term.

Behavioral Changes in Physical Activity

It has frequently been assumed that a behavioral reduction in the energy expended on physical activity helps to counteract the increases in expenditure due to increased body weight, and in some women this leads to saving of energy that largely meets the costs of pregnancy. However, although relatively small changes in activity patterns can potentially result in significant energy savings, there is little evidence that this occurs to a large extent. A possible reason for this is that affluent women are habitually so sedentary that there is little scope for further reduction. In contrast, in developing countries habitual levels of physical activity are high and there is therefore more potential for behavioral reductions. However, many women are likely to be unable to reduce their physical activity because of the constraints imposed by a subsistence livelihood, where farm work is obligatory for survival.

This topic has been one of considerable debate in recent years, particularly since longitudinal studies that have measured total energy expenditure with doubly labeled water have shown that many women increase the energy expended on physical activity during pregnancy, and that any decreases are not sufficient to counterbalance the energy costs of pregnancy due to tissue (fat) deposition and maintenance energy metabolism. It has been recommended that the data used by the World Health Organization should be revised to take account of changes in energy expended on physical activity and to separate these energy costs from those of maintenance and tissue deposition. The Dietary Reference Intakes for the United States and Canada have already incorporated these changes (**Table 3**).

Between-Country Comparison of the Metabolic Costs of Pregnancy

The average costs across different populations result in a wide range of energy needs from −30 MJ (−7000 kcal) to 523 MJ (125 000 kcal). Studies found that the average costs in the well-nourished groups were similar to the current international assumption of 336 MJ (80 000 kcal). These studies have also shown that the amount of prepregnancy body fat is strongly correlated with both the maintenance costs and the total metabolic costs of pregnancy. The combined costs of maintenance, fat deposition, and conceptus across studies from different countries drawn from emerging and affluent nations show that the energy cost of fat deposition also varies according to the state of affluence and is positively correlated with variations in maintenance requirements.

This flexibility in energy metabolism acts in a protective manner, with undernourished women showing significant energy-sparing adaptive strategies that tend to normalize energy balance. Body fat content is one of the measures of fitness for reproduction; fertility is suppressed in undernourished women. However, future unfavorable conditions cannot be anticipated and pre- or early pregnant fatness may be indicative of overall nutritional status and energy balance during pregnancy.

These relationships suggested the existence of a mechanism that can monitor the mother's prepregnancy energy status and adjust the homeorrhetic changes in maternal metabolism accordingly. The discovery of leptin provides a plausible mechanism by which peripheral energy status can be centrally monitored and may coordinate the metabolic responses to pregnancy. It is clear that in addition to its role in the regulation of adipose tissue, appetite, and metabolic rate, leptin plays a significant role in several components of the reproductive axis. Evidence suggests that it plays a key role in pregnancy, including the modulation of fetal growth.

Individual Variability in the Total Energy Costs of Pregnancy

Because of the marked differences between individuals in the different components of the energy costs of pregnancy (changes in BMR, body fat, and energy expended on physical activity), the total energy costs, and therefore energy requirements, are also variable. Studies of well-nourished women indicate that the total extra energy costs of pregnancy average 418 MJ (100 000 kcal), considerably higher than the estimates in **Table 3**, and there is a large range from 34 to 1200 MJ (8000–287 000 kcal). These values are probably representative of many women in developed countries. They show that it is impossible to prescribe energy intakes for individual women since it cannot be predicted how they will respond metabolically (BMR and fat) or behaviorally (physical activity and food intake) to pregnancy.

Implications of Energy-Sparing Adaptations for Mother and Infant

Human energy metabolism is particularly adaptable during pregnancy, with early/prepregnancy body 'fatness' being a major determinant. The adaptive strategies that maintain energy balance seem to be a coordinated biological system in which energy-sensitive modulations in metabolism help to sustain human pregnancies and protect fetal growth in highly marginal environmental circumstances. However, the existence of such mechanisms should not be misinterpreted as suggesting that maintenance of optimal nutritional status in pregnant women is not a priority because the adaptive mechanisms of the women will cope. It cannot be assumed that pregnant women will have energy-sparing alterations in metabolism and/or that physical activity decreases. Any adaptations that do occur should not be over-interpreted as suggesting that this is the case. The possible long-term detrimental effects must also be considered. The biochemical and physiological processes that are downregulated in the mother causing the suppression in BMR are unknown and there may be long-term consequences to her health and that of her infant.

The associations between maintenance needs, pregnancy weight gain, and prepregnant fatness indicate that a target weight gain of 12.5 kg is associated with maintenance costs of approximately 160 MJ (38 000 kcal). Although individual women or populations may have lower maintenance requirements, these may be associated with inadequate weight gain and low-birth-weight infants. A major determinant of birth weight is maternal weight gain, and the single most important determinant of infant survival is birth weight. Although birth weight is relatively well preserved at different planes of nutrition, weight alone is an inadequate measure of an infant's overall condition at birth. Even subtle nutritional influences on the fetal environment may have long-term consequences.

As mentioned previously, pregnancy weight gain is a critical component of the overall energy costs of pregnancy. The issue of whether pregnancy weight gain drives, or is driven by, the metabolic changes is interesting, but it is clear that women who consume marginal diets have small weight gains and that women from poorer countries have much lower percentage weight gains despite having lower initial body weights. Extremes of weight gains during pregnancy may have several consequences, which may or may not be mediated directly through an effect on birth weight. Other effects of weight gain may be more subtle and may be mediated through qualitative effects on fetal growth and development at different stages of intrauterine growth. There is a considerable body of evidence that suggests that many chronic adult diseases have their origins in fetal and infant nutrition, which has refocused attention on early life as a critical period in human development.

See also: **Energy**: Metabolism; Balance; Requirements. **Energy Expenditure**: Indirect Calorimetry; Doubly Labeled Water. **Pregnancy**: Nutrient Requirements; Weight Gain.

Further Reading

Barash IA, Cheung CC, Weigle DS *et al.* (1996) Leptin is a metabolic signal to the reproductive system. *Endocrinology* **137**: 3144–3147.

Butte N, Hopkinson J, and Nicholson M (1997) Leptin in human reproduction: Serum leptin levels in pregnant and lactating women. *Journal of Clinical Endocrinology and Metabolism* **82**: 585–589.

Butte N, Treuth M, Mehta N *et al.* (2003) Energy requirements of women of reproductive age. *American Journal of Clinical Nutrition* **77**: 630–638.

Department of Health (1991) *Dietary Reference Values for Food Energy and Nutrients for the United Kingdom*, Report on Health and Social Subjects No. 41. London: HMSO.

FAO/WHO/UNU (1985) *Report of a Joint Expert Consultation: Energy and Protein Requirements*, Technical Report Series 724. Geneva: WHO.

Forsum E (2004) Energy requirements during pregnancy: Old questions and new findings. *American Journal of Clinical Nutrition* **79**: 933–934.

Goldberg GR (1997) Reproduction: A global nutritional challenge. *Proceedings of the Nutrition Society* **56**: 319–333.

Goldberg GR, Prentice AM, Coward WA *et al.* (1993) Longitudinal assessment of energy expenditure in pregnancy by the doubly-labelled water method. *American Journal of Clinical Nutrition* **57**: 494–505.

Harigaya A, Nagashima K, Nako Y *et al.* (1997) Relationship between concentration of serum leptin and fetal growth. *Journal of Clinical Endocrinology and Metabolism* **82**: 3281–3284.

Hytten FE (1991) Nutrition; Weight gain in pregnancy. In: Hytten F and Chamberlain G (eds.) *Clinical Physiology in Obstetrics*, 2nd edn. Oxford: Blackwell Scientific.

Kopp-Hoolihan LE, Loan MV, Wong WW *et al.* (1999) Longitudinal assessment of energy balance in well nourished, pregnant women. *American Journal of Clinical Nutrition* **69**: 697–704.

National Academy of Sciences (2002) *Dietary Reference Intakes for Energy, Carbohydrates, Fiber, Fat, Protein and Amino Acids (Macronutrients)*. Washington, DC: National Academy Press.

Poppitt SD, Prentice AM, Goldberg GR *et al.* (1994) Energy-sparing strategies to protect human fetal growth. *American Journal of Obstetrics and Gynecology* **171**: 118–125.

Poppitt SD, Prentice AM, Jequier E *et al.* (1993) Evidence of energy-sparing in Gambian women during pregnancy: A longitudinal study using whole-body calorimetry. *American Journal of Clinical Nutrition* **57**: 353–364.

Prentice AM and Goldberg GR (2000) Energy adaptations in human pregnancy: Limits and long-term consequences. *American Journal of Clinical Nutrition* **71**(supplement): 1226S–1232S.

Prentice AM, Spaaij CJK, Goldberg GR *et al.* (1996) Energy requirements of pregnant and lactating women. *European Journal of Clinical Nutrition* **50**(supplement 1): S82–S111.

Scrimshaw NS, Waterlow JC, and Schurch B (1996) Energy and protein requirements. Proceedings of an IDECG Workshop. *European Journal of Clinical Nutrition* **50**(supplement 1): S1–S197.

Weight Gain

L H Allen and J M Graham, University of California at Davis, Davis, CA, USA

During the past 40 years, there have been dramatic changes in the recommendations for optimal maternal weight gain during pregnancy. In the past, it was thought that it was necessary to restrict the diet of many pregnant women in order to reduce the perceived risks associated with higher weight gains. The fetus was thought to be relatively unaffected by this advice. In contrast, the current recommendations in the United States are based on weight changes in pregnancy that have been taken from records and known to be compatible with a healthy pregnancy outcome. The US recommendations have been widely accepted by many other Western countries. Because several maternal factors influence the amount of weight gained in pregnancy, these factors have to be taken into consideration when basing recommendations on actual weight gain. The result has been the development of more realistic weight gain guidelines that are based to some extent on the characteristics of the mother. Additional experience has been gained since these guidelines were developed that encompasses a variety of subpopulations including different ethnic groups and overweight women, and the knowledge gained broadens the scope of these recommendations among modern diverse populations. However, there is still much to be learned about the determinants of, and variability in, energy requirements and balance of pregnant women.

Pregnancy Weight Gain Recommendations

In 1970, the US National Academy of Sciences published guidelines for weight gain during pregnancy in the report, Maternal Nutrition and the Course of Pregnancy. The recommended pregnancy gain was 24 lb (10.9 kg), with a range of 10–25 lb (9.1–11.4 kg). The report advised health care providers and pregnant women not to restrict weight gain—a practice that had been fairly widespread during the previous decade in order to reduce the perceived risks of labor complications, preeclampsia, and excess weight retention postpartum. In fact, many obstetricians had been recommending gains of only 15–20 lb (6.8–9.1 kg).

Even with the more generous recommendations set in 1970, by the 1980s it had become clear that average gains of women in the United States far exceeded these guidelines. An analysis of data from the National Natality Survey in 1980 showed the average pregnancy weight gain to be 29 lb (13.2 kg), and by the time of the National Maternal Infant Health Survey in 1988 the average had increased to 32 lb (14.5 kg). The range of gain was very wide, from no gain to more than 75 lb (34.1 kg).

Based on this realization, in 1990 the weight gain recommendations were revised completely by a committee established by the Institute of Medicine (IOM) of the National Academy of Sciences. Existing data from a national survey were analyzed to determine the weight gain that was compatible with a normal pregnancy outcome. The latter was defined as the infant being born full term and of normal birth weight and the absence of pregnancy or delivery complications. It became apparent from these analyses that maternal weight-for-height at conception, expressed as body mass index (BMI; weight in kilograms and height in meters squared), was an important predictor of actual weight gain. Thin women (with a low BMI) gained more weight than fatter women. Different weight gain recommendations were therefore developed for women entering pregnancy with different BMIs (**Table 1**). For thinner women (BMI <19.8 or <90% of ideal body weight), recommended gains are 28–40 lb (12.7–18.2 kg); for women with a normal BMI (19.8–25.9), gain should be 25–35 lb (11.4–15.9 kg) or 1 lb (0.45 kg) per week; and for overweight women (BMI >29.0 or >135% ideal body weight), gain should be at least 15 lb (6.8 kg) or 0.7 lb (0.32 kg) per week. New weight gain grids were constructed that showed the

Table 1 Recommendations for pregnancy weight gain by body mass index (BMI) at conception

BMI category	Recommended total gain	
	Kilograms	Pounds
Low (BMI <19.8)	12.8–18.0	28–40
Normal (BMI >19.8–26.0)	11.5–16.0	25–35
High (BMI >26.0–29.0)	7.0–11.5	15–25
Obese (BMI >29.0)	≤6.0	≤13

Modified from Institute of Medicine, Committee on Nutritional Status during Pregnancy and Lactation (1990) Nutrition During Pregnancy. Weight Gain. Nutrient Supplements. Food and Nutrition Board. Washington, DC: National Academy Press.

recommended gains over the course of pregnancy for each BMI group (**Figure 1**), enabling the adequacy of weight gain to be tracked for individual women. To use the chart, women's height and weight should be measured as near to the time of conception as possible (because pregnancy causes a temporary reduction in height) and used to obtain their BMI from a table. The US recommendations are deemed to be appropriate for women in developed countries worldwide.

Pattern of Weight Gain

Relatively little (1–2.5 kg) of the total weight gain during pregnancy occurs during the first trimester, whereas gain in the last two trimesters is relatively linear. Nevertheless, it is important to pay attention to the quality of pregnant women's diets during the first trimester and to ensure that they do not restrict their intake during this time, when there is the

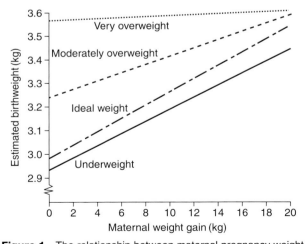

Figure 1 The relationship between maternal pregnancy weight gain and birth weight. (Reproduced with permission from the Institute of Medicine, Committee on Nutritional Status during Pregnancy and Lactation (1990) *Nutrition during Pregnancy. Weight Gain. Nutrient Supplements. Food and Nutrition Board.* Washington, DC: National Academy Press.)

strongest risk of nutrition-related birth defects and spontaneous abortions. In some studies, an association has been noted between low weight gain in the first trimester and increased risk of spontaneous preterm delivery.

Variability in Weight Gain

The BMI-specific target ranges for pregnancy weight gain are relatively narrow, but a very wide range of gain actually occurs. In a California study, for example, only 50% of the mothers who had an uncomplicated pregnancy with a normal birth-weight infant gained the recommended 12.5–18 kg, with the remainder gaining more or less. Since a substantial amount of the variation in weight gain is due to physiological variability and prepregnancy BMI, deviation from the recommended range may not necessarily be cause for concern. However, it is especially important to assess the dietary patterns and other behaviors of women whose weight gain is unexpectedly high or low. The IOM *Implementation Guide* for weight gain recommendations provides helpful information on the assessments that should be used.

Maternal Weight Gain and Birth Weight

Inadequate weight gain is associated with poor fetal growth even when the contribution of fetal weight and factors such as length of gestation are taken into consideration. Birth weight is an important determinant of child health and survival; low-birth-weight (<2.5 kg) infants are 40 times more likely to die in the neonatal period. Low weight-for-length at birth may be a risk factor for chronic disease in later life. It has been estimated that in women with a normal prepregnancy BMI, each kilogram of total pregnancy weight gain has an average effect on birth weight of 20 g. In California, women with pregnancy weight gains below recommendations had a 78% higher risk of the infant being born small, whereas women who gained in excess of recommendations were twice as likely to give birth to a large infant.

As noted previously, maternal BMI at conception is strongly inversely related to expected pregnancy weight gain. Nevertheless, heavier women still tend to deliver heavier infants (**Figure 2**) and thinner women tend to have smaller infants. In thinner women, birth weight is more strongly related to pregnancy weight gain. Thus, as is evident from

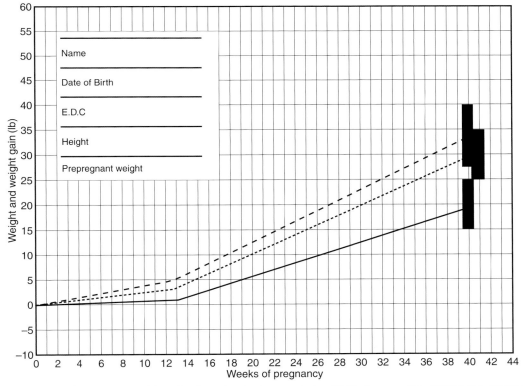

Figure 2 Recommended pregnancy weight gains based on body mass index (BMI) at conception. Dotted line, prepregnancy BMI <19.8 lbs; dashed line, prepregnancy BMI 19.8–26.0 lbs (normal); solid line, prepregnancy BMI >26.0 lbs. (Reproduced with permission from the Institute of Medicine, Committee on Nutritional Status during Pregnancy and Lactation (1992) *Nutrition during Pregnancy and Lactation. An Implementation Guide. Food and Nutrition Board.* Washington, DC: National Academy Press.)

Figure 2, the greatest risk of low birth weight is for thin women with a low pregnancy weight gain. It is crucial that thin women gain adequate amounts of weight. These associations are not explained by other risk factors associated with thinness, such as smoking.

Changes in Body Composition and Maternal Energy Status

It used to be assumed that maternal energy intake during pregnancy was the main determinant of the amount of weight gained. Although our knowledge of this relationship is still inadequate, newer information indicates that other maternal factors, and especially body composition, are more important predictors.

The weight gained during pregnancy can be roughly divided into the weight of the fetus, placenta, and amniotic fluid (a total of approximately 5 kg), maternal gain in the uterus, breasts, blood, and fluid (approximately 4 kg), and maternal fat. The latter component is the most variable, accounting for approximately 70% of the variability in pregnancy weight gain. Although average fat gain in different studies is approximately 2–5 kg, values for individual women range from a loss of several kilograms to a gain of approximately 12 kg. Even in a group of women with normal BMIs at conception, the range of fat gain was 0.5–9.5 kg. Fatter women at conception gained less fat during pregnancy, as would be expected from their lower weight gains. The greater fat gain of thinner women is a potential energy store for the fetus and would afford some protection against maternal malnutrition in late pregnancy—a situation that is not uncommon in some economically disadvantaged countries.

Maternal BMI at conception influences not only the amount of maternal weight and fat gained during pregnancy but also changes in maternal basal metabolic rate (BMR). In studies of well-nourished pregnant women, BMR has been reported to increase by approximately 20–30%. For undernourished women, however, the increment in BMR may be only 20% of that seen in those who are well nourished. In contrast, in a group of well-nourished Californian women weighing 55–116 kg, the BMR of those with higher BMIs was almost twice that of the thinnest women in the group.

Overall, it is clear that heavier women gain less weight and fat during pregnancy and have a larger increase in BMR. It has not been determined how these changes translate into energy requirements for women in the different BMI groups used to predict weight gains. Therefore, a single value for energy requirements is used for all pregnant women regardless of their BMI at conception.

Weight Gain for Special Population Groups

Adolescents

Well-nourished adolescents tend to gain at least as much, if not more, weight than adult women. The relationship between BMI, pregnancy weight gain, and birth weight is probably no different in this group, but to ensure adequate nutrition for those who are still growing, weight gain in the upper range of BMI-specific recommendations is advised. The effects of this recommendation on weight retention postpartum have not been evaluated adequately.

Short Women

Women who are less than 157 cm tall tend to give birth to infants who are large relative to maternal pelvic size, with a subsequently slightly greater risk of a more difficult delivery. These women are therefore advised to gain near the lower end of the weight gain range that is compatible with their BMI.

Ethnic Groups

Black women in the United States tend to gain less weight in pregnancy and to produce lower birthweight infants. The reasons for this are not known, but it could not be explained by differences in gestational age or other factors that were measured. Adequate weight gain in this group is known to be especially important for the prevention of fetal growth retardation. In one study, 18% of nonobese black women who gained less than the IOM recommendations gave birth to low-birth-weight infants compared to 10% whose gain was in the ideal range and 4% who gained more than the recommendations. In obese black women, the low birth weight prevalence was approximately six times higher than that for those who gained less than the recommendations.

Most surveys indicate that Hispanics seem to gain approximately the same amount of weight as Anglo women. In the 1980 National Natality Survey, Hispanic and non-Hispanic white women gained a similar amount of pregnancy weight, but the risk of low birth weight was twice as high in Hispanics. Surveillance of a predominantly Hispanic population indicated that half of the underweight women and one-third of the normal weight women gained the recommended amount of weight, whereas more than half and three-fourths of overweight and obese women, respectively, had excessive gains. Inadequate weight gain during the third trimester was predictive of preterm birth. Underweight Hispanic women had nearly twice the risk of premature delivery.

The maternal weight gain recommendations have been evaluated in a group of Chinese women with good pregnancy outcomes ($N = 504$) to assess the need for an ethnic-specific recommendation for this group. The BMI categories were used at different levels. The recommended total pregnancy weight gain ranges according to BMI for Chinese women were 13–16.7 kg for BMI <19, 11–16.4 kg for BMI 19–23.5, and 7.1–14.4 kg for BMI >23.5. Women with weight gain in the lowest quartile had twice the risk of having a low-birth-weight infant, and those with excessive weight gain were in need of assisted delivery (either vaginal or cesarean delivery).

Substance Abusers

Cigarette smokers tend to gain less weight during pregnancy and to produce smaller infants. This effect is not explained by a lower food intake of smokers. Alcohol and drug use have similar effects. Simply gaining more weight during pregnancy will not compensate for the adverse effects of these practices on fetal outcome or pregnancy complications.

Multiple Births

Relatively few data are available from national surveys on which to base weight gain recommendations for women with twins. A weight gain of 15.9–20.5 kg or 0.7 kg per week in the second and third trimesters is usually consistent with a healthy pregnancy outcome for these women. No recommendations are available for women carrying more than two fetuses, but it is reasonable to expect that they will increase by 3.5 kg for each additional infant.

Obese and Overweight Women

Obesity during pregnancy is associated with higher morbidity for both the mother and the child. Higher prepregnancy weights have been shown to increase the risk of late (>28 weeks of gestation) fetal deaths. In addition, the prevalence of gestational hypertension increases 3-fold and there is a 3–4 times greater risk of gestational diabetes in obese pregnant women.

Exercising Women

Women who are physically fit at conception appear to be able to continue to exercise during pregnancy without harm to themselves or the fetuses, as long as the activity is not too strenuous or prolonged. In

several studies it was observed that exercising women gained 2 or 3 kg less than those who were more sedentary.

Pregnancy Weight Gain and Postpartum Risk of Obesity

On average, well-nourished women retain relatively little weight approximately 1 year postpartum (approximately 0.5–1.5 kg). Delivery is followed by a rapid loss of weight in the subsequent 2 weeks due to fluid loss. This is followed by a slower rate of loss for the next 6 months, so a complete return to preconception weight should not be expected in less time than this. In general, weight still retained at 1 year postpartum is unlikely to be lost without lowering intake and/or increasing physical activity. If weight retention is substantial, it can add to the risk of obesity in the longer term, and obesity is a major public health concern in many countries.

The relatively low average weight retention postpartum obscures the fact that many women do retain an excessive amount of weight. Those who retain most are likely to have gained large amounts of weight during pregnancy. At 10–18 months postpartum, weight retention was 2.5 kg for women who gained more than the IOM recommendation compared to 0.7 kg for white women and 3.2 kg for black women who gained the advised amount. These large racial differences in weight retention have not been explained and certainly may be a risk factor for the higher prevalence of later obesity in this group.

Most women breast-feed their infants exclusively or partially for a relatively short time. There is little difference in weight loss between women who breast-feed and those who do not for periods up to 6 months postpartum. This is presumably due to the greater appetite and energy intake of women who are breast-feeding and perhaps to dieting on the part of non-breast-feeders. One study of women who breast-fed until 12 months postpartum did report a 2-kg greater weight loss compared to women who stopped breast feeding before 3 months. Even more weight was lost by those who breast-fed more often and gave longer feeds.

Women with a high BMI at conception tend to either lose or gain more weight postpartum than those with a normal BMI; approximately one-third end up weighing less than at conception, and one-third weigh substantially more. The reasons for the highly variable weight retention in this group are not known.

Although inadequate intake of nutrients during lactation can lead to maternal nutrient depletion and lower breast milk content of some nutrients and especially vitamins, breast feeding women who choose to lose weight can do so by exercising and/or reasonable restriction of energy intake. Exercising by jogging, biking, and aerobics for 45 minutes, four or five times per week for 12 weeks did not affect well-nourished mothers' ability to lactate or influence their milk composition. However, it is possible that severe energy deficit in lactation, especially of thinner women, will reduce breast milk volume.

Impact of Supplementation

Numerous investigators have explored the benefits of energy and/or protein supplementation for pregnancy weight gain and other outcomes. However, relatively few trials have randomly assigned these supplements and used control diets. A statistical analysis was conducted of the 10 such studies that met this criterion in 1995. Most, but not all, of these studies were performed in developing countries. A 5-year controlled trial in The Gambia provided daily prenatal dietary supplements (two biscuits) that contained 4250 kJ energy and 22 g protein. This supplement increased pregnancy weight gain and birth weight during the hungry and harvest seasons. There was a significant but very small increase in head circumference and a significant reduction in perinatal mortality.

It was originally thought that timing of supplementation during later gestation would be most likely to increase birth weight. This hypothesis was supported by data from the Dutch famine, during which women in their third trimester had infants with the lowest birth weights. An increase in low birth weight prevalence was also observed in The Gambia when third-trimester gestation overlapped with the hungry season. Nonetheless, research suggests nutrition interventions initiated earlier in pregnancy will have the strongest effect on birth weight. There are enduring advantages to continued supplementation postpartum (during lactation) and into the ensuing pregnancy. A longitudinal study in Guatemala reported a significant increase (approximately 350 g) in birth weight in the second pregnancy when the mother was supplemented during the previous pregnancy and throughout subsequent lactation and the second pregnancy compared to those who were not supplemented during the prior pregnancy. Overall, it is appropriate for supplementation to begin as early in the pregnancy as possible so that both mother and fetus receive the maximum benefits for optimal health and development. However, this advice is tempered by concerns that supplementation of short Asian women may increase their offspring's risk of diabetes in later life.

See also: **Adolescents**: Nutritional Requirements. **Breast Feeding**. **Lactation**: Physiology; Dietary Requirements. **Obesity**: Complications. **Pregnancy**: Role of Placenta in Nutrient Transfer; Nutrient Requirements; Energy Requirements and Metabolic Adaptations; Safe Diet for Pregnancy; Dietary Guidelines and Safe Supplement Use; Prevention of Neural Tube Defects; Pre-eclampsia and Diet.

Further Reading

Ceesay SM, Prentice AM, Cole TJ *et al.* (1997) Effects on birth weight and perinatal mortality of maternal dietary supplements in rural Gambia: 5 year randomised controlled trial. *British Medical Journal* 315: 786–790.

Cnattingius S, Bergstrom R, Lipworth L, and Kramer MS (1998) Prepregnancy weight and the risk of adverse pregnancy outcomes. *New England Journal of Medicine* 338: 147–152.

Dewey KG and McCrory M (1994) Effects of dieting and physical activity on pregnancy and lactation. *American Journal of Clinical Nutrition* 59(supplement): 439–445.

Hickey C, Cliver S, Goldenberg R, Kohatsu J, and Hoffman H (1993) Prenatal weight gain, term birth weight, and fetal growth retardation among high risk multiparous black and white women. *Obstetrics and Gynecology* 81: 529–535.

Institute of Medicine, Committee on Nutritional Status during Pregnancy and Lactation (1990) *Nutrition during Pregnancy. Weight Gain. Nutrient Supplements. Food and Nutrition Board.* Washington, DC: National Academy Press.

Institute of Medicine, Committee on Nutritional Status during Pregnancy and Lactation (1992) *Nutrition during Pregnancy and Lactation. An Implementation Guide. Food and Nutrition Board.* Washington, DC: National Academy Press.

Keppel K and Taffel S (1993) Pregnancy-related weight gain and retention: Implications of the 1990 Institute of Medicine Guidelines. *American Journal of Public Health* 83: 1100–1103.

King JC, Butte NF, Bronstein MN, Kopp LE, and Lindquist SA (1994) Energy metabolism during pregnancy: Influence of maternal energy status. *American Journal of Clinical Nutrition* 59(supplement): 439S–445S.

Kramer M (1993) Effects of energy and protein intakes on pregnancy outcome: An overview of the research evidence from controlled clinical trials. *American Journal of Clinical Nutrition* 58: 627–635.

Luke B, Minogue J, Witter F, Keith LG, and Johnson TRB (1993) The ideal twin pregnancy: Patterns of weight gain, discordancy, and length of gestation. *American Journal of Obstetrics and Gynecology* 169: 588–597.

Parker J and Abrams B (1992) Prenatal weight gain advice: An examination of the recent prenatal weight gain recommendation of the Institute of Medicine. *Obstetrics and Gynecology* 79: 664–669.

Siega-Riz AM, Adair LS, and Hobel CJ (1994) Institute of Medicine maternal weight gain recommendations and pregnancy outcome in a predominantly Hispanic population. *Obstetrics and Gynecology* 84: 565–573.

Wong W, Tang NL, Lau TK, and Wong TW (2000) A new recommendation for maternal weight gain in Chinese women. *Journal of the American Dietetic Association* 100: 791–796.

ISBN 0-12-150110-8

9 780121 501105